Pediatric Surgical Oncology

Under the Aegis of the Indian Association of Pediatric Surgeons

Pediatric Surgical Oncology

Editors

Devendra K Gupta

MBBS, MS, MCh, FICS, FAMS, FAMS (Hony), FRCSG (Hony), DSc (Honoris Causa)
Professor and Head, Department of Pediatric Surgery
All India Institute of Medical Sciences, Ansari Nagar, New Delhi, INDIA

Robert Carachi

MD, PhD, FRCS (Glasgow), FRCS (Eng)
Professor and Head, Section of Surgical Paediatrics
Royal Hospital for Sick Children
Yorkhill, Glasgow, Scotland, UK

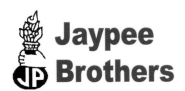

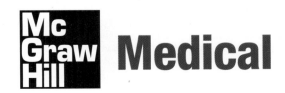

© 2008, Devendra K Gupta, Robert Carachi

First published in India in 2008 by

Corporate Office
4838/24 Ansari Road, Daryaganj, **New Delhi** - 110002, India, +91-11-43574357
Registered Office
B-3 EMCA House, 23/23B Ansari Road, Daryaganj, **New Delhi** 110 002, India
Phones: +91-11-23272143, +91-11-23272703, +91-11-23282021,
+91-11-23245672, Rel: +91-11-32558559 Fax: +91-11-23276490, +91-11-23245683
e-mail: jaypee@jaypeebrothers.com, Visit our website: www.jaypeebrothers.com

First published in USA by The McGraw-Hill Companies, 2 Penn Plaza, New York, NY 10121.
Exclusively worldwide distributor except South Asia (India, Nepal, Sri Lanka, Bhutan, Pakistan, Bangladesh, Malaysia).

ISBN-13: 978-0-07-160190-0
ISBN-10: 0-07-160190-2

CONTRIBUTORS

Akira Nakagawara MD, PhD
Director, Chiba Cancer Center
Research Institute
Chiba Cancer Center
Professor, Department of Molecular
Biology and Oncology
Chiba University School of Medicine
662-2 Nitona, Chuob-ku
Chiba 260-8717, Japan

Akshay Pratap Chauhan MCh
Assistant Professor
Department of Pediatric Surgery
Daran Medical College
Nepal

Amulya K Saxena MD
Consultant Pediatric Surgeon
Department of Pediatric Surgery
Medical University of Graz
Auenbruggerplatz 34
Graz
A-8036
Austria

Andrew B Pinter MD
Professor of Pediatric Surgery
Pecs University, Faculty of Medicine
Department of Pediatrics – surgrical
unit, H- 7623, Jozsef A. Str. 7, Pecs
Hungary

Arun Malhotra MD
Professor and Head
Department of Nuclear Medicine
All India Institute of Medical
Sciences
New Delhi-110029, India

Arvind Bagga MD, FIAP, FAMS
Professor
Dept of Pediatrics
All India Institute of Medical
Sciences, Ansari Nagar
New Delhi-110029 India

Bharat R Agarwal MD, DCH (BOM),
DNB (MNAMS)
Head of Department
Pediatric Hematology and Oncology
BJ Wadia Hospital for Children
Parel, Mumbai-400012, India

Bhaskar N Rao MD
Senior Oncology Surgeon
Department of Surgery
St Jude Children's Research Hospital
Memphis, TN 38105, USA

Brijesh Arora MD, DM
Assistant Professor
Pediatric Oncology
Tata Memorial Hospital
E. Borges Marg, Parel
Mumbai-400012, India

Chan Hon Chui MBBS, FRCS (Glasg)
Senior Surgical Oncology Fellow
Department of Surgery
St Jude Children's Research
Hospital
Memphis, TN 38105, USA

Chantal Rodary
Biostatistics, Bellon Nicolas
Institut Gustave Roussy
Villejuif, France

Chittaranjan Joshi MD
Senior Resident
Department of Anaesthesia
All India Institute of Medical
Sciences
New Delhi-110029, India

C van den Bos MD, PhD
Dept of Pediatric Oncology
Late Effects Outpatient Clinic
EKZ-AMC
Emma Children's Hospital AMC
Amsterdam, Holland

Deepika Gupta BA (Hons.)
Intern (MA Hons.)
Department of Psychology
University of Delhi
New Delhi

Devendra K Gupta MBBS, MS, MCh,
FICS, FAMS, FAMS (Hony), FRCSG
(Hony), DSc (Honoris Causa)
Professor and Head
Department of Pediatric Surgery
All India Institute of Medical
Sciences, Ansari Nagar
New Delhi
India

Ernst Horcher MD
Professor and Head
Department of Paediatric Surgery
University of Vienna Medical School
Vienna
Austria

Franz Xaver Felberbauer MD
Department of Paediatric Surgery
University of Vienna Medical School
Vienna
Austria

Gauri Kapoor MD, PhD
Sr Consultant and Incharge
Division of Pediatric Hematology
and Oncology
Rajiv Gandhi Cancer Institute and
Research Centre
Sector 5, Rohini
Delhi-10085
India

Gautam Agarwal MS, MCh
Senior Research Associate
Department of Pediatric Surgery
All India Institute of Medical
Sciences, New Delhi
India

GK Rath MD
Professor and Head
Department of Radiotherapy
Institute Rotary Cancer Hospital
All India Institute of Medical
Sciences
New Delhi-110029, India

GP Hadley MB, ChB, FRCSEd
Professor and Head
Department of Pediatric Oncology
Faculty of Health Science
Nelson R Mandela School of
Medicine
University of KwaZulu-Natal
KwaZulu-Natal
Durban, 4013
Republic of South Africa

HA Heij MD, PhD
Pediatric Surgical Center of
Amsterdam
Emma Children's Hospital AMC
and VU University Medical Center
Amsterdam, Holland

Hidetaka Niizuma MD, PhD
Biochemistry
Chiba Cancer Center Research
Institute
666-2 Nitonu, Chuoh-ku
Chiba 260-8717
Japan

Hitoshi Ikeda MD, PhD
Professor
Department of Pediatric Surgery
Dokkyo Medical University
Koshigaya Hospital
2-1-50, Minami-Koshigaya
Koshigaya
Saitama-343-8555
Japan

HJH van der Pal MD
Department of Medical Oncology
Late Effects Outpatient Clinic
EKZ-AMC
Emma Children's Hospital AMC
Amsterdam, Holland

Jaun A Tovar MD, PhD
Professor and Head
Department of Pediatric Surgery
Hospital Universitario La Paz
Madrid, Spain

Kalinga K Naik MD
Senior Resident
Department of Radiotherapy
Institute Rotary Cancer Hospital
All India Institute of Medical
Sciences
New Delhi-110029, India

K Ganessan MD
Senior Resident,
Department of Medical Oncology
Institute Rotary Cancer Hospital
All India Institute of Medical
Sciences
New Delhi-110029, India

Kenneth W Gow MSc, MD, FRCSC
Junior Attending Pediatric Surgeon
Department of Surgery
St Jude Children's Research Hospital
Memphis, TN 38105, USA

KH Reeta MD
Assistant Professor
Department of Pharmacology
All India Institute of Medical
Sciences, Ansari Nagar
New Delhi-110029, India

Kiran Mishra MBBS, MD
Professor
Department of Pathology
University College of Medical
Sciences and GTB Hospital
Shahdara
Delhi-110095, India

Lalit Kumar MD
Professor
Department of Medical Oncology
Institute Rotary Cancer Hospital
All India Institute of Medical
Sciences
New Delhi-110029, India

LS Arya MD
Former Professor and Head
Department of Pediatrics
All India Institute of Medical
Sciences
New Delhi-110029, India

Madhu Bhardwaj
Former Clinical Psychologist
Department of Pediatric Surgery
All India Institute of Medical
Sciences
New Delhi-110029, India

MA Skinner MD
Department of Surgery
Washington University School of
Medicine
St Louis, MO
USA

Mark D Stringer BSc, MBBS, FRCP,
FRCS, MS, FRCS (Paed.), FRCS (Ed.)
Consultant Paediatric
Hepatobiliary/Transplant Surgeon
and Professor of Paediatric Surgery
Children's Liver and GI Unit
Gledhow Wing
St. James's University Hospital
Beckett Street, Leeds
West Yorkshire
LS9 7TF, UK

MK Arora MD
Professor
Department of Anaesthiology and
Intensive Care, AIIMS
New Delhi-110029, India

M Ragavan MS, MRCS
Senior Resident
Department of Pediatric Surgery
AIIMS, New Delhi-110029, India

Mridula Mehta MS, DNB
Senior Resident
Ophthalmology
Dr RP Centre for Ophthalmic
Sciences, AIIMS
New Delhi-110029, India

PA Kurkure MD, DCH
Professor/Incharge
Pediatric Oncology
Department of Medical Oncology
Tata Memorial Hospital
Parel, Mumbai-400012

Partha Mukhopadhyay MD
Department of Radiotherapy
Institute Rotary Cancer Hospital
All India Institute of Medical
Sciences, New Delhi

Piotr Czauderna MD, PhD
Head of the Department
Department of Surgery and Urology
for Children and Adolescents
Medical University of Gdansk
Poland
UI. Nowe Ogrody 1-6
Gdansk-80-803
Poland

PK Julka MD
Professor
Department of Radiotherapy
Institute Rotary Cancer Hospital
All India Institute of Medical
Sciences, New Delhi

P Sarat Chandra MCh
Assistant Professor
Department of Neurosurgery
Cardio Neuro Center
All India Institute of Medical
Sciences, New Delhi

Rakesh Kumar MD
Associate professor
Department of Nuclear Medicine
All India Institute of Medical
Sciences
New Delhi-110029, India

R Jagarlamudi MD
Department of Medical Oncology
Institute Rotary Cancer Hospital
All India Institute of Medical
Sciences
New Delhi-110029, India

RK Minkes MD
Department of Surgery
Washington University School of
Medicine
St Louis, MO, USA

Robert Carachi MD, PhD, FRCS
(Glasgow), FRCS (Eng)
Professor and Head
Section of Surgical Paediatrics
Royal Hospital for Sick Children
Yorkhill, Glasgow, Scotland, UK

Sameer Bakhshi MD
Diplomate of American Board of
Pediatrics, Fellowship in Pediatric
Hematology Oncology (USA)
Assistant Professor of Pediatric
Oncology
Department of Medical Oncology
Dr BRA Institute Rotary Cancer
Hospital
All India Institute of Medical
Sciences, New Delhi

Sandeep Agarwala MCh
Associate Professor
Department of Pediatric Surgery
All India Institute of Medical
Sciences, New Delhi

Sandeep Guleria MS, DNB, FRCS,
FRCS (Ed) MNAMS
Additional Professor
Surgery
All India Institute of Medical
Sciences, New Delhi-110029

Sani Molagool MD
Surgical Oncology Fellow
Department of Surgery
St Jude Children's Research
Hospital
Memphis, TN 38105, USA

Sanjiv Nainiwal MD, DNB, MNAMS
Senior Resident
Ophthalmology
Dr RP Centre for Ophthalmic
Science, AIIMS, New Delhi

Savita Sapra
Clinical Psychologist
Department of Pediatrics
All India Institute of Medical
Sciences, New Delhi

Seema Briyal PhD
Senior Research Fellow
Department of Pharmacology
All India Institute of Medical
Sciences, Ansari Nagar
New Delhi-110029, India

Seong Min Kim MD
Division of Pediatric Surgery
Department of Surgery
Yonsei University College of
Medicine
Seoul, Korea

Seung Hoon Choi MD
Division of Pediatric Surgery
Department of Surgery
Yonsei University College of
Medicine
146-92, Dokok-dong
Kangnam-Gu
Seoul
Korea-135-752

Shilpa Sharma MS, MCh, DNB
Senior Research Associate
Department of Pediatric Surgery
All India Institute of Medical
Sciences, New Delhi

Shinitsu Hatakeyama MD
Director Radiology
Gunma Children's Medical Center
Hokkitsu, Shibukawa
Gunma, Japan

Spencer W Beasley MB ChB (Otago),
MS (Melb), FRACS
Chief, Child Health Service and
Clinical Director
Department of Pediatric Surgery
Christchurch Hospital
Canterbury District Health Board
New Zealand

Subhash C Gulati MD
Department of Medical Oncology
Institute Rotary Cancer Hospital
All India Institute of Medical
Sciences, New Delhi

Sudeep Gupta MD
Department of Medical Oncology
Institute Rotary Cancer Hospital
All India Institute of Medical
Sciences, New Delhi

Sunil Narain
Senior Resident
Department of Pediatrics
All India Institute of Medical
Sciences
New Delhi-110029, India

Supriyo Ghose MD, MNAMS
Chief Ophthalmology
Dr RP Centre for Ophthalmic
Sciences, AIIMS
Ansari Nagar
New Delhi-110029, India

Tatsuo Kuroda MD, PhD
Chief
Surgery
National Center for Child Health
and Development
2-10-1 Okura, Setagaya-ku
Tokyo
Japan-157-8535

TD Chugh MD, FRC Path, FAAH
Director of Laboratories and
Sr. Consultant Microbiology
Sir Ganga Ram Hospital
New Delhi, India

Tulika Seth MD
Fellowship Pediatric Hematology
and Oncology
Assistant Professor
Department of Hematology
All India Institute of Medical
Sciences, Ansari Nagar
New Delhi-110029, India

Veena Gupta MD
Department of Radio Therapy
Safdarjung Hospital
Ansari Nagar
New Delhi-110029, India

Venkateswaran K Iyer MD
Associate Professor
Department of Pathology
AIIMS, Ansari Nagar
New Delhi-110029, India

Vinod Kochupillai MD
Professor and Head
Department of Medical Oncology
Chief, Dr B R Ambedkar Institute
Rotary Cancer Hospital
All India Institute of Medical
Sciences, New Delhi-110029

VS Mehta MCh
Professor and Head
Department of Neurosurgery
Cardio Neuro Center
All India Institute of Medical
Sciences, New Delhi-110029

VT Joseph MD
Professor and Chairman
Department of Pediatric Surgery
KK Women's and Children's
Hospital
Singapore 229889

Winfried Rebhandl MD
Department of Paediatric Surgery
University of Vienna Medical School
Vienna, Austria

Yogendra K Gupta MD
Professor and Head
Pharmacology
All India Institute of Medical
Sciences, Ansari Nagar
New Delhi-110029, India

(Late) Yoshiaki Tsuchida MD, PhD,
FACS
Director
Department of Surgery
Gunma Children's Medical Center
779, Shimo-hakota, Hokkitsu
Seta-gun, Gunma 377-8577
Japan

FOREWORD

"Twenty years from now you will be disappointed by the things you did not do rather than by the things you did. Catch the trade winds. Explore. Dream. Discover." – Mark Twain

This multiauthor text on pediatric oncology edited by Prof. Devendra K Gupta and Prof. Robert Carachi fulfills an important need in the assessment, management, and long-term follow-up of children with cancer. Modern oncology has evolved remarkably over the past two decades, so that we are now able to treat the unique pathology and disease processes associated with pediatric tumors. Clinicians increasingly must have a comprehensive background in the molecular basis of cancer, as it takes a leading role in determining diagnosis and treatment.

Since 1960, overall survival has increased from 20 to 70 percent for most pediatric cancers. This stunning progress has been made through strict adherence to investigational protocols conducted by single institutions and multi-institutional study groups. These multidisciplinary protocols have made multi-agent chemotherapy, newer and more effective radiation therapy, and improved surgical techniques the standard of care. These improvements, combined with progress in diagnostic imaging (MRI, PET scans) and supportive care (antibiotics, nutrition, blood products, rehabilitation, pain control), have made treatment planning for childhood cancer safe, innovative, and effective.

The logical conclusion of improved long-term survival has been a shift in philosophy. The primary aim of treatment is now to reduce morbidity while maintaining disease-free survival. Modifications aimed at achieving that goal include: (a) decreased chemotherapy and radiation therapy for localized disease, (b) use of preoperative therapy to decrease the size of bulky tumors, and (c) changes in the role of surgery in relation to other therapies. The rapid pace of growth in knowledge, plus greater understanding of the molecular basis of cellular processes, improved biotechnology, and refinement of treatment modalities, has advanced every phase of care.

The 21st century may hold great opportunities and challenges in the care of children with cancer. The practicing oncologist—whether his specialty is medicine, radiation, or surgery—must be able to command a formidable knowledge base and to interact with colleagues in a wide range of disciplines. This text, written by multiple investigators and innovative oncologists, should be of value to all students, faculty members, and physicians, regardless of their years in practice.

Although it is gratifying to see how far the practice of pediatric oncology has come, it is also daunting to recognize how far it has yet to go.

"Once you start studying medicine you will never get through." – CH Mayo

Bhaskar N Rao MD, FACS
Member, Department of Surgery
Director, Surgical Training Program
International Outreach Program
322 N. Lauderdale St.
Memphis, TN38105-2794, USA

FOREWORD

Significant improvements in survival have been achieved for children with malignant solid tumors during the past three decades. This no doubt has been influenced by the establishment of multidisciplinary cancer treatment programs following carefully designed protocols as part of cooperative cancer group studies. Most of the research and progress in childhood cancer has occurred in developed countries, mainly in the West where a health care infrastructure can support these endeavors. Unfortunately, 60 percent of the children with cancer in the world have limited access to effective cancer care and their survival is significantly less than children residing in developed countries. Cancer has emerged as a major cause of childhood mortality of Asia, South and Central America, northwest and Sub-Saharan Africa, and the Middle East. For example, it is estimated that in China alone, a country with 300 million children, 45,000 new pediatric cancer cases will occur annually. It is therefore appropriate and timely that a textbook concerning childhood cancer be forthcoming from this region of the world. *Pediatric Oncology (Surgical and Medical Aspects)* is edited by Professors Devendra K Gupta and Robert Carachi.

The content of the book is exhaustive and covers a wide spectrum of both pediatric medical and surgical oncologic topics. Most of the contributors are cancer experts from Asian countries including India, Japan, China and Korea. Some of the contributors from Europe have been active in the SIOP study groups and a sparse number from the US and Africa involved with COG studies and similar cancer protocols. The content focuses mainly on surgical oncologic care. The text is divided into seven sections: the scientific basis of pediatric surgical oncology, clinical pediatric surgical and medical oncology, subspecialty tumors, endocrine and other rare tumors, therapeutic strategies (including chemotherapy, radiation therapy and some novel treatments) and long-term outcomes. The latter area is of special importance since a considerable number of pediatric cancer survivors experience adverse long-term side-effects related to intensive treatment and quality of life is an important parameter.

In regard to solid tumors, the pediatric surgical oncologist still plays a vital role in the care of the cancer patient. The survival of children with most solid malignancies is enhanced by complete removal of the primary tumor. The text carefully covers the surgical management of each of the major childhood tumors and the multimodal neoadjuvant or adjuvant therapy that results in improved survival. The editors have also included useful appendices that provide details regarding tumor protocols and chemotherapy schedules.

The textbook, originating in Asia, should provide a unique perspective for pediatric surgical oncologic care to the readers in India and other parts of Asia. Hopefully, this will also stimulate an improved understanding of the surgical aspects of pediatric cancer and nurture the development of cancer programs in less developed areas of the world. I congratulate the editors for putting together a very contemporary and informative textbook that should be a useful addition to the surgeon's library.

Jay L Grosfeld MD
Lafayette F Page Professor of Pediatric Surgery, Emeritus
Indiana University School of Medicine
Indianapolis, Indiana, USA

PREFACE

Dealing with young children suffering from the most dreaded disease of malignancy has never been a pleasant experience. It requires tremendous zeal of courage to deal with the parents and help them cope up with the reality to put a brave front forward to win the battle. This is followed by an array of investigations in the right direction and then the appropriate treatment as decided by the cancer board. There are various gray areas in between the diagnosis and cure.

The incidence of cancer worldwide for age matched controls for all sites varies between 220 and 320 per 100,000 populations. The highest incidence is in the South American continent followed by Australia, Europe, Africa, North America and Asia in the decreasing order. The term 'childhood cancer' describes cancer diagnosed before the age of 15. This includes 30 percent of the total cases of cancer. About half of these die each year.

The cancers found in children are completely different from those seen in adults and these include leukemia, lymphomas, brain tumors, nephroblastoma, neuroblastoma and others and forms one of the leading causes of mortality the world over. It is the third main cause of deaths in children, after infections and malnutrition in developing countries and second most common cause in developed countries after trauma.

The treatment for pediatric cancer as in adults is multispecialty, involving pediatric surgeons, oncologists, radiotherapist, radiologist, pathologist and nuclear medicine specialist. An expert in the field of pain relief and nutrition is also needed for the terminally ill patients with incurable diseases. Though, a steady progress has been made over the past 40 years resulting in substantial improvement in the comprehensive medical and surgical care resulting in better quality of life of children suffering with malignancy yet, the children from developing world present very late with advanced stage of the disease, suffer from poor nutrition, anemia and bulky tumors. The resources are limited. The workload is too much. Also the expertise and the facilities remain limited and available mostly to the urban population.

There are presently about 40 pediatric centers in India providing surgical care to the children with various types of pediatric cancers. The number is grossly inadequate keeping in mind the massive workload from 400 million children in India alone. Chemotherapy drugs, though available, are expensive and toxic to our children. The facility for radiotherapy is available only at a few places. The overall cancer treatment is very expensive and remains beyond the reach of the common man. Though, a support from the Government, NGOs and philanthropists is made available from time to time, yet it remains inadequate and insufficient.

The Department of Pediatric Surgery at All India Institute of Medical Sciences, New Delhi has been actively involved with the pediatric cancer patients, providing surgery, chemotherapy, radiotherapy and other support. Many academic activities including the Pediatric Cancer Awareness Day and an International Symposium on Pediatric Oncology have been organized from time to time with the objectives to create awareness among the general public and to share the scientific knowledge with the experts. This recent symposium held during the Golden Jubilee of AIIMS, laid the foundation to publish this book on Pediatric Malignancies to serve as a reference point for various institutions and the teaching community, especially those serving in the developing world. AIIMS has developed a telemedicine link with the Royal Hospital for Sick Children, Yolkhill, Glasgow. This has led to various discussions on difficult tumor cases between the two institutions.

The book has been divided into seven sections for easy understanding and smooth flow of ideas from one section to the other. Section 1 on Basic Sciences provides an insight into the epidemiology, genetics, pathology and recent developments in the diagnosis of the various tumors. Section 2 on Clinical Basis deals with the major tumors dealt by pediatric surgeons in great depth and deals with all minute details of handling these cases. Section 3 on Medical Oncology deals with the thee major malignancies in children as dealt by the experts in their field would be beneficial to medical oncologists. The sections 4 and 5 on Subspecialities and Rare Tumors make this book complete in itself on all types of malignancies in children including bone, brain and eye. Sections 6 and 7 deal with Therapeutic Strategies and Long-term Results in Pediatric Surgical Oncology.

We warmly acknowledge the support received from the faculty and the staff of our departments, in particular Dr Shilpa Sharma, Senior Research Associate, who has been working very hard, almost single handedly, reviewing and scrutinizing the manuscripts in detail before sending these to print.

It was a pleasant experience to work with M/s Jaypee Brothers Medical Publishers (P) Ltd, New Delhi, who agreed to publish this book at a reasonable cost. It is hoped that it would be useful to the students, teachers and the experts dealing with various types of cancers in children, working under suboptimal facilities.

Devendra K Gupta
Robert Carachi

CONTENTS

SECTION FIVE: ENDOCRINE TUMORS AND RARE PEDIATRIC SURGICAL TUMORS

SECTION SIX: THERAPEUTIC STRATEGIES IN PEDIATRIC SURGICAL ONCOLOGY

SECTION SEVEN: LONG-TERM RESULTS IN PEDIATRIC SURGICAL ONCOLOGY

The Scientific Basis of
Pediatric Surgical Oncology

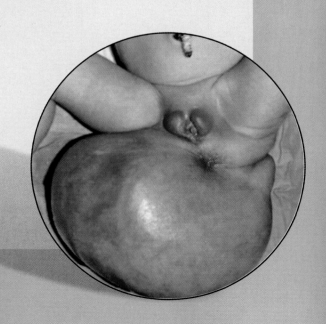

CHAPTER 1

Chantal Rodary
Robert Carachi
Devendra K Gupta

Epidemiology of Childhood Tumors

Epidemiology is the study of the frequency and distribution of malignant tumors. The two frequency parameters most employed are incidence and mortality. These will be presented globally for the five continents, and also individually for certain countries, and according to the main characteristics of the subjects (age, sex, etc.) and of the type of cancers, without neglecting the dynamic nature of these parameters over time.

Unlike those found in adults, childhood cancers are particular in many respects: they are rare with the overall cumulative incidence up to 15 years varying only slightly from one country to another (roughly 1.0-2.5 per 1000). The incidence rate standardized on the age distribution of the world population ranges from 75 to 140 per million.[1] Furthermore, the histology of these tumors differs considerably and carcinomas are infrequent among the histologic types.

Many childhood cancers have histological features that resemble fetal tissues at various stages of development and are therefore designated as embryonal. Childhood cancers tend to have short latent periods, but are more responsive to chemotherapy than the tumors typically occurring in adults. Prospective epidemiological studies on childhood cancers need to be conducted to allow for uniform treatment policies.

Pediatric tumors should be classified by histology rather than primary site of the tumor. The incidence of childhood cancer is only 2 percent of that in adults in developed countries and about 3 percent in developing countries. It is likely that genetic predisposition has a greater role in the etiology. In the developing countries, reliable data on incidence and mortality of childhood cancers are available from only a few areas. Analysis of specific tumor types show more striking geographic

variations of rates that are not readily explained by deficiencies in the data. It is essential that childhood tumors than those of adults, and thus comparisons between different ethnic groups living in the same area or between similar ethnic groups in different environments may be particularly relevant.

In this chapter, frequency parameters, the age of the children (0-14 years), age categories and the classification of tumors are those defined by the International Agency for Research on Cancer (IARC, Lyon, France) in its publications.[2-6]

CLASSIFICATION OF CHILDHOOD TUMORS

Due to the diversity of the histologic types of childhood tumors, the *International Classification of Disease for Oncology* (ICDO) used for adults, cannot be applied.[7] The Birch and Marsden Classification, recognized by the World Health Organization (WHO) is the classification most often used.[8] It is based on histology and the site of the tumors that are divided into 12 diagnostic groups:

I. Leukemias
II. Lymphomas and other reticuloendothelial neoplasms
III. Central nervous system and miscellaneous intracranial and intraspinal neoplasms (including non-malignant tumors, recorded in many cancer registries)
IV. Sympathetic nervous system tumors
V. Retinoblastomas
VI. Renal tumors
VII. Hepatic tumors
VIII. Malignant bone tumors
IX. Soft tissue sarcomas

X. Germ-cell trophoblastic and other gonadal neoplasms

XI. Carcinomas and other malignant epithelial neoplasms

XII. Other and unspecified malignant neoplasms

Each of these groups is further subdivided. This classification was revised and modified in 1996 to incorporate recent developments in pathology and epidemiology.[9] This work was conducted in collaboration with the IARC and the International Society of Pediatric Oncology (SIOP). The modifications are only applicable to the subgroups. Among them, the subgroup of renal tumors now comprises three categories:

a. Wilms' tumor, clear-cell sarcoma and rhabdoid tumors

b. Renal carcinoma

c. Unspecified malignant renal tumors

The histiocytosis X category, part of group II, has been totally excluded from the classification. Non-malignant intracranial and intraspinal germ-cell tumors are no longer in group III but are now in group X.

A correspondence table has been established with ICD, but this presents some imperfections especially for neoplasms of the nervous system: for instance neuroblastoma is occasionally coded with the organ affected or with connective and soft tissue sarcomas and with the nervous system.[10]

MORBIDITY REGISTRIES

The objective is to compile a registry of all the new cancer cases. If a registry is to be of good quality, it must have an underlying epidemiological structure that conti-nuously and exhaustively records new cancer cases occurring in the population in a given region. These registries are called population-based registries. As childhood cancers are rare, it is important that the population on which the registry is based is sufficiently large to accommodate an adequate number of events permitting reliable estimations.

Currently, few countries are entirely covered by cancer morbidity registries. Denmark was among the first to start a registry (1942), then the Nordic countries (Sweden, Finland, Norway, from 1952), the UK (since 1962) and more recently Canada and Australia (1977). In the USA, the National Cancer Institute (NCI) SEER (Surveillance, Epidemiology and End-Results) program registries cover roughly 10 percent of the population. In African and certain Asian countries, only hospital-based or histopathology-based registries are available

and these sources contain information of dubious precision on the size of the population at risk and the number of new cases in the population.

Quality of diagnosis and classification of tumor site also need to be evaluated in each registry, to determine reliability of data.

An International Association of Cancer Registries (IACR) was created in 1966 to support members interested in the development and applications of cancer registration and morbidity survey techniques to studies on well-defined populations. The statistics published by the IARC in 1982 are based on registries of approxi-mately 50 countries. More recent data have been published in other registries.[11-15]

Cancer Mortality Data

Since the 1950s, data on mortality have been available in numerous countries. They are published annually for each country by the WHO in the World Health Statistics Directory.

In reality, registration of deaths is not always all-embracing. WHO recommendations concerning registration of deaths are not complied with everywhere and certain procedures can vary between countries often resulting in inaccurate or even unavailable information on the causes of deaths.

Survival Data

Some morbidity registries also record data on survival, thus allowing survival rates to be compared by type of cancer. A European study (EUROCARE), which began in 1990, has compiled data from 30 European registries (approximately 800000 patients - of whom just under 8000 are children) to compare survival rates between countries.[6]

MORBIDITY AND MORTALITY PARAMETERS
Crude Rate

Crude Incidence Rate (IR)

This quantitates new cases over a given period, in a given population. Most often, annual figures are provided per million persons. Data abstracted from the cancer morbidity registries that exist in each country are used to calculate this rate. The denominator, also known as the total number of person-years, is the time accumulated for a subject exposed to a risk of developing a cancer during the period under consideration. The quality of these estimations is obviously contingent upon that of the registries.

Crude Mortality Rate (MR)

This is calculated in a similar manner to that used to calculate the incidence rate, but taking into account the number of deaths. Here, the denominator is the number of individuals at risk of death due to cancer, accumulated for the periods considered (person-years). The calculation of mortality rates is exhaustive, since all the deaths are recorded and the size of the population at risk is counted at the census.

Specific Rates

It is possible to calculate specific rates by age categories, site, geographic location, etc. Thus, if we consider age-specific morbidity, four rates, IR0, IR1, IR2, IR3, will be obtained for children aged < 1 year, 1-4 years, 5-9 years, and 10-14 years respectively.

Standardized Rates

In order to be able to compare cancer incidence or mortality rates between populations, the effect of confounding factors such as age, sex, site, etc. must be eliminated with standardization methods.

DIRECT STANDARDIZATION (STANDARD POPULATION METHOD)

The procedure is based on the calculation of the expected number of cases in each age group of a standard population by applying to the corresponding person-years, the estimated rate of the population under study. The total number of expected cases is then divided by the total number of person-years in the theoretical population and yields an age standardized rate (ASR). This method, used by Parkin can also be used for incidence and mortality rates.[2] A cumulated incidence rate (CUM) can also be calculated using the corresponding specific rates for each year by summing the total of each year (0-14).

INDIRECT STANDARDIZATION

Standardized incidence rates (SIR) are defined as the ratio between the total number of new cases and the number of new cases expected if the population was subject to the specific incidence rates of the standard population for each age group. The same procedure is applied for the calculation of the Standardized mortality rate (SMR).

INCIDENCE RATE FOR TOTAL CHILDHOOD CANCERS WORLDWIDE

The IARC study which essentially covers the decade around 1975, provides the ASR and CUM for certain countries.[2] Worldwide ASR vary from 75 to 140 per million population, whereas CUM vary from 1000 to 25000 per million population.

Regarding sex, ASR vary by a ratio of 1:2 (86.3-164.1 per million for boys and 34.5-130.4 for girls). The rates are on average higher among boys than among girls, whatever the country considered.

Concerning race, ASR are higher among whites than among blacks of whatever sex.[17]

Variations in Incidence Rates

The distribution of types of childhood cancers is practically identical worldwide, the most frequent cancers being leukemias (30%) followed by brain tumors and tumors of the central nervous system (20%), lymphomas (14%) and neuroblastomas (8%) (Fig. 1.1). In certain developing countries the relative frequency of lymphomas, retinoblastomas and Wilms' tumors is higher.

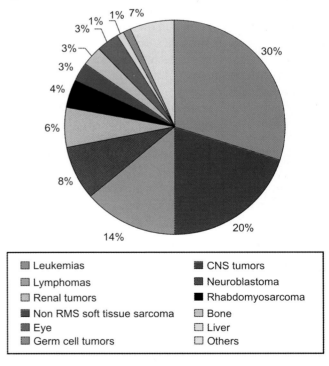

Figure 1.1: Chart showing frequency distribution of the incidence of pediatric malignancies in percentage

The total crude incidence rates in India per 1,000,000 populations were 100 for males and 68 for females.[16] Age adjusted incidence rate for world population and crude rates for both the sexes for total childhood cancers did not show any differences. Leukemias showed the highest incidence rate followed by CNS tumors in both the sexes. Male preponderance was observed at all sites and was most marked in the leukemias and lymphomas.

Stiller and Parkin1 have synthesized IARC data having compared the results for countries where the type of cancer was known.[2] They found that lymphoblastic acute leukemias, especially during early childhood, are more frequent in countries with a high standard of living and that they represent approximately 80 percent of childhood leukemias in the industrialized countries.

In Hodgkin's disease, the variations between countries and ethnic groups are complex and imply the existence of various etiological factors linked to age or to the histologic subtype. It is well known that Burkitt's lymphoma, identified to have originated in Tropical Africa, is particularly frequent on both sides of the Equator. Socioeconomic factors have been suggested in the causation in these areas. In Nigeria (Ibadan), between 1960 and 1984, almost half of the cancers were Burkitt's lymphomas and the ASR was approximately 80 per million. In high risk areas, Burkitt's lymphoma occur in the head and neck. In most of these countries, the incidence is decreasing as a result of malaria eradication programs. The new histological and immunological data on lymphomas should shed light in the coming years on specific geographical variations of certain forms of lymphoma.

Brain tumors rank second after leukemias in industrialized countries, with the ASR between 20 and 30 per million. In decreasing order of frequency, astrocytomas and medulloblastomas are to be found (included in the 1996 modifications among the primitive neuroectodermal tumors (PNET). It is noteworthy that in developing countries where neurosurgical facilities are lacking and where the number of autopsies is low, the number of new cases is undoubtedly underestimated.

Neuroblastomas account for the quasi-totality of childhood sympathetic central nervous system tumors. During the 1970s, the ASR varied from 7 to 12 per million for populations in Europe, North America and Oceania, with an extremely elevated rate for the first year of life. This rate has risen considerably in Japan since the introduction of early screening in the 1980s: between 1971 and 1980, it varied from 27.1 to 34.1 per million in the first year of life. Since then, it has approached the 100 per million.[18] It is widely admitted that many of the neuroblastomas among those screened would never have been clinically detectable and would never have led to fatal oucome.

The retinoblastomas (non-inherited) (which make up 60 percent of the total) are more frequent in the less affluent countries. It has been hypothesized that poor living conditions could be at the origin of infections or that environmental factors may lead to a mutation *in utero* or during childhood.

The great majority of renal tumors are Wilms' tumors. The highest ASR are observed in black populations regardless of whether Africa or the USA. Age distribution is the same as that of the white populations. The lowest ASR are observed in East Asia.

Hepatoblastoma is one of the least common embryonal tumors whose incidence worldwide is stable (ASR H" 1 per million). Hepatocellular carcinoma is even more rare than hepatoblastoma. It mainly occurs among children suffering from chronic hepatitis B, in regions in Africa or Asia where the rate of liver cancer is elevated among adults.

Concerning bone tumors, slight variations are noted in the incidence of osteosarcomas from one country to another.[19] Such is not the case for Ewing's tumors whose incidence rates vary by a ratio of roughly 1:3 with the lowest rates being observed in Africa and in East and South-East Asia and the highest rates in Australia.

Soft tissue sarcomas comprise numerous histologically heterogeneous tumors, the most common among them being rhabdomyosarcoma. France and the Jewish population in Israel have the highest ASR for all of these tumors. The lowest rates are in Asia, but the difference observed may be related to the difficulty in the accurate histologic diagnoses of these tumors where more sophisticated diagnostic techniques are required. Given their limited number, the incidence rates of germ-cell trophoblastic and other gonadal tumors are rather stable. However, the ASR is elevated in East Asia.

Worldwide Temporal Trends in Cancer Incidence

The publications are based on the works of the IARC.[5,10,20,21] Numerous problems are encountered when attempts are made to establish these estimations over time: rareness of the disease, the calendar period during which these data are available and the grouping together of regions according to geographical or economic development criteria are some of the many factors and sources of heterogeneity that need to be taken into account. For instance, Europe is divided into four regions consisting of the following countries: Central Europe (Hungary, Germany (former GDR), Poland, Slovenia); Nordic (Denmark, Finland, Norway, Sweden); Western (France, Germany (former FRG), Italy, Spain, Switzerland); United Kingdom (UK) and Southern Ireland.

In the Nordic region and the UK, the registries cover all the countries concerned, which is not the case for the other regions. To these difficulties must be added the quality of the registries that vary markedly from one country to another.

Coleman uses the linear trend (LT) which is the percentage change in risk every 5 years over the entire data period to express these variations.[5] For example, for leukemias, the most frequent cancer in childhood whose diagnosis is the least problematic, he observed the following: the incidence has risen significantly from 1965 to 1985 among boys in central Europe (LT: 3.7%) and for both sexes in the UK (LT: 5.2 and 7.3% respectively for boys and girls). Among girls, it has increased in the Nordic countries (LT: 5.2%) and declined in Western Europe (LT: 22.8%). In Asia and Oceania, although the incidence rates are very heterogeneous, a significant increase is observed among boys in Bombay, Hong Kong and New Zealand (LT respectively: 12.2, 18.1, 8.0%). In the USA, the CUM are stable among blacks as well as among whites.

If these estimations are limited to countries with a population-based registry, the information is more complete and the diagnosis of the type of tumor is more accurate.[22-25] It should nonetheless be noted that the significant decline in unspecified malignant neoplasms attributable to an increased number of biopsies and progress in histological diagnoses, is at the origin of part of the increase observed.

Gurney found an annual increase of 1 percent in the SIR in the USA (95% confidence interval: 0.6-1.3) between 1974 and 1991 for all the cancers registered by the SEER program.[23] This increase is 2 percent per annum or more for tumors of the central nervous system (CNS), rhabdomyosarcomas, germ-cell tumors and osteosarcomas.

Bunin also observed an annual increase of 1 percent for all the cancers registered in the Greater Delaware Valley Registry (USA) between 1970 and 1989.[22] This increase essentially concerns CNS tumors (2.7%).

MORTALITY RATE

Mortality Rate for Total Childhood Cancers Worldwide

Between 1985 and 1990,[10,21] the age standardized mortality rates (ASRM) of the world population were based on WHO mortality data. In Europe they range from 42.4 in Austria to 82.3 in Bulgaria per 1000000 boys and 30.2 in Finland to 59.7 in Portugal per 1000000 girls.

Variations in Mortality Rates

Role of Cancer in Infant Mortality

If the first year of life is excluded, because of the extent of neonatal mortality after accidents, deaths due to cancer are the second highest cause of death between 1 and 14 years of age.[26]

Temporal Trends in Cancer Mortality

In the worldwide study conducted by Levi based on WHO mortality data a general decline in age standardized mortality rates is observed between 1950 and 1989 for all cancer.[10,21] Temporal trends vary from one country to another. Thus in Europe, these declines were generally earlier and larger in Northern Europe compared with Southern Europe, and mostly with Eastern European countries; this reduction in mortality is still evident over the most recent calendar periods. The range of variation in total childhood cancer mortality was around a factor of 2 in both sexes, with the highest rates in Bulgaria, Portugal, Hungary, Czechoslovakia and Poland, and the lowest rates in Austria, UK, Germany, The Netherlands and Finland.

In the majority of European countries, these declines are sharp for leukemias, Wilms' tumors, Hodgkin's disease and other lymphomas. It is more difficult to interpret data from the American continent or Oceania because of the dubious reliability of death certificates in certain countries in Latin America and Asia. It can however be stated, beyond reasonable doubt, that the highest mortality rates for all types of cancer are in certain Latin American countries, in Kuwait, New Zealand and Singapore (between 65 and 75 per 1000000 among boys and between 50 and 65 per 1000000 among girls). When compared with the developed countries where mortality rates are low: Canada, USA, Australia, Japan and Israel (roughly 45 per 1000000 among boys and between 35 and 40 per 1000000 among girls) the ratio between sexes is 1:8.

In a study from developing countries, the death rate per 1,000,000 population in pediatric malignancies in decreasing order of death rate was leukemia (20), CNS tumors (10), lymphoma (5) and others (1 each).[16]

A study concerning the entire US population provides accurate results for the period 1950-80. For the period 1965-79, standardized mortality rates were obtained by using data for the 1950-54 period as a reference. The decline in mortality was marked from 1965, and during 1965 through 1979, the number of deaths observed was 44 percent below the expected number at the 1950 rate. With respect to the type of tumor, the decline in mortality was 50 percent for leukemia, 32 percent for non-Hodgkin's lymphoma (NHL), 80 percent for Hodgkin's disease, 50 percent for bone sarcomas, 68 percent for kidney cancer and 31 percent for all other cancers.

SURVIVAL RATES

Recorded survival data allow a more detailed assessment of the temporal evolution of cancers.[17,27-32]

Among these studies, Stiller's report analyzed 5-year survival rates in the UK in a series of 15000 children suffering from a cancer diagnosed between 1971 and 1985, with a follow-up of at least 3 years.[30] A notable improvement was observed in survival rates except for those regarding brain tumors (excepting medullo-blastomas), Ewing's tumors, fibrosarcomas, neuro-fibrosarcomas and other soft tissue sarcomas for which progress is minimal. The most spectacular improvements (as regards the c2 test for linear trends) between 1971-73 and 1983-85 concerned ALL (acute lymphoblastic leukemia), NHL and neuroblastomas (localized forms). They were also marked for ANLL (acute non-lymphoblastic leukemia), rhabdomyosarcomas and Wilms' tumors.

In 1994, Stiller continued the same study including children suffering from a cancer diagnosed between 1980 and 1991, in order to assess the impact of recent developments in medical care since 1985.[31] Compared with the results published in 1990, the notable findings since 1985 were an improvement in ANLL and in short-term (1-year) survival of Ewing's sarcomas. No progress was observed for neuroblastomas. Stiller concluded: 'The projections of 10-year survival for children who had cancer diagnosed in 1989-91 suggested an overall

increase in survival of 19 percent since 1980-82.' This suggests that nearly two-thirds of children who have cancer diagnosed can expect to survive at least 10 years.[31]

The significant advances achieved during the past 30 years are due to the multidisciplinary care, the employment of new treatments administered within the framework of standardized protocols, and in hospitals specializing in childhood cancer. The creation of an international organization such as the International Society of Pediatric Oncology in 1969 and the establishment of different cooperative groups have permitted better coordinated research programs (Children's Cancer Group, Pediatric Oncology Group in the USA and United Kingdom Children's Cancer Study Group in the UK).

Further progress will undoubtedly ensue through analytical and experimental epidemiology. To this end, more reliable descriptive data are required. The problems with the reliability of the diagnosis on death certificates and completeness of data have been alluded to in this chapter. Draper underscored the risks of misinterpreting the results of mortality data.[33]

1. Tumor can be misclassified at diagnosis (e.g. neuroblastoma when using the ICDO code).
2. Random fluctuations (especially if rates are based on small numbers).
3. Trends in mortality may be the results of, or may be obscured by underlying incidence rates.

If epidemiology is to fulfill its objectives then accurate data of good quality should be obtained and studies should use population-based registries as a source of solid, reliable data.

AGE AND SEX DISTRIBUTION

Most of the tumors in children occur more frequently in boys than girls. However, for acute nonlymphatic leukemia, osteosarcoma, retinoblastoma and melanoma the sex ratio is around unity. The tumors more frequent in girls are Wilms' tumor, carcinomas of the adrenal cortex and thyroid.

Tumors more common in infants include neuroblastoma, retinoblastoma, soft tissue sarcoma and hepatic tumors. The incidence of hepatic tumors is highest in children aged under 1 years. Acute lymphatic leukemia is well documented for distinctive peak in the age range of 1-5 years. Wilms' tumor and germ cell tumor are more common in children under 5 years than in older age groups.

Wilms' tumor comprises approximately 95 percent of all renal neoplasms. Sixty five percent Wilms' tumors occur in children under 5 years of age, 35 percent in children aged 5-9 years and 10 percent in 10-14 children aged years.

Osteosarcoma is very rare below the age of 5 years, but increases steeply thereafter. Ewing's sarcoma is also very rare under 5 years and the incidence increases with age, but less markedly than for osteosarcoma.

Retinoblastoma has the lowest median age of all childhood cancers (approximately 15 months) and bilateral cases tend to be diagnosed at a younger age than unilateral cases. Incidence peaks in the first year of life and declines gradually with age thereafter.

To summarize, childhood cancers are much more in boys than in girls. Leukemias are the most common cancers affecting children followed by CNS tumors and lymphomas. Fatality from cancer in children appears to be of the same order in both the sexes. There is no significant change in incidence patterns of childhood cancer worldwide and over time.

REFERENCES

1. Stiller CA, Parkin DM. Geographic and ethnic variation in the incidence of childhood cancer. Brit Med Bull 1996;52:682-703.
2. Parkin DM, Stiller CA, Draper GJ, et al. (Eds). International Incidence of Childhood Cancer. Lyon, France: IARC Scientific Publications No 87, 1988.
3. Parkin DM, Stiller CA, Draper GJ, et al. The international incidence of childhood cancer. Int J Cancer 1988; 42: 511-20.
4. Parkin DM, Muir CS, Whelan SL, et al. Cancer Incidence in Five Continents Vol 6. Lyon, France: IARC Scientific Publications No 120, 1992.
5. Coleman MP, Estève J, Damiecki P, Arslan A, Renard H. Trends in Cancer Incidence and Mortality. Lyon, France: IARC Scientific Publications No 121, 1993.
6. Berrino F, Sant H, Verdecchia A, Capocaccia R, Hakulinen T, Estève J. Survival of Cancer Patients in Europe. The EUROCARE Study. Lyon, France: IARC Scientific Publications No 132, 1995.
7. World Health Organization. International Classification of Diseases for Oncology. Geneva: WHO, 1976.
8. Percy C, Van Holten V, Muir C. ICD-0. International Classification of Diseases for Oncology (2nd edn). Geneva: World Health Organization, 1990.
9. Kramarova E. The international classification of childhood cancer. Int J Cancer 1996; 68: 759-65.
10. Levi F, La Vecchia C, Lucchini F, Negni E, Boyle P. Patterns of childhood cancer incidence and mortality in Europe. Eur J Cancer 1992;28A:2028-49.
11. Gurney JG, Severson RK, David S, Robison LL. Incidence of cancer in children in the United States: sex-, race-, and 1-year age-specific rates by histologic type. Cancer 1995;75:2186-95.
12. Stiller CA, Allen MB, Eatock EM. Childhood cancer in Britain: The National Registry of childhood tumours and incidence rates 1978-1987. Eur J Cancer 1995;31A:2028-34.
13. Kaatsch P, Haaf G, Michaelis J. Childhood malignancies in Germany. Methods and results of a nationwide registry. Eur J Cancer 1995;31A:993-9.
14. Ross JA, Severson RK, Pollock BH, Robison LL. Childhood cancer in the United States. A geographical analysis of cases from the Pediatric Cooperative Clinical Trials Groups. Cancer 1996; 77:201-7.
15. McWhirter WR, Dobson C, Ring I. Childhood cancer incidence in Australia. 1982-91. Int J Cancer 1996;65:34-8.
16. Yeole BB, Advani SH, Sunny Lizzy. Epidemiological Features of Childhood Cancers in Greater Mumbai. Indian Pediatrics 2001;38:1270-7.
17. Miller BA, Ries Lag, Hankey BF, et al (Eds): SEER Cancer Statistics Review: 1973-1990. National Cancer Institute. NIH Pub 1993; 92: 2789.
18. Sawada T, Kidowaki T, Sugimoto T, Kusunaki T. Incidence of Neuroblastoma in infancy in Japan. Med Pediatr Oncol 1984;12:101-3.
19. Parkin DM, Stiller CA, Nectoux J. International variations in the incidence of childhood bone tumors. Int J Cancer 1993;53:371-6.
20. Draper GJ, Kroll ME, Stiller CA. Childhood cancer. In: Doll R, Fraumeni JF Jr, Muir CS (Eds): Trends in Cancer Incidence and Mortality. Cancer Surveys 19/20. New-York: Cold Spring Harbor Laboratory Press 1994;493-517.
21. Levi F. La Vecchia C, Lucchini F, Negni E. Boyle P. Patterns of childhood cancer mortality: America, Asia and Oceania. Eur J Cancer 1995;31A:771-82.
22. Bunin GR. Increasing incidence of childhood cancer: report of 20 years experience from the Greater Delaware Valley Pediatric Tumor Registry. Paediatr Perinat Epidemiol 1996;10:319-38.
23. Gurney JG, Davis S, Severson RK, Fang JY, Ross JA, Robison LL. Trends in cancer incidence among children in the US. Cancer 1996;78:532-41.
24. Blair V, Birch JM, Patterns and temporal trends in the incidence of malignant disease in children. Leukaemia and lymphoma. Eur J Cancer 1994;30A:1490-97.
25. Blair V, Birch JM. Patterns and temporal trends in the incidence of malignant disease in children II. Solid tumours of childhood. Eur J Cancer 1994;30A:1498-1511.
26. Higginson J, Muir CS, Munoz N. Human Cancer: Epidemiology and Environmental Causes. Cambridge: Cambridge University Press, 1992;58:439-96.
27. Miller RW, McKay FW. Decline in US Childhood cancer mortality, 1950 through 1980. J Am Med Assoc 1984;251:1567-70.
28. Young JL, Gloeckler Ries L, Silverberg E, Horm JW, Miller RW. Cancer incidence, survival and mortality for children younger than age 15 years. Cancer 1986;58(Suppl 2):598-602
29. Birch JM, Marsden HB, Morris Jones PH et al. Improvements in survival from childhood cancer: Result of a population based survey over 30 years. Brit Med J 1988;296:1372-6.
30. Stiller CA, Bunch KJ. Trends in survival for childhood cancer in Britain diagnosed 1971-85. Brit J Cancer 1990;62:806-15.
31. Stiller CA. Population based survival rates for childhood cancer in Britain, 1980-91. Brit Med J 1994;309:1612-16.
32. Adami HO, Glimelius B, Sparen P, Holmberg L, Krusemo UB, Poten J. Trends in childhood and adolescent cancer survival in Sweden: 1960 through 1984. Acta Oncol 1992;31:1-10.
33. Draper GJ. Childhood cancer: Trends in incidence, survival and mortality. Eur J Cancer 1995; 31A:653-4.
34. Birch JM, Marsden HB. A classification scheme for childhood cancer. Int J Cancer 1987;40:620-4.

CHAPTER 2

Hidetaka Niizuma
Akira Nakagawara

Genetics and Molecular Biology of Pediatric Tumors

INTRODUCTION

"Cancer is a genetic disease." This grim principle, that everyone knows now, has made oncology one of the most progressed fields of medicine both in basic research and in clinics. Cancer cells present very different biological properties from normal cells in many aspects, including accelerated proliferation, resistance to apoptosis, limitless dividing, sustained angiogenesis, capability of invasion and metastasis, and instability of genome.[1,2] Such alterations in tumor biology, in theory, are due to genetic alterations which result from somatic and germ-line mutations. Genetic alterations have a fundamental role in the development of cancer, not only in adults but also in children. Actually, the number of children with cancer is much less than that of adult patients. However, research in pediatric cancer has provided many important basic insights into genetic mechanisms of tumorigenesis, as infant patients are usually exposed to less environmental oncogenic factors, such as mutagens and viruses than adults, thus pediatric tumors are more simply governed by genetic factors.

Over the past decades, fabulous findings in cancer genetics have been accumulated, which are supported by databases of human genomic information, and the amazing progress in microarray techniques both for gene expression analysis in tumor cells and for genomic analysis. Unfortunately, this advance in cancer genetics has not led to the entire understanding of tumor biology that contributes to tumor development, but some key mechanisms in molecular biology are being unveiled.[3] This chapter will show major concepts of the role of genetic alterations in tumorigenesis and subsequent modifications in molecular biology, both in general and

in children, and will present some established concepts of individual solid tumor of childhood.

ONCOGENES AND TUMOR-SUPPRESSOR GENES

There are two classes of genes which can be targets for genetic damage leading to tumorigenesis: (proto-)oncogenes and tumor-suppressor genes. Both are by origin normal genes involved in the regulation of cellular behavior.

An oncogene is a gene that promotes cellular growth, and often dominantly exerts its power through a single alteration in one allele. There are three possible ways in which the oncogene can be made overactive (Fig. 2.1). Firstly, a deletion or a point mutation in the coding sequence that makes a small but significant change in protein function. The resultant mutant protein would be constitutively active, or in a stable form that interrupts downregulating activities. Activating mutations in the *ras* gene is a frequent and well-established example in adult cancers,[4] though it is much rarer in pediatric tumors. Secondly, gene amplification, which results in the acquisition of extra copies of a normal single gene, leading to a proportional increase in protein production. This event may be caused by errors in DNA replication. One of the most famous example of oncogene amplification is that of *MYCN*, which is frequently observed in aggressive neuroblastomas.[5] The *MYCN* gene codes for N-myc, which is a member of Myc transcription factor family and acts for promoting cell proliferation. *MYCN* amplification is important for the diagnosis and evaluation of the prognosis of neuroblastoma, and examined routinely in most

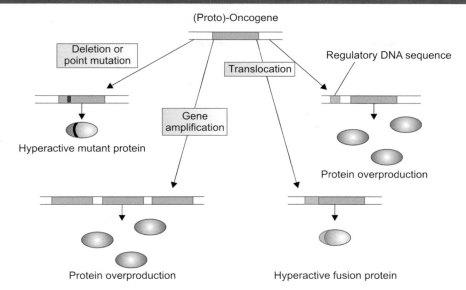

Figure 2.1: Activation of oncogenes. Both overproduction of normal protein and alteration in protein structure which leads to hyperactivity of the molecule contributes to tumorigenesis

institutions. Additionally, whole chromosome amplifications, another mode of gene amplification, results in an altered status of ploidy (aneuploidy). The implication of aneuploidy is antithetic between adult and pediatric cancers; aneuploidy in adult tumors is invariably associated with poor prognosis,[6-8] in contrast, aneuploidy is not an unfavorable factor in pediatric solid tumors like neuroblastoma, rhabdomyosarcoma and retinoblastoma,[9] and moreover, neuroblastomas with aneuploidy are expected to have a favorable prognosis.[5] The mechanism of how aneuploidy affects prognosis is not understood well. Lastly, translocation, this involves the breakage and rejoining of the DNA helix to make altered gene structures at the breakpoint. Accelerated expression of an oncogene, or creation of a fusion gene encoding an active chimeric protein can happen. Lymphoid cells have greater susceptibility for translocations because of their potential for gene rearrangement. Translocations involving chromosomes 2, 14 or 22, carrying the genes for immunoglobulin heavy and light chains, are frequently observed in B-lineage lymphomas.[10] In these cases, c-myc on chromosome 8 and bcl-2 on chromosome 18 are preferred partners in translocations that leads to aberrant regulation of these oncogenic genes. Similarly, T cell leukemia and lymphoma are frequently associated with translocations involving T cell receptor genes and oncogenes.[11] Tumor-specific translocations also occur in solid tumors. A well-known example is EWS-FLI1

fusion gene which is detected in 90 percent of Ewing's sarcoma and produces a chimeric protein that act as a transcription factor.[12] Most fusion proteins originating from translocations in tumor cells, appear to be protein kinases or transcription factors that control proliferation and differentiation.

In contrast, tumor-suppressor genes, which normally act for tumor suppression, contribute to tumorigenesis when their functions are suppressed or abolished. Because every cell possesses two copies of each gene, inactivation of both copy of the gene is required to lose its tumor-suppressing activity. Thus tumor-suppressor genes act recessively at the cellular level. The loss of function of a tumor-suppressor gene on each allele can be attained by point mutation, deletion or translocation (Fig. 2.2). Even epigenetic alteration such as hypermethylation of the promoter region would inactivate the tumor-suppressor gene. The first gene loss on one allele often occurs by deletion of a relatively large segment of a chromosome, where polymorphic differences between two allelic loci disappears. Such a change is detected as a loss of heterozygosity. And then, the other copy of the gene may undergo an inactivating point mutation as a second hit. Constant detection of loss of heterozygosity in some kind of tumor suggests the existence of important tumor-suppressor genes in the region. For example, aggressive neuroblastoma often presents the loss of heterozygosity of the distal part of chromosome 1p, where tumor-suppressor gene(s) for neuroblastoma might be present.[5]

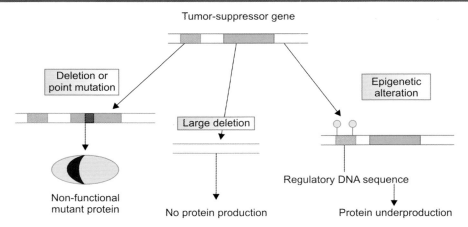

Figure 2.2: Inactivation of tumor-suppressor genes. Not only genetic abnormalities in coding sequence, but also regulatory sequence of the gene, can inactivate the function of the gene. Damages on two alleles are required for complete inactivation of a tumor-suppressor gene

SOMATIC AND GERM-LINE MUTATIONS

Genetic damage can occur at two different levels in the human genome; somatic mutation and germ-line mutation.[3] As to tumorigenesis, however, most tumors are developed through the accumulation of somatic mutations, which are alterations restricted to the genome of the affected somatic cell. In contrast, the other mode of genetic damage, germ-line mutation, affects a germ cell and will be inherited by posterity to represent the starting point for a family afflicted with cancer. The target of such germ-line damage for tumorigenesis is usually a tumor-suppressor gene which causes high susceptibility

to cancer. In the case where the target gene on one allele is already inherited in a damaged state, the chance of the second damage to the gene on the other allele will be far much greater than that in normal cells with two gene copies intact. Such second hit of genetic damage in the tumor-suppressor gene tend to happen early in life, and most cancers originating from germ-line mutations are recognized as pediatric cancers.[2] This model was first established after investigation of familial retinoblastoma, in which double inactivation of retinoblastoma gene (*RB*) were observed (Fig. 2.3). This mode of inheritance is not usually applicable to

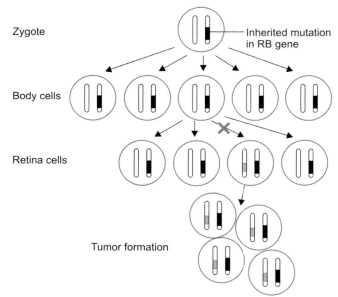

Figure 2.3: Two-hit model for the inactivation of two alleles of *RB* gene. The first mutation of *RB* gene occurs in a germ-line cell, and as a consequence, all somatic cells of the next generation carry only one intact allele. The second mutation of *RB* on the intact allele will happen in a somatic cell, which is likely to be a retina cell

alterations in oncogenes. The activation of oncogenes, due to their dominant character, would deregulate cellular growth at an early stage of development and not allow embryonic growth. An exception may be the activating mutation in *RET* oncogene, which can be inherited and causes tumorigenic sydromes called multiple endocrine neoplasia (MEN) type 2A and 2B.[13]

MULTISTEP NATURE OF CANCER DEVELOPMENT

Several lines of evidences indicate that tumorigenesis in humans is a multistep process.[1] Alterations in a single gene is not usually sufficient for making a malignant cell, but some changes in sequence, occurred together in a cell, would drive the cell to be cancerous. Many kinds of genetic aberrations have been identified in a number of tumors, both of adults and of children, on the contrary, subsequent changes in tumor cell biology are much less known. It is not hard, however, to imagine that such genetic damages might give tumor cells the capabilities of rapid proliferation and resistance to death. And some important principles of the molecular biology involved in tumorigenesis, driven by genetic changes, are being unveiled. Moreover, all of these principles are shared with both adult and pediatric tumors.

Activation and Self Maintenance of Growth Signals

Normal cells require mitogenic growth signals for proliferation. These signals are mediated by extracellular molecules and their appropriate receptors on cell membrane, and relayed by intracellular messengers to promote transcription of genes involved in proliferation. The proliferation of *every* normal cell is dependent on growth signals which usually are supplied by neighbor cells. Many oncogenes are associated with this growth signaling pathway, and by activating those oncogenes, cancer cells reduce their dependence on stimulation from outside, and acquire self-sufficiency in growth signals.

Activation of growth signals can be achieved by three common strategies. Firstly, by making growth-stimulating ligands by themselves, that stimulate cell membrane receptors after being secreted out of the cell (Fig. 2.4A). This signaling loop is termed autocrine stimulation. For instance, aggressive neuroblastomas frequently express TrkB tyrosine kinases, and also produces its ligand BDNF at the same time. TrkB bound to BDNF fires growh signals, which makes an autocrine signaling loop.[14] Secondly, altering membrane receptors for extracellular growth-stimulating signaling molecules. Tumor cells can activate growth signaling pathway irrespective of extracellular growth signals, by structural alterations of growth factor receptors into a constitutively active form (Fig. 2.4B). In addition, cells could be hyperresponsive to extracellular ligands by overexpressing receptors (Fig. 2.4C). Indeed, many types of cancers carry over-expressed growth factor receptors on their cell membrane which have tyrosine kinase activities in their cytoplasmic domains.[15] And lastly, alterations of intracellular circuits that translate those growth signals into action (Fig. 2.4D). One of the most profoundly investigated alterations of this group is the mutation of the *ras* gene.[4] Ras protein is involved in the SOS-Ras-Raf-MAPK intracellular cascade, which relays growth signals from receptor tyrosine kinases on cell membrane to the nuclear transcription machinery. In many adult cancers, Ras proteins are structurally altered and activated, to release mitogenic signals continuously

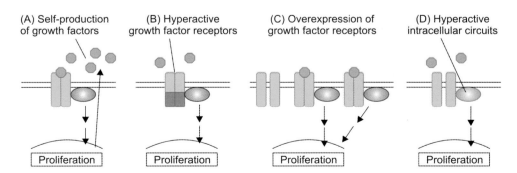

Figure 2.4A to D: Activation of growth signaling pathway. Activation of any of components involved in the pathway will give the cell self-sufficiency in growth signaling

irrespective of their upstream regulators. This mutation of *ras* oncogene, however, is highly associated with exposure to environmental carcinogens, and thus the frequency of *ras* mutation is much lower in pediatric cancers than in adults. Instead, one of the characteristics of growth stimulating mechanisms in pediatric tumors is active concernment of *c-myc*. This gene tends to be highly expressed physiologically in embryonic tissues, and is frequently involved in many pediatric tumors.[16,17] The growth stimulatory mechanisms in pediatric cancers are due to embryonic pattern of gene expression, rather than to exposure to environmental carcinogenic factors.

Insensitivity to Antigrowth Signals and Deregulation of Cell Cycle

Opposite to growth-stimulatory mechanisms, it is as much important for cancer cells to block the antigrowth signals that retard cell cycle or induce differentiation. Antigrowth signals are also received by receptor molecules on the cell membrane and transferred to intracellular circuits. The consequent effect of this signaling pathway is stopping the active proliferative cell cycle. Alternatively, such signals may induce target cells to enter into postmitotic states that are associated with differentiation. There are some checkpoints in the cell cycle control system (Fig. 2.5), and the most important phase of the cell cycle for responding to antigrowth signals is G1 phase,[18,19] when cells check external environment during this period and decide whether to proliferate, to be quiescent or to enter into a postmitotic state.

Growth-inhibiting signals in G1 phase are ultimately integrated into the modification of the retinoblastoma protein (pRb) and its family molecules (Fig. 2.6). pRb is the critical determinant of cell cycle progression from G1 to S phase,[19,20] and its activity is post-translationally regulated by phosphorylation. The hypophosphorylated form of pRb binds with and inhibit the E2F transcription factor, which acitivates transcription of target genes for cell cycle progression. Oppositely, when hyperphosphorylated by cyclin-dependent kinases (CDKs), pRb releases E2F to promote transition into S phase. Thus pRb is a key player in the growth-inhibitory signaling pathway, and all of antigrowth signals finally act for the maintenance of pRb as a hypophosphorylated form. In most cancer cells, the pRb pathway is disrupted, in order to acquire the insensitivity to antigrowth signals. In some cancers, pRb itself is mutated and has lost its function to inhibit E2F. Such loss of function would occur only if *RB* gene on both allele are deleted or mutated, in other words, *RB* is a tumor-suppressor gene. While in other tumors, the surrounding molecules are altered to inhibit pRb, including activation of cyclins and CDKs, and inactivation of CDK-inhibitors.[19] In certain virus-induced tumors, though they are rather rare in childhood, pRb function is eliminated by viral oncoproteins such as the E7 oncoprotein of human papillomavirus that causes cervical cancer.[21]

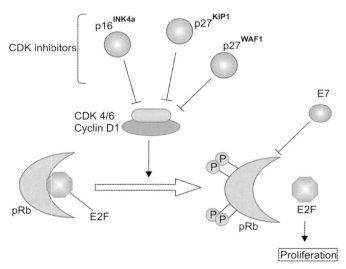

Figure 2.6: pRb and its regulators. Hypophosphorylated pRb binds with and inhibits E2F transcription factor, while phosphorylation of pRb by cyclin/CDK complex releases E2F to promote transcription for proliferation. In normal cells, antigrowth signals act to maintain pRb in hypophosphorylated state, through increasing CDK-inhibitors. In tumor cells, pRb is inactivated or kept hyperphosphorylated

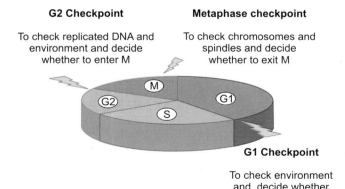

Figure 2.5: Checkpoints in the cell cycle. Extracellular antigrowth signals work at G1 checkpoint, to prevent entering S phase

Resistance Toward Apoptosis

Cancer is a proliferative disease. It is necessary for increasing the number of cells comprising tumor mass, not only to accelerate cell division, but also to inhibit cell death.[22] The most important mode of cell death that determines attrition of tumor cells is programmed cell death, or apoptosis. Most tumors are thought to have acquired the resistance toward apoptosis, by activating a class of oncogenes which regulates survival rather than proliferation, and/or by inactivating tumor-suppressor genes that induces apoptosis. Activation of Bcl-2 was the first reported case;[23] it is an anti-apoptotic protein which suppresses apoptotic signals from several kinds of apoptotic stimuli by inhibiting the release of cytochrome *c* from mitochondria into cytoplasm and the activation of caspase-9[24] (Fig. 2.7). In non-Hodgkin's lymphoma, translocation 14;18 deregulates the *bcl-2* gene, and overexpresses Bcl-2 protein.[25] In this tumor, *c-myc* is also frequently activated to promote cell proliferation.[26] Interestingly, when *c-myc* alone is overexpressed in a normal cell, it triggers apoptosis to eliminate the cell.[22] In general, activation of oncogenes that accelerate proliferation is often apoptotic to the cell, and thus a cancer cell inevitably needs another biological alteration for resistance to apoptosis.

There are barriers to apoptosis in many other strategies. The most commonly occuring one is the functional loss of *p53* tumor-suppressor gene, which is seen in as many as more than a half of all human cancers.[27] The p53 protein is a key component in monitoring DNA damage, hypoxia, oncogene

hyperexpression and other abnormalities.[28] Upon DNA damage, p53 is phosphorylated, stabilized and activated in the nucleus, then transactivates its target genes that act for cell cycle arrest and/or apoptosis (Fig. 2.8A). When p53 is functionally lost by mutation of both alleles, such stimuli cannot elicit apoptosis (Fig. 2.8B). Functional loss of p53 is due not only to genetic alteration of *p53* itself. For example, in human neuroblastoma, *p53* gene is very rarely mutated or deleted, and is expressed abundantly as its wild-type form.[29] However, interestingly, p53 is accumulated in the cytoplasm by binding with an anchor protein Parc,[30] and would not exert its normal function in the nucleus of neuroblastomas (Fig. 2.8C). Additionally, there are still other mechanisms of resistance to apoptosis including the activation of PI3 kinase-Akt survival signaling pathway typically in association with activation of some receptor tyrosine kinases or their ligands,[31] and the production of decoy receptors for FAS ligand which stimulates extrinsic pathway of apoptosis through FAS on the cell membrane and consequent activation of caspase-8.[32]

The gene that inhibits apoptosis is recognized as an oncogene. In some pediatric tumors, however, there is a discrepancy between the expression levels of such gene and the prognosis. For instance, in childhood acute lymphoblastic leukemia, highest levels of anti-apoptotic Bcl-2 are found in the most favorable prognostic group of patients.[33] There is not a satisfying account for this descrepancy. However, it is still an attractive strategy for novel cancer therapy to stimulate apoptosis of cancer cells by targeting apoptosis-related molecules more specifically.

Limitless Replicative Potential

Every mammalian cell is thought to have a limit to the number of times it can multiply, and after a certain number of divisions, cells stop growing and enter into a state termed senescence. Cancer cells need to overcome this limit, in addition to proliferative and anti-apoptotic properties. The senescence of cultured human fibroblasts can be overcome by suppressing their pRb and p53 tumor-suppressor proteins. After some more doubling, however, they would face a second state called crisis, that attends massive cell death with aberrant chromosomal change including end-to-end fusion.[34] The lifetime of a cell, or how many times it can divide, is determined by telomeres at the ends of chromosomes, which are made of a short 6 bp nucleotides repeats[35]

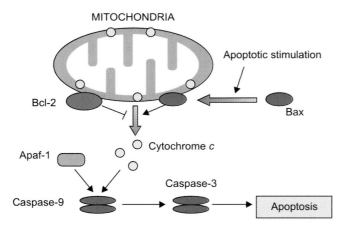

MITOCHONDRIA

Apoptotic stimulation

Bcl-2

Bax

Apaf-1

Cytochrome *c*

Caspase-3

Caspase-9

Apoptosis

Figure 2.7: Bcl-2 and apoptotic pathway in the cell. Bcl-2 and Bax, both of which is a member of Bcl-2 family, control the cytoplasmic release of cytochrome *c* from mitochondria. Released cytochrome *c*, in concert with Apaf-1, activates caspases and finally induces apoptosis

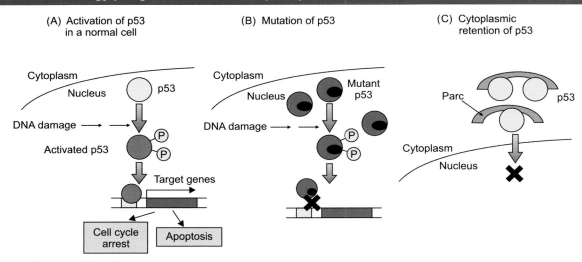

Figures 2.8A to C: Activation of p53. Normal p53 protein is accumulated and activated in the nucleus upon DNA damage, and induces cell cycle arrest and/or apoptosis **(A)**. This system is abrogated in some ways including mutation of p53 in DNA-binding domain **(B)**, and cytoplasmic retention of normal p53 protein **(C)**.

(Fig. 2.9A). Initially cells have telomeres with several thousand repeats, 50-100 bp of which are lost in each cell division (Fig. 2.9B). The regular loss of telomeric DNA serve as a mitotic clock in the senescence program, and if all of the telomeres are gone and the ends of chromosomes are denuded, the cell would finally enter into the crisis.[36]

The loss of telomeres is countered by the activity of an enzyme telomerase, which extend telomeres of chromosomes by adding 6 bp nucleotides.[37] Telomerase is functionally active in as many as 85-90 percent of cancer cells,[38] while it is inactivated in normal cells to inhibit limitless and uncontrolled division. Malignant cells have acquired the limitless replicative potential not only

by accelerating cell cycle, but also by the maintenance of telomeres.

Sustained Angiogenesis

Mammalian cells needs oxygen and nutrients to live and to proliferate, and require blood vessels through which they are supplied *in vivo*. It seems very reasonable that cancer cells induce blood vessels in order to obtain blood supply enough for rapid growth. At the early stage of cancer, however, malignant cells do not possess the angiogenic ability, that is acquired at a certain stage of tumor progression.[39] This step may play quite an important role in progression of a tumor to a larger size, that demands more blood supply, at an early to midstage. Angiogenesis is controlled by the balance of stimulatory factors and inhibitory factors. The angiogenesis-initiating signals are exemplified by vascular endothelial growth factor (VEGF) and fibroblast growth factors (FGF1/2), and they all bind with transmembrane receptor tyrosine kinases expressed on endothelial cells.[40] In contrast, counteracting inhibitory molecules are thrombospondin-1 and β-interferon.[41] Tumor cells activate angiogenesis by altering the balance of these stimulatory and inhibitory factors; some tumors increase expression of VEGF and/or FGFs, while others transcriptionally downregulate thrombospondin-1 or β-interferon.[42]

The control of angiogenesis is not tissue-specific; every kind of malignant tumor needs promotion of angiogenesis. A novel therapy which targets angiogenesis is a hopeful strategy to treat cancers.

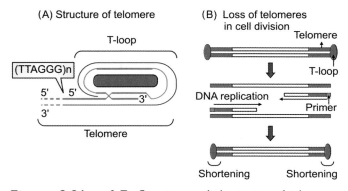

Figures 2.9A and B: Structure and shortening of telomere. The ends of chromosomes are protected by making coiled structure termed T-loop of telomeres **(A)**. Every T-loop is lost in S phase of cell cycle, when DNA double strands are denatured and replicated, thus telomeres are gradually lost **(B)**

Invasion and Metastasis

Initially, in the primary site of tumor origin, the space there tumor cells can grow is limited. Malignant tumors grow to larger sizes and expand their territories, invading adjacent tissues, and finally move to distant sites to make new colonies. This phenomenon is termed metastasis, which is actually the cause of 90 percent of human cancer deaths.[43] The capabilities of invasion and metastasis are not basically carried by all cancer cells, and through tumor progression, they acquire these abilities and can move out of the primary site to find other places to grow.

Invasion and metastasis are very complicated processes and the molecular mechanisms involved are not precisely understood. However, two classes of molecules are considered important for these steps (Fig. 2.10). First, cell-cell adhesion molecules (CAMs), the inactivation of which contributes to promoting invasion and metastasis. This group contains E-cadherin, N-CAM and integrin. Among them, N-CAM is reported to be altered to a poorly adhesive form in Wilms' tumor and neuroblastoma of children.[44] The other group is extracellular matrix metalloproteases (MMPs). Both upregulation of proteases and downregulation of protease inhibitors stimulates destruction of extracellular matrix,[45] and facilitate invasion and metastasis by cancer cells into normal structures including stroma, blood vessels and epithelial cell layers. This system is very complex and it is still not clear which enzyme of this class is critical for invasion and metastasis. In addition,

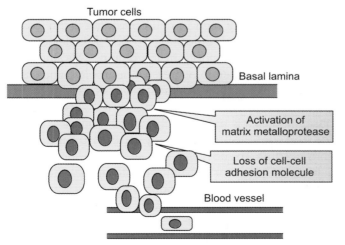

Figure 2.10: Key steps in the process of invasion and metastasis. Tumor cells abrogate cell-cell adhesion and activate extra cellular matrix metalloproteases, to expand out of their primary site

such proteases may be produced not only by tumor cells but normal neighbor cells like stromal or inflammatory cells.[46]

Invasion and metastasis are distinctive hallmarks of cancer, and it is no doubt that both CAMs and MMPs have important roles to play. The precise molecular mechanisms, however, are mostly veiled. Understanding these phenomena is desirable for the development of new therapeutic strategies of cancers.

Genomic Instability

All of the hallmarks of cancer mentioned above are quite essential for malignant tumor cells, and most, if not all, tumors need to acquire all these capabilities for further progression. It is almost impossible, however, that as many as at least six genetic alterations happen in a single cell, because there are caretakers such as DNA monitor and repair enzymes, whose functions are DNA damage sensing, base and nucleotide excision repair, mismatch repair of spontaneous or adduct-induced replication errors, and repair of double strand breaks induced by radiation or by drugs. These molecules assure genomic integrity, and multiple mutations enough for tumorigenesis of a cell is unlikely to happen within a lifetime. Adversely, such sequence of multiple genetic damages in a cell can occur, if such caretakers are disabled. The normal function of caretaker, to monitor and repair damaged DNA, are lost in cases where both alleles of the gene are altered; they are tumor-suppressor genes. This is another integral feature of cancer, which causes genomic instability to increase the mutability of genome.

The most prominent member of the caretaker system is p53 tumor-suppressor protein. p53 is a guardian of the genome that senses DNA damage and other abnormalities, as already mentioned (Figs 2.8A to C). The mutation of *p53* is very popular among various tumors, which is observed in as many as more than a half of all tumors.[27] Even in most tumors carrying wild-type p53, some other molecule is wrong within the p53-related system. Additionally, there are other caretaker genes that play roles in DNA damage sensing, DNA repair and chromosomal segregation in mitotic process. All of them are tumor-suppressor genes, the dysfunction of which deteriorate the stability of the genome and induce the accumulation of genomic mutations. At a certain stage of tumor progression, tumor cells are likely to disable these caretaker systems.

In children of a certain family, some deficient caretaker genes are inherited through the germ-line.

Such patients are exposed to an increased possibility of a tumor occuring, due to deficiency in repairing capability. For instance, germ-line mutations of *ATM* and *p53*, that are DNA repair enzymes, present dysregulation of the cell cycle and cause hereditary syndromes carrying tumors: ataxia telangiectasia syndrome and Li-Fraumeni syndromes, respectively.[47] Xeroderma pigmentosum is also one of such repair-deficient syndromes derived from mutations in both copies of a gene coding for a DNA repair enzyme.[48]

GENETICS AND MOLECULAR BIOLOGY OF EACH PEDIATRIC SOLID TUMOR

Retinoblastoma

Retinoblastoma is a malignant endo-ocular tumor of children arising in the embryonic neural retina.[49] Ten percent or less of retinoblastoma cases occur in a familial form, and most of familial cases are bilateral.[50] This tumor is historically of particular importance though it is rare. In 1971, Knudson suggested a concept which explained the heredity of retinoblastoma, saying that two hits on a gene are required for the development of retinoblastoma[50] (Fig. 2.3). Later the retinoblastoma gene (*RB*) was isolated at chromosome 13q14 as Knudson expected, which was the first isolated human tumor-suppressor gene.

In familial cases, the first hit on *RB* gene is a germ-line damage which patients already possess hereditarily (in an autosomal dominant way). This first change is usually a deletion or translocation at the *RB* gene on one allele. The second hit happens as a somatic mutation, which leads to retinoblastoma. In sporadic cases, both hits occur at the somatic level by chance, and all cases are unilateral.

The product of *RB* gene, pRb, is now recognized as one of the most important tumor-suppressor proteins.[19] The activity of pRb is regulated by phosphorylation, and pRb plays a critical role in the cell cycle transition from G1 phase to S phase in all types of cells (Fig. 2.6). It is still unknown why congenital inactivation of *RB* specifically elicits retinoblastoma. Some common adult cancers, including osteosarcoma, small-cell lung cancers and breast cancers, carries inactivation of the *RB* gene on the somatic level. Such tumors, however, are not always likely to happen in patients with germ-line mutation of *RB*, in addition to retinoblastoma. However, hereditarily affected patients of retinoblastoma tend to develop a second malignancy at the rate of more than 30 percent, irrespective of the therapy received, and most of them are osteosarcomas of the irradiated part,[51] suggesting that radiotherapy may increase the risk of a second hit on the intact *RB* on the other allele.

Neuroblastoma

Neuroblastoma, arising from the sympathetic nervous system derived from the primitive neural crest, is the most frequent solid tumor of children.[5] Neuroblastoma has the greatest diversity in clinical features; most infant patients experience complete regression of the disease without given therapy, while older patients have metastatic and chemoresistant tumors with the poorest prognosis of all pediatric malignancies.[5] These two subsets of neuroblastoma are also different in alterations in genetics and molecular biology. A number of findings have been accumulated which greatly contribute to the diagnosis and risk assessment of neuroblastoma, though the molecular mechanisms of the genesis of neuroblastoma are still not clear.

There are two typical genetic damages that appear centrally involved in neuroblastoma development. One is the amplification of the *N-myc* gene, that is a specific change in neurobal tumors. Aggressive neuroblastoma cells often carry hundreds of extra copies of the gene. The *N-myc* amplification results in proportional overexpression of the gene and the protein product. N-myc is a transcription factor of myc family,[52] thus this protein is thought to contribute to the aggressiveness of the tumor through its transcriptional activity. The target gene of N-myc which is critical for neuroblastoma development, however, has not been determined. The other abnormality seen in neuroblastoma is the loss of the distal part of chromosome 1p, which is detected as the *loss of heterozygosity* in the region. This finding is also frequently seen in aggressive neuroblastomas, and *N-myc*-amplified tumors almost always carry the loss of chromosome 1p at the same time.[5] From these observations, it is supposed that tumor-suppressor gene for the development of neuroblastoma lies in chromosome 1p, however, any such gene identified as a tumor-suppressor for neuroblastoma has not been determined. In addition, though there are a few reports of familial neuroblastoma with earlier onset of the disease, a specific locus of genetic predisposition for neuroblastoma has not been revealed.

Additionally, the expression levels of several genes have been shown to be associated with prognosis, though their genomic DNAs are not damaged. Among them, the most significant prognostic factors are the expression levels of *trk-A* and *trk-B* that code for transmembrane receptors for NGF and BDNF, respectively. The high expression of *trk-A* is strongly correlated with good prognosis,[53] in contrast, *trk-B* is expressed at high levels in aggressive cases with *N-myc* amplification and loss of chromosome 1p.[14] Though the molecular mechanisms of how the expression of these genes are upregulated in favorable or unfavorable groups are unknown, the product of both genes has tyrosine kinase activity at the cytoplasmic part and activate signaling pathway for cell survival when neurotrophic ligands bind. The difference between them, however, is whether they produce ligands or not. Favorable neuroblastomas expressing high Trk-A are dependent on survival stimulation by its specific ligand NGF from outside, and when NGF is relatively insufficient for tumor cells, they tend to undergo massive apoptosis, that is thought to play at least in part an important role in spontaneous regression of such tumors.[54] On the other hand, neuroblastomas with unfavorable prognosis often express both Trk-B and its ligand BDNF, making an autocrine stimulation loop independent of surrounding cells, offering self-sufficiency in growth signals[14] (Fig. 2.4A).

Hepatoblastoma

Hepatoblastoma is the commonest malignant hepatic tumor in children. Because of its low incidence, basic research on hepatoblastoma has a rather short history. Some hepatoblastomas occur in association with Beckwith-Wiedemann syndrome and hemihypertrophy,[55] which also increases the risk of Wilms' tumor and rhabdomyosarcoma. In line with that, the *loss of heterozygosity* of chromosome 11p15 is frequently found in both Beckwith-Wiedemann syndrome and hepatoblastoma, suggesting the existence of a tumor-suppressor gene at the locus.[56]

The link between hepatoblastoma and familial adenomatous polyposis was also reported.[57] Inactivation of the adenomatous polyposis coli (*APC*) gene, that is hereditarily mutated in familial adenomatous polyposis patients, was found mutated in some hepatoblastoma patients, though not frequent. However, interestingly, the mutation of *CTNNB1* gene coding for β-catenin, which is a key player of Wnt signaling pathway where APC also functions, was found with quite high frequency. Actually, more than a half of all hepatoblastomas carry mutant *CTNNB1* by deletion or point mutation.[58] Wild-type β-catenin is controlled by a proteasome-dependent degradation system in which APC and Axin participate, and not accumulated in the nucleus (Fig. 2.11A). In contrast, the mutant β-catenin is much more stable than wild-type form, and is detected in the nucleus of hepatoblastoma cells to act as an oncogenic transcription factor (Fig. 2.11B). This nuclear translocation of β-catenin is detected in almost all hepatoblastoma cells, even in cells with wild-type β-catenin.[59] Such cells may carry another genetic aberrations in Wnt signaling pathway, including that of *APC*. Thus abnormal signaling of Wnt pathway, mostly brought by *CTNNB1* mutation, seems to play a critical role in the genesis and progression of hepatoblastoma.

Wilms' Tumor

Wilms' tumor or nephroblastoma is the most frequently seen renal tumor in children. Wilms' tumor often appears in association with some congenital anomalies including aniridia, hemihypertrophy, and genitourinary anomalies, and with some congenital systemic syndromes such as Beckwith-Wiedemann syndrome, Denys-Drash syndrome and WAGR (Wilms' tumor, aniridia, genitourinary abnormalities, mental retardation) syndrome.[60] Account for these observations was again successfully made by Knudson's two-hit theory. The model suggests that Wilms' tumor is due to loss of both alleles of a certain tumor-suppressor gene, and patients with a genetic susceptibility have a germ-line genetic damage of one allele, thus such children develop Wilms'

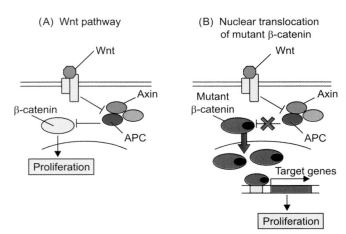

Figure 2.11A and B: Wnt signal pathway and mutation of β-catenin. β-catenin is usually maintained at low levels by APC and Axin, and is accumulated only when Wnt pathway is activated **(A)**. In many hepatoblastomas, mutant β-catenin escapes from interaction with APC and Axin, and it is accumulated in the nucleus to be hyperactive in proliferative transcription **(B)**.

tumor more easily with one more hit. Analyzing the karyotypes of WAGR syndrome patients revealed a deletion in one allele of chromosome 11p13.[61] The predisposed damage in the region actually induces not only other anomalies (aniridia and genitourinary abnormalities), but also Wilms' tumor. Then *PAX6* gene whose mutation is responsible for aniridia, and *WT1*, for Wilms' tumor, were cloned from chromosome 11p13, both of them was altered in WAGR syndrome.[61] WT1 protein seems to act as a transcriptional down-regulator and is important for normal renal and genital development.[62] Functional loss of this protein may deregulate gene expression pattern in renal cells, leading to tumorigenesis.

Since sporadic Wilms' tumors do not frequently carry *WT1* mutation, seen in about 10-20 percent,[63] another suppressor gene was sought. The second putative suppressor gene for Wilms' tumor, *WT2*, was assumed to lie on chromosome 11q15, where frequent *loss of heterozygosity* is found in Beckwith-Wiedemann syndrome.[64] *WT2* seems to be involved more commonly in Wilms' tumor than *WT1*, though the gene has not yet been localized to chromosome position 11q15.

Ewing's Sarcoma

Ewing's sarcoma is a malignant bone tumor that belongs to a group of small round cell tumors. The concept of Ewing's tumor is supported by the discovery of a specific chromosome translocation 11;22.[65] Two genes disrupted by this translocation have already been cloned.[66] One is Ewing's sarcoma gene (*EWS*) located on chromosome 22q12, which encodes a putative RNA-binding protein. The other is *FLI1* on 11q24, which codes for a transcription factor of the ETS family. Translocation involving these two genes results in the production of a chimeric gene, and it is detected in as many as about 90 percent of histologically defined Ewing's sarcoma.[67] Another kind of translocation 21;22 involves *EWS* gene and *ERG* gene on chromosome 21q12, which is also a member of the ETS family, and account for most of the remaining cases of Ewing's tumor.[68] The diagnosis of Ewing's sarcoma have been much improved by the identification of these chimeric genes. FISH (fluorescence *in situ* hybridization) and PCR (polymerase chain reaction) techniques are major approaches, which contribute not only to initial diagnosis, but also to chasing tumor cells remaining in the blood or bone marrow in a low number.

The molecular mechanisms of how these specific genetic alterations are related to the genesis of Ewing's

sarcoma are still not clear. So far, several kinds of different fusion transcripts of *EWS-FLI1* have been reported, and the association between the heterogeneity of these fusion transcripts and the difference in clinical outcome is still controversial.

CONCLUSIONS

Genetic alterations, that are found in virtually all cancer cells of both children and adults, have been identified at an incredible speed. Such findings are now providing us with great advantages in diagnosis, and also in judging the prognosis of certain tumors. Following these advances in translational studies from genetics into clinics, the molecular biology of tumor cells are gradually being disclosed. However, the biochemical mechanisms involved in critical parts of tumorigenesis have not yet been satisfactorily understood.

Hopefully, in the next decades, the biochemical functions of oncogenes and tumor-suppressor genes altered in each cancer will be identified, and novel therapeutic approaches can be designed in association with central players in the tumorigenesis of each tumor. Such a therapeutic strategy, targetting molecules specifically, in addition to non-specific chemotherapy, will unequivocally provide patients with great benefits.

ACKNOWLEDGEMENT

We thank Thanh D Phan for valuable discussion.

REFERENCES

1. Hanahan D, Weinberg RA. The hallmarks of cancer. Cell 2000;100:57-70.
2. Smets LA. Molecular basis of childhood cancer. In: Voute PA, Kalifa C, Barrett A, (Eds). Cancer in children: clinical management. New York: Oxford University Press; 1998. pp. 31-43.
3. Schwab M. Genetic elements of childhood cancer. In: Voute PA, Kalifa C, Barrett A, (Eds): Cancer in children: clinical management. New York: Oxford University Press; 1998. pp. 21-30.
4. Medema RH, de Vries-Smits AM, van der Zon GC, Maassen JA, Bos JL. Ras activation by insulin and epidermal growth factor through enhanced exchange of guanine nucleotides on p21ras. Mol Cell Biol 1993; 13:155-62.
5. Brodeur GM. Neuroblastoma: biological insights into a clinical enigma. Nat Rev Cancer 2003;3:203-16.
6. Sciallero S, Giaretti W, Geido E, Bonelli L, Zhankui L, Saccomanno S, Zeraschi E, Pugliese V. DNA aneuploidy is an independent factor of poor prognosis in pancreatic and peripancreatic cancer. Int J Pancreatol 1993;14:21-8.
7. Ikeguchi M, Ohfuji S, Oka A, Tsujitani S, Maeta M, Kaibara N. Aneuploidy of tumor cells in cases of gastric cancer with esophageal invasion: another indicator of poor prognosis. J Surg Oncol 1995;58:83-90.
8. Nakopoulou L, Tsirmpa I, Giannopoulou I, Trafalis D, Katsarou S, Davaris P. Aneuploidy of chromosome 20 in invasive breast

cancer correlates with poor outcome. Cancer Genet Cytogenet 2002;134:127-32.

9. Dias P, Kumar P, Marsden HB, Gattamaneni HR, Kumar S. Prognostic relevance of DNA ploidy in rhabdomyo-sarcomas and other sarcomas of childhood. Anticancer Res 1992;12:1173-7.

10. Arber DA. Molecular diagnostic approach to non-Hodgkin's lymphoma. J Mol Diagn 2000;2: 178-90.

11. Falini D, Mason DY. Proteins encoded by genes involved in chromosomal alterations in lymphoma and leukemia: clinical value of their detection by immunocytochemistry. Blood 2002;99:409-26.

12. Zucman J, Delattre O, Desmaze C, Plougastel B, Joubert I, Melot T, Peter M, de Jong P, Rouleau G, Aurias A, et al. Cloning and characterization of the Ewing's sarcoma and peripheral neuroepithelioma t(11;22) translocation break points. Genes Chromosomes Cancer 1992;5:271-7.

13. Santoro M, Carlomagno F, Romano A, Bottaro DP, Dathan NA, Grieco M, Fusco A, Vecchio G, Matoskova B, Kraus MH, et al. Activation of RET as a dominant transforming gene by germline mutations of MEN2A and MEN2B. Science 1995;267:381-3.

14. Nakagawara A, Azar CG, Scavarda NJ, Brodeur GM. Expression and function of TRK-B and BDNF in human neuroblastomas. Mol Cell Biol 1994;14:759-67.

15. Di Fiore PP, Pierce JH, Kraus MH, Segatto O, King CR, Aaronson SA. ErbB-2 is a potent oncogene when over-expressed in NIH/3T3 cells. Science 1987;237:178-82.

16. Raetz EA, Perkins SL, Carlson MA, Schooler KP, Carroll WL, Virshup DM. The nucleophosmin-anaplastic lymphoma kinase fusion protein induces c-Myc expression in pediatric anaplastic large cell lymphomas. Am J Pathol 2002;61:875-83.

17. Korshunov A, Savostikova M, Ozerov S. Immuno-histochemical markers for prognosis of average-risk pediatric medulloblastomas. The effect of apoptotic index, TrkC, and c-myc expression. J Neurooncol 2002;58:271-9.

18. Massague J. G1 cell-cycle control and cancer. Nature 2004;432:298-306.

19. Sherr CJ. The pezcoller lecture: cancer cell cycles revisited. Cancer Res 2000;60:3689-95.

20. Hatakeyama M, Weinberg RA. The role of RB in cell cycle control. Prog Cell Cycle Res 1995;1:9-19.

21. Dyson N, Howley PM, Munger K, Harlow E. The human papilloma virus-16 E7 oncoprotein is able to bind to the retinoblastoma gene product. Science 1989;243:943-7.

22. Cory S, Vaux DL, Strasser A, Harris AW, Adams JM. Insights from Bcl-2 and Myc: malignancy involves abrogation of apoptosis as well as sustained proliferation. Cancer Res 1999;59:1685s-92s.

23. Korsmeyer SJ. Chromosomal translocations in lymphoid malignancies reveal novel proto-oncogenes. Annu Rev Immunol 1992;10:785-807.

24. Cory S, Huang DC, Adams JM. The Bcl-2 family: roles in cell survival and oncogenesis. Oncogene 2003;22:8590-607.

25. McDonnell TJ, Korsmeyer SJ. Progression from lymphoid hyperplasia to high-grade malignant lymphoma in mice transgenic for the t(14; 18). Nature 1991;349:254-6.

26. Strasser A, Harris AW, Bath ML, Cory S. Novel primitive lymphoid tumours induced in transgenic mice by cooperation between myc and bcl-2. Nature 1990; 348:331-3.

27. Harris CC. p53 tumor suppressor gene: from the basic research laboratory to the clinic—an abridged historical perspective. Carcinogenesis 1996;17:1187-98.

28. Levine AJ. p53, the cellular gatekeeper for growth and division. Cell 1997;88:323-31.

29. Hosoi G, Hara J, Okamura T, Osugi Y, Ishihara S, Fukuzawa M, Okada A, Okada S, Tawa A. Low frequency of the p53 gene mutations in neuroblastoma. Cancer 1994;73:3087-93.

30. Nikolaev AY, Li M, Puskas N, Qin J, Gu W. Parc: a cytoplasmic anchor for p53. Cell 2003;112:29-40.

31. Blume-Jensen P, Hunter T. Oncogenic kinase signalling. Nature 2001;411:355-65.

32. Pitti RM, Marsters SA, Lawrence DA, Roy M, Kischkel FC, Dowd P, Huang A, Donahue CJ, Sherwood SW, Baldwin DT, et al. Genomic amplification of a decoy receptor for Fas ligand in lung and colon cancer. Nature 1998; 396:699-703.

33. Tsurusawa M, Saeki K, Katano N, Fujimoto T. Bcl-2 expression and prognosis in childhood acute leukemia. Children's Cancer and Leukemia Study Group. Pediatr Hematol Oncol 1998;15:143-55.

34. Wright WE, Pereira-Smith OM, Shay JW. Reversible cellular senescence: implications for immortalization of normal human diploid fibroblasts. Mol Cell Biol 1989;9:3088-92.

35. Counter CM, Hahn WC, Wei W, Caddle SD, Beijersbergen RL, Lansdorp PM, Sedivy JM, Weinberg RA. Dissociation among in vitro telomerase activity, telomere maintenance, and cellular immortalization. Proc Natl Acad Sci USA 1998;95:14723-8.

36. Counter CM. The roles of telomeres and telomerase in cell life span. Mutat Res 1996;366:45-63.

37. Bryan TM, Cech TR. Telomerase and the maintenance of chromosome ends. Curr Opin Cell Biol 1999;11:318-24.

38. Shay JW, Bacchetti S. A survey of telomerase activity in human cancer. Eur J Cancer 1997;33:787-91.

39. Hunahan D, Folkman J. Patterns and emerging mecha-nisms of the angiogenic switch during tumorigenesis. Cell 1996;86:353-64.

40. Veikkola T, Karkkainen M, Claesson-Welsh L, Alitalo K. Regulation of angiogenesis via vascular endothelial growth factor receptors. Cancer Res 2000;60:203-12.

41. Singh RK, Gutman M, Bucana CD, Sanchez R, Llansa N, Fidler IJ. Interferons alpha and beta down-regulate the expression of basic fibroblast growth factor in human carcinomas. Proc Natl Acad Sci U S A 1995;92:4562-6.

42. Volpert OV, Dameron KM, Bouck N. Sequential development of an angiogenic phenotype by human fibroblasts progressing to tumorigenicity. Oncogene 1997;14:1495-502.

43. Sporn MB. The war on cancer. Lancet 1996;347:1377-81.

44. Johnson JP. Cell adhesion molecules of the immuno-globulin supergene family and their role in malignant transformation and progression to metastatic disease. Cancer Metastasis Rev 1991;10:11-22.

45. Chambers AF, Matrisian LM. Changing views of the role of matrix metalloproteinases in metastasis. J Natl Cancer Inst 1997;89:1260-70.

46. Werb Z. ECM and cell surface proteolysis: regulating cellular ecology. Cell 1997;91:439-42.

47. Westphal CH, Rowan S, Schmaltz C, Elson A, Fisher DE, Leder P. ATM and p53 cooperate in apoptosis and suppression of tumorigenesis, but not in resistance to acute radiation toxicity. Nat Genet 1997;16:397-401.

48. Cleaver JE. Xeroderma pigmentosum: a human disease in which an initial stage of DNA repair is defective. Proc Natl Acad Sci U S A 1969;63:428-35.

49. Schvartzman E, Chantada G. Retinoblastoma. In: Voute PA, Kalifa C, Barrett A, editors. Cancer in children: clinical management. New York: Oxford University Press; 1998. pp. 324-37.

50. Knudson AG. Mutation and cancer: statistical study of retinoblastoma. Proc Nat Acad Sci U S A 1971;68:820-3.

51. Roarty JD, McLean IW, Zimmermann LE. Incidence of second neoplasms in patients with bilateral retino-blastomas. Ophthalmology 1988;95:1583-7.

52. Hermeking H. The MYC oncogene as a cancer drug target. Curr Cancer Drug Targets 2003;3:163-75.

53. Nakagawara A, Arima-Nakagawara M, Scavarda NJ, Azar CG, Cantor AB, Brodeur GM. Association between high levels of expression of the TRK gene and favorable outcome in human neuroblastoma. N Engl J Med 1993; 328:847-54.

54. Nakagawara A. Molecular basis of spontaneous regression of neuroblastoma: role of neurotrophic signals and genetic abnormalities. Hum Cell 1998;11:115-24.

55. Steenman M, Westerveld A, Mannens M. Genetics of Beckwith-Wiedemann syndrome-associated tumors: common genetic pathways. Genes Chromosomes Cancer 2000;28:1-13.

56. Albrecht S, von Schweinitz D, Waha A, Kraus JA, von Deimling A, Pietsch T. Loss of maternal alleles on chromo-some arm 11p in hepatoblastoma. Cancer Res 1994; 54:5041-4.

57. Kingston JE, Draper GJ, Mann JR. Hepatoblastoma and polyposis coli. Lancet 1982;1:457.

58. Koch A, Denkhaus D, Albrecht S, Leuschner I, von Schweinitz D, Pietsch T. Childhood hepatoblastomas frequently carry a mutated degradation targeting box of the beta-catenin gene. Cancer Res 1999;59:269-73.

59. Blaker H, Hofmann WJ, Rieker RJ, Penzel R, Graf M, Otto HF. Beta-catenin accumulation and mutation of the CTNNB1 gene in hepatoblastoma. Genes Chromosomes Cancer 1999;25:399-402.

60. de Camargo B, Weitzman S. Nephroblastoma. In: Voute PA, Kalifa C, Barrett A, editors. Cancer in children: clinical management. New York: Oxford University Press; 1998. pp. 259-73.

61. Coppes MJ, Haber DA, Grundy PE. Genetic events in the development of Wilms' tumor. N Engl J Med 1994; 331:586-90.

62. Rivera MN, Haber DA. Wilms' tumour: connecting tumorigenesis and organ development in the kidney. Nat Rev Cancer 2005;5:699-712.

63. Madden SL, Cook DM, Morris JF, Gashler A, Sukhatme VP, Rauscher FJ III. Transcriptional repression mediated by the WT1 Wilms tumor gene product. Science 1991;253:1550-3.

64. Feinberg AP. Multiple genetic abnormalities of 11p15 in Wilms' tumor. Med Pediatr Oncol 1996;27:484-9.

65. Jurgens H, Barrett A, Dockhorn-Dworniczak B, Winkelmann W. Ewing's sarcoma. In: Voute PA, Kalifa C, Barrett A, editors. Cancer in children: clinical management. New York: Oxford University Press; 1998. pp. 232-58.

66. Zucman J, Delattre O, Desmaze C, Plougastel B, Joubert I, Melot T, Peter M, de Jong P, Rouleau G, Aurias A, et al. Cloning and characterization of the Ewing's sarcoma and peripheral neuroepithelioma t(11;22) translocation breakpoints. Genes Chromosomes Cancer 1992;5:271-7.

67. Delattre O, Zucman J, Melot T, Garau XS, Zucker JM, Lenoir GM, Ambros PF, Sheer D, Turc-Carel C, Triche TJ, et al. The Ewing family of tumors—a subgroup of small-round-cell tumors defined by specific chimeric transcripts. N Engl J Med 1994;331:294-9.

68. Im YH, Kim HT, Lee C, Poulin D, Welford S, Sorensen PH, Denny CT, Kim SJ. EWS-FLI1, EWS-ERG, and EWS-ETV1 oncoproteins of Ewing tumor family all suppress transcription of transforming growth factor beta type II receptor gene. Cancer Res 2000;60:1536-40.

Fine Needle Aspiration Cytology of Pediatric Tumors

Tissue diagnosis is the essential key to guide the events of further investigations and needful management for pediatric tumors. Fine needle aspiration cytology (FNAC) is a very useful technique in the initial assessment of pediatric tumors.[1] Proof of malignancy is mandatory to institute therapy for cancer. A positive report is helpful but a negative report does not rule out malignancy.

ADVANTAGES AND LIMITATIONS OF FINE NEEDLE ASPIRATION CYTOLOGY (FNAC)

A number of advantages make FNAC an attractive investigational modality. The single biggest advantage of FNAC in comparison to biopsy is that it does not require anesthesia, an important benefit in pediatric patients. FNAC is safe, does not harm the patient, gives quick results and importantly, does not upstage a tumor. In a majority of instances, the treating physician gets the answer he is looking for from FNAC, thereby obviating the need for biopsy.

It is important to be aware of the limitations of FNAC as well. In general, FNAC is usually indicative and not the final diagnostic modality that is histopathology. In many situations, FNAC may give a diagnosis of malignancy without being specific regarding subtype, which is essential for starting therapy. Since a subsequent biopsy becomes necessary, the physician becomes discouraged regarding the effectiveness of FNAC. However, one must remember that if 60 to 80 percent of tumor patients can be managed without the requirement of anesthesia for biopsy, the purpose of cytology has been served. Cytology is a very subjective science and only an experienced cytopathologist will be able to adequately assist the pediatric surgeon. Cytology cannot be effectively practiced by general histopathologists and the physician must be aware of this limitation.

PREREQUISITES FOR FNAC

There are only a few prerequisites for performing fine needle aspiration cytology

1. Coagulation disorders should be ruled out. It may be worthwhile getting the Prothrombin time done in sick children with advanced tumors that may have involved the liver with metastasis. In cases of hepatoblastoma , it is mandatory to have a normal prothrombin time.

2. Adequate knowledge of the surface anatomy is important especially in neck masses as the normal anatomical structures may be displaced due to the mass lesion.

3. The mass may need to be fixed in cases with associated ascites so that the material aspirated is from the mass and not an ascitic tap.

4. Minimal investigations like an ultrasound is essential before an attempt is made for FNAC. An ultrasound helps to delineate the organ of origin and is helpful to avoid the catastrophy of puncturing a vascular lesion. Also the role of FNAC for cystic lesions is less defined.

5. Smaller deep-seated swellings or thoracic swellings may require ultrasound or rarely other imaging guidance for aspiration.

THE PROCEDURE

The child should be made comfortable by making him lie down with gentle restriction to avoid unnecessary movement of the needle.

FNAC is performed using a 22 to 26 gauge needle of adequate length to reach the mass. For superficial swellings a one inch or one and a half inch needle is used, fitted on a 10 or 20 ml syringe. Using a specially constructed syringe holder permits one handed operation, freeing up the other hand for localizing and stabilizing the swelling. The needle is introduced into the swelling without suction, then 5 to 10 ml of suction pressure is applied. 3 to 5 passes of the needle, traversing through the substance of the swelling are made. Then suction is completely released after which the needle is withdrawn. All material collected within the needle is expelled onto a small area of a slide. A second slide is used as a spreader to spread the material on to one or more slides. Spreading should evenly spread the material without causing crushing. Smears should ideally be subjected to both alcohol and air dried fixation. The smear should be immersed immediately in alcohol before the material dries in the air. Such smears are suitable for Papanicolaou staining (or Haematoxylin and Eosin in some centers). Airdried smears are suitable for Giemsa (May Grunwald Giemsa) staining.

Papanicolaou stained smears are ideal for evaluating nuclear features and making a diagnosis of malignancy as well as the architectural features for subtyping the tumor. Giemsa stained smears provide additional details regarding cytoplasmic features which may help in subtyping in some cases.

Deep seated swellings which cannot be reached with an ordinary one and a half inch needle require ultrasound guidance and a 22 or 23 gauge LP needle. However, the majority of childhood intra-abdominal masses are large and can be aspirated without guidance using ordinary needles in an outpatient setting.

COMPLICATIONS

Complications of FNAC are unusual. However a little caution is advocated for their identification in the rare instance of their occurrence so that timely management can be instituted. The only real complication is hemorrhage, which can be problematic in abdominal masses. The incidence of this complication is around 1 percent, making it very rare. Ideally overnight observation of the patient should be done. If the patient is going home, the parents should be explained the circumstances for which they should return immediately to the hospital. In an experience of over 1000 pediatric FNACs in our institution (and innumerably more adult FNACs), complications have virtually never occurred.

Needle track tumor seedling has been over-emphasized in the past as a complication. Vast worldwide experience has not substantiated initial fears of tumor dissemination along needle track and it is now definitely accepted that FNAC does not upstage a tumor.

RADIOLOGICAL CORRELATION

Any amount of emphasis is not enough to reinforce the importance of radiological information in interpretation of FNAC slides. The exact site and extent of tumor will help the cytologist to decide on how much importance and weight is to be given for the observed cytological feature. For example, if an intra-abdominal round cell tumor has cytoplasm, if the tumor is in the lower pole of the kidney then clear cell sarcoma is a possibility. A similar morphology in a tumor from the upper pole should prompt a differential diagnosis with suprarenal tumors like primitive neuroectodermal tumor, paraganglioma and neuroblastoma, which can look similar. Similarly a morphological feature like rosettes in a round cell tumor of bone can be metastatic neuroblastoma or a primary Ewings sarcoma, which have different radiological appearance. It is the role of the cytologist to weigh clinical information (like age and presentation), biochemical, radiological and morphological features to arrive at a best fit diagnosis. Reliance on cytological features alone can result in a misdiagnosis, which is of no service to the patient.

PEDIATRIC SOLID TUMORS

The majority of pediatric solid tumors belong to a morphological group known as malignant round cell tumors. Most of them have a similar morphological appearance of monotonous round cells with scant cytoplasm, on histopathology and on cytopathology.[2] The neuroblastomas, Ewings sarcoma, Primitive neuroectodermal tumors, rhabdomyosarcomas, Wilms' tumor with blastemal predominance (on FNAC) and most lymphomas all belong to this broad category of tumors. Central nervous system tumors like medulloblastoma and retinoblastoma among others also belong to this group. Rarely tumors which are otherwise of different morphology can take on a malignant round cell tumor appearance like small cell carcinomas, small cell osteosarcomas, round cell liposarcomas, etc. Since morphologically these are similar, immnohistochemistry in biopsies and immunocytochemistry on FNAC is almost mandatory for proper diagnosis. Hence in the discussion of these tumors, adequate attention to immuno-cytochemical details is included in all instances.

The second group of pediatric tumors are epithelial in origin. These include pediatric primary hepatic tumors like hepatoblastoma and hepatocellular carcinoma as well as pediatric germ cell tumors. On FNAC they are not classified with malignant epithelial tumors and are morphologically very different.

SUPRARENAL TUMORS

Neuroblastoma

The most commont adrenal tumor in the pediatric age group is neuroblastoma. This tumor has enough clinical, radiological and biochemical features to make for a strong clinical suspicion. The role of FNAC is to confirm the diagnosis on the basis of which chemotherapy can be started.

Aspirates from neuroblastoma show a malignant round cell tumor morphology in which tumor cells have round nuclei with scant cytoplasm.[3] Neuroblastoma classically has abundant neuropil, seen in aspirates as fibrillary material (Fig. 3.1). Rosettes are seen with the same fibrillary material in their center (Fig. 3.1 arrow). When this morphology is seen in an aspirate, in the presence of supporting radiological, clinical and biochemical features, an FNAC diagnosis of neuro-blastoma can be made.

Some aspirates do not show the characteristic neuropil and rosettes. In this situation, immuno-cytochemistry performed on aspirated smears can help. Tumor cells of neuroblastoma are positive for neural markers like neurofilament, synaptophysin (Fig. 3.2), neuron specific enolase, PGP 9.5 and chromogrannin. The most important differential diagnosis is with primitive neuroectodermal tumor (PNET), which can also be positive for the same markers. Hence negativity for Mic-2 (a specific PNET marker) should be demonstrated. NB 84 is a specific marker for neuroblastoma which is negative in PNET, and can be done. Negativity for desmin, a marker for rhabdomyosarcoma should also ideally be demonstrated. With the help of immuno-cytochemistry, the majority of neublastomas can be adequately diagnosed on FNAC on the basis of which treatment can be started.

Many centers also test for n-myc amplification in neuroblastoma. This can be performed on FNAC smears using FISH (Fluorescence *in situ* hybridization). DNA from aspirates can also be extracted and used for PCR detection of n-myc amplification as well as for other chromosomal studies like 1p deletion, which are of prognostic importance.

Pheochromocytoma and adrenocortical tumors are rare in the pediatric age group. FNAC is contrain-dicated in pheochromocytoma. **Adrenocortical tumors** can be diagnosed on FNAC. Aspirates typically show a cytoplasmic syncytium in which nuclei of varying sizes are embedded. However, it is very difficult to differentiate adrenocortical tumors from pheo-chromocytoma in some instances and histopathology is indicated for proper evaluation.

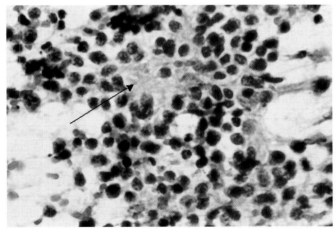

Figure 3.1: Aspirate from neuroblastoma showing a round cell tumor with scant cytoplasm. Rosette arrangement with fibrillary neurophil material in the center is seen (arrow) **(Papanicolaou, X400)**

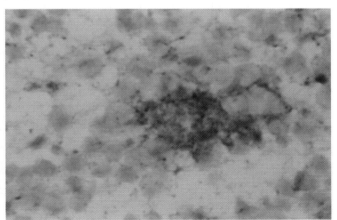

Figure 3.2: Aspirate from neuroblastoma on which immuno-cytochemistry for synaptophysin has been performed, showing positivity in a rosette with fibrillary neurophil material in the center staining positive

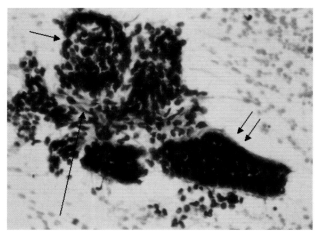

Figure 3.3: Aspirate from Wilms' tumor showing blastema (arrow), tubules (double arrow) and mesenchymal cells which are spindle shaped (long arrow) (**Papanicolaou, X200)**

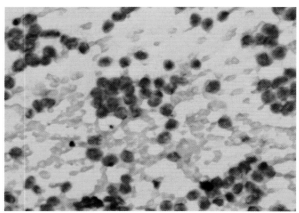

Figure 3.4: Aspirate from Wilms' tumor showing blastemal cells with strong nuclear positivity for WT-1 with immunocytochemistry

RENAL TUMORS

Wilms' tumor is the commonest pediatric renal tumor. Aspirates from Wilms' tumor show a classical triphasic appearance in one-third of cases.[4] In these, small round cells with scant cytoplasm (blastemal cells), tubular epithelial cells and spindle shaped mesenchymal cells are identified in aspirates (Fig. 3.3) and biphasic with blastema and tubules in another one third of aspirates. Therefore two thirds of aspirates can be diagnosed on FNAC on the basis of light microscopic evaluation. However, one-third of total cases with consist of only blastema on FNAC. Blastemal cells have a round cell morphology with scant cytoplasm, similar to all other round cell tumors (Fig. 3.2). In the absence of tubular differentiation, such cases cannot be diagnosed on FNAC, resulting in a nonspecific designation as malignant round cell tumor, which does not help the treating physician.

Immunocytochemistry for cytokeratin can demonstrate epithelial islands in blastema predominant aspirates of Wilms tumor in upto one-third of patients. Immunocytochemistry for WT-1 is strongly positive in Wilms' tumor and is a good positive marker (Fig. 3.4). With the help of these two antibodies and with negativity for neural markers listed above for neuroblastoma as well as for Mic-2 being demonstrated, a definite diagnosis of Wilms' tumor can be rendered in the vast majority of cases.

The exact role of FNAC in evaluation of renal masses of children is unclear. Primary renal neoplasms on radiology which are amenable to surgery require primary resection. This makes the entire specimen available for histopathological evaluation, thereby obviating the need for FNAC prior to operation. Inoperable renal tumors on the other hand require FNAC or biopsy for diagnosis before starting chemotherapy.[5]

A policy of performing FNAC in all pediatric renal tumors has several advantages. FNAC can detect unusual morphological features like anaplastic Wilms[6,7] (unfavorable histology) and clear cell sarcoma before surgery is done. More intensive investigation of these patients, especially for bony metastasis from clear cell sarcoma, can be done with such early warning.

Clear cell sarcoma constitutes 5-7 percent of pediatric renal tumors and can be diagnosed or suspected when aspirates show tumor cells with cytoplasm.[8] There is eccentric placement of nucleus (Fig. 3.5). Myxoid matrix can be seen. There is no tubular differentiation and immunocytochemistry for WT-1 and cytokeratin are negative. Clear cell sarcoma is also known as bone metastasizing tumor because of its propensity for bony metastasis.[9] FNAC can be an early indication for searching for bone metastasis in this tumor.

Rhabdoid tumor of kidney is much rarer (around 1% of renal tumors). Aspirates show dyscohesive cells with round nuclei and a large cytoplasmic hyaline inclusion. Nucleoli are large and prominent. **Renal cell carcinoma** rarely occurs in pediatric age group and shows cytological features similar to those seen in adults. Aspirates show perivascular clustering of large cells with abundant vacuolated cytoplasm. **Mesoblastic nephroma** is another rare renal tumor which shows aspirates with predominantly spindle shaped cells.

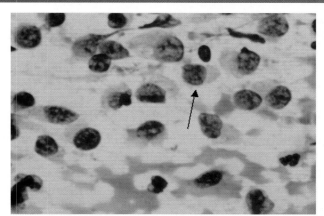

Figure 3.5: Aspirate from clear cell sarcoma showing cells with cytoplasm and eccentric placement of nucleus (arrow) **(Papanicolaou, X400)**

HEPATIC TUMORS

Hepatoblastoma is the commonest primary pediatric liver tumor. Tumors like neuroblastoma, rhabdomyosarcoma and Wilms' tumor frequently metastasize to the liver, but do not present as large primary liver masses. The primary site can be clearly made out in the majority and the liver involvement is in the form of multiple small deposits. Excluding such metastasis, large primary liver masses are rare and of these, hepatoblastoma constitutes nearly 90 percent of cases. Hepatoblastoma can be diagnosed on FNAC. Aspirates show a tumor of clearly epithelial nature with moderate to abundant cytoplasm and epithelial cell grouping.[10] Acinar arrangement of tumor cells is typical (Fig. 3.6) and helps in differentiating tumor cells from normal liver cells.

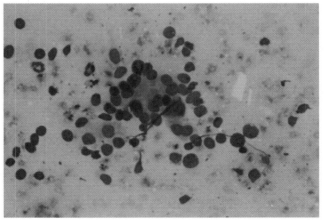

Figure 3.6: Aspirate from hepatoblastoma showing epithelial grouping and acinar arrangement (**May Grunwald Giemsa, X200**)

Table 3.1: Histological classification of hepatoblastoma	
Epithelial	Fetal
	Embryonal
	Macrotrabecular
Mixed epithelial and mesenchymal	Epithelial component subdivided as above
	Teratoid
Small cell undifferentiated	Mucoid anaplastic

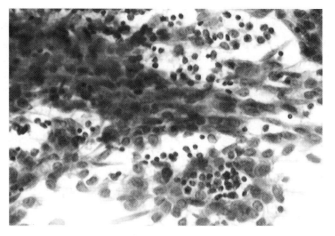

Figure 3.7: Aspirate from hepatoblastoma showing tumor cells between which hemopoietic cells of erythroid series are seen (**Papanicolaou, X400**)

Extramedullary hemopoiesis is seen in a majority of aspirates (Fig. 3.7). It is important to note that hepatoblastoma is an epithelial and not a malignant round cell tumor and hence can be easily differentiated on cytology from other metastatic round cell tumors.

On histology, hepatoblastomas are classified as per schema given in Table 3.1.[11] There is a variability of cytological features depending upon whether fetal areas or embryonal areas have been sampled by the needle. Fetal cells resemble normal fetal liver with small round nuclei and abundant cytoplasm. They have to be differentiated from normal liver cells and very well differentiated hepatocellular carcinoma. Embryonal cells are larger with high nuclear cytoplasmic ratio, but continue to have epithelial grouping and acinar arrangement. These have to be differentiated from usual hepatocellular carcinomas which have pleomorphic nuclei. The distinction between fetal and embryonal cells is not necessary in FNAC, although awareness of the morphological differences is useful when the cytopathologist is trying to differentiate the tumor from hepatocellular carcinoma. Presence of extramedullary hemopoiesis in hepatoblastoma is a useful feature in this distinction. Small cell undifferentiated (or anaplastic) hepatoblastoma is an extremely rare variety of hepatoblastoma which takes on a malignant round cell tumor morphology. Alpha fetoprotein levels are more frequently normal in this variant. This tumor cannot be diagnosed on cytology and a biopsy with a battery immunohistochemical stains are necessary before making a definite diagnosis.

Hepatocellular carcinoma is rare in the pediatric population and when seen occurs at a much later age group than hepatoblastoma. On aspirates they can be well differentiated or usual trabecular types (Fig. 3.8). Presence of intranuclear cytoplasmic inclusions, prominent central nucleoli and trabecular arrangement characterize the majority of hepatocellular carcinomas.[12] Acinar arrangement and extramedullary hemopoiesis are extremely rare, and when seen point towards hepatoblastoma. Since alpha fetoprotein can be elevated in hepatocellular carcinomas, careful consideration of morphological features by the cytopathologist is needed to set apart the rare hepatocellular carcinomas from the more common hepatoblastomas.

Embryonal sarcoma of the liver is a rare tumor. Aspirates show a pleomorphic spindle cell tumor with presence of mucoid material. **Infantile hemangio-endothelioma** has characteristic radiological features. Aspirates show heavy admixture with normal hepatocytes and the tumor cells have elongated nuclei with scant cytoplasm. It is easy to misdiagnose this tumor as hepatoblastoma, especially since extramedullary haemopoiesis is sometimes present and hence careful

attention to radiological and cytological features is essential. **Mesenchymal hamartoma** is an exceptionally rare pediatric liver tumor and aspirates show an admixture of epithelioid and spindle shaped cells with minimal pleomorphism.

SOFT TISSUE AND BONE TUMORS

Rhabdomyosarcoma is the most important soft tissue tumor in childhood. FNAC from this tumor shows a round cell tumor morphology. In alveolar rhabdomyosarcoma of the limbs, minimal or no differentiation is appreciated on cytology. In embryonal rhabdomyosarcoma, differentiation in the form of rhabdomyoblasts and strap cells are frequently seen (Fig. 3.9). Rhabdomyoblasts are polygonal cells with abundant dense cytoplasm and an eccentric nucleus with nucleolus. Strap cells have elongated cytoplasmic projections which rarely may show cross striations. In the presence of such differentiation, a morphological diagnosis of rhabdomyosarcoma can be made and is possible in around half of the patients.[13] In the rest the aspirate is like that of any other round cell tumor and requires immunocytochemistry for diagnosis.

Rhabdomyosarcoma shows immunocytochemical positivity for muscle related proteins like actin and myoglobin. In tumors exhibiting earlier developmental stages, muscle related intermediate filaments like desmin are positive while actin and other muscle proteins may be negative. The most primitive rhabdomyosarcomas are negative even for desmin, but show nuclear positivity for muscle development related proteins like myo D1 and myogenin. In most instances, for FNAC, immunocytochemistry for desmin works well and desmin

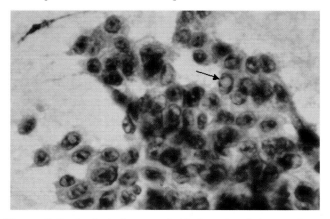

Figure 3.8: Aspirate from pediatric hepatocellular carcinoma showing pleomorphic tumor cells with prominent central nucleoli and intranuclear cytoplasmic inclusions (arrow) **(Papanicolaou, X400)**

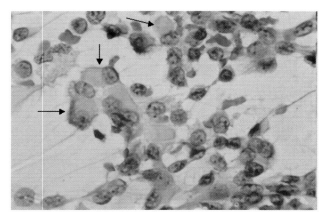

Figure 3.9: Aspirate from rhabdomyosarcoma showing polygonal cells with abundant dense cytoplasm, termed rhabdomyoblasts (arrows) **(Papanicolaou, X400)**

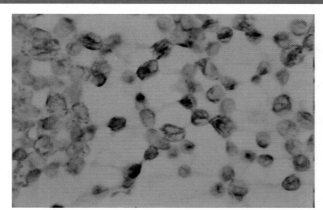

Figure 3.10: Aspirate from rhabdomyosarcoma immunocytochemical positivity for desmin

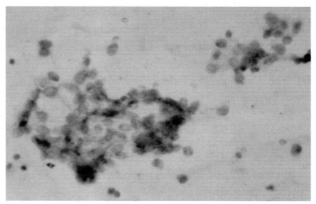

Figure 3.12: Aspirate from primitive neuroectodermal tumor showing immunopositivity for Mic-2

positivity helps to make a positive diagnosis of rhabdomyosarcoma (Fig. 3.10). It is equally important to demonstrate negativity for other markers like Mic-2 for PNET/Ewings sarcoma and synaptophysin for neural differentiation. On electron microscopy, cross striations can be identified in this tumor.

Ewing's sarcoma and Primitive neuroectodermal tumor (PNET) are now considered to be tumors originating from the same primitive neuroectodermal progenitor cell and both tumors have the same translocation (t11,22) involving EWS/FLI-1 fusion gene formation. Both tumors look similar on FNAC and share similar immunocytochemical profiles. Aspirates usually show a malignant round cell tumor with minimal to no differentiation.[14] Sometimes rosettes may be seen, like in neuroblastoma (Fig. 3.11). In this situation immunocytochemistry for Mic-2 is necessary differentiate it from neuroblastoma. Mic-2 is strongly positive in Ewing's sarcoma/PNET (Fig. 3.12). In tumors without

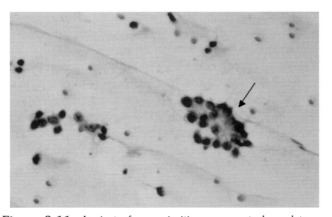

Figure 3.11: Aspirate from primitive neuroectodermal tumor showing rosette formation (arrow) (**Papanicolaou, X400**)

rosette formation or any evidence of differentiation, it is necessary to demonstrate Mic-2 positivity on cytochemistry or evidence of neural differentiation in the form of immunopositivity for synaptophysin, chromigrannin, neuron specific enolase (NSE), etc. Electron microscopy may show neurosecretory granules.

LYMPHOHEMOPOIETIC MALIGNANCIES

FNAC is useful as a screening technique in childhood lymph node enlargement. The purpose of FNAC is not to diagnose lymphoma but to screen large numbers of patients with lymphadenopathy and select out those patients in whom a biopsy is necessary. **Hodgkin's lymphoma** on FNAC shows infiltration of lymphoid tissue by eosinophils, plasma cells and large atypical cells including typical Reed Sternberg cells. Although similar cells can be seen in T cell lymphomas, the vast majority of aspirates showing the above classical features will turn out to be Hodgkins lymphoma. Despite this, most cytopathologists are cautious in giving a diagnosis of Hodgkin's lymphoma on fine needle aspiration cytology and the treating physician should understand the limitations of cytology in this diagnosis. Even if a definite diagnosis of Hodgkin's lymphoma is given on FNAC, the physician should correlate with clinical and radiological findings and be circumspect about initiating therapy based on FNAC report of Hodgkin's lymphoma. Any unusual findings like bony mass or involvement of unusual sites, atypical physical symptoms or inappropriate age should promt a histopathological confirmation before initiating treatment. **Anaplastic large cell lymphoma** and **T cell lymphomas** are differential diagnoses which may be difficult to distinguish from Hodgkin's lymphoma on FNAC alone.

There are certain situations where FNAC diagnosis of Hodgkin's lymphoma is acceptable. When patient has a mediastinal mass or retroperitoneal lymph node which is difficult to access except through FNAC, then treatment can be initiated based on FNAC diagnosis. However a proper clinicopathological correlation of clinical radiological findings is mandatory prior to taking such a decision. It is also understood that it is a consultative clinical decision rather than a pathological diagnosis which is being rendered on FNAC.,

Non-Hodgkin's lymphoma in childhood are mostly of high grade type. Burkitt's lymphoma, Lymphoblastic lymphoma and large B cell lymphomas are the most common types. FNAC diagnosis in deep seated inaccessible swellings and in large tumorous masses requiring immediate treatment is useful. However, most centers prefer to follow-up FNAC with a biopsy so that a battery of immunohistochemical stains for phenotyping as well as material for molecular genetic studies can be done. Pediatric lymphoma responds well to therapy and this requires tailoring based on accurate histopathological evaluation. Basing clinical decisions on FNAC would be a compromise.

Most lymphomas on aspirates are clearly lymphoid in origin, with dyscohesive individual blast like cells. Sometimes differentiation of NHL from other malignant round cell tumors becomes difficult and immuno-cytochemical positivity for leukocyte common antigen with negativity for other antigens seen in malignant round cell tumors elaborated above is needed for diagnosis. **Burkitt's lymphoma** has a classical appearance with starry sky macrophages dispersed in between the immature lymphoid (blast like) cells. Immunocytochemistry for leukocyte common antigen and B cell markers like CD 20 is positive. High proliferation in the form of very high MiB-1 nuclear immunopositivity is another useful diagnostic feature, since proliferation in Burkitt's lymphoma is much higher than in other lymphomas. Most other high grade and lymphoblastic lymphomas look rather similar to each other with monotonous immature lymphoid cells (blast like) and are difficult to distinguish from leukemias.

GERM CELL TUMORS

Fine needle aspiration cytology is able to distinguish the seminomas from non seminomatous germ cell tumors.[15] **Seminomas** are more usually seen in adults than children. On aspirates they have a typical tigroid pattern of cytoplasmic processes and pleomorphic nuclei with

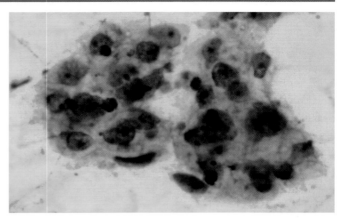

Figure 3.13: Aspirate from embryonal carcinoma showing an epithelial tumor with large nuclei having prominent nucleoli (**Papanicolaou, X400**)

prominent single nucleoli. Non-seminomatous germ cell tumors like **Embryonal carcinoma** as well as **Endodermal sinus tumors** are more common in childhood. Clear distinction of these two types with each other is not always possible. Aspirates show a highly pleomorphic epithelial tumor composed of large cells with moderate cytoplasm and very large nuclei with multiple angulated nucleoli (Fig. 3.13).

Other germ cell tumors are rare in childhood except **teratomas**. These tumors have a complex histology but on aspirates usually show squames from keratin filled cysts. Sometimes intra-abdominal teratomas bleed after FNAC.

SUMMARY

To summarize, FNAC has a definite role in pre-operative evaluation of pediatric tumors. The small round cell tumor group includes Ewing's sarcoma/PNET, neuroblastoma, rhabdomyosarcoma and Wilms' tumor of blastemal type. Differential diagnosis with the help of immunocytochemistry is possible within this group, with radiological correlation being mandatory in every case. Tumors of the liver and germ cell tumors are of epithelial origin and can be evaluated only on morphological basis without immunocytochemistry being required. The role of FNAC in renal tumors is mainly the early detection of unusual variants like clear cell sarcoma and to have a safely achieved positive diagnosis before initiation of therapy. Evaluation of FNAC from pediatric tumors is a specialized area and should be attempted by experienced cytopathologists and not by general histopathologists.

REFERENCES

1. Cohen MB, Bottles K, Ablin AR, Miller TR. The use of fine needle aspiration biopsy in children. West J Med 1989;150:665-7.
2. McGahey BE, Moriarty AT, Nelson WA, Hull MT. Fine needle aspiration biopsy of small round blue cell tumors of childhood. Cancer 1992;69:1067-73.
3. Akhta M, Ali MA, Sabbah R, Bakry M, Sackey J, Nash NJ. Aspiration cytology of neuroblastoma. Light and electron microscopic correlations.
4. Quijano D, Drut R. Cytologic characteristics of Wilms' tumors in fine needle aspirates. A study of ten cases. Acta Cytol. 1989;33:263-6.
5. Schmidt D, Beckwith JB. Histopathology of childhood renal tumors. Hematol Oncol Clin North Am 1995;9:1179-200.
6. Iyer VK, Kapila K, Agarwal S, Dinda AK, Verma K. Role of fine needle aspiration and ploidy by image analysis in the prognostication of Wilms tumour. Analyt Quant Cytol Histol 1999;21:505-11.
7. Drut R, Pollono D. Anaplastic Wilms' tumor. Initial diagnosis by fine needle aspiration. Acta Cytol. 1987; 31:774-6.
8. Iyer VK, Agarwala S, Verma K. Fine needle aspiration cytology of clear cell sarcoma of the kidney: Study of eight cases. Diagn Cytopathol 2005;33:83-9.
9. Argani P, Perlman EJ, Breslow NE, Browning NG, Green DM, D'Angio GJ, Beckwith JB. Clear cell sarcoma of the kidney. A review of 351 cases from the National Wilms' Tumor Study Group pathology center. Am J Surg Path. 2000;24:4-18.
10. Iyer VK, Kapila K, Agarwala S, Verma K. Fine Needle Aspiration Cytology of Hepatoblastoma: Recognition of Subtypes on Cytomorphology. Acta Cytol 2005;49:355–64.
11. Ishak KG, Glunz PR: Hepatoblastoma and hepato-carcinoma in infancy and childhood: Report of 47 cases. Cancer 1967;20:396-422.
12. Dekmezian R, Sneige N, Popok S, Ordonez NF. Fine needle aspiration cytology of pediatric patients with primary hepatic tumors. A comparative study of two hepatoblastomas and a liver cell carcinoma.
13. Seidal T, Walaas L, Kindblom LG, Angervall L. Cytology of embryonal rhabdomyosarcoma. A cytologic, light micro-scopic, electron microscopic and immunohistochemical study of seven cases. Diagn Cytopathol 1988;4:292-300.
14. Silverman JF, Berns LA, Holbrook CT, Neill JSA, Joshi VV. Fine needle aspiration cytology of primitive neuro-ectodermal tumors. A report of three cases. Acta Cytol 1992;36:541-50.
15. Akhtar M, Dayel FA. Is it feasible to diagnose germ cell tumors by fine needle aspiration biopsy? Diagn Cytopathol 1997;16:72-7.

Pathology of Renal Tumors and the Indian Scenario

The phenotypic and genotypic features of a disease are influenced to a large extent by the hereditary, social, cultural and ethnic environment. These features play a great role in its management and prognosis. The study of Wilms' tumor and other renal tumors in children is a prototype of this.

In 1978 Beckwith and Palmer classified kidney tumors in children into Wilms' tumor (Nephroblastoma) and the renal sarcomas.[1] Wilms' tumor, which constitutes approximately 80 percent of the childhood renal tumors, has different morphologic patterns mimicking various stages in the developing kidney. The chief histologic patterns noted in this tumor are stromal, blastemal, epithelial and mixed/triphasic (Fig. 4.1). A pattern is said to predominate when it represents more than 65 percent of the tumor area. Based on its prognosis, the tumor is further typed as non-anaplastic or favorable histology and anaplastic or unfavorable histology, the latter having nuclear pleomorphism, hyperchromasia and multipolar or abnormal mitotic figures that are more than 3 times the size of normal mitosis (Fig. 4.2). The histologic classification and sub-classification along with stage of the tumor has formed a strong basis for therapy and improved the overall survival of the disease over the years to more than 95 percent for favorable histology Wilms' tumor.

The common tumors amongst non-Wilms' tumors are the two sarcomas, clear cell sarcoma of the kidney (CCSK) or the bone metastasizing tumor and malignant rhabdoid tumor (MRT) (Fig. 4.3). Other tumors like neuroblastoma, primitive neuroectodermal tumor (PNET) and lymphoma form a small percentage.

Congenital mesoblastic nephroma (CMN) is a benign tumor that occurs below the age of one year.

In the year 1990 Beckwith et al in their seminal paper described in detail an important concept of precursor lesions (nephrogenic rests) of Wilms' tumor.[2] Several important aspects in the biology of the tumor were explained in this paper. A nephrogenic rest was defined as a focus of abnormal nephrogenesis containing embryonal cell types, in which nephroblastoma may arise. It was divided into intralobar and perilobar nephrogenic rest, depending on its location in the renal lobe (Fig. 4.4). The differences between the two types of rests were elaborated and these were modified and refined over the years, shown in Table 4.1.

Intralobar nephrogenic rests are present deep within the renal lobe and arise early in nephrogenesis. This explains an early age of onset in the tumors associated with them, distinctive age distribution that peaks in the second year and a morphology consisting of the more undifferentiated stroma (Triphasic and stromal pattern in Fig. 4.1).

Perilobar nephrogenic rests on the other hand are present at the periphery of the renal lobe, occur late in embryogenesis and may present in the kidney without the association of Wilms' tumor. The tumors arising from these have an equally distinctive age distribution, with a peak at four years and a median of 46 months;[3] and consist of blastemal or the more differentiated epithelial elements (Tubular and blastemal pattern in Fig. 4.1). The differences in the time of tumor occurrence in the two types of rests support Knudson's two hit theory of tumorigenesis.[4]

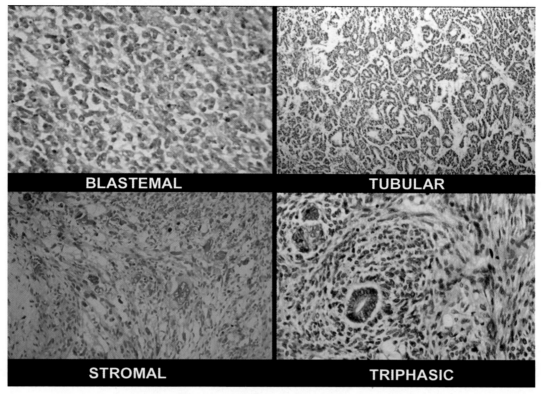

Figure 4.1: Histologic types of Wilms' tumor

The nephrogenic rests and the tumors associated with them have a different genetic basis as has been proven by several past and ongoing studies. The intralobar rests are associated with mutations at 11p13 locus or the WT1 gene present near the PAX6 or aniridia gene and the perilobar are associated with 11p15.5 locus placed near the IGF2 or the hypertrophy gene. The frequent association of WT1 mutations in WAGR (Wilms' tumor,

ANAPLASIA

• Markedly enlarged nuclei with increased chromatin

and / or

• Polypoid (usually multipolar mitotic figures)

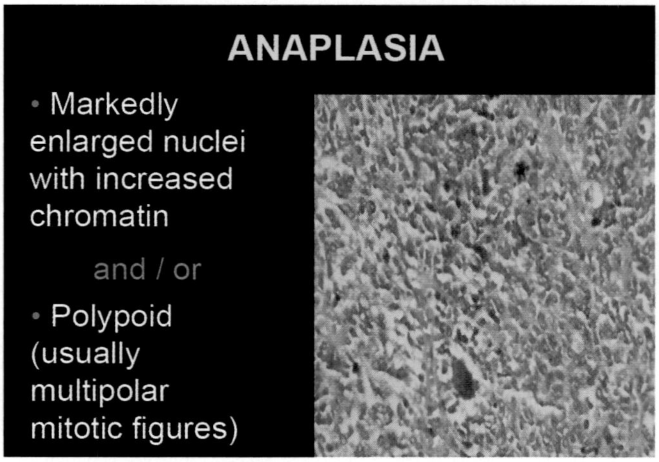

Figure 4.2: Histology of anaplastic Wilms' tumor

aniridia, genital anomalies mental retardation) and Denys Drash syndrome (>30% and 90% respectively), both of which have intralobar nephrogenic rests and Wilms' tumor as their component initiated further work on WT1 gene in this tumor.[5] Beckwith Wiedemann syndrome on the other hand is associated with perilobar nephrogenic rests, Wilms' tumor, hemihypertrophy and mutations at 11p15.5 or the WT2 locus.[6]

Epidemiological studies published from NWTS at the USA brought out several differences between the age of occurrence and tumor morphology of Caucasian, Black, Hispanic and Asian children.[3,7] However, these characteristics were noted on a small population of migrant population in the country and needed further studies on people in their own physical and cultural environment.

THE INDIAN SCENARIO

A multi-institutional study from four institutions in North India published by us in 1998 clearly brought out various differences between the tumors in the West and our country.[8] These are discussed in detail in the following text.

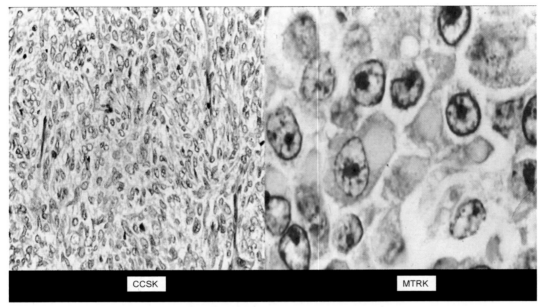

Figure 4.3: Sarcomatous renal tumors

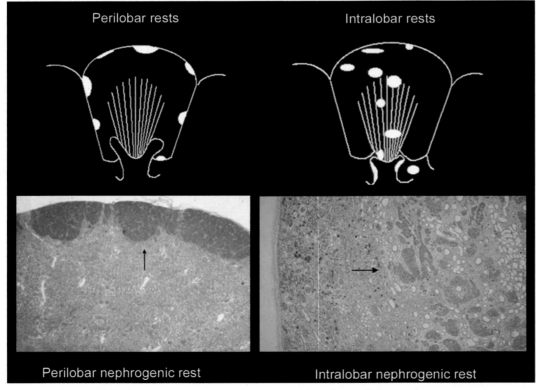

Figure 4.4: Diagrammatic representation and histology of the nephrogenic rests

PATTERN OF RENAL TUMORS

A total of 154 tumors were reviewed histologically. Of these 80 percent were Wilms' tumors and the remaining were sarcomas and others (Table 4.2).

The relative frequency of Wilms' tumor was the same as that reported in the West, however, significant difference was a less frequent presence of anaplasia (1.5% vs 5%) and a higher frequency of Clear cell sarcoma (7% vs 4%) and MRT (4% vs 2%).

Table 4.1: Differences between the two types of nephrogenic rests

Features	Perilobar rests	Intralobar rests
Position in lobe	Periphery	Random, interstitial
Margins	Demarcated, pushing	Interdigitating
Number	Usually numerous	Often single or usually sparse
Stroma	Sparse or sclerotic	Usually prominent
Relation to adjacent nephrons	Demarcated, no nephrons inside rest	Interstitial, nephrons intermingled with rest cells

NEPHROGENIC RESTS

The study comprised of a review of 127 Wilms' tumors that met the evaluation criteria (2 cm^2 of normal kidney adjacent to the tumor) for assessing the nephrogenic rests. Surprisingly, the only types seen in our study were *Intralobar nephrogenic rests*. They were associated with 41 percent of the tumors, being definite in 21 percent and probable in the remaining. Figure 4.5 shows definite ILNRs and Wilms' tumor on gross specimens. Figure 4.6 shows a bilateral tumor with nephrogenic rests.

None of the tumors was associated with perilobar nephrogenic rests.

There are no other studies from India or other parts of Asia on the precursor lesions of Wilms' tumor except for a few studies from Japan[9,10] that have also shown a predominance of ILNRs in their children with Wilms' tumor.

AGE OF THE PATIENTS

The age range of children in our study is depicted in Figure 4.7. The median age of children in our population was much less than that reported in the Caucasians[7] (24 months as against 32 months). This corroborates with the fact that the tumors arose mostly from the ILNRs.

Table 4.2: Primary renal tumors in children

Diagnosis	Relative % (Indian)	(Caucasian)
• Nephroblastoma		
Nonanaplastic	80	80
Anaplastic	1.6	5
• Clear cell sarcoma	7	4
• Malignant rhabdoid tumor	4	2
• Mesoblastic nephroma	5	5
• Miscellaneous	2.5	4

Lymphoma, Neurogenic tumors, Angiomyolipoma, Renal cell carcinoma and others

TUMOR HISTOLOGY

The histologic pattern of tumors and the percentage of rest association in our study are shown in Table 4.3. Majority of the tumors was triphasic (67%) and a significant number were stroma predominant, tumors with heterologous element and botryoid tumors (Fig. 4.8). All these tumors are central in origin and known to be associated with ILNRs.

ANAPLASIA

Only 2/127 (1.5%) of our children were seen to have anaplastic Wilms as against 5 percent in the white population. Both the cases in our study were associated with blastemal histology. This finding also supports the fact that our tumors arise from ILNRs as the tumors arising from PLNRs occur at a later age, have more of blastemal morphology and anaplasia that is most frequently seen between 4 and 5 years.

Studies from other parts of India[11] on the histological review of Wilms' tumor are few but the findings in these coordinate well with our study and show a lesser incidence of anaplasia than the Caucasian population.

GENETICS

There are no studies on the genetics of Wilms' tumor from our country. We have an ongoing study where abnormalities have been seen in 8/24 children at the WT1 locus and none at the WT2 locus (unpublished data}. The fact that there are reports of Denys Drash syndrome and WAGR from our country[12,13] and none on Beckwith Wiedemann syndrome also supports the view that the genetic abnormalities in Wilms' tumor in Indian children are located at the WT1 locus.

The hypothesis that genetic composition of Wilms' tumor in Asian children is different from the Caucasians is supported by the few studies from Japan[9,10] that have also shown deletions, mutations and loss of heterozygosity at 11p13 locus and none at 11p15.5 locus.

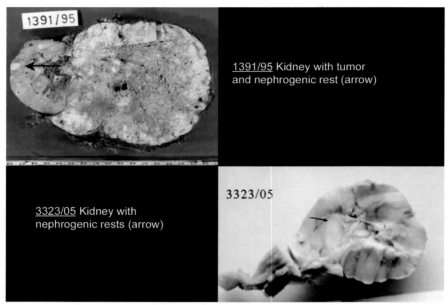

Figure 4.5: Gross photographs of kidney with Wilms' tumor and nephrogenic rests

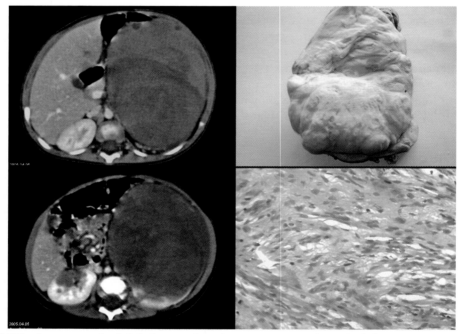

Figure 4.6: MRI of Wilms' tumor in the left kidney and nephrogenic rests in the right kidney. Right side shows the gross and microscopic features of the tumor. The kidney labeled 3323/05 in Figure 4.5 belongs to the case shown here

CLINICAL IMPLICATIONS OF TUMORS ARISING FROM INTRALOBAR NEPHROGENIC RESTS

There are several clinical implications of tumors arising from a particular type of precursor lesion. Those arising from ILNRs present at a younger age group, as large

sized but low stage tumors. FNAC is quite useful as ILNRs rarely occur without an associated tumor and differentiation of tumor from the mere presence of rest is not an issue. On the other hand PLNRs may present with or without an associated tumor and differentiation is not possible on morphology alone. Also, the presence

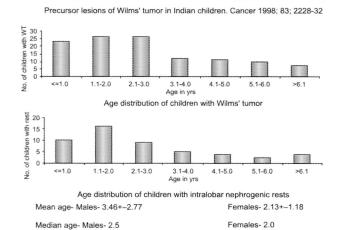

Precursor lesions of Wilms' tumor in Indian children. Cancer 1998; 83; 2228-32

Age distribution of children with Wilms' tumor

Age distribution of children with intralobar nephrogenic rests

Mean age- Males- 3.46+–2.77   Females- 2.13+–1.18

Median age- Males- 2.5   Females- 2.0

Figure 4.7: Age range of Indian children with Wilms' tumor

Table 4.3: Pattern of nephrogenic rests in Indian children		
All were ILNRs present in 50.127 (39.4%)		
Histologic pattern		*Association with rests*
Triphasic	83	42 (84%)
Blastemic	23	2 (4%)
Epithelial	8	2 (4%)
Stromal	4	1 (2%)
Biphasic	5	1 (2%)
Teratoid	4	2 (4%)

of a triphasic or stromal pattern associated with ILNRs is easier to type on cytology smears as Wilms' tumor as against blastemal histology where the other round cell tumors also form a differential diagnosis. Imaging studies have a definite role in diagnosis and follow-up, as 5-10 percent of tumors arising from a rest are bilateral. Metachronous bilaterality is more common in ILNRs as against PLNRs where it is synchronous. Triphasic and stroma rich tumors show a poor response to chemotherapy because of the presence of diploid cells with fewer mitosis but they are not as aggressive as

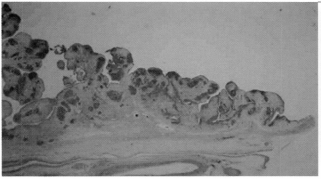
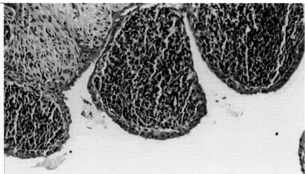

Botryoid

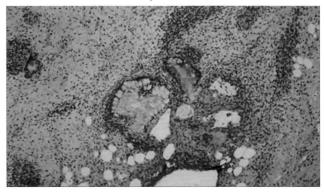

Teratoid

Figure 4.8: Botryoid tumor shows grape like structures hanging into the pelvis. Teratoid tumor has heterologous elements like fat and columnar epithelium

blastemal tumors and respond well to surgical excision. Their association with WT1 gene and the relative paucity of 16q connotes a better prognosis for these tumors. Although the prognosis after regular surgery should be good, the role of nephron saving surgery appears to be limited in the tumors associated with ILNRs as these lesions are located deep within the substance of the kidney.

The hypothesis of different histogenesis of Wilms' tumor in Indian population appears to be very promising and attractive. However, prospective clinico-pathologic and radiologic collaborative studies are needed to substantiate this and thereby modify the treatment modalities.

ACKNOWLEDGEMENT

The author is indebted to Dr Bruce Beckwith, a great teacher, scientist and a great human being for inspiring her to work on the subject. The photographs and figures in the first section are borrowed from his extensive work on Wilms' tumor.

REFERENCES

1. Beckwith JB, Palmer NF. Histopathology and prognosis of Wilms' tumor. Cancer 1978;41:1937-48.
2. Beckwith JB, Kiviat NB, Bonadio JF. Nephrogenic Rests, nephroblastomatosis and the pathogenesis of Wilms' Tumor: Pediatr Pathol 1990;10:1-36.
3. Breslow N, Olshan A, Beckwith JB, Green DM. Epidemiology of Wilms' Tumor. Medical and Pediatric Oncology 1993;21:172-81.
4. Knudson AG, Strong LC. Mutation and cancer: A model of Wilms' tumor of the kidney. J Natl Cancer Inst 1972;48:313-24.
5. Pelletier J, BrueningW, Kashtan CE, Mauer CM, Manievel JC, Striegel JE, Houghton DC, et al. Germline mutations in Wilms' tumor suppressor gene are associated with abnormal urogenital development in Denys Drash syndrome Cell. 1991;67:437-47.
6. Koufos A, Grundy P, Morgan K, Aleck KA, Hadro T, Lampkin BC, et al. Familial Wiedemann- Beckwith syndrome and a second Wilms' tumor locus both map to 11p15.5. Am J Human Genet 1991;44:711-9.
7. Breslow N, Olshan A, Beckwith JB, Moksness J, Feigl P, Green D. Ethnic variation in the incidence, diagnosis, prognosis and follow up of children with Wilms' tumor. J Natnl Cancer Inst. 1994;86:49-51.
8. Mishra KM, Mathur M, Logani KB, Kakkar N, Krishna A. Precursor Lesions of Wilms' tumor in Indian children – A multi-institutional study. Cancer 1998;83:2228-32.
9. Nakadate H, Yokomori K, Watanabe N, Tsuchya T, Namik T, KobayashiH, Suita S, Tsunematsu Y, et al. Mutations/Deletions of the WT1 gene, loss of heterozygosity on chromosome arm 11p and 11q, chromosome ploidy and histology in Wilma tumor in Japan. Int J Cancer 2001;94:396-400.
10. Fukuzava R, Breslow NE, Morison IA, Dwyer P, Kusafuka T, Kobayashi Y, Becroft DM, Beckwith JB, et al. Epigenetic differences between Wilma tumor in White and East Asian children. Lancet 2004;363:446-51.
11. Sharma S, Nath P, Srivastava AN, and Singh KM. Wilms' Tumor: A clinico- pathologic study with special reference to morphologic variants: Indian J Pathol Microbiol 1995;38:55-62.
12. Rao SR, Athale UH, Kadam PH, Nair CN, Pai SK, Kurkure PA, Advani SH. Aniridia- Wilms' tumor association- A case with 11p13. 14.1 deletion and ventricular septal defect: Indian J Cancer 1992;29:117-21.
13. Suri M, Kabra M, Kataria et al. Denys Drash Syndrome. Indian Pediatr 1995;32:1310-3.

CHAPTER 5

Vinod Kochupillai
Sudeep Gupta

Tumor Markers

INTRODUCTION

Broadly, tumor marker is defined as a substance detected in a tissue, giving useful information about the biology of a particular tumor, or a family of tumors. With this broad definition, the field of tumor markers encompasses a variety of disciplines and techniques including serology, histopathology, cytopathology, immunohistochemistry, flow cytometry, molecular genetics, immunoscintigraphy and many others. However, in a more restricted and traditional sense (which will be used in this chapter), tumor markers refer to biologic or biochemical substances produced by tumors and secreted into blood or other body fluids in detectable amounts. Estimation of these markers may provide useful information about the risk, presence, status, or future behavior of malignant disorders.

The history of tumor markers dates back to the nineteenth century when Bence Jones first described abnormal proteins (now known to be monoclonal immunoglobulins) in myeloma in 1848. Another landmark in this field was the description of elevated levels of human chorionic gonadotropin (hCG) in trophoblastic tumors by Ascheim and Zondek in 1928.[1] The second half of twentieth century saw rapid advances in all oncology disciplines and tumor markers were no exception. Abelev discovered alpha fetoprotein (AFP) in 1963[2] and Gold and Freedman[3] in 1965 provided the description of carcinoembryonic antigen (CEA) in colorectal cancers.

Till 1970s most tumor markers were estimated by serologic techniques using polyclonal antibodies. These techniques often led to problems of cross reactivity and the consequent loss of specificity. Manufacture of monoclonal antibodies using hybridoma technology by Kohler and Milstien in 1975,[4] made it easier to identify antigens in various malignancies. Some of these markers have withstood the test of time and are routinely used by clinicians for diagnosis and management. These markers are most often estimated in blood or serum; other body fluids like pleural, peritoneal, and cerebrospinal. Urine and sputum however can also be assayed for some relevant markers. Biochemically and functionally, tumor markers can be classified into circulating proteins, enzymes, hormones, antigens, growth factors and cell surface mucins.

ASSOCIATION OF MARKERS WITH TUMORS

An important underlying theme in tumor markers has been the unique and specific association of a particular marker with a particular malignancy. However, many tumor markers do not fulfill these criterion. Possible reasons include: (i) Many tumor markers are proteins, overexpressed by cancer cells, but also produced by normal tissues. Thus elevation of these markers may occur in non-neoplastic conditions affecting the tissues of origin. An obvious example is elevation of CA-125 levels in conditions like endometriosis and non-malignant ascites in addition to epithelial ovarian cancer, (ii) Some markers are elevated in more than one type of cancer, thereby decreasing their diagnostic accuracy. For example, elevated CEA levels are found in multiple malignancies of gastrointestinal origin, and (iii) Many markers share cross-reacting epitopes with products of normal tissues, which leads to errors in their quantitative estimation. Despite these reservations, the appropriate use of tumor markers with an appreciation of their limitations can greatly aid in the diagnosis of many cancers.

USES OF TUMOR MARKERS

Tumor markers have been used by oncologists, epidemiologists, preventive health specialists, clinicians and basic scientists and have the following applications:
1. Screening of asymptomatic but high-risk individuals to detect cancers at early stage.
2. As an aid in the diagnosis of some cancers.
3. Providing prognostic information at diagnosis. A good example is the use of markers to prognosticate patients with testicular germ cell tumors and manage them accordingly.
4. Monitoring response to treatment including surgery, radiation and chemotherapy. The persistent elevation of tumor markers after curative therapy beyond the period predicted by its half-life (see below) is an indication of residual disease, and may signal the need for additional treatment.
5. Detection of early relapse. Elevation of a tumor marker during the follow-up of patients may be the first evidence of relapse. Therapeutic intervention at the stage of biochemical relapse is beneficial in some malignancies like testicular germ cell tumors.
6. Recently, tumor markers have been used as targets for antibody based immunotherapy. For example, monoclonal anti-CD 20 antibody is used in the treatment of some types of non-Hodgkin's lymphomas.

Many of these uses will be alluded to in the discussion of individual markers. However, the use of tumor markers in the early diagnosis of cancers needs some clarifications and will be discussed next.

USE OF MARKERS FOR EARLY DIAGNOSIS OF CANCERS

An important theme in the use of tumor markers is the hope that they would allow early detection of cancers when they are still potentially curable. This is however possible only if a tumor marker is relatively specific for a particular malignancy, so that it can be applied to populations at high risk for that cancer. This entails considerations of Bayesian analysis, which will be discussed in greater detail below. Also, a relationship between tumor burden and marker levels is important. Since the concentration of a marker may vary widely between patients for a given tumor burden, serial values in the same patient reflect a more regular relationship. Tumors that produce a greater amount of marker per mean tumor cell mass are more amenable to early diagnosis. Methodological issues also used to be taken into consideration. The assay used to estimate the marker should be sensitive and able to distinguish the marker from cross-reacting substances, i.e. the 'background noise' should be filtered. In view of these considerations, only few markers are currently in use for diagnosis of early asymptomatic cancers.

STATISTICAL CONSIDERATIONS IN THE USE OF TUMOR MARKERS

For optimal use of tumor markers, a basic understanding of the statistical issues involved is important. Some important terms are defined in Table 5.1.

Table 5.1: Definition of statistical terms	
Term	*Definition*
Sensitivity	Proportion of persons with the disease who test positive: a / (a+c)
Specificity	Proportion of persons without the disease who test negative: d / (b+d)
Positive predictive value	Proportion of persons with a positive test who have the disease: a / (a+b)
Negative predictive value	Proportion of persons with a negative test who do not have the disease: d / (c+d)

	Disease present	Disease absent
Positive test	a	b
Negative test	c	d

a = True positive
b = False positive
c = False negative
d = True negative

Sensitivity and specificity imply the ability of the test to correctly identify persons with or without the disease when applied to a population. Positive and negative predictive values, on the other hand, refer to the chance that any individual with a positive or negative test has or does not have the disease, respectively. One important aspect that is often overlooked is the influence of disease prevalence on predictive values, also known as the *Bayes* theorem. According to this theorem the probability of having the disease after the test result (the posttest or posterior probability) is directly influenced by the pretest probability of that disease (prior probability). The pretest probability, as is obvious, refers to the prevalence of the disease in the population from which that individual is derived. Formally, the *Bayes* theorem can be expressed in the following terms:

$$\text{Post test probability of having the disease} = \frac{\text{Sensitivity} \times \text{Prevalence}}{(\text{Sensitivity} \times \text{Prevalence}) + (1 - \text{Specificity}) \times (1 - \text{Prevalence})}$$

A practical example can be used to illustrate this concept. Fecal occult blood testing is used to screen for colorectal cancer. A positive test is much more likely to be due to colorectal cancer in an elderly, anemic man with new onset bowel symptoms (a high prevalence group) than in a young asymptomatic woman (a low prevalence group). Thus clinicians should always interpret positive (and negative) tumor marker tests in the light of clinical and epidemiological context in which those tests are ordered.

Tumor Marker Methodologies

The methods to assay tumor markers, often requiring sophisticated equipment, have evolved over the past few decades. Accurate and reproducible results depend upon standardization of instruments, reagents and processes, including the use of appropriate controls. Tumor markers are estimated by the following methods
1. Antigen–antibody based techniques like enzyme linked immunosorbent assay (ELISA), radio-immunoassay (RIA), precipitin tests, flowcytometry, immunohistochemistry, immunoscintigraphy, etc.
2. Spectrophotometry
3. Chromatographic techniques like HPLC
4. Molecular genetic methods like polymerase chain reaction (PCR), fluorescent in site hybridization (FISH) etc.

An ideal tumor marker is required to have high sensitivity, specificity, predictive values, estimation at low cost, and subject to very little variability when tested at different laboratories. Some markers possess some of these qualities but no known marker can stand strict scrutiny on all these counts.

Serial Monitoring of Tumor Marker Levels and the Concept of Half-life

Some malignancies such as trophoblastic and germ cell tumors exhibit a good correlation between changes in marker levels and response or progression of the tumor. A defined change in marker levels can therefore be used as a measure of the response to therapy. A marker response can be defined as complete (fall to within the normal range), greater than a log (ten-fold) fall, less than a log fall, or progression.

A related concept is that of 'half-life', originally borrowed from radioactive decay times in nuclear physics. A half-life is defined as the time needed for a particular tumor marker to fall to half its initial level. Assuming no further production of the tumor marker (for e.g. after complete surgical removal of the tumor) its half-life is determined by the rate of its catabolism, and can be calculated by the following formula:

$$\text{Half-life} = \frac{\text{Time interval between two estimations}}{\sqrt{(\text{Initial value} / \text{final value})}}$$

Using experimental data, the half-lives of many tumor markers have been determined with a fair degree of accuracy. Using known values of half-life, the time taken for any tumor marker level to fall to its normal range can be calculated and persistence of elevated levels beyond this period may indicate residual disease. For example, using a half-life of β-hCG of 24-48 hours, a level of 100 iu/ml should fall to the normal range (<5 iu/ml) within 6 half-lives, i.e. 6-12 days. Conversely, in any particular patient the half-life of tumor marker fall may be calculated from serial values using the above formula. Prolongation beyond the normal range may have adverse prognostic implications as has been shown for βhCG and AFP in germ cell tumors.[5]

Having reviewed some of the general principles involved, the subsequent discussion will involve the characteristics and uses of some important tumor markers. This list is not complete and undoubtedly new markers will be added with continuing advances in this area.

ALPHA FETOPROTEIN

It is a single chain sialated glycoprotein with a molecular weight of 67,500 daltons. AFP is the major serum protein in fetal serum. It is synthesized initially by fetal liver and yolk sac and by 11 weeks gestation exclusively in the liver. Peak levels occur at 14 weeks followed by a rapid decline in levels until term, when it is found at a concentration of 20 to 120 μg/ml. Higher levels at birth are found in premature infants.[6] The levels are elevated throughout the first year of life: 30 to 400 ng/ml in first 2 months and 15 to 30 ng/ml during the remainder of that period. At one year adult levels of 3 to 15 ng/ml are reached.[7] AFP is somewhat similar in size, structure and amino acid sequence to albumin[8,9] and possibly serves the same osmotic and carrier functions in the fetus as albumin does in the adult.[7,8] The half-life in serum has been estimated to be 5 to 7 days.

Increased levels are most commonly associated with hepatoblastoma, non-seminomatous germ cell tumors (NSGCT) of testis, non-dysgerminomatous germ cell tumors of ovary and hepatocellular carcinoma (HCC). Elevated levels may be found in other malignancies like gastric, pancreatic, and lung carcinomas. In addition, levels are elevated in early pregnancy, and in some cases of cirrhosis and hepatitis. After complete resection of AFP producing tumors, an exponential fall to normal range is expected. AFP is a valuable tool for the diagnosis and monitoring of hepatic tumors. In hepatoblastoma, raised levels are found in 80 to 90 percent of patients presumably reflecting the recapitulation of foetal liver development by the tumor. Hepatoblastomas with a preponderance of embryonal elements produce AFP less frequently. Elevated levels are found in about 50 percent of childhood hepatocellular carcinomas[7] and about two thirds of adult patients.[10] Since chronic hepatitis itself can cause elevations of AFP (usually less than 400 ng/ ml), care is needed to interpret levels in these patients who are at high risk of HCC. About 36 to 63 percent of patients with large HCC show marked elevations of AFP of more than 1000 ng/ ml.[10] On the other hand upto 40 percent of patients with smaller resectable tumors have normal values.[10] Thus, a markedly elevated AFP value is helpful in the diagnosis of HCC in the appropriate clinical context, but a normal value does not rule it out. Borderline elevations need to be interpreted with caution.

The other important application of AFP is in the diagnosis and management of germ cell tumors of testes, ovaries, and extragonadal sites.[11] It is most often elevated in yolk sac tumors (80-90%) embryonal cell carcinomas and mixed germ cell tumors. Less frequently, elevated levels may be found in immature teratoma and polyembryomas. Overall about 40 percent of patients with non-seminomatous germ cell tumors will be associated with elevated AFP. Similar considerations apply to patients with non-dysgerminomatous germ cell tumors of the ovary. It is important to note that elevated levels of AFP are inconsistent with the diagnosis of pure seminoma and dygerminoma. The use of AFP in various aspects of management of GCTs is considered together with human chorionic gonadotropin below.

HUMAN CHORIONIC GONADOTROPIN (hCG)

hCG is a glycoprotein whose α and β subunits are normal products of the placental trophoblast and particularly the syncitiotrophoblast. The α-subunit structure is shared with the corresponding subunits of leutenizing hormone, follicle stimulating hormone, and thyroid stimulating hormone. The β-subunit is unique and used as a tumor marker primarily in tumors of trophoblastic origin. The normal level in non-pregnant adults is less than 5 miu/ml. Elevated levels are normally found upto 20 weeks of gestation with peak levels at 10 weeks. The serum half-life of β-hCG is 18 to 48 hours.

The most important use of β-hCG is in the diagnosis and monitoring of response in trophoblastic tumors. Typically, high levels ($>10^3$ μ/ml) are found in choriocarcinoma (gestational and non-gestational) and hydatiform mole. Lesser elevations are found in placental site trophoblastic tumors. In these tumors, the rate of fall of β-hCG is used to assess the adequacy of response to treatment. The lower limit of detection (<5 miu/ml) corresponds to approximately 10^5 viable tumor cells. Therefore, treatment of choriocarcinoma is continued for several weeks after achievement of these levels. The pretreatment levels of hCG correlates quite well with prognosis and is incorporated in the risk stratification of both gestational trophoblastic neoplasms (GTN) and testicular germ cell tumors (along with AFP in the latter). Estimation of β-hCG in spinal fluid has some diagnostic utility. Serum/spinal fluid concentration ratios of less than 60 indicate the presence of brain metastases. In hydatiform mole, the continued elevation of β-hCG after 5 to 6 weeks of evacuation is an indication of persistent disease and indicates the need for additional treatment. It should be noted that transient elevation of β-hCG and AFP might occur immediately after chemotherapy, due to cell lysis.[12]

Seminomas and dysgerminomas are associated with minor elevations of β-hCG (usually < 100 miu/ml) in about 10 percent of cases. These cases are due to the presence of syncitiotrophoblastic giant cells and probably do not indicate a worse prognosis.[13] It is important to note that elevations of β-hCG can be encountered in other neoplastic and non-neoplastic conditions like cancers of the bladder, prostate and kidney and states of hypogonadism. The latter leads to compensatory hypersecretion of luteinizing hormone which can cross-react with β-hCG. However in a patient with documented GCT or GTN with elevated markers at baseline (β-hCG and/or AFP) any elevation after attainment of normal levels is highly predictive of relapsed or progressive disease. It is therefore recommended that patients of GCT should be followed up after successful treatment with periodic estimation of β-hCG and AFP. Thus β-hCG and AFP are together used in various aspects of the management of germ cell tumors including diagnosis, prognostication and follow-up.

PLACENTAL ALKALINE PHOSPHATASE (PLAP)

This is the foetal isoenzyme of alkaline phosphatase which is found to be elevated in about 30 percent of early stage and almost all cases of advanced seminoma.[14] Immunohistochemical staining for PLAP is sometimes used to determine the origin of histologically undifferentiated tumors.

Table 5.2 shows the incidence of elevated levels of β-hCG and AFP in various types of testicular germ cell tumors.

Table 5.2: Tumor markers in testicular germ cell tumors			
	Raised β-hCG (%)	Raised AFP (%)	Marker negative (%)
Seminoma	<10	0	>90
NSGCT	50	40	15
Embryonal	0	10	40
Folk sac	Rare	90	
Choriocarcinoma	>90	0	

LACTATE DEHYDROGENASE (LDH)

This is an important enzyme that catalyzes the oxidation of lactic to pyruvic acid. It is composed of five isoenzymes with the same molecular weight but different charges. It is widely distributed in mammalian tissues, being found in myocardium, kidney, bone, muscle and red cells. Because of its wide distribution, elevation of LDH is non-specific, being found in conditions like leukemias, lymphomas, Ewing's sarcoma, rhabdomyosarcoma and neuroblastoma. In some malignancies like non-Hodgkin's lymphoma (NHL) and germ cell tumors pretreatment LDH level has been found to be of independent prognostic significance and has been formally incorporated in prognostic indices.[15,16]

CATECHOLAMINES

The precursor amino acids for catecholamine synthesis are phenylalanine and tyrosine. By a series of enzymatic steps these aminoacids are converted into the catecholamines dopamine, norepinephrine and epinephrine. The catecholamines are metabolized primarily by two enzymes: catechol-o-methyl transferase (COMT) and monoamine oxidase (MAO). Dopamine is converted into homovanillic acid (HVA) and norepinephrine and epinephrine are converted to vanillylmandelic acid (VMA), through an intermediate step involving the formation of metanephrines. The levels of catecholamines in plasma and of their metabolites in urine are found to be elevated in various tumors derived from neural crest cells, i.e. neuroblastomas, ganglioneuromas and pheochromocytomas.

Most laboratories estimate the levels of VMA, HVA and metanephrines in a 24 hour urine collection. During and prior to the urine collection drugs and foods that stimulate catecholamine secretion or interfere with catecholamine assays must be avoided. Neuroblastomas primarily produce dopamine, whose metabolite HVA is found to be elevated in 80 to 90 percent of patients when sensitive techniques are used. Urinary catecholamine levels are used both for diagnosis and monitoring the response to therapy in this disease since they are sensitive indicators of disease status.[17] Elevated urinary levels of HVA, VMA and metanephrines are also found in the majority of patients with pheochromocytomas, where it is used as one of the initial tests in the diagnostic work-up.

NEURON SPECIFIC ENOLASE (NSE)

NSE is the neuronal isomer of a widely distributed glycolytic enzyme. NSE is not as neuron specific as once thought and mild to moderate elevation in serum levels have been noted in many pediatric tumors. However, marked elevations are primarily seen in neuroblastoma and small cell lung cancer. High serum levels have been shown to be associated with worse prognosis in patients with neuroblastoma and it may be useful to follow disease activity in some patients with this marker. The principal use of this enzyme is as an immunohistochemical marker for tumors derived from neural cells. Recently serum NSE levels have been shown to correlate with the presence and natural history of gastrointestinal endocrine tumors.[18]

THYROGLOBULIN

Elevated levels of thyroglobulin in the serum are found in patients of differentiated thyroid cancer but also in benign thyroid disorders. Therefore it is not used for diagnostic purposes but is useful in the follow-up of patients who have undergone thyroid resection for thyroid cancers and are on thyroxine treatment. In such patients low or undetectable levels correlate with a low probability of recurrent disease. Whole body ^{131}I scans may be avoided in many such patients. On the other hand elevated levels during follow-up are usually a sensitive indicator of recurrence and may antedate clinical and radiologic detection. It must be remembered, however, that patients whose metastases are confined to neck nodes may show very little or no increase in thyroglobulin levels, i.e. false negative tests.

CALCITONIN

Calcitonin is a polypeptide hormone produced by the parafollicular 'C' cells of thyroid, which inhibits bone resorption. It is used as a tumor marker in medullary thyroid carcinoma (MTC), an uncommon cancer arising from C cells. About one-fourth of cases of MTC are part of the dominantly inherited multiple endocrine neoplasia type 2 (MEN 2A and MEN 2B)and rare cases have the MTC only phenotype. Patients with hereditary disease present at a younger age compared to non-hereditary cases; MEN 2B earlier than MEN 2A. Since surgery of localized disease is the only curative treatment, calcitonin is used as a marker for screening families with affected members. The simplest screening test is a basal calcitonin measurement, which is however, not sensitive enough to detect all MTC at a curable stage. Therefore it is preferable to use a stimulated calcitonin test. The most commonly used procedure is the calcium-pentagastrin stimulation test. A two fold increase in baseline levels is usually taken as a positive result. Although recommendations vary, many authorities recommend yearly screening from the age of 5 years for MEN 2A and the age of 1 to 2 years for MEN 2B. Recently the genetic

basis of MEN 2 syndromes has been established with the discovery of mutations in the *ret* proto-oncogene. Genetic testing at birth is now possible and this has implications for calcitonin based screening in the future. Calcitonin levels should also be measured postoperatively both in hereditary and non-hereditary cases of MTC. Stable or rising values have implications for subsequent management including surgical reexploration.

5-HYDROXYINDOLEACETIC ACID (5-HIAA)

5-HIAA is a very useful diagnostic marker for carcinoid tumors, which arise from the enterochromaffin cells in gastrointestinal tract and lungs. The carcinoid tumor cells synthesize serotonin (5 hydroxytryptamine) from the amino acid tryptophan. Serotonin is later metabolized to 5-HIAA, which in turn is excreted in the urine. Measurement of 24 hour 5-HIAA urinary excretion (normal upper limit 6 to 10 mg) is the most common and reproducible test for the carcinoid syndrome. Although this estimation has a very high specificity (>95%) and high sensitivity (>70%) for the presence of carcinoid syndrome, its sensitivity is lower for the presence of carcinoid tumor without the syndrome. Borderline elevations of 5-HIAA urinary levels (<30 mg/24 hours) may be seen in noncarcinoid tumors, after intake of certain foods (e.g. bananas), medications (e.g. acetaminophen) and in patients with diarrhea and malabsorption due to any cause. Urinary 5-HIAA levels usually decline in patients of carcinoid syndrome whose symptoms are effectively palliated with the somatostatin analogue octreotide.

OTHER HORMONES USED AS TUMOR MARKERS

Many other hormones act as reliable indicators of neoplasms of endocrine origin. These include the adrenocorticotrophic hormone (ACTH), cortisol, insulin, glucagon, somatostatin and vasoactive intestinal peptide (VIP). Occasionally these hormones can be produced in an ectopic manner by an unrelated tumor, most commonly small cell lung cancer, and may be associated with well defined paraneoplastic syndromes.

Next, some markers useful in the management of epithelial tumors will be discussed.

CARCINOEMBRYONIC ANTIGEN (CEA)

CEA is an oncofetal antigen belonging to the immunoglobulin superfamily. The normal level in adults is less than 5 ng/ml and it has a half life of approximately 2 weeks in the circulation. This protein has been used mainly in the evaluation and follow-up of patients with colorectal cancer. However, elevated levels are found in many other tumors like breast cancers, choloangiocarcinoma, gastric carcinoma, liver metastases, malignant ascites and pleural effusion. Borderline elevations (usually <10 ng/ml) are also found in smokers, fatty infiltration of liver, hepatitis and in 3 percent of normal adult population. Among colorectal cancers, more than 90 percent of tumors produce CEA, but elevated levels are found only in 20 to 60 percent of patients depending on the stage. Thus CEA is neither sensitive not specific for the diagnosis of colorectal cancer. Elevated serum levels usually return to normal levels within 3 to 4 weeks after complete resection. Persistently elevated levels after surgery reliably predict residual disease. Many clinicians advocate the use of regular CEA levels to follow-up patients in complete remission, although this is the subject of much controversy.[19] Regular CEA is advocated with the idea of detecting relapses early when some of them may be potentially curable by surgical resection. However, the lack of effective treatment for most metastatic colorectal cancers means that this goal has not yet been realized. It has been estimated that if all patients were submitted to CEA surveillance after resection, less than 1 percent would be cured by CEA directed second surgery. Therefore, routine postoperative CEA monitoring is currently not the standard of care in colorectal cancer. One situation where serial CEA estimations have been found to be useful is in monitoring the response to treatment of metastatic disease with second and third line regimens. Two consecutive elevations of CEA over the baseline value predict progressive disease with high accuracy such that further treatment with the same regimen can be discontinued. One recent advance in this field has been the use of [99m]-Tc radiolabelled anti-CEA Fab monoclonal antibody fragment for radioimmuno-imaging of recurrent disease[20] using single photon emission computerized tomography (SPECT). It has been shown that this procedure improves the sensitivity of detection of resectable metastases.

CA 19-9

CA 19-9 is a glycoprotein that results from glycosylation of proteins found in the circulation of patients with certain malignancies. It was first defined by a monoclonal antibody developed from mice immunized with colorectal carcinoma cells.[21] Approximately 5 to 10 percent of the adult population lacks the enzyme required for CA 19-9 production and are constitutively negative. The CA 19-9 epitope is normally present within the cells of the biliary tract. The half-life of this marker has not been definitively characterized but serum levels should fall to normal within one month of complete removal of the primary tumor.

CA 19-9 is most commonly used as an aid in the diagnosis and follow-up of patients with pancreatic carcinoma but it can be elevated in other malignancies like gastric carcinoma, colorectal carcinoma, cholangiocarcinoma and occasionally breast and lung cancers. In addition, it can also be elevated in certain benign disorders of the biliary tract like acute cholangitis. In pancreatic cancer, elevated CA 19-9 has a sensitivity of about 80 percent for the diagnosis of this malignancy, particularly in patients with a high pretest probability. Some studies have suggested that higher levels are associated with advanced disease and poor prognosis.[22] Failure to attain normal level within one month of a curative resection predicts a poor prognosis and elevated levels in patients who had previously achieved normal values is a reliable indicator of relapse. However, because of the limited therapeutic options available in advanced and recurrent pancreatic cancer, monitoring with CA 19-9 after curative resection currently has very limited impact on patient outcome.

CA-125

CA-125 is a glycoprotein with N-linked glycosylation, which is distributed on the endothelium of fallopian tubes, endometrium, endocervix, in normal ovary and on the mesothelial cells of pleura, pericardium and peritoneum. Although CA-125 has been most frequently used in the diagnosis and follow-up of epithelial ovarian cancer, it is quite non-specific. Elevated levels above the normal value of 35 U/ml, can be found in upto 40 percent of patients with advanced intra-abdominal malignancy,[23] and in certain benign conditions like pregnancy, menstruation, endometriosis, ascites and pleural effusion. The half-life of this marker is about 6 days. After complete removal of the primary tumor, levels should fall to normal within several weeks depending on the initial values.

For the diagnosis of epithelial ovarian cancer, the sensitivity of elevated CA-125 is more than 90 percent in advanced stage disease, but only about 50 percent in stage 1. This fact limits its use as a screening tool for this malignancy.[24] Although marked elevation above 500 U/ml are most often found in ovarian cancer, the non-specificity of this marker also limits its role in the initial diagnosis of an individual patient. It has been shown that rising CA-125 values in patients who had previously been in remission following therapy, predicts clinical relapse with high accuracy and antedates it by a median of four months.[25] However the value of monitoring with CA-125 during routine follow-up is limited by the fact that relapsed disease is generally incurable and it is yet to be proven that therapeutic intervention at the stage of biochemical relapse (versus clinical relapse) has any impact on outcome. This issue is being looked at in a current MRC/EORTC randomized trial. Perhaps the most useful role of CA-125 is in the follow-up of patients during frontline and salvage chemotherapy. In this setting, a rising CA-125 (by 25% above the previous value, confirmed by repeat testing) defines progressive disease with a specificity of more than 90 percent and a sensitivity of 40 percent.[26] Such patients can be spared further therapy with the same regimen, which is ineffective as defined by marker levels. The value of CA-125 as a prognostic indicator is also controversial. However some studies show that it may provide useful prognostic information in patients with early stage disease.[27]

CA 15-3

This is a circulating glycoprotein which has been defined by a monoclonal antibody and has been used in patients with breast cancer. It is elevated in about 80 percent of patients with metastatic breast cancer but only about 10 percent of patients with localized disease. Although serial measurements of CA 15-3 correlate with clinical response in patients with metastatic disease, CA 15-3 is not routinely recommended either in the initial or follow-up evaluation of patients with breast cancer, since it has no impact on the outcome.

PROSTATE SPECIFIC ANTIGEN (PSA)

PSA is a serine protease which is produced by both benign and malignant prostate epithelium, i.e. it is prostate specific but not cancer specific. It is most commonly measured by radioimmunoassay and the normal serum values range from 0 to 4 ng/ml. It has a half-life of approximately 3 days. Apart from prostate cancer, PSA can be elevated in prostatitis, benign prostatic hyperplasia (BPH) and prostatic manipulation, which has implications for its use in screening, diagnosis, staging and post treatment follow-up of prostate cancer.[28]

RENIN AND PRORENIN

Renin and prorenin are both secreted from normal kidneys. Renin is synthesized as an enzymatically inactive prorenin is split by limited proteolysis to give the active enzyme. Circulating renin concentrations are occasionally raised in nephroblastoma. Plasma prorenin concentrations have been found to be raised in patients with nephroblastoma. Normal renin values are 192.1 ± 26.5 microunits/ml.[29]

USE OF TUMOR MARKERS IN CANCERS WITH UNKNOWN PRIMARY

Tumor markers have been used in the diagnostic work-up of patients with metatstatic cancers with unknown primary. Appropriately ordered tumor markers can be helpful in this evaluation. However, with few exceptions like β-hCG and AFP (in germ cell tumors) most tumor markers are not sufficiently sensitive or specific to be of unique diagnostic value.

CONCLUSIONS

The field of tumor markers has witnessed rapid progress in the past two decades with many new candidate markers either in clinical use or under active evaluation. As is evident from the preceding sections, many markers have failed to live up to the initial expectations, particularly in their use for screening asymptomatic individuals and follow-up of treated cancer patients. While some of this failure may be attributed to the characteristics of particular markers themselves, it can also be ascribed in a large measure to the biological nature of the underlying malignancy. For example, it may not be of much benefit to use markers to detect a relapse early, if the ultimate outcome is unchanged by therapeutic intervention at this stage. On the other hand appropriate use of tumor markers, integrated with other data, can provide valuable input in the clinical management of many malignancies. For this it is essential that clinicians possess a sound understanding of the statistical and biochemical considerations underlying the use of each tumor marker. It is possible and likely that existing tumor markers will find new uses in the future due to advances in cancer therapeutics, and new markers with greater sensitivity and specificity will be discovered.

REFERENCES

1. Ascheim S. Early diagnosis of pregnancy, chorio-nepithelioma and hydatiform mole by the Ascheim-Zondek test. Am J Obstet Gynecol 1930;19:335.
2. Abelev GI. a-Fetoprotein in oncogenesis and in association with malignant tumors. Adv Cancer Res 1971;14:295.
3. Gold P, Freedman SO. Specific carcinoembryonic antigens of the human digestive system. J Exp Med 1965;122:467.

4. Kohler G, Milstein C. Continuous culture of fused cells secreting antibodies of predefined specificities. Nature 1975;256:495.

5. Toner GC, Geller NL, Lin S-Y, et al. Extragonadal and poor-risk non-seminomatous germ cell tumors. Survival and prognostic features. Cancer 1991 ;67:2049.

6. Goraya SS, Smythe PJ, Walker V. Plasma alpha-fetoprotein concentrations in preterm neonates. Ann Clin Biochem 1985;22:650.

7. Yachnin S. The clinical significance of human alpha-fetoprotein. Ann Clin Lab Sci 8: 84, 1978

8. Rouslahti E, Terry WD. a-Fetoprotein and serum albumin show sequence homology. Nature 1976; 260:804.

9. Ruoslahti E, Pihko H, Seppala M. a-Fetoprotein: Immunochemical purification and chemical properties, expression in normal state and in malignant and non-malignant liver disease. Transplant Rev 1974;20:39.

10. Nomura F, Ohrushi K, Tanabe Y. Clinical features and prognosis of hepatocellular carcinoma with reference to serum alpha-fetoprotein levels. Analysis of 606 patients. Cancer 1989;64:1700.

11. Sesterhenn IA, Weiss RB, Mostofi FK, et al. Prognosis and other clinical correlates of pathologic review in stage 2 and 22 testicular carcinoma: a report feom the testicular cancer intergroup study. J Clin Oncol 1992;10:69.

12. Vogelzang NJ, Longe PH, Goldman A, et al. Acute change of alpha-fetoprotein and human chorionic gonadotropin during induction chemotherapy of germ cell tumor. Cancer Res 1982;42:4855.

13. Butcher DN, Gregory WM, Gunter PA, et al. The biological and clinical significance of HCG- containing cells in seminoma. Br J Cancer 1985;51:473.

14. Koshida K, Nishino A, Yamamoto H, et al. The role of alkaline phosphatase isoenzymes as tumor markers for testicular germ cell tumors. J Urol 1991;146:57.

15. Voneyben FE, Blaabjerg O, Madsen EL, et al. Serum lactate dehydrogenase isoenzyme and tumor volume are indicators of response to treatment and predictors of prognosis in metastatic testicular germ cell tumors. Eur J Cancer 1992;28:410.

16. Shipp M, Harrington D, Anderson J, et al. Development of a predictive model for aggressive lymphoma: the international NHL prognostic factors project. N Engl J Med 1993;329:997.

17. Protchard J, Berthold F, et al. Revisions in the international criteria for neuroblastoma diagnosis, staging and response to treatment. J Clin Oncol 1993;11:1466.

18. D' Alessandro M, Mariani P, Lomanto D. Serum neuron-specific enolase in diagnosis and follow-up of gastrointestinal neuroendocrine tumors. Tumor Biol 1992;13:352.

19. Nelson RL. Postoperative evaluation of patients with colorectal cancer. Sem Oncol 1995 ;22:488.

20. Moffat FL, Pinsky CM, Hammershaimb L, et al. Clinical utility of external immunoscintigraphy with the IMMU –4 technetium – 99m Fab' antibody fragment in patients undergoing surgery for carcinoma of the colon and rectum: Results of a pivotal, phase-III trial – The Immunomedics Study Group. J Clin Oncol 1996; 14:2995.

21. Ritts RE, Del Villano BC, Go VLW, et al. Initial clinical evaluation of an immunoradiometric assay for CA 19-9 using the NCI serum bank. Int J Cancer 1984;33:339.

22. Sakahara H, Nakajima K, Nakashima T, et al. Serum CA 19-9 concentrations and computed tomography findings in patients with pancreatic carcinoma. Cancer 1986;57:1324.

23. Meyer T, Rustin GJ. Role of tumor markers in monitoring epithelial ovarian cancer. Br J Cancer 2000;82:1535.

24. Jacobs IJ, Skates SJ, MacDonald N, et al. Screening for ovarian cancer: a pilot randomised study. Lancet 1999; 353:1207.

25. Rustin GJ, Nelstrop AE, Tuxen MK, et al. Defining progression of ovarian carcinoma during follow-up according to CA 125: a North Thames Ovary Group Study. Ann Oncol 1996;7:361.

26. Rustin GJ, Nelstrop A, Stilwell J, et al. Savings obtained by CA 125 measurements during therapy for ovarian carcinoma. The North Thames Ovary Group. Eur J Cancer 1992;28:79.

27. Nagele F, Petru E, Medl M, et al. Preoperative CA 125: an independent prognostic factor in patients with stage I epithelial ovarian cancer. Obstet Gynecol 1995;86:259.

28. Catalona WJ, Ritchie JP, Ahmann FR, et al. Comparison of digital rectal examination and serum prostate specific antigen in the early detection of prostate cancer: results of a multicenter clinical trial of 6,630 men. J Urol 1994; 151:1283.

29. BJ Leckie, G Birnie, and R Carachi. Renin in Wilms' Tumor: Prorenin as an Indicator. J Clin Endocriml Metab 1994;79: 1742-6.

CHAPTER 6

Devendra K Gupta
Shilpa Sharma

Surgical Principles of Management of Common Pediatric Solid Tumors

Surgical techniques in a child for pediatric tumors are important to ensure proper removal of tumor for long-term survival and good quality of life. Solid abdominal tumors are of special importance in the field of pediatric surgery. To avoid dangers of cumulative irradiation and improved delineation of soft parts, MRI is usually employed in children for diagnostic assessment. Compiling the radiologic information for surgical planning is often difficult by conventional methods. Newly improved and efficient 3-D volume rendering software is now available for visual reconstruction of tumor anatomy utilising segmentation and other special techniques.[1] A better understanding of the surgical anatomy, particularly regarding the surrounding organs and vasculature, can be helpful in decreasing the incidence of inadvertent intraoperative injuries to these structures. Unresectable intraabdominal tumors pose a challenge to the pediatric oncology team. Tumor tissue is needed for diagnostic and prognostic analyses. Laparoscopy is a valuable technique in the management of pediatric intraabdominal tumors. It allows for tumor biopsy under direct vision, and adequate tissue is procured for all analyses. Moreover, it allows the surgeon to dissect the tumor and determine resectability.[2] The surgical aspects for Wilms' tumor are consistent but the procedures for difficult cases of neuroblastomas differ depending on the surgeons preference and expertise. This chapter will discuss the surgical principles of Wilms' tumor, Neuroblastoma and Liver tumors.

WILMS' TUMOR

According to the NWTSG protocol, the first step in the treatment of Wilms tumor is surgical staging followed by radical nephrectomy, if possible. The authors do not follow this aspect of NWTS and give upfront chemotherapy in clinically unresectable tumors based on assessment of mobility in a calm or sleeping child.[3] A few cycles of chemotherapy are given and then the tumor is reassessed for mobility. If mobile, surgical intervention is planned (Fig. 6.1). All tumors given preoperative/upfront/neoadjuvant chemotherapy are taken as minimum stage III for planning further treatment. Cases with distant metastasis are taken as stage IV.

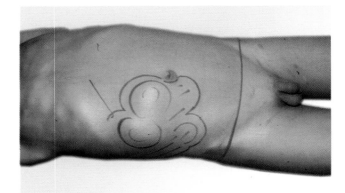

Figure 6.1: Right Wilms' tumor in a child that decresed in size after chemotherapy

Surgical Technique

A folded towel under the flank helps to bring the tumor forward towards the operative field (Fig. 6.2). The tumor is palpated and the incision is planned. A big transverse upper abdominal incision is made that crosses the midline to the opposite side cutting both the recti abdominis. Adequate exposure is vital for performing the surgery (Fig. 6.3). The incision is made over the midpoint of the palpable lump or 1-2 cm above the umbilicus in cases where the lump has decreased in size after chemotherapy. The liver is examined and palpated for any secondaries. Abdominal Exploration of the contralateral kidney is currently being questioned because of the improvement in imaging techniques (CT scan, MRI) (Figs 6.4 and 6.5). Convention holds that the contralateral kidney can be explored by mobilizing the ipsilateral colon and opening the Gerota fascia. However, the authors rely on the current imaging techniques and do not open the Gerota fascia. The contralateral kidney is palpated through the peritoneum and the Gerota fascia. If bilateral disease is diagnosed, nephrectomy is not performed but biopsy specimens are obtained. If the disease is unilateral, radical nephrectomy and regional lymph node dissection or sampling are performed.

Minimum tumor handling is done. The lateral peritoneum is incised. The dissection is begun by mobilization of the mesocolon taking care to preserve the vascularity of the colon (Fig. 6.6). Gerota's fascia is mobilized along with the kidney. If the tumor is small and the access to the renal vessels is defined, the vessels are approached first, renal vein followed by renal artery

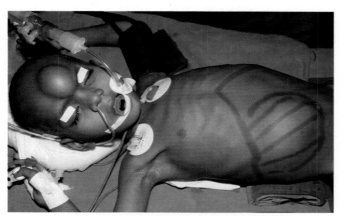

Figure 6.2: Preoperative photograph of a child with a right renal tumor and cranial metastasis. Note the folded towel under the right flank

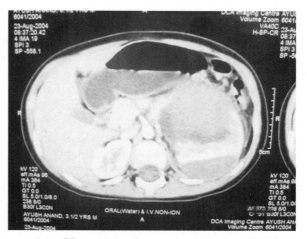

Figure 6.4: CT scan showing a resectable left Wilms' tumor

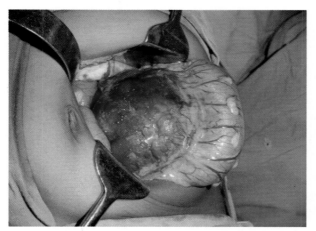

Figure 6.3: Adequate exposure for performing the surgery is essential

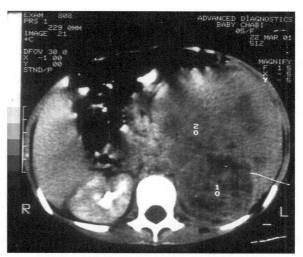

Figure 6.5: CT scan showing an inoperable left Wilms' tumor

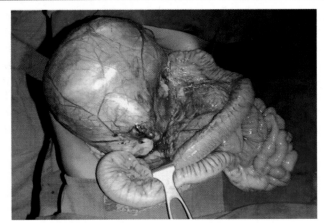

Figure 6.6: The mesocolon and the colon are dissected off the tumor very carefully preserving the vasculature

to avoid tumor embolization. The ureter is mobilized upto the entry in bladder and ligated and cut. If the tumor is large so as to distort the normal anatomy, the authors begin with dissection of the tumor on the lateral and inferior aspect. The ureter is handled as it comes along, clamped as low as possible and ligated after tumor removal to ensure better ligation upto the lowest end after adequate space is created. The vessels come into view after the inferior aspect is mobilized proceeding medially and are then tackled appropriately.

There are controversies regarding the tackling of vessels. Some feel the renal vein should be tackled first to avoid tumor embolization, others feel the renal artery should be tackled first to avoid tumor congestion. The authors feel the time period between ligating either of the vessels is too less to effect either of these reasons and the vessels should be tackled meticulously as they present, the vessel presenting first to the surgeon should be tackled first to avoid unnecessary tumor manipulation.

The kidney is then mobilized along with the Gerota's fascia and adherent lymphnodes in close proximity. The adrenal gland is usually removed along with the kidney except in cases of lower pole tumors where the adrenal gland may be spared.

After removal of the tumor, the remaining lymph nodes are palpated and sampling is done. Haemostasis of the tumor bed is assured. Ligature clips are applied to mark the tumor bed for radiation in future if needed.

In rare instances of misjudging resectability or in cases with poor response to chemotherapy, the tumor may involve adjacent structures that need to be tacked. These include the mesocolon, diaphragm, transverse colon and posterior abdominal wall (Fig. 6.7). The tumor may be adherent to the liver, this may need seperation.

If the tumor is unresectable, biopsies are performed and the nephrectomy is deferred until after chemotherapy, which will shrink the tumor in most cases. If IVC thrombus is present, preoperative chemotherapy will reduce the cavotomy rate by 50 percent.

In cases with tumor extension into the ureter, a cystoscopic examination in recommended. In cases with intravesical extension, that is rare after preoperative chemotherapy, a cut of the bladder 1 cm beyond the tumor should be resected. This makes the tumor stage III. Tumor extension into the ureter without extension into the bladder is considered as stage II.

With bilateral Wilms' tumor, surgical exploration, biopsies from both sides, and accurate surgical staging (including lymph node biopsy of both sides) are performed. A generous trans-abdominal incision is made (Fig. 6.8). This is followed by 6 weeks of chemotherapy that is appropriate to the stage and histology of the

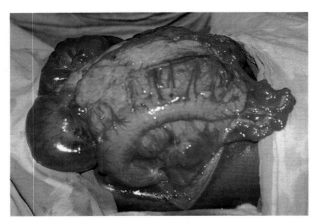

Figure 6.7: Extensive Wilm's tumor

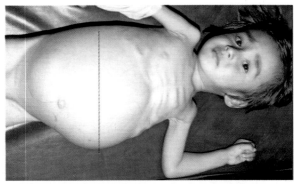

Figure 6.8: A generous incision (marked) has to be given for bilateral Wilms' tumor

tumor. Then, reassessment is performed using imaging studies, followed by definitive surgery with (i) unilateral radical nephrectomy and partial nephrectomy on the contralateral side; (ii) bilateral partial nephrectomy; and (iii) unilateral nephrectomias only, if the response was complete on the opposite side. This approach dramatically reduces the renal failure rate following bilateral Wilms' tumor therapy.

Multimodal therapy (i.e. surgery, radiation, and chemotherapy) is the key to success when treating Wilms' tumor.

The NWTSG recommends preoperative chemotherapy (after initial exploratory laparotomy and biopsy) in the following situations:

- Intracaval tumor extension: This occurs in 5 percent of cases of Wilms' tumor. It is associated with a 40 percent rate of surgical complications, even in experienced hands. Upfront chemotherapy after staging and biopsy reduces tumor and thrombus size, which account for 25 percent of surgical complications.
- Inoperable tumors: Large tumors that involve vital structures, make resection difficult. The complication rate is high, and the incidence of tumor spill soilage also is high. Upfront chemotherapy reduces soilage by 50 percent.
- Bilateral Wilms' tumor.

SIOP advocates upfront chemotherapy without previous laparotomy and biopsy. The NWTSG suggests that this approach comprises a 1-5 percent risk of treating a benign disease.

Chemotherapy without proper surgical staging (e.g. staging by means of imaging studies only) may alter the actual initial stage of the disease by the time of surgery and may subsequently alter decisions regarding the adjuvant chemotherapy and radiation therapy, which is based on the surgical staging.

In cases of bilateral disease, excisional biopsy of visible tumor is indicated, followed by re-resection with nephron preservation after chemotherapy. The involved nodes should be marked with clips to facilitate postoperative radiation therapy.

Preoperative angiographic embolization of the renal artery has been used for large vascular tumors with preoperative hemorrhage in which the risk of embolization is likely to outweigh the risk of intraoperative disruption and hemorrhage.[4]

Surgical Complications

- Small bowel obstruction (7%)
- Hemorrhage (6%)
- Wound infection, hernia (4%)
- Vascular complications (2%)
- Splenic and intestinal injury (1.5%).

Surgical data derived from the 606 patients in the National Wilms' Tumor Study were analyzed in 1978.[5] Certain aspects of surgical technique that have traditionally been thought to be important for success appear to be irrelevant. Physical characteristics of the tumor, preoperative rupture and vascular invasion by tumor were not associated with higher relapse rates. Large tumors, those with capsular infiltrations, and tumors with spread to lymph nodes were associated with higher recurrence rate.[5] Operative spill increased the chance of abdominal recurrence. There was no evidence that early ligation of the renal vein was of value in prevention of recurrence, nor was incomplete removal of tumor associated with an increase in relapse rate.[5]

Laparoscopic nephrectomy is contraindicated in Wilms' tumor.

Emergency Nephrectomy

Emergency nephrectomy may be essential for cases with intratumoral bleed. Adequate arrangement of blood and platelets should be made. Bare minimum to prevent loss of life due to massive bleeding should be done. Even debulking of the tumor may benefit the child in such a scenario to save life without attempting complete removal.

IVC and Intra-atrial Thrombus

The management of these has been detailed in a separate chapter.

Lung Metastasis

Thirty to forty percent of the oncologic patients have pulmonary metastases. The common primary tumors include Wilms' tumors and bone tumors (Ewing and osteosarcoma) (Fig. 6.9). Two-third cases may present as a solitary nodule.[6] Pulmonary resection in selected patients can offer better survival. Surgical techniques include metastasectomy, wedge resection and lobectomy. The patients with a Disease Free Interval of less than 2

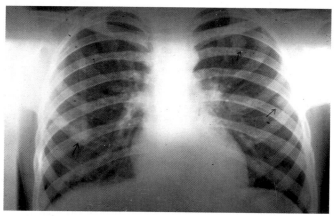

Figure 6.9: Skiagram chest showing lung metastasis in a child with Wilms' tumor (stage IV)

years have been found to have a survival of 25 percent compared with 100 percent for patients with a Disease Free Interval of more than 2 years. In experienced hands, a thoracoscopic removal of a nodule/nodules may be considered.

Secondary Liver Tumors

Cure can be achieved in patients with Wilms' tumor or renal cell carcinoma with secondaries in the liver.[7] In the few symptomatic patients in whom extrahepatic disease is excluded, symptomatic treatment has failed, and the lesions are not resectable, liver transplantation can provide a reasonable therapeutic choice (Fig. 6.10).

The risk of fatal hemorrhage may limit the completeness of resection in hepatic malignancies. Ein's technique of deep hypothermia (average 17 degrees C) with cardiac arrest (average 39 minutes) and exsanguination has been used for performing hepatic resections.[4] The initial hepatic resection took less than 15 minutes to perform in a bloodless field and the specimen was immediately examined by frozen section for determination of adequacy of margin.

NEUROBLASTOMA

Neuroblastoma is one of the most difficult tumors to tackle amongst pediatric tumors due its varied location, engulfment around major vessels and intraspinal extension (Fig. 6.11). Anatomic evaluation may be performed preoperatively with angio-magnetic resonance imaging. CT scan is also sufficient to assess resectability (Fig. 6.12).

Abdominal neuroblastoma is approached through a transverse upper abdominal incision 1-2 cm below the lateral costal margin crossing the midline (Fig. 6.13). An extension into the lateral flank laterally gives adequate exposure. The liver is examined and palpated for any metastatic lesions. An assessment is made for resectability though the tumor is almost always adherent in the midline posteriorly with the major vessels. The dissection begins with mobilization of the mesocolon and colon after an incision along the lateral parietal wall to reflect the peritoneum and expose the retroperitoneal space.

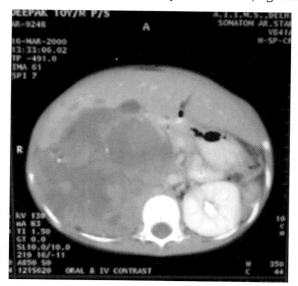

Figure 6.10: CT scan image of a child with recurrent Wilms' tumor and secondaries liver

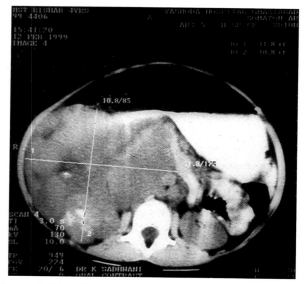

Figure 6.11: CT scan image of a calcified neuroblastoma involving kidney, aorta and inferior vena cava

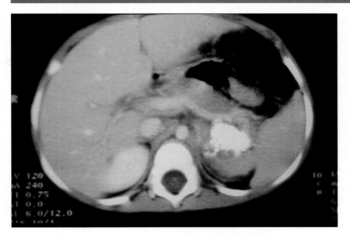

Figure 6.12: CT scan showing a calcified adrenal neuroblastoma

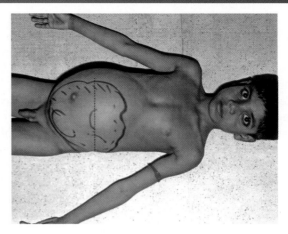

Figure 6.13: A supraumbilical transverse incision (marked) crossing the midline with extension into the flank laterally provides adequate exposure for operating neuroblastoma

The tumor is then reassessed for resectability sparing the kidney or whether nephrectomy is inevitable for complete excision. Mobilization of the tumor is then begun laterally and then anteriorly and posteriorly. Meticulous dissection is then begun medially starting from the inferior aspect. The vessels are tackled one by one staying close to the tumor without jeopardizing the vital structures. The course of the vessels is short so in some cases the tunica adventitia is incised and left adherent to the tumor and the tunica media is ligated and cut. This dissection proceeds upwards for the complete length of the tumor. After the tumor is excised, a reassessment is done for the tumor bed and the residual tumor is excavated out from behind the aorta and inferior vena cava.

The advantage of using an Cavitron ultrasonic surgical aspirator (CUSA) is well emphasized as it makes it possible to remove residues of the tumor without damaging the large blood vessels.[8] Lymphnodes are then sampled from each region- above and below the renal veins, left of aorta, between the aorta and vena cava and right of the vena cava, as divided into six sections.[9] Laparoscopic adrenalectomy has been done successfully for neuroblastoma in children.[10] It gives a very good exposure of the retroperitoneal area, small scars and reduces the hospital stay.

Mediastinal neuroblastomas are tackled by thoracotomy. The intraspinal extensions through the intervertebral foramina are cut flush without brave attempts to remove the intraspinal components, as there is risk of nerve damage. The residual tissue can be treated with chemotherapy or radiotherapy.

Thoracoscopic surgery has been described as a feasible, safe, and effective technique in the treatment for children with neurogenic mediastinal tumors like neuroblastoma, ganglioneuroblastoma and ganglioneuroma with successful removal without any evidence of tumor recurrence.[11] General anesthesia using a Fogarty catheter as an ipsilateral bronchial blocker was utilized. Four 5-mm ports were placed in all patients The tumor was captured in an extraction bag, fragmented, and then removed through the trocar site, which had been enlarged up to 2.0-2.5 cm.[11]

Cervicothoracic neuroblastoma originates from the cervical sympathetic nerves and ganglia and thus presents a problem when dissecting the vascular and nervous elements of the subclavian region. The standard operation is based on thoracotomy or dual cervicotomy/thoracotomy, but these approaches do not provide optimal control of the subclavian vessels.

Transmanubrial approach, performed through a manubrial L-shaped transection and first costal cartilage resection, affords excellent access to the subclavian region with safe control of the vessels and nerves and exposure of the first 4 thoracic intervertebral foramina.[12] Removal of more than 90 percent of the tumor was possible in 4 cases with no recurrence during the follow-up period of 8 to 32 months.[12] The transmanubrial approach is an osteomuscular-sparing technique that seems particularly suitable for the treatment of these tumors, which require a resection that is as complete as possible to avoid postoperative chemotherapy and tumor relapse.

The transcranial surgical technique for olfactory neuroblastoma consists of a bicoronal incision, followed by a standard frontal craniotomy with or without a separated orbital bar osteotomy.[13] The tumor could be removed en bloc transcranially after the cranial base osteotomy according to the tumor extent delineated by preoperative magnetic resonance imaging and intraoperative findings. The defect in the floor of the anterior cranial fossa can be reconstructed with a galeopericranial flap.[13] With thorough knowledge of the basic topographic anatomy of the anterior cranial base, transcranial resection can provide adequate surgical exposure to facilitate oncologically sound resection and to execute reliable skull base reconstruction in selected patients with an olfactory neuroblastoma. A transcranial approach alone may further decrease the rate of surgical morbidity by omitting the facial incision and osteotomy.

HEPATOBLASTOMA

Despite the success of chemotherapy in the treatment of hepatoblastoma (HB), the complete surgical resection of the primary liver tumour and metastases is the most important factor for survival. The tumor is usually chemoresponsive and decreases in size following adequate chemotherapy (Fig. 6.14). Hepatic resection is the main treatment modality for hepatic tumors in childhood. Resection of hepatic malignancies in childhood has been facilitated greatly by an understanding of hepatic segmental anatomy. Anatomic hepatic resection is dependent on the segmental infrastructure of the liver, whereas nonanatomic resection is independent of structural planes and is often fraught with excessive bleeding. Hepatic lobectomy is a major operation, which is feasible yielding curative results in children. Safe hepatic resections with acceptable blood loss can be performed by a technique relying on good anatomic dissection and surgical control.[14]

With diagnostic imaging, the resection is planned ahead of surgery. 85 percent of the liver may be safely resected in pediatric patients with rest of the liver being healthy. The vascular anatomy and extent of resection should be studied. Standard anatomic resections based on the segmental distributions can be planned. With smaller lesions, a segmental resection can be achieved. However, usually the resection required is extensive. Left lateral segmentectomy includes the liver substance to the left of the falciform ligament (segments II and III) (Fig. 6.15). Left medial segmentectomy consists of resection of liver parenchyma right to the falciform ligament and medial to the right lobe (segment IV). Left and right lobectomies consist of removal of the liver tissue on either side of the anatomic plane that runs from the gallbladder bed to the suprahepatic vena cava. An extended right lobectomy (right trisegmentectomy) consists of the complete removal of the right lobe (segments V-VIII) plus the medial segment of the left lobe (segment IV). An extended left lobectomy (left trisegmentectomy) is the complete removal of the left lobe (segments II-IV) plus the anterior segment of the right lobe (segments V and VIII). Hepatoblastoma usually expands without breaching the umbilical fissure. Therefore, although the tumor may be large, successful extended resection may still be possible.

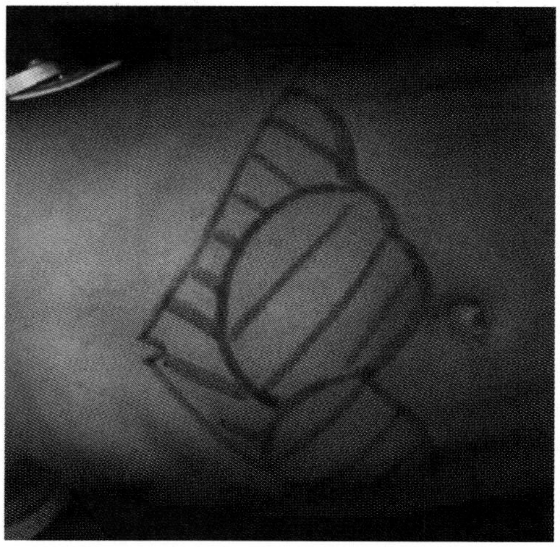

Figure 6.14: A hepatoblastoma that decreased in size following chemotherapy

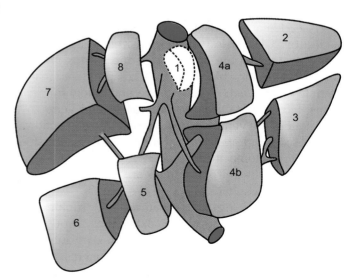

Figure 6.15: Couinaud's segmental anatomy of the liver

Resection is usually performed from a standard transabdominal Chevron incision (Fig. 6.16). Some may also adapt a thoracoabdominal incision for higher lesions. The tumor is inspected for margins of resection (Figs 6.17A and B). The vascular inflow and outflow are exposed for adequate vascular control to avoid any catastrophy (Fig. 6.18). The liver is mobilized by taking down the diaphragmatic ligamentous attachments, thereby exposing the suprahepatic vena cava. The porta hepatis is then dissected, and the vessels and bile ducts to the involved lobe are ligated and divided. A slight Trendelenberg position maintains a low central venous pressure during this portion of the procedure and helps to minimize blood loss. The liver capsule is incised in an area demarcated by division of the hepatic artery and the portal vein. Intraoperative ultrasonography may assist complete resection and guide the operator to the exact location of vascular structures whose location may be distorted by the tumor. The liver parenchyma may be dissected by various methods including finger fracture, suction knife, ultrasonic dissector, harmonic scalpel, or laser. These expose the bridging vessels so that they can be ligated or clipped to limit hemorrhage. After dissection through the liver substance, the hepatic veins must be ligated. These veins are quite short in children so they may be dissected through the liver substance. After removal of the affected lobe, hemostasis must be achieved. Argon beam coagulation is helpful for cauterizing the large raw surface that sometimes results after extensive resections.

Normothermic total vascular exclusion of the liver, although used in the adult population, has not been commonly used to treat pediatric patients. Total vascular exclusion is most useful for central lesions involving the hepatic veins or IVC. Ein's technique of profound hypothermia and circulatory arrest to achieve a

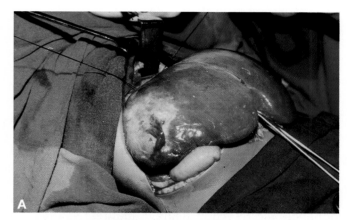

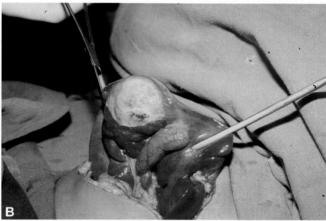

Figure 6.17A and B: **(A)** Anterior inspection of the tumor, **(B)** Posterior inspection of the tumor

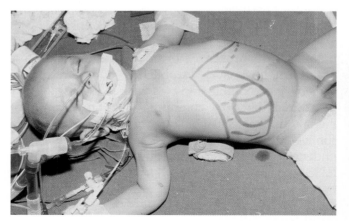

Figure 6.16: Outline of a hepatoblastoma and the costal margin in a child. The Chevron incision is given above the most prominent part of the mass depending upon the amount of resection planned

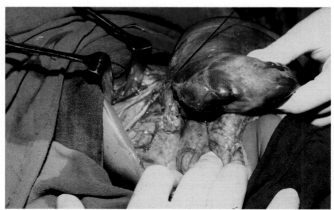

Figure 6.18: The tumor being seperated from inferior vena cava and the hepatic veins being tackled

bloodless operative field and minimize blood loss has been described. However, this may prolong operative time, and the coagulopathy that may develop as the result of hypothermia may in fact increase the likelihood of hemorrhage. Alternatively, standard cardiopulmonary bypass may be quicker and does not cause the coagulopathy that is associated with hypothermia.

Other Techniques

New technique for liver resection include use of heat coagulative necrosis and banding method. Segmental liver resection using ultrasound-guided selective portal venous occlusion has also been described.

In lesions considered unresectable by segmental anatomy, a surgical technique has been described in which nonabsorbable 2-0 Teflon felt pledgetted sutures were placed through the liver parenchyma in a nonanatomic resection plane.[15] Mattress sutures are sequentially tied until the resection plane is defined. The resection is sharply completed with a scalpel along the line of pledgetted sutures, independent of hepatic segmental anatomy. The pledgetted suturing technique for hepatic resection is relatively bloodless, safe, easy to perform, and may enable a complete surgical resection of otherwise unresectable lesions.[15] This technique may be used when approaching a large hepatic lesion that would entail a difficult or incomplete anatomic resection in infants.

Nonanatomic Hepatic Resection may also be required for secondary hepatic tumors. Liver tumors that surround the three major hepatic veins traditionally have been considered unresectable. Extended left hepatectomy, also referred to as left hepatic trisegmentectomy, in which segments II, III, IV, V, and VIII are excised, is rarely performed in children. Although technically challenging and rarely performed, extended resection of the left hepatic lobe is feasible in children and can yield curative results with minimal morbidity.[16] Central hepatic resection (mesohepatectomy) of malignant tumors involving segments IV, V, and VIII is feasible and effective in childhood.[17]

Extended atypical left hepatectomy technique for tumors around the major hepatic veins has been described. The left hepatic artery, left branch of the portal vein, and the 3 hepatic veins are occluded with vascular clamps.[18] Perfusion of the remaining liver is through the right hepatic artery and portal vein into the retrohepatic vena cava via the retro hepatic veins. If the liver remains soft and does not become mottled, division

of the 3 hepatic veins and resection of the tumor are carried out. Successful extended atypical left hepatectomy depends on the ability of the retro hepatic veins to adequately drain blood into the vena cava after interruption (clamping) of the main hepatic veins.[18] If the liver becomes mottled and tense, the procedure must be abandoned and the patient should be considered for hepatic transplantation.

Complications

The most common intraoperative complication is hemorrhage. Other complications include air embolism, tumor embolus, hyperkalemia resulting from tumor lysis, and primary or secondary (ischemic) bile duct injury. Postoperative complications include bile leak (caused by parenchymal transection and resolving spontaneously with drainage), subphrenic abscesses, pulmonary complications, adhesive bowel obstruction, and wound problems. Posthepatectomy liver failure is unusual except for patients with cirrhosis. Surgical mortality rates have been reported to be 0 to 3 percent.

Thirty eight percent cases with atypical tumor resection and only 18 percent cases with anatomical liver resection had residual tumors in the liver (p < 0.019).[19] These results underline the necessity for preoperative chemotherapy in all HB Atypical tumour resection should be avoided because of the higher rate of incomplete tumor resections and local relapse compared to the group with anatomical tumor resection.

The survival of children with hepatoblastoma, the most common malignant tumor of the liver in children, has improved dramatically over the past 20 years. This progress has been made with advances in surgical technique and improved chemotherapy, primarily with adriamycin and cisplatin. Despite these advances, those patients who present with advanced disease have unsatisfactory survival.[20] Continued refinement of liver surgery and chemotherapy, as well as the use of new techniques such as chemoembolization, immunotherapy, and molecular biology, should lead to improved survival in patients with advanced disease. The work is underway with the use of single drug (cisplatin) to reduce toxicity specially in children with small tumors and poor nutritional status.

REFERENCES

1. Gunther P, Schenk JP, Wunsch R, Troger J, Waag KL. Abdominal tumours in children: 3-D visualisation and surgical planning. Eur J Pediatr Surg 2004;14:316-21.

2. Sandoval C, Strom K, Stringel G. Laparoscopy in the management of pediatric intraabdominal tumors. JSLS 2004;8:115-8.

3. Gupta DK, Sharma S, Agarwala S, Carachi R. Saga of wilms' tumor, lessions learnt from the past. Journal of Indian Association of Pediatric Surgeons 2005;10:217-28.

4. Harrison MR, de Lorimier AA, Boswell WO. Preoperative angiographic embolization for large hemorrhagic Wilms' tumor J Pediatr Surg 1978;13:757-8.

5. Leape LL, Breslow NE, Bishop HC. The surgical treatment of Wilms' tumor: results of the National Wilms' Tumor Study Ann Surg 1978;187:351-6.

6. Delgado Munoz MD, Anton-Pacheco JL, Matute JA, Cuadros J, Aguado P, Vivanco JL, Berchi FJ. Surgery of lung metastasis Cir Pediatr 2000;13:7-10

7. Broelsch CE, Knoefel WT, Gundlach M, et al. Surgical therapy of primary and secondary liver tumors Schweiz Rundsch Med Prax 1997;86:91-3.

8. Snajdauf J, Zeman L, Horn M, Koutecky J, Smelhaus V, Horak J, Kodet R. Surgical methods in the treatment of retroperitoneal neuroblastoma. Rozhl Chir 1994;73:31-3.

9. Tsuchida Y, Iwanaka T. Neuroblastoma-general consi-derations In Atlas of Children's surgery. Eds. GH Willital, E Keily, AM Gohary,DK Gupta, M Li,Y Tsuchida.2005 Germany. Chap18.3. pp400-4.

10. de Mingo Misena L, Rollan Villamarin V, Chaves Pecero F, Jimenez Lorente A, Morales Conde S. Laparoscopic adrenalectomy for neuroblastoma in children] Cir Pediatr. 2004 Oct;17(4):199-201.

11. Nio M, Nakamura M, Yoshida S, Ishii T, Amae S, Hayashi Y. Thoracoscopic removal of neurogenic mediastinal tumors in children. J Laparoendosc Adv Surg Tech A 2005;15:80-3.

12. Sauvat F, Brisse H, Magdeleinat P, Lopez M, Philippe-Chomette P, Orbach D, Aerts I, Brugieres L, Revillon Y, Sarnacki S. The transmanubrial approach: a new operative approach to cervicothoracic neuroblastoma in children Surgery. 2006; 139:109-14.

13. Wang CC, Chen YL, Hsu YS, Jung SM, Hao SP. Transcranial resection of olfactory neuroblastoma. Skull Base. 2005;15:163-71; discussion 171.

14. Ekinci S, Karnak I, Tanyel FC, Senocak ME, Kutluk T, Buyukpamukcu M, Buyukpamukcu N. Hepatic lobectomies in children: experience of a center in the light of changing management of malignant liver tumors. Pediatr Surg Int. 2006;22:228-32. Epub 2006 Jan 3.

19. Fuchs J, Rydzynski J, Hecker H, Mildenberger H, Burger D, Harms D, V Schweinitz D; German Cooperative Liver Tumour Studies HB 89 and HB 94. The influence of preoperative chemotherapy and surgical technique in the treatment of hepatoblastoma—a report from the German Cooperative Liver Tumour Studies HB 89 and HB 94. Eur J Pediatr Surg 2002 Aug;12(4):255-61.

15. Sandler A, Kimura K, Soper R. Nonanatomic hepatic resection with a pledgetted suturing technique J Pediatr Surg 2001;36:209-12.

16. Glick RD, Nadler EP, Blumgart LH, La Quaglia MP. Extended left hepatectomy (left hepatic trisegmentectomy) in childhood. J Pediatr Surg. 2000;35:303-7; discussion 308.

17. La Quaglia MP, Shorter NA, Blumgart LH. Central hepatic resection for pediatric tumors J Pediatr Surg 2002 Jul;37(7):986-9.

18. Superina RA, Bambini D, Filler RM, Almond PS, Geissler G. A new technique for resecting 'unresectable' liver tumors. J Pediatr Surg 2000 Sep;35(9):1294-9.

20. Geiger JD. Surgery for hepatoblastoma in children. Curr Opin Pediatr 1996;8:276-82.

CHAPTER 7

TD Chugh

Infections in Pediatric Oncology Patients

Since the introduction of antineoplastic therapy and consequent myelosuppression, mucosal injury, infections and complications have been found to be the major limitation to treatment. However, the development of effective antimicrobial strategies for their management led to a dramatic decline in mortality and thus paved the way for significant strides in the development of effective antineoplastic regimens for various tumors in all age groups. The combination cancer chemotherapy protocols were introduced to avoid excessive toxicity and minimize infections. The introduction of new antibacterial, antifungal and antiviral therapeutics, development of hematopoietic growth factors and various molecular and immunodiagnostic techniques for the early and specific diagnosis of infections have been major contributions to the advancement of care of cancer patients.[1]

IMPACT ON HOST DEFENSES

The impact on host defenses may be attributed to disease or therapy. In hematopoietic malignancies, disease-related factors play a major role due to depletion of marrow and lymphoid cells while in solid tumors; therapy-related effects are the primary determinants of the status of host defenses. The spectrum of changes in host defenses is shown in Figure 7.1.

Corticosteroids are a major determinant of abnormal functions of cellular elements of host immune system. There is a marked alteration in the functions of neutrophils, monocytes, lymphocytes and macrophages that enhance host susceptibility to infection. IL – 2 therapy for malignant melanoma and renal cell carcinoma has been associated with defect in neutrophil chemotaxis and an increased incidence of staphylococcal infections. Patients on dose -intensive cyclophosphamide and/or corticosteriods are at increased risk of viral and opportunistic infections.[2]

INFECTIONS IN HEMATOLOGICAL MALIGNANCIES

Fever and Infection

A large retrospective study of 1894 febrile episodes in acute leukemics from 1966-74 from MD Anderson Hospital showed that 64 percent were microbiologically

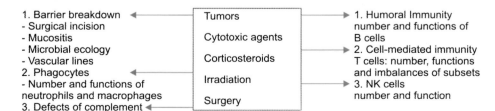

Figure 7.1: Effect of tumor and treatment on host defenses

documented infections, 35 percent were unexplained fevers and only 1 percent were non-infectious. One-third were bacteremics. The major bacterial isolates were gram-negative bacilli (72%), of which *E.coli* was 33 percent. *Klebsiella* spp (25%) and *Ps. aeruginosa* (24%). Anaerobic bacteria were 3 percent and fungi 5 percent. However, marked shift in the bacterial pathogens from gram-negative bacilli to gram-positive cocci has occurred. This is due to the marked increase in the use of indwelling vascular devices, use of antibacterial chemoprophylaxis which suppress aerobic gram-negative bacilli and use of antacids and H_2 receptor blockers which allow oropharyngeal gram-positive microflora to overgrow. The clinically important gram-positive pathogens are viridans streptococci, coagulase – negative staphylococci and enterococci.[3-5]

Fungal Infections[6-9]

Candida spp. is a common cause of infections in patients with neoplastic diseases. The manifestations range from generally benign, oropharyngeal and vaginal candidiasis to life-threatening invasive blood stream and visceral infections. Invasion can occur through an intravascular catheter or through translocation from the gastrointestinal tract. Typically, the highest risk for invasion is during neutropenic period. Historically, *C. albicans* and *C. tropicalis* have been the major pathogens but the emergence of non-albicans candida spp. has made the management more difficult. It is likely that *C. glabrata* and *C. krusei* have emerged in association with use of azoles for prophylaxis or empiric therapy.

Invasive aspergillosis (IA) is an important cause of morbidity and mortality in such patients and the ones with allogeneic hematopoietic stem cell transplantation (HSCT). The burden of IA has increased significantly in recent years. The incidence of IA has increased from 7.9 percent in 1992 to 16.9 percent in 1998 at one of the large HSCT Centers in the USA and mortality has increased to 35 percent since 1980. There has been a recent expansion of the antifungal therapy against IA but the optimal treatment is still elusive. Some aspects of IA in children are quite different to those in adults. There have been two published reviews of childhood IA, the first one of 39 cases from the Hospital for Sick Children in Toronto (1979-1988) and second one of 66 cases (1962-1996) from St. Jude's Children's Hospital in Memphis. Although new diagnostic tools hold great promise for adult patient, it appears that they have limited usefulness in children without the appropriate testing as yet. Antifungal management of pediatric aspergillosis also requires unique domain regimens that are not used in adult patients. In adult series of pulmonary aspergillosis, around 50 percent of cases show cavitation and 40 percent air- crescent formation. In a review of 27 consecutive pediatric patients, cavitation was seen in 25 percent and no evidence of a crescent was seen. Diagnosis with galactomannan assay has shown repeated differences in pediatric and adult values. There has been no dedicated, prospective, large study into treatment of pediatric IA.

Apart from Candida and Aspergillus as the principal systemic fungal pathogens, *Trichosporon, M. furfur, Rhodotorula, Saccharomyces* and *Fusarium* has been encountered in immunocompromised hosts.

Viral Infections

Lower respiratory tract infections are leading cause of infections in neutropenic patients and viruses are responsible for a substantial number of these cases.[10] Respiratory viruses (Influenza A and B, respiratory syncitial virus, parainfluenza viruses, rhinoviruses and adenoviruses) may cause a self-limited runny nose in previously healthy subjects to severe pneumonia in immunocompromised hosts. In addition, herpes viruses (cytomegalovirus, herpes simplex virus) are the most frequent viruses recovered from respiratory specimens in such patients. In a study of 800 such patients with suspected respiratory infection, viruses were recognized in bronchoalveolar lavage from 182 subjects. CMV (66% cases) and HSV (16%) accounted for the majority of cases. In immunocompetent patients, respiratory virus infections are generally limited to the upper respiratory tract and tracheobronchial tree. In immunocom-promised patients, the risk of developing lower respiratory tract infections, especially pneumonia, is extremely high (10-40%) and may be upto 80 percent for RSV infections in recipients of HSCT. Respiratory failure is frequent and mortality rates are high.

Hepatitis virus infections in patients with cancer are common and liver-related morbidity and mortality is high especially in countries where viral hepatitis is endemic. Hematologic malignancy, highly immuno-suppressive therapy and use of corticosteriods are risk factors for hepatitis B leading to increased serum ALT (50%), increased serum bilirubin (10%) and liver failure (5%). Serum titres of hepatitis B and C virus rise during periods of immunosuppression but little clinical hepatitis is seen due to lack of T-Cell response. However, when immunity returns following recovery from chemotherapy, clinical hepatitis may manifest. In contrast to the normal adults, where antibodies against structural and non-structural HCV proteins develop during acute HCV infection, pediatric cancer patients do not develop this antibody response.

In cancer patients, Epstein–Barr Virus (EBV) plays two major roles. Firstly, it is found in association with malignant tumors (Nasopharyngeal carcinoma, Burkitt's lymphoma and Hodgkin's lymphoma). Secondly, in severely immunocompromised patients, EBV is responsible for severe post transplant lymphoproliferative disease.

Human CMV remains a significant cause of morbidity and mortality in such patients. The disease has lately increased after day 100 and an increase in early disease after post transplantation immunosuppression (with high doses of corticosteroids, use of antithymocyte globulin and CD34 depletion). Reactivation of CMV occurs in around 70-80 percent of seropositive recipients of allogeneic HSCT and without prophylaxis 20-35 percent of these progress to CMV disease. The risks to immunocompromised patients with Varicella – Zoster virus infection are primary viral pneumonia, encephalitis, disseminated intravascular coagulation, generalized rash and death. Reactivation of Herpes simplex virus is enhanced by immunosuppression and is clinically more severe in cancer patients. Both adult and children with cancer may have clinically severe, chronic and frequent recurrences of either oral or genital herpes. The severity of infection is usually a function of the degree of immunosuppression or the resistance of HSV to an antiviral therapeutic. The disease in such patients may result in extensive tissue destruction with prolonged virus shedding.

INFECTIONS IN PATIENTS WITH SOLID TUMORS

The chances of infection vary with the physical extent of the disease, and effects of treatment that the patient is undergoing especially chemotherapy induced immunosuppression. During immunosuppression, the signs and symptoms of infection are attenuated making diagnosis a formidable challenge.

The causes of pulmonary infiltrates in such patients are varied (Table 7.1).

Table 7.1: Causes of pulmonary infiltrates in solid tumor patients

		Diffuse infiltrates	*Localized infiltrates*
A.	Infections	Pneumocystis carinii	Bacteria
		Legionella spp.	(Klebsiella,
		Cytomegalovirus	Pseudomonas,
		Influenza virus	Staphylococcus aureus)
		Respiratory syncitial virus	Aspergillus
			Nocardia
			Mycobacteria
B.	Non-infectious	Radiation	
		Chemotherapy	Tumor infarct
		Acute respiratory distress syndrome	

Catheter – Associated Infections

Overall infection rates vary widely; the infections are more with external devices (Hickmann, Broviac) than with implanted ports. The risk is higher with infant and young children. The infections may be exit-site, tunnel, or systemic. The mainstay of infection prevention is the catheter insertion technique and maintenance practices of catheter care.

Febrile Neutropenia

In general, a specific infectious etiology can be established in nearly two-thirds of febrile episodes. The most common sites of infection are oral cavity, lungs, skin, anal fissure and indwelling intravascular catheters. The signs and symptoms of infection are often attenuated during myelosuppression. Neutropenic enterocolitis must be suspected in patients with fever, diarrhea or abdominal pain.

There is a distinct change in the pattern of infectious agents from gram-negative bacilli to gram-positive cocci. Laboratory investigations should include urine analysis, two sets of blood cultures, respiratory secretions and biopsy or aspiration of any accessible sites suggestive of infection.

Nosocomial Infections[11-14]

The greatest risk of exogenous source of microbial pathogens comes from within the hospital environment-hospital ventilation system, ventilator equipment, showers, flowers, bedpans, food, healthcare workers and visitors. Construction and hospital renovations pose major challenges especially Aspergillus dissemination.

Acquisition of *Clostridium difficile* during long hospital stay of upto 50 percent has been reported with symptomatic diarrhea in 9-13 percent in pediatric and 7-12 percent in adult oncology units. Case fatality rate in neutropenic patients may be as high as 48 percent. Intestinal colonization with nosocomial pathogens from food is common and may frequently translocate to cause bacteremia in neutropenics.

A coordinated, multidisciplinary approach involving all hospital services is essential to minimize patient risk. Published CDC guidelines and individual hospital policies should be followed to ensure that proper infection control practices are maintained.

REFERENCES

1. Wingard JR, Bowden RA. Management of Infection in Oncology Patients. Publisher MD Martin Duritzm, London 2003.
2. De Pauw BE, Donnelly JP, Kullberg BJ. Host impairments in patients with neoplastic diseases. Cancer Treat Res 1998;96:1-32.
3. Shenep JL. Viridans-group streptococcal infections in immunocompromised hosts Int. J. Antimicrob Agent 2000;14:129-35.
4. Kremery V, Spanik S, Mrazova M, et al. Bacteremias caused by *E. coli* in cancer patients – analysis of 65 episodes. Int J Infect Dis 2002;6:69-73.
5. Tunkel AR, Sepkowitz KA. Infections caused by viridans streptococci in patients with neutropenia. Clin Infect Dis 2002;34:1524-9.
6. Auner HW, Sill H, Mulabecirovic A, et al. Infectious complications after autologous hematopoeitic stem cell transplantation: Comparison of patients with acute myeloid leukaemia, malignant lymphoma, and multiple myeloma. Ann Hemabol 2002;81:374-7.
7. Stenbach WJ. Pediatric aspergillosis. Pediat Infect Dis J 2004;24:358-64.
8. Anaissie E, Rex J, Uzun O, et al. Predictors of adverse outcome in cancer patients with candidemia. Am J Med 1998;104:238-45.
9. Hall CB. Respiratory syncitial virus and parainfluenza virus. N Eng J Med 2001;344:1917-28.
10. Schuller J, Saha V, Lin L, et al. Investigation and management of *Clostridium difficile* colonization in pediatric oncology unit. Arch Dis Child 1995;72:219-22.
11. Burgner D, Siavakas S, Eagles Cs, et al. A prospective study of *Clostridium difficile* infection and colonisation in pediatric oncology patients. Pediatr. Infect Dis J. 1997; 16:1131-4.
12. Herbrecht R, Letscher – Bru V, Opera C, et al. Aspergillus galactomannan detection in the diagnosis of invasive aspergillosis in cancer patients. J Clin Oncol 2002; 20:1898-906.
13. Garner JS. Guidelines for isolation precautions in hospitals. Infect Control Hosp Epidemiol. 1996;17:53-80.
14. Anaissie EJ, Penzak SR, Dignani MC. The hospital water supply as a source of nosocomial infections: a plea for action. Arch Intern Med 2002;162:1483-92.

CHAPTER 8

Lalit Kumar
R Jagarlamudi
V Kochupillai
Subhash C Gulati

Fungal Infections in Hematological Malignancies

INTRODUCTION

The prospects of survival have improved with the use of aggressive chemotherapy for the treatment of malignancies, but this approach has increased the risk of infection in these patients due to significant myelosuppression. Neutropenia is the most important predisposing factor to such infections. Infections generally occur when the absolute neutrophil count (ANC) is less than 500/cmm; patients with a count below 100/cmm being at greater risk.[1] During the neutropenic phase, the patient is prone to develop bacterial and fungal infections; occasionally mycobacterial, viral and protozoal organisms may also cause infections. There could be a change in pattern of microorganisms causing the infection and also in their sensitivity and resistance pattern, depending upon hospital flora and extensive use of antibiotics. In addition, cost of therapy has become a major issue in designing therapeutic strategies for a large number of patients. This necessitates a periodic update on febrile neutropenia and associated infections as our armamentarium and techniques evolve.

RISK FACTORS

Patients of acute leukemia on induction and/or consolidation chemotherapy or those undergoing allogeneic or autologous bone marrow/stem cell transplantation are at greatest risk of having severe (ANC<100/cmm) and prolonged neutropenia (> 10 days) and consequently at greatest risk of fungal infection. Up to 60 percent of febrile episodes are due to clinically or microbiologically documented infections.[2]

Generally gram-positive (*Staphylococcus epidermidis, Streptococcus viridans, Staphylococcus aureus*) and gram-negative rods (*Pseudomonas aeruginosa, Klebsiella* and *Escherichia coli*) are the common cause of initial infections in neutropenic patients.[3-4] Fungal infections are increasingly being recognized as an important medical problem in these patients in recent years. Though fungal infections are seen in <10 percent of acute leukemia patients at diagnosis, they may occur in more than 50-60 percent of patients following intensive chemotherapy.[5-6] An International autopsy survey on patients with malignant diseases showed a total of 455 fungal infections in 4096 (11%) post-mortem examinations; 25 percent of these were seen in leukemia patients and bone marrow transplant (BMT) recipients.[5] The incidence of invasive fungal infections (IFI) varies with the underlying diagnosis and phase of treatment. Patients with hematological malignancies have significantly higher risk of IFI than those with solid tumours. In a multicentric study, IFI were documented in 19 percent of acute lymphoblastic leukemia and 47 percent of acute myeloid leukemia patients undergoing remission induction therapy. Further IFI were documented in 12 percent of post-remission induction chemotherapy recipients.[7] Similarly, the incidence of IFI ranges from 5 percent in autologous stem cell transplant recipients to 18-45 percent in mismatched or unrelated allogeneic BMT recipients. Risk of IFI increases upto 85 percent in patients receiving immunosuppressive therapy for acute graft versus host disease (GVHD).[8] The risk of IFI is low, being <5 percent in patients receiving chemotherapy for solid tumors.

ascending loop of Henle and distal tubule and is best replaced by adding magnesium sulfate to pre- and post-hydration fluids. A further advantage of zinc supplementation is that it helps to reduce mucositis and improve wound healing.[15]

Fruit does not need to be eliminated from the diet during chemotherapy. Only during stem cell transplant is a special neutropenic diet required. Usually during routine chemotherapy, all foods are allowed when counts are normal, and avoidance of thin peel fruits and raw vegetables during severe Neutropenia, is sufficient to prevent dietary deficiency and reduce infections. Local, seasonal, fresh food should be used as much as possible. It is important to emphasize that during intervals of low dose therapy or when discharged home a good diet of fresh vegetables and fruits along with unprocessed cereals, lentils and other protein sources should be consumed.

Many parents feel guilty about not providing expensive food and spend money they can ill afford in their attempt to provide pomegranate juice, dry fruits and other perceived "good food" for their child. Though these items are not detrimental to health, however for poor patients alternative foodstuffs are cheaper and may be even more nutritious.[12] But since basic nutritional awareness is lacking, it is important for the physician to either provide a handout or talk about how to improve the diet using local, seasonal foodstuffs.

CRITERIA FOR NUTRITIONAL INTERVENTION

1. Interval or total weight loss >5 percent
2. Arm fat <5th percentile

   Skin fold <10th percentile } for age and sex

3. Inability to eat normal diet due to prolonged nausea, vomiting or mucositis
4. Weight/height <10th percentile.
5. Fall in height by 2 percentile channels, (if prior records are available)
6. Recurrent infections
7. Fall in serum albumin.

If any of the above features are present then nutritional intervention is urgently required. Repeated assessments are required during different stages of cancer treatment.

METHODS OF INTERVENTION

The enteral route is preferred as it is physiological, economical and maintains gut integrity. This results in a decreased risk of infection. If the first stage of intervention does not improve nutritional status, then the next stage should be resorted to.

Dietary Advice

Due to chemotherapy and radiation there is nausea and altered taste perception. Many favorite foods are now disliked due to their altered taste. Children become irritable and may use food as a tool to get what they want. Meal times should be relaxed, too much parental concern may be counter productive.

Practical Tips for Parents to Improve Dietary Compliance

1. Avoid food which child dislikes
2. Serve small portions
3. Try different dishes, something not previously tasted (likes and dislikes may be altered due to medicines)
4. Give frequent snacks, allow small amounts of junk food (to increase patient co-operation)
5. Prepare food with fresh herbs and extra salt if taste is decreased
6. Calorie dense foods should be used, so that even small portions are effective
7. Fruit and vegetables if eaten raw, should be washed repeatedly in running water and cut fresh. Avoid eating stored cut fruit
8. Yoghurt and cottage cheese (*paneer*) may be more easily digestible than milk
9. Milk if taken can be fortified with over the counter supplements if tolerated. Care needs to be taken that diarrhoea does not occur; otherwise the intervention is not effective. Lactose free supplements are better tolerated
10. If severe nausea is present, take medications for nausea. Non-medical management for nausea includes not offering medicines and food immediately upon waking up
11. Avoid cooking smells, strongly flavoured foods and fried food
12. Eat outdoors (this avoids the smell of cooking and gives a new environment)
13. Give encouragement for every bite consumed.

Oral Supplements and Enteral Feeds

These can be used orally as an adjunct to the diet, or used via nasogastric tube (NG)/gastrostomy to provide the total caloric intake for a child refusing or unable to eat.

Use formula feeds, which are low in lactose and have medium chain triglycerides as the fat source. This will usually be sufficient to prevent diarrhoea. The feeds should gradually be built up in volume and concentration initiate with small amounts of supplement for the first 3-4 days so the patient can digest it, and the volume does not cause bloating. This is also important to prevent hyperglycemia.

Children with food aversion often benefit from a short course of NG feeds. Care to avoid sinus and middle ear infections; during such feeds is needed. Prompt treatment of mucositis and ulcers should be done. Good oral hygiene should always be maintained. Proper storage of feeds is necessary so that they do not get contaminated. The time which the feed can be left at room temperature, before spoiling should be clearly explained to the parents. The parents must be counseled not to panic if the NG tube accidentally comes out, and it is advised, to return to the clinic the next day for replacement of the tube. If the parents do not live near the hospital they can be taught to replace the NG tube.

Gastric motility agents may be needed, e.g. metoclopromide, cisapride or low dose erythromycin. They prevent retching, reflux and aid in the passage of the feed through the gastrointestinal tract. If severe vomiting persists in a child, work up for its etiology is required, e.g. Hiatal hernia, raised ICP, obstruction etc. If the Nasogastric feed is not tolerated then Nasoduodenal/Jejunal feeds may be tried. In some cases a gastrostomy tube may need to be placed for nutritional support of the child.[16,17]

Parenteral Nutrition

Parenteral Nutrition is expensive and has many side effects, e.g. hepatotoxicity and increased risk of infections. In certain situations, it may be required for short periods, e.g. child on a ventilator, post major surgery, if oral intake not possible for more than 4 days or more, and during stem cell transplantation.

TPN CALCULATION

	10 kg	10-20 kg	>20 kg
Volume (cc/kg/day)	100–125 cc	1000+50 cc/kg	1500+20 cc/kg
Calories (kcal/kg/day)	90	80	60-70
Protein (g/kg/day)	2–2.5	1.5–2.5	1.5–2.5

Intralipid—Max. 60 percent of total calories 0.5 g/kg/day or 2g/kg twice weekly.

GUIDELINES FOR TOTAL PARENTERAL NUTRITION (TPN)

Begin only when oral and enteral routes not possible. Estimate calorie, protein requirements. Baseline electrolyte, triglycerides albumin, bilirubin and creatinine should be done along with weekly monitoring of above. In acutely ill children electrolytes should be monitored every day, while for chronic TPN in stable children; they may be monitored once a week.

Many commercial TPN solutions are now available, which have essential nutrients in the required concentrations. They take into account calcium/phosphorus solubility, dextrose (D) and amino acid ratio for optimal utilization. For liver dysfunction, trace elements should be used with caution. Initial TPN should be started with D10 and gradually increased.

Intralipids should be used to prevent fatty acid deficiency if long term TPN is planned. 2 g/kg twice weekly will prevent fatty acid deficiency. If using peripheral venous access, then maximum dextrose concentration, which can be used, is D12.5 percent and maximum protein concentration is 2.5 g/kg/day. With central venous access, D30 percent and protein concentration up to 3 g/kg/day may be delivered.

With all of these above measures the nutrition of the child may be improved. Understanding on the part of the parent and physician is required as well as a great deal of patience. However the effort is beneficial, as an improvement in the nutritional status of the child will improve tolerance to therapy, result in less infections and may improve the final height of the child. In developing countries, there are studies to show that outcome of acute lymphoblastic leukemia in poor children may be dependent on their nutritional status.[18,19] Obesity in children is increasing even in India, and children who are overweight and have cancer will require care for drug dosing, and monitoring of hyperglycemia. Further studies on specific nutritional deficiencies and innovative repletion strategies for malnourished patients are required from India.

REFERENCES

1. Sherry Mary Ellen, Aker N. Saundra, Cheney Carrie. Nutrition assessment and management of the pediatric cancer patient. Top Clin Nutr 1987;2(1):38-48.
2. Chandra RK. Nutrition and the Immune System. Proc Nutr Soc. 1993;52(1):77-84.
3. Sala A, Pencharz P, Barr RD. Children, cancer, and nutrition—A dynamic triangle in review. Cancer 2004; 15;100(4):677-87.
4. Viana MB, Fernandes RA, de Carvalho RI, Murao M. Low socioeconomic status is a strong independent predictor of relapse inchildhood acute lymphoblastic leukemia. Int J Cancer Suppl 1998;11:56-61.
5. Pedrosa F, Bonilla M, Liu A, Smith K, Davis D, Ribeiro RC, et al. Effect of malnutrition at the time of diagnosis on the survival of children treated for cancer in El Salvador and Northern Brazil. J Pediatr Hematol Oncol 2000; 22(6):502-5.
6. Principles and Practice of Pediatric Oncology, Lippincott Raven. 3rd Edition.
7. Yu LC, Kuvibidila S, Ducos R, Warrier RP. Nutritional status of children with leukemia.Med Pediatr Oncol 1994; 22(2):73-7.
8. Mercadante S. Nutrition in cancer patients. Cancer 1996; 4(1):10-20.
9. Kumar RV, Gokhale SV, Ambaye RY, Shetty PA. Pharmacokinetics of methotrexate in Indian children and its relationship to nutritional status. Chemotherapy 1987;33(4):234-9.
10. Coassolo P, Valintin M, Bourdeaux M, Briand C. Modification of human serum albumin binding of methotrexate by folinic acid and certain drugs used in cancer chemotherapy. Eur J Clin Pharmacol 1980; 17(2):123-7.
11. Halton JM, Nazir DJ, McQueen MJ, Barr RD. Blood lipid profiles in children with acute lymphoblastic leukemia. Cancer 1998;83(2):379-84.
12. Gopalan C, Rama Sastri BV, Balasubramanian SC. Nutritive Value of Indian Foods. National Institute of Nutrition, Indian Council of Medical Research, Hyderabad, India. Reprinted 1999.
13. Nutrient Requirements and Recommended Dietary Allowances for Indians. Indian Council of Medical Research. (A Report of the Expert Group of the Indian Council of Medical Research), Reprinted 2000.
14. Sahin G, Ertem U, Duru F, Birgen D, Yuksek N. High prevelance of chronic magnesium deficiency in T-cell lymphoblastic leukemia and chronic zinc deficiency in children with acute lymphoblastic leukemia and malignant lymphoma. Leuk Lymphoma 2000;39(5-6):555-62.
15. Chandra RK, McBean LD. Zinc and Immunity, Nutrition, 1994;10(1):79-80.
16. Aquino M Victor, Smyri CB, Hagg R, et al. Enteral Nutritional Support by Gastrostomy Tube in Children with Cancer. The Journal of Pediatrics 1995;58-62.
17. Harrison Lawrence E, Fong Yuman. Enteral Nutrition in the Cancer Patient. Clinical Nutrition-Enteral and Tube feeding, 3rd edition, Rombeaujl, Rolandelli RH, 1997.
18. Lobato-Mendizabal E, Lopez-Martinez B, Ruiz-Arguelles GJ. A critical review of the prognostic value of the nutritional status at diagnosis in the outcome of therapy of children with acute lymphoblastic leukemia. Rev Invest Clin 2003;55(1):31-5.
19. Viana MB, Fernandes RA, deOliveira BM, Murao M, et al. Nutritional and socio-economic status in the progress of childhood acute lymphoblastic leukemia Hematologica 2001;86(2):113-20.

CHAPTER 10

Rakesh Kumar
A Malhotra

PET and PET-CT in Pediatric Oncology

Diagnostic nuclear medicine procedures are well suited for the evaluation of pediatric patients as these are highly sensitive, non-invasive, simple, rapid, and non-toxic and provide qualitative and quantitative information often unavailable from other sources. The practice of pediatric nuclear medicine includes patients from infants to adolescents and young adults. The increasing availability of positron emission tomography (PET) scanner and high quality radiopharmaceuticals has greatly facilitated the advances in radionuclide studies. During the past decade, the PET has remarkably improved the management of cancer patients including children.[1,2] Modern-day PET cameras are considerably more "pediatric friendly" than their predecessors; additional efforts are required to ensure safety, comfort of the patient and quality of the imaging data. PET has been used in oncology for detecting and grading tumors, monitoring response and distinguishing between residual tumors and scarring. Much work has been done regarding PET/PET-CT in the adults but there is paucity in the same in pediatric group. Child must receive special attention when embarking on what is uncertain and often a frightening procedure; a set of protocols encompassing issues relevant to pediatrics should be implemented. While performing PET in pediatric patients emphasis given to patient consent, intravenous access, bladder catheterization, and sedation. [^{18}F]fluoro-2-deoxy-D-glucose ^{18}F-FDG which is glucose analogue is the most widely used radiotracer in clinical practice of oncology. Recently, use of PET in conjunction with CT has been found to be more useful as it provides enhanced view of the anatomical details and metabolic status of lesions with highest accuracy.

PRINCIPLE AND TECHNIQUE

PET imaging utilizes positron-emitting radionuclides such as ^{11}C, ^{13}N, ^{15}O and ^{18}F, which can replace their respective stable nuclei respectively in biologically active molecules. These radionuclides decay by positron emission, which combine with a nearby electron through a process known as annihilation. This process of annihilation emits two antiparallel 511 keV gamma rays. The PET detectors are arranged in a ring in order to detect these gamma rays.

At present, ^{18}F-FDG is the most commonly used positron-emitting radiopharmaceutical used for PET imaging. FDG is an analog of glucose and is taken up by the cell in a similar manner as that of normal glucose and therefore, is able to detect altered glucose metabolism in diseases processes. Like glucose, FDG is transported into cells by means of a glucose transporter protein and begins to follow the glycolytic pathway.[3] Once inside the cell, ^{18}F- FDG is phosphorylated into ^{18}F-FDG-6-phosphate. However, ^{18}F-FDG-6-phosphate cannot continue through glycolysis because it is not a substrate for enzyme glucose-6-phosphate isomerase. As a result, ^{18}F-FDG-6-phosphate is biochemically trapped within the cell and that constitutes the basis of PET imaging. PET imaging makes, it possible to calculate a specific uptake value, normalized to the injected dose, which is known as "standardized uptake value" (SUV). The SUV provide an approximate indicator that correlates with FDG metabolism. A lesion with an SUV greater than 2.5 is considered to be malignant. Higher values of SUV are associated with poor prognosis.

PATIENT PREPARATION AND ACQUISITION

All children should be fasted for a minimum of 4 hours before the study, and blood glucose level should be less than 140 mg/dl. Normal blood glucose level is very important as increased glucose level can alter distribution of ^{18}F-FDG. All the younger children who cannot follow the instructions should be sedated before the procedure. The older children who can follow instructions are asked to refrain from talking, walking and any other muscular activity after FDG injection. Most of the time no contrast is used for the CT portion of the PET/CT study, therefore no additional patient preparation is required. However, if contrast is used for PET/CT study, the precautions normally taken for contrast CT should be observed. Sequential overlapping emission scans of the neck, chest, abdomen, and pelvis should be acquired on PET or PET/CT scanner 60 minutes after injection of ^{18}F-FDG.

CLINICAL INDICATIONS

PET scanning is considered to be useful for the following indications: (a) the distinction of benign from malignant neoplasms; (b) staging of the malignancy; (c) determination of the response to therapy; and (d) distinguishing scar from residual neoplasm in children who have completed therapy. Commoner malignancies in children, which have been studied with PET-CT, are brain tumors, lymphomas, neuroblastomas and soft tissue sarcomas, etc. PET scanning can also be quite useful in the evaluation of uncommon tumors, such as the peripheral nerve sheath tumor, and hepato-blastomas, which have not yet been well characterized with regard to FDG uptake and retention. There are relatively few FDG-PET reports describing its role in assessing primary urologic tumors at their sites of origin due to the potential problem of tracer excretion through the kidneys. That is why FDG-PET is not explored in children with Wilms' tumor. However, the usefulness of FDG-PET has been documented in the detection of distant metastasis from urologic malignancies in adults.

LYMPHOMAS

Lymphoma is a common malignancy in children and account for 6 percent of childhood cancers. Accurate staging of Hodgkin's disease and non-Hodgkin's lymphoma is essential to achieve a high cure rate. The main aims of various imaging techniques in these patients are to accurately identify all disease sites, to monitor the therapy response and differentiate scar tissue from

residual disease.[4] Usually, conventional CT is used for these indications. However, CT might not be always correct to detect the presence or absence of disease as it is based on the criteria of size of the lymph nodes, which may sometimes be inaccurate.[5] When CT used along with PET it provides the functional activity within the lymph nodes, thereby leads to correct diagnosis. Miller et al, performed the study regarding the role of FDG-PET/CT in staging and follow-up of lymphoma in pediatric and young patients.[4] They studied on 31 patients. PET/CT findings provided the data that staging of the disease has been changed in 10 patients (32%), upstaging occurred in 7 (23%), and down staging occurred in 3 (10%) patients (Fig. 10.1). Analysis of lesions revealed that 164 sites were detected by PET/CT of which CT overlooked 38 lesions. In the middle of treatment, PET was negative in 28 out of 31 patients with NPV of 96 percent as all latter patients were disease-free except one. PPV was 100 percent as rest of three had active disease. Of the 164 lesions only 149 were true positives and the rest 15 were non-lympha-tomatous. Thirty-eight lesions were overlooked by the diagnostic CT, located in normal size lymph nodes, bone marrow, thymus, spleen, bone, liver, pancreas and ascending colon. Various studies have shown the superiority of PET/PET-CT in the detection of the unexpected extra-nodal sites of disease. It has been well established that PET/CT detect unexpected lesions, both nodal and extra-nodal, and exclude disease involvement in false-positive CT lesions. PET has been used to predict disease relapse in pediatric patients (Fig. 10.2).[6] False-positive results with PET in pediatric patients are inflammation, infection, and effects of therapy such as radiation or physiologic uptake associated with brown fat, muscle tension or post-treatment thymic hyperplasia (Fig. 10.3).

HEPATOBLASTOMA

Hepatoblastoma is the most common primary liver tumor in children, which accounts for around 79 percent of pediatric liver malignancies in children younger than 15 years. Many techniques have been used for the detection of tumor recurrence. These are tumor markers, different imaging techniques such as CT and MRI. An elevated level of AFP is considered as gold standard to find out the hepatoblastoma recurrence.[7] PET has been shown to be superior for detection of recurrent disease when compared with conventional imaging modalities like CT and MRI.[8,9] Wong et al, performed FDG-PET

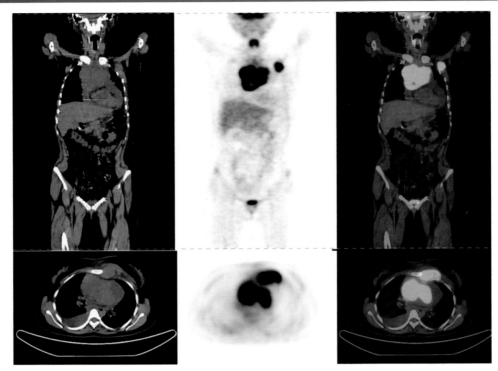

Figure 10.1: Non-Hodgkin's lymphoma for staging: Coronal and axial section CT shows mediastinal mass and left axillary mass. Intense FDG uptake was seen in PET and PET-CT images in mediastinal mass and left axillary lymph nodes

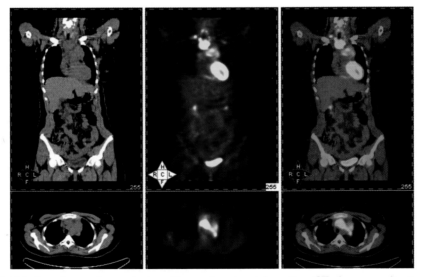

Figure 10.2: Non-Hodgkin's lymphoma for restaging: Coronal and axial section CT shows mediastinal mass and left axillary mass. Intense FDG uptake was seen in PET and PET-CT images in mediastinal mass and right supraclavicular lymph nodes

imaging along with measurement of AFP during post-treatment follow-up in 16 patients.[7] Three patients had positive PET results suggesting the tumor recurrence. One of these patients had normal AFP levels but the PET results were positive. The other 2 patients had raised AFP levels as well as abnormal uptake on PET during postoperative period. The CT and MRI for these 3 patients were normal. PET is also useful in detection of residual tumor after surgical resection.[9] It has been found to have good correlation with tumor marker levels in follow-up of these patients and can be used for determining the recurrent disease.

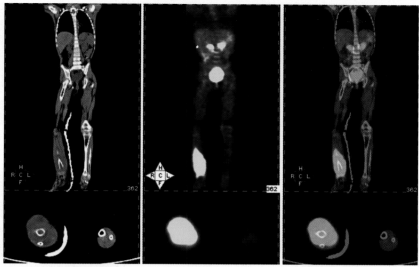

Figure 10.3: Ewing's sarcoma right tibia: Whole body coronal, and axial sections of CT shows soft tissue mass with right tibia involvement. Intense FDG uptake was seen in PET and PET-CT images in soft tissue mass and right tibia

SARCOMAS

In musculoskeletal cancers, osteosarcoma (OS) and the Ewing's sarcoma family of tumors (ESFT) are the most common childhood primary bone cancers. A tumor's histologic response, i.e. the percent necrosis of the resected specimen, to neoadjuvant therapy is predictive of prognosis. Tumors may respond well to therapy without substantial change in size.[10] So conventional imaging like MRI can not assess it well. Fall in SUV in post-treatment PET study when compared to pretreatment SUV are predictive of tumor response. Hawkins et al, evaluated 33 pediatric patients with OS and ESFT using FDG-PET. FDG-PET uptake values before (SUV1) and after (SUV2) chemotherapy were analyzed and correlated with chemotherapy response.[11] Mean SUV1 in patients with OS and ESFT were similar (8.2 vs 5.3, p = 0.13). Mean SUV2 for OS patients was higher than for ESFT patients (3.3 vs 1.5, p = 0.01). All ESFT patients and 28 percent of OS patients had a favorable histologic response to chemotherapy. SUV2 and the ratio of SUV2 to SUV1 when correlated with histologic response, provided the similar results and also their correlation is very significant statistically (p = 0.01). Therefore, PET-CT/ PET can be used as a noninvasive surrogate to predict response to chemotherapy.

PET is useful not only for detection of extent of the primary bone tumor but also useful in detection of the soft tissue, lymph nodes and bone metastases (Fig. 10.3). Although detection of the primary site of disease can be well established with the help of conventional imaging techniques but it is difficult to find out clinically occult metastasis with these modalities. Bone scan has been used to detect distant bone metastases in these patients before surgery and during follow up. However, bone scan has low specificity. PET is more specific in detection of bone metastases when compared with bone scan.[12] Alveolar rhabdomyosarcoma accounts for 20 to 30 percent of childhood rhabdomyosarcoma and have worse prognosis than embryonal rhabdomyosarcoma as metastatic disease is more common in the former. Hematogenous spread to the lung is the most frequent route of spread (Fig. 10.4). Arush et al, assessed the use of PET in the detection of regional and metastatic nodes in alveolar rhabdomyosarcoma of extremities[13] (Fig. 10.5).

ENDOCRINE TUMORS

PET scanning is now widely accepted imaging approach in clinical oncology. However, FDG-PET is only useful in some endocrine tumors as glucose metabolism is not much altered in most of these tumors.[14] Newly developed PET radiopharmaceuticals with specific cellular targets for example receptors, transporters, etc. are more trustworthy than FDG in endocrine oncology. Other positron-emitting radionuclides, such as ^{11}C, can be incorporated without changing the molecular structure or characteristics, e.g.[11]C-Hydroxyephedrine, ^{11}C-Epinephrine, ^{11}C-Etomidate and ^{11}C-Metomidate, etc. Pheochromocytomas are chromaffin cell tumors usually arising in the adrenal gland. For their initial

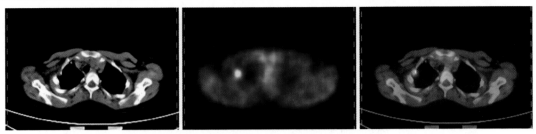

Figure 10.4: Lung metastasis: Axial sections of CT shows subpleural nodule in right lung upper lobe. Intense FDG uptake was seen in PET and PET-CT images in subpleural nodule suggestive of metastasis

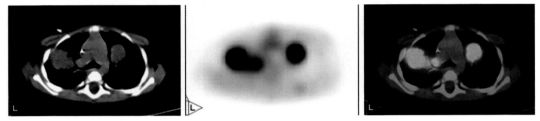

Figure 10.5: ^{18}F-FDG positron emission tomography (PET/CT) demonstrating intense FDG concentration in the masses in bilateral lung parenchyma suggestive of pulomonary metastases in patient with rhabdomyosarcoma

localization CT and MRI can be used. Their sensitivities vary between 75 and 100 percent but specificity is very poor. Because of rapid uptake of circulating catecholamines by chromaffin cells and rapid loss of their metabolites from the circulation, PET scanning can visualize a pheochromocytoma almost immediately after administration of ^{18}F-Fluorodopamine (FDA). Pacak et al, have put some light on the usefulness of PET scanning for diagnostic localization of pheochromocytoma[15] (Fig. 10.6). In the study, 9 out of 28 patients who had surgical confirmation of tumor also showed abnormal uptake of FDA-PET scans. Another 8 patients who were previously diagnosed with metastatic pheochromocytoma had extra-adrenal sites of FDA activity. Another 11 patients with normal metanephrine levels, 9 of them had negative FDA-PET scans, 1 had extra-adrenal foci of activity and 1 had symmetric uptake of FDA in the region of adrenal glands. So PET scanning can detect and localize pheochromocytomas with high sensitivity and these findings suggests that FDA-PET scanning is a diagnostic tool in endocrine tumors. In recurrent or metastatic thyroid cancer degree of accumulation of radiotracer has prognostic value. CT, MRI, ultrasound and radioiodine scanning are currently the preferred first-line imaging modalities. But on recurrence radioiodine scanning fails to detect 1/3rd to ½ of the cases due to poor iodine uptake or small tumor size.[16] Armstrong et al, evaluated the papillary thyroid carcinoma recurrence through PET.[17] It is a case history of 12-year-old girl who had past history of ALL 9 years

ago. An incidental large thyroid nodule along with neck lymphadenopathy and pharyngitis was found on ultrasound scan. Nodule was papillary carcinoma as identified on histology. The PET was performed. PET scan identified a solitary focus of glucose analog hypermetabolism representing the recurrent thyroid papillary carcinoma. ^{18}F-FDG PET scanning has established its value for detecting recurrence of papillary and follicular thyroid cancer, but this is limited to patients with increased thyroglobulin levels and negative radioiodine scanning. High uptake of ^{18}F-FDG carries a poor prognosis.[18]

Neuroblastomas are tumors derived from neural crest cells of the sympatho-adrenal system. They are the most common solid extracranial tumor in children and are found most often in the abdomen. Early detection of metastatic neuroblastoma by sufficiently specific and sensitive scanning may reveal otherwise unsuspected and still resectable tumors, facilitating staging and prognosis (Fig. 10.7).[19] ^{18}F-FDG scanning has overall similar sensitivity but may be superior to metaiodobenzylguanidine scintigraphy for locating neuroblastoma in certain tissues or when a tumor becomes less differentiated or loses the noradrenergic transporter system.[20] ^{11}C-Hydroxyephedrine represents another PET imaging agent for localization of neuroblastoma. Overall, PET scanning should be reserved for situations in which there is high suspicion of neuroblastoma and when metaiodobenzylguanidine scintigraphy is negative (Fig. 10.8).

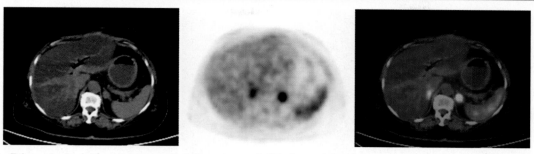

Figure 10.6: Bilateral pheochromocytoma: Axial sections of CT shows bilateral adrenal masses. ^{18}F-FDG positron emission tomography (PET/CT) images demonstrate intense FDG concentration in the masses in bilateral adrenal masses

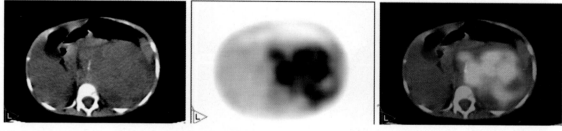

Figure 10.7: Left suprarenal neuroblastoma: Axial sections of CT shows left suprarenal mass with areas of calcification. ^{18}F-FDG positron emission tomography (PET/CT) demonstrating intense FDG concentration in the left suprarenal mass. In homogeneous pattern suggestive of areas of necrosis in a patient of neuroblastoma

BRAIN TUMORS

Brain tumors represent 1/5th of all childhood malignancies. Early detection and their treatment is essential to avoid mortality or any long-term morbidity. Many imaging techniques are there to evaluate brain tumors but we are here to discuss the usefulness of PET as functional imaging technique. PET as an important functional imaging technique is useful in measuring the regional blood flow of the CNS of visual, sensory, motor, auditory, memory, attention, and language areas.[21] And this very ability of PET to localize and identify the functional cortical areas in patients having brain tumors provide the neurosurgeon important information about how to approach the tumor so that it could be resected with no residue left and simultaneously saving the functional areas. Kaplan et al, studied 5 children patients, age ranging from 3 to 13 yrs, with hemispheric brain tumors.[21] Their objective was to plan neurosurgery preoperatively to make an approach to the tumor. So they used PET scanning for functional imaging and concluded that PET scans and co-registered MR images provided the exact location of tumor and functional cortical areas and this thing altered surgical management in terms of from where the tumor should be accessed so that the resection become complete leaving the cortical functional areas fully safe. In 1 of their case PET

revealed that right hemispheric expressive and receptive speech areas are there adjacent to the neoplastic lesion. Then the craniotomy was performed through lateral and inferior approach which allowed cortical entry outside the language and speech areas and gross total resection of the tumor. Pirotte et al, evaluated the role of PET for the early post-surgical evaluation of pediatric brain tumors. It is important and essential to assess the completeness of tumor resection at an early postoperative stage.[22] In their study 20 children were operated for the total resection of glial tumors. These all children postoperatively showed some signals on MR imaging for a possible tumor residue. Then they performed PET on all ^{18}F-FDG in 1, ^{11}C-methionine in 16, and both in rest 3. Increased tracer uptake was found in 14 children, which led to reoperation of 11 of them after confirming the tumor histologically. And no ^{11}C-methionine uptake led to conservative treatment in 6 of them which were also showing abnormality on MR imaging earlier. So PET saved the unnecessary surgical intervention in these children. So they concluded from their study that early postoperative PET with ^{11}C-methionine is valid for complementary therapeutic basis. Now also the metabolic activity of brain cells is good indicator of whether the cells have turned malignant or not. It is also useful indicator to comment on the therapy response. Rate of decrease in the metabolic activity of

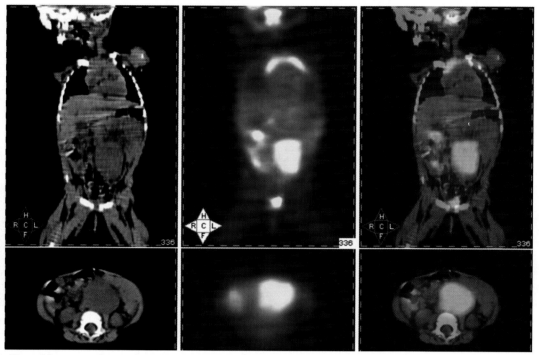

Figure 10.8: Neuroblastoma: Coronal and axial section CT shows left abdominal mass. Intense FDG uptake was seen in PET and PET-CT images in left abdominal mass

the tumor cells tells better about the initial response to the therapy used. PET is useful to evaluate metabolic activity of the tumor cells. One study is there on pediatric group regarding the *in vivo* metabolism of brain tumors before and after treatment which was conducted by Holthoff et al.[23] The author measured the metabolic activity of the brain tumor cells using the PET with FDG. The activity was different for different types of brain tumors; primary medulloblastoma (42.8 ± 14.0 micromol/100 g/min), PNET (17.3 ± 4.51 micromol/100 g/min), glioma lesions (21.8 ± 4.22 micromol/100 g/min). They found that more marked the decrease in tumor metabolism after chemotherapy, longer the period of initial clinical improvement lasted. So the PET is useful in pediatric brain tumors preoperatively as well as postoperatively for planning the surgery and for better management of the patients by predicting the prognosis.

REFERENCES

1. Kumar R, Nadig M, Chauhan A. Positron emission tomography: clinical application in oncology: part I. Expert Rev Anticancer Ther 2005;5:1079-94.
2. Kumar R, Chauhan A. Positron emission tomography: clinical applications in oncology. part 2. Expert Rev Anticancer Ther 2006;6:625-40.
3. Mochizuki T, Tsukamoto E, Kuge Y, et al. FDG uptake and glucose transporter subtype expressions in experimental tumor and inflammation models. J Nucl Med 2001;42:1551-5.
4. Miller E, Metser U, Avrahami G. Role of ^{18}F-FDG PET/CT in staging and follow-up of lymphoma in pediatric and young adult patients. J Comput Assist Tomogr 2006; 30(4):689-94.
5. Kumar R, Maillard I, Schuster SJ, Alavi A. Utility of fluorodeoxyglucose-PET imaging in the management of patients with Hodgkin's and non-Hodgkin's lymphomas. Radiol Clin North Am 2004;42:1083-100.
6. Meany HJ, Gidvani VK, Minniti CP. Utility of PET scans to predict disease relapse in pediatric patients with Hodgkin's lymphoma. Pediatr Blood Cancer 2006; [Epub ahead of print].
7. Wong KK, Lan LC, Lin SC. The use of positron emission tomography in detecting hepatoblastoma recurrence—a cautionary tale. J Pediatr Surg 2004;39:1779-81.
8. Philip I, Shun A, McCowage G, Howman-Giles R. Positron emission tomography in recurrent hepatoblastoma. Pediatr Surg Int 2005;21:341-5.
9. Figarola MS, McQuiston SA, Wilson F, Powell R. Recurrent hepatoblastoma with localization by PET-CT. Pediatr Radiol 2005;35:1254-8.
10. McCarville B. The role of positron emission tomography in pediatric musculoskeletal oncology. Skeletal Radiol 2006;35:553-4.

11. Hawkins DS, Rajendran JG. Conrad EU 3rd evaluation of chemotherapy response in pediatric bone sarcomas by ^{18}F-fluorodeoxy-D-glucose positron emission tomography. Cancer 2002;94:3277-84.

12. Kato H, Miyazaki T, Nakajima M, et al. Comparison between whole body positron emission tomography and bone scintigraphy in evaluating bony metastases of esophageal carcinomas. Anticancer Research 2005; 25:4439-44.

13. Ben Arush MW, Bar Shalom R, Postovsky S. Assessing the use of FDG-PET in the detection of regional and metastatic nodes in alveolar rhabdomyosarcoma of extremities. J Pediatr Hematol Oncol 2006;28:440-5.

14. Kumar R, Xiu Y, Yu JQ, et al. ^{18}F-FDG-PET in evaluation of adrenal lesions in patients with lung cancer. J Nucl Med 2004;45:2058-62.

15. Pacak K, Eisenhofer G, Carrasquillo JA. 6-[^{18}F]-fluoro-dopamine positron emission tomographic (PET) scanning for diagnostic localization of pheochromocytoma. Hypertension 2001;38:6-8.

16. Pacak K, Eisenhofer G, Goldstein DS. Functional imaging of endocrine tumors: role of positron emission tomography. Endocr Rev 2004;25:568-80.

17. Armstrong S, Worsley D, Blair GK. Pediatric surgical images: PET evaluation of papillary thyroid carcinoma recurrence. J Pediatr Surg 2002;37:1648-9.

18. Karel Pacak, Graeme Eisenhofer, David S Goldstein. Functional imaging of endocrine tumors: Role of positron emission tomography. Endocrine Reviews 2004;25:568-80.

19. Sisson JC, Shulkin BL. Nuclear medicine imaging of pheochromocytoma and neuroblastoma. Q J Nucl Med 1999;43:217-23.

20. Kushner BH, Yeung HW, Larson SM, et al. Extending positron emission tomography scan utility to high-risk neuroblastoma: fluorine-18-fluorodeoxyglucose positron emission tomography as sole imaging modality in follow-up of patients. J Clin Oncol 2001;19:3397-405.

21. Kaplan AM, Bandy DJ, Manwaring KH. Functional brain mapping using positron emission tomography scanning in preoperative neurosurgical planning for pediatric brain tumors. J Neurosurg. 1999;91:797-803.

22. Pirotte B, Levivier M, Morelli D. Positron emission tomography for the early postsurgical evaluation of pediatric brain tumors. Childs Nerv Syst 2005;21:294-300.

23. Holthoff VA, Herholz K, Berthold F. *In vivo* metabolism of childhood posterior fossa tumors and primitive neuro-ectodermal tumors before and after treatment. Cancer 199315;72:1394-403.

Section Two

The Clinical Basis of
Pediatric Surgical Oncology

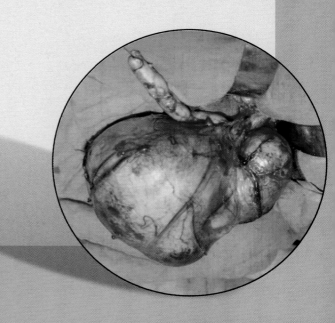

CHAPTER 11

Devendra K Gupta
Shilpa Sharma
Robert Carachi

Neonatal Tumors

Neonatal tumors are those tumors which occur within the first 28 days of neonatal life or to be more accurate are diagnosed at less than 44 weeks of gestational age.[1] They provide an opportunity to investigate tumors in which minimal environmental interference has occurred.

INCIDENCE

Neonatal tumors comprise 2 percent of childhood malignancies with a reported incidence of approximately 1:12,500-27,500 live births in UK and USA respectively.[2] The highest reported incidence is in Japan.[3] The male to female ratio is equal in the majority of cases[4] with the exception of teratoma (female preponderance, excluding teratoma of the pericardium and stomach).

EPIDEMIOLOGY

  i. **Congenital defects**: The association of congenital abnormalities and tumors has been reported to vary between 9.6 and 15 percent of neonatal tumors.[5] Most of these are related to chromosomal abnormalities, particularly trisomies 13,18 and 21. Leukemia and retroperitoneal teratomas have an increased incidence in patients with Down syndrome.[5] Trisomy 18 has a particular association with hepatoblastoma and nephro-blastoma. Teratomas may be associated with regional abnormalities like cloaca, limb hypoplasia and spina bifida as well as distal abnormalities suggesting a congenital association.[6]

  ii. **Genetic factors**: These comprise of three groups[1]

  a. Chromosomal abnormalities—resulting in an increased risk of malignancy, e.g. RB-1 gene in retinoblastoma, Li-Fraumeni syndrome—association of rhabdomyosarcoma, soft tissue tumors, breast and adrenocortical carcinomas, brain tumors and leukemia.

  b. Genetically determined syndromes—which confer an increased risk of malignancy. This includes Mendelian gene-related syndromes, the familial association of tumors and loss of heterozygosity of tumor suppressor genes.

  c. Genes conferring higher risk and increased susceptibility to environmental factors, but are of little importance to neonatal tumors, e.g. WAGR and Denys-Drash syndromes (Wilms' tumor), Beckwith-Wiedemann syndrome (Fig. 11.1), Down syndrome, MEN II (RET proto-oncogene), congenital adrenal hyperplasia and basal cell nevus.

  There is some evidence for the 2 hit theory with a small deletion of primary DNA sequence (first hit) and a gross deletion with loss of heterozygosity later on (second hit), but even multistep models exist.[1] There is hope that these tumors could be prevented by gene therapy.

  iii. **Environmental factors**: Their role is much less in the development of neonatal tumors compared to older age groups though events during pregnancy or prenatal parental exposure could theoretically be of significance.

  a. Ionizing radiation—There is a dose-related increase in tumor incidence at a younger age

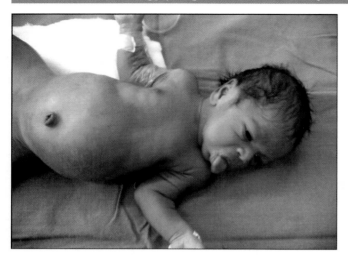

Figure 11.1: Neonate with Beckwith-Wiedemann syndrome needs to be screened for malignancy

following prenatal or neonatal radiation exposure[7] and internally deposited radionuclides administration.[8]

b. Drugs taken during pregnancy—The established link between diethylstilbestrol and adenocarcinoma of the vagina and cervix demonstrates that drugs taken during pregnancy may act as carcinogens.[9] Transplacental oncogenesis has been suspected in the context of fetal hydantoin syndrome and neuroblastoma[10] but is still open to debate.[11] Neonatal neoplasms mainly neural tumors and leukemias have occurred after treatment for infertility.[12,13] Solid tumors and leukemias have been identified in neonates whose mothers took medical treatment during gestation.[14] Links between sex hormones and neonatal vascular neoplasms and antibiotics and neonatal leukemia has been suggested.[14]

c. Environmental exposure—Neonatal neoplasms have occurred after exposure to hydrocarbons, dyes or heptachlor. An excess risk with parental occupational exposure to metals, oil, paints, coal and coal products has been reported.[15] Parental smoking may induce prezygotic genetic damage that predisposes to tumor formation.[16]

d. Infectious agents—Maternal infections like influenza, varicella, mumps and chickenpox during pregnancy have been associated with childhood leukemia but rarely in neonates.[17] Human immunodeficiency virus (HIV-1) infection has been associated with CNS lymphoma and Kaposi's sarcoma in newborns.[18,19] These reports suggest HIV causing viral oncogenesis *in utero*. Congenital infilterating lipomatosis of the face and callosal lipoma have been associated with congenital CMV infection.[20,21]

CLASSIFICATION

The Society of Paediatric Pathology in the United Kingdom identified teratoma (23.5%) and neuroblastoma (22.5%) as being the leading neonatal tumors with soft tissue sarcoma (8.1%), renal tumors (7.1%), CNS tumors (5.9%) and leukemia (5.9%) being the next common types.[22] Plaschkes[23] described at least four clinical groupings of neonatal tumors (Table 11.1).

NEONATAL NEUROBLASTOMA

Neonatal neuroblastomas are one of the most common tumors in the neonatal period, and represent 28-39 percent of all neuroblastomas.[24] Neuroblastoma is the most common extra-cranial solid tumor of children, with an overall incidence of 1:100,000. The tumor is derived from neural crest cells; 70 percent arise in the abdomen, 45 percent being of adrenal origin.

Neuroblastomas often present in children less than 2 years of age with an abdominal mass, fever and/or weight loss. Stage I involves localized tumor with clear margins, and no lymph nodes. Stage II involves localized tumor that is incompletely resected, +/– positive lymph nodes. Survival rates for stages I and II are 85 percent. In stage III, the tumor has crossed the midline and is unresectable. Stage IV involves distant metastases. Stage IV-S is a special category reserved for children less than one year of age, and is important in demonstrating the difference between neonatal neuroblastoma and infantile neuroblastoma. Stage IV-S describes a localized tumor, otherwise classified as stage I or II with the presence of metastases in infants < 1 year. Metastatic sites commonly include the liver, skin, bone and bone marrow.

With increasing antenatal imaging, neuroblastoma may be detected antenatally (Figs 11.2 and 11.3). Neonatal neuroblastomas behave differently than neuroblastomas of older children. The incidence of neonatal neuroblastomas has been documented to be as high as 1:200 by neonatal autopsy. These tumors often regress spontaneously, with survival rates up to 91 percent. Even in disseminated disease, considered to be stage IV-S, neonates have a survival rate greater than 80 percent. The neonatal neuroblastomas vary

Table 11.1: Types of neonatal tumors

Benign	Locally invasive	Malignant	Extremely rare
a. Life-threatening due to size and location—Cervical teratoma	Congenital fibrosarcoma, Fibromatosis	a. Behave as in older children	Carcinoma, Lymphoma, Hodgkin's disease, Kaposi's sarcoma
b. Tendency towards malignant transformation— Sacrococcygeal teratoma, giant nevus		b. Behave better than expected— Hepatoblastoma, neuroblastoma	
c. Neither a or b— Mesoblastic nephroma		c. Behave worse than expected— Congenital alveolar rhabdomyosarcoma, leukemia	
		d. Unpredictable behavior	

radiologically; many have a mixed echogenic pattern on ultrasound and are vascular. CT is used to further evaluate the mass, looking for a site of origin, relationship to other abdominal organs and metastases. Eighty percent of neuroblastomas have calcifications and 50 percent of neuroblastomas are calcified.

Neuroblastomas can cause hemorrhage, mimicking an adrenal hemorrhage. The treatment of neuroblastoma depends on the age of the child and the stage of the tumor. Surgery is indicated for stages I and II tumors while chemotherapy and radiation are the primary treatment modalities for advanced tumors. Neonatal neuroblastomas in the early stages can be followed with serial imaging to watch for spontaneous regression.

PERINATAL (FETAL AND NEONATAL) GERM CELL TUMORS

Germ cell tumors are relatively common in the fetus and neonate and are the leading neoplasms in some perinatal reviews.

The most common initial finding reported is a mass, noted either by antenatal sonography or by physical examination during the neonatal period, with signs and symptoms referable to the site of origin. Overall polyhydramnios is next followed by respiratory distress and stillbirth. The number of mature and immature teratomas is almost similar.

The incidence of teratoma with yolk sac tumor either at presentation or at recurrence is reported as 5.8 percent, and the survival rate as 39 percent.[25]

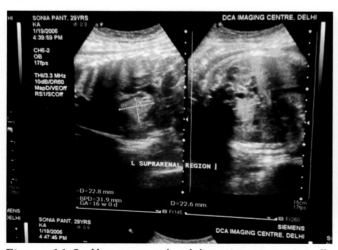

Figure 11.2: Utrasonography delineating an antenatally diagnosed neuroblastoma

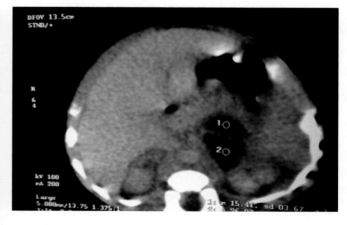

Figure 11.3: CT scan on day 2 of an antenatally diagnosed neuroblastoma showing a hypodense lesion that disappeared at 1 month of life

Sacrococcygeal teratomas have the highest incidence of yolk sac tumor at 10 percent.

Recurrent disease in the form of either teratoma or yolk sac tumor has been found to develop in 5 percent of patients.[25]

Treatment

Surgical resection alone may be adequate therapy for teratomas with nonmetastatic, microscopic foci of yolk sac tumor.

Prognosis

Some germ cell tumors of the fetus and neonate have a better prognosis than others. Neonates with gastric teratomas have the best survival rates, and those with intracranial germ cell tumors the worst. Fetuses with teratomas detected antenatally have 3 times the mortality rate compared with postnatally diagnosed neonates. Although perinatal teratomas have a relatively low recurrence rate of 5 percent, close follow-up with imaging studies and serum alpha-fetoprotein determinations is strongly recommended. In the nonteratoma group, patients with pure yolk sac tumor and gonadoblastoma have a much better outcome than those with choriocarcinoma, which has a very low survival rate of 12 percent. Currently, the use of platinum-based combination chemotherapy has significantly improved the survival rate of infants with advanced malignant germ cell tumor disease.

ORONASOPHARYNGEAL TERATOID TUMORS

Ninety percent of head and neck teratomas present during the neonatal and infantile period, predominantly involving the neck and nasopharynx and occurring only once in every 20,000-40,000 births.[26] Female predominance has been reported.

Ewing[27] classified oronasopharyngeal teratoid tumors into three types:

Type I: Dermoid tumors, the most common form, composed of ectoderm and mesoderm. These tumors are often pedunculated and are covered with skin and hair.

Type II: Teratoma, composed of tissues derived from all three germ layers. They have more marked structural differentiation and larger size. Skull deformities are often associated.

Type III: Epignathus. These are highly organized teratomas containing recognizable organs. *Epignathus* has also been called as "fetus in fetu" or "parasitic fetus" as it contains fetal organs. It is a misnomer meaning "upon the jaw "which has been used for almost *every* teratoma of the oral cavity, pharynx and for teratomas protruding from the mouth.

In Arnold's system of classification, another type known as Teratoid tumor is included describing poorly differentiated lesions that are composed of all three germ layers.

Oronasopharyngeal tumors typically arise from the wall of the nasopharynx above the level of soft palate, but may also arise from the soft or hard palate, uvula or the tonsillar area[28] (Fig 11.4).

The mass may prevent palatal fusion resulting in an associated cleft palate.[29] The tumor is often a pedunculated, rounded nodular whitish mass which is only a few centimeters in diameter. A giant epignathus has been described as one that fills the mouth and protudes from it.[30] Rarely, it may extend into the neck or cranium. Pure oral teratomas are rare with only 14 cases described till date, seven originating from the tongue and seven from the hard palate.[31]

Clinical Picture

Large teratomas and epignathi may result in stillbirth or death at delivery.[29] The usual presenting symptom is dyspnoea which may be present at birth or occur after a change in posture causing airway obstruction. The sudden onset and relief of obstruction related to changes in posture should suggest the diagnosis.[32] Excessive nasal

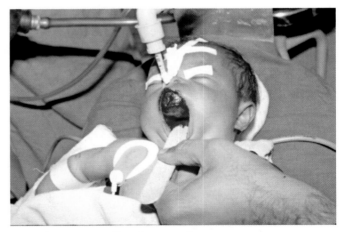

Figure 11.4: Oropharangeal teratoma in a neonate

mucus and feeding problems may also occur. Forward displacement or absence of soft palate or replacement of hard palate by the tumor has been described. Pure oral teratomas have less dramatic respiratory behavior as they tend to grow outside and newborn being obligate nasal breathers, oral obstruction usually causes less urgent feeding problems.[33] A small nasopharyngeal mass missed on routine visual examination can be diagnosed on palpation or by radiography.

Investigations

It is reported that more than 90 percent of oral teratomas are diagnosed during the perinatal period. Ultrasonography is useful in prenatal diagnosis,[34] particularly for oropharyngeal teratomas that interfere with fetal swallowing of amniotic fluid. Polyhydramnious is the most characteristic finding associated with large cervical and nasopharyngeal teratomas.

Ultrasonography establishes the presence of solid and cystic tissue components. Plain lateral skiagrams are useful in demonstrating virtually diagnostic calcifications. Non-calcified masses can also be delineated as filling defects in the nasopharyngeal air shadow. CT scan can be helpful in defining bony defects. Teratomas do not enhance with administration of contrast material due to their avascular character, and hence can cause diagnostic confusion with choristomas, endodermal sinus tumors and granular cell tumors.[35] Teratomas of the floor of the mouth may imitate thyroglossal duct cysts.[35] The diagnosis is sometimes possible only after histopathological examination.

Treatment

When a congenital oronasopharyngeal teratoma is suspected, the baby should be electively delivered by cesarean section. The airway must be secured by an airway, oral or nasal endotracheal intubation or, if necessary by tracheotomy. Early resection is advised, especially for airway obstructing teratomas. Removal of pedunculated tumors is relatively easy, a snare can be used for a narrow pedicle, but excision with diathermy is necessary to minimize blood loss. Giant tumors necessitate extensive dissection of the tumor from soft tissues, jaws, and base of skull. Failing to diagnose or treat head and neck teratoma until late adolescence or adulthood causes a risk of malignant degeneration up to 90 percent.[36] In malignant teratomas, radiotherapy and chemotherapy are recommended after complete extirpation.[35] AFP has been shown to be a reliable indicator of disease activity, thus serial measurements are advocated to detect recurrences.[26] Long-term follow-up has been advocated in all cases—benign or malignant.

CERVICAL TERATOMA

Cervical teratomas are rare tumors that result from abnormal prenatal development. They are usually detected at birth, but can occasionally remain silent until adulthood. They are usually large, partly cystic and partly solid and well encapsulated. They are true neoplasms, composed of tissues foreign to the site of origin, with derivatives of all three germ layers, often with a preponderance of central nervous tissue. Most of them are associated with the thyroid gland, either in direct continuity with it or replacing part of the gland.[37] A common origin from totipotential cells in the thyroid gland has been proposed.[37]

Clinical Picture

Maternal polyhydramnios is a common feature. Large tumors may cause dystocia. The tumor is a firm well-defined mass with multiple bosselations. It is mobile from side to side, is situated anteriorly or to one side of the neck and may extend from the mandible to the clavicle, with rare extension into the superior mediastinum or floor of the mouth.

Obstruction of the airway is the major challenge in the neonatal period. The differential diagnosis includes cystic hygroma (Fig. 11.5).

Investigations

Prenatal diagnosis by ultrasonography allows for early consultation with paediatric surgical specialists, so that

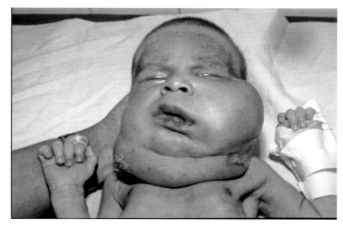

Figure 11.5: Huge cystic hygroma in a neonate

the time and place of delivery can be addressed, and planning for resuscitative efforts can be organized in advance.

Postnatal ultrasonography demonstrates the mixture of solid and cystic components and differentiates from cystic hygroma if doubt exists on clinical grounds. Skiagram helps to demonstrates presence of calcification and tracheal compression and deviation.

Rapidly growing embryonal tissue within these tumors could increase serum AFP levels.[38]

Treatment

If the airway is quickly stabilized and resection of the tumor is not delayed, the prognosis is good.[39] The excision is carried out through a cervical skin crease incision usually with division of the strap muscles. The tumor may be connected by flimsy pedicle to the thyroid gland, or may be more intimately connected to the thyroid, necessitating partial thyroidectomy.

Cervical teratomas in neonates are usually benign; however, malignant transformation and metastasis can occur as a rare event,[40] influencing long-term survival and prognosis. No developmental or neurological deficit has been detected on long-term follow-up at 5 years of age in benign cases.[39]

GASTRIC TERATOMA

Gastric teratoma is an extremely rare embryonic neoplasm containing tissue from all three germ layers (ectoderm, endoderm, and mesoderm) comprising less than 1 percent of all teratomas in children. Male predominance is well documented (9:1) in contrast to teratomas at other sites that are more common in girls.

Majority of the cases (90%) have occurred in neonatal and infancy.[41,42] Cases of congenital gastric teratomas have been described which were detected prenatally by ultrasound as abdominal calcifications when investigated for maternal polyhydramnios.[43,44] It has been hypothesized that gastric teratomas may actually originate in the gestational period and reflect a growth disturbance causing an early arrest in the normal process of differentiation and organogenesis. The tumor has been described as being essentially benign though few cases with presence of immature neuroepithelial elements have been reported.

Clinical Picture

The presenting clinical features include abdominal mass (75%), progressive abdominal distension (56%), tarry stools, failure to thrive, and anemia. Endogastric teratoma may present with vomiting, haemetemesis, or malena.[45,46] Rarely, difficulty during childbirth[46] and respiratory distress[47] has been reported.

Investigations

A plain skiagram of the abdomen may demonstrate irregular, coarse calcifications in the left upper quadrant. The calcification can be picked up on plain radiographs in approximately 60 percent of patients with teratomas.[41] The presence of teeth or bone is pathognomonic of teratomas but are less frequently seen in teratomas of gastrointestinal region and never in gastric teratoma. Ultrasonography and computerized tomography of the abdomen reveal the large heterogeneous tumor with calcified parts in the left hemiabdomen. The differential diagnosis of gastric teratomas include congenital neuroblastoma, infantile haemangioepithelioma, hepatoblastoma, Wilm's tumor, mesoblastic nephroma, mesenteric lymphangiomas and GI duplication cyst, all of which can show calcification and cysts.[48]

The tumor is generally found in relation to the greater curvature though occasional cases arising from lesser curvature have been reported.[41] The tumor may be predominantly exogastric, predominantly endogastric or multilobular, being exogastric and endogastric, including a portion of the wall of the stomach.[49] Exogastric growths (58-70%) are more common than endogastric tumors (30%). The tumor has variable attachment to the stomach wall, sometimes just attached to the serosa. Endogastric growths occur commonly on the posterior gastric wall along the greater curvature of the stomach.

Treatment

The treatment modalities described include simple total excision of tumor along with the adherent stomach wall with primary closure of the defect, enucleation of the mass, partial gastrectomy and total gastrectomy.[42,47] Complete excision has usually been accomplished. Misdiagnosis and complications like haemorrhage have been the usual causes of rare fatal cases.

Both the mature and immature types of GT have an excellent prognosis after complete excision of the tumor. Even when the immature type infiltrates surrounding structures, complete excision offers recurrence-free survival without requiring chemo- or radiotherapy.[50] However, an occasional case of peritoneal gliomatosis after surgical removal of gastric teratoma has been reported.[51] Malignancy in gastric teratoma is extremely rare.[52] Both the cases reported were treated by total excision of the tumor. A careful follow up of the patients by clinical evaluation, radiological imaging and tumor marker monitoring is recommended.

RETROPERITONEAL TERATOMA

Retroperitoneal teratoma presents as a large, partly solid and partly cystic mass which may originate in the abdomen or pelvis. The tumor contains derivatives of all three embryonic layers, mature tissues such as brain; bone and skin are commonly present. Most cases present at birth or in early infancy, with abdominal distension or palpable mass. Skiagram demonstrates a soft tissue mass, often with calcification or ossification. Ultrasonography is useful in demonstrating the solid and cystic components of the complex mass and associated urinary tract displacement and dilatation. The treatment is complete surgical excision as the possibility of later malignant change is always present. Chemotherapy is indicated in cases with histological evidence of malignancy.

SACROCOCCYGEAL TERATOMA

These tumors can occur at any age but are most common during the neonatal period. Rather, they rank as the most common neonatal tumor. The incidence is 1; 40,000 with female predominance. A high proportion of fetuses with this tumor die in utero or at birth. Prenatal diagnostic studies include ultrasound scan, magnetic resonance imaging (MRI), and echocardiography. The mean gestational age at presentation is reported as 23.9 weeks (range, 19 to 38.5).[53] Significant obstetric complications include polyhydramnios, oligohydramnios, preterm labor and preeclampsia. These complications along with fetal exsanguination due to massive haemorrhage into the tumor, tumor rupture, placentomegaly along with hydrops fetalis account for causes of fetal demise. Fetal interventions reported include cyst aspiration, amnioreduction, amnioinfusion and open fetal surgical resection. Indications for cyst aspiration and amnioreduction include maternal discomfort, preterm labor, and prevention of tumor rupture at delivery. Intraoperative events reported include maternal blood transfusion, fetal blood transfusion, chorioamniotic membrane separation and fetal arrest. For fetal SCT, the rapidity at which cardiac compromise can develop and the high incidence of obstetric complications warrant close prenatal surveillance. Amnioreduction, cyst aspiration, and surgical debulking are described as potentially life-saving interventions.

Clinical Picture

In 75 percent cases, the baby is born with a rounded, often bossed cystic or solid mass overlying the sacrum and coccyx usually large in size. The tumor is usually in the midline but may be paramedian. The overlying skin is normal with occasional port-wine staining and necrotic patches. If there is an intrapelvic extension the anus is pushed anteriorly and the mass is palpable on rectal examination. An abdominal mass may be felt in cases with intra-abdominal extension. Tumors that are predominantly presacral in location are rare in the neonatal period being diagnosed as a rule at a later age with bowel or urinary obstructive symptoms. Associated anomalies are present in 20 percent of the cases and include most commonly musculoskeletal anomalies followed by renal, CNS, cardiac and GIT anomalies.

Classification

Altmann et al (AAPSS, 1974)[54] classified SCT according to the anatomical site as;

Type I (47%): Predominantly external with minimal presacral component.

Type II (34%): Presenting externally with significant intrapelvic extension.

Type III: Apparent externally but are predominantly pelvic with abdominal extension.

Type IV: Presacral with no external presentation.

Investigations

Anteroposterior and lateral skiagrams of pelvis and sacrum may demonstrate calcification in either diffuse form or in the form of incompletely formed bones or toothbuds (Fig. 11.6). It is less frequent in malignant lesions in comparison to benign ones. Concave defects of the posterior aspects of the vertebral bodies and neural arch defects that are suggestive of intraspinal extension are unusually seen in the neonatal period. Soft tissue mass with displacement of bowel gas may be seen.

Ultrasonography determines the predominantly solid or cystic nature, pelvic or abdominal extension and evidence of obstructive uropathy. CTscan aids in determining the pelvic, abdominal, intraspinal extension and integrity of the sacrum. Serum alpha-fetoprotein

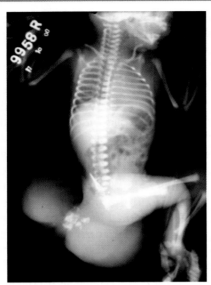

Figure 11.6: Skiagram lateral view delineating calcification in a case of sacrococcygeal teratoma

(AFP) is a useful serum marker as an indicator of malignancy and for monitoring malignant recurrence. The most important differential diagnoses include sacral meningocele and chordoma (Fig. 11.6).

Treatment

The treatment of choice is complete operative removal of the tumor en bloc with the coccyx as early as possible as most tumors are benign in the neonatal period with the incidence of malignant changes increasing with age. The incidence of malignancy has been reported as 3 percent at less than 1-month age and 38 percent over the age of 1 month.[55]

FETUS-IN-FETU

A fetus-in-fetu is an encapsulated, pedunculated vertebrate tumor. It is described as a condition in which a malformed monozygotic, monochorionic diamniotic parasitic twin lies within the body of its fellow (or autosite) twin. It was earlier hypothesised that FIF results from a modified process of twinning and with a natural progression from normal to conjoined symmetrical twins through parasitic fetus and fetal inclusion and finally to teratoma.[56]

Characteristically the fetus-in-fetu complex is composed of a fibrous membrane (equivalent to the chorioamniotic complex) that contains some fluid (equivalent to the amniotic fluid) and a fetus suspended by a *cord* or pedicle The enclosed parasite is distinguished

from a teratoma by its possession of a spinal column and of limbs and organs arranged appropriately to the spinal axis. The presence of a rudimentary spinal architecture is used to differentiate a fetus-in-fetu from a teratoma, since teratomas are not supposed to develop through the primitive streak stage (12-15 days). This last criterion has been considered too stringent by many authors who regard a rudimentary body architecture (metameric segmentation, craniocaudal and lateral differentiation, body coelom, "gestational sac"), or the presence of an associated fetus-in-fetu as equivalent criteria. Although teratomas can achieve striking degrees of differentiation by the inductive effect of adjacent tissues on one another, they do not present the criteria mentioned above.

Clinical Picture

The clinical presentation is that of an abdominal mass usually in the upper retroperitoneum.[57,58] They may be totally asymptomatic.[59] Symptoms, if present, are related to mass effect and include abdominal distension, feeding difficulties, emesis, jaundice and dyspnoea.[59] Rare locations like cranial cavity, pelvis, scrotal sac, sacrococcygeal region, mesentery and right iliac fossa are also reported.[60]

The fetus-in-fetu is usually single but rarely multiple fetuses have been reported.[61,62] Chromosome studies of the fetus show normal chromosomes identical to the host and the same blood group as their bearer.[60] Serum alpha feto protein (AFP) levels may be elevated or may be normal.

Investigations

FIF has characteristic imaging features. The few cases detected prenatally on ultrasonography presented as a complex mass. The general appearance is a well-delineated capsule, with an echogenic mass suspended in fluid or partially surrounded by fluid. Occasionally, the diagnosis can be suggested by the recognition of a rudimentary spine.

Plain abdominal radiographs may show a vertebral column and/or bony structures within a soft tissue mass.[58] CT features are diagnostic of this entity. A mass comprising of round or tubular collection of fat around a central bony structure are typical CT findings in FIF.[58] The identification of vertebrae or long bones within the lesion is essential for establishing the diagnosis. The exact extent of the mass and its relations with other abdominal structures are well elucidated on a contrast enhanced

CT scan. This information aids in surgery, which is the treatment of choice for this condition. FIF shows varying degrees of organ system differentiation and deformity. Symmetric arrangement of the vertebral axis is required for diagnosis. Frequently vascular anastomoses with the host vessels are identified.[59]

When discovered in a newborn child during physical examination, the differential diagnosis includes all the common masses such as Wilms' tumor, hydronephrosis, and neuroblastomas. Prenatally, the main differential diagnosis is with teratoma.

Teratomas have a definite malignant potential, a feature that has been rarely reported in fetus-in-fetu. Teratomas occur predominantly in the lower abdomen, not the upper retroperitoneum. Yet, the coexistence of a fetus-in-fetu and a teratoma as well as the occurrence of a teratoma 14 years after removal of a twin fetus-in-fetu have been reported, supporting the older hypothesis of a continuum between twin and teratoma. Cases of sacrococcygeal fetus-in-fetu should probably be regarded and treated as teratoma, because of the high incidence of teratoma in this region.

Ectopic testicles have a higher incidence of germ cell tumors, and the differentiation between fetus-in-fetu and teratoma is particularly important.

The treatment of choice is complete surgical excision. Fetus-in-fetu is a histologically proven benign entity but one case of malignant transformation and recurrence has been reported.[59]

CONGENITAL MESOBLASTIC NEPHROMA

It is the most common renal tumor in infants, with a mean age at diagnosis of 3.5 months. The tumor occurs more commonly in males and is usually unilateral. The typical presentation is a newborn with an abdominal mass, but the tumor can be detected prenatally. The tumor induction is postulated to occur at a time when the multipotent blastema is predominantly stromagenic.[63] No cytogenic or molecular markers have been found that are unique to CMN. Associated congenital anomalies were found in 14 percent of children with CMN that is comparable to the incidence in Wilm's tumor.[64] Imaging studies cannot reliably distinguish CMN from other renal mass lesions. Abdominal CT scan shows a heterogenous mass arising from the kidney.

CMN is a very firm tumor on gross examination, and the cut surface has a yellowish gray trabeculated appearance. The tumor tends to demonstrate local infiltration into the surrounding perirenal connective tissue lacking the pseudocapsule typically seen in Wilms' tumor. The neoplasm is histologically distinct from Wilms' tumor. The cell population is characterized by interlacing sheets of connective cells. An atypical or cellular variant has been reported. This lesion is characterized by a high mitotic index and dense cellularity, but these features are seen in 25 percent of CMN cases.[65]

Treatment

Complete excision is curative for most cases. The growth pattern is one of local invasion and extension through the capsule.[64] Local recurrence has been reported in several patients with a cellular variant. Adequacy of surgical resection and age at diagnosis are more important predictors of relapse than histology.[65] The risk of recurrence is less in cases younger than 3 months of age at diagnosis, but metastasis has been reported in few infants. Neither chemotherapy nor radiotherapy is routinely recommended,[64] but adjuvant treatment should be considered in cases with cellular variants that are incompletely resected.[66]

RHABDOMYOSARCOMA

Sarcoma botryoides is a highly malignant, embryonic mesenchymal tumor. It is multicentric in its viscus of origin. The authors have managed a rare case of neonatal rhabdomyosarcoma in the paraspinal location (Fig. 11.7). The common sites of origin are the bladder and prostate in the male and the vagina in females. The tumor consists of polypoid masses projecting into the lumen of the viscus. Histologically, fusiform or stellate cells, striated muscle fibres or multinucleated rhabdomyoblasts may be identified in a loose or myxomatous matrix. The neoplasm infiltrates the wall of the viscus to invade the pelvic cellular tissues but distant

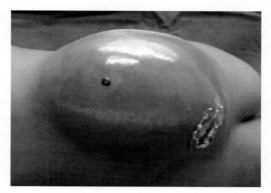

Figure 11.7: Rhabdomyosarcoma of the paraspinal region that presented at birth

metastases occur late. Rare cases of congenital rhabdomyosarcoma of the bladder have been described presenting with dysuria, palpable bladder, infection and haematuria. Neonatal sarcoma botryoides of the vagina have presented as solitary vaginal polyps and diagnosed on histopathological examination[67] thus warranting careful follow-up of such cases though benign polyps have regressed spontaneously.[68] Fourteen cases of neonatal rhabdomyosarcoma out of 1561 cases were registered in the IRS by Ragab.[69] Infants younger than one year had a higher rate of bladder-prostate-vagina primary tumor than older children (26% versus 10%). Excellent results have been obtained in vaginal tumors, which respond to chemotherapy.[70] The prognosis is worse in infants than in older children in primary bladder-prostate tumors.

OVARIAN TUMORS AND CYSTS

The widespread use of antenatal ultrasonography has led to an increase in the detection of large ovarian cysts in the neonatal period though true neoplasms of the ovary are rare Fig. 11.8.

The cyst may be follicular arising from a graafian follicle or, less commonly, luteal from a corpus luteum. It is usually unilateral and unilocular. The presenting feature is abdominal distention in most of the cases. The cyst is palpable as a mobile mass in the lower abdomen which may be displaceable upto the epigastrium. Complications include rupture leading to hemorrhage or torsion causing shock, intestinal obstruction or peritonitis. Resolution of the cysts has been studied by serial ultrasonography. Conservative

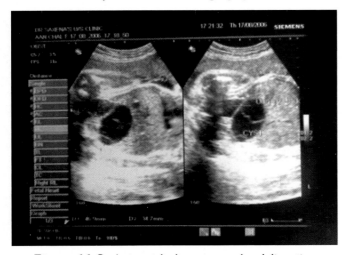

Figure 11.8: Antenatal ultrasonography delineating an ovarian cyst with multiple septae

management has been suggested for cysts less than 4 cm in size.[71] Surgical intervention is indicated in large cysts and in those showing evidence of complications. The treatment options include preferably cystectomy with preservation of the ovary that is difficult in neonates as the normal ovarian tissue may be splayed out over the cyst. The alternative approach is to aspirate the cyst and resect its wall.

TESTICULAR TUMORS

Congenital testicular tumors are extremely rare but few cases of benign Sertoli cell tumor, benign teratoma and endodermal sinus tumor (malignant yolk cell tumor) have been described.

AFP is produced by 90 percent of endodermal sinus tumor. Hematogenous spread to the lung is common but no cases of metastasis in neonates have been described.

Congenital testicular tumor usually present as a painless, firm testicular enlargement.

Treatment consists of orchidectomy through an inguinal incision with high ligation of the cord. Cases of malignant yolk cell tumor are followed up with serial serum AFP measurements. Routine retroperitoneal lymph node dissection is not required but may be needed in cases with high serum AFP levels and involved retroperitoneal lymph nodes on ultrasonography or CTscan followed by chemotherapy.[72]

NASAL GLIOMA

Nasal gliomas are uncommon lesions, with approximately 100 cases reported in the literature.[73] Nasal gliomas occur sporadically with no familial tendency or sex predilection.[74]

This tumor consists of astrocytic neuroglial tissue separated into islets by dense fibrous tissue trabeculae. There is no capsule and no covering of meninges. The overlying skin is usually normal but may be atrophic. About 60 percent cases are entirely extranasal, 30 percent intranasal and 10 percent are combined defects. A fibrous intracranial connection through a bony defect in the cribriform plate has been reported in 20 percent cases.[75] The tumor has been described as a choristoma, a tumor-like malformation composed of tissue not normally found in the affected part. It has been thought to be a sequestrated encephalocele separated from the frontal lobes by closure of the cranial sutures, completely or partially. About 90 percent of the reported nasal gliomas do not contain neurones, explained by either insufficient supply of oxygen to support the neurons or failure of the neurons to differentiate from the embryonic neuroectoderm in an intranasal glioma or both.[76]

Clinical Picture

Extranasal glioma present at birth as a firm subcutaneous lump with red or bluish discoloration, lying on one side of the nasal bridge. Hypertelorism or widening of the nasal bridge may be seen. Obstruction of the nasal passage and nasolacrimal duct can lead to respiratory distress and epiphora on the affected side. Complications like CSF rhinorrhea, meningitis or epistaxis can also develop in these patients.[76] The tumor is firmly attached to the overlying skin. It is nonpulsatile and does not increase in size on crying. The average lesion is 2-3 cm. in size. Intranasal lesions present at or shortly after birth as a polyp-like mass causing unilateral nasal obstruction.

Investigations

Skiagram skull and CT scan are useful to evaluate intranasal lesions. On MRI, nasal gliomas are usually hyperintense on T2WI. They may appear hypo-, iso- or hyper-intense to the grey matter on T1WI. Adjacent CSF space may be shown by MRI in encephaloceles.[77] Encephaloceles usually retain connection with the brain parenchyma whereas nasal gliomas do not. Using MRI, nasal dermoids (which appear strikingly hyperintense on T1WI due to fat content) and epidermoids (which appear marginally hyperintense to the CSF on both T1 and T2WI) can easily be differentiated from nasal gliomas. Other less common causes of intranasal mass lesions in an infant include inclusion cysts. haemangiomas and aberrant ethmoid sinuses.[77] Unlike inflammatory polyps, nasal gliomas typically lie medial to the middle turbinate, occur in infancy, are less translucent and firm in consistency. Inflammatory polyps usually lie inferolateral to the middle turbinate

Treatment

Simple excision with skin flaps can be done safely for extranasal gliomas but removal of intranasal and combined lesions requires greater expertise. Nasal gliomas are benign lesions with recurrence reported only following incomplete excision.[75]

FETAL AND NEONATAL CARDIAC TUMORS

Primary tumors of the heart are uncommon in the fetus and neonate. Nevertheless, the widespread use of new imaging techniques has contributed significantly to earlier diagnosis, treatment, and thus improved survival. Most tumors have been reported to be benign, rhabdomyoma being the most common, followed by teratoma, fibroma, oncocytic cardiomyopathy, vascular tumors, and myxoma.[78] Malignant and metastatic tumors are described but are rare. Herniation of liver (left lobe usually) through the defect in the central tendon of diaphragm may mimic as the tumor arising from the heart or the pericardium.

Murmurs, arrhythmias, cyanosis, respiratory distress, and cardiac failure are the main presenting signs of cardiac tumors in the perinatal period. Disturbances in hemodynamic function are correlated with the size and location of the tumor. Cardiac vascular tumors have the best outcome, whereas malignant tumors have the worst.

NEONATAL LIVER TUMORS

Primary liver tumors are very rare during the neonatal period, but increasing numbers of them are now diagnosed prenatally by routine ultrasound scan.[79] A precise diagnosis is sometimes problematic because of nonspecific clinical symptoms, misleading imaging and difficulties with histological interpretation.

Benign infantile haemangioendothelioma usually undergoes spontaneous regression, but may be life-threatening due to congestive heart failure and/or consumptive coagulopathy when treatment with resection, embolization or arterial ligation is necessary. Mesenchymal hamartoma is a benign cystic lesion that should be resected whenever possible. Malignant hepatoblastoma may occur in the newborn, and often has to be treated with chemotherapy to achieve resectability. Symptoms are less specific and the prognosis is worse than in older children.

Rarely, germ cell tumors occur in the neonatal liver. Benign teratomas have to be resected, while malignant choriocarcinomas may respond to chemotherapy and can be cured in some cases.

HEPATIC HEMANIOMA

Hepatic vascular hamartomas usually occur as multiple hemangioendotheliomas (MHE) but may occur as localized single cavernous hemangiomas. The condition is potentially lethal in the neonates due to the serious complications associated with it.

Clinical Picture

The presenting feature in neonates is usually hepatomegaly or less commonly localized upper abdominal mass. Complicated cases with rupture may present with shock or hemoperitoneum. Multiple cutaneous hemangiomas are present in 25 percent cases of hepatic hemangioendothelioma and are a valuable clue to the diagnosis.[80]

Hepatic hemangiomas may cause death by necrosis with rupture and fatal hemorrhage, platelet trapping and thrombocytopenia, or high output cardiac failure due to large AV shunt. Regression before the age of 1 year has been reported.[81]

Investigations

Skiagram abdomen may show hepatomegaly. Ultrasonography is useful in locating the lesion. Technetium-99m scanning will show areas of decreased activity that will appear as fluid filled on ultrasonography.[82] Selective angiography is the most valuable investigation. It shows the vascular character of the lesion, its early venous drainage and tortuosity of the vessels and gives an indication of whether the lesion is resectable. However, being invasive, it should be reserved for cases in which surgery or hepatic embolization is planned. CECT has also been found as specific as selective angiography.[83]

MHE appear grossly as multiple circumscribed lesions and may involve whole of the liver. On microscopic examination, the nodules are composed of cellular capillary hemangiomas.

Treatment

Close observation is advised in asymptomatic cases for evidence of increasing hepatic enlargement, cardiac failure, respiratory distress, thrombocytopenia and anemia. Medical treatment in form of digitalis, diuretics and steroids is the first line of treatment in such cases. Failure of response necessitates intervention in form of hepatic resection in localized tumors or hepatic arterial ligation or embolization.

Although hepatic hemangioma remains a potentially lethal condition, the recent literature shows an improved survival rate from 12 percent in past[84] to 78 percent.[85] The improvement has been contributed by both conservative and aggressive management.[81,85]

MESENCHYMAL HAMARTOMA OF LIVER

It is a benign cystic tumor-like malformation that usually presents in the first year of life and has been described in the fetus and neonate.[86] It is postulated that these tumors arise in areas of focal intrahepatic biliary atresia.[87] Another hypothesis is that these lesions arise in conjunction with vascular anomalies, which explains the occurrence of small hemangiomas in close proximity.[88]

Clinical Picture

Mesenchymal hamartoma make up 6 percent of primary liver tumors in children. There is a male predominance. Two-thirds of these tumors occur in infants and the mean age at diagnosis is 16 months.[89] The typical features include an asymptomatic palpable mass or rapid abdominal enlargement. The tumor may present as a predominantly cystic structure which may enlarge rapidly due to fluid accumulation[88] or one that is vascular and presents with CHF.[90] The large size may produce respiratory distress or vena caval obstruction.

Investigations

Serum AFP is usually normal but may be mildly raised. Predominance of cysts on ultrasonography indicates the benign nature of the lesion. CT scan and MRI are other diagnostic modalities. The tumor that is usually solitary may be pedunculated or deeply embedded in the liver substance. An open biopsy is frequently required to confirm the diagnosis. The multiple cysts are filled with clear or mucoid fluid. The histopathological examination shows loose myxoid tissue containing branching bile ducts, hepatocytes and angiomatous elements.

Treatment

The treatment of choice is surgical resection that may include lobectomy or enucleation of the mass that is facilitated by its capsule. Marsupialization of a large hamartoma may be done if enucleation is not feasible. The overall prognosis is good and most patients do well with all forms of therapy.[89]

MALIGNANT TUMORS OF THE LIVER

Congenital and neonatal cases that have been rarely reported include mostly hepatoblastoma and few cases of hepatocarcinoma.[91,92]

The usual presentation in the neonatal period is an abdominal mass. Skiagram abdomen shows hepatomegaly and displacement of colonic or stomach gas in right or left lobe lesions respectively but calcification is rarely seen. Ultrasonography is useful in locating the lesion as an intrahepatic solid mass and differentiating it from hydronephrosis, choledochal cyst or mesenchymal hamartoma. Technetium-99m scanning will delineate the exact site and size of the lesion. CT scan identifies multifocal tumor formation within the liver parenchyma.[93]

Angiography, preferably via an umbilical artery is essential if resection is being considered, but should be done only if the possibility of resection has not been excluded by other modalities. Liver Function Tests are usually normal. Serum AFP is raised in about 90 percent of liver carcinoma cases and serves as a useful tumor marker.

The only curative treatment is surgical resection by lobectomy, hemihepatectomy or extended right hepatectomy. In the neonatal period, radiotherapy is inappropriate and chemotherapy should be considered only in unresectable cases due to the severe side effects. Thus, the primary treatment of choice remains surgical.

NEONATAL CRANIOPHARYNGIOMA

Craniopharyngioma is a rare neonatal tumor, although it is the most common tumor of the parasellar region in childhood. Only a few cases have been diagnosed antenatally. Ultrasonography may reveal a high echoic mass at the center of the head in the fetus.[94] Hypotonicity of the lower limbs has been observed. The tumor may be excised by an interhemispheric trans-lamina-terminalis approach.

CONGENITAL ALVEOLAR RHABDOMYOSARCOMA

Congenital alveolar rhabdomyosarcoma is a highly malignant tumor with no record of long-term survivors. Malignancy in the neonatal period is uncommon and the clinical management presents considerable challenges. A rare case of solid alveolar type of rhabdomyosarcoma presenting as a solitary skin lesion on the right upper lip of a 2-week-old infant boy has been reported.[95] Treatment options include chemotherapy, excision, and radiotherapy.

CONGENITAL SALIVARY GLAND ANLAGE TUMOR OF THE NASOPHARYNX

A rare case of congenital salivary gland anlage tumor of the nasopharynx presenting with complaints of nasal obstruction and feeding difficulties in the neonate has been described.[96] Cannulation of the nasal cavity to rule out choanal atresia resulted in a burst of bleeding from the nose and mouth. A finger sweep of the oropharynx dislodged the mass lesion.

CONGENITAL FIBROSARCOMA OF THE JEJUNUM

Rupture of a malignant tumor is an extremely rare cause of peritonitis in the fetus and neonate. An unusual case of perforation of a congenital fibrosarcoma of the jejunum in utero and secondary meconium peritonitis has been reported.[97] Prenatal ultrasound showed polyhydramnios and fetal ascites from 25 gestational weeks in the absence of other fetal congenital anomalies. The baby presented with severe generalized edema and respiratory distress immediately after birth. The treatment consisted of resection and anastomosis of the involved segment of the bowel.

REFERENCES

1. SW Moore, D Satge, AJ Sasco, A Zimmermann, J Plaschkes. The epidemiology of neonatal tumors. Pediatr. Surg Int 2003;19:509-19.
2. Bader JL, Miller RW. US Cancer incidence and mortality in the 1st year of life. Am J Dis Child 1979;133:157-9.
3. Birch JM, Marsden HB, Swindell R. Pre-natal factors in the origin of germ cell tumors of childhood. Carcinogenesis 1982;3:75-80.
4. Gurney JG, Severson RK, Davis S, Robison LL. Incidence of cancer in children in the United States; sex-race-and 1-year age specific rates by histological type. Cancer 1995;75:2186-95.
5. Altmann AE, Halliday JL, Giles GG. Associations between congenital malformations and childhood cancer: a register-based case-control study. Br J Cancer 1998;78:1244-9.
6. Rao S, Azmy A, Carachi R. Neonatal tumors: a single centre experience. Pediatr. Surg Int 2002;18:306-9.
7. Doll R, Wakeford R. Risks of childhood cancer from fetal irradiation. Br J Radiol 1997;70:130-9.
8. Sikov MR. Tumor development following internal exposures radionuclides during the perinatal period. IARC Sci Publ 1989;96:403-19.
9. Potter EL. A historical view: diethylstilbesterol use during pregnancy: a 30-year historical perspective. Pediatr Pathol.1991;11:781-9.
10. Sherman S, Roizen N. Fetal hydantoin syndrome and neuroblastoma. Lancet 1976;1:517.
11. Little J. Epidemology of childhood cancer. IARC scientific publication No.149 International Agency for Research on Cancer. Lyon, France, 1999;206-41.
12. Bruisma F, Venn A, Lancaster P, Speirs A, Healy D. Incidence of cancer in children born after in vitro fertilization. Hum Reprod.2000;15:604-7.
13. Rizk T, Nabbout R, Koussa S, Akatcherian C. Congenital brain tumor in a neonate conceived by in vitro fertilization. Childs Nerv Syst 2000;16:502.
14. Satge D, Sasco AJ, Little J. Antenatal therapeutic drug exposure and fetal/neonatal tumors: review of 89 cases. Paediat Perinat Epidemiol 1998;12:84-117.
15. Chadduck WM, Gollin SM, Gray BA, Norris JS, Araoz CA, TRyka Af. Gliosarcoma with chromosomal abnormalities in a neonate exposed to heptachlor. Neurosurgery 1987;21:557-9.
16. Boffetta P, Tredaniel J, Greco A. Risk of childhood cancer and adult lung cancer after childhood exposure to passive smoke; a meta-analysis. Environ Health Perspect 2000;108:73-82.

17. Naumburg E, Bellocco R, Cnattingius S, Jonzon A, Ekbom A. Pernatal exposure to infection and risk of childhood leukemia. Med Pediatr Oncol 2002;38:391-7.

18. Capelli A, Familiari U, Fundaro C, Segni G, Carbone A, Larocca LM. CNS lymphoma in a newborn infant with HIV-1 infection. Path Res Pract 1989;185:A29.

19. Gutierrez-Ortega P, Hierro-Orozo S, Sanchez-Cisneros R, Montano LF. Kaposi's sarcoma in a 6-day-old infant with human immunodeficiency virus. Arch Dermatol 1989;125:432-3.

20. Aydingoz U, Emir S, Karli-Oguz K, Kose G, Buyukpamukcu M. Congenital infilterating lipomatosis of the face with ipsilateral hemimegalencephaly. Pediatr radiol 2002;32:106-9.

21. Mehta NM, Hartnoll G. Congenital CMV with callosal lipoma and agenesis. Pediatr Neurol 2001;24:222-4.

22. Barson AJ. Congenital neoplasia; The Society's experience. Arch Dis Child 1978;53:436.

23. Plauschkes J. Epidemiology of neonatal tumors. In P Puri (Ed.): Neonatal tumors. Spinger– Verleg, Heidelberg Berlin New York, 1996;11-22.

24. Becker JM. Schneider KM. Krasna IH. Neonatal Neuroblastoma. Progress in Clinical Cancer 1970;4:382-6.

25. Isaacs H Jr. Perinatal (fetal and neonatal) germ cell tumors. J Pediatr Surg. 2004;39:1003-13.

26. Azizkhan RG, Haase GM, Applebaum H, Dillon PW, Coran AG, King DR, Hodge DS. Diagnosis, management and outcome of cervicofacial teratomas in neonates: a Children's Cancer Group study.. J Pediatr Surg. 1995;30:312-6.

27. Ewing J. Neoplastic diseases. 4th edn. W. B. Saunders, Philadelphia 1940.

28. Valente A, Grant C, Orr JD, Brereton RJ. J Pediatr Surg 1988;33:364-6.

29. Rintala A, Ranta R. Separate epignathi of the mandible and the nasopharynx with cleft palate: case report. Br. J. Plast. Surg 1974;27:103-6.

30. Hatzihaberis F, Stamatis D, Staurinos D. Giant epignathus. J Pediatr Surg 1978;13:517-8.

31. Cay A, Bektas D, Imamoglu M, Bahadir O, Cobanoglu U. Sarihan H. Oral teratoma: a case report and literature review. Pediatr Surg Int 2004;20:304-8.

32. Jones PG, Campbell PE. Tumors of infancy and childhood. Blackwell Scientific Publications, Oxford 1976;348-50.

33. Uchida K, Urata H, Suzuki H. Teratoma of the tongue in neonates: report of a case and review of literature. Pediatr Surg Int 1998;14:79-81.

34. Raveh E, Papsin BC, Farine D, Kelly EN, Forte V. The outcome after perinatal management of infants with potential airway obstruction. Int J Pediatr Otorhino-laryngol 1998;46:207-14.

35. Lack EE. Extragonadal germ cell tumors of the head and neck region: review of 16 cases. Hum Pathol 1985;16:56-64.

36. Buckley NJ, Burch WM, Leight GS. Malignant teratoma in the thyroid gland of an adult: case report and a review of the literature.Surgery 1986;100:932-7.

37. Roediger WE, Spitz L, Schmaman A. Histogenesis of benign cervical teratomas. Teratology 1974;10:111-8.

38. Jordan RB, Gauderer MWL. Cervical teratomas: an analysis. Literature review and proposed classification. J Pediatr Surg. 1988;23:583-91.

39. Kerner B, Flaum E, Mathews H, Carlson DE, Pepkowitz SH, Hixon H, Graham JM Jr. Cervical teratoma: prenatal diagnosis and long-term follow-up. Prenat Diagn 1998;18:51-9.

40. Touran T, Applebaum H, Frost DB, Richardson R, Taber P, Rowland J. Congenital metastatic cervical teratoma: diagnostic and management considerations. J Pediatr Surg 1989; 24:21-3.

41. Basak D, Das A, Chatterjee SK, Mukherjee P. Gastric teratoma in children. Ind Pediatr 1992;29:231-4.

42. Purvis JM, Miller RC, Bernard. Gastric teratoma-First reported case in a female. J Pediatr Surg 1979;14:86-8.

43. Falik-Borenstein TC, Korenberg JR, Davos I, Platt LD, Gans S, Goodman B, Schreck R, Graham JM Jr. Congenital gastric teratoma in Wiedmann-Beckwith syndrome. Am J Med genet 1991;3:52-7.

44. Henderson P, Lake Y. An unusual case of polyhydramnios: Congenital Gastric teratoma. NZ Med J.1994;107:133-4.

45. Gangopadhyay AN, Pandit SK, Gopal SC. Gastric teratoma revealed by gastrointestinal haemorrhage. Ind Pediatr 1992;29:1145-7.

46. Matias IC, Huang YC. Gastric teratoma in infancy: Report of a case and review of world literature. Ann Surg 1973;170:631-6.

47. Senokak ME, Kale G, Buyukpakcu N, Hicsonmez A, Ceglar M.Gastric teratoma in children including the third reported female case. J Pediatr Surg 1990;25:681-4.

48. Niedzwicki G, Wood BP. Radiological case of the month-Gastric teratoma. Am J Dis Child 1990;114:1147-8.

49. Munoz NA, Takehara H, Komi N, Hizawa K. Immature gastric teratoma in an infant. Acta Paediatr Jpn 1992;34:483-8.

50. Gupta DK, Srinivas M, Dave S, Agarwala S, Bajpai M, Mitra DK. Gastric teratoma in children. : Pediatr Surg Int 2000;16:329-32.

51. Couson WF. Peritoneal gliomatosis from a gastric teratoma. Am J Clin Pathol 1990;94(1):87-89.

52. Balk E, Tuncyurek M, Sayan A, Avanoglu A, Ulman I, Cetinkursun S. Malignant gastric teratoma in an infant. Z Kinderchir 1990;45(6):383-5.

53. Hedrick HL, Flake AW, Crombleholme TM, Howell LJ, Johnson MP, Wilson RD, Adzick NS. Sacrococcygeal teratoma: prenatal assessment, fetal intervention, and outcome. J Pediatr Surg. 2004 Mar; 39(3):430-8; discussion 430-8.

54. Altman RP, Randolph JG, Lilly JR. Sacrococcygeal teratoma: American Academy of Pediatrics Surgical Section Survey-1973. J Pediat. Surg 1974;9:389-98.

55. Billmire DF, Grosfeld JL. Teratomas in childhood: analysis of 142 cases. J Pediat. Surg.1986;21:548-51.

56. Gross RE, Clatworthy HW. Twin foetus in fetu. J Pediatr 1951;38:502-8.

57. Galatius-Jensen F, Rah DH, Uhm IK. Foetus in fetu. Br J Radiology 1965;38:305.

58. Lord JM. Intra-abdominal foetus in foetu. J Pathol Bacteriol 1956;72:627-41.

59. Hopkin KL, Dickson PK, Ball TI, Ricketts RR, O'Shea PA, Abramovosky CR. Fetus in fetu with malignant recurrence. J Pediatr Surg 1997;32:1476-9.

60. Eng HL, Chuang JH, Lee TY, Chen WJ. Fetus in fetu: a case report and review of the literature. J Pediatr Surg 1989;24:296-9.

61. Gross RE, Clatworthy HW. Twin fetuses in fetu. J. Pediat.1951;38:502-8.

62. Lee EYC. Foetus in foetu. Arch. Dis. Child.1965;40:689-93.

63. Tournade MF, Com-Nougue C, Voute PA, et al. Results of the sixth International Society of Paediatric Oncology Wilms' Tumor Trial and Study: a risk adapted therapeutic approach in Wilms' tumor. J Clin Oncol.1993;11:1014.

64. Howell CJ, Othersen HB, Kiviat NE, et al. Therapy and outcome in 51 children with mesoblastic nephroma: a report of the National Wilms' Tumor Study. J Pediatr Surg. 1982;17:826.

65. Beckwith JB. Congenital Mesoblastic Nephroma. When should we worry? Arch Pathol Lab Med. 1986;110:98.

66. Gormley TS, Skoog SJ, Jones RV, et al. Cellular congenital mesoblastic nephroma: what are the options? J Urol. 1989;142:479.

67. Ober WB, Smith JA, Rouillard FC. Congenital sarcoma botryoides of the vagina; report of two cases.Cancer. 1958;11:620-3.

68. Norris HJ, Taylor HB. Polyps of the vagina.Cancer 1966;19:227-32.

69. Rhagab AH, Heyn R, Tefft M, Hays DN, Newton WA, Beltangady M.Infants younger than 1 year of age with rhabdomyosarcoma. Cancer 1986;58:2606-10.

70. Hays DN, Shimada H, Raney RB, Tefft M, Newton WA, Crist WM, et al. Sarcoma of the vagina and uterus: The Intergroup Rhabdomyosarcoma Study. J Pediatr Surg. 1985;20:718-24.

71. Ikeda K, Suita S, Nakano H. Management of ovarian cyst detected antenatally. J Pediatr Surg. 1988;23:432-5.

72. Flamant F, Nihoul-Fekete C, Patte C, Lemerle J. Optimal treatment of stage I yolk sac tumor of the testis in children. J Pediatr Surg. 1968;21:108-11.

73. Naldich TP, Zimmerman RA, Bauer BS. Midface: Embryology and congenital lesions. In: Som PM, Curtin HD, (Eds): Head and Neck Imaging, Vol. 1, St. Louise Mosby; 1996;1-45.

74. Gorenstein A, Kern EB, Facer GW, Lows ER Jr. Nasal gliomas. Arch Otolaryngol 1980;106:536-40.

75. Karma P, Rasanen O and Karja J. Nasal gliomas. A review and report of two cases. Laryngoscope 1977;73:93-107.

76. Harley EH. Pediatric congenital nasal masses. Ear Nose Throat J 1991; 70:28-32.

77. Barkowich AJ, Vandermarck P, Edwards MSB. Congenital nasal masses: CT and MR imaging features in 16 cases. Am J Neuroradiol 1991;12:105-116.

78. Isaacs H Jr. Fetal and Neonatal Cardiac Tumors. Pediatr Cardiol. 2004 Apr 19 [Epub ahead of print]

79. Von Schweinitz D. Neonatal liver tumors. Semin Neonatol. 2003 Oct;8(5):403-10.

80. Dachman AH, Lichtenstein JE, Friedman AC, Hartman DS. Infantile haemangioendothelioma of the liver. Am J Roent 1983;140:1091-6.

81. Nguyen B, Shandling B, Elin S, Stephens C. Hepatic haemangioma in childhood: medical management or surgical management. J Pediat Surg 1982;17:576-9.

82. Larcher VF, Howard ER, Mowat AP. Hepatic haemangiomata: diagnosis and management. Arch Dis Child.1981;56:14.

83. Holcomb GW III, O'NeillJA, Mahboubi S, Bishop HC. Experience with hepatic haemangioendothelioma in infancy and childhood. J Pediat Surg 1988;23:661-6.

84. Delorimer AA, Simpson EB, Baum RS, Carlson E. Hepatic artery ligation for hepatic haemangiomatosis. New Engl T Med 1967;227:333-6.

85. Burrows PE, Rosenberg HC, Chuang HS. Diffuse hepatic haemangiomas: percutaneous transcatheter embolization with detachable silicone balloons. Radiology 1985;156:85-8.

86. Foucar E, Williamson RA, Yiu-Chiu V. Mesenchymal hamartoma of the liver identified by fetal sonography. Am J Roent 1982;140:970-2.

87. Dehner LP, Ewing SI, Sumner HW. Infantile mesenchymal hamartoma of the liver. Histologic and ultrastructural observations. Arch Pathol 1975;99:379-82.

88. Srouji MN, Chatten J, Schulman WM, et al. Mesenchymal hamartoma of the liver in infants. Cancer 1978; 42:2483-9.

89. Demarioribus CA, Lally KP, Sim K, et al. Mesenchymal hamartoma of the liver; A 35-year review. Arch Surg 1990;125:598-600.

90. Smith WL, Ballantine TVN, Gonzalez- Crussi F. Hepatic mesenchymal hamartoma causing heart failure in the neonate. J Pediat Surg 1978;13:183.

91. Gauthier F, Valayer J, Le Thai B, Sinico M, Kalifa C. Hepatoblastoma and hepatocarcinoma in children: analysis of a series of 29 cases. J Pediat Surg. 1986; 21:424-9.

92. Fraumeni JF, Miller RW, Hill JA. Primary carcinoma of the liver in children: an epidemiological study. J. Nat Cancer Inst.1968;40:1087-99.

93. Snow JH, Goldstein HM, Wallace S. Comparison of scintigraphy, sonography and computed tomography in the evaluation of hepatic neoplasms. Am J Roent. 1979;132:915-8

94. Arai T, Ohno K, Takada Y, Aoyagi M, Hirakawa K. Neonatal craniopharyngioma and inference of tumor inception time: case report and review of the literature.Surg Neurol. 2003;60:254-9; discussion 259.

95. Brecher AR, Reyes-Mugica M, Kamino H, Chang MW, Ronald O Perelman. Congenital primary cutaneous rhabdomyosarcoma in a neonate. Pediatr Dermatol. 2003;20:335-8.

96. Shima Y, Ikegami E, Takechi N, Migita M, Hayashi Z, Araki T, Tanaka Y, Sugiyama M, Hashizume K. Congenital fibrosarcoma of the jejunum in a premature infant with meconium peritonitis. Eur J Pediatr Surg. 2003;13:134-6.

97. Cohen EG, Yoder M, Thomas RM, Salerno D, Isaacson G. Congenital salivary gland anlage tumor of the nasopharynx. Pediatrics 2003;112:66-9.

CHAPTER 12

Winfried Rebhandl
Franz Xaver Felberbauer
Ernst Horcher

Pediatric Renal Tumors

WILMS' TUMOR

HISTORY

It was in 1899 when Max Wilms, a German surgeon and pathologist, described a group of children with kidney tumors and since that time his name has been applied to pediatric nephroblastoma.[1] Although adjuvant radiation treatment had been introduced in 1916, in 1938 the overall survival rate was still only 8 to 20 percent.[2] Addition of radiotherapy and improvement of surgical techniques resulted in a survival of 22 percent by 1954. In 1956, actinomycin and in 1963 vincristine were added as chemotherapeutic agents.

The dramatic improvement in overall cure we experience lately resulted from the coordinated use of modern surgical technique and anesthesia, multiple drug chemotherapy, and radiation therapy. Today, standardized treatment of patients in accordance with the guidelines of large cooperative cancer groups, especially the National Wilms' Tumor Study (NWTS), and the Société Internationale d'Oncologie Pédiatrique (SIOP) achieves a 5-year survival rate of more than 90 percent.

In the early 1960s, a genetic basis of Wilms' tumor was suggested for the first time. From retrospective analysis of the first (NWTS-1) in the mid-1970s, anaplasia was initially recognized as an adverse prognostic feature.

EPIDEMIOLOGY, INCIDENCE, AND AGE AT ONSET

Wilms' tumor is the most common abdominal malignancy observed in children and affects approximately 1 in 10, 000 children before the age of 15 worldwide.[3] Wilms' tumor is only exceptionally congenital but primarily seen in infants, with 50 percent of cases occurring before the age of 3 years and 90 percent before the age of 6.[4] Rarely, it is seen in adults aged 50 or older. The incidence in European populations ranges above Asian but below Africans. The frequency in females may be slightly higher.

Wilms' tumor is primarily a disease of the kidney, but occasionally extrarenal locations have been reported, especially in the retroperitoneum, the sacrococcygeal region, testis, uterus, inguinal canal, and mediastinum.[5]

CLINICAL PRESENTATION

Patients usually present with a large (12 cm on average), smooth, and non-tender flank mass on palpation, usually noted by a parent. About 25 percent of cases experience (microscopic) hematuria, dysuria, malaise, weight loss, anemia, or hypertension.

The tumor can rupture with or without abdominal trauma and these patients present with acute abdominal pain. Obstruction of the left spermatic vein by the mass can result in a left-sided varicocele.

INVESTIGATIONS

Routine sonographic imaging of the abdomen for unspecific abdominal discomfort usually allows the diagnosis even of small, non-palpable Wilms' tumors. A detailed description of anomalies of the urinary tract and a check for the presence of aniridia should be done.

Laboratory Tests

A clinically useful biological serum marker specific for Wilms' tumors providing early diagnosis, accurate therapy monitoring, or both, has not been found yet. Lin and coworkers described a correlation between preoperative hyaluronic acid levels and clinical tumor staging[6] but this awaits further evaluation.

Recently, urinary basic Fibroblast Growth Factor (βFGF) has been reported to be elevated preoperatively in patients with Wilms' tumor.[7] Rebhandl et al described the Tissue Polypeptide Specific antigen (TPS), a cytokeratin-18 derived marker, which might be of clinical value in monitoring the therapy of nephroblastoma.[8]

Hypertension is a well-known clinical manifestation of Wilms' tumor. Increased plasma prorenin and renin levels, found by several investigators, could be the cause.

In a murine model of human anaplastic Wilms' tumor, vascular endothelial growth factor (VEGF) production correlated with tumor metastasis and therapy with anti-VEGF antibodies suppressed both primary tumor growth and the establishment of metastases.[9] Other putative serum markers and paraneoplastic syndromes have been extensively reviewed by MJ Coppes.[10] One of the goals of the current NWTS-5 is to assess the ability of tumor markers in defining specific risk groups.

The serum level of Neuron-Specific Enolase (NSE) and urinary catechol levels should routinely be measured to exclude neuroblastoma.

Imaging Studies

Today, advances in radiological techniques are able to detect non-palpable Wilms' tumors, nephroblastomatosis, and tumor spread much earlier and in a less invasive manner than in the past. Still, considerable disagreement remains in choosing the optimal method of evaluating children with renal masses. Initially a multiplanar abdominal ultrasound study of the mass, volumetry of the tumor and color-duplex investigation of the renal vessels should be performed. Thus, the extent of renal involvement (contralateral kidney), the renal vein, the inferior vena cava (IVC) and the liver can be assessed. Additionally, high-resolution sonography may detect areas of nephroblastomatosis usually presenting as multiple solid, subcapsular, hypovascular and hypoechogenic nodules or cysts.

Most centers further use chest radiograph (p.a. and lateral), CT scans of the chest (spiral technique without intravenous contrast medium, collimation of 5-mm or less) and the abdomen (oral and intravenous contrast), or MRI as baseline diagnostic procedures (Figs 12.1 and 12.2). Following the NWTS-5 recommendations,

positive findings seen in chest CT but not on chest radiograph should be ignored.[11] Whether the accuracy of CT or MRI obviates the need for surgical exploration of the contralateral kidney remains controversial. The sensitivity and specificity of CT-scans for detecting contralateral lesions of 55 bilateral tumors were described as 98 percent and 100 percent, respectively. However, other studies reported correct staging by CT-scans in 38 percent only (10 of 26 patients; overstaging in 75% and understaging in 40%, respectively).[12] Intraoperative sonography is still under evaluation.

MRI (native and with intravenous contrast) studies have a predominant role in demonstrating the relation of the tumor to other organs. Because of long scan times, in children sedation is usually required. Like sonography, MRI is more sensitive than CT for assessing extension of a tumor thrombus into the inferior vena cava (IVC) with the additional possibility of MR-venography. Nephrogenic rests (NRs) as small as 4 mm typically appear as homogeneous lesions after Gado-

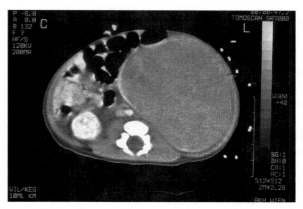

Figure 12.1: Computed tomography scan demonstrating a large Wilms' tumor originating from the left kidney

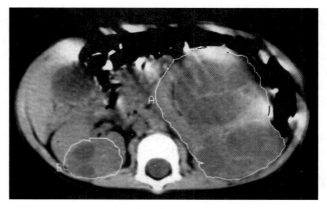

Figure 12.2: Computed tomography scan showing a bilateral Wilms' tumor

linium enhancement, different from the heterogeneous appearance of Wilms' tumor. The sensitivity for NRs was reported to be 58 percent.

SIOP-investigators strongly recommend a judgment by a reference radiologist because in these studies preoperative chemotherapy without histopathological diagnosis is favored.

Angiography is nowadays rarely performed and excretory urography provides only little information. If there is no clear discrimination from neuroblastoma, a J-metaiodobenzylguanidine-scan has to be performed.

Pre-treatment kidney scintigraphy, echocardiography and an audiogram should be performed in patients planned to receive cardio-, nephro- or ototoxic chemotherapy.

Patients with clear cell sarcoma or rhabdoid tumor of the kidney additionally need skeletal radiographs, radionuclide bone scans, and MRIs of the cranium.

MOLECULAR BIOLOGY

The first report suggesting a genetic basis for Wilms' tumor was written by Miller and co-workers in the early 1960s.[13] Wilms' tumor specimens have been noted to include numerous karyotypic abnormalities. Tumors occur bilaterally in approximately 5 to 10 percent of affected children. *Nephrogenic rests*, potentially premalignant lesions, are found in the kidneys of 30 to 40 percent of children with Wilms' tumors.[14] Children with various congenital abnormalities have an increased predisposition for the development of a Wilms' tumor.

In 1984, the loss of heterozygosity (LOH) on chromosome 11p alleles was described in up to 40 percent of Wilms' tumors. A "two hit model" similar to that of retinoblastoma was proposed, indicating a recessive mutation in the etiology of Wilms' tumor. The inherited susceptibility in Wilms' tumor families is explained by the inactivation of a critical oncosuppressor gene in the short arm of one copy of chromosome 11 at band 13. The subsequent loss of the normal alleles (somatic event) in susceptible tissues results in the development of a Wilms' tumor. Today it is estimated that approximately 7 to 10 percent of Wilms' tumors and virtually all bilateral cases are inherited. Sporadic cases are thought to occur when both of the inherited normal alleles were lost by somatic events.

Tumor Suppressor Genes

These genes act in a recessive manner and their absence or inactivity allows the manifestation of cancer. The loss of both the maternal and the paternal allele copies results in complete loss of the gene's function and contributes to tumorigenesis. Usually, one allele is inactivated by inherited mutation in the gene itself (genetic predisposition), whereas the other allele is inactivated by a loss of heterozygosity (LOH).

WT1

The *Wilms' tumor gene 1* (*WT1*, on chromosome 11p13) was isolated in 1989, is regulated during kidney development and inactivated by mutation in a subset of Wilms' tumors.[15] Even though the function of WT1 is not entirely clear, experiments involving WT1 knockout mice suggest that *WT1* is necessary for normal kidney development. It encodes a tumor suppressor gene product (zinc finger transcription factor). It has been shown to downregulate several growth factors and cognate receptor genes, however it still remains unclear whether endogenous *WT1* acts as a tumor *suppressor* or as an *oncogene* in nephroblastomas.

WT1 is biallelically expressed in normal kidney, heart, lung, and liver tissue, but is expressed largely or exclusively from the maternal allele in fetal brain (genomic imprinting, see below).

It has become obvious that mutations in WT1 form only part of the genetic complexity of Wilms' tumors. Loss of one copy of WT1 allele may confer genitourinary defects in addition to constituting the first hit required for the development of Wilms' tumor.[16] The protein motif of *WT1* is known to facilitate binding to DNA. It regulates the expression of other genes such as IGF2 epidermal growth factor receptor (EGFR), and the early growth response gene, PAX2. It also modulates apoptosis by inhibiting *p53*-dependent apoptosis.[17] However, biallelic inactivation of *WT1* appears to account for only a small fraction (10%) of unilateral Wilms' tumors not associated with congenital syndromes.

WT1 mutations are not a general feature of embryonal tumors. Some authors showed that *WT1* might not display growth inhibitory function, but instead may provide a cell survival advantage to tumors that express this transcription factor. *WT1* seems to correlate with increased Bcl-2-expression and thus may be required to overcome apoptosis and pro-apoptotic stimuli, which is crucial for tumorigenesis and potentiates proliferation by clonal expansion due to reduced cell death.[18]

WT2

The majority of Wilms' tumors continue to express normal wildtype *WT1* and these tumors seem to have developed by the inactivation of genes different from WT1. DNA loss on 11p15 has been designated as *WT2* and seems to be involved much more commonly that *WT1* in Wilms' tumor but also in other embryonal tumors.[19] The locus has been linked to the familial form of the Beckwith-Wiedemann Syndrome.

p53

The presence of structural anomalies of the chromosome 17 in approximately 15 percent of tumors and the observation of an individual with Wilms' tumor in a Li-Fraumeni family (a cancer susceptibility syndrome with germline mutations of *p53*) suggested a role for the *p53* tumor suppressor gene.[70] The p53-encoded protein appears to act as a cell cycle checkpoint protein that arrests cell growth in G1. Inactivation by mutation or alteration results in genomic instability and cytogenetic aberrations, (e.g. aneuploidy, translocations, deletions, and gene amplification).[20]

Advanced stage tumors displaying diffuse anaplasia also display increased resistance to therapy. This histological subtype commonly shows mutations in the *p53* allele, and the loss of functional *p53* tumor suppressor protein seems to contribute to chemoresistance. However, considering that *p53* alterations have been reported in almost every type of sporadic neoplasm, the reported incidence in Wilms' tumor is low. Since *p53* mutations were preferentially found in anaplastic tumors, it has been speculated that its role is restricted rather to a histopathological variant of Wilms' tumor with poor prognosis than to the overall development of these tumors. *p53* alterations have also been reported in tumors of favorable histology so prognostic significance remains unclear so far.

Other Wilms' Tumor Loci

Somatic alteration of the long arm of chromosome 16, as a 16q23 deletion or LOH for 16q or both was found in approximately 20 percent of Wilms' tumor patients.[21] These patients had significantly higher relapse rates, consistent with the hypothesis that a locus at 16q is important in malignant progression rather than tumor initiation. These alterations have also been found in other cancers.

In Wilms' tumor patients, approximately 10 percent of cases are reported to have LOH at chromosome 1p and 7p (15%). Up to now the prognostic significance of

these changes remains unclear. In familial Wilms' tumor, three different genetic loci have been implicated: *WT1* located on chromosome 11p13, *FWT1* on 17q12-q21, and *FWT2* on 19q13.

Genomic Imprinting

Although one of the assumptions of the "two-hit model" is that chromosome 11p LOH should occur randomly, LOH for the maternal allele on chromosome 11p was reported to occur preferentially.

Although we inherit two copies of all genes (except those on the sex chromosomes), in certain genes only the maternal or paternal allele is functional. This phenomenon of mono-allelic, parent-of-origin expression of genes is termed *genomic imprinting* and constitutes an epigenetic form of gene regulation resulting in the silencing of either the maternally or the paternally inherited gene.[22] Imprinted genes are normally involved in growth control but they occasionally function also inappropriately as oncogenes or tumor-suppressor genes. LOH or *uniparental disomy* (denotes a situation when an individual has inherited two copies of a specific chromosome from a single parent) at an imprinted locus may result in the loss of the only functional copy of an imprinted tumor-suppressor gene. Biallelic expression of *IGF2* and *H19* gene inactivation were found in 70 percent of Wilms' tumor patients.[23] IGF2 encodes for a growth factor known to be oncogenic when over-expressed. These findings suggested that this coupling (maternal chromosome: H19 is turned on and IGF2 is turned off; maternal IGF2 and the paternal H19 genes are silenced) is closely linked and occurs early in tumor development. Imprinted genes implicated in carcinogenesis include *WT1*, *IGF2*, *mannose 6-phosphate (M6P)/IGF2 receptor* (in 50% of Wilms' tumor patients) and cyclin-dependent kinase inhibitor *p57*[KIP2] (11p15.5, in 10% of BWS patients).[88]

DNA Content

Some studies suggested that flow cytometric evaluation of DNA-ploidy is a useful predictor of outcome and response to therapy. Diploid and aneuploid tumors are reported to have better long-term survival when compared with tetraploid tumors. However, other studies evaluating nuclear morphometric techniques reported that this factor is not superior compared to histology and staging. Ongoing studies try to determine the clinical usefulness of DNA-ploidy.

CONGENITAL ANOMALIES AND SYNDROMES ASSOCIATED WITH WILMS' TUMOR

Most of the patients display a sporadic type of Wilms' tumor; patients with genetic syndromes (Table 12.1) are at a much higher risk for the development of Wilms' tumor.[24]

Aniridia is a congenital abnormality of the iris; approximately one third of these patients have other associated defects that form part of the **WAGR syndrome** (Wilms' tumor, aniridia, genitourinary anomalies, mental retardation.[25] In these patients a deletion at chromosome 11p13 is often found. The aniridia gene has been identified as *PAX-6*.[26]

Hemihypertrophy is extremely rare and normally seen in only 3 per 100,000 children.

Genitourinary anomalies such as hypospadia or cryptorchidism are frequently seen in boys with Wilms' tumor.[27]

Beckwith-Wiedemann Syndrome (BWS) is an overgrowth syndrome characterized by neonatal hypoglycemia, abdominal wall defects (such as hernia or omphalocele), organomegaly, macroglossia, hemihypertrophy, and renal medullary dysplasia. The incidence of BWS in children with Wilms' tumor is 1.1 percent (NWTS-3 and 4: 53 of 4669 patients).[28] Conversely, children with BWS are at an increased risk for developing embryonal tumors. There is an overall incidence of abdominal tumors of 4 to 7 percent, especially neuroblastomas, hepatoblastomas, rhabdomyosarcomas, and adrenocortical carcinomas, but preferentially (in 60%) Wilms' tumors. BWS is associated with a dysregulation of genomic imprinting at chromosomal locus 11p15. It is hypothesized that increased expression of Insulin-like growth factor II *(IGF2)* gene (chromosome 11p15), but also *p57^{KIP2}*, *H19* and *KVLQT1* may be responsible for somatic overgrowth in the BWS. Twenty-one percent of the patients with BWS (NWTS-4) had bilateral disease, either at diagnosis or as metachronous contralateral recurrence. BWS patients enrolled onto NWTS 4 were younger (mean age at diagnosis: 28 months) and tended to present with an earlier-stage disease (51% stage I) than those enrolled onto NWTS 3, a trend not seen in the non-BWS patients (34% stage I). In addition, they are more likely to have tumors with favorable histology (2% anaplasia vs. 6% in the non-BWS population).

The Denys-Drash Syndrome includes male pseudohermaphroditism, progressive renal insufficiency and Wilms' tumor.[29]

Septal defects: There may be also an excess of congenital heart defects, particularly septal defects (normal frequency in children 2-4 per 1,000).

Other associated malformations include **microcephalus, hyperinsulinism**, and **von Willebrand's disease (8%)**

PATHOLOGY

Morphology

Grossly, most tumors are solitary, well circumscribed masses with predominantly solid and pale gray or tanned cut surfaces and a median weight of 550 g (Fig. 12.3). Areas of cystic changes, necrosis, and hemorrhage are frequent, especially after neoadjuvant chemotherapy.

Table 12.1: Congenital abnormalities with predisposition to Wilms' tumor[17]			
	Frequency (%)		
Congenital abnormality or syndrome	NWTS (1969-1992) n=5871	UK (1971-1977) n=549	France (1955-1989) n=501
Hemihypertrophy	2.9	2.9	5.2
Aniridia	0.6	2.2	0.8
Genitourinary malformations		1.8	2.2
— Cryptorchism	4.5*	–	–
— Hypospadias	2.4*	–	–
Beckwith-Wiedemann syndrome	0.8	0.7	0.6
Denys-Drash syndrome	0.3**	–	–
Septal defect	0.7	1.8	1.0

*% of males; **since 1980

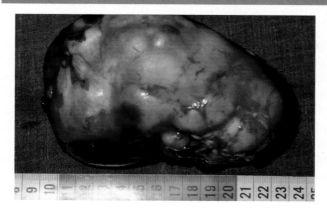

Figure 12.3: Gross appearance of Wilms' tumor after complete excision

Histology as a Prognostic Indicator

Histologically, Wilms' tumor, derived from the metanephric blastema, has been found to reveal a disorganized renal developmental process in which neoplastic blastema and epithelia are randomly interspersed in varying amounts of stroma. All these components are seen in normal kidney differentiation. The classic microscopic appearance is one of triphasic differentiation, sometimes there are fewer than three elements or there may be predominance of a single element (monophasic Wilms' tumor). The tumor may contain heterologous elements such as skeletal muscle, adipose tissue, cartilage and bone.

Anaplasia is the only criterion for assigning a Wilms' tumor as having an "unfavorable histology" (UFH), which beside advanced tumor stage constitutes the most important indicator for poor prognosis. Whereas anaplasia seems to be associated with resistance to therapy, but not increased aggressiveness, a predominantly blastemal pattern, although usually markedly aggressive, suggests a high responsiveness to chemotherapy. In contrast, epithelial-predominant WTs usually exhibit a low degree of aggressiveness but may be quite therapy-resistant.

Judgment of histology by a reference pathologist is strongly recommended.

Anaplasia in Wilms' Tumor

Anaplasia (extreme polyploidy or aneuploidy) is found in approximately 5 percent (3.2 to 7.3%) of Wilms' tumors and is believed to be the product of continued genetic instability.[30] It is rare during the first 2 years of life but present in approximately 10 percent of Wilms' tumors diagnosed at age 6 or later. It is two to three times more common in blacks than in whites, but is encountered only slightly more frequently in higher stage tumors. A female preponderance for anaplasia has been reported. Anaplasia seems to be associated with resistance to adjuvant therapy, rather than increased aggressiveness.

There are three main cytopathologic features of anaplasia: (a) a threefold or greater nuclear enlargement, compared to nearby nuclei of the same cell type, (e.g. stromal or epithelial; (b) hyperchromatism (indicating that the nuclear enlargement is attributable to gross polyploidy and not to hydrophic swelling or poor fixation); and (c) enlarged abnormal (usually multipolar) mitotic figures, which is regarded as the most quintessential criterion.[31] All three features must be present and can be seen in all three compartments of the tumor. The presence of sub-anaplastic degrees of nuclear enlargement (2 to 3 times with hyperchromasia) and atypism (so-called "nuclear unrest") indicate that thorough sampling of the primary tumor for these poor prognostic features of anaplasia is warranted.

Focal versus Diffuse Anaplasia

The criteria for "focal anaplasia" are fulfilled if the mentioned changes are confined to one or a few clearly localized foci. If this criterion is not met or anaplasia is present in tumor outside kidney capsule, the renal sinus, or in resected metastases, the tumor is designated as showing "diffuse anaplasia". Marked "subanaplastic" nuclear changes are subjected to the same limitations. Anaplasia found in small biopsy specimens is also designated as diffuse. The 4-year survival rate of patients with diffuse anaplastic tumors is 50 percent compared to 90 percent survival in patients with focal anaplasia. It is of note that these unfavorable prognostic implications of anaplasia do not have any significance for stage I tumors.

Precursor Lesions and Pathogenesis

In the normal infant, primitive metanephric blastema has largely differentiated into mature renal tissue by 34 weeks' gestation and, in general, no primitive blastema should remain after this time.

Nephrogenic rests (NR) or nephroblastomatosis are foci of persistent primitive blastemal cells, which are normally found in neonatal kidneys (approximately 1% of newborn infants have NRs at autopsy) but also in 30 to 40 percent of adjacent normal renal tissue removed together with a Wilms' tumor.[14] NRs may be microscopic or grossly visible, single or multiple. Patients with NRs (in particular perilobar NRs), have a significantly increased risk of metachronous bilateral Wilms' tumor. In NWTS-3 this was found to be particularly true for young children (20 of 206 children aged < 12 months compared with 0 of 304 children aged > 12 months). It is intriguing that virtually all kidneys of children with inherited susceptibility for Wilms' tumor contain NRs, providing evidence that these premalignant lesions represent a constitutional defect in nephrogenesis. Anatomical location of NRs may reflect the genetic and pathogenic heterogeneity of Wilms' tumor precursor lesions.[32]

Perilobar and Intralobar Nephrogenic Rests

A renal lobe consists of a medullary pyramid composed of collecting ducts, surrounded by a mantle of nephrons. According to their position within the lobe, the "perilobar (PLNR)" located at the periphery of the renal lobe are differentiated from the "intralobar (ILNR)" nephrogenic rests.[14] It is of interest that ILNR are consistently present in patients with deleted or mutated *WT1*-associated syndromes (WAGR complex–11p13 locus, Denys-Drash syndrome), whereas PLNR are usually found in children with BWS (11p15 locus).[32] These observations provide evidence of distinct pathways of normal kidney development resulting from inactivation of various involved Wilms' tumor genes. Multiple or diffuse NRs found in a kidney suggest the diagnosis of nephroblastomatosis. Multifocal NRs found in a removed kidney for Wilms' tumor are of clinical importance. In these instances the contralateral kidney is likely to contain NRs as well and careful imaging during follow-up to detect metachronous disease is warranted. The same is recommended for patients suspected to have NR in the remaining renal tissue.

Hyperplastic versus Neoplastic Rests

According to size, structure, and histology, various fates of NR have been recognized. Most NRs undergo regressive changes (involution or sclerosis) or stay dormant for many years. Hyperplasia of NRs, as defined by synchronous proliferation of many or all cells of a given rest, can occur and can be easily mistaken for a small Wilms' tumor. However neoplastic induction is presumed to occur in a single cell of the NR and tends to form a spherical expanding mass. The same therapy as for stage I Wilms' tumor is recommended for hyperplastic NRs.

SPREAD AND METASTASES

Expanding growth of the tumor usually leads to the formation of a pseudocapsule. Although rare, Wilms' tumor has the capability of infiltration into adjacent organs. Initially, invasion most often occurs into the renal hilum. Hematogenous spread might proceed along vascular paths from the renal vein to the IVC and rarely up into the right atrium. The lung is the most common site of metastases in Wilms' tumor (>80% of patients with stage IV disease); followed by lymph-node involvement (15 to 20%) and liver metastases (5 to 10%). Lymphatic spread progresses from the renal hilum, along the renal vessels to the paraaortic, paracaval nodes (see Fig. 12.1). Transperitoneal seeding, due either to rupture or direct extension of the tumor, is rarely seen (1%). Bone metastases are only exceptionally encountered.[33]

STAGING

Staging and histopathology represent the most import determinators of outcome in Wilms' tumor. Pediatric surgeons and pathologists are responsible for exact assessment of the extent of disease. Capsular invasion, rupture during surgery, invasion of extrarenal veins, tumor implants, lymph node metastases, distant metastases, and bilaterality are the main criteria used. Nowadays, the renal sinus has been included for microsubstaging with the following variables: inflammatory pseudocapsule, renal sinus invasion, and tumor in the intrarenal veins. According to NWTS-5, the distinction between stages 1 and 2 in the renal sinus is no longer defined by the hilar plane but by the presence or absence of venous or lymphatic invasion.

NWTS

Stage I: The tumor is limited to the kidney and has been completely excised. The renal capsule and the tumor were not ruptured. The vessels of the renal sinus are not involved and there is no residual tumor.

Stage II: The tumor extends beyond the kidney but was completely resected. There is regional extension of the tumor (i.e., penetration of the renal capsule, extensive invasion of the renal sinus). Blood vessels outside the renal sinus may contain tumor (tumor thrombus or infiltration). The tumor may have been biopsied, or there was local spillage of tumor confined to the flank. There is no evidence of tumor at or beyond the margins of resection.

Stage III: Residual nonhematogenous tumor confined to the abdomen or any of the following:
1. Lymph node involvement in the hilum or pelvis
2. Diffuse peritoneal spillage either before or during surgery
3. Peritoneal implants
4. Tumor beyond the surgical margin either grossly or microscopically
5. Tumor not completely resected because of local infiltration into vital structures.

Stage IV: Hematogenous metastases to lung, liver, bone, brain, or lymph node metastases outside the abdomen or pelvis. Pulmonary nodules seen on CT must undergo biopsy for definitive diagnosis of stage IV.

Stage V: Bilateral renal involvement at diagnosis. Each side must be staged individually according to the criteria mentioned above.

SIOP

The staging criteria of the SIOP protocol differ only slightly from NWTS-staging (Table 12.2).[34]

SURGERY FOR WILMS' TUMOR

Preoperative Preparation

Laboratory evaluation should include kidney function tests, complete peripheral blood count, electrolytes, liver function tests, and blood-clotting profile. Szintigraphic evaluation of kidney function should be performed and blood typing and cross-match should be obtained. A 24-hr urine sample for analysis of vanylmandelic acid, as well as serum NSE should be obtained in order to exclude neuroblastoma. In some cases it might be necessary to perform a J-metaiodobenzylguanidine-scan. Therapy for elevated blood pressure may be necessary. In case of significant anemia, a preoperative transfusion may be required. Erythropoetin substitution during preoperative chemotherapy can decrease the need for transfusion. There is no need for emergent operation unless there is evidence of active bleeding. The child is kept without oral intake (except tea) for 6 to 8 hours before the operation. Older children should receive an oral bowel flush.

Anesthetic Management

Standard monitoring of blood pressure, temperature, ECG, and O_2-saturation are accomplished. An arterial line is optional. An indwelling urethral catheter is placed to control urinary output. A reliable venous access is established in the neck or upper extremities (manipulation of inferior vena cava).

Surgical Technique

Radical transperitoneal nephrectomy remains the cornerstone of the management of Wilms' tumor. As the prognosis is determined by histology and stage of disease, the role of surgery is threefold: 1) radical resection of the tumor, 2) definition of a post-surgical stage and 3) establishment of an accurate histological diagnosis. The surgeon has to assess the extent of local tumor spread. Since tumors are generally large, the gross appearance of the tumor at the time of surgery can be misleading in interpreting tumor extent. Radical en bloc resection of tumors that compress and adhere to adjacent visceral organs is generally not justified since it increases morbidity.

Incision and Exposure

The patient is in a supine position, tilt to the tumor side at approximately 30 degrees. A generous transverse transperitoneal incision 2 fingerbreadths above the umbilicus is required to facilitate complete exposure of both kidneys (Fig. 12.4). The anterior rectus sheath on the side of the tumor is incised. The incision is extended laterally to open the external oblique fascia and muscle and similarly the internal oblique fascia. Then, the

Table 12.2: Wilms' tumor staging according to SIOP[9]	
Stage I	Tumor limited to kidney and completely excised
Stage II	Tumor extending outside kidney, but completely excised with negative or invaded regional lymph nodes
Stage III	Incomplete excision, without hematogenous metastases, extraregional lymph node infiltration, peritoneal metastases, tumor rupture, or biopsy before or at surgery
Stage IV	Distant metastases.
Stage V	Bilateral tumor

posterior rectus sheath, transversalis fascia and peritoneum are opened. The falciform ligament with umbilical veins is divided between ligatures. The peritoneum is entered with care to avoid breaching the anterior surface of the tumor and the incision is extended laterally under direct vision. The liver and abdominal contents should be inspected and palpated for secondaries. Before tumornephrectomy, the contra-lateral kidney is carefully examined on both anterior and posterior surfaces in order to detect previously unsuspected bilateral disease or the presence of nephrogenic rests. Only biopsies from the main tumor and opposite lesion are performed under these circumstances. The colon is dissected free from the white line and reflected medially together with its mesentery; care is taken to preserve the colonic blood supply (Fig. 12.5).

A plane adjacent to the great vessels is developed posteriorly of these structures by gently inserting a finger into the paravertebral space. The tumor itself is not mobilized at this stage and gentle handling throughout the procedure is mandatory in order to prevent rupture of the tumor capsule and spillage, which is associated with upstaging of the tumor and increased risk for local recurrence.

Resection

After assessing the extent of the tumor, vascular and/or nodal involvement and/or metastases, the possibility of a primary excision has to be determined. The dissection is begun caudally, sweeping adventitial tissue and lymph nodes lateral to the great vessels. The renal vein and its branches are gently exposed and carefully palpated to exclude intravascular extension of the tumor. Early mobilization of the IVC and renal vein may be required

to prevent embolization of the tumor into the IVC, heart, and pulmonary artery. A caval thrombus below the level of the hepatic veins can be removed via cavotomy after proximal and distal vascular control is obtained. On the right side, exposure of the tumor necessitates separation of the hepatic flexure, the right and transverse colon from the liver. The gallbladder and the second part of the duodenum are retracted medially. The renal vein (note: the left renal vein crosses the aorta ventrally) is gently mobilized and elevated using a vascular sling to expose the renal artery, which should be ligated and divided before the renal vein to prevent swelling of the kidney. Subsequently, the gonadal vessels are ligated. Occasionally, tumor vessels directly draining into the IVC are encountered and have to be identified. A dissection plane should afterwards be established outside Gerota's fascia (see Fig. 12.5). The posterior aspect of the kidney is partially mobilized by sharp dissection.

Superior dissection is hazardous on the left side and damage to the spleen and tail of the pancreas must be avoided. The adrenal gland is removed in case of adherent upper-pole Wilms' tumor. Identification of the adrenal artery is important to avoid bleeding. A generous segment of the ureter should be resected after double ligation. The kidney within Gerota's fascia is lifted out of the abdomen and the posterior dissection is inspected following removal of the kidney (Fig. 12.6). Any suspicious lymph nodes near the great vessels are removed. For exact staging, excision of lymph nodes

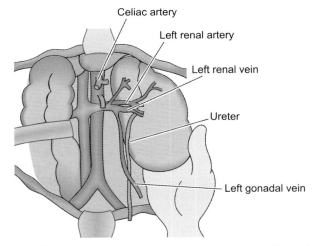

Figure 12.5: Excision of left-sided Wilms' tumor: The colon and mesocolon have been dissected free from the tumor's anterior surface and reflected over the opposite kidney. The renal vein and artery are identified and ligated. Then the posterior aspect of the kidney is mobilized by establishing a retro-renal plane of dissection

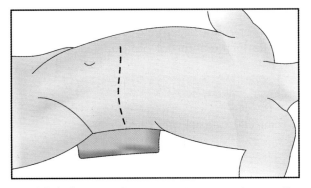

Figure 12.4: Incision: A generous transverse transperitoneal incision 2 fingerbreadths above the umbilicus facilitates exposure and resection

should include at least hilar and periaortic samples (Fig. 12.7). Absence of lymph node biopsy may result in understaging and inadequate adjuvant treatment and may cause an increased risk of local recurrence. Titanium clips can be used to delineate the tumor bed for radiation therapy. After irrigation with physiologic saline and insertion of a Penrose drain retroperitoneally, the colon is replaced and the wound closed in layers.

Partial Nephrectomy

The role of partial nephrectomy (nephron-sparing surgery) remains controversial.[35] Several studies reported an increased incidence of hypertension, proteinuria and decreased renal function, even renal failure, in patients who underwent unilateral nephrectomy for Wilms' tumor. Total tumor nephrectomy might potentially be harmful to the patient due to the substantial risk of renal function loss of a solitary kidney caused by the consecutive hypertrophy of the remaining contralateral kidney as well as to the probability of a primary malformation, metachronous tumor occurrence (1.5% in NWTS, 2–3% in SIOP studies), accidental damage, or other superimposed renal injury. The currently reported poor evidence of a marked risk of renal failure following unilateral nephrectomy however might be due to the lack of long-term follow-up studies. Some investigators report an 87 percent accuracy of predicting the possibility of partial nephrectomy. According to the SIOP treatment strategy (SIOP-9 65% stage I,) partial nephrectomy can be considered more often. Surgical (radiological and pathological) selection criteria for partial nephrectomy should include functioning kidney, tumor confined to one pole occupying less than one third of

the kidney, no invasion of the renal vein or collecting system, and clear margins between tumor, kidney, and surrounding structures. Most studies concur that safe partial nephrectomy is applicable in approximately 5 percent of tumors at diagnosis (10% of patients after preoperative chemotherapy) without violating oncological principles. The local recurrence rate for partial nephrectomy in patients with bilateral tumors was found to be 8.2 percent (NWTS-4, 4-year survival rate: 81.7%).[36]

Surgical Complications

In NWTS-3, the incidence of surgical complications was found to be 19 percent, most often hemorrhage, small bowel obstruction, vascular injury, and tumor embolus. The SIOP studies reported a lower incidence of surgical complications (SIOP-9: 8%) presumably since preoperative chemotherapy facilitates tumor resection.[37] NWTS-4 investigators have demonstrated that the surgeon must avoid rupture of the tumor, because spills produce an increased risk of local relapse, associated with a far poorer outcome. From results of NWTS-4 it was concluded that Stage II children with local spill require more aggressive therapy.

Postoperative Treatment

The removed specimen forms the backbone of further therapy planning. Subsequent adjuvant radio- and/or chemotherapy are determined by the pathological stage and tumor type (FH/UFH). It is important to recognize that in the SIOP series, tumors were stratified to 3 different pathological groups: favorable histology (multicystic type, fibroadenomatous structures), standard

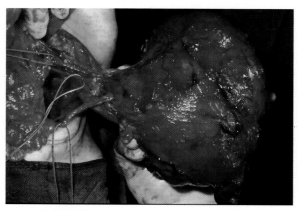

Figure 12.6: Left-sided Wilms' tumor: The kidney is fully mobilized and lifted out of the abdomen; the ureter, left renal artery and vein are identified and elevated with vascular slings

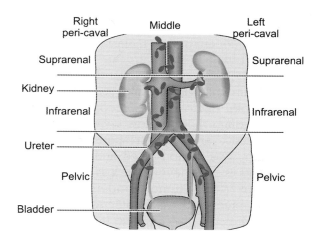

Figure 12.7: Lymphatic drainage of the kidneys

histology (epithelial, blastematous regular and irregular, mixed epithelial with regular or irregular blastema) and unfavorable histology (with anaplasia).[38]

CHEMOTHERAPY AND RADIOTHERAPY

The goal of both study groups is to improve survival by identifying high-risk patients for more intense therapy while minimizing therapy and thus short- and long-term side effects for low-risk patients.

Except for patients younger than 6 months, SIOP therapeutic protocols include a 4-week-period of preoperative chemotherapy (vincristine and actinomycin D), followed by nephrectomy and postoperative chemotherapy.[39] Stage IV Wilms' tumors receive 6 weeks of pre-treatment and epirubicin is additionally administered.[40] Diagnosis is based on imaging analysis and metabolic exclusion of neuroblastoma and currently is reported to be correct in 99 percent of cases (initial SIOP studies suggested a 5% misdiagnosis rate). SIOP investigators use the post-treatment stage to determine further therapy. The SIOP studies have demonstrated that neoadjuvant therapy will make the tumor less prone to intraoperative rupture or spillage and reduces surgical complications. Since benign tumors represent less than 1 percent of cases, avoiding an up-front biopsy but treatment with neoadjuvant chemotherapy outweighs the increased risk for tumor rupture in case of primary excision, converting a stage I to a stage III tumor.[34] This protocol leads to an increased number of postchemotherapy stage I tumors (downstaging: SIOP-1, no pre-treatment: 20%, against SIOP-9: 65%), resulting in a smaller number of patients receiving adjuvant radiotherapy and aggressive postoperative chemotherapy. However, NWTS studies also showed that radiation therapy is unnecessary for stage II patients with favorable histology. In case of advanced disease at diagnosis, pulmonary or liver metastases can disappear after neoadjuvant therapy. In the SIOP-9 nephroblastoma trial, investigators recently described a group of patients with unilateral nonanaplastic Wilms' tumors displaying total necrosis after preoperative chemotherapy. Although these tumors were reported to be initially aggressive, an excellent response to preoperative chemotherapy was demonstrated and the outcome of these patients is most favorable. It is concluded, that patients with Wilms' tumors undergoing complete necrosis after preoperative chemotherapy should benefit from less aggressive postoperative treatment.

The NWTS studies rely on surgical and pathological staging, stratifying patients into high-risk and low-risk groups.[41] After adverse prognostic factors are identified, treatment of children with Wilms' tumor is tailored based on these factors (Table 12.3). A major concern of NWTS is that staging the patient after preoperative chemotherapy can destroy the evidence of extrarenal spread of disease and therefore the risk of relapse or recurrence is inadequately defined.[42] Few studies have documented modifications of the tumor after chemotherapy. According to NWTS, preoperative chemotherapy is done only in patients with very large, initially inoperable tumors, or bilateral Wilms' tumors and some patients with suprahepatic IVC thrombus. NWTS-5 recommends that any patient undergoing preoperative chemotherapy should first undergo surgical staging. To avoid undertreatment, any patient without surgical staging should be treated as stage III. Based on the positive experience of SIOP studies with preoperative chemotherapy in reducing tumor bulk and facilitating surgical intervention, individual surgeons may offer this protocol as an alternative in selected patients (e.g. infrahepatic IVC thrombus).

The results of preoperative chemotherapy used in Europe (SIOP) are similar to those noted in the NWTS (USA).[43]

Previously it was thought that size of tumor represents a predictor of outcome and a special class of tumors (Cassady tumor: <550 g and age <24 months with FH) could be treated with surgery only.[44] This approach was recently abandoned because of high recurrence rates.

According to NWTS-5, radiotherapy is not used for patients with stages I or II/FH (see Table 12.3). Patients with stage II/diffuse anaplasia are treated with flank radiotherapy and intensified chemotherapy. Patients with stage III and IV/FH as well as all patients with unfavorable histology additionally receive radiation.[45] In patients with other aggressive tumors, like clear cell sarcoma and rhabdoid tumors of the kidney, postoperative flank irradiation is also recommended. Patients with involvement of the vena cava or inoperable patients, where neoadjuvant chemotherapy fails to reduce tumor size significantly, should also receive additional radiotherapy. Bilateral pulmonary radiation of lung metastases (stage IV) is performed only if the nodules appear also in chest radiograph.

The current SIOP protocol does not recommend radiotherapy for stage I patients, but provides postoperative randomization in patients with intermediate or high-risk tumors. Stages II and III are treated with postoperative flank irradiation.[46]

	Table 12.3: NWTS-5 chemotherapy schedules for each stage			
Stage	*Histology*	*Surgery*	*Radiotherapy*	*Chemotherapy*
I	FH/anaplasia	Nephrectomy	None AMD (18 wk)	VCR, Pulse-intensive
II	FH	Nephrectomy	None	VCR, Pulse-intensive AMD (18 wk)
II-IV	Focal anaplasia	Nephrectomy	10.8 Gy	VCR, Pulse-intensive AMD and DOX (24 wk)
III/IV	FH	Nephrectomy	10.8 Gy	VCR, Pulse-intensive AMD and DOX (24 wk)
II-IV	Diffuse anaplasia, CCSK	Nephrectomy	Yes	VCR, DOX, CPP and ETP
I-IV	RTK	Nephrectomy	Yes	CP, ETP and CPP

FH, favorable histology, AMD, dactinomycin; VCR, vincristine; DOX, doxorubicin; CPP, cyclophosphamide; ETP, etoposide (VP16); CP, carboplatin; RTK, rhabdoid tumor of the kidney; CCSK, clear cell sarcoma; Note: Radiation is given to all clear cell sarcoma patients. Stage IV FH patients are given irradiation based on the local tumor stage. For further information consult protocol.

LONG-TERM COMPLICATIONS

Fortunately Wilms' tumor is a curable malignancy in most patients, so limiting iatrogenic sequelae is essential wherever possible. Paulino et al. reported late effects of therapy in more than two thirds of children treated for Wilms' tumor.[47] Beside morbidity from chemotherapeutic agents, potential side effects of radiotherapy like intestinal strictures, ulceration, perforation, hematochezia, growth arrest and osteonecrosis have to be considered.[48]

Renal Function

NWTS and SIOP studies showed that the risk of renal failure for patients with unilateral Wilms' tumor and a normal opposite kidney is very low (0.25%). Most of these children had unrecognized renal disease (Denys-Drash syndrome) followed by radiation nephritis. In patients with nephrectomy and abdominal irradiation, renal dysfunction is more common. However, the development of compensatory postnephrectomy hypertrophy of the contralateral kidney is obvious and proteinurea and hypertension may occur long after tumornephrectomy.

Of 5823 registered patients in the NWTS trials (1969–1993) a total of 55 patients (1%) developed renal failure. Seventy-one percent[39] of the 55 had either synchronous or metachronous bilateral disease. "Renal failure" in these patients was most often caused by bilateral nephrectomy (24 patients of 39), followed by radiation nephritis and surgical complications.

Congestive Heart Failure

The administration of anthracyclines has improved the survival of stage III and IV Wilms' tumor patients because of its significant single-agent activity against Wilms' tumor. Congestive heart failure is typically seen after administration of anthracyclines. Reported cardiotoxicity includes electrocardiographic changes, changes in myocyte morphology (necrosis and fibrosis), decreased cardiac function, and congestive heart failure.

Dose related cardiomyopathy caused by doxorubicin is a well-known complication, reported for approximately 5 percent of patients receiving a cumulative dose of 400 to 500 mg/m^2. There is evidence of considerable additive risk factors, like mediastinal radiation, young age at the time of treatment, and female sex. The cumulative rate of patients treated with doxorubicin in NWTS 2/3 that developed cardiac disease at 15 years after diagnosis is 1.7 percent.[49]

Lung Damage

Both chemotherapeutic agents and total lung-irradiation can cause severe changes in pulmonary function. Radiation pneumonitis is dose dependent, and is reported from 13 percent (NWTS-3) up to 23 and 25 percent, respectively, in patients receiving actinomycin D. Prophylaxis against *Pneumocystis carinii* is recommended for patients receiving pulmonary irradiation.

Liver Damage

The liver was originally considered to be a radio-resistant organ. In 1965, Ingold et al.[50] were the first to describe the clinicopathologic findings of radiation hepatitis. Normal hepatic function is essential for the inactivation and excretion of vincristine and actinomycin D. NWTS-4 studies reported a dose-related incidence of hepatotoxicity in patients receiving chemotherapy (especially vincristine and actinomycin D) ranging from 3 to 14 percent, however, hepatic irradiation (above 30 Gy) also increases the risk for hepatotoxicity and veno-occlusive disease as characterized by hepato-megaly, elevated liver enzymes, hyperbilirubinemia, and ascites.[51] Investigators reported the overall incidence of veno-occlusive disease in patients treated according SIOP-9 trial to be 8 percent (3% during preoperative chemotherapy).

Infertility

Damage to the reproductive systems may represent one of the main late sequelae of both, gonadal radiation or chemotherapeutic agents. Radiation effect even on prepubertal germ cells may lead to hormonal dysfunction (hypogonadism) or infertility.[52] Abdominal irradiation in females has been reported to be significantly associated with an increased risk for perinatal mortality rate and low-birth-weight infants.[53] As with the testis, the effect on the ovaries (ovarian failure in 75 percent where the ovaries were included in the treatment field) is dose-dependent.

Alkylating chemotherapeutic agents more often affect dividing cells, which may be the reason that impaired gonadal function is preferentially seen in males. Vincristine has been described as a major risk factor for azoospermia.

Musculoskeletal Function

Ionizing radiation (megavoltage/orthovoltage) has well been documented to interfere with epipyseal growth. Soft tissue hypoplasia and diminished bone growth is followed by scoliosis and other orthopedic abnormalities with a frequency of 60 to 80 percent of patients treated with radiation.

Second Malignant Neoplasms

NWTS studies reported that the risk of developing a second malignant neoplasm in patients with successfully treated Wilms' tumors is 1.6 to 5.6 percent at 15, respectively 25 years after diagnosis.[54] The cumulative incidence of a second cancer reported by SIOP investigators observed at 15 years after Wilms' tumor diagnosis was 0.65 percent.[55] Most solid tumors (73%) arise in the irradiated areas.[56] All patients with hepatocellular carcinoma had received flank irradiation. Other reported tumors mainly seen in the irradiated field are bone, breast and thyroid malignancies. The risk of developing leukemia or lymphoma because of the topoisomerase II inhibiting activity of anthracyclines and other agents is highest in the first 8 years after treatment. The risk of developing a second tumor in the opposite kidney is about 1.2 percent, depending on the presence of nephrogenic rests. Generally, it is believed, that children with a history of malignancy have a 10-20 times higher risk of developing a second malignancy, indicating the need for careful follow-up of these patients.

RECURRENCE

In the NWTS-4 study a total of 2482 randomized or followed patients were identified. Local recurrence, defined as recurrence in the original tumor bed, retroperitoneum, or within the abdominal cavity or pelvis, occurred in 100 children. The largest relative risks for local recurrence were observed in patients with stage III disease, those with unfavorable histology (especially diffuse anaplasia), and those where tumor spillage occurred during surgery. The relative risk of local recurrence from spill was largest in children with stage II disease. The absence of lymph node biopsy was also associated with an increased relative risk of recurrence, which was largest in children with stage I disease. The survival of children after local recurrence is poor, especially if the recurrence occurs early and follows triple-drug chemotherapy and radiotherapy. The average survival rate at 2 years is only 43 percent.[57] The role of high-dose therapy with autologous stem cell transfusion or marrow reconstitution is still under investigation by various national groups.[58]

TREATMENT OF METASTATIC DISEASE

Bilateral tumors have been dealt with in detail in a seperate chapter.

Intravascular Extension

Infradiaphragmatic Infrahepatic Extension

An adherent caval vein thrombus generally can be removed by cavotomy or using a Fogarty or Foley balloon catheter. Patients with intravascular extension above the level of the hepatic veins should receive preoperative chemotherapy.

Supradiaphragmatic Intrapericardial or Suprahepatic Extension and Supradiaphragmatic Intracardiac Extension

Recent reports showed that preoperative therapy in patients with suprahepatic caval or atrial extension led to a marked decrease in size of tumor thrombus and even complete regression of thrombus without embolization. As an alternative in adverse cases embolectomy under cardiopulmonary bypass is required.

Lung Metastases

Pulmonary nodules seen on chest CT and not on chest radiograph *("CT only" metastases)* do not mandate treatment with whole-lung irradiation in NWTS-5. NWTS-4 data raise the possibility that children with CT-only pulmonary nodules who receive whole lung irradiation have fewer pulmonary relapses than those who were treated less aggressively (based on the extent of locoregional disease with 2 or 3 drugs), but a greater number of deaths due to treatment toxicity (4-year event-free 89 vs. 80%, overall survival 91 vs. 85%). The role of whole lung irradiation in the treatment of this group of patients cannot be definitively determined as yet. The nodules should be removed to confirm diagnosis.

Advanced Local Tumors, Inoperable Tumors

Since imaging studies alone carry the risk of overstaging, NWTS recommends determining "inoperability" at surgical exploration. In our experience, nephrectomy is often technically easier than the imaging studies would suggest. In rare cases, advanced right-sided tumors may extend into the liver and wedge resection *en bloc* or even hepatic lobectomy may be necessary in these patients. If the diaphragm has been infiltrated by tumor, it should also be partially excised *en bloc*. Patients considered to have unresectable tumor based on imaging studies only should be considered stage III and treated accordingly.

PROGNOSIS

Two-year relapse-free survival of children in the fourth NWTS study exceeded 91 percent. The disease-free survival (SIOP) for stage I is 85 percent, IINO, 84 percent,

IIN+ and III, 75 percent at 2 years and a 3 year disease-free survival for all patients of 81 percent (crude survival of 90%).

The 4-year relapse-free survival (NWTS-4) and overall survival rates for patients with Wilms' tumor were reported to be 84 and 90 percent, respectively (Patients with BWS: 81 and 89 percent respectively; outcome analysis excluded contralateral recurrences: 18 percent for BWS and 3 percent for non-BWS patients).[59] The cumulative survival rate for infants with bilateral tumors is approximately 65 to 70 percent at 10 years. However, Paulino *et al.* reported the overall survival of metachronous bilateral Wilms' tumor to be only 49.1 and 47.2 percent at 5 and 10 years, respectively.[60]

FUTURE DIRECTIONS

Recent advances in understanding the molecular biology of the tumorigenesis of Wilms' tumor have provided significant implications for the clinical management. Thus, both large study groups currently aim to intensify treatment for patients with poor prognosticators while reducing therapy and subsequent long-term complications, for those with favorable prognostic features.

Parenchymal sparing renal surgery for patients with small unilateral Wilms' tumor remains controversial.

Treatment of children with Wilms' tumor should certainly involve a team of specialized pediatric physicians consisting of surgeons, oncologists, radiologists, pathologists, and radiotherapists.

RENAL CELL CARCINOMA

Compared to Wilms' tumor, Renal Cell Carcinoma (RCC) rarely presents in childhood. It comprises only 2 to 6 percent of primary renal neoplasms in the pediatric population with a mean age of 8 to 9 years at presentation.

Renal cell carcinoma occurs rather in the second than in the first decade of life.

An analysis of the genetics of pediatric renal cell carcinoma leads to the assumption that renal cell carcinomas in children and young adults represent a distinct group. These tumors have unique genetic findings (most commonly t(x;1)(p11:q21)[61] in comparison to the anomalies (translocation and deletion) of the chromosome 3p in adult renal cell carcinomas.

Besides the classical triad of abdominal or flank pain, hematuria and a palpable mass, presenting complaints include also weight loss, fever, and gastrointestinal distress. A palpable mass is thought to be slightly more common than hematuria or flank pain and the complete triad has only been reported in 6 to 8 percent of affected children[62] compared to 10 percent of adults. Although the preoperative diagnosis of renal cell carcinoma in children and its distinguishing of Wilms' tumor is difficult, the preoperative evaluation offers a range of methods including plain abdominal and chest x-rays, excretory urography, ultrasonography, CT, angiography and isotope bone scan. The abdominal x-ray and CT reveal abnormal calcification, excretory urography demonstrates filling defects or caliceal distortion, indicating an intrinsic renal mass, ultrasonography shows an echogenic mass and angiography confirms a well defined hypervascular mass. Despite the fact that Castellanos et al.[63] reported that tumor calcification and high density areas are more common in renal cell carcinoma (approximately 25% of cases) than in Wilms' tumor (approximately 5%) and angiography reveals less vascularity in Wilms' tumor than in renal cell carcinoma, the preoperative differential diagnosis of renal tumors remains unsure. Certainty can only be gained definitively by radical nephrectomy.

The current SIOP-10 protocol does not allow pretreatment histological classification of renal tumors in children for fear of needle tract recurrences but a retrospective study by Skoldenberg et al. proves that ultrasound-guided cutting needle biopsy is a method of high sensitivity (76%) without any major complications.[64]

Histopathology reveals a clear cell pattern with low-grade nuclear cytology and papillary or mixed tubular and papillary features are the principal findings. Immunohistology show a varying intensity of cytokeratin expression.

Tumor classification according to the pathological staging system modified by Robson et al. is described as follows—stage 1: tumor confined to the kidney with no perirenal fat involvement—stage 2: tumor extension into the perirenal fat but within Gerota's fascia- stage 3: regional lymph node metastases or gross involvement of the inferior vena cava- stage 4: adjacent organ involvement other than that of the adrenal glands or distant metastases (concerning most of all the lung, liver and bone).

As in adults, the primary and only effective mode of treatment is radical nephrectomy with regional lymphadenectomy. Regional lymphadenectomy in adults with renal cell carcinoma has been questioned lately, but it may be advantageous for the pediatric population. Pediatric patients with isolated regional lymph node metastasis have significantly better expected survival than adults. Although radiation and chemotherapy may provide a slight benefit in selected patients, their efficacy remains unproven and uncertain.

Common combinations of chemotherapeutic agents are vincristine and actinomycin D. doxorubicin, methotrexate and cyclophosophamide; bleomycin and vinblastine sulphate. Immunotherapy has shown promise for treating children who have advanced renal cell carcinoma mainly using interferon-alpha and interleukin 2.

The overall 5-year survival rate in children with renal cell carcinoma has been estimated to be between 56 to 64 percent.[65] A number of features have been investigated as potential prognostic factors in renal cell carcinoma. These include stage, vascular invasion, tumor size, nuclear grade, cell type, immunohistochemical staining pattern, location, and age. However in most published series, tumor size, cell type, cellular pattern, location or age did not correlate with outcome. Nuclear grade is reportedly a good prognostic predictor, especially for patients with stage 1 tumors, as is increased vimentin expression in immunohistochemical studies.[66] Thus, of all the proposed prognostic factors, tumor stage appears to be the most important, and may even be the only meaningful one.

STROMAL TUMORS OF THE KIDNEY

About 15 percent of all renal neoplasms are stromal tumors. These include clear cell sarcoma of the kidney, rhabdoid tumor, congenital mesoblastic nephroma, and metanephric stromal tumor.

Clear Cell Sarcoma of the Kidney

CCSK accounts for about 3 percent of renal tumors reported to the NWTS. Since CCSK displays the same location, clinical presentation, gross appearance and age at diagnosis as Wilms' tumor, it was formerly regarded as an unfavorable histologic variant of Wilms' tumor with poor prognosis and was called "bone metastasizing renal tumor" (Figs 12.8A to C). Its incidence peaks during the second year of life (NWTS mean age at clinical presentation 36 months, range, 2 months to 14 years). The male to female ratio is 2:1. Kidd and co-workers in 1970 were the first to report its propensity to metastasize to bone.[67]

Several other investigators later on described distinctive histopathologic features, a much higher rate of relapse and death than in favorable histology Wilms'

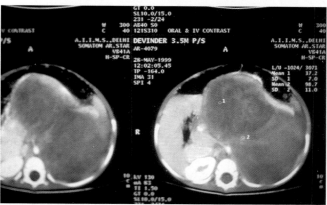

Figure 12.8A: CT scan abdomen of a left clear cell sarcoma of the kidney

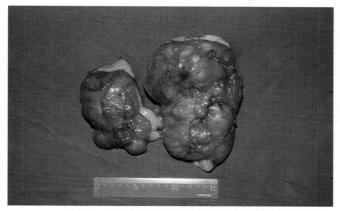

Figure 12.8B: Gross aperrence of the excised specimen of CCSK

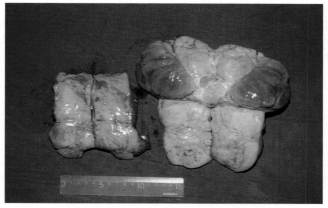

Figure 12.8C: Cut section of the excised specimen

tumor. Only recently CCSK has been recognized as a distinct clinicopathologic entity.

The histopathologic characteristics include a wide diversity of morphologic features, ranging from spindle cell to epitheloid patterns. The largest series has recently been reported by Argani et al and included 351 patients

from NWTS-1 to 5.[68] Most tumors show the classic histological picture, i.e. multiple blended patterns. The following histopathologic variants were described: myxoid (50%), sclerosing (35%), cellular (26%), epitheloid (13%), palisading (11%), spindle cell (7%), storiform (4%), and anaplastic pattern (2.6% vs. about 5% in Wilms' tumor).

In this cumulative report, 29 percent of patients showed lymph node involvement at the time of presentation. Bone metastases were the most common mode of relapse (49 cases), followed by lung metastases (37 cases), local (abdominal/retroperitoneal) recurrence (25 cases), and brain metastases (16 cases). It is of note that CCSK metastases were frequently encountered in unusual soft tissue, (e.g. scalp, epidural, nasopharynx) and other sites (orbital). The time interval to relapse in the NWTS patient group ranged from <16 months to 4 years. Although the overall relapse rate is significantly lower for patients treated with doxorubicin, the risk of recurrence is prolonged.

Currently (NWTS-5), patients with CCSK are treated with initial nephrectomy regardless of stage, abdominal radiation (10.8 Gy), combined chemotherapy with actinomycin D, vincristine, and doxorubicin (Table 12.3). The main prognosticators for favorable outcome in CCSK are revised stage 1, age at diagnosis (2–4 years), therapy with doxorubicin and absence of tumor necrosis.[68] Except for the presence of necrosis, which seems to be a feature of aggressive high-grade sarcomas, no other histopathologic pattern in CCSK appears to be of prognostic significance. The reported 6-year survival rates (therapy with vs. therapy without doxorubicin) are 98 vs. 100 percent (revised stage I), 75 vs. 31 percent (stage II), 77 vs. 30 percent (stage III) and 50 vs. 0 percent (stage IV), respectively.

Rhabdoid Tumor

Formerly, rhabdoid tumor of the kidney (RTK) was regard as a solid monophasic, or rhabdomyo-sarcomatoid variant of unfavorable histology Wilms' tumor. Nowadays, it is recognized as a separate highly malignant entity. RTK represents only 1.8 percent of cases entered into NWTS since 1969, with a median age at presentation of 17 months and a slight male preponderance (male-to-female, 1.5:1).[69]

Some of the patients have hypercalcemia. In about 15 percent of RTK, patients develop other primary embryonal tumors in the midline posterior fossa, particularly medulloblastoma. These intracranial tumors are histologically distinct from the primary renal lesion. In contrast to Wilms' tumor, about 80 percent of RTKs have stage III or IV disease at presentation. Grossly, RTK typically appears as a bulky, solid, and relatively well-circumscribed lesion. The histiogenesis remains controversial, the tumor may not even be renal-specific since morphologically indistinguishable rhabdoid tumors occur in many other sites, (e.g. pelvis, soft tissue, bladder) and deletion of the hSNF5/INI1 gene on chromosome 22 has been found in all these tumors.[70]

Light-microscopic and ultrastuctural features have been defined.

The tumor behavior is extremely aggressive and clinical management (triple chemotherapy) has not proven successful. So far, male sex and high tumor stage are the only identified unfavorable prognosticators. Metastases occur most frequently in the lung (70%) and most patients with relapse die from tumor progression (NWTS 96%). The reported survival rate at 3 years is less than 20 percent.

Congenital Mesoblastic Nephroma

Congenital mesoblastic nephroma (CMN), also known as fetal renal hamartoma, leiomyomatous hamartoma, and mesenchymal hamartoma of infancy, seems to be a low grade spindle cell tumor originating in the renal medulla. Bolande and coworkers established it as a distinct renal tumor in 1967.[71] It constitutes the most common benign renal tumor in the neonate. Nearly all solid renal tumors presenting in the first weeks of life are mesoblastic nephromas (note: the most common neonatal abdominal masses are hydronephrosis and multicystic dysplastic kidney disease). However, a few cases of mesoblastic nephroma have been reported in older children, and rare adult cases exist. NWTS reported a mean age of diagnosis of 3.4 months with a male preponderance (male-to-female ratio 1.8:1).[72] About 2.8 percent of all renal neoplasms in children are CMNs. About 14 percent of cases are associated with prematurity and polyhydramnion. The precise association between mesoblastic nephroma and polyhydramnion remains uncertain. Hypertension and increased renin concentration and skeletal fibromatosis have been reported. On ultrasound, mesoblastic nephroma is an evenly echogenic mass with concentric echogenic and hypoechoic rings resembling uterine fibroids. It may in time form a heterogeneous mass with hemorrhage and cyst formation secondary to central regions of necrosis. Calcification is rare. In one series of 20 cases, all were unilateral. Grossly, the tumor is usually of a light tan, fleshy with a whorled configuration and has ill-defined peripheral borders, blending into the adjacent renal parenchyma and even the perirenal fat. Most are centered near the hilus of the kidney.

Microscopically CMN consists of monomorphic spindle-shaped cells, resembling fibroblasts with scant interstitial collagen. Two morphological subtypes are distinguished: the classical or leiomyomatous type and the atypical or cellular type. Mixed forms have also been described.

In a series of 51 cases, 50 patients survived and only one patient experienced local recurrence.[72] Despite this excellent prognosis, local recurrence and even tumor-related death have been described and were always related to the cellular (atypical) form or to the mixed form, particularly in patients aged more than 3 months and in those cases where surgical removal was not complete.

Cytogenetic studies have reported common trisomies in cellular CMN, particularly of chromosome 11 and t(12;15) (p13;q25)-associated ETV6-NTRK3 gene fusions.[73] These fusions have also been demonstrated in infantile fibrosarcoma[74] and cellular CMN is probably the renal presentation of this neoplasm.

Except for these unfavorable variants that may require adjuvant therapy, total surgical excision independent of histological type without further therapy is recommended for most patients as the treatment of choice. Tumor rupture and difficulties in achieving clear surgical margins have been frequently reported but did not affect the excellent prognosis.

ANGIOMYOLIPOMA OF THE KIDNEY

This benign tumor is often associated with Tuberous sclerosis; sporadic cases can be associated with von Recklinghausen's disease or autosomal dominant polycystic kidney disease. Usually, flank pain or acute abdomen due to hemorrhage is the presenting symptom and the indication for surgical treatment. Although the mean age at diagnosis is 41 years, the tumor may be discovered in children or adolescents. The tumor contains thick-walled vessels, smooth muscle cells, and maturated adipose tissue. Hemorrhage and necrosis are common. Malignant transformation has been described but is extremely rare,[75] so nephron-sparing surgery should be attempted whenever possible.

Table 12.4: Other renal neoplasms in children

	Cases described	Age at presentation	Clinical presentation	Gross pathology	Microscopic features	Treatment	Prognosis	Note
Metanephric stromal tumor (MST[78]	31	24 mo (newborn to 11y)	Mass, hematuria	Tan, lobulated, partially cystic fibrous mass	Cellular stromal tumor, collarettes around entrapped tubules and vessels	Nephrectomy	Good	Must be distinguished from CCSK, stromal variant of MAF
Metanephric adenofibroma (MAF)[79]	5	13.3 y (3.5 to 23)	Abdominal mass, polycythemia, hematuria	Homogeneous, bosselated, firm, gray-white, yellow, or tan, nonencapsulated	Spindled cells encasing immature epithelium, small RCC in 2 cases	Nephrectomy	Good	
Ossifying renal tumor of infancy[80]	9	6 d to 14 m	Gross hematuria	Tumor attached to renal papilla spindle cells.	Osteoid and osteoblastic cells mixed with	Nephrectomy	Good	
Multicystic Nephroma[81]	>100	3 m to 4 y	Same as Wilms' Tumor	Solitary, well-circumscribed, multiseptated mass surrounded by a thick fibrous capsule	Septa contain no blastemal cells	Surgery (partial nephrectomy)	Excellent	Predominantly found in boys (m:f 7:1)
Cystic partially differentiated nephroma	>100	3 m to 4 y	Same as Wilms' Tumor	Solitary, well-circumscribed, multiseptated mass surrounded by a thick fibrous capsule	Similar to multicystic nephroma but blastemal elements in septa	Nephrectomy	Good	
Cystic embryonal sarcoma of kidney[82]	28		Abdominal mass	Multilocular, friable tumor	Mesenchymal tumor cells in myxoid stroma	Nephrectomy and high-dose chemotherapy	Poor	

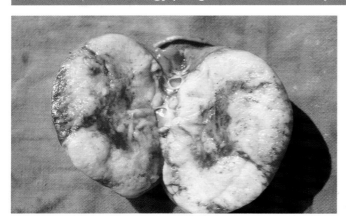

Figure 12.9: Bisected specimen of a neuroblastoma of the kidney

INTRARENAL NEUROBLASTOMA AND INTRARENAL TERATOMA

Occasionally, *neuroblastomas* may be clinically and radiologically undistinguishable from Wilms' tumors (Fig. 12.9). Elevated urinary vanillin mandelic acid levels and serum NSE should allow a differential diagnosis before surgery. In a recent series the prognosis was found to be very poor.

While sacrococcygeal *teratomas* can contain elements of Wilms' tumors and Wilms tumors have been found to produce Alpha-fetoprotein (AFP),[76] about ten cases of intrarenal teratomas have been described.[77] Assessments of AFP and β-human chorionic gonadotropin (β-hCG) are usually not performed during evaluation of a renal mass, so the diagnosis relies on histological examination. After complete resection, the prognosis should be excellent provided the tumor does not contain yolk sac elements.

OTHER RENAL NEOPLASMS IN CHILDREN

These are summarized in Table 12.4.

REFERENCES

1. Wilms M. Die Mischgeschwulste der Nieren. Leipzig, Arthur Georgi, 1899.
2. Ladd W. Embryoma of the kidney (Wilms' tumor). Ann surg 1938;108:885.
3. Breslow NE, Olshan A, Beckwith JB, et al. Ethnic variation in the incidence, diagnosis, prognosis, and follow-up of children with Wilms' tumor. J Natl Cancer Inst 1994;86: 49-51.
4. Breslow NE, Beckwith JB, Ciol M, et al. Age distribution of Wilms' tumor: report from the National Wilms' Tumor Study. Cancer Res 1988;48:1653-7.
5. Roberts DJ, Haber D, Sklar J, et al. Extrarenal Wilms' tumors. A study of their relationship with classical renal Wilms' tumor using expression of WT1 as a molecular marker. Lab Invest 1993;68:528-36.
6. Lin RY, Argenta PA, Sullivan KM, et al. Urinary hyaluronic acid is a Wilms' tumor marker. J Pediatr Surg 1995;30: 304-8.
7. Lin RY, Argenta PA, Sullivan KM, et al. Diagnostic and prognostic role of basic fibroblast growth factor in Wilms' tumor patients. Clin Cancer Res 1995;1:327-31.
8. Rebhandl W, Rami B, Turnbull J, et al. Diagnostic value of tissue polypeptide-specific antigen (TPS) in neuroblastoma and Wilms' tumour [see comments]. Br J Cancer 1998;78:1503-6.
9. Kayton ML, Rowe DH, O'Toole KM, et al. Metastasis correlates with production of vascular endothelial growth factor in a murine model of human Wilms' tumor. J Pediatr Surg 34:743-747; discussion 1999;747-8.
10. Coppes MJ. Serum biological markers and paraneoplastic syndromes in Wilms' tumor. Med Pediatr Oncol 1993;21:213-21.
11. Meisel JA, Guthrie KA, Breslow NE, et al. Significance and management of computed tomography detected pulmonary nodules: a report from the National Wilms' Tumor Study Group. Int J Radiat Oncol Biol Phys 1999;44:579-85.
12. Gow KW, Roberts IF, Jamieson DH, et al. Local staging of Wilms' tumor—computerized tomography correlation with histological findings. J Pediatr Surg 2000;35:677-9.
13. Miller RW, Fraumeni JF, Manning MD. Association of Wilms' tumor with aniridia, hemihypertrophy and other congenital malformations. N Engl J Med 1964;270: 922-7.
14. Beckwith JB. Precursor lesions of Wilms' tumor: clinical and biological implications. Med Pediatr Oncol 1993;21:158-68.
15. Huang A, Campbell CE, Bonetta L, et al. Tissue, developmental, and tumor-specific expression of divergent transcripts in Wilms' tumor. Science 1990;250:991-4.
16. Re GG, Hazen-Martin DJ, Sens DA, et al. Nephroblastoma (Wilms' tumor): a model system of aberrant renal development. Semin Diagn Pathol 1994;11:126-35.
17. Maheswaran S, Englert C, Bennett P, et al. The WT1 gene product stabilizes p53 and inhibits p53-mediated apoptosis. Genes Dev 1995;9:2143-56.
18. Bardeesy N, Beckwith JB, Pelletier J. Clonal expansion and attenuated apoptosis in Wilms' tumors are associated with p53 gene mutations. Cancer Res 1995;55:215-9.
19. Dowdy SF, Fasching CL, Araujo D, et al. Suppression of tumorigenicity in Wilms' tumor by the p15.5-p14 region of chromosome 11. Science 1991;254:293-5.
20. Soussi T. The p53 tumor suppressor gene: from molecular biology to clinical investigation. Ann N Y Acad Sci 910:121-137; discussion 2000;137-129.
21. Austruy E, Candon S, Henry I, et al. Characterization of regions of chromosomes 12 and 16 involved in nephroblastoma tumorigenesis. Genes Chromosomes Cancer 1995;14:285-94.
22. Reeve AE. Role of genomic imprinting in Wilms' tumor and overgrowth disorders. Med Pediatr Oncol 1996; 27:470-5.
23. Dao D, Walsh CP, Yuan L, et al. Multipoint analysis of human chromosome 11p15/mouse distal chromosome 7: inclusion of H19/IGF2 in the minimal WT2 region, gene specificity of H19 silencing in Wilms' tumorigenesis and methylation hyperdependence of H19 imprinting. Hum Mol Genet 1999;8:1337-52.
24. Bonaiti-Pellie C, Chompret A, Tournade MF, et al. Genetics and epidemiology of Wilms' tumor: the French Wilms' tumor study. Med Pediatr Oncol 1992;20:284-91.
25. Park S, Tomlinson G, Nisen P, et al. Altered trans-activational properties of a mutated WT1 gene product in a WAGR-associated Wilms' tumor. Cancer Res 1993;53:4757-60.

26. Jordan T, Hanson I, Zaletayev D, et al. The human PAX6 gene is mutated in two patients with aniridia. Nat Genet 1992;1:328-32.

27. Huff V. Genotype/phenotype correlations in Wilms' tumor. Med Pediatr Oncol 1996;27:408-14.

28. Porteus MH, Narkool P, Neuberg D, et al. Characteristics and outcome of children with Beckwith-Wiedemann syndrome and Wilms' tumor: a report from the National Wilms' Tumor Study Group. J Clin Oncol 2000;18:2026-31.

29. Poulat F, Morin D, Konig A, et al. Distinct molecular origins for Denys-Drash and Frasier syndromes. Hum Genet 1993;91:285-86.

30. Zuppan CW, Beckwith JB, Luckey DW. Anaplasia in unilateral Wilms' tumor: a report from the National Wilms' Tumor Study Pathology Center. Hum Pathol 1988; 19:1199-1209.

31. Zuppan CW. Handling and evaluation of pediatric renal tumors. Am J Clin Pathol 1998;109:S31-37.

32. Beckwith JB, Kiviat NB, Bonadio JF. Nephrogenic rests, nephroblastomatosis, and the pathogenesis of Wilms' tumor. Pediatr Pathol 1990;10:1-36.

33. Gururangan S, Wilimas JA, Fletcher BD. Bone metastases in Wilms' tumor—report of three cases and review of literature. Pediatr Radiol 1994;24:85-87.

34. Godzinski J, Tournade MF, De Kraker J, et al. The role of preoperative chemotherapy in the treatment of nephro-blastoma: the SIOP experience. Societe Internationale d'Oncologie Pediatrique. Semin Urol Oncol 1999;17:28-32.

35. Cooper CS, Jaffe WI, Huff DS, et al. The role of renal salvage procedures for bilateral Wilms' tumor: a 15-year review. J Urol 2000;163:265-268.

36. Horwitz JR, Ritchey ML, Moksness J, et al. Renal salvage procedures in patients with synchronous bilateral Wilms' tumors: a report from the National Wilms' Tumor Study Group. J Pediatr Surg 1996;31:1020-25.

37. Godzinski J, Tournade MF, deKraker J, et al. Rarity of surgical complications after postchemotherapy nephrec-tomy for nephroblastoma. Experience of the International Society of Pediatric Oncology-Trial and Study "SIOP-9". International Society of Pediatric Oncology Nephro-blastoma Trial and Study Committee. Eur J Pediatr Surg 1998;8:83-6.

38. Delemarre JF, Sandstedt B, Harms D, et al. The new SIOP (Stockholm) working classification of renal tumors of childhood. International Society of Pediatric Oncology [letter]. Med Pediatr Oncol 1996;26:145-6.

39. Ludwig R, Weirich A, Potter R, et al. [Preoperative chemotherapy of nephroblastoma. Preliminary results of the SIOP-9/GPO therapy study]. Klin Pediatr 1992; 204:204-13.

40. Tournade MF, Com-Nougue C, Voute PA, et al. Results of the Sixth International Society of Pediatric Oncology Wilms' Tumor Trial and Study: a risk-adapted therapeutic approach in Wilms' tumor [see comments]. J Clin Oncol 1993;11:1014-23.

41. Ritchey ML. Primary nephrectomy for Wilms' tumor: approach of the National Wilms' Tumor Study Group [editorial]. Urology 1996;47:787-91.

42. Zoeller G, Pekrun A, Lakomek M, et al. Staging problems in the pre-operative chemotherapy of Wilms' tumour [see comments]. Br J Urol 1995;76:501-03.

43. Montgomery BT, Kelalis PP, Blute ML, et al. Extended followup of bilateral Wilms' tumor: results of the National Wilms' Tumor Study. J Urol 1991;146:514-18.

44. Larsen E, Perez-Atayde A, Green DM, et al. Surgery only for the treatment of patients with stage I (Cassady) Wilms' tumor. Cancer 1990;66:264-6.

45. Davies-Johns T, Chidel M, Macklis RM. The role of radiation therapy in the management of Wilms' tumor. Semin Urol Oncol 1999;17:46-54.

46. Flentje M, Weirich A, Graf N, et al. Abdominal irradiation in unilateral nephroblastoma and its impact on local control and survival. Int J Radiat Oncol Biol Phys 1998;40:163-9.

47. Paulino AC, Wen BC, Brown CK, et al. Late effects in children treated with radiation therapy for Wilms' tumor. Int J Radiat Oncol Biol Phys 2000;46:1239-46.

48. Egeler RM, Wolff JE, Anderson RA, et al. Long-term complications and post-treatment follow-up of patients with Wilms' tumor. Semin Urol Oncol 1999;17:55-61.

49. Green DM, Donckerwolcke R, Evans AE, et al. Late effects of treatment for Wilms' tumor. Hematol Oncol Clin North Am 1995;9:1317-27.

50. Ingold J, Reed G, Kaplan H, et al. Radiation hepatitis. Am J Roentgenol 1965;200.

51. Bisogno G, de Kraker J, Weirich A, et al. Veno-occlusive disease of the liver in children treated for Wilms' tumor. Med Pediatr Oncol 1997;29:245-51.

52. Blumenfeld Z, Haim N. Prevention of gonadal damage during cytotoxic therapy. Ann Med 1997;29:199-206.

53. Li FP, Gimbrere K, Gelber RD, et al. Outcome of pregnancy in survivors of Wilms' tumor. Jama 1987;257:216-9.

54. Ritchey M, Petruzzi M. Wilms' Tumor: US Perspective, in Pediatric Surgery and Urology: Long Term Outcomes, edited by Stringer MD. MP, Oldham KT., Howard ER, London, WB Saunders Company Ltd, 1998;pp 665-75.

55. Carli M, Frascella E, Tournade MF, et al. Second malignant neoplasms in patients treated on SIOP Wilms tumour studies and trials 1, 2, 5, and 6. Med Pediatr Oncol 1997; 29:239-44.

56. Breslow NE, Takashima JR, Whitton JA, et al. Second malignant neoplasms following treatment for Wilms' tumor: a report from the National Wilms' Tumor Study Group. J Clin Oncol 1995;13:1851-9.

57. Grundy P, Breslow N, Green DM, et al. Prognostic factors for children with recurrent Wilms' tumor: results from the Second and Third National Wilms' Tumor Study. J Clin Oncol 1989;7:638-47.

58. Dagher R, Kreissman S, Robertson KA, et al. High dose chemotherapy with autologous peripheral blood progenitor cell transplantation in an anephric child with multiply recurrent Wilms' tumor. J Pediatr Hematol Oncol 1998;20:357-60.

59. Biemann Othersen H. TE, Garvin AJ. Wilms' Tumor, in Pediatric Surgery (vol One), edited by O'Neill JA. RM, Grossfeld JL., Fonkalsrud EW., Coran AG., Fifth Edition ed, St. Louis, Missouri, Mosby, 1998;pp 391-403.

60. Paulino AC, Thakkar B, Henderson WG. Metachronous bilateral Wilms' tumor: the importance of time interval to the development of a second tumor. Cancer 1998;82:415-20.

61. Renshaw AA. Pediatric renal cell carcinomas: where do they fit in the new histologic classification of renal cell carcinoma? Adv Anat Pathol 2000;7:135-40.

62. Carcao MD, Taylor GP, Greenberg ML, et al. Renal-cell carcinoma in children: a different disorder from its adult counterpart? Med Pediatr Oncol 1998;31:153-8.

63. Castellanos RD, Aron BS, Evans AT. Renal adeno-carcinoma in children: incidence, therapy and prognosis. J Urol 1974;111:534-7.

64. Skoldenberg EG, Jakobson A, Elvin A, et al. Pretreatment, ultrasound-guided cutting needle biopsies in childhood renal tumors. Med Pediatr Oncol 1999;32:283-8.

65. Dehner LP, Leestma JE, Price EB, Jr. Renal cell carcinoma in children: a clinicopathologic study of 15 cases and review of the literature. J Pediatr 1970;76:358-68.

66. O'Toole KM, Brown M, Hoffmann P. Pathology of benign and malignant kidney tumors. Urol Clin North Am 1993; 20:193-205.

67. Argani P, Beckwith JB. Metanephric stromal tumor: report of 31 cases of a distinctive pediatric renal neoplasm. Am J Surg Pathol 2000;24:917-26.

68. Kidd J. Exclusion of certain neoplasms from the category of Wilms' Tumor [abstract]. Am J Pathol 1970;59:16.

69. Weeks DA, Beckwith JB, Mierau GW, et al. Rhabdoid tumor of kidney. A report of 111 cases from the National Wilms' Tumor Study Pathology Center. Am J Surg Pathol 1989;13:439-58.

70. Versteege I, Sevenet N, Lange J, et al. Truncating mutations of hSNF5/INI1 in aggressive pediatric cancer. Nature 1998;394:203-6.

71. Bolande RP, Brough AJ, Izant RJ, Jr. Congenital meso-blastic nephroma of infancy. A report of eight cases and the relationship to Wilms' tumor. Pediatrics 1967;40:272-8.

72. Howell CG, Othersen HB, Kiviat NE, et al. Therapy and outcome in 51 children with mesoblastic nephroma: a report of the National Wilms' Tumor Study. J Pediatr Surg 1982;17:826-31.

73. Knezevich SR, Garnett MJ, Pysher TJ, et al. ETV6-NTRK3 gene fusions and trisomy 11 establish a histogenetic link between mesoblastic nephroma and congenital fibro-sarcoma. Cancer Res 1998;58:5046-8.

74. Rubin BP, Chen CJ, Morgan TW, et al. Congenital mesoblastic nephroma t(12;15) is associated with ETV6-NTRK3 gene fusion: cytogenetic and molecular relationship to congenital (infantile) fibrosarcoma. Am J Pathol 1998;153:1451-8.

75. Martignoni G, Pea M, Rigaud G, et al. Renal angio-myolipoma with epithelioid sarcomatous transformation and metastases: demonstration of the same genetic defects in the primary and metastatic lesions. Am J Surg Pathol 2000;24:889-94.

76. Patriarca C, Orazi A, Massimino M, et al. A cystic partially differentiated nephroblastoma producing alpha-fetoprotein. Am J Pediatr Hematol Oncol 1992;14:352-5.

77. Argani P, Beckwith JB. Metanephric stromal tumor: report of 31 cases of a distinctive pediatric renal neoplasm. Am J Surg Pathol 2000;24:917-26.

78. Aubert J, Casamayou J, Denis P, et al. Intrarenal teratoma in a newborn child. Eur Urol 1978;4:306-8.

79. Hennigar RA, Beckwith JB. Nephrogenic adenofibroma. A novel kidney tumor of young people. Am J Surg Pathol 1992;16:325-34.

80. Sotelo-Avila C, Beckwith JB, Johnson JE. Ossifying renal tumor of infancy: a clinicopathologic study of nine cases [see comments]. Pediatr Pathol Lab Med 1995;15:745-62.

81. Sacher P, Willi UV, Niggli F, et al. Cystic nephroma: a rare benign renal tumor. Pediatr Surg Int 1998;13:197-9.

82. Delahunt B, Beckwith JB, Eble JN, et al. Cystic embryonal sarcoma of kidney: a case report. Cancer 1998;82:2427-33.

Wilms' Tumor in South Africa

In the Western World the problems of Wilms' tumor have to a large extent been solved.[1] Research effort can now be directed towards reducing the intensity of treatment and refining nosology to incorporate an ever increasing and bewildering array of genes and gene products.[2] The aim in developed countries is to reduce the long-term toxicity of treatment and more precisely identify risk.[3] Survival is virtually assured.[4]

In Africa, and indeed throughout much of the Third World, this is not the case. The management of children with Wilms' tumor is complicated by the Third World Triad of late presentation, advanced disease and associated illnesses.[5,6] Each element of this triad presents the clinician with a number of challenges. The biggest challenge of all is to achieve survival.

As international migrations present First World physicians with increasing numbers of immigrants from former colonies, a deeper interest may develop in the problems encountered in countries such as South Africa and India, and the approaches that have been developed.

Having a Wilms' tumor does not protect the child from the environment. Poverty, poor nutrition (Fig. 13.1), infections and infestations, social deprivation and poor education affect those children with tumors just as intensely as those without.[7] Protocols that have been demonstrated to be effective in Europe and America may be inappropriate in a setting where patients cannot afford to travel to a treatment center on a regular basis, cannot afford drugs and there is competition for limited family resources from unaffected siblings.

Mothers may be unable to accompany the patient when there are siblings that require attention at home and patients may therefore be abandoned at the treatment center. Protocols must accommodate the severely malnourished, those with HIV disease (Fig. 13.2), tuberculosis and a myriad of other disorders that would alarm those who have been brought up to think of Wilms' tumor as something that occurs in the otherwise healthy child.

Each comorbidity has a mortality of its own and can reasonably be considered a poor prognostic factor. It is

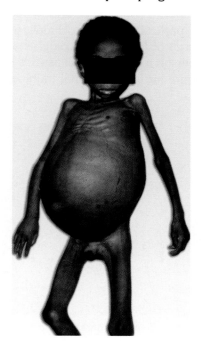

Figure 13.1: Child with Wilms' tumor at presentation. Wasting due to a poor premorbid diet, rapid tumor growth and anorexia, is evident

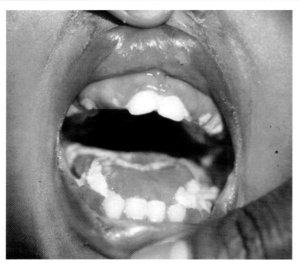

Figure 13.2: Oral candidiasis in a patient with Wilms' tumor. As HIV screening is not considered ethically justifiable diagnosis is often based on clinical findings

the child that needs management, not the Wilms' tumor. Compounding variables such as the availability of chemotherapy, blood and blood products, antibiotics and other medications become the legitimate concern of the surgeon. In addition, over-riding these variables, is the faith of many communities in traditional healers and healing methods that can delay presentation (Fig. 13.3), interfere with compliance and preclude essential interventions, particularly surgery.[8] Finally in many areas there is a dearth of Pediatric Oncologists and often the best placed person to supervise all aspects of care is the surgeon, despite his lack of formal training in pediatric oncology.[5]

INCIDENCE

Statistics from the Third World can be difficult to interpret as population data are either incomplete or not available. In US studies the incidence of Wilms' tumor is appreciably higher in patients of African origin. In South Africa the Children's Cancer Registry has recorded an annual incidence of 4.7 per 100,000 children. This is certainly a low estimate and does not include patients treated outside the state sector. The Registry estimates that it records just over half of the childhood tumors occurring in the country. Six state hospitals in South Africa treat approximately 100 new patients per annum.

PRESENTATION

Delay in presentation is manifest in the size of tumors at presentation and the advanced age and stage at which patients are first seen (Fig. 13.4).

Emphasis on advanced local disease must not obscure the high incidence of metastatic disease at presentation (Fig. 13.5).

The frequency of locally advanced and metastatic disease in patients presenting to a unit in Durban can be appreciated graphically (Fig. 13.6). As staging is a postoperative exercise, unstaged patients represent those who died before operation or refused surgery.

Advanced disease can also be manifest by intracaval and intracardiac extension of the tumor (Fig. 13.7). Although some such extensions respond to neoadjuvant chemotherapy approximately half will require excision under cardiac bypass.[9] Surgery of such tumors should be planned with this possibility in mind. More typical caval extension (Fig. 13.8) can be approached through

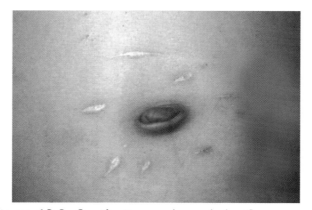

Figure 13.3: Scarification marks made by iSangoma, or traditional healer, in a child with Wilms' tumor. Note that the marks have healed indicating the delay in presentation

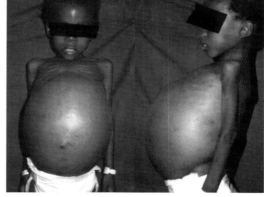

Figure 13.4: Advanced local disease at presentation. The large abdominal tumor, muscle wasting and restriction of chest movement is evident

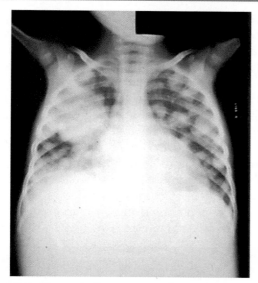

Figure 13.5: Cannonball metastases of Wilms' tumor in a child presenting for treatment

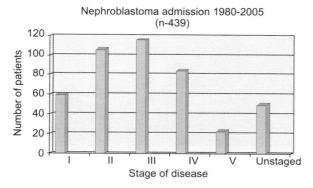

Figure 13.6: Stage-wise distribution of 439 cases of nephroblastoma seen from 1980-2005

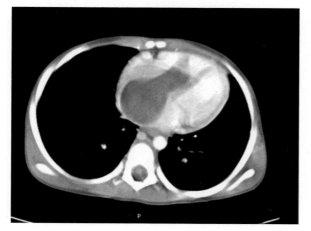

Figure 13.7: Intracardiac extension of Wilms' tumor which, having filled the right atrium has herniated through the tricuspid valve to compromise function of the right ventricle

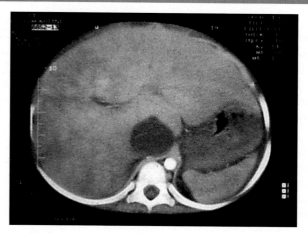

Figure 13.8: Intracaval extension into the retrohepatic inferior vena cava

the abdomen if the proximal extent of the thrombus lies below the hepatic veins (Fig. 13.9). In a series of 383 children with Wilms' tumor caval extension was identified in 33 (9%) but not all was identified preoperatively. Ultrasound evaluation of the cava can define flow, or an absence of flow, but cannot distinguish between compression by tumor or intravascular thrombus.[10] The surgeon is still ultimately responsible for identifying intracaval tumor at operation.

These manifestations of advanced disease simply reflect the rapidity of growth of Wilms' tumor. A tumor doubling time in the region of 28 days must emphasise that any delay in presentation or investigation prior to starting effective therapy is unjustifiable.[11]

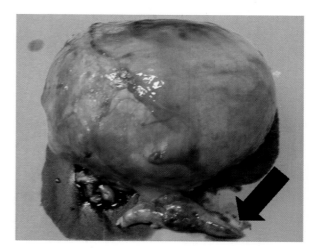

Figure 13.9: Right Wilms' tumor removed *en bloc* with caval extension (arrow). Note that tumor extends both proximally and distally within the cava

Paraneoplastic effects of Wilms' tumor must be sought and identified at presentation. 51 percent of 383 consecutive children presenting with Wilms' tumor were hypertensive and complications including stroke (Fig. 13.10), cerebral atrophy, hypertensive encephalopathy and left ventricular failure were identified, each requiring specific non-oncological intervention.[12]

At presentation care should be taken to assess the patients' socioeconomic status. In South Africa all treatment for children under the age of six years is free. This relieves the clinician of the anxieties of attracting funding. For children over the age of six care is usually provided free of charge unless the parents have medical insurance. This is rare. Radiotherapy is readily available at all major treatment centers.

INVESTIGATION

It should be clear from the above that a full range of laboratory services is essential to the primary assessment of the child with Wilms' tumor and these are usually only available at tertiary institutions. For this reason, if for no other, treatment of childhood solid tumors should be centralized.

In our practice following clinical assessment, including blood pressure measurement, simple anthropometric measurements such as height, weight, triceps skin-fold thickness and mid-arm circumference are taken. Blood is taken for a complete blood count, assessment of renal function, liver function, serum renin if the initial blood pressure was elevated, and estimation of calcium and phosphate levels.

Stools are sent for parasitology and urine is sent for definition of microscopic hematuria as well as culture.

Imaging starts with ultrasound examination not to identify the tumor, that is usually all too obvious, but to assess the contralateral kidney, retroperitoneal lymph nodes and the inferior vena cava. CT scan is routine and allows more precise definition of the contralateral kidney (Fig. 13.11), liver and lung.

In our practice 6 percent of patients have synchronous occult disease in the contralateral kidney.

CT also forms the basis for objective assessment of the initial response to treatment (Fig. 13.12), and is essential when planning nephron-sparing surgery in patients with bilateral tumors (Fig. 13.13). The proximal

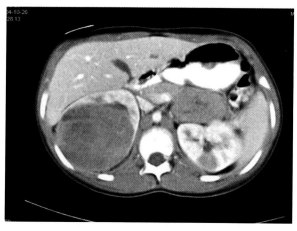

Figure 13.11: Transverse CT scan of child who presented for repair of hypospadias. The right-sided tumor was palpable. Biopsies confirmed bilateral Wilms' tumor

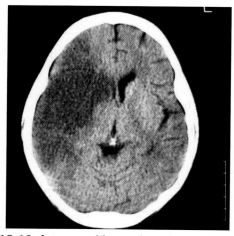

Figure 13.10: Intracranial hemorrhage in a patient presenting with Wilms' tumor and hemiplegia. There was remarkable neurological recovery following removal of the kidney and postoperative chemotherapy

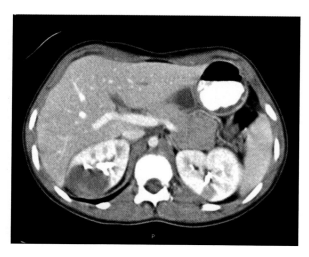

Figure 13.12: Transverse CT scan of the same patient shown in Figure 13.11 demonstrating the response to four weeks' neoadjuvant chemotherapy

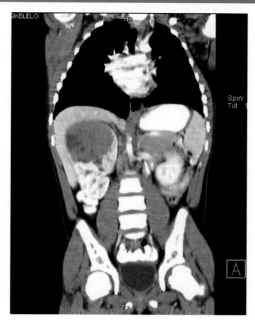

Figure 13.13: Coronal CT image of the same patient demonstrating the potential for an upper pole nephrectomy on the left

extent of caval thrombus is best defined by echocardiography (Fig. 13.14).

Preoperative fine needle aspiration cytology or core needle biopsy reduces the risk of diagnostic error.

PRIMARY TREATMENT

In America it has long been assumed that early removal of the primary tumor is essential to survival.[13] This has been challenged by the European group who have demonstrated results that are at least as good as the

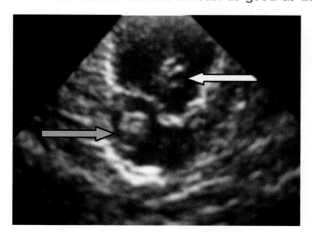

Figure 13.14: Echocardiograph showing thrombus in the right atrium (gray arrow) as well as within the right ventricle (white arrow)

American results using neoadjuvant chemotherapy.[14] Following chemotherapy tumors are smaller, of lower stage and more easily removed.[15] This is now accepted also by the NWTS protocol that advises neoadjuvant chemotherapy whenever preoperative imaging suggests that a "formidable" operation would be necessary.[16] In the Third World a period of chemotherapy allows nutritional status to be improved and acute comorbidities, e.g. hypertension, to be treated as well as improving the surgical risk. Neoadjuvant chemotherapy has therefore been adopted as the norm in our environment.

In neonates, where there is a greater likelihood of a benign renal tumor such as mesoblastic nephroma, primary surgery is offered.

OPERATIVE MANAGEMENT

Surgeons operating on patients with Wilms' tumor should follow a strict surgical protocol that recognizes the dual function of the operation; complete removal of the tumor and accurate staging of the disease. It is not an area for the occasional pediatric oncolgical surgeon.[15]

Accurate staging should include cytological examination of peritoneal fluid retrieved prior to mobilization of abdominal structures. Sixteen percent of our patients have been upstaged following the finding of malignant cells in peritoneal fluid in the absence of positive lymph nodes.[17] Additionally the contralateral kidney must be exposed and inspected and the liver carefully palpated. Para-aortic lymph node biopsy is essential.

It is important to review recent imaging before starting an operation in order to enhance safety. Displacement of the great vessels and their branches predisposes them to injury by the unwary (Fig. 13.15).

Surgery also has a role to play in the management of solitary lung and liver metastases. Peripheral lesions can readily be removed thoracoscopically. Multiple lesions are probably best treated with radiotherapy.

POSTOPERATIVE MANAGEMENT

Complications are related to the extent of the primary surgery.[15] Despite tumor reduction by neoadjuvant chemotherapy, in 25 percent of our patients the resected specimen weighed more than 1.0 kg and represented a median of 12 percent of the patient's pre-operative mass. In such large tumors there is an increased risk to neighboring viscera and to the sequelae of increased blood loss (Table 13.1).

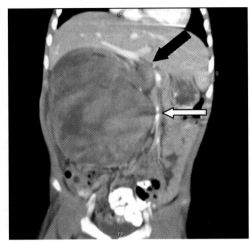

Figure 13.15: Coronal CT scan showing typical displacement of the inferior vena cava (white arrow) by a right-sided Wilms' tumor. Thrombus within the cava is evident (black arrow)

Postoperative analgesia is best provided by a continuous epidural infusion of local anesthetic with or without the addition of regional opioids.

It is impossible to overemphasize the importance of nutritional support in these children. Caloric intake must be maintained despite chemotherapy induced anorexia and nausea, and we aim to provide 120-150 percent of the estimated energy requirement. Overnight tube feeds are a useful supplement to a hospital diet. Nutrition is directly related to survival. This relationship in our own patients is described graphically in Figure 13.16, wherein ponderal index is derived from anthropometric data gathered at the time of admission.[18]

Given the limited resources of many Third World countries attention must be paid to those available

criteria that indicate a poor prognosis. Prime amongst these is the histological appearance of the tumor. Unfavorable histology, beyond tumor limited to the kidney, has such a poor prognosis that the yield of treatment is negligible.[19] Every patient deserves to be treated according to a protocol of proven value and in Africa that means following the precepts of SIOP.

RESULTS

Despite the many negative factors impinging on care of the child with Wilms' tumor in the Third World, clinicians' efforts are rewarded with generally satisfactory long-term survival. By any measure the resources allocated to the care of these children can be shown to be a worthwhile investment.[20,21]

In Durban, of 460 children presenting between 1976 and 2004, the two year survival is reflected in Table 13.2.

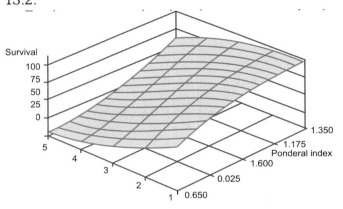

Figure 13.16: The relationship between ponderal index and survival for each stage of Wilms' tumor. Data derived from 47 consecutive patients[17]

Table 13.1: Intra- and postoperative complications in 64 patients with resected tumors greater than 1.0 kg	
Cardiac arrest	2
Resection adjacent organs	15 (22%)
Diaphragm (6), Spleen (3), Pancreas (4), Colon (2), Jejunum (1), Liver (2)	
Tumor spillage	14
Localized (4), Generalized (10)	
Intestinal obstruction	9
Intussusception (2), Adhesions (8), Volvulus (1)	
Bleeding	2 (requiring re-operation)
Wound complications	8
Dehiscence (2), Infection (4), Hernia (2)	
Death	1
Abdominal compartment syndrome	

Table 13.2: Survival of 460 children related to stage of disease

Stage I	(n=67)	93 percent
Stage II	(n=110)	85 percent
Stage III	(n=126)	72 percent
Stage IV	(n=88)	31 percent
Stage V	(n=21)	33 percent
Unstaged	(n=47)	

presentation. Although the majority of patients present with advanced disease, the survival rate for early stage disease is comparable to First World centers. There is clearly room for improvement in the management of metastatic disease.

REFERENCES

1. Metzger ML, Dome JS. Current therapy for Wilms' tumour. The Oncologist 2005;10:815-26.
2. Takahashi M, Yang XJ, Lavry TT, Furge KA, Williams BO, et al. Gene expression profiling of favourable histology Wilms' tumors and its correlation with clinical features. Cancer Res 2002; 62(22):6598-605.
3. Coppes MJ, Egeler RM. Genetics of Wilms' tumour. Seminars in Urol Oncol 1999; 17(1): 2-10.
4. Pritchard-Jones K. Controversies and advances in the management of Wilms' tumour. Arch Dis Childh 2002; 87:241-4.
5. Hadley GP. The Paediatric Surgeon in Africa: Luxury or necessity. East and Central Afr J Surg 2004;9(2):104-9.
6. Abdallah FK, Macharia WM. Clinical presentation and treatment outcome in children with nephroblastoma in Kenya. E Afr Med J 2001;78(7)S:S43-7.
7. Hadley GP, Jacobs C. The clinical presentation of Wilms' tumour in black children. S Afr Med J 1990;77:565-7.
8. Lusu T, Buhlungu N, Grant HW. The attitudes of parents to traditional medicine and the surgeon. S Afr Med J 2001;91:270-1.
9. Giannoulia-Karadana A, Moschovi M, Koutsovitis P, et al. Inferior vena cava and right atrial thrombosis in children with nephroblastoma: Diagnostic and therapeutic problems. J Pediatr Surg 2000;35(10):1459-61.
10. Solwa Y, Sanyika C, Hadley GP, Corr P. Colour Doppler ultrasound assessment of the inferior vena cava in patients with Wilms' tumour. Clin Radiol 1999;54(12):811-4.
11. Zoubek A, Slavc I, Mann G, Trittenwein G, Gadner H. Natural course of a Wilms' tumour. The Lancet 1999; 354:344.
12. Hadley GP, Mars M. Hypertension in a cohort of African children with renal tumours. Pediatr Surg Int 2006 (in Press).
13. Ross JH, Kay R. Surgical considerations for patients with Wilms' tumor. Seminar in Urol Oncol 1999;17(1):33-9.
14. Tournade MF, Com-Nougué C, de Kraker J, et al. Optimal duration of pre-operative therapy in unilateral and non-metastatic Wilms' tumour in children older than 6 months: Results of the Ninth International Society of Pediatric Oncology Wilms' tumour trial and study. J Clin Oncol 2001;19(2):488-500.
15. Hadley GP, Bösenberg AT. Surgery for Wilms' tumour. Paediatr Surg Int 1995;10:362-5.
16. Ritchey ML. The role of pre-operative chemotherapy for Wilms' tumor: The NWTSG perspective. Sem Urol Oncol 1999;17(1): 21-7.
17. Hadley GP, Steenhuisen K. Peritoneal fluid cytology in Wilms' tumour: A staging investigation Proceedings of the 2nd Meeting of SIOP in Africa 1996.
18. Hadley GP, Gouws E. Nutritional indices and treatment outcome in children with Wilms' tumour in the Third World. Med and Ped Oncol 1991;19(5):348.
19. Hadley GP, Landers G, Govender D. Wilms' tumour with unfavourable histology, implications for clinicians in the Third World. Med and Ped Oncol 2001;36;652-3.
20. Madani A, Zafod S, Harif M, et al. Treatment of Wilms' tumour according to SIOP 9 protocol in Casablanca, Morocco. Pediatr Blood Cancer 2005; July epub.
21. Nkrumah FK, Danzo AK, Kumar R. Wilms' tumour (nephroblastoma) in Zimbabwe. Ann Trop Paediatr 1998;44(10):242-5.

CHAPTER 14

Devendra K Gupta
Shilpa Sharma

Bilateral Wilms' Tumor

Bilateral Wilms' tumors present a therapeutic challenge for the pediatric surgeon. Delayed presentation, poor response to chemotherapy and associated nephro-blastomatosis contribute to the multifold difficulties in proper management.

The primary aim of treatment is eradication of neoplasm with preservation of the renal function. Achieving curative resection of such tumors by partial nephrectomy or tumor enucleation while maintaining sufficient renal function represents a surgical challenge. Effective preoperative chemotherapy facilitates this aim considerably. With the modern diagnostic facilities, synchronous bilateral Wilms' tumors have been reported to be successfully managed in a neonate.[1] However, a case of bilateral Wilms' tumor in a stillborn fetus who could not be saved despite monitoring pregnancy by frequent sonography has also been reported.[2]

INCIDENCE

Bilateral Wilms' tumor occurs in 5-10 percent of all cases of nephroblastoma. In the NWTS studies, approximately 4-6 percent of children registered presented with synchronous bilateral tumors. The metachronous form represents 2-3 percent of cases.

The male-to-female ratio is 1:2, and the patients are usually younger at diagnosis. It was found that more bilateral or multifocal tumors occur at an earlier age (2 years versus 3.6 years in sporadic tumors). Some have reported an even lower median age of 1.1 years for bilateral tumors compared with 3.5 years for unilateral tumors.[3]

A high frequency of bilaterality as well as the male preponderance has been reported in some parts of the world like UAE, different from that reported in other parts of the world; reflecting regional variations of Wilms' tumor.[4]

ETIOLOGY

Familial WT

Wilms' tumor (WT) is an embryonic tumor arising from undifferentiated renal mesenchyme and has been a productive model for understanding the role of genes in both tumorigenesis and normal organogenesis. Approximately 2 percent of WT patients have a family history of WT, and even sporadic WT is thought to have a strong genetic component to its etiology. Familial WT cases generally have an earlier age of onset and an increased frequency of bilateral disease, although there is variability among WT families, with some families displaying later than average ages at diagnosis. Two familial WT genes have been localized, FWT1 at 17q12-q21 and FWT2 at 19q13.4; lack of linkage in some WT families to either of these loci implies the existence of at least one additional familial WT gene.[5]

It has also been seen that early age of diagnosis and bilaterality are not by themselves efficient predictors of germline WT1 alterations in WT patients without associated abnormalities.[6]

In newborns with severe urogenital malformations, not due to known chromosomal or endocrine disorders, mutational screening of the WT1 gene should be performed, to evaluate the high risk of developing a

Wilms' tumor. Mutational screening in these patients may be an easy tool for investigation.[7] Bilateral Wilms' tumor has also been reported in brothers pointing to a genetic basis.[8]

Among 6,209 patients with Wilms' tumor entered on the National Wilms' Tumor Study (NWTS), 1.5 percent had a positive family history. 16.1 percent of the familial, but only 7.1 percent of sporadic cases had bilateral disease.[9] Mean ages at diagnosis were 15.8 vs 35.2 months (p = 0.012) for bilateral vs unilateral familial cases. Intralobar nephrogenic rests were found twice as frequently in association with the tumors of familial than as with those of sporadic cases. Cases of bilateral and metastatic disease tended to cluster within specific families, suggesting heterogeneity in the genetic etiology.[9] The number and age distribution of familial cases transmitted through the father were about the same as those of cases transmitted through the mother. This finding is inconsistent with models of genomic imprinting that involve familial transmission of a tumor-suppressor gene and it casts further doubt on the hypothesis that all bilateral cases are hereditary.[9]

Wilms' tumor develops from nephrogenic blastema rests that usually disappear after 34 weeks of gestation. Pediatric autopsies show that blastematous foci may persist after birth without necessarily forming nephroblastomas. Their frequency is one hundred times higher than that of nephroblastomas although they are often associated. Wilms' tumors are hereditary and more frequent in patients with congenital malformations related to genetic disorders.[2]

Nephroblastomatosis

Nephroblastomatosis is the persistence of embryonal renal tissue, a facultatively precancerous lesion, which requires quarterly sonographic controls and which can induce a second metachronous contralateral Wilms' tumor.

Nephroblastomatosis was identified in 95 percent patients in a series of 19 patients of bilateral Wilms' tumor.[10] Nephroblastomatosis requires close monitoring because Wilms' tumors develop in residual suspect areas. Revision tumorectomy for recurrence in areas of nephroblastomatosis has been found effective.[10] Hyperplastic perilobar nephroblastomatosis (HPLN) is a self-limited, pre-neoplastic proliferative process associated with a high risk of developing WT. Ninety-four percent lesions have been found to be bilateral and the mean age at diagnosis is 16 months. The

accurate diagnosis and the choices of therapy during the often-complex course of HPLN depend on the availability and accurate interpretation of a combination of pathologic, radiologic, and clinical information. When such information is appropriately obtained, the long-term survival of patients with HPLN is excellent.[11]

Nephrogenic Rests (NRs)

A significantly increased risk of metachronous bilateral Wilms' tumor has been reported in patients with nephrogenic rests (NRs).[12] It has also been confirmed there is an increased relative risk associated with younger age and presence of NRs.[12] Children younger than 12 months diagnosed with Wilms' tumor who also have NRs, in particular perilobar NRs, have a markedly increased risk of developing contralateral disease and require frequent and regular surveillance for several years. Surveillance is also recommended for those with NRs who are diagnosed after the age of 12 months.[12] Given the high incidence of coexisting nephrogenic rests in bilateral Wilms' tumor, careful follow-up is required, as these potentially premalignant rests may resist chemotherapy.[13]

ASSOCIATED ANOMALIES

Some of the clinical stigmata known to be associated with Wlms' tumors are especially linked with bilaterality—mainly cryptorchidism and hypospadias.[14] 17.5 percent of 108 cases of metachronous bilateral Wilms' tumor in a series had a congenital anomaly.[15] The frequency of genitourinary anomalies (16%) and hemihypertrophy (5.4%) has been found to be higher compared to unilateral disease.[8] Beckwith-Wiedemann syndrome has also been reported in association with bilateral Wilms'.[13,16]

SYNCHRONOUS, METACHRONOUS AND EXTRARENAL RELAPSES

The metachronous form represents 2-3 percent of cases. Metachronous bilateral tumors have been reported in about 1.5 percent of NWTS patients (58 of 4,669 registered children). Since many of these lesions appear to be overlooked at initial laparotomy, a thorough investigation of the opposite kidney remains crucial. The cumulative risk of contralateral disease as a function of time since initial presentation has been calculated as 1 minus the Kaplan-Meier estimate of remaining free of contralateral disease.[12] The median interval of diagnosis of metachronous Wilms' tumor ranges from 1.37 (NWTS) to 3.29 (SIOP) years. The appearance of a metachronous Wilms' tumor 5 years after that of the primary tumor is rare but a metachronous relapse of Wilms' tumor 7 years after the first diagnosis has been reported.[17]

Synchronous tumors are those appearing at the same time and require proper evaluation and planning of the treatment options for maximal retention of renal function for the particular case (Fig. 14.1).

There may be extrarenal relapses.[10] A nephroblastoma was diagnosed in the retroperitoneal space 14 years after the patient had completed a complex therapy for bilateral Wilms' tumor. This has been related to the survival of metanephros located outside the kidney.[18] Metastatic spread outside the kidney has a poor prognosis.

INVESTIGATIONS

Investigations are required to make the diagnosis, determine the tumor volume, follow the response to chemotherapy, and determine the operability of the tumor.
1. Ultrasonography is good for diagnosis and to see the state of the venacaval involvement.
2. Skiagram abdomen may be done for any evidence of calcification.
3. Fine needle aspiration cytology (FNAC) is helpful for tissue diagnosis.

4. CT scan of abdomen and chest is important to look for metastasis and lymph node involvement (Fig. 14.2).
5. Positron emission tomography (PET). Wilms tumors can concentrate 18F-FDG thus evaluation of the metabolic activity of these neoplasms can be done with PET with 2-[fluorine-18]-fluoro-2-deoxy-D-glucose (FDG) scanning. PET can be used to search for skeletal metastases, evaluate renal function and influence the therapeutic decisions in patients with bilateral Wilms'.[19]

While in earlier days, surgical exploration of the contralateral kidney was the only method to detect a contralateral tumor; the necessity of this method of assessment has been questioned with introduction of modern imaging techniques like CT scan and NMR.[20] However, some have reported that imaging may still miss upto 50 percent of the lesions below 1 cm in its greatest dimension.[14,21]

DIFFERENTIAL DIAGNOSIS

1. *Non-Hodgkin's lymphoma:* Bilateral renal involvement is present in 25-50 percent of children with B-cell non-Hodgkin's lymphoma.[22] Pediatric oncologists therefore encounter bilateral renal disease relatively frequently. Renal failure due to the infiltration of both kidneys by lymphoma may be treated successfully by chemotherapy. There is

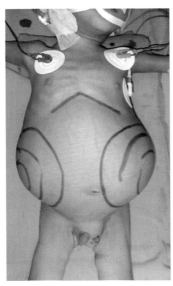

Figure 14.1: Synchronous bilateral Wilms' tumor in a child presenting with abdominal masses

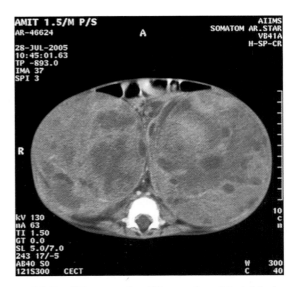

Figure 14.2: CT scan of a 22 months old child showing bilateral Wilms' tumor. There was not much response after 2 cycles of chemotherapy. Right partial lower pole nephrectomy and left nephroureterectomy were done simultaneously

complete reversibility of the damage up to some critical point, beyond which, failure and atrophy result.

2. *Pyonephroma:* Multiple intrarenal abscesses may simulate multiple necrotic tumor masses.

MANAGEMENT

Management of stage V Wilms' tumor is tailored to the individual case, being as conservative as possible to spare renal parenchyma. The assessment of resectability may become particularly problematic in bilateral or multifocal Wilms' tumors and in nephroblastomatosis.[23]

Management of Synchronous Wilms' Tumor

The management of children with synchronous BWT still needs standardization. The presence of synchronous bilateral disease requires alteration of management.

It is not recommended to perform unilateral nephrectomy and contralateral biopsy or heminephrectomy. Initial attempts at radical surgery have given way to the current use of preoperative chemotherapy to preserve as much kidney tissue as possible. For staging, biopsies of both lesions are taken, especially when both kidneys contain a large tumor. Preoperative chemotherapy (vincristine and actinomycin-D in case of FH) may facilitate subsequent second look.

If the histology is unfavorable, intensive chemotherapy (addition of doxorubicin and cyclophosphamide) is followed by radiation. After chemotherapy, the patient is reassessed with abdominal CT to determine the feasibility of resection. For small synchronous bilateral lesions at the poles, bilateral partial nephrectomies or wedge resections can be performed. Excisional biopsy or partial nephrectomy is regarded as appropriate only if radical tumor resection is not compromised, negative margins can be obtained and if two-thirds of the renal parenchyma can be preserved. The goal is to achieve survival and at the same time to preserve an adequate amount of renal parenchyma. In case of a large tumor on one side and a contralateral small one, radical tumor nephrectomy on the extensively involved site and partial nephrectomy on the opposite side is done (Figs 14.3A to C). A third look may be indicated; bilateral nephrectomy and subsequent renal transplantation remain the last issue. With preoperative treatment, usually chemotherapy only, overall survival has become quite favorable in this group of patients, approaching 83 percent at 2 years.[24] This has facilitated the use of parenchymal-sparing operations, with the potential

advantage of decreasing the incidence of end-stage renal disease (Fig. 14.4).

Bilateral multiple small tumors have been treated successfully with chemotherapy with normal renal function and no evidence of disease 3 years after diagnosis.[13] Synchronous tumors have been found to have a better prognosis than metachronous tumors.[25]

Unfortunately, due to immunosuppression, recurrence of disease occurs frequently. Before considering bilateral nephrectomy, bench surgery with autotransplantation and intraoperative radiotherapy may be performed. Current recommendation is to wait at least 1-2 yr after completion of chemotherapy for Wilms' tumor before renal transplantation. Most children dialyzed because of Wilms' tumor and Denys-Drash syndrome who did not receive a renal transplant died of Wilms' tumor. However, current practices in children with Wilms' tumor and Denys-Drash syndrome appear to show good outcome following renal transplantation comparable with children with other diagnoses undergoing renal transplantation.[26]

Management of Metachronous Wilms' Tumor

The median time interval to the development of a second tumor was 23.1 months on analysis of metachronous bilateral Wilms' tumor from 30 studies.[27] Screening by abdominal ultrasound of the contralateral kidney for ≤ 5 years after initial diagnosis of Wilms' tumor may not be necessary because 96.2 percent of children had a time interval to the development of a second tumor of ≤ or = 60 months.[27] When a contralateral tumour develops, chemotherapy must be given until the size of the tumor is reduced in order to preserve renal function and avoid dialysis. Nephrectomy may be needed in only a few complicated cases leading to anephria and chronic renal failure with dependency on dialysis.

Partial nephrectomy in unilateral Wilms' tumor is recommended by some in patients who present with known risk factors for bilaterality.[14]

Chemotherapy

Neoadjuvant chemotherapy has become an acceptable and mainstay of treatment for cases of bilateral Wilms' tumor. Reduction of tumor volume of upto 50 percent on an average has been reported. This results in converting primarily inoperable tumors to become suitable for parenchymal-sparing procedures. The added advantage includes reduced incidence of intraoperative tumor rupture that also results in decreased need for

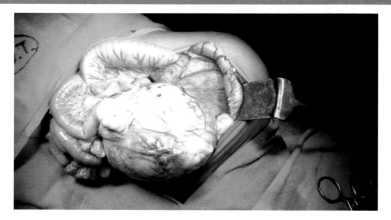

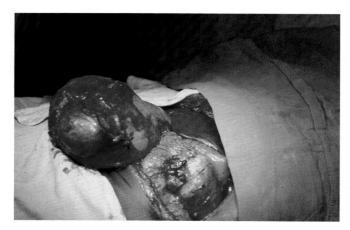

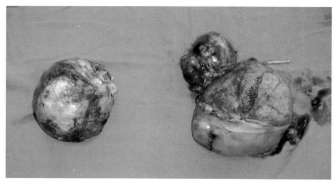

Figures 14.3A to C: (A) Operative photograph showing bilateral Wilms' tumor in a child. **(B)** Operative photograph showing the bigger tumor in a case of bilateral Wilms' tumor. **(C)** Resected specimens of partial nephrectomy and nephroureterectomy

radiotherapy with its harmful effects in young children.

For patients with tumors with favorable histology, two drugs actinomycin-D and vincristine are given. For

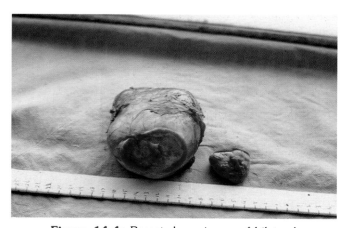

Figure 14.4: Resected specimens of bilateral tumorectomies in a case of bilateral Wilms' tumor

unfavorable histology and advanced inoperable tumors, three drugs, actinomycin-D, adriamycin and vincristine are given. The duration of neo-adjuvant chemotherapy may be prolonged in cases with bilateral Wilms' tumor till there is tumor response as evaluated by serial imaging modalities. The operation is planned at the time there is no more tumor response. This may range from a period of 4 weeks to 12 weeks. Too prolonged chemotherapy beyond cessation of good response may result in tumor progression. Also, the adverse effects and complications of chemotherapy like veno-occlussive disease may preclude its continuation and delay surgical treatment leading to tumor progression.

Conservative surgery and simple outpatient-based, low toxicity chemotherapy has been found to be curative in most patients.[3] Univariate Cox Regression analysis demonstrated that sites receiving two drugs had a statistically significant increase in loco-regional relapse when compared to sites receiving three drugs (p = 0.004).[28]

Salvage chemotherapy regimens using cis-plantinum, ifosphamide and VP-16 has also been found useful.[29] Spectacular cure rates can be achieved in BWT by renal conservation surgeries and effective chemotherapy.[29]

Renal Salvage Surgery

Several kidneys, which would have been sacrificed by application of traditional criteria, could be salvaged by atypical and unconventional tumor resections and by superficial dissection and enucleation of supposed nephroblastomatosis. Atypical resections of localized lesions and superficial dissections of suspected nephroblastomatosis appeared as valid surgical treatment options for patients who would otherwise have been candidates for nephrectomy. Nephrectomy appeared unavoidable with hilar invasion by tumor.[30] Renal salvage surgery can maintain satisfactory renal function in the majority of these patients without an increased risk of local recurrence.[31] When transplantation is required, the remaining native kidney should be removed to prevent tumor recurrence.[31]

Renal salvage procedure has also been performed with bilateral renal tumors comprising of a multilocular, cystic tumor of one kidney and a solid and cystic nephroblastoma of the other kidney after chemotherapy.[32] Surgery was performed because the multilocular, cystic kidney became hydronephrotic due to compression by the enlarged cysts, while the tumor showed only minimal shrinkage even after three courses of chemotherapy. The cysts may be simply unroofed if the pathological features of the tumor are relatively favorable.[32]

In a multicenter study involving United Kingdom Children's Cancer Study Group analyzing the records of 71 children with bilateral Wilms' tumor diagnosed over 15 years the overall survival was 69 percent with similar survival in the conservatively treated and initial surgical resection groups. At the last follow-up renal function was normal in 80-percent of the patients in each group.[33] Mean preserved renal mass was 45 and 35 percent in the conservatively treated and initial resection groups, respectively, with a trend toward better preservation in those treated conservatively.[33] Bilateral Wilms' tumor with an unfavorable histology was associated with a poor prognosis.[33]

Conservative surgical treatment of favorable histology bilateral Wilms' tumor may improve the preservation of renal mass and function without impairing patient survival.[33] The tumor may be extirpated by partial nephrectomy.

Renal salvage procedures (partial nephrectomy and enucleation) have been recommended to conserve renal parenchyma. On reviewing the records of 98 children enrolled in the Fourth National Wilms' Tumor Study who had synchronous bilateral tumors and underwent renal salvage procedures, complete excision of gross disease was accomplished in 88 percent.[34] Local tumor recurrence in the remnant kidney or tumor bed occurred in 8.2 percent. Overall, 72 percent of the kidneys were preserved, and the 4-year survival rate was 81.7 percent.[34] The surgical morbidity after a salvage procedure was comparable to that of a complete nephrectomy in patients with unilateral Wilms' tumor. Although the incidence of positive surgical margins is worrisome, it did not invariably lead to local recurrence in the remnant kidney or the tumor bed.[34] However, nephron-sparing surgery is contraindicated in diffuse anaplasia.[35] A patient with bilateral Wilms' tumor has been reported in whom at least 16 synchronous tumors in the kidneys were treated successfully by primary chemotherapy and 'nephron-sparing' surgery, without renal radiotherapy. Some believe the successful treatment without radiotherapy will allow greater potential for normal growth in the future.[22] Local control does not seem to be compromised by renal conservation therapy.

Adjuvant Methods Used for Preserving Renal Function

Techniques used to minimize blood loss included erythropoietin, hemodilution, and the argon beam coagulator.[36] Nephrectomy (partial or complete) using ice dam topical cooling and vascular control; bench surgery and extensive renal reconstruction with orthotopic autotransplantation have been described.[10]

Ex vivo tumor dissection followed by autotransplantation in an attempt to preserve functioning renal tissue with good outcome and as an acceptable alternative to bilateral nephrectomy and transplantation has been described.[37]

Removal of six subcapsular tumors has been described from a kidney that had been protected from ischemia by *in situ* cooling with UW-Belzer solution and by surface cooling. This technique was safe, easy to perform, and allowed all the time required to resect the tumors under adequate visual control and to wait for analysis of the frozen sections. It might be a useful alternative to the more complicated "bench" technique.[38]

Radiotherapy

Radiotherapy may be required for margins showing microscopic residual in an attempt to preserve maximal renal parenchyma for adequate renal function to take care of any recurrence. Radiotherapy is also required for gross tumor spill and metastatic disease.

Brachytherapy should be considered for treating local disease involving chemoresistant tumors.[35] Local control is excellent in sites treated with radiation therapy in combination with three-drug chemotherapy.[25]

However, local radiotherapy has been considered to give rise to second malignant neoplasms and impair renal function.[39]

Bone Marrow Transplant Program

After a period of conventional chemotherapy, the patients may be consolidated with high-dose (HD) melphalan and autologous bone marrow transplant (ABMT).[39]

The toxicity of the ABMT procedure is mild, the patients engraft promptly and good preservation of renal parenchyma and normal function has been achieved. The risk of ABMT program is considered smaller than the late consequences of local radiotherapy for children with bilateral Wilms' tumor.[39]

Renal Transplantation

In some patients, complete surgical removal of the malignant tissue cannot be achieved without bilateral total nephrectomy. Advances in dialysis and transplantation programs for young children offer the potential for a marked improvement in the prognosis for patients with BWT and for those with DDS.[40]

PROGNOSIS

The cumulative survival rate for infants with bilateral tumors is approximately 65 to 70 percent at 10 years. Some authors have reported that synchronous bilateral Wilms' tumor, stage V, have an excellent prognosis: over 87 percent survival, compared to 40 percent of the metachronous bilateral Wilms' tumors.[25]

Analysis of overall survival of patients with a time interval of < 18 months and ≥ 18 months showed a 10-year survival of 39.6 and 55.2 percent, respectively. Kaplan-Meier analysis rates of overall survival for metachronous bilateral Wilms' tumor were 49.1 and 47.2 percent at 5 and 10 years, respectively.[27]

Mortality is common in children presenting with stage IV tumors and high-grade malignancy.[8]

LATE SEQUELAE OF TREATMENT

Renal Function

The treatment of bilateral Wilms' tumor (BWT) involves a multidisciplinary approach including surgery, chemotherapy, and radiation therapy. The long-term renal function in patients receiving all three treatment modalities needs to be evaluated. The development of renal insufficiency in children with synchronous BWT nonetheless remains a concern. It is important that long-term survivors have systematic follow-up, with measurements of blood pressure, urine protein, serum creatinine, renal clearance, and renal size.[24] Renal function may be assessed by measuring blood urea nitrogen (BUN) and serum creatinine (Cr). 34.6 percent children had elevated BUN and/or Cr levels during the post-treatment follow-up period in a study evaluating long-term renal function in 81 children with synchronous BWT who received radiation therapy as part of their treatment.[41] No dose-response relationship was established when comparing the radiation doses of those with elevated values to those with normal values. The elevations could be attributed to tumor recurrence in some cases.[41]

The median interval from diagnosis to the onset of renal failure has been reported as around 21 months. The incidence of RF in bilateral WT was 16.4 percent for NWTS-1 and -2, 9.9 percent for NWTS-3, and 3.8 percent for NWTS-4.[42] On the other hand the risk of end-stage renal failure lay between 0.2 and 0.4 percent in unilateral Wilms' tumor. The risk is higher in bilateral disease due to two stage bilateral nephrectomy thus warranting attempts to preserve renal parenchyma in their management.

Small Bowel Obstruction

Major morbidities related to multimodality therapy have also included small bowel obstruction requiring lysis of adhesions.[28]

Malignant Neoplasms

Malignant neoplasms after treatment for metachronous bilateral Wilms' tumor can occur.[15] Health care professionals caring for these patients should be aware of this late sequelae of treatment. 3.7 percent patients have been found to develop a malignant neoplasm after treatment of a metachronous bilateral Wilms' tumor.[15] Three out of 18 patients followed for at least 10 years developed a solid tumor, including two sarcomas in the irradiated areas.[15] Fifty percent of the children who developed a malignant neoplasm on follow up had a congenital anomaly.[15]

REFERENCES

1. Gordon B, Manivel JC, Gonzalez R, Reinberg Y. Synchronous bilateral Wilms' tumor in a neonate. Urology. 1996;47:409-11.
2. Kalifat R. Bilateral Wilms' tumor in the fetus. Ann Urol (Paris). 1999;33:37-41.
3. Tomlinson GS, Cole CH, Smith NM. Bilateral Wilms' tumor: a clinicopathologic review. Pathology 1999;31:12-6.
4. Nawaz A, Mpofu C, Shawis R, Matta H, Jacobsz A, Kassir S, Al Salem A. Synchronous bilateral Wilms' tumor. Pediatr Surg Int 1999;15:42-5.
5. Ruteshouser EC, Huff V. Familial Wilms' tumor. Am J Med Genet C Semin Med Genet 2004;129:29-34.
6. Perotti D, Mondini P, Terenziani M, Spreafico F, Collini P, Fossati-Bellani F, Radice P. WT1 gene analysis in sporadic early-onset and bilateral Wilms' tumor patients without associated abnormalities. J Pediatr Hematol Oncol 2005;27:197-201.
7. Kohler B, Schumacher V, Schulte-Overberg U, Biewald W, Lennert T, l'Allemand D, Royer-Pokora B, Gruters A. Bilateral Wilms' tumor in a boy with severe hypospadias and cryptochidism due to a heterozygous mutation in the WT1 gene. Pediatr Res 1999;45:187-90.
8. Presedo A, Martinez Ibanez V, Marques A, Sanchez de Toledo J, Boix Ochoa J. Bilateral Wilms' tumor. Cir Pediatr 1997;10:108-11.
9. Breslow NE, Olson J, Moksness J, Beckwith JB, Grundy P. Familial Wilms' tumor: a descriptive study. Med Pediatr Oncol 1996; 27:398-403.
10. Millar AJ, Davidson A, Rode H, Numanoglu A, Hartley PS, Daubenton JD, Desai F. Bilateral Wilms' tumors: a single-center experience with 19 cases. J Pediatr Surg 2005;40:1289-94.
11. Perlman EJ, Faria P, Soares A, Hoffer F, Sredni S, Ritchey M, Shamberger RC, Green D, Beckwith JB. Hyperplastic perilobar nephroblastomatosis: Long-term survival of 52 patients. Pediatr Blood Cancer. 2005 Apr 6 [Epub].
12. Coppes MJ, Arnold M, Beckwith JB, Ritchey ML, D'Angio GJ, Green DM, Breslow NE. Factors affecting the risk of contralateral Wilms' tumor development: a report from the National Wilms' Tumor Study Group. Cancer. 1999; 85:1616-25.
13. Regalado JJ, Rodriguez MM, Toledano S. Bilaterally multicentric synchronous Wilms' tumor: successful conservative treatment despite persistence of nephrogenic rests. Med Pediatr Oncol. 1997;28:420-3
14. Paya K, Horcher E, Lawrenz K, Rebhandl W, Zoubek A. Bilateral Wilms' tumor—surgical aspects. Eur J Pediatr Surg 2001;11:99-104.
15. Paulino AC. Malignant neoplasms after treatment for metachronous bilateral Wilms' tumor: a literature review. Pediatr Hematol Oncol 1999;16:533-8.
16. Breslow N, Olshan A, Beckwith JB, Green DM. Epidemiology of Wilms' Tumor. Med Ped Oncol 1993; 21:172-81.
17. Mambie Melendez M, Guibelalde Del Castillo M, Nieto Del Rincon N, Rodrigo Jimenez D, Femenia Reus A, Roman Pinana JM. Metachronous bilateral Wilms' tumor. An Esp Pediatr. 2002 Mar;56(3):247-50.
18. Apoznanski W, Sawicz-Birkowska K, Pietras W, Dorobisz U, Szydelko T. Extrarenal Wilms' tumour. Eur J Pediatr Surg 2005 Feb;15(1):53-5.
19. Shulkin BL, Chang E, Strouse PJ, Bloom DA, Hutchinson RJ. PET-FDG studies of Wilms' tumors. J Pediatr Hematol Oncol. 1997 Jul-Aug;19(4):334-8.
20. Ross JH, Kay R. Surgical considerations for patients with Wilms' tumor. Semin Urol Oncol 1999;17:33-9.
21. Ritchey ML, Green DM, Breslow NE, Moksness J, Norkool P. Accuracy of current imaging modalities in the diagnosis of synchronous bilateral Wilms' tumor. Cancer 1995; 75:600-4.
22. Abdel Hamid AM, Rogers PB, Sibtain A, Plowman PN. Bilateral renal cancer in children: a difficult, challenging and changing management problem. Clin Oncol (R Coll Radiol). 1999;11(3):200-4.
23. Schaarschmidt K, Ritter J, Willital GH, Olesczcuk-Raschke K, Kindhauser V, Stratmann U. Assessment of the resectability of Wilms' tumors in childhood: Langenbecks Arch Chir Suppl Kongressbd 1996;113:1084-90.
24. Ritchey ML, Coppes MJ. The management of synchronous bilateral Wilms' tumor. Hematol Oncol Clin North Am 1995;9:1303-15.
25. Delgado G, Viluce C, Fletcher E, de Espinosa H, Del Rio B, Chen LN. Bilateral Wilms' tumor. Current treatment] Rev Med Panama 1996;21:93-101.
26. Kist-van Holthe JE, Ho PL, Stablein D, Harmon WE, Baum MA. Outcome of renal transplantation for Wilms' tumor and Denys-Drash syndrome: a report of the North American Pediatric Renal Transplant Cooperative Study. Pediatr Transplant 2005;9:305-10.
27. Paulino AC, Thakkar B, Henderson WG. Metachronous bilateral Wilms' tumor: the importance of time interval to the development of a second tumor. Cancer 1998;82:415-20.
28. Paulino AC, Wiliams J, Marina N, Jones D, Kumar M, Greenwald C, Chen G, Kun LE. Local control in synchronous bilateral Wilms' tumor. Int J Radiat Oncol Biol Phys 1996;36:541-8.
29. Misra D, Gupta DK, Bajpai M, Bhatnagar V, Mitra DK. Bilateral Wilms' tumor: an eleven-year experience. Indian J Cancer 1998;35:42-6.
30. Fuchs J, Wunsch L, Flemming P, Weinel P, Mildenberger H. Nephron-sparing surgery in synchronous bilateral Wilms' tumors. J Pediatr Surg 1999 Oct;34(10):1505-9.
31. Kubiak R, Gundeti M, Duffy PG, Ransley PG, Wilcox DT. Renal function and outcome following salvage surgery for bilateral Wilms' tumor. J Pediatr Surg 2004 Nov;39(11):1667-72.
32. Nakada K, Kitagawa H, Wakisaka M, Chihara H, Koike J. Renal salvage procedure for synchronous bilateral Wilms' tumor. Pediatr Surg Int 2000;16(3):222-5.
33. Kumar R, Fitzgerald R, Breatnach F. Conservative surgical management of bilateral Wilms' tumor: results of the United Kingdom Children's Cancer Study Group. J Urol. 1998;160:1450-3. Comment in: J Urol 1999;162:167.
34. Horwitz JR, Ritchey ML, Moksness J, Breslow NE, Smith GR, Thomas PR, Haase G, Shamberger RC, Beckwith JB. Renal salvage procedures in patients with synchronous bilateral Wilms' tumors: a report from the National Wilms' Tumor Study Group: J Pediatr Surg 1996;31:1020-5.
35. Cooper CS, Jaffe WI, Huff DS, Canning DA, Zderic SA, Meadows AT, D'Angio GJ, Snyder HM 3rd. The role of renal salvage procedures for bilateral Wilms' tumor: a 15-year review. J Urol 2000;163:265-8.
36. Ross JH, Kay R, Alexander F. Management of bilateral Wilms' tumors in the daughter of Jehovah's Witnesses. J Pediatr Surg 1997;32:1759-60.

37. Desai D, Nicholls G, Duffy PG. Bench surgery with autotransplantation for bilateral synchronous Wilms' tumor: a report of three cases. J Pediatr Surg 1999;34: 632-4.

38. De Backer A, Lamote J, Keuppens F, Willems G, Otten J. Bilateral Wilms' tumor: *in situ* cooling of the kidney facilitates curative excision of tumors, with preservation of renal function. J Pediatr Surg 1995;30:1338-40.

39. Saarinen-Pihkala UM, Wikstrom S, Vettenranta K. Maximal preservation of renal function in patients with bilateral Wilms' tumor: therapeutic strategy of late kidney-sparing surgery and replacement of radiotherapy by high-dose melphalan and stem cell rescue. Bone Marrow Transplant 1998;22:53-9.

40. Rudin C, Pritchard J, Fernando ON, Duffy PG, Trompeter RS. Renal transplantation in the management of bilateral Wilms' tumour (BWT) and of Denys-Drash syndrome (DDS). Nephrol Dial Transplant 1998;13:1506-10.

41. Smith GR, Thomas PR, Ritchey M, Norkool P. Long-term renal function in patients with irradiated bilateral Wilms' tumor. National Wilms' Tumor Study Group. Am J Clin Oncol 1998;21:58-63.

42. Ritchey ML, Green DM, Thomas PR, Smith GR, Haase G, Shochat S, Moksness J, Breslow NE. Renal failure in Wilms' tumor patients: a report from the National Wilms' Tumor Study Group. Med Pediatr Oncol. 1996; 26:75-80. Comment in: Med Pediatr Oncol 1997;28:239-40.

CHAPTER 15

Robert Carachi
Devendra K Gupta

Management of Wilms' Tumor with Intracaval Thrombus

Wilms' tumor is the most common childhood renal tumor and has an excellent prognosis, with over 85 percent long-term survival using chemotherapy and nephrectomy, and radiotherapy in the minority of cases. The focus of current research is improved patient selection for risk-adapted stratification of treatment intensity. Minimizing surgical morbidity and mortality is a crucial component of such an approach.

Vascular extension to the vena cava occurs in 4 percent of Wilms' tumor cases and can reach the right atrium in up to 1 percent. The thrombus is usually not adherent to the vessel wall, and there is blood flow around it. Some have reported an incidence of up to 10 percent of patients undergoing nephrectomy for Wilms' tumor having intracaval tumor extension. Thus the incidence reported is in 4-10 percent of Wilms' tumor cases, mostly into the infrahepatic portion but it may extend into the right atrium.[1-4]

8.1 percent out of 730 cases of Wilms' tumor in third UK Children's Cancer Study Group (UKCCSG) had evidence of intracaval extension, either documented at diagnosis (53) or found unexpectedly at nephrectomy (6). Out of 59 cases, the level of thrombus was intra-atrial (10), suprahepatic (9), retrohepatic (8), infrahepatic (26) and unknown (6).

CLINICAL FEATURES

Most patients with tumor thrombus in the IVC are asymptomatic and diagnosis is only made on imaging investigations. The median age at diagnosis has been reported as 3.75 years compared to 2.97 years in patients without IVC thrombus (p < 0.0001). The most common presenting symptom is as an abdominal mass in 90 percent cases, followed by gross hematuria in 25 percent cases. Hypertension, which corrected after nephrectomy, may be seen in 10 percent cases. Occasionally, patients may present acutely after trauma, severe hematuria, acute abdomen, with varicocele or evidence of pulmonary embolus.

INVESTIGATIONS

Due to a variety of uniformity of imaging modalities used, it is not possible to comment on their relative merits. IVC involvement was found in 59 percent of the right-sided Wilms' tumors in this study. It has been reported to be more common (59-85%) in right-sided tumors because of the shorter right renal vein.[2]

The useful modalities of investigation have included vena cavagram, contrast enhanced CT scan, MRI scan and echocardiogram.[4] 8.3 percent cases of Wilms' tumor in a series were diagnosed preoperatively as having intracaval tumor thrombus using ultrasound as the most sensitive non-invasive diagnostic technique.[4] Imaging by ultrasound and CT scans is routine in most centers and where there is any suspicion of caval extension then an echocardiogram should be performed to detect atrial extension of the thrombus.

Transesophageal echocardiography to localize the tumor thrombus and detect any tumor or air embolization and a minimal lower sternotomy to obtain intrapericardial control of the inferior vena cava has also been used as an alternative to median sternotomy and use of cardiopulmonary bypass.[5]

MANAGEMENT

The traditional approach to extension of Wilms' tumor into IVC used to be primary surgical resection, which often required sternotomy and cardiopulmonary bypass with the thrombus extending above the diaphragm.[6] This was associated with significant morbidity and mortality. In the UKW-3 trial, elective preoperative chemotherapy was the preferred approach for IVC thrombus. Thus the routine use of preoperative chemotherapy continues to be the mainstay in the management of such patients. Primary surgery would only be indicated in a patient who is unstable due to thrombus that might dislodge and cause acute symptoms.

Preoperative Chemotherapy

Preoperative chemotherapy can cause thrombus regression and even resolution. If the thrombus persists after chemotherapy, surgery will be a challenge.

Nearly all patients (52/59) with IVC involvement in the third UK Children's Cancer Study Group (UKCCSG) received preoperative chemotherapy.

Significant shrinkage of the thrombus and tumor was demonstrated in 35 out of 49 patients in whom comparable pre- and post-chemotherapy imaging was available. In 8 cases no response was seen after preoperative chemotherapy in either the size of the tumor or the thrombus All ten patients with intra-atrial extension at diagnosis received preoperative chemotherapy and only three (30%) required sternotomy and cardiopulmonary bypass.

Wagget and Koop first advocated the precedent of preoperative chemotherapy and radiation therapy in Wilms' tumor in 1970.[7] Thereafter many authors have reported resolution of the intracaval extension of thrombus by using chemotherapy.[8-13]

Preoperative chemotherapy is useful adjunct to shrink the tumor and thrombus. This reduces the requirement for cavotomy and cardiopulmonary bypass. Intraoperative hemorrhage remains a significant cause of operative morbidity and mortality.

Elective preoperative chemotherapy with "intensive AVA" vincristine (1.5 mg/m^2 weekly) together with actinomycin D (1.5 mg/m^2) and adriamycin (30 mg/m^2) every 3 weeks was recommended for all patients with suspected tumor extension into the IVC on diagnostic imaging. Preoperative chemotherapy was continued until the tumor was deemed resectable by the treating surgeon. Recommended postoperative treatment was continuing chemotherapy with "intensive

AVA" and flank radiotherapy only if the local tumor stage defined at time of delayed nephrectomy was stage III.

Concerns regarding dense adherence of tumor thrombus to the cava resulting from preoperative therapy has been reported during the early use of preoperative therapy.[14] Following preoperative chemotherapy, the IVC was found to be fibrosed and calcified in eight cases in the UKW-3 trial. However, this did not make surgery difficult and no recurrence at the local site was seen in any of the cases.

Surgical Intervention

Although operative treatment of Wilms' tumors has become more straightforward as a result of advances in preoperative treatment and precise diagnosis, vascular involvement by the tumor can cause serious problems at operation. These problems can be more easily managed if they have been identified preoperatively and the level of the intravascular tumor thrombus has been defined (Figs 15.1A and B).[4] At operation, the IVC may be documented to be patent and free of tumor.

Milking Out the Thrombus

The thrombus is palpated for the upper extent (Fig. 15.2). If it has been found to be reduced to the renal vein with patent flow on color Doppler, the thrombus may be milked into the renal vein and removed *en bloc* with the tumor (Fig. 15.3).

Cavotomy

The upper end of the thrombus is palpated within the IVC. An incision is made in the IVC vertically after applying vascular clamps above and below the thrombus retrieved and the repair of the IVC done 52 percent of

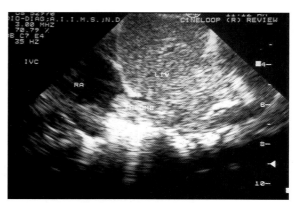

Figure 15.1A: An ultrasonogram documenting the presence of an IVC thrombus in a case of Wilms' tumor

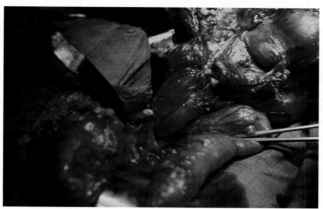

Figure 15.1B: Operative photograph of the same patient confirming the preoperative findings of left Wilms' tumor with thrombus in the inferior vena cava

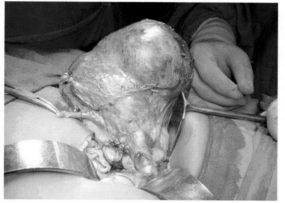

Figure 15.2: Operative photograph of a tumor thrombus in renal vein causing the vein to stretch upto 5 cm

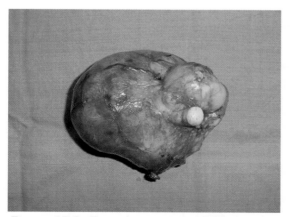

Figure 15.3: Excised specimen of Wilms' tumor with calcified thrombus in renal vein

the patients in the UKW-3 trial needed cavotomy. Ein's technique comprising of deep hypothermia (average 17°C) with cardiac arrest (average 39 minutes) and

exsanguination has been used in performing intravenous Wilms' tumor resections. The initial hepatic resection takes less than 15 minutes to perform in a bloodless field and the specimen is immediately examined by frozen section for determination of adequacy of margin. Additional resection can be easily performed if required. Mattress sutures can be used to control hemorrhage during recirculation.

Cavectomy

If the thrombus invades the vessel wall, its removal may not be feasible. In this situation cavectomy is a good surgical strategy because it provides complete resection. The prerequisite for cavectomy is the absence of blood flow in the vena cava on preoperative Doppler ultrasonography. Cavectomy is a safe procedure for treating pediatric patients with Wilms' tumor when there is extension and invasion of the vena cava wall without blood flow.[15]

Intra-atrial Extension

The tumor may have varied extensions from the iliac vein into the right atrium, from the right renal vein to the right atrium with extensions into the hepatic and lumbar veins. The atria and inferior vena cava can be opened and the tumor can be extracted under direct vision.[16] Intravascular extension of thrombus within the right atrium is treated with extracorporeal circulation, cardiac arrest and profound hypothermia.[15,17] Cardiopulmonary by-pass, hypothermia and cardiac arrest facilitates surgery with wide exposure of the IVC in a bloodless field permitted complete removal of all visible tumor in each case.[18] This provides good local control of the tumor and offers the only hope of cure in patients with this disease. Cardiopulmonary bypass with profound hypothermia and circulation simplifies tumor excision.[19]

The use of extracorporeal circulation and deep circulatory arrest provides the safest and optimal technique for removing intracardiac thrombus extension in a bloodless field, even in the presence of metastatic disease, with acceptable morbidity and mortality and has good early and long-term results.[17,19,20]

Tumor thrombus extending into the right atrium can also be removed using a normothermic cardiopulmonary bypass circuit connected with a vacuum-assisted venous drainage giving a negative pressure of 20 to 40 mm Hg without circulatory arrest or hypothermia.[21] This avoids the potential complications associated with these procedures. Tumor thrombus can be extracted through a longitudinal "cavotomy" and removed along with the kidney. With respect to veno-venous shunts this technique guarantees complete surgical control of the thrombus and avoids the need for extensive dissection of the retrohepatic vena cava and Pringle maneuver.[21]

In cases of suprahepatic Wilms' tumor thrombus that may extend into the right atrium, a median sternotomy and cardiopulmonary bypass are used to facilitate tumor resection.[6] However, if the tumor can be localized and controlled below the atrium, resection without the use of cardiopulmonary bypass may limit morbidity.

A new radiological technique has been described utilizing a temporary occlusion balloon inserted via an open venotomy of the left internal jugular vein into the retrohepatic cava to create a bloodless field to facilitate surgery.[22]

The risk of fatal hemorrhage may limit the completeness of resection in hepatic malignancies and in vascular extensions of Wilms' tumors.

COMPLICATIONS

The most common operative complication is significant hemorrhage and may even result in mortality in few cases. A surgical complication rate of 43 percent was found in patients with intracaval extension treated in the NWTS-3 study.[2] Massive hemorrhage was the most common and the next was tumor embolization with acute cardiac decompensation or arrest, following manipulation of the thrombus if it was not adherent to the vessel wall.[2] Preoperative chemotherapy and delayed surgery is often recommended to reduce the anticipated surgical risks in such cases.[7-13]

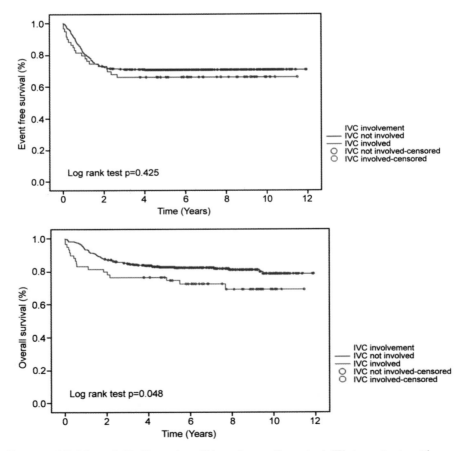

Figures 15.4A and B: Event-free **(A)** and overall survival **(B)** in patients with Wilms' tumor (stage II – IV) with or without vascular extension in UKW-3

Table 15.1: Overall survival according to presence of intravascular extension in patients with stage II–IV Wilms' tumor in UKW-3

IVC involvement	Survival rate at 5 years	Survival rate at 10 years
IVC not involved (n= 379)	78.8%	78.6%
IVC involved (n= 59)	74.3%	68.8%

PROGNOSIS

The poor prognostic factors include poor response to chemotherapy and unfavorable histology. Among patients with favorable histology tumors, the causes of death include pulmonary embolism, severe respiratory distress or uncontrollable hemorrhage at operation, tumor recurrence or progression.

Intravascular extension makes a tumor at least stage II. Survival analyses should be adjusted for age at diagnosis, since patients with intracaval extension of their tumor are older than patients without this finding and older age is an adverse prognostic factor in Wilms' tumor.[23] Patients with intravascular involvement have a slightly worse overall survival but not event-free survival (Figs 15.4A and B, Table 15.1). Overall survival is defined as time to mortality for all cause death and event-free survival is defined as time to relapse or death.

The operative morbidity and mortality reported in NWTS-3 study in which all the 77 patients were treated with primary surgery was 43 percent. The most frequent complication was major intraoperative bleeding. There were no operative deaths but cardiac arrest due to profound hypotension occurred in 3 patients. IVC occlusion was found in follow-up in 5 patients. In NWTS-4 study complications in the primary surgical group were 26 percent and in the preoperative therapy group were 13 percent. The difference was at the margins of stastical significance (p= 0.053).

The survival for patients with IVC extension does appear slightly worse, even after adjustment for age. Avoidance of early events due to operative mortality is an important consideration in the management of these patients.

Much of the morbidity is due to under-diagnosing of intracaval extension. Better imaging and echocardiography would pick up more of these patients.

REFERENCES

1. Clayman RV, Sheldon CA, Gonzalez RA. Wilms' tumor: An approach to vena cava intrusion. Prog Pediatr Surg 1980;15:285-9.
2. Ritchey ML, Kelalis PP, Breslow N, et al. Intracaval and atrial involvement with nephroblastoma: review of National Wilms Tumor Study 3. J Urol 1988;140:1113-8.
3. Nakayama DK, deLorimier AA, O'Neill JA, et al. Intracardiac extension of Wilms' tumor: A report of the National Wilms Tumor study. Ann Surg 1986;204:693-7.
4. Daum R, Roth H and Zachariou Z. Tumor infiltration of the vena cava in nephroblastoma. Eur J Pediatr Surg 1994;4:16-20.
5. Lodge AJ, Jaggers J, Adams D, Rice HE. Vascular control for resection of suprahepatic intracaval Wilms' tumor: technical considerations J Pediatr Surg. 2000 Dec;35(12):1836-7.
6. Luck SR, DeLeon S, Shkolnik A, et al. Intracardiac Wilms' tumor: Diagnosis and management. J Pediatr Surg 1982;17(5):551-4.
7. Wagget J, Koop CE. Wilms' tumor: Preoperative radio-therapy and chemotherapy in the management of massive tumors. Cancer 1970;26:338-40.
8. Sullivan MP, Sutow WW, Cangir A, et al. Vincristine sulfate in management of Wilms' tumor. JAMA 1967;202:381-4.
9. Lemerle J, Voute PA, Tournade MF, et al. Effectiveness of preoperative chemotherapy in Wilms' tumor: Results of an Interational Society of Pediatric Oncology (SIOP) clinical trial. J Clin Oncol 1983;1:604-10.
10. Oberholzer HF, Falkson G, DeJager LC. Successful management of IVC and right atrial nephroblastoma tumor thrombus with preoperative therapy. Med Pediatr Oncol 1992;20:61-3.
11. Crombleholme TM, Jacir NN, Rosenfield CG, et al. Preoperative hemotherapy in the management of intracaval extention of Wilms' tumor. J Paediatr Surg 1994;29:229-31.
12. Mushtaq I, Carachi R, Roy G, Azmy A. Childhood renal tumors with intracaval extension. Br J Urol 1996;78:772-6.
13. Shamberger RC, Ritchey ML, Haase GM, et al. Intra-vascular extension of Wilms' tumor. Ann Surg 2001; 234(1):116-21.
14. DeLorimier AA. Surgical treatment of Wilms' tumor. In: Pochedly C, Miller D, (Eds). Wilms' tumor. New York: John Wiley and Sons: 1976;167-88.
15. Ribeiro RC, Schettini ST, Abib Sde C, da Fonseca JH, Cypriano M, da Silva NS. Cavectomy for the treatment of Wilms' tumor with vascular extension J Urol. 2006; 176:279-83; discussion 283-4.
16. Chang JH, Janik JS, Burrington JD, Clark DR, Campbell DN, Pappas G. Extensive tumor resection under deep hypothermia and circulatory arrest. J Pediatr Surg. 1988;23:254-8.
17. Almassi GH. Surgery for tumors with cavoatrial extension. Semin Thorac Cardiovasc Surg. 2000;12:111-8.
18. Matthews PN, Evans C, Breckenridge IM. Involvement of the inferior vena cava by renal tumour: surgical excision using hypothermic circulatory arrest Br J Urol. 1995; 75:441-4.
19. Theman T, Williams WG, Simpson JS, Radford D, Rubin S, Stephens CA. Tumor invasion of the upper inferior vena cava: the use of profound hypothermia and circulation arrest as a surgical adjunct. J Pediatr Surg. 1978;13:331-4.
20. Chiappini B, Savini C, Marinelli G, Suarez SM, Di Eusanio M, Fiorani V, Pierangeli A. Cavoatrial tumor thrombus: single-stage

surgical approach with profound hypothermia and circulatory arrest, including a review of the literature. J Thorac Cardiovasc Surg. 2002 Oct;124(4):684-8. Comment In: J Thorac Cardiovasc Surg. 2004;127:301-2; author reply 302.

21. Tasca A, Abatangelo G, Ferrarese P, Piccin C, Fabbri A, Musi L. Experience with an elective vacuum assisted cardiopulmonary bypass in the surgical treatment of renal neoplasms extending into the right atrium. J Urol 2003;169:75-8; discussion 78.

22. Adams WM, Huskisson L, Gornall P, John PR. Temporary balloon occlusion of the inferior vena cava as an alternative to cardiopulmonary bypass in resection of Wilms' tumour with vena cava extension. Pediatr Radiol 1997;27:236-8.

23. Breslow N, Sharples K, Beckwith JB, et al. Prognostic Factors in Nonmetastatic, Favourable Histology Wilms' Tumor: Results of the Third National Wilms' Tumor Study. Cancer 1991;68: 2345-53.

CHAPTER 16

Yoshiaki Tsuchida
Hitoshi Ikeda
Shin Itsu Hatakeyama

Neuroblastoma

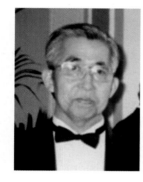

In remembrance

Prof. Yoshiaki Tsuchida (25-10-36 to 28-06-05) was a renowned pediatric surgeon, who devoted most of his life to basic and clinical research. He has contributed to the International Society of Pediatric Oncologists with various academic achievements in the field of pediatric oncology. This is probably the last chapter by him on his favourite subject.

Neuroblastoma is the second most common solid tumor in infancy and childhood after brain tumors. It accounts for 7 to 10 percent of cancers of childhood, and the annual incidence is 1 per 100,000 children under the age of 15 years in the United States[1] and 1 per 76,000 in Japan where mass screening is carried out.[2]

The history of neuroblastoma dates to 1864 when Virchow first described its typical histological features.[3] In 1901, Pepper reported autopsy findings of 6 infants with suprarenal and liver tumors, which were probably the first patients with the disease type now called stage IV-S neuroblastoma.[4] In 1907, Huntington recorded older patients with "sarcoma" of the adrenal gland and metastases to the skull.[5] In 1910, Wright first used the term neuroblastoma by likening the rosettes and neural fibrils of such tumors to the developing adrenals,[6] and since then the term neuroblastoma has been widely used.

The biology of neuroblastoma is enigmatic and it is important to understand it to the extent possible in order to improve its treatment and clinical results further. It is widely accepted that neuroblastoma is a tumor of the sympathetic nervous system. While neuroblastoma may produce catecholamines, this is not always true in advanced neuroblastoma. Le Douarin and her associates have shown that the fate of neural crest-derived cells is highly dependent upon environmental causes.[7] That is, neural crest cells that are supposed to produce catecholamines may begin to synthesize acetylcholine under specific conditions[8] and vice versa.[9] Cloned adrenergic neuroblastoma cells may even become cholinergic after serial transplantation.[10] In addition, we have confirmed that only 75 percent of clinically detected neuroblastomas have the key enzyme, i.e. tyrosine hydroxylase, required to produce catecholamines.[11]

Cytogenetically, chromosome 1p deletions, extrachromosomal double minutes, and homogeneously staining regions (HSRs) are commonly observed in neuroblastoma cell lines and advanced-stage neuroblastoma tumors. It was also recently found that an HSR represents genomic amplification of *MYCN*, which plays a key role in determining the aggressiveness of neuroblastoma.[12,13] However, stage IV neuroblastomas or cell lines that lack *MYCN* amplification are also progressive, and some of them show evidence of *MYCN* expression in terms of mRNA and/or *MYCN* oncoprotein.[14,15] It was also recently shown that a small proximal locus mapped between 1p35-36.1 and 1p36.23 may function as a suppressor gene of *MYCN* amplification.[16] However, the relation is not simple,[17] because it has been reported that chromosome 17q gain may also be associated with *MYCN* amplification.[18] In addition, loss of heterozygosity on chromosomes 2q, 9p, 11q, 14q, and 18q has been reported in some patients with advanced neuroblastoma.[19,20]

Cellular DNA content or ploidy is relevant to clinical outcome.[21] Hyperploidy is closely associated with a favorable patient outcome, while diploidy usually predicts poor patient prognosis. Ploidy analysis using *in situ* hybridization showed that numeric chromosome aberrations are found in neuroblastic/ganglionic cells, but not in the Schwann cells which have long been thought to be neoplastic in origin.[22] This led to the hypothesis that Schwann cells in neuroblastoma are infiltrating normal cells that are responsible for the differentiation of neuroblastoma cells.[22]

In sympathoadrenal lineage cells in the later stages of neural crest development, the *Trk-A* tyrosine kinase receptor for which nerve growth factor (NGF) is a ligand is expressed.[23] While NGF binding to the receptor transmits a signal that leads immature sympathetic neurons to differentiate into mature ganglion cells, deprivation of NGF results in apoptosis, or programmed cell death, of the neurons. In neuroblastoma, *Trk-A* is expressed in tumors with a favorable prognosis, and tumor cells expressing high levels of *Trk-A* differentiate in response to NGF.[23,24] The NGF that is produced by schwannian stromal cells may regulate the differentiation and survival of neuroblastoma cells.[25] *MYCN* amplification downregulates *Trk-A* expression and low or absent expression of *Trk-A* is associated with an unfavorable prognosis.[23,24] *Trk-B*, a high-affinity receptor for brain-derived neurotrophic factor (BDNF), also is expressed in aggressive neuroblastoma.[26]

The presence of cells with characteristic features of apoptosis (e.g. condensed nuclear fragments and eosinophilic cytoplasm) and the demonstration of a ladder of DNA fragments indicate that apoptosis is involved in the process of neuroblastoma cell death.[27] A number of studies showed that neuroblastoma expresses Bcl-2 which inhibits apoptosis, but there is no definitive evidence regarding the relationship between Bcl-2 and other prognostic factors.[28] Expression of proteases involved in the process of apoptosis, caspase-1 and caspase-3, is high in the nuclei of neuroblastoma with favorable prognostic characteristics.[29,30]

Telomerases are DNA-protein structures at the ends of eukaryotic chromosomes and are thought to be important in the positioning, protection, and replication of chromosomes.[31] Telomerase, an RNA-dependent DNA polymerase, stabilizes telomeres and the telomere maintenance is essential for attainment of immortality in tumor cells. Several studies have shown that telomerase activity is detectable in neuroblastomas, except for stage IV-S tumors.[31-33] High telomerase activity is associated with advanced stage or *MYCN* amplification, while neuroblastomas with low or undetectable telomerase activity are usually tumors that are diagnosed in infants and have favorable prognostic characteristics.[31]

Ha-*ras* p21, a product of the Ha-*ras* gene, is expressed in normal neuronal cells and participates in the signal transduction pathway relating to NGF.[34] Expression of Ha-*ras* p21 is significantly associated with patient prognosis and higher expression predicts a favorable patient outcome.[35] Prognostic discrimination based on Ha-*ras* and *Trk-A* gene expression in patients with stage III and IV diseases therefore appears useful, and the survival rate of patients with neuroblastoma highly expressing both genes is significantly better than that of patients with tumors with low expression of the genes.[36]

P-glycoprotein, a plasma membrane efflux pump, plays a role in drug resistance and is responsible for multidrug resistance against the vinca alkaloids, anthracyclines, and epipodophyllotoxins. However, the role of P-glycoprotein in predicting prognosis in neuroblastoma is controversial.[37,38] Expression of the *MDR*1 gene that encodes P-glycoprotein is correlated with *MYCN* gene expression in neuroblastoma without *MYCN* amplification, and high expression of *MDR*1 is significantly associated with poor outcome.[39] High expression of the *MRP* gene that encodes multidrug resistance-associated protein (MRP) is also associated with poor survival in patients with neuroblastoma and in subgroups of patients without *MYCN* gene amplification and those with localized disease.[40]

The genetic and molecular analyses described above not only have revealed biological differences between neuroblastomas with favorable prognosis and those with aggressive biological behaviors, but also have provided insight into both tumorigenesis and spontaneous regression of neuroblastoma. It is generally accepted that there are at least two types of neuroblastoma: one seen mainly in infancy and associated with particularly good prognosis; and the other usually encountered in older children with an extremely poor prognosis, often associated with MYCN amplification. Brodeur and others place an intermediate group[41] between these two groups, but identification of the intermediate group is equivocal because the prognosis of patients with neuroblastoma is not determined by MYCN amplification alone. Furthermore, the prognosis of stage IV neuroblastoma patients older than 12 months of age does not differ greatly whether MYCN is amplified or not.[42]

CLINICAL SYMPTOMS

Neuroblastoma may diagnosed prenatally. Seventeen patients with prenatally diagnosed neuroblastoma were identified in a cohort of 591 patients in the Italian Neuroblastoma Registry.[43] It was reported that the tumor was solid in 13 patients (76.5%) and cystic in 4 (23.5%). The tumor occurred in the adrenal gland in 16 and in the retroperitoneal sympathetic ganglion in one. Fifteen patients were in stage I or II, and the remaining 2 patients had stage IV-S disease.[43] The treatment strategy is controversial, but it is generally considered that it should not differ much from that in infantile neuroblasoma identified by mass screening.[43]

Clinical symptoms of postnatally diagnosed neuroblastoma differ based on the mode of diagnosis and the stage/age of the disease. Infants with neuroblastoma identified by mass screening usually present with a small tumor mass in the adrenal glands or paravertebral sympathetic ganglia, or less frequently with multiple hepatic metastases together with a small primary tumor mass. The distribution of tumor masses diagnosed in mass screening is thus similar to that of neuroblastomas identified by antenatal diagnosis. The primary tumors in the adrenal glands or paravertebral sympathetic ganglia are usually not palpable in patients diagnosed by mass screening. On the other hand, multiple hepatic metastases cause significant liver enlargement. Infantile neuroblastoma may also metastasize to the skin and bone marrow.

Some tumors can develop intra- and extraspinally, and can be of the dumbbell or hourglass shape. The site of origin of neuroblastoma varies with age, since adrenal tumors are more common in children than in infants.[44] In children, a fixed, hard, irregular mass is frequently palpable. Tumors originating in the pelvis may cause mechanical obstruction and result in difficulties in defecation or urination. A dumbbell-type tumor can cause paraplegia or fecal/urinary incontinence. Larger thoracic tumors may cause dyspnea or dysphagia, and may also cause superior vena cava syndrome.[44] Upper thoracic and cervical neuroblastomas are sometimes associated with Horner's syndrome. It has been presumed that neuroblastoma of adrenal origin may leads to renovascular hypertension, but the serum renin level is usually normal, and if elevated serum active or inactive renin levels are associated with neuroblastoma, anomalies of the vascular system such as middle aortic syndrome should be considered, as observed in one of the authors' patients or reported by others.[45]

Neuroblastomas in children older than 12 months of age often metastasize to the lymph nodes, bone, and bone marrow. Neuroblastomas have a predilection for the bones of the skull, orbit, jaw, and long bones, and metastases to the orbit produce the characteristic unilateral or bilateral periorbital ecchymosis and exophthalmos. Metastases to the bone marrow are so common that routine examination of bone marrow is essential. Lung and brain metastases are rare at diagnosis.

Hypertension, diarrhea, and opsoclonus-myoclonus syndrome are important paraneoplastic syndromes of neuroblastoma. Excretion of catecholamines and stretching (constriction) of the renal arteries are possible causes of hypertension in neuroblastoma, but the latter is less plausible because serum total rennin is usually within the normal ranges. Neuroblastomas are known to produce vasoactive intestinal peptide (VIP), which causes intractable diarrhea. Interestingly, the VIP-producing tumors are mature ganglioneuroblastomas or ganglioneuromas.[46] Opsoclonus-myoclonus syndrome has been observed in up to 4 percent of neuroblastoma patients.[47] This syndrome is neither due to direct involvement of the brain by tumor, nor to the production of catecholamines. While the mechanism is unclear, this syndrome may respond to high doses of corticosteroids.[44,47]

ASSOCIATED ANOMALIES AND FAMILIAL OCCURRENCE

In contrast to Wilms' tumor and acute leukemia in childhood, neuroblastomas are associated less frequently with combined congenital abnormalities. Nishi and coworkers found no Down's syndrome and no undescended testicle but 5 cases of mental retardation in 288 patients with neuroblastoma.[48] Familial occurrence of neuroblastoma is rare.[49]

DIAGNOSIS, STAGING, AND HISTOLOGICAL CLASSIFICATION

The diagnosis of neuroblastoma should be established histologically.[50,51] Characteristic histological features of neuroblastoma are described below. In most cases, a tissue diagnosis of neuroblastoma based upon hematoxylin and eosin staining is not difficult, especially if features suggestive of neuronal differentiation are present (Figs 16.1A to D). However, in some cases neuroblastomas are characterized by densely packed, small blue cells with little differentiation. Electron microscopy and implementation of immunohisto-chemical methods are recommended to confirm the diagnosis.[50] Core-needle biopsy or fine-needle aspiration is recommended to make the diagnosis by some but discouraged by others because of the small amounts of tissue obtained using these methods (Fig. 16.2). The diagnosis is also established if bone marrow aspirates or trephine biopsy contain unequivocal tumor cells (i.e. syncytia or immunocytologically positive clumps of cells)

and increased urine or serum levels of catecholamines or metabolites >3.0 SD above the mean are seen.[50] Serum neuron-specific enolase (NSE) is not decisive of diagnosis, but is of value in monitoring the clinical course.[52]

Evans' staging system[53] has long been used for neuroblastoma. However, the International Neuroblastoma Staging System (INSS) was first proposed in 1988, and after revisions in 1993[50] is currently used worldwide (Table 16.1). Before the INNS, the staging system of the Children's Cancer Group of the United States, its modification by the Japanese Society of Pediatric Surgeons, and that of the Pediatric Oncology Group of the United States were used. Each system had its strengths, but the differences made it difficult to compare the results of clinical trials and biologic studies

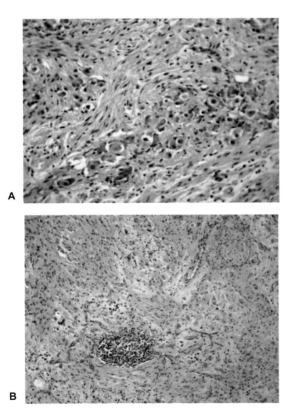

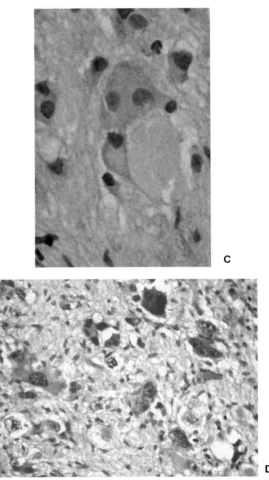

Figures 16.1A to D: Histopathological features of neuroblastoma are shown: **(A)** Small uniform cells with dense darkly staining nuclei and scant cytoplasm. **(B)** Rosette formation is seen. **(C)** Photomicrograph depicting a histopathological diagnosis of ganglioneuroma. **(D)** Photomicrograph depicting a histopathological diagnosis of ganglioneuroblastoma with islands of neuroblastoma cells and fibrous stroma

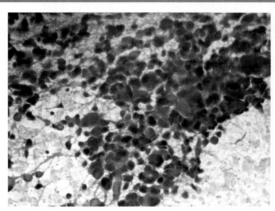

Figure 16.2: Photomicrograph showing the round cell appearance on fine-needle aspiration cytology in a case of neuroblastoma

performed by different groups and in different countries. The tests recommended for the assessment of extent of disease are well outlined in the report by Brodeur and his associates.[50]

It is tempting to consider that the histopathology of neuroblastomas, ganglioneuroblastomas, and ganglioneuromas parallels the pattern of differentiation expressed by the developing sympathetic nervous system.[54] Typical neuroblasts are small uniform cells with dense, hyperchromatic nuclei and a paucity of cytoplasm. The neuritic process or neuropil is noted, and pseudorosettes consisting of neuroblasts surrounding areas of eosinophilic neuropil are seen in a majority of cases. Tumors such as primitive neuroectodermal tumors, undifferentiated soft tissue sarcoma, Ewing's sarcoma, and non-Hodgkin's lymphoma should be carefully differentiated from neuroblastoma. The International Neuroblastoma Pathology Classification (INPC) was recently established.[51] Originally, Shimada and colleagues[55] established a classification in which the presence of Schwann's cells, degree of cellular differentiation, and mitosis-karyorrhexis index are determined to define favorable or unfavorable histologic types. The original Shimada classification was reviewed by an international panel of six member pathologists, and the INPC was approved.[51] In both the Shimada classification and INPC, the age of the patient at diagnosis is one of the factors predicting favorable or unfavorable prognosis.

IMAGING OF NEUROBLASTOMA

As neuroblastoma originates from the sympathetic ganglia and adrenal medulla, imaging investigation must focus on the pertinent area. However, it should be remembered that it is not uncommon for neuroblastoma to present first with the symptoms produced by metastases or even with peculiar clinical manifestations before the actual tumor is detected (Fig. 16.3). Although the imaging evaluation of a child with a presumed neuroblastoma varies from institution to institution, our routine procedures are as follows: plain radiograph of the chest and abdomen; abdominal sonography (US); magnetic resonance (MR) imaging; and bone scintigraphy with ^{99m}Tc MDP (methylendiphosphonate)

Table 16.1: International Neuroblastoma Staging System[50]	
Stage	Definition
I.	Localized tumor with complete gross excision, with or without microscopic residual disease; representative ipsilateral lymph nodes negative for tumor microscopically (nodes attached to and removed with the primary tumor may be positive)
IIA.	Localized tumor with incomplete gross excision; representative ipsilateral nonadherent lymph nodes negative for tumor microscopically
IIB.	Localized tumor with or without complete gross excision, with ipsilateral nonadherent lymph nodes positive for tumor; enlarged contralateral lymph nodes must be negative microscopically
III.	Unresectable unilateral tumor infiltrating across the midline, with or without regional lymph node involvement; or localized unilateral tumor with contralateral regional lymph node involvement; or midline tumor with bilateral extension by infiltration (unresectable) or by lymph node involvement
IV.	Any primary tumor with dissemination to distant lymph nodes, bone, bone marrow, liver, skin and/or other organs (except as defined for stage IV-S)
IV-S.	Localized primary tumor (as defined for stage I, IIA or IIB), with dissemination limited to skin, liver, and/or bone marrow (limited to infants < 1 year of age)

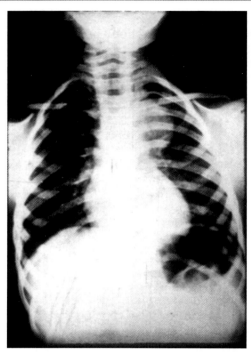

Figure 16.3: Skiagram chest outlining mediastinal deposits in a case of neuroblastoma

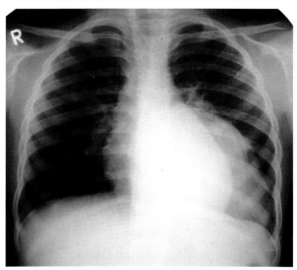

Figure 16.4: Skiagram chest showing a space occupying lesion in the left hemithorax that turned out to be a neuroblastoma of the posterior mediastinum

and metaiodobenzylguanidine (^{123}I MIBG) scintigraphy, if indicated. In Japan, neuroblastoma is not indicated in the application list of ^{123}I MIBG scintigraphy.

In the case of a thoracic neuroblastoma, imaging is 100 percent sensitive in suggesting the diagnosis[56] (Fig. 16.4). The mass is well defined and mediastinal based, associated with widening of the paraspinal line and rib erosion adjacent to the mass. On the other hand, plain abdominal radiography is less sensitive and often superfluous in terms of detection of the mass and intratumoral calcification. Thus the investigation should be followed with US regardless of the findings on abdominal radiograph.

On US, neuroblastoma is heterogeneously echogenic with poorly defined margins, and calcification, which is frequent, is identified as bright echoes with or without acoustic shadowing.[57] Most neuroblastomas demonstrate a "globular" region of increased echogenicity within the mass, which is regarded as an aggregate of uniform neuroblastoma cells marginated by reticulum and collagen.[58] The cystic form of neuroblastoma is rare, and located almost exclusively in the adrenal gland. This could be easily confused with adrenal hemorrhage as both have mainly been identified in neonates. Serial US imaging can resolve this problem as adrenal

hemorrhage changes in its echo pattern and size over a period of days. Adrenal hemorrhage is rare *in utero* and any adrenal mass seen *in utero*, whether cystic or solid, is likely to be a neuroblastoma.[59] Careful US examination can demonstrate the origin and extent of the tumor, and the relationship of the tumor to the adjacent organs and major abdominal vessels. However, it is difficult to obtain or propose a convincing anatomic delineation for surgeons in planning surgery and predicting tumor resectability. Intravenous urography may show displaced renal calyces (Fig. 16.5).

Computed tomography (CT) is comparable to MR imaging as a cross-sectional imaging modality and both can demonstrate the presence and extent of neuroblastoma (Fig. 16.6). Although unenhanced CT is very sensitive in demonstrating intratumoral calcification and is advised for the evaluation of adjacent bones,[60] the additional information from MR imaging makes findings of less importance than was true previously (Figs 16.7A to C).

Because of its sensitivity to tissue characteristics and multiplanar and angiographic capability, MR has the advantage of distinguishing the tumor from other surrounding soft tissues, defining the tumor extent from the wide view or on any plane, showing its relationship to adjacent vessels without contrast medium, and demonstrating intraspinal spread, as well as accuracy in the recognition of bone marrow involvement (Figs 16.8A to C and 16.9).[61] There is a limitation, however, in

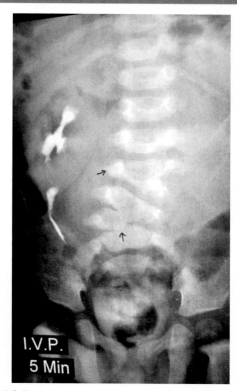

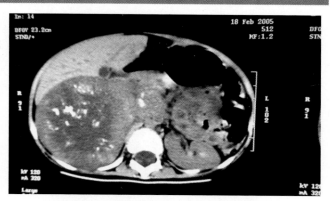

Figure 16.7A: Prechemotherapy CT scan image in axial section showing calcification in a case of neuroblastoma

Figure 16.5: Intravenous urogram in a child with a huge neuroblastoma showing displayed renal calyces and vertebral anomalies

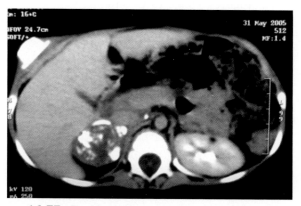

Figure 16.7B: Postchemotherapy CT scan image showing the residual tumor in axial section

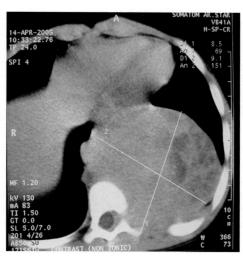

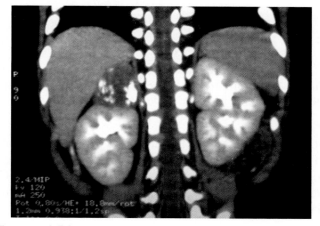

Figure 16.6: CT scan showing a posterior mediastinal neuroblastoma

Figure 16.7C: Postchemotherapy CT scan image showing the residual tumor in coronal section

differentiating residual tumor from ongoing fibrosis or scar tissue after chemotherapy, and differential criteria remains to be established.

Bone scintigraphy with ^{99m}TC MDP is well established and more sensitive than radiographic bone survey for the diagnosis of skeletal metastases of neuroblastoma (Fig. 16.10). In addition, this radiotracer can accumulate in the tumor itself. MIBG scintigraphy is also able to detect primary tumor and metastases. As a positive finding on MIBG scintigraphy is more specific, it can

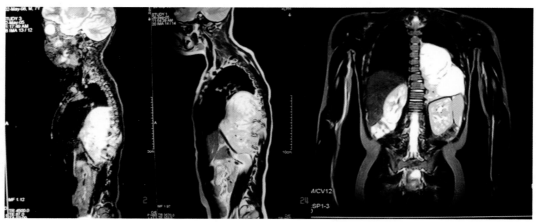

Figures 16.8A to C: MRI images in sagittal (**A** and **B**) and coronal sections (**C**) in a case of posterior mediastinal neuroblastoma with intraspinal extension

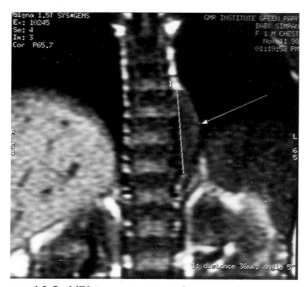

Figure 16.9: MRI image in coronal section showing a small mediastinal neuroblastoma

noninvasively establish the diagnosis of neuroblastoma in a child with a tumor of unknown origin. Cumulative results of MIBG scintigraphy indicate that MIBG scintigraphy should be used initially, followed by bone scintigraphy, if necessary.[62]

TUMOR MARKERS

The implication of determining tumor markers is two-fold. One is to make a definitive diagnosis and monitor patients during the course of treatment, and the other is to predict prognosis. The most definitive diagnostic markers are catecholamines and their metabolites in serum and urine, although the positivity is approximately

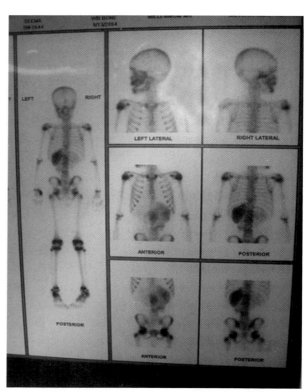

Figure 16.10: Bone scan images in a case of neuroblastoma showing thoracic and abdominal vertebrae involved with metastasis

75 to 80 percent in clinically diagnosed patients with neuroblastoma. Elevated neuron-specific enolase (NSE) levels are seen not only in the sera of patients with neuroblastoma but also in those with other pediatric tumors. However, serum NSE levels are elevated in all types of neuroblastoma whether or not the metabolic

pathways of catecholamines are present, and NSE serves as a good tumor marker in monitoring the disease course of neuroblastoma.[52,63]

A serum ferritin level > 142 ng/ml is found in many patients with advanced-stage neuroblastoma but rarely in low-stage disease, and it was reported that increased levels of ferritin are associated with a poorer progression-free survival rate.[64] Similarly, serum lactic dehydrogenase (LDH) levels > 1,500 U/ml are associated with a poorer prognosis in neuroblastoma,[65] and a serum NSE level elevated > 100 ng/ml is associated with poor survival in advanced-stage patients with neuroblastoma.[54]

The roles of CD44, ganglioside GD2, chromogranin A, neuropeptide Y (NPY), and proliferating cell nuclear antigen (PCNA) have been studied.[54] CD44 is a glycoprotein found in the cell surface of many tumors and is associated with aggressive behavior. Interestingly, expression of CD44 in neuroblastomas correlates with less aggressive behavior and has been highly predictive of favorable outcome.[66] Ganglioside GD2 is the characteristic ganglioside on human neuroblastoma cell membranes and increased plasma levels of GD2 have been found in patients with neuroblastoma. Shed ganglioside may accelerate tumor progression,[67] and human-type anti-GD2 monoclonal antibody combined with interleukin-2 is currently undergoing clinical trials in the United States.[68] Chromogranin A is an acidic protein present in the neurosecretary granules of neuroendocrine tumor cells, and has been identified as a marker possibly indicative of neuronal differentiation.[69] NPY is another neurosecretory protein, and its plasma levels may also indicate the level of neuronal differentiation in neuroblastoma.[70] PCNA correlates with the level of cell proliferation. The PCNA index in neuroblastoma is closely related to *MYCN* amplification and to poor prognosis.[71]

MASS SCREENING

The purpose of screening infants for neuroblastoma is to reduce the number of advanced-stage neuroblastomas in older children by identifying more number of infants with the favorable type of neuroblastoma. The concept of detecting catecholamine metabolites in urine dates back to LaBrosse, who first used spot tests of catecholamine metabolites for infants with neuro-blastoma in 1968.[72,73] In 1972 Sawada started to screen infants for neuroblastoma in Kyoto using a quantitative vanillylmandelic (VMA) test (VMA spot test).[74] This test was changed to quantitative measurements of urinary VMA and homovanillic acid (HVA), mass screening of neuroblastoma was introduced in all prefectures in Japan in 1985, and the methods for the measurement of urinary VMA and HVA were refined to sensitive high-performance liquid chromatography (HPLC) in 1988.[75] As a result, the incidence of neuroblastoma changed after the introduction of nationwide mass screening. Between 1980 and 1985, approximately 120 patients with neuroblastoma were registered yearly, while the number of annual neuroblastoma patients increased to about 250 during the period from 1991 to 1995.[2,75] Neuroblastomas identified in infancy through mass screening were exclusively of the favorable types, and roughly 99 percent of such infants have been cured, some of whom were only observed.

It must be remembered that the purpose of mass screening is to decrease the number of older children with advanced neuroblastoma. Some questions have been raised in this respect,[76] and it was shown that the absolute number of stage IV (excluding stage IV-S) neuroblastoma patients older than 12 months of age was not decreasing significantly when the number of live births was taken into account (Table 16.2).[2] Not all neuroblastoma, perhaps only 75 to 80 percent, possess the metabolic pathways of catecholamines.[11] Overdiagnosis of infant neuroblastoma which otherwise might have regressed spontaneously has also been pointed out.[76,77] A consensus conference to discuss the true value of mass screening was held in Lyon, France, in December 1998. Investigators from North America reported that they were negative toward mass screening based upon their own data,[77] and the majority of European researchers agreed with the contention of the North American group,[78] but the German group emphasized that one must consider the results of the German mass screening conducted at the age of 12 months[79] and which may reduce overdiagnosis of infant neuroblastoma.

TREATMENT OF LOW-RISK NEUROBLASTOMA

The treatment of neuroblastoma should be planned individually according to the risk group. There has been argument over whether neuroblastoma consists of two or three types of tumor. Brodeur and Ambros[41] consider that it consists of three types, low risk (type 1), intermediate risk (type 2A), and high risk (type 2B), but the differentiation between their type 2A and type 2B is difficult from a clinical viewpoint, and it should be

Table 16.2: The incidence of stage IV neuroblastoma in Japan, according to Tsuchida et al[2]

Year	Number of neuroblastoma cases*	Number of stage IV neuroblastoma patients older than 12 months of age	Number of live births
1981	107 (1)	55	1,529,455
1982	139 (4)	63	1,515,392
1983	152 (8)	62	1,508,687
1984	136 (12)	46	1,489,780
1985	142 (32)	40	1,431,577
1986	162 (39)	56	1,382,946
1987	143 (49)	30	1,346,658
1988	198 (88)	57	1,314,006
1989	179 (90)	33	1,246,802
1990	190 (108)	40	1,221,585
1991	238 (138)	51	1,223,245
1992	229 (121)	54	1,208,989
1993	207 (135)	32	1,188,282
1994	298 (208)	41	1,238,328
1995	222 (140)	32	1,187,064
1996	238 (162)	28	1,206,555
1997	276 (164)	47	1,191,665
1998	229 (147)	29	1,203,147

*Numbers in parentheses represent cases identified by mass screening and are part of the total. Cases with incomplete data with regard to patient age and disease stage are excluded.[61]

taken into account that prognosis is not determined by *MYCN* amplification alone. Therefore, division into two types, as proposed by Tsuchida and La Quaglia,[80] appears to be more reasonable (Table 16.3).

Low-risk neuroblastomas here denote those occurring in infants younger than 12 months of age in INSS stage I, II, III, and IV-S and without *MYCN* amplification. These tumors should be treated less intensively compared with high-risk tumors.[81] Some neuroblastomas found by mass screening at about 6 or 7 months of age may be treated by observation only if the mass is less than 3 to 4 cm in diameter and does not show any signs of enlargement during the observation period.[82] Nevertheless, in the majority of institutions, the tumor is excised and less aggressive surgery is recommended.[83] Original tumors in stage I, II, and IV-S are excised at the start of treatment, but they should be removed after chemotherapy when they are in stage III.

Chemotherapy for low-risk neuroblastoma should not be aggressive. In Japan, no chemotherapy is administered for stage I and II tumors after complete resection. The recommended preoperative chemotherapy for infant neuroblastoma in stage III consists of alternating weekly administration of vincristine 1.5 mg/ m^2 iv and cyclophosphamide 300 mg/m^2 iv, repeated

six times. For stage IV without bone cortex metastases, regimen C2 consisting of vincristine 1.5 mg/m^2 on day 1, cyclophosphamide 600 mg/m^2 on day 1 and pirarubicin (THP-adriamycin, Nihon Kayaku, Tokyo) 30 mg/m^2 on day 3 is given nine times at 4-week intervals.[81]

When the tumor is associated with *MYCN* amplification and/or 1p-deletion and/or bone cortex metastases, the infants are treated with a modification of the regimens for advanced neuroblastoma.

TREATMENT OF HIGH-RISK NEUROBLASTOMA

High-risk neuroblastomas here denote those occurring in children older than 12 months of age, in INSS stage III and IV, and with/without *MYCN* amplification. Reports[84,85] show that the results of treatment of stage III and IV disease in older children are still not very good, and are poorer when associated with *MYCN* amplification. Yet it is generally agreed that these two groups, *MYCN* amplified and unamplified, should be given the same consideration as high-risk neuroblastoma. The prognostic significance of *MYCN* amplification is very clear in low-stage patients, but not as clear in stage IV patients.[42,85,86] In the treatment of high-risk neuroblastoma, chemotherapy is vitally important.

Table 16.3: A simplified comparison of risk factors for high- and low-risk neuroblastoma by Tsuchida and La Quaglia[80]

Parameter	High-risk	Low-risk
Age	> 1 year, especially > 2 years	< 1 year
Stage	INSS IV, some III	INSS I, II, III, IV-S
MYCN status	> 10 copies	9 copies, especially < 3 copies
1p36 deletion	Present	Absent
Shimada classification	Unfavorable	Favorable
Ploidy	Diploid	Hyperploid
Trk-A expression	Absent	Present
Ferritin at diagnosis	> 143-150 ng/ml	< 143-150 ng/ml

Chemotherapy

Numerous chemotherapeutic protocols have been proposed and utilized worldwide for advanced neuroblastoma.[86]

Different induction chemotherapeutic regimens were used in Japan from March 1991 to May 1998 based on MYCN amplification status (Table 16.4).[87] Researchers were requested to perform a biopsy before treatment and to treat all stage IV patients with one cycle of regimen new A_1 while awaiting the results of Southern blot analysis of the MYCN oncogene. When the tumor was found to contain more than 10 copies of MYCN, patients received five courses of regimen A_3 until a total of six cycles was reached. On the other hand, if it was found to contain fewer than 9 copies of MYCN, patients received further courses of regimen new A_1 until a total six cycles was reached. Both regimen new A_1 and

Table 16.4: Induction chemotherapy regimens (Kaneko et al. from 1991 to 1998[87])

Regimen new A_1
  Cyclophosphamide 1,200 mg/m^2 day 1
  THP-adriamycin 40 mg/m^2 day 3
  Etoposide 100 mg/m^2/day days 1, 2, 3, 4, 5
  Cisplatin 90 mg/m^2 day 5

Regimen A_3
  Cyclophosphamide 1,200 mg/m^2/day days 1, 2
  THP-adriamycin 40 mg/m^2 day 3
  Etoposide 100 mg/m^2/day days 1, 2, 3, 4, 5
  Cisplatin 25 mg/m^2/day days 1, 2, 3, 4, 5 (continuous)
  Matthay et al from 1991 to 1996[88]

Regimen
  Cisplatin 60 mg/m^2 day 1
  Adriamycin 30 mg/m^2 day 3
  Etoposide 100 mg/m^2/day days 3, 6
  Cyclophosphamide 1,200 mg/m^2/day days 4, 5

regimen A_3 were well tolerated with acceptable complications.[87] Matthay and her associates used an induction chemotherapeutic regimen similar to this (Table 16.4),[88] but they used a single regimen for both MYCN-amplified and unamplified neuroblastomas.

Surgery

Radical surgery is performed during the first six cycles of induction chemotherapy. It seems ideal to operate after the fourth or fifth cycle of intensive induction chemotherapy. There are some controversies regarding the timing of surgery, operative methods, and value of surgical resection in high-risk neuroblastoma.[80]

Excision of the primary tumor and retroperitoneal lymph node dissection are carried out systematically in the six sections defined by the authors, as shown in Figure 16.11.[89] These include areas to the left of the abdominal aorta (1+2); between the aorta and vena cava (3+4); and to the right of the vena cava (5+6); with further subdivision according to the level of the renal vein. When the tumor occurs on the left, dissection begins at the common iliac lymph nodes and moves upward after exploring the left common or external iliac artery and dissecting its adventitia longitudinally along the middle (section 1). During this process, neuroblastoma in the left adrenal gland is removed, but every effort should be made to preserve the left kidney.

The inferior and superior mesenteric arteries and the celiac axis are encountered in that order during dissection. Lymph nodes located on the right side of these arteries are not removed at this time, but are left in place for the following step. During dissection, care is taken not to damage the left renal artery and its adventitia; dissection stops at the outer sheath and a small sponge soaked in procaine chloride is left in place during the procedure. Next, the dissection proceeds to the suprarenal region (section 2).

14. Cohn SL, Salwen H, Quasney NW, et al. Prolonged N-myc protein halflife in a neuroblastoma cell line lacking N-myc amplification. Oncogene 1990;5:1821-27.

15. Wada RK, Seeger RC, Brodeur GM, et al. Human neuroblastoma cell lines that express N-myc without gene amplification. Cancer 1993;72:3346-54.

16. Tsuchida Y, Hemmi H, Inoue A, et al. Genetic clinical markers of human neuroblastoma with special reference to N-myc oncogene: Amplified or not amplified? Tumor Biol 1996;17:65-74.

17. Marris J, Matthay KK. Molecular biology of neuroblastoma. J Clin Oncol 1999;17:2264-79.

18. Speleman F, Bown N. 17q gain in neuroblastoma. In Brodeur GM, Sawada T, Tsuchida Y, Voûte PA (Eds): Neuroblastoma. Amsterdam, Elsevier, 2000;113-24.

19. Suzuki T, Yokota J, Mugishima H, et al. Frequent loss of heterozygosity on chromosome 14q in neuroblastoma. Cancer Res 1989;49:1095-8.

20. Takita J, Hayashi Y, Takei K, et al. Allelic imbalance on chromosome 18 in neuroblastoma. Eur J Cancer 2000; 36:508-13.

21. Look AT, Hayes FA, Shuster JJ, et al. Clinical relevance of tumor cell ploidy and N-myc gene amplification in childhood neuroblastoma: A Pediatric Oncology Group study. J Clin Oncol 1991;9:581-91.

22. Ambros IM, Zellner A, Roald B, et al. Role of ploidy, chromosome 1p, and Schwann cells in the maturation of neuroblastoma. N Engl J Med 1996;334:1505-11.

23. Nakagawara A, Kogner P. Expression and function of Trk and its related genes in human neuroblastoma. In Brodeur GM, Sawada T, Tsuchida Y, Voûte PA, (Eds): Neuroblastoma. Amsterdam, Elsevier, 2000, pp 147-157.

24. Nakagawara A, Arima-Nakagawara M, Scavarda NJ, et al. Association between high levels of expression of the TRK gene and favorable outcome in human neuroblastoma. N Engl J Med 1993;328:847-54.

25. Kwiatkowski JL, Rutkowski JL, Yamashiro DJ, et al. Schwann cell-conditioned medium promotes neuro-blastoma survival and differentiation. Cancer Res 1998; 58:4602-6.

26. Nakagawara A, Azar CG, Scavarda NJ, et al. Expression and function of TRK-B and BDNF in human neuroblastoma. Mol Cell Biol 1994;14:759-67.

27. Ikeda H, Hirato J, Akami M, et al. Massive apoptosis detected by in situ DNA nick end labeling in neuroblastoma. Am J Surg Pathol 1996;20:649-55.

28. Ikeda H, Castle VP. Apoptosis in neuroblastoma and pathways involving bcl-2 and caspases, in Brodeur GM, Sawada T, Tsuchida Y, Voûte PA, (Eds): Neuroblastoma. Amsterdam, Elsevier, 2000, pp 197-205.

29. Nakagawara A, Nakamura Y, Ikeda H, et al. High levels of expression and nuclear localization of interleukin-1β converting enzyme (ICE) and CPP32 in favorable human neuroblastoma. Cancer Res 1997;57:4578-84.

30. Ikeda H, Nakamura Y, Hiwasa T, et al. Interleukin-1β converting enzyme (ICE) is preferentially expressed in neuroblastoma with favourable prognosis. Eur J Cancer 1997;33:2081-3.

31. Hiyama E, Reynolds CP. Telomerase as a biological and prognostic marker in neuroblastoma. In Brodeur GM, Sawada T, Tsuchida Y, Voûte PA, (Eds): Neuroblastoma. Amsterdam, Elsevier, 2000; 159-74.

32. Hiyama E, Hiyama K, Yokoyama T, et al. Correlating telomerase activity levels with human neuroblastoma outcomes. Nat Med 1995;1:249-55.

33. Reynolds CP, Zuo JJ, Kim NW, et al. Telomerase expression in primary neuroblastomas. Eur J Cancer 1997;33:1929-31.

34. Thomas SM, DeMarco M, D'Arcangelo G, et al. Ras is essential for nerve growth factor- and phorbolester-induced tyrosine phosphorylation of MAP kinases. Cell 1992;68:1031-40.

35. Tanaka T, Slamon DJ, Shimada H, et al. A significant association of Ha-ras p21 in neuroblastoma cells with patient prognosis: A retrospective study of 103 cases. Cancer 1991;68:1296-302.

36. Tanaka T, Sugimoto T, Sawada T. Prognostic discrimination among neuroblastomas according to Ha-ras/trkA gene expression. Cancer 1998;83:1626-33.

37. Chan HSL, Haddad G, Thorner PS, et al. P-glycoprotein expression as a predictor of the outcome of therapy for neuroblastoma. N Engl J Med 1991;325:1608-14

38. Obana K, Hashizume K. Expression of multidrug resistance-related P-glycoprotein shows good prognosis in neuroblastoma. J Pediatr Surg 1997;32:420-22.

39. Haber M, Bordow SB, Haber PS, et al. The prognostic value of MDR1 gene expression in primary untreated neuroblastoma. Eur J Cancer 1997;33:2031-6.

40. Norris MD, Bordow SB, Marshall GM, et al. Expression of the gene for multidrug-resistance-associated protein and outcome in patients with neuroblastoma. N Engl J Med 1996;334:231-8.

41. Brodeur GM, Ambros PF. Genetic and biological markers of prognosis in neuroblastoma. In Brodeur GM, Sawada T, Tsuchida Y, Voûte PA, (Eds): Neuroblastoma. Amsterdam, Elsevier, 2000; 355-69.

42. Kaneko M, Tsuchida Y, Mugishima H, et al. Higher doses in chemotherapy may treat away the effect of MYCN amplification in patients with high-risk neuroblastoma. Int J Cancer (submitted).

43. Granata C, Fagnani AM, Gambini C, et al. Features and outcome of neruroblastoma detected before birth. J Pediatr Surg 2000;35:88-91.

44. Mugishima H, Sakurai M. Symptoms of neuroblastoma: Paraneoplastic syndromes. In Brodeur GM, Sawada T, Tsuchida Y, Voûte PA (Eds): Neuroblastoma. Amsterdam, Elsevier, 2000;293-301.

45. Lee LCL, Broadbent V, Kelsall W. Neuroblastoma in an infant revealing middle aortic syndrome. Med Pediatr Oncol 2000;35:150-2.

46. Bjellerup P, Theodorsson E, Kogner P. Somatostatin and vasoactive intestinal peptide (VIP) in neuroblastoma and ganglioneuroma: Chromatographic characterisation and release during surgery. Eur J Cancer 1995;31:481-5.

47. Shapiro B, Shulkin BL, Hutchinson RJ, et al. Location of neuroblastoma in the opsoclonus-myoclonus sindrome. J Nucl Biol Med 1994;38:545-55.

48. Nishi M, Miyake H, Takeda T, et al. Congenital malformations and childhood cancer. Med Pediatr Oncol 2000;34:250-4.

49. Robertson CM, Tyrrell JC, Pritchard J. Familial neural crest tumors. Eur J Pediatr 1991;150:789-92.

50. Brodeur GM, Pritchard J, Berthold F, et al. Revisions of the international criteria for neuroblastoma diagnosis, staging, and response to treatment. J Clin Oncol 1993;11:1466-77.

51. Shimada H, Ambros IM, Dehner LP, et al. The international neuroblastoma pathology classification (the Shimada system). Cancer 1999;86:364-72.

52. Tsuchida Y, Honna T, Iwanaka T, et al. Serial determination of serum neuron-specific enolase in patients with neuroblastoma and other pediatric tumors. J Pediatr Surg 1987;22:419-24.

53. Evans AE, D'Angio GJ, Randolph J. A proposed staging for children with neuroblastoma: Children's Cancer Study Group A. Cancer 1971;27:374-8.

54. Black CT, Haase GM. Neuroblastoma and other adrenal tumors. In Carachi R, Azmy A, Grosfeld JL, (Eds): The Surgery of Childhood Tumors. London, Arnold, 1999; 140-77.

55. Shimada H, Chatten J, Newton WA, et al. Histopathologic prognostic factors in neuroblastic tumors: definition of subtypes of ganglioneuroblastoma and an age-linked classification of neuroblastomas. J Natl Cancer Inst 1984;73:405-16.

56. Slovis TL, Meza MP, Cushing B, et al. Thoracic neuroblastoma: what is the best imaging modality for evaluating extent of disease? Pediatr Radiol 1997;27:273-5.

57. Bousvaros A, Kirks DR, Grosman H. Imaging of neuro-blastoma: an overview. Pediatr Radiol 1986;16:89-106.

58. Amundson GM, Trevenen CL, Mueller DL, et al. Neuroblastoma: a specific sonographic tissue pattern. Am J Roentgenol 1987;148:943-5.

59. Leonidas JC, Berdon W. The adrenal gland: the neonate and young infant. In Silverman HN, Ku HN, (Eds): Caffey's Pediatric X-ray Diagnosis, 9th ed, Vol 2. St. Louis, Mosby, 1993;2141-4.

60. Vazquez E, Enriquez G, Castellote A, et al. US, CT, and MR imaging of neck lesions in children. Radiographics 1995;15:105-22.

61. Tanabe M, Ohnuma N, Iwai J, et al. Bone marrow metastasis of neuroblastoma analyzed by MRI and its influence on prognosis. Med Pediatr Oncol 1995;24:292-9.

62. Staalman CR, Hoefnagel CA. Imaging of neuroblastoma and metastasis. In Brodeur GM, Sawada T, Tsuchida Y, Voûte PA, (Eds): Neuroblastoma. Amsterdam, Elsevier, 2000;303-32.

63. Massaron S, Seregni E, Luksch R, et al. Neuron-specific enolase evaluation in patients with neuroblastoma. Tumor Biol 1998;19:261-8.

64. Hann HWL, Bombardieri E. Serum markers and prognosis in neuroblastoma: Ferritin, LDH, and NSE. In Brodeur GM, Sawada T, Tsuchida Y, Voûte PA, (Eds): Neuroblastoma. Amsterdam, Elsevier, 2000;371-81.

65. Joshi VV, Cantor AB, Brodeur GM, et al. Correlation between morphologic and other prognostic markers of neuroblastoma: A study of histologic grade, DNA index, N-myc gene copy number, and lactic dehydrogenase in patients in the Pediatric Oncology Group. Cancer 1993;71:3173-81.

66. Combaret V, Lasset C, Frappez D, et al. Evaluation of CD44 prognostic value in neuroblastoma: Comparison with the other prognostic factors. Eur J Cancer 1995;31A:545-9.

67. Valentino L, Moss T, Olson E, et al. Shed tumor gangliosides and progression of human neuroblastoma. Blood 1990;75:1564-7.

68. Handgretinger R, Anderson K, Lang P, et al. A phase 1 study of human/mouse chimeric anti-ganglioside GD2 antibody ch14.18 in patients with neuroblastoma. Eur J Cancer 1995;31A:261-7.

69. Schmid KW, Dockhorn-Dworniczak S, Fahrenkamp A. Chromogranin A, secreto-granina II and vasoactive intestinal peptide in phaeochromocytomas and ganglioneuromas. Histopathology 1993;22:527-33.

70. Rascher W, Kremens B, Wagner S, et al. Serial measurements of neuropeptide Y in plasma for monitoring neuroblastoma in children. J Pediatr 1993;122:914-6.

71. Kawasaki H, Mukai K, Yajima S, et al. Prognostic value of proliferating cell nuclear antigen (PCNA) immunostaining in neuroblastoma. Med Pediatr Oncol 1995;25:300-4.

72. LaBrosse EH. Biochemical diagnosis of neuroblastoma: Use of new urine spot test. Proc Am Assoc Cancer Res 1968;9:39.

73. LaBrosse EH, Com-Nougue C, Zucker JM, et al. Urinary excretion of 3-methoxy-4-hydroxymandelic acid and 3-methoxy-4-hydroxyphenylacetic acid by 288 patients with neuroblastoma and related neural crest tumors. Cancer Res 1980;40:1995-2001.

74. Sawada T, Imashuku S, Takada H, et al. Screening of random urine specimens with use of VMA spot test. J Jpn Soc Pediatr Surg 1975;11:49-52.

75. Sawada T, Takeda T. Screening for neuroblasoma in infancy in Japan. In Brodeur GM, Sawada T, Tsuchida Y, Voûte PA, (Eds): Neuroblastoma. Amsterdam, Elsevier, 2000;245-64.

76. Bessho F. Effects of mass screening on age-specific incidence of neuroblastoma. Int J Cancer 1996;67:520-2.

77. Lemieux B, Woods WG. Mass screening for neuro-blastoma: The North American experience. In Brodeur GM, Sawada T, Tsuchida Y, Voûte PA, (Eds): Neuro-blastoma. Amsterdam, Elsevier, 2000; 265-79.

78. Schilling FH, Parker L. Mass screening for neuroblastoma: The European experience. In Brodeur GM, Sawada T, Tsuchida Y, Voûte PA, (Eds): Neuroblastoma. Amsterdam, Elsevier, 2000; 281-92.

79. Berthold F, Baillot A, Laioum H, et al. Neuroblastoma screening at 12 months may reduce overdiagnosis. Med Pediatr Oncol 1994;23:208.

80. Tsuchida Y, La Quaglia MP. Surgery for neuroblastoma. In Brodeur GM, Sawada T, Tsuchida Y, Voûte PA, (Eds): Neuroblastoma. Amsterdam, Elsevier, 2000;497-517.

81. Matsumura T, Michon J. Treatment of localized neuro-blasoma. In Brodeur GM, Sawada T, Tsuchida Y, Voûte PA, (Eds): Neuroblastoma. Amsterdam, Elsevier, 2000; 403-15.

82. Yamamoto K, Hanada R, Tanimura M, et al. Natural history of neuroblastoma found by mass screening. Lancet 1997;349:1102.

83. Ikeda H, Suzuki N, Takahashi A, et al. Surgical treatment of neuroblastomas in infants under 12 months of age. J Pediatr Surg 1998;33:1246-50.

84. Hartmann O, Berthold F. Treatment of advanced neuroblastoma: The European experience. In Brodeur GM, Sawada T, Tsuchida Y, Voûte PA (Eds): Neuroblastoma. Amsterdam, Elsevier, 2000; 437-52.

85. Kaneko M, Tsuchida Y, Uchino J, et al. Treatment results of advanced neuroblastoma with the First Japanese Study Group Protocol. J Pediatr Hematol Oncol 1999;21:190-7.

86. Berthold F, Hero B. Neuroblastoma: Current drug therapy recommendations as part of the total treatment approach. Drug Management 2000;59:1261-77.

87. Kaneko M, Nishihira H, Mugishima H, et al. Stratification of treatment of stage 4 neuroblastoma patients based on N-myc amplification status. Med Pediatr Oncol 1998;31:1-7.

88. Matthay KK, Villablanca JG, Seeger RC, et al. Treatment of high-risk neuroblastoma with intensive chemotherapy, radiotherapy, autologous bone marrow transplantation, and 13-cis-retinoic acid. N Engl J Med 1999;341:1165-73.

89. Tsuchida Y, Honna T, Kamii Y, et al. Radical excision of primary tumor and lymph nodes in advanced neuroblastoma: Combination with intensive induction chemotherapy. Pediatr Surg Int 1991;6:22-7.

90. Miyauchi J, Matsuoka K, Oka T, et al. Histopathological findings in advanced neuroblastoma after intensive induction chemotherapy. J Pediatr Surg 1997;32:1620-23.

91. Tsuchida Y, Yokoyama J, Kaneko M, et al. Therapeutic significance of surgery in advanced neuroblastoma: A report from the Study Group of Japan. J Pediatr Surg 1992;27:616-22.

92. Ikeda H, August CS, Goldwein N, et al. Sites of relapse in patients with neuroblastoma following bone marrow transplantation in relation to preparatory "debulking" treatment. J Pediatr Surg 1992;27:1438-41.

93. Habrand JP, D'Angio GJ. Radiotherapy in neuroblastoma. In Brodeur GM, Sawada T, Tsuchida Y, Voûte PA (Eds): Neuroblastoma. Amsterdam, Elsevier, 2000; 479-96.

94. Kushner BH, O'Reilly RJ, Mandell LR, et al. Myeloablative combination chemotherapy without total body irradiation for neuroblastoma. J Clin Oncol 1991;9:274-9.

95. Leavy PJ, Odom LF, Poole M, et al. Intraoperative radiation therapy in pediatric neuroblastoma. Med Pediatr Oncol 1997;28:424-8.

96. Seeger RC, Reynolds CP. Treatment of high-risk solid tumors of childhood with intensive therapy and autologous bone marrow transplantation. Pediatr Clin North Am 1991;38:393-424.

97. Ohnuma N, Takahashi H, Kaneko M, et al. Treatment combined with bone marrow transplantation for advanced neuroblastoma: An analysis of patients who were pretreated intensively with the protocol of the Study Group of Japan. Med Pediatr Oncol 1995;25:181-7.

98. Kawa K, Ohnuma N, Kaneko M, et al. Long-term survivors of advanced neuroblastoma with *MYCN* amplification: A report of 19 patients surviving disease-free for more than 66 months. J Clin Oncol 1999;17:3216-20.

99. Gaze MN, Wheldon TE. Radiolabelled MIBG in the treatment of neuroblastoma. Eur J Cancer 1996;32A:93-6.

100. Mastrangelo R, Tornesello, Riccardi R, et al. A new approach in the treatment of stage IV neuroblastoma using a combination of ^{131}I-meta-iodobenzylguanidine (MIBG) and cisplatin. Eur J Cancer 1995;31A:606-11.

101. van Hasselt EJ, Heij HA, de Kraker J, et al. Pretreatment with ^{131}I]metaiodobenzylguanidine and surgical resection of advanced neuroblastoma. Eur J Pediatr Surg 1996;6:155-8.

102. Furman WL, Stewart CF, Poquette CA, et al. Direct translation of a protracted irinotecan schdule from a xenograft model to a phase I trial in children. J Clin Oncol 1999;17:1815-24.

103. Mugishima H, Matsunaga T, Yagi K, et al. Phase I study of irinotecan in pediatric patients with malignant solid tumors. J Pediatr Hematol Oncol (submitted).

104. O'Reilly MS, Boehm T, Shing Y, et al. Endostatin: An endogenous inhibitor of angiogenesis and tumor growth. Cell 1997;88:277-85.

105. Nagabuchi E, VanderKolk WE, Une Y, et al. TNP-470 antiangiogenic therapy for advanced murine neuro-blastoma. J Pediatr Surg 1997;32:287-93.

106. Katzenstein HM, Rademaker AW, Senger C, et al. Effectiveness of the angiogenesis inhibitor TNP-470 in reducing the growth of human neuroblastoma in nude mice inversely correlates with tumor burden. Clin Cancer Res 1999;5:4273-8.

107. Meadows AT, Tsunematsu Y. Late effects of treatment of neuroblastoma. In Brodeur GM, Sawada T, Tsuchida Y, Voûte PA, (Eds): Neuroblastoma. Amsterdam, Elsevier, 2000; pp 561-70.

CHAPTER 17

Devendra K Gupta
Shilpa Sharma

Recent Advances in Neuroblastoma

Neuroblastoma is the third most common neoplasm of childhood and the most common solid tumor in infancy. About 70 percent of cases occur by 5 years age and around 95 percent cases are in the patients younger than 10 years old.

Neuroblastoma is a tumor of mystery from all aspects, symptomatology, diagnosis, behavior and response to treatment. Specific areas of interest include prognostic factors and approaches for therapy; biochemistry—neuropeptides, retinoic acid and cell adhesion molecules; the role of N-Myc oncogene amplification; and chromosome 1p alterations as an indicator for the role of a cancer preventing gene.

Spontaneous regression is more common in neuroblastomas than in any other tumor type, especially in young patients under 12 months. Unfortunately, the full clinical spectrum of neuroblastomas also includes very aggressive tumors, unresponsive to multi-modality treatment and accounting for most of the pediatric cancer mortalities less than 5 years of age.

Neuroblastoma has received particular attention as a model to describe the role of cellular differentiation in context with genetic alterations during tumorigenesis. Neuroblastoma is part of the spectrum of the family of neuroblastic tumors, consisting of neuroblastoma, ganglioneuroblastoma and ganglioneuroma. In recent years there has been considerable development in the classification concepts from purely histological to clinico-pathological one.

It is a tumor with varied histological features and prognosis in different age groups. It is generally emphasized that more than one biological entity of neuroblastoma exists. Structural genetic defects such as amplification of N-Myc, gain of chromosome 17q and LOH of 1p and several other chromosomal regions have proven to be valuable as prognostic factors and will be discussed in relation to their clinical relevance. Recent research is starting to uncover important molecular pathways involved in the pathogenesis of neuroblastomas.Numerous biological factors have been identified to have a role in determining the prognosis, yet the facilities differ from place to place. The treatment instituted also differs from center to center.

The most important fact to be faced by treating surgeons is the unpredictable behavior of the tumor. The tumor may remain silent for a long time and then just present with secondaries in the eye making the tumor stage IV at diagnosis.

As far as surgery is concerned, the tumor may at times be difficult to eradicate completely especially in cases with intraspinal extention. The response of the tumor to chemotherapy is also unpredictable depending upon the maturity of the tumor. The role of radiotherapy in gross residual tumors has also been evaluated time and again due to the initial fear of side effects of radiotherapy on the growing child.

Neuroblastoma is the only tumor in which ongoing research still continues to identify factors to determine the treatment strategy. It is thus vital to stay in touch with the recent advances and identify useful modifications in the management depending upon the facilities available. The chapter includes present in-depth, up-to-date information and continued progress in understanding and treatment of this enigmatic tumor

HUMAN NEUROBLASTOMA STEM CELLS

Human neuroblastoma is an embryonic cancer of the neural crest. Cellular heterogeneity is a characteristic feature of both tumors and derived cell lines. Recent studies have revealed that both cell lines and tumors contain cancer stem cells.[1] In culture, these cells are self-renewing, multipotent, and highly malignant; in tumors their frequency correlates with a worse prognosis.[1] Their identification and characterization should now permit a targeted approach to more effective treatment of this often fatal childhood cancer.

SPONTANEOUS REGRESSION

Neuroblastoma frequently shows spontaneous regression in which two distinct types of programmed cell death, i.e. caspase-dependent apoptosis and H-Ras-mediated autophagic degeneration, have been suggested to play a key role. However, in a recent study conducted to determine which of these cell suicide pathways predominated in this tumor regression, it was concluded that that neither caspase-dependent apoptosis nor autophagic degeneration may be involved in spontaneous neuroblastoma regression.[2] Other mechanisms, such as tumor maturation have been suggested to be responsible for this phenomenon. The incidence of caspase-dependent apoptosis was significantly correlated with indicators of a poor prognosis in these tumors, including Shimada's unfavorable histology, N-Myc amplification, and a higher mitosis-karyorrhexis index, but not with factors related to tumor regression such as clinical stage and mass screening.[2]

HEREDITARY PREDISPOSITION TO NEUROBLASTOMA

Hereditary predisposition to neuroblastoma accounts for less than 5 percent of neuroblastomas and is probably heterogeneous. Recently, a predisposition gene has been mapped to 16p12-p13, but has not yet been identified. Occurrence of neuroblastoma in association with congenital central hypoventilation and Hirschsprung's disease suggests that genes, involved in the development of neural-crest-derived cells, may be altered in these conditions. A constitutional R100L PHOX2B mutation was identified in a family with three first-degree relatives with neuroblastic tumors in all three patients and a germline PHOX2B mutation was identified in one patient treated for Hirschsprung's disease who subsequently developed a multifocal neuroblastoma in infancy.[3] Both mutations disrupt the homeodomain of the PHOX2B protein. No loss of heterozygosity at the PHOX2B locus was observed in the tumor, suggesting that haploinsufficiency, gain of function or dominant negative effects may account for the oncogenic effects of these mutations. PHOX2B has thus been identified as the first predisposing gene to hereditary neuroblastic tumors.[3]

The biologic basis of neuroblastoma has come into clearer focus. PHOX2B is the first bonafide neuroblastoma predisposition gene identified, but is mutated in only a small subset of cases.[4] Somatically acquired alterations at chromosome arms 3p and 11q are highly correlated with acquisition of metastases in the absence of N-Myc amplification and may be useful as prognostic markers.[4] The Children's Oncology Group risk classification system has been validated, with current emphasis on further refinement such as reevaluation of the age cut-off used to stratify therapy, and incorporation of additional molecular genetic markers is being studied prospectively. High-throughput genome scale analyses of neuroblastomas are further clarifying the genetic basis of this heterogeneous disease.[4]

There is remarkable heterogeneity observed in tumor phenotype, ranging from spontaneous regression to relentless progression. There are multiple clinical and biologic markers that have been proposed as being predictive of disease outcome, but large clinical correlative studies are sharpening the focus of which markers can be used by the clinician to optimize therapy for an individual patient.[4]

PTPN11 has been identified as a causative gene in for about 50 percent of cases of Noonan syndrome. Given the association between Noonan syndrome and an increased risk of some malignancies, notably leukemia and probably some solid tumors including neuroblastoma and rhabdomyosarcoma, recent studies have reported that gain-of-function somatic mutations in PTPN11 occur in some hematological malignancies and in some solid tumors such as neuroblastoma, although at a low frequency. However, no mutations of PTPN11 were detected in neuroblastoma in a recent study.[5]

ENVIRONMENTAL FACTORS

As neuroblastoma is a tumor of infancy, an environmental factor as a causative agent is sought. A decrease in incidence before and after folic acid fortification has been observed though long-term studies into the role of folate metabolism in neuroblastoma are neccesary.[6] Breastfeeding has been reported as a protective agent against neuroblastoma.[7]

BIOLOGICAL AND CLINICAL ROLES OF p73 IN NEUROBLASTOMA

The p73 gene is a p53 homologue localized at 1p36.3, a chromosomal region frequently deleted in neuroblastoma. p73 was originally considered an oncosuppressor gene. However, it was soon realized that its mode of action did not resemble that of a classic anti-oncogene. The recent discovery of N-terminal truncated isoforms, with oncogenic properties, showed that p73 has a 'two in one' structure. Indeed, the full-length variants are strong inducers of apoptosis while the truncated isoforms inhibit the pro-apoptotic activity of p53 and of the full-length p73.[8]

TP73, as a TP53 homologue, drew the attention of tumor biologists because it is rarely mutated in human cancers and can induce cell cycle arrest and apoptosis by activating genes also regulated by p53. However, TP73 harbors an additional promoter that produces a dominant negative p73 protein (deltaNp73) having the opposite effect of the TAp73 protein.[9] Thus, the regulation of p53 responsive genes in the absence of p53 relies on a critical balance between different p73 gene-derived proteins. The molecular mechanism through which p73 induces apoptosis involves (i) expression and changes in subcellular localization of scotin, producing an endoplasmic reticulum (ER) stress; and (ii) transactivation of PUMA and Bax, thus determining cell fate.[9] On the contrary, deltaNp73 inhibits apoptosis, thus contributing to the oncogenic potential of neuroblastoma cells.[9]

NEUROBLASTOMA AS AN EXPERIMENTAL MODEL

Neuroblastoma has been used as an experimental model for neuronal differentiation and hypoxia-induced tumor cell dedifferentiation.[10] Neuroblastoma is a childhood tumor derived from precursor or immature cells of the sympathetic nervous system. Neuroblastomas show a tremendous clinical heterogeneity, encompassing truly benign as well as extremely aggressive forms. *In vivo* as well as *in vitro* data have shown that the degree of sympathetic neuronal tumor cell differentiation influences patient outcome. Oxygen shortage and hypoxia have been found to shift neuroblastoma cells toward an immature, stem cell-like phenotype.[10]

Endothelin-converting enzyme (ECE-1) has been suggested to play an important role in amyloid-beta peptide metabolism as one of the amyloid-degrading enzymes.[11] The analysis of the levels of expression and distribution of ECE-1 in the brain under effects of hypoxia and oxidative stress on ECE-1 in human neuroblastoma NB7 cells was studied and it was found that chronic (24 hr) hypoxia and oxidative stress resulted in 30 and 20 percent decrease in expression of ECE-1 at the protein level, respectively, although at the level of ECE-1 mRNA there were no statistically significant changes.[11]

The vitamin A metabolite, all-trans retinoic acid (ATRA) plays essential roles in nervous system development, including neuronal patterning, survival, and neurite outgrowth.[12] Our understanding of how the vitamin A acid functions in neurite outgrowth comes largely from cultured embryonic neurons and model neuronal cell systems including human neuroblastoma cells. Human neuroblastoma cells also show enhanced numbers of neurites and longer processes in response to ATRA.[12] Recent data indicate that isomerization to all-trans retinoic acid (ATRA) is the key mechanism underlying the favorable clinical properties of 13-cis-retinoic acid (13cisRA) in the treatment of neuroblastoma. Retinoic acid (RA) metabolism is thought to contribute to resistance, and strategies to modulate this may increase the clinical efficacy of 13cisRA. Iinhibition of RA metabolism may further optimize retinoid treatment in neuroblastoma.[13]

5-S-cysteinyl-dopamine, a catechol-thioether metabolite of dopamine, has been identified in certain dopaminergic regions of the brain, notably the Substantia Nigra. The effect of 5-S-cysteinyl-dopamine on human dopaminergic neuroblastoma SH-SY5Y cells was investigated and it was found that the substance is highly cytotoxic and induced a decrease of the mitochondrial transmembrane potential, an increase in reactive oxygen species such as superoxide anion and peroxides, a marked decrease of reduced glutathione and an inhibition of the complex I activity.[14] Caspase-3-like protease activation and oligonucleosomal DNA fragmentation were also observed. Thus 5-S-cysteinyl-dopamine induces onset of apoptotic processes.[14]

Molecular morphology and toxicity of cytoplasmic prion protein aggregates (PrP) in neuronal and non-neuronal cells has been studied in human neuroblastoma BE2-M17 cells and mouse neuroblastoma N2a cells.[15] Transient expression of cytoplasmic PrP produced juxtanuclear aggregates reminiscent of aggresomes in human neuroblastoma BE2-M17 cells and mouse neuroblastoma N2a cells. Time course studies revealed that discrete aggregates form first throughout the cytoplasm, and then coalesce to form an aggresome. Aggresomes containing cytoplasmic PrP were 1-5-microm inclusion bodies and were filled with electron-dense particles. Cytoplasmic PrP aggregates induced mitochondrial clustering, reorganization of intermediate filaments, prevented the secretion of wild-type PrP molecules and diverted these molecules to the cytoplasm.[15] Cytoplasmic PrP decreased the viability of neuronal and non-neuronal cells and led to cell death.[15]

Studies in advanced-stage neuroblastoma have shown a link between the silencing of caspase-8 and methylation of a regulatory region at the boundary between caspase-8 exon 3 and intron 3. However, a number of recent studies from neuroblastoma cell lines have shown that the transcriptional regulation of caspase-8 may reside with interferon gamma-sensitive promoters through the action of transcription factors, such as signal transducer and activator of transcription 1 (STAT-1). A strong correlation was observed between STAT-1 levels and caspase-8 levels in clinical stage IV neuroblastoma.[16] This suggests that STAT-1 or similar transcription factors, and not methylation, may play a role in controlling caspase-8 levels in stage IV neuroblastoma.[16] No evidence of such a correlation between caspase-8 and STAT-1 levels was observed in lower clinical stages, suggesting that mechanisms controlling caspase-8 expression in neuroblastoma vary with clinical stage.

Recent studies indicate that NF-E2 related factor 2 (Nrf2) is a substrate for the ubiquitin-proteasome pathway. It has been found that identified antioxidant genes, which were upregulated through tBHQ induced that NF-E2 related factor 2 Nrf2 stabilization, confer protection on target cells against H_2O_2-induced apoptotic cell death in neuroblastoma cells as well as the necrotic cell death in the human neural stem cells hNSC.[17] NF-E2 related factor 2 stabilization by pharmacological modulation or adenovirus-mediated Nrf2 overexpression, therefore, might be viable strategies to prevent a wide-spectrum of oxidative stress-related neuronal cell injuries.[17]

Neuroblastoma is unique for its broad spectrum of clinical virulence from spontaneous remission to rapid and fatal progression despite intensive multimodality therapy. To a large extent, outcome could be predicted by the stage of disease and the age at diagnosis. However, a number of molecular events in neuro-blastoma tumors, accounting for the variability of outcome and response to therapy, have been identified over the past decades. Among these, N-Myc amplification is the most relevant prognostic factor and was the first genetic marker, in pediatric oncology, to be included in clinical strategies as a guide for therapeutic decision. This has allowed the most suitable intensity of therapy to be delivered according to a risk-stratified strategy, from observation to megadose chemotherapy with stem cell transplantation. Recent advances in understanding the biology and genetics of neuroblastoma will ultimately allow to select poor-risk patients for appropriate future biologically based therapies.[18]

The Trk family consists of three receptor tyrosine kinases, each of which can be activated by one or more of four neurotrophins-NGF, BDNF, NT3 and NT4. Neurotrophins mediate their multiple effects through a number of distinct intracellular signaling cascades regulating such diverse biological responses as cell survival, proliferation and differentiation in normal and neoplastic neuronal cells. Expression of Trk receptors also plays an important role in the biology and clinical behavior of neuroblastomas. High expression of TrkA was found in neuroblastomas with favorable biological features and highly correlated with patient survival, whereas TrkB was mainly expressed on unfavorable, aggressive neuroblastomas.[19]

CD40 expression by dendritic cells (DCs) critically regulates their maturation/antitumor activity. CD40-CD40 ligand (CD40L) signaling stimulates DC-mediated IL-12 production/cytotoxicity. Recent studies suggest that neuroblastoma derived gangliosides impair DC maturation, IL-12 secretion, and NK/T-cell activity. In a mice model, it was concluded that neuroblastoma-induced inhibition of dendritic cell function may result from ganglioside-mediated CD40 signaling deficiency.[20] Strategies to bypass/augment CD40-CD40L signaling may improve current neuroblastoma immuno-therapies.[20] Recent findings link increased expression of the structurally complex 'b' pathway gangliosides GD1b, GT1b, GQ1b (CbG) to a favorable clinical and biological behavior in human neuroblastoma. Very low CbG content (4-10%) in three of the four human NB cell lines (LAN-5, LAN-1, SMS-KCNR) reflected the ganglioside pattern observed in the most aggressive NB tumors.[21] Pharmacological alterations of complex ganglioside synthesis in vitro by a 5-7 day exposure to 5-10 microM retinoic acid, which is employed in maintenance therapy of disseminated neuroblastoma, included markedly increased (i) relative expression of

CbG (6.6+/–2.0-fold increase, p=0.037), (ii) relative expression of the analogous 'a' pathway gangliosides, termed CaG (6.4+/–1.4-fold increase in GM1a and GD1a; p=0.010), and (iii) total cellular ganglioside content (2.0-6.3-fold), which in turn amplified the accumulation of structurally complex gangliosides.[21] Substantial increases (2.7-2.9-fold) in the activity of GD1b/GM1a synthase (beta-1, 3-galactosyltransferase), which initiates the synthesis of CbG and CaG, accompanied the ATRA induced ganglioside changes. Thus, increased CbG synthesis in neuroblastoma cell lines was attributable to a specific effect of ATRA, namely induction of GD1b/GM1a synthase activity. Since the shift towards higher expression of CbG and CaG during RA-induced cellular differentiation reflects a ganglioside pattern found in clinically less-aggressive tumors, it was suggested that complex gangliosides may play a role in the biological and clinical behavior of neuroblastoma.[21]

RECENT ADVANCES IN DIAGNOSIS

Recent advances have developed in the molecular biology and diagnosis of various small blue round cell tumors. Though a recent study (Schilling et al 2002) concluded that the mass screening for neuroblastoma targeting children age 12 months was ineffective.[22] However, Nishi M et al reestimated this study for its effectiveness and it was concluded that the original study had underestimated the effectiveness of the mass screening. The percentage of spontaneous regression cases among the true positives was estimated to be about 40 percent.[23]

Small blue round cell tumors may be successfully differentiated from one another using immunoperoxidase staining, reverse transcriptase polymerase chain reaction and fluorescence *in situ* hybridization techniques.[24]

Fetal neuroblastomas are usually detected by routine prenatal sonography between 26 and 39 weeks gestation.[25] Around 90 percent are adrenal tumors with occasional cervical and thoracic ones. Most have stage I or II disease, though few cases may have advanced disease. Twenty percent of the mothers may have hypertension or pre-eclampsia. These usually include neonates with stage IV or IV-S disease with liver metastases and fetal hydrops.[25] Ten percent cases may have with large tumors resulting in dystocia and fetal dismemberment. Metastases have been described to placenta and umbilical cord with subsequent fetal death. Accurate staging of fetal neuroblastoma is difficult by sonography, but in mothers with no pre-eclampsia symptoms the chance of widely disseminated disease is less.[25]

Detailed ultrasound and MRI of fetal neck and liver, in conjunction with amniocentesis for measurement of homovanillic acid levels, should enable considering the diagnosis of fetal cervical neuroblastoma.[26]

Neuroblastoma is an enigmatic tumor with heterogeneous clinical behaviors including maturation, regression, and aggressive growth. Despite recent progress in therapeutic strategies against advanced neuroblastoma, long-term outcomes still remain very poor. The prediction of cancer prognosis is one of the most urgent demands to initiate the suitable treatment of neuroblastoma.

Molecular profiling of neuroblastoma has become a feasible tool for clinical applications.[27] The genes differentially expressed between favorable and unfavorable neuroblastomas have been identified to make an neuroblastoma-proper cDNA chip for large-scale analysis of neuroblastoma tumors.[27] Computational analysis of gene expression data in neuroblastomas identified many prognosis-related genes and provided a classifier to predict the patient prognosis with high efficiency.[27]

Nuclear medicine modalities use radiolabeled ligands that either follow metabolic pathways or act on cellular receptors. Thus, they permit functional imaging of physiological processes and help to localize sites such as tumors that harbor pathological events.

MIBG scintigraphy has added a new dimension in diagnosis in patients with high-risk neuroblastoma by picking up bone marrow or cortical bone disease[28] (Fig. 17.1).

A new phenotype of neuroblastoma has been identified with aggressive clinical behavior termed a large cell neuroblastoma. It is a poorly differentiated Schwannian stroma-poor tumor composed of large cells with sharply outlined nuclear membranes and one to four prominent nucleoli.[29]

The application of positron emission tomography (PET) ligands to the specific pathways of synthesis, metabolism and inactivation of catecholamines found in chromaffin tumors, neuroblastomas and ganglioneuromas can be used to provide a more thorough localization of these types of tumor.[30] Recent advances have been made in functional imaging to localize pheochromocytomas, paragangliomas, neuroblastomas and ganglioneuromas, including approaches based on

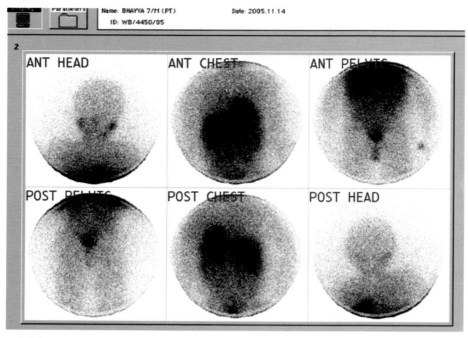

Name: BHAYYA 7/M (PT)   Date: 2005.11.14
ID: WB/4450/05

Figure 17.1: MIBG scan in a case of mediastinal ganglioneuroblastoma showing positive uptake

PET with [^{18}F] fluorodopamine, [^{18}F] fluorohydroxy-phenylalanine, [^{11}C] epinephrine or [^{11}C] hydroxy-ephedrine.[30] Such functional imaging can complement computed tomography or magnetic resonance imaging and other scintigraphic techniques to localize these tumors before surgical or medical therapeutic approaches are considered[30] (Figs 17.2 and 17.3A to C).

Three basic types of neuroblastic tumors are recognized: neuroblastoma (NBs) and ganglio-neuroblastomas (GNBs) and ganglioneuromas (GNs).[31] Neuroblastomas can be undifferentiated, poorly differentiated or differentiating; ganglioneuroblastomas have the following three subtypes: (i) nodular, (ii) intermixed, and (iii) borderline.

THE INTERNATIONAL NEUROBLASTOMA PATHOLOGY CLASSIFICATION (THE SHIMADA SYSTEM)

As part of the international cooperative effort to develop a complete set of International Neuroblastoma Risk Groups, the International Neuroblastoma Pathology Committee (INPC) initiated activities in 1994 to devise a morphologic classification of neuroblastic tumors (NTs; neuroblastoma, ganglioneuroblastoma, and ganglio-neuroma). Six member pathologists discussed and defined morphologically based classifications (Shimada classification; risk group and modified risk group proposed by Joshi et al) on the basis of a review of 227 cases, using various pathologic characteristics of the NTs. The classification is given as Table 17.1.[32] The classification-grading system was evaluated for prognostic significance and biologic relevance.[32, 33] The INPC

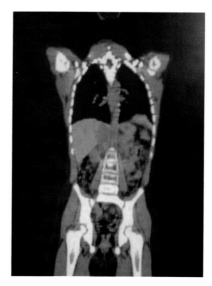

Figure 17.2: PET scan in a case of neuroblastoma stage IV showing increased uptake in the cervical and lumbar vertebrae

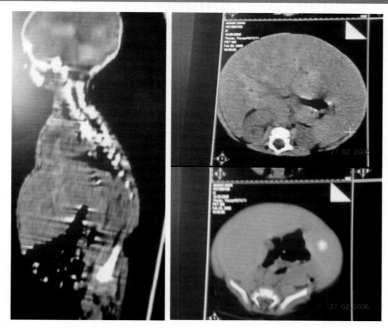

Figures 17.3A to C: PET scan in a case of neuroblastoma IV-S showing irregular uptake in the liver, increased uptake in the spleen, left adrenal and lymph nodes in the porta

adopted a prognostic system modeled on one proposed by Shimada et al. It is an age-linked classification dependent on the differentiation grade of the neuroblasts, their cellular turnover index, and the presence or absence of Schwannian stromal develo3epment. Based on morphologic criteria defined, NTs were classified into four categories and their subtypes: i) neuroblastoma (Schwannian stroma-poor), undifferentiated, poorly differentiated, and differentiating; ii) ganglioneuroblastoma, intermixed (Schwannian stroma-rich); iii) ganglioneuroma (Schwannian stromadominant), maturing and mature; and iv) ganglioneuroblastoma, nodular (composite Schwannian stroma-rich, stroma-dominant and stroma-poor). Specific features, such as the mitosis-karyorrhexis index, the mitotic rate, and calcification, were also included to allow the prognostic significance of the classification to be tested. Recommendations are made regarding the surgical materials to use for an optimal pathobiologic assessment and the practical handling of samples.

PROGNOSTIC FACTORS

Neuroblastoma serves as the paradigm for the clinical utility of tumor-specific biologic data for prognostication.

The continued investigation into prognostic genetic markers for neuroblastoma has been augmented by gene array analysis. Using this technology, a number of novel candidate prognostic markers for neuroblastoma have been identified including BIRC (associated with apoptosis), CDKN2D (associated with cell cycle), and SMARCD3 (associated with transcriptional activation).[34] Genes involved with differentiation/growth arrest have been found to be closely related to low telomerase activity in neuroblastoma, whereas overexpression cell-cycle-related genes and transcriptional factors were associated with high telomerase activity.[35] Finally, full-length telomerase reverse transcriptase messenger RNA was found to be an independent prognostic factor in neuroblastoma.[36]

New chromosomal abnormalities reported include a mosaicism for monosomy 22, 11q interstitial deletion, and a Robertson translocation t(13;14).[37]

Univariate analysis found N-Myc amplification, chromosome 1p deletion, recurrence within 12 months of diagnosis, and recurrence within 6 months of stem cell transplant all to be significant factors in decreasing survival time after relapse in patients with recurrent neuroblastoma.[38]

In the Children's Oncology Group, risk group assignment for neuroblastoma is critical for therapeutic decisions, and patients are stratified by International Neuroblastoma Staging System stage, N-Myc status, ploidy, Shimada histopathology, and diagnosis age. Age less than 365 days has been associated with favorable

Table 17.1: Prognostic evaluation of neuroblastic tumors according to the International Neuroblastoma Pathology Classification (Shimada system)*

International neuroblastoma pathology classification		Original Shimada classification	Prognostic group
Neuroblastoma Favorable	(Schwanian stroma-poor)[a]	Stroma-poor Favorable	Favorable
<1.5 yr	Poorly differentiated or differentiating and low or intermediate MKI tumor		
1.5-5 yr Unfavorable	Differentiating and low MKI tumor	Unfavorable	Unfavorable
<1.5 yr	a) undifferentiated tumor[b] b) high MKI tumor		
1.5-5 yr	a) undifferentiated or poorly differentiated tumor b) intermediate or high MKI tumor		
>5 yr	All tumors		
Ganglioneuroblastoma intermixed	(Schwanian stroma-rich)	Stroma-rich intermixed (favorable)	Favorable[c]
Ganglioneuroma Maturing Mature	(Schwanian stroma-dominant)	Well differentiated (favorable) Ganglioneuroma	Favorable[c]
Ganglioneuroma, nodular	(composite Schwanian stroma-rich/stroma-dominate and stroma-poor	Stroma-rich nodular (unfavorable)	

MKI: mitosis-karyorrhexis index
[a] Subtypes of neuroblastoma were described in detail elsewhere.[10]
[b] Rare subtype, especially diagnosed in this age group. Further investiagtion and analysis required
[c] Prognostic grouping for these tumor categories is not related to patient age.
* This table has been cited from Shimada H, Ambros IM, Dehren LP, et al from the International Neuroblastoma Pathology Classification (the Shimada system). Cancer 1999;86:364-72.

outcome, but recent studies suggest that older age cutoff may improve prognostic precision. The prognostic contribution of age to outcome is continuous in nature. Within clinically relevant risk stratification, statistical support has been reported for an age cut-off of 460 days.[39]

The outcome for patients with stage A neuroblastoma treated with surgery alone is excellent. Although event free survival and survival rates were significantly worse for patients with N-Myc -amplified tumors, a subset achieved long-term remission after surgery alone. For patients with stage A and N-Myc amplification, additional factors are needed to distinguish the patients who will achieve long-term remission with surgery alone from those who will develop recurrent disease.[40]

In a recent series, ten of 14 morphologic features, including nuclear size, cellularity, prominent nucleoli in undifferentiated or poorly differentiated neuroblasts, and the number of mitotic and karyorrhectic cells (MKI), showed a significant correlation with the clinical groups (ORs between 36.9 and 10.5 and p values between < 0.001 and 0.002).[41] This study confirmed the prognostic impact of the criteria used in the Shimada system and revealed that some other morphologic features, such as prominent nucleoli in undifferentiated and poorly differentiated neuroblasts, identify unfavorable tumor biology, partly independent from the patient's age at diagnosis.[41]

In another recent series, the outcomes for patients with N-Myc-nonamplified, hyperdiploid tumors was reported as excellent.[42] A trend toward less favorable outcome for patients with N-Myc-nonamplified, diploid tumors was observed; more children may need to be evaluated before therapy is reduced for this subgroup. For patients with N-Myc-amplified tumors, new strategies are needed.[42]

A statistically significant association of low Histologic grades HG (1 and 2) was found with DNA index (DI) of more than 1 (hyperdiploid), single copy of N-Myc gene per haploid genome, and an serum lactic dehydrogenase (LDH) of less than 1500 IU/l (p value for each, < 0.001), factors that are associated with better prognosis. High HG was associated with DI of 1 (diploidy), amplified N-Myc gene, and an LDH of 1500 or more, factors that are associated with aggressive behavior.[43] The presence of N-Myc amplification in localized neuroblastoma does not necessarily portend an adverse outcome.[44] Furthermore, the biological features of this subset of N-Myc-amplified neuroblastoma has been reported to differ from those of more advanced N-Myc-amplified tumors.

Histologic grading (HG) of neuroblastomas of prognostic significance is based on the presence of absence of calcification and low mitotic rate ($\leq$ or = 10/ 10 high power fields). Mitosis karyorrhexis index (MKI) is the main feature used for prognostic categorization in Shimada classification and can be determined more readily than mitotic rate (MR). Joishi et al lumped together low and intermediate MKI as low MKI and replaced MR with the modified MKI categories.[45] Histologic grades were defined as follows: HG 1 = calcification + low MKI, HG 2 = calcification or low MKI, HG 3 = high MKI and absence of calcification. HGs were linked with age: low risk (LR) = HG 1 in all age groups + HG 2 in patients age younger than 1 year; high risk (HR) = HG 2 in patients age 1 year of older + HG 3 in all age groups.

Advantages of Joshi's modified Histologic grading HGs include: (i) familiarity and reproducibility of MKI; (ii) no need for linkage with age; and (iii) a combination of features used in original HGs and Shimada classification.

Morphologic (Shimada classification—SC, original and modified histologic grades—OHG and MHG) and nonmorphologic (serum LDH, 1 p del, DNA index, N-Myc copy number, telomerase activity, and expression of MRP, MDR1, and TRK) prognostic markers for neuroblastoma were reviewed.[46] The functional role of these nonmorphologic markers in the development and progression of this disease include abnormal cell proliferation, resistance to chemotherapeutic agents, and induction of apoptosis. A statistically significant association between high OHG/MHG (grade 3), DNA index of 1 (diploidy), > 1 copy of N-Myc per haploid genome and serum LDH of $\geq$ or = 1500 IU/1 (p < 0.001 for each) has been described.[46]

In SC, undifferentiated histology and high MKI are associated with N-Myc amplification. However, a lack of correlation between morphology and N-Myc amplification has been found in localized neuroblastomas.

Ganglioneuroblastoma (GNB) diagnosed by conventional criteria included tumors showing more than 5 percent ganglion cells but no predominant ganglioneuromatous component, as well as tumors containing predominant ganglioneuromatous component. By modified criteria, the former would be considered differentiating neuroblastoma, and only the latter would be considered GNB.

Ganglioneuroblastoma (GNB) diagnosed by conventional and modified criteria were divided into low-risk and high-risk histology subgroups as follows:[47] (i) GNB by conventional criteria: low-risk group, differentiating neuroblastoma of histologic grades 1 and 2 and GNB of intermixed and borderline subtypes; high-risk group, differentiating neuroblastoma of histologic grade 3 and GNB of nodular subtype; (ii) GNB by modified criteria: low-risk group, GNB of intermixed and borderline subtypes; high-risk group, GNB of nodular subtype. The low- and high-risk subgroups of GNBs diagnosed by conventional (69 cases) and modified (36 cases) criteria showed statistically significant differences in survival (p = 0.03 and 0.01, respectively).

NEW PERSPECTIVES IN TREATMENT

Neuroblastoma is one of the most common extracranial solid tumors in childhood with a poor prognosis in its advanced stage. Treatment failure is often associated to the occurrence of drug resistance. To date, treatment of pediatric neuroblastoma is still dismal, and therefore novel effective drugs are awaited. Retinoid therapy, new forms of drug delivery, and immunologic therapies are the newest weapons under investigation.

Research into the use of retinoids in the treatment of neuroblastoma has remained a major focus of current investigations.[48] A phase III randomized trial has shown that high-dose, pulse therapy with 13-cis-retinoic acid given after intensive chemoradiotherapy significantly improved event-free survival in high-risk neuroblastoma. Using Microarray technology to screen for genes that are important in neuroblastoma differentiation induced by 13-cis-retinoic acid, a number of genes have been found to be either up- or down-regulated in this process.[49] These genes interfere with cell growth by inducing neuronal differentiation in N-type neuroblastoma cells and apoptosis in S-type neuroblastoma cell lines.[50] Fenretinide, a synthetic retinoid has been shown to induce apoptosis in neuroblastoma cell lines and up-regulate the stress-induced transcription factor GADD153 and the Bcl-2-related protein Bak.[51] The targeting of GADD153 and Bak in neuroblastoma cells may provide novel pathways for the development of drugs inducing apoptosis of neuroblastoma with improved specificity.[52]

Recombinant Antibodies in the Immunotherapy of Neuroblastoma

The impact of monoclonal antibodies (mAbs) in the treatment of human tumors has greatly increased in recent years. mAb engineering has allowed reducing the immunogenicity of therapeutic antibodies as well as improving their biodistribution. Furthermore, engineered mAbs have been used to vehiculate toxins, drugs and other antineoplastic agents to the tumor site. In the case of neuroblastoma, both murine and chimeric antibodies against the tumor associated antigen GD2 have been tested in clinical trials, either alone or in combination with cytokines. A novel promising approach to mAb engineering is the small immuno-protein (SIP) technique, whereby the variable regions of heavy and light chains of a mAb with a given specificity are connected to the dimerizing CH(3) domain of an immunoglobulin molecule. Novel anti-GD2 molecules using the SIP technique have been explored as immunotherapy for neuroblastoma.[53] Another novel form of therapy for neuroblastoma that has recently been investigated is the targeted delivery of antisense oligonucleotides.

C-myb antisense oligonucleotides have been encapsulated within liposomes to take care of rapid degradation by cellular nucleases.[54] These liposomes were then externally coupled to a monoclonal antibody specific for the neuroectodermal antigen disialoganglioside GD2 resulting in creation of anti-GD2-targeted liposomes. These liposomes were characterized by high loading efficiency, small particle size, and good stability. *In vitro*, they were able to be selectively delivered to neuroblastoma cells and inhibit cell proliferation by down-modulation of c-myb protein expression.

Efforts to develop immunotherapy for neuroblastoma resulted in the development of a DNA vaccine that induces protection against metastatic neuroblastoma in a mouse model.[55]

Half of neuroblastoma cases present with metastatic disease at diagnosis and have a poor prognosis, in spite of the most advanced chemotherapeutic protocols combined with autologous hematopoietic stem cell transplantation.[56] Among the new avenues for neuroblastoma treatment that are being explored, immunotherapy has attracted much interest.[56] Emphasis has been placed on monoclonal antibodies directed to tumor-associated antigens—in particular the disialoganglioside GD2—that have been tested in the clinical setting with promising results. In addition, stimulation of cell-mediated antitumor effector mechanisms have been attempted—for example, by recombinant interleukin (IL)-2 administration. NB cells express tumor-associated antigens, such as MAGE-3, but lack constitutive expression of costimulatory molecules and surface HLA class I and II molecules. As such, NB cells are likely to be ignored by the host T cell compartment, since expression of HLA and costimulatory molecules on antigen presenting cells are sine qua non conditions for efficient peptide presentation to T cells and for the subsequent activation and clonal expansion of the latter cells. Notably, *in vitro* experiments with NB cell lines demonstrated that surface HLA class I molecules and the CD40 costimulatory molecule were upregulated following cell incubation with recombinant interferon-gamma. Interaction of CD40 with recombinant CD40 ligand induced apoptosis of NB cells through a caspase 8-dependent mechanism. Immunogenicity of human NB cells is very low but suggest that manipulation by cytokine administration or gene transfer can increase their immunogenic potentia.[56] On the other hand, NB cells represent an excellent target for natural killer cells, the potential role of which in immunotherapy of NB is now being investigated.[56]

Chemotherapy—Camptothecin Analogs

In recent years, an increasing interest has concentrated on camptothecin analogs. Topotecan and irinotecan, the only two clinically relevant camptothecin derivatives to date, have entered clinical trials in neuroblastoma with varying results.

In 1966 the plant alkaloid camptothecin was isolated and identified as an agent with promising anticancer properties. Insolubility was an initial impediment to the clinical development of this agent. Phase I studies of the sodium salt of camptothecin, reported in the early 1970s, showed impressive antitumor activity, but also showed severe and unpredictable toxicities. As a result, camptothecin was effectively shelved for a decade and a half, until the identification of topoisomerase I as the target for camptothecin renewed interest in its clinical development. Just over a decade ago, researchers at a Japanese company reported that the eleventh in a series of semi-synthetic, soluble derivatives of camptothecin, (CPT-11, in company shorthand) was demonstrating important activity in a number of refractory tumor models. Since its approval in the United States in 1996, irinotecan (CPT-11, Camptosar®, Pharmacia Corp.; Peapack, NJ) has undergone extensive clinical evaluation.

Irinotecan is a water-soluble derivative of camptothecin, which is isolated from a Chinese tree, Camptotheca acuminata; Its effectiveness against neuroblastoma was confirmed by *in vivo* preclinical studies, and phase I clinical trials in Japan concluded the maximum tolerated dose of this agent is 160-180 mg/m^2/day for 3 consecutive days repeated after 25 days.[5,7]

Short courses of irinotecan have been given for palliative therapy in patients with neuroblastoma A retrospective review was conducted of patients treated for resistant NB with irinotecan at 50 mg/m^2 per day for 5 days as a 1-hour intravenous infusion. Of 23 patients, 15 patients had stable disease, 7 were not evaluable for response because of concurrent radiotherapy, and 1 patient had a major response.[58] A recommended phase II dose of irinotecan administered weekly 4x, *every 6 weeks* in children with solid tumors is 125 mg/m^2/dose for heavily pretreated patients and 160 mg/m^2/dose for less heavily pretreated patients.[59] A phase I study was performed to determine the maximum-tolerated dose (MTD) and safety profile of irinotecan (CPT-11) administered as a single intravenous infusion *every 3 weeks* in children with recurrent or refractory solid tumors. Another recommended phase II dose of CPT-11 in a 3-week schedule was 600 mg/m^2 in less heavily, and heavily pretreated children with solid tumors.[60]

Dramatic efficacy of irinotecan in the treatment of chemoresistant neuroblastoma without the use of other antitumor agents has been reported in few cases.[61]

Despite promising antitumor activity, the combination of topotecan and irinotecan given on a protracted schedule has been found to have unacceptable toxicity like neutropenia, typhlitis, and skin rash.[62] Neutropenia and diarrhea were the dose-limiting toxicities in heavily pretreated patients.[58]

Prospects for irinotecan and recombinant human endostatin (rhEndostatin) were studied experimentally and clinically. rhEndostatin was studied in *in vivo* experimental models. The action of rhEndostatin was quite different from those of other cytotoxic chemotherapeutic agents, and continuous administration of this substance showed a more marked anti-effect than its intermittent use. Irinotecan appeared promising when it is given to the patients neuroblastoma, whereas rhEndostatin was thought to have more preclinical studies before it is used in patients.[58]

A Temozolomide, a new dacarbazine analog with optimal oral bioavailability, is being used in an ongoing phase II study as an alternative to oral etoposide.

A phase II multicenter Study of Irinotecan Hydrochloride and Temozolomide in Pediatric Patients With Recurrent Neuroblastoma is currently underway by the National Cancer Institute. The patients receive irinotecan hydrochloride IV over 1 hour on days 1-5 and 8-12 and oral temozolomide on days 1-5. Treatment repeats every 3 weeks for up to 6 courses in the absence of disease progression or unacceptable toxicity.

In one trial, high-dose cyclophosphamide plus topotecan/vincristine CTV or irinotecan C/I were used in patients with resistant neuroblastoma.: CTV and C/I included cyclophosphamide 140 mg/kg (approximately 4200 mg/m^2). With CTV, topotecan 2 mg/m^2 was infused IV (30 min) on days 1-4 (total, 8 mg/m^2), and vincristine 0.067 mg/kg was injected on day 1. With C/I, irinotecan, 50 mg/m^2 was infused IV (1 h) on days 1-5 (total, 250 mg/m^2).[63]

Mesna and granulocyte colony-stimulating factor were used. Major responses were seen in 15 percent of CTV and 17 percent C/I-treated patients with assessable disease. Bone marrow disease resolved in 28 percent CTV-treated patients and 27 percent 15 C/I-treated patients. 3F8 after CTV or C/I was not blocked by neutralizing antibodies, consistent with the desired immunosuppressive effect of high-dose cyclophosphamide. Thus, it was concluded that CTV and C/I entail tolerable morbidity, have modest antineuroblastoma activity in heavily treated patients and are good preparative regimens for passive immunotherapy with monoclonal antibodies.

In a prospective phase II trial, topotecan was administered intravenously daily for 5 days for each of 2 consecutive weeks for two cycles.[64] On the basis of

CHAPTER 18

Shilpa Sharma
Devendra K Gupta

Stage IV-S Neuroblastoma

Stage IV-S Neuroblastoma has behaved as a mystery disease involving malignancy from derivatives of the neural crest cells involving multiple sites yet having a better prognosis than other widespread similar disease like stage IV. Thus it was seperated from the other stage IV counterparts by making it stage IV-S as it is a metastatic disease associated with a high likelihood of spontaneous regression and good survival, though about 10 to 20 percent of infants die from early complications.

Case Report

A three months old male child presented with history of generalized abdominal distension noticed since 1 month of age that was progressively increasing. There was no history of fever/loss of weight/loss of apetite. The bowel and urinary habits were normal. The child was active with preserved general condition and mild pallor. On examination, there was no icterus or subcutaneous nodules. His respiration was normal. The abdomen was grossly distended with visible dilated veins and a small umbilical hernia. The liver was grossly enlarged (15 cm below the costal margin), firm in consistency with smooth surface and sharp margin and mobile with respiration (Fig. 18.1). There were no signs of free fluid in the abdomen.

The biochemical and blood investigations were Hb-15.9 gm percent, TLC- 29200, PLT- 672000, urea/creatinine – 14/0.7, T. Prot/Alb/Glob – 5.6/3.2/2.4, Total Bil – 0.7, SGOT/SGPT/SALP – 88/31/550. The ultrasonographic examination delineated hepatosplenomegaly with heterogenous echotexture of the liver. A solid mass, 5 × 5 × 3.6 cm in size with central

calcific foci was picked up in right suprarenal area. The left adrenal gland was also enlarged. The CECT of the abdomen showed a grossly enlarged liver (22 cms in superoinferior span) with normal attenuation. There were two focal hypodense lesions one in each lobe of liver. There was a right adrenal mass with calcific specs (Fig. 18.2). The left adrenal and spleen were also enlarged. There was no free fluid or retroperitoneal lymphadenopathy in the abdomen.

The urinary VMA/HVA were raised. USG-guided fine needle aspiration cytology was suggestive of neuroblastoma. Bone marrow aspirate and biopsy were normal. The skeletal survey and bone scan were normal. Positron Emission Tomography (PET) showed irregular uptake in the liver, increased uptake in the spleen with a hot spot and increased uptake in the left adrenal and lymph nodes in the portal area.

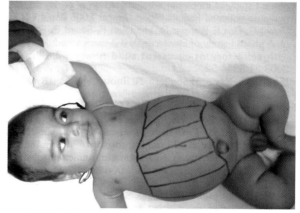

Figure 18.1: A baby with neuroblastoma IV-S presenting with hepatomegaly

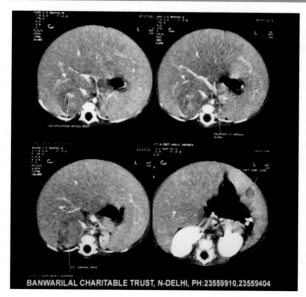

Figure 18.2: CECT of the abdomen showing a grossly enlarged liver and a right adrenal mass with calcific specs

The baby was given cyclophosphamide 5 mg/kg/day for 5 days at 3 weeks interval for 3 cycles. There was good response and the liver decreased in size.

DEFINITION

It was originally defined in 1971 and incorporated in the Evans' classification.[1,2] As per the international neuroblastoms staging, it is defined as a localized primary tumor (as defined for stage I, IIA or IIB), with dissemination limited to skin, liver, and/or bone marrow (< 10% tumor) but not to bone limited to infants < 1 year of age with no infiltration across the midline or contralateral lymph node involvement.[3] The two added features in addition to Evans' staging include age less than 1 year and < 10 percent of bone marrow involvement. However, it has been reported that stage IV-S and International Neuroblastoma Staging System stage IV-S are 98 percent concordant.[4] Bilateral synchronous tumors have not previously been included in the definitions, but in INSS stage IV-S, multifocal tumors have been included.[2]

AGE AT PRESENTATION

Most of the patients present during the first few months of life. The average age at diagnosis is around 3 months.[5] Seventy percent patients in a series of 97 patients were younger than 4 months.[6] Mortality is common in infants younger than 2 months of age at diagnosis and is due to complications of extensive abdominal involvement with respiratory compromise or disseminated intravascular coagulation.[4] Thus infants younger than 2 months old at diagnosis with rapidly progressive abdominal disease require cytotoxic therapy twice as frequently as older infants and may benefit from earlier and more intensive treatment.[4,7] It has been reported that for infants with disease diagnosed before they are 2 months old, stage IV-S disease may have an even worse prognosis than stage IV disease.[7]

SITE OF INVOLVEMENT

Though it is difficult to identify the primary site of the tumor in stage IV-S disease, adrenal is the most common primary tumor site.[5,6,8] Other sites of primary tumor include abdominal paravertebral region, mediastinum, retroperitoneum, pelvis, kidney and unknown site.[5,8,9] Liver is most often infiltrated by the tumor, followed by bone marrow and then skin.[6,9] Other sites that have been affected are pancreas, pleura, peritoneum, and regional nodes.[9]

Metastatic pattern in neuroblastoma differs with age and correlates with tumor biological features and event-free survival (EFS). These correlations could reflect changes in host or tumor biological features with age resulting in differences in metastatic capacity or tumor affinity for specific sites. Event-free survival (EFS) was decreased in patients with bone, bone marrow, CNS, intracranial/orbital, lung, and pleural metastases, and improved in those with liver and skin metastases. In infants, N-Myc amplification and unfavorable Shimada histopathology correlated with increased frequencies of bone and intracranial or orbital metastases. In older patients, N-Myc amplification correlated with increased frequencies of intracranial or orbital, liver, and lung metastases.[10]

CLINICAL PRESENTATION

The most common presentation is with distention of the abdomen due to hepatomegaly. Upto 69 percent cases may present with massive hepatomegaly.[11] The massive hepatomegaly may extend below the umbilicus.[8] Symptoms may be referable to the enlarged liver size including respiratory distress, gastroesophageal reflux, or decreased urine output.[11] Other presenting features include subcutaneous nodules and fever.

An acute clinical course may be seen in some patients.[5] Acute cases may present with jaundice, refusal to feed, hematemesis due to portal hypertension and hepatosplenomegaly or massive abdominal distention, umbilical hernia and bilateral hydroceles due to ascitis. The findings may also be picked up on routine ultrasonography for excessive crying or incidently for some other cause in a healthy baby or during screening for neuroblastoma as was done in Japan.

INVESTIGATIONS

Liver function may be normal or only mildly abnormal.[11] Urine catecholamines need to be done to establish a diagnosis. Serum ferritin may be determined by radioimmunoassay. Serum LDH may be done. The N-Myc gene copy number may be determined by using Southern analysis of DNA or analysis of N-Myc protein expression by semiquantitative polymerase chain reaction and immunoperoxidase stain.

The radiological investigations include skiagram chest and abdomen, ultrasound, computed tomography, or magnetic resonance imaging.

Bilateral bone marrow aspirate and biopsy may be done along with either skeletal survey or bone scan. Bone marrow immunocytology is more sensitive method of detection depicting the sensitivity of one tumor cell per 10^5 nucleated bone marrow cells. Positive bone marrow immunocytology was a more significant factor for EFS ($p = 0.049$) than was light microscopic bone marrow examination suggesting that infants with bone marrow involvement by the more sensitive detection method may have a worse outcome. However, neither method of bone marrow examination is predictive of overall survival.

Staging may be done on clinical and radiological basis and with the help of needle biopsy of the liver, primary tumor or by biopsy of skin lesions when present. However, in case adequate specimen cannot be obtained for biologic studies by needle biopsy, INSS staging by rigorous surgical exploration has been recommend by some authors. Infants less than 2 months of age with massive liver enlargement are considered poor surgical candidates, and diagnostic material may be obtained only by percutaneous needle biopsy in such cases.

BIOLOGICAL FACTORS

Elucidation of the biochemical and genetic mechanisms leading to spontaneous maturation of neuroblastoma may obviate the need for precise anatomic staging. Majority of patients of stage IV-S fall into low-risk group. The intrinsically biologically favorable nature of stage IV-S neuroblastoma is further supported by the lack of effect of primary tumor resection on EFS or survival.

Biological variables and markers include: genetic (cytogenetics [1p deletions], nuclear genomic content), molecular biologic (N-Myc oncogene amplification, mdr-1, ras, and trk, gene expression), immunological (major histocompatibility antigen density, cellular and humoral immunity), and biochemical (creatine kinase isoenzyme profile, neuron specific enolase, ferritin, chromatograffin, lactic acid dehydrogenase and catecholamine levels).[12] Other biologic factors include tumor suppressor genes, expression of nerve growth factor and low telomerase activity.

Hyperdiploidy is a favorable prognostic factor in infants with stage IV-S disease.[13] Elevated ferritin levels and E-rosette inhibitory factor appear to distinguish stage IV neuroblastoma from stage IV-S. Stage IV disease (metastases to bone), which is usually fatal shows elevated serum ferritin levels and presence of E-rosette inhibitory factor in contrast to stage IV-S.[14] Elevated serum ferritin levels above 143 ng/ml is a poor prognostic factor in stage IV-S neuroblastoma.[4] However, elevated serum ferritin serum levels are normally present in the first few months of life.

Whereas stages I to IV neuroblastoma expressed low levels of class I (MHC) surface antigen, stage IV-S tumor cells expressed normal levels, similar to control tissues.[15] Tumors comprised predominantly of ganglion cells expressed significantly more class I antigen than neuroblasts.[15] Thus it has been suggested that class I MHC expression may play a role in the natural history of human neuroblastoma.[15] High levels of serum LDH and low urinary excretion of vanillylmandelic acid were associated with worse prognosis.[7]

N-Myc is usually not amplified in these tumors and Shimada histopathologic classification is favorable in 96 percent.[4] Occasionally, stage IV-S patient may show mild N-Myc gene amplification.[16] N-Myc amplification is found in less than 10 percent of infants with stage IV-S disease. Fluorescent *in situ* hybridization for detection of N-Myc amplification will allow measurement from touch preparations in future studies. The presence of N-Myc amplification in neuroblasts has been associated with a poor outcome in the late stages of disease. N-Myc gene amplification has been associated with lower survival ($p < .001$) late disease progression and death.[13,17] The vanillylmandelic acid (VMA) to homovanillic acid (HVA) ratio was low in tumors with an increased number of copies of N-Myc.[18] Serum lactate dehydrogenase (LDH) levels have been found to be increased in stage IV-S patients with N-Myc amplification but not in those with regressing tumors and without N-Myc amplification.[18] It has been suggested that N-Myc amplification may affect the final outcome in the patient classified as stage IV-S, but tumor regression can occur early after birth and appears to be independent of N-Myc amplification.[18]

TREATMENT

There is a lot of heterogeneity in stage IV-S neuroblastoma and thus, its management cannot be uniform and pediatric oncologists are regularly confronted with a decision whether or not to treat a newly presenting patient that fits into the the definition of clinical IV-S. It has been suggested that further development of a subclassification, or a reclassification based on molecular biologic markers may help overcome this issue.[17] Some authors have distinguished two groups were according to the initial clinical presentation: one with life-threatening symptoms and needing immediate treatment, and one with no life-threatening symptoms.[19] Rare stage IV-S patients with unfavorable biologic features should be considered for either intermediate risk (diploid) or high risk (N-Myc amplification) treatment stategy.

Supportive Care

Supportive care is still taken as the cornerstone of therapy by majority of the pediatric surgeons not mandating resection of the primary tumor. Many investigators have recommended minimal or no therapeutic intervention for asymptomatic patients as it has been well appreciated that stage IV-S patients have frequent spontaneous remissions and a 60 to 90 percent survival rate. Close observation is thus warranted for the common presentation of massive hepatomegaly in an infant, unless life-threatening complications occur. Patients with favorable biologic features should be observed for symptomatology from tumor expansion. Serial monitoring by ultrasonography, urinary catecholamines and serum LDH may suffice in centers where facilities for N-Myc amplification are not available. Upto 50 percent sites of disease that regressed spontaneously have been noticed.[9]

Role of Treatment

The role of radiation therapy, surgery, and chemotherapy for those infants with progressive or symptomatic disease remains controversial, combined modality therapy (CMT) being more effective than single modality treatment.[17] Initial therapeutic intervention may be indicated in those patients with life-threatening presentations.

Surgery

In cases where the primary site is resectable, surgical intervention may be considered. Extirpation of the primary tumor has been accomplished in upto 65 percent.[8] However, it has been seen that resection of the primary tumor does not influence the outcome.[6] Other indications for surgery include excision biopsy for subcutaneous nodules. Silastic abdominal pouches for rapidly expanding abdominal disease have also been described though they could not prevent mortality.[4]

Chemotherapy

The treatment policies in general are a combination of radiotherapy and chemotherapy or infrequently one modality alone. If respiratory compromise occurs then moderately intensive chemotherapy is started. Cyclophosphamide 5 mg/kg/d either orally or intravenously for 5 days with or without hepatic radiation is given.[4] Chemotherapy may be repeated at 2-3 week intervals if the absolute neutrophil count was greater than $1,000/\mu l$. Cyclophosphamide can be discontinued at the first indication of tumor regression or resolution of symptoms. Only a single course of cyclophosphamide may be enough for some patients though majority may require more than two courses. The course of chemotherapy may vary between 1 month and 1 year.[9] More intensive chemotherapy may obviate the need for radiation, as was used in a POG study of stage IV-S infants, where only 6 percent needed radiation in addition to chemotherapy.[13]

Radiotherapy

Symptomatic patients with hepatomegaly may be given radiotherapy directly though some authors reserve radiotherapy for chemo non-responsive patients.

Prompt subjective response has been noticed with low doses of radiation in quantities less than or equal to 600 rad without chemotherapy. The liver may be irradiated with a median dose of 450 rad.[9] The radiation dose of 450 rad has also been spread over 3 days in combination with chemotherapy.[4] Follow-up at 18 years from diagnosis has shown 80 percent survival with resolved or resolving hepatomegaly.[11] Thus low dose radiotherapy should be considered for symptomatic hepatomegaly.[11] The side effects of radiotherapy include asymptomatic scoliosis or kyphoscoliosis. High dose (greater than or equal to 3,300 rad) radiation-related side effects included multiple rib chondromas, chest- and pelvic-wall hypoplasia and radiation nephritis with hepatic fibrosis resulting in death.[11]

RESULTS

Progressive disease is defined as an increase in tumor size or development of new tumors. The sites of progression described have been liver, adrenals, lymph nodes, bone marrow and the lung, neck, chest, and bone. Mortality may be related to mechanical complications related to progressive disease with massive hepatomegaly, late recurrence and unresponsive abdominal disease.[17,20] Death may also occur due to skeletal dissemination.[21] Disseminated intravascular coagulation may be a terminal event. The overall survival (OS) rate at 5 years is 80-92 percent and event-free survival (EFS) rate 68- 86 percent.[4,6]

Five-year survival rate was 100 percent for those requiring supportive care compared with 81 percent survival for those requiring cytotoxic therapy for symptoms Nickerson HJ.

The only other significant factor predictive for improved survival has been favorable Shimada histopathologic classification.[4] Sites of metastatic involvement (liver, skin, or bone marrow) and surgical resection of the primary tumor were not significant for survival. Reports have confirmed the high probability of survival with bilateral adrenal neuroblastoma.

FETAL NEUROBLASTOMA

Obstetrical sonography has helped diagnose and define the features of fetal neuroblastomas detected by routine prenatal sonography. Most of the tumors are adrenal tumors diagnosed between 26 and 39 weeks gestation.[22] Most are in Evans' stage I or II though few cases may be in advanced stage. Most of these tumors do not have N-Myc amplification. The mothers may have hypertension or pre-eclampsia during the pregnancy in neonates with stage IV or IV-S disease with liver metastases.[22] Fetal hydrops is a serious complication in stage IV or IV-S disease. Tumors have been reported to metastasize to the placenta and umbilical cord with subsequent fetal demise.

REFERENCES

1. D'Angio G, Evans A, Koop C. Special pattern of widespread neuroblastoma with a favourable prognosis. Lancet 1971;1:1046-9.
2. Evans AE, D'Angio GJ, Randolph J. A proposed staging for children with neuroblastoma: Children's Cancer Study Group A. Cancer 1971;27:374-8.
3. Brodeur GM, Pritchard J, Berthold F, et al. Revisions of the international criteria for neuroblastoma diagnosis, staging, and response to treatment. J Clin Oncol 1993;11:1466-77.
4. Nickerson HJ, Matthay KK, Seeger RC, Brodeur GM, Shimada H, Perez C, et al. Favorable biology and outcome of stage IV-S neuroblastoma with supportive care or minimal therapy: a Children's Cancer Group study. J Clin Oncol 2000;18:477-86.
5. Rollan Villamarin V, Garcia Aroca J, Costa Borras E, Cuadros Garcia J, Jimenez Alvarez C, Martinez-Caro A, et al. Neuroblastoma IV-S. A multicenter study. Work Group of Pediatric Oncology. Spanish Society of Pediatric Surgery: Cir Pediatr 1994;7:167-70.
6. M Guglielmi, B De Bernardi, A Rizzo, S Federici, C Boglino, F Siracusa, et al. Resection of primary tumor at diagnosis in stage IV-S neuroblastoma: does it affect the clinical course? Journal of Clinical Oncology 1996;14:1537-44.
7. De Bernardi B, Pianca C, Boni L, et al. Disseminated neuroblastoma (stage IV and IV-S) in the first year of life: outcome related to age and stage. Italian Cooperative Group on Neuroblastoma. Cancer 1992;70:1625-33.
8. Martinez DA, King DR, Ginn-Pease ME, Haase GM, Wiener ES. Resection of the primary tumor is appropriate for children with stage IV-S neuroblastoma: an analysis of 37 patients. J Pediatr Surg. 1992;27:1016-20; discussion 1020-1.
9. Evans AE, Baum E, Chard R. Do infants with stage IV-S neuroblastoma need treatment? Arch Dis Child 1981;56:271-4.
10. DuBois SG, Kalika Y, Lukens JN, Brodeur GM, Seeger RC, Atkinson JB, et al. Metastatic sites in stage IV and IV-S neuroblastoma correlate with age, tumor biology, and survival. J Pediatr Hematol Oncol. 1999; 21:181-9. Comment In: J Pediatr Hematol Oncol 1999;21:178-80.
11. Blatt J, Deutsch M, Wollman MR. Results of therapy in stage IV-S neuroblastoma with massive hepatomegaly. Int J Radiat Oncol Biol Phys 1987;13:1467-71.
12. Miale TD, Kirpekar K. Neuroblastoma stage IV-S. Med Oncol 1994;11:89-100.
13. Katzenstein HM, Bowman LC, Brodeur GM, et al. Prognostic significance of age, MYCN oncogene amplification, tumor cell ploidy, and histology in 110 infants with stage D-S neuroblastoma: The Pediatric Oncology Group experience—A Pediatric Oncology Group study. J Clin Oncol 1998;16: 2007-17.
14. Hann HW, Evans AE, Cohen IJ, Leitmeyer JE. Biologic differences between neuroblastoma stages IV-S and IV. Measurement of serum ferritin and E-rosette inhibition in 30 children. N Engl J Med 1981;305:425-9.
15. Squire R, Fowler CL, Brooks SP, Rich GA, Cooney DR. The relationship of class I MHC antigen expression to stage IV-S disease and survival in neuroblastoma. J Pediatr Surg 1990;25:381-6.

16. Tonini GP, Verdona G, De Bernardi B, Sansone R, Massimo L, Cornaglia-Ferraris P. N-myc oncogene amplification in a patient with IV-S neuroblastoma. Am J Pediatr Hematol Oncol. 1987 Spring;9:8-10.

17. Wilson PC, Coppes MJ, Solh H, Chan HS, Jenkin D, Greenberg ML, Weitzman S. Neuroblastoma stage IV-S: a heterogeneous disease. Med Pediatr Oncol 1991;19:467-72.

18. Nakagawara A, Sasazuki T, Akiyama H, Kawakami K, Kuwano A, Yokoyama T, Kume K. N-myc oncogene and stage IV-S neuroblastoma. Preliminary observations on ten cases. Cancer 1990;65:1960-7.

19. Suarez A, Hartmann O, Vassal G, Giron A, Habrand JL, Valteau D, et al. Treatment of stage IV-S neuroblastoma: a study of 34 cases treated between 1982 and 1987. Med Pediatr Oncol 1991;19:473-7.

20. Stephenson SR, Cook BA, Mease AD, Ruymann FB. The prognostic significance of age and pattern of metastases in stage IV-S neuroblastoma. Cancer 1986;58:372-5.

21. Stokes SH, Thomas PR, Perez CA, Vietti TJ. Stage IV-S neuroblastoma. Results with definitive therapy. Cancer 1984;53:2083-6.

22. Jennings RW, LaQuaglia MP, Leong K, Hendren WH, Adzick NS. Fetal neuroblastoma: prenatal diagnosis and natural history. J Pediatr Surg 1993;28:1168-74.

Tatsuo Kuroda

CHAPTER 19

Intraoperative Radiation Therapy in Advanced Neuroblastoma

INTRODUCTION

Patients with advanced neuroblastoma often revealed systemically disseminated metastasis at their first appearance at the hospital. Since the disease is no longer localized in most of the advanced cases, treatment for advanced neuroblastoma should be directed to manage the two different aspects of the disease, local growth of the primary tumor and systemic metastasis. Therefore, the role of surgery in neuroblastoma has been controversial, especially in the era of micrometastasis exploration using highly sensitive methods. In this chapter, experience of intraoperative radiation in our institution is presented, and the role of surgery and the clinical impact of intensive local management with intraoperative radiation in advanced neuroblastoma are discussed.

THE ROLE OF LOCAL MANAGEMENT IN NEUROBLASTOMA WITH SYSTEMIC METASTASES

Some studies back in 1980s reported the improved survival rate in the patients with metastatic neuroblastoma by total resection of the primary tumor,[1,2] whereas some studies demonstrated the opposed conclusion.[3,4] Thereafter, several study groups including the Children's Cancer Study Group (CCSG) in the United States[5] and the Japanese group[6] insisted the importance of local control in the stage IV disease, but subsequent studies reported that gross total resection did not improve the survival.[7-9] Recent studies from Germany,[10] Spain,[11] Memorial Sloan-Kettering[12] and CCSG[13] in the United

States, and our own[14] again aimed to assess the clinical significance of local radicality in advanced neuroblastoma with metastasis, however, no consensus has been obtained on this issue. Nevertheless, the method of local management has been one of the biggest concern in the treatment of stage IV neuroblastoma. Several alterations are still proposed recently regarding the surgery such as primary radical surgery[20] and a trial of super-delayed surgery after mega-chemotherapy with stem cell rescue in stage IV neuroblastoma.

On the other hand, radiation is another strong means to manage the local lesion, and indispensable for the treatment of childhood malignancies. Radiation therapy is given sequentially from outside of the body more often, but direct irradiation to the lesion through the operative wound is sometimes applied as an alternative option in the selected malignancies. Efficacy of intraoperative irradiation therapy (IORT) was reported in advanced neuroblastoma.[16-19] Extensive surgery followed by IORT is considered to provide most intensive local treatment. However, the clinical impact of this intensive local therapy has been rarely assessed in neuroblastoma in the large series yet.

PRACTICAL PROCEDURES OF INTRAOPERATIVE RADIATION

Indication and Decision of Radiation Dose

Intraoperative radiation therapy (IORT) is indicated for the patients who have advanced solid malignancy and are older than 1 year at surgery, in our institution. In neuroblastoma, patients who have stage 3 or 4 disease

CHAPTER 21

Sani Molagool
Bhaskar Rao
Chen Hon Chui
Kenneth W Gow

Benign Liver Tumors

INTRODUCTION

Benign liver tumors are uncommon in pediatric patients; primary liver tumors account for only 1 to 2 percent of all pediatric tumors and only about one-third of these are benign.[1-4] Benign tumors are usually vascular in origin but may also be epithelial (focal nodular hyperplasia, hepatocellular adenoma) or mesenchymal (infantile hemangioendothelioma, mesenchymal hamartoma, cavernous hemangioma); some may be teratomas (Table 21.1). Treatment is conservative and seldom surgical except for symptomatic hemangioendothelioma in infants, for which multiple approaches have been recommended. Differentiating benign tumor from malignant tumor may be difficult, but a reliable diagnosis is very important for treatment decisions.

CLINICAL EVALUATION

A detailed history and a complete physical examination are always necessary for the assessment of patients with newly discovered liver lesions. Often, the clinical presentation points to a specific diagnosis, because benign liver tumors tend to occur in patients with other underlying conditions. Pediatric patients are at risk of hepatocellular adenoma if they have received androgen therapy for aplastic anemia, have chronic iron overload as the result of β-thalassemia, or have received steroids after renal transplantation.[5] Liver hamartoma may occur in children with tuberous sclerosis.[6] Patients with type I glycogen storage disease are at increased risk of focal nodular hyperplasia and hepatocellular adenoma.[7]

The most common symptom of pediatric benign liver tumors at the time of diagnosis is a painless right upper quadrant abdominal mass or abdominal distention. Clinical symptoms due to mass effect, such as constipation, anorexia, or vomiting, may also be present. Dull, aching pain is sometimes present and is caused by expansion of the liver capsule or compression of surrounding structures. Acute abdominal pain can result from bleeding into the mass or into the peritoneum, especially in the case of hepatocellular adenoma. Jaundice and weight loss are rare except in patients with large hemangioendotheliomas; if these symptoms are present, malignancy should be suspected.

Patients with large hemangioendotheliomas can exhibit the Kasabach-Merritt syndrome, which consists of the triad of congestive heart failure (CHF), thrombocytopenia, and a large vascular lesion.[8] The high-output congestive heart failure is caused by the shunting of blood through the liver. Thrombocytopenia is caused by the trapping of platelets within the tumor. High-output CHF without thrombocytopenia can also be seen in patients with arteriovenous malformation (AVM)[9] of the liver or with mesenchymal hamartoma.[10] In the case of large or diffuse hemangioendotheliomas, rapid enlargement of the liver can cause elevation of the diaphragm and, when combined with CHF, can lead to respiratory distress or even apnea.

Because most pediatric patients with hepatic hemangioendothelioma and hemangioma also have cutaneous hemangiomas,[11] a thorough physical examination should always be conducted so that the tell-tale vascular lesions can be detected.

	HCA	FNH	Mesenchymal hamartoma	Hemangio-endothelioma	Hemangioma
Symptoms	None	None	Mass effect	Mass effect, CHF, KM syndrome	Mass effect
Sex ratio	F=M	F-M, 4:1	M>F	F>M	F>M
Age of patient at the time of diagnosis	> 5 years	> 5 years	< 2 years	2-6 months	< 6 months
Site	Right lobe?	Left lobe?	Right lobe?	Bilateral	Right lobe?
Multifocal	Often	15-20%	10%	< 10%	< 20%
Hemorrhage	Yes	Rare	Rare	Yes	Yes

Table 21.1: Differentiating features of benign liver tumors

HCA, hepatocellular adenoma; FNH, focal nodular hyperplasia; CHF, congestive heart failure; KM, Kasabach-Merritt syndrome

LABORATORY STUDIES

Benign liver tumors rarely cause substantial abnormalities in liver function. A markedly elevated serum α-fetoprotein (AFP) concentration in a child with a liver mass almost certainly means that the mass is malignant, although a slight elevation may be associated with benign lesions. However, the results of laboratory tests must be interpreted in relationship to the normal AFP concentration for age, because this concentration is very high at birth but declines rapidly to the normal adult level of less than 40 ng/ml by the time the patient reaches the age of 8 months.[12] Thrombocytopenia associated with a liver mass is usually a part of the Kasabach-Merritt syndrome.

RADIOLOGIC STUDIES

Several imaging methods have been used to visualize pediatric hepatic masses; these include ultrasonography, computed tomography (CT), magnetic resonance (MR) imaging, angiography, and radionuclide techniques. The role of imaging in cases of pediatric liver tumors is four-fold: characterization of the mass, localization, determination of resectability, and follow-up monitoring.

In pediatric patients with abdominal masses, the organ of origin can often not be determined without imaging studies. Ultrasonography is usually used first;[13] it can accurately rule out the presence of a mass and can identify the organ of origin when a mass is present. Ultrasonography can also determine whether a mass is cystic or solid, can assess vascular flow, can screen the rest of the abdomen, can document the patency of the portal vein and the inferior vena cava, and can detect AVM. Ultrasonography is also used intraoperatively to guide resection.[14]

When ultrasonography confirms the presence of a liver lesion, additional images are obtained with CT or MR imaging because these techniques are more accurate than ultrasonography in predicting the type or resectability of the tumor. Whether CT or MR imaging is the technique of choice for definitive imaging of liver masses is still controversial.[15-17] MR imaging depicts exquisite anatomic detail in multiple planes, does not rely on contrast administration, and does not require radiation. On the other hand, CT is more sensitive than MR imaging in detecting regional lymphadenopathy because oral contrast can be used to opacify the bowel. The choice between CT and MR imaging is usually based on institutional experience and the availability of each technique.[13]

Radionuclide studies, such as liver-spleen scanning and labeled red blood cell scanning, can be used in conjunction with other imaging techniques to differentiate liver masses, especially those tumors with atypical appearance on CT or MR images.[18] Angiography is rarely indicated for benign liver tumors, except those for which percutaneous embolization is a part of the treatment plan.

HEMANGIOENDOTHELIOMA

Infantile hemangioendothelioma is the most common benign tumor of the liver in pediatric patients. The female-male ratio is 1.5:1 to 2:1.[19] The tumor is most commonly detected before the patient reaches the age of 6 months; 85 percent of the lesions are detected by the time patients are 2 months old.[20] Tumors in older children should be suspected of being malignant lesions such as angiosarcoma rather than benign lesions.[21] The most common physical finding associated with hemangioendothelioma is hepatomegaly. At the time of diagnosis, patients may exhibit no symptoms and minimal hepatomegaly, or they may exhibit massive hepatomegaly together with life-threatening high-output CHF and respiratory compromise; in such cases, the mortality rate is as high as 90 percent.[22] Hemangioendothelioma has also been associated with Kasabach-Meritt syndrome, anemia, intraperitoneal hemorrhage secondary to rupture, consumptive coagulopathy, and vascular malformations involving the brain, skin, gastrointestinal tract, and other organs.

Lesions are usually found throughout the liver but may be localized to one hepatic lobe. Radiographic features include punctate calcification in as many as 50 percent of cases.[20] The sonographic appearance is variable, but the presence of small, multifocal, hypoechoic lesions scattered throughout the liver of a child without an extrahepatic mass strongly suggests multifocal hepatic hemangioendothelioma. The sonographic appearance of large solitary lesions may differ and is therefore nondiagnostic. The tumor may be hypoechoic but is usually heterogeneous with focal areas of increased echogenicity caused by thrombosis and calcification.[23] Duplex and color Doppler ultrasonography show prominent hepatic arteries, the portal vein, and arterial-venous shunting.

CT images obtained without the use of a contrast agent most commonly show a hypodense mass with or without calcification. In the early phase after the administration of an intravenous contrast agent, images show preferential enhancement of the peripheral edge of the mass with a variable degree of central enhancement (Fig. 21.1).[23] On delayed images, multinodular lesions become isodense in comparison with normal liver, whereas solitary lesions may show variable degrees of centripetal enhancement and persistent central unenhanced regions.

On MR images, lesions usually appear hypointense on T1-weighted images and hyperintense on T2-weighted images, although these findings are nonspecific. T1-weighted images may show focal areas of hypointensity or hyperintensity that suggest fibrosis, hemosiderin deposition, or more acute hemorrhage. On all types of images, the descending aorta above the level of the celiac artery may appear abnormally enlarged in comparison with the infrahepatic aorta;[22] this enlargement is related to an increase in blood flow caused by intratumoral shunting.

Static and dynamic hepatic scintigraphy, although not frequently used, can elucidate the nature, size, and vascularity of hemangioendothelioma. Other characteristics of this tumor include the detection of abnormal persistence during the dynamic phase of scintigraphy and focal central defects during the static phase. Hepatic angiography, which is rarely required for diagnostic purposes, shows enlarged and tortuous feeding arteries, dilation in the aorta proximal to the hepatic artery, and a decrease in size in the aorta distal to the hepatic artery. Angiography also shows enlarged, early draining hepatic veins with large, vascular lakes.

Dehner and Ishak identified two microscopic patterns of hemangioendothelioma.[24] The more common pattern, type 1, exhibits a dilated and compressed vascular channel lined by plump endothelial cells that are arranged in an orderly fashion; cytologic analysis demonstrates that these cells are benign. The type 2 pattern exhibits irregularly branched vascular channels that are lined by tufted hyperchromatic, pleomorphic endothelial cells with papillary structures budding into the vessels. Lesions with a type 2 pattern may resemble angiosarcoma, and small-needle biopsy may produce results that are indistinguishable from those produced by small-needle biopsy of sarcoma. Hemangioendothelioma cells lack mitotic activity; microscopic examination of the tumor shows that there is no giant cell formation, no solid sarcomatous area, and no invasion of sinusoids or hepatic and portal veins (Fig. 21.2). Dehner and Ishak reported that the mortality rate associated with the type 2 pattern was higher than that associated with the type 1 pattern, but more recent series report a favorable outcome regardless of type.

Once identified, asymptomatic lesions can be managed conservatively as long as the diagnosis can be made with a high degree of certainty on the basis of noninvasive radiographic studies. Because of the risk of hemorrhage percutaneous or open biopsy of the lesion is discouraged unless there is serious concern that the lesion is malignant. Spontaneous resolution is likely to occur within months or years. Sequential sonography is often used to monitor lesions and usually demonstrates a progressive decrease in size and an increase in the degree of calcification.

Symptomatic lesions are treated first by pharmacological control of the tumor and its symptoms. Aggressive therapy is necessary, especially in cases of Kasabach-Merritt syndrome, because the symptoms can progress rapidly. Several studies have reported estimated survival rates of 12 to 40 percent if symptoms alone are treated and of 70 percent if specific therapy with steroids or resection is undertaken.[25] Medical management of

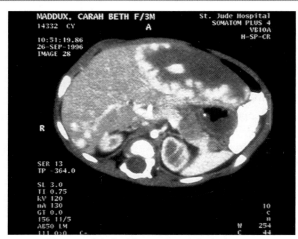

Figure 21.1: Hemangioendothelioma: appearance on CT scan

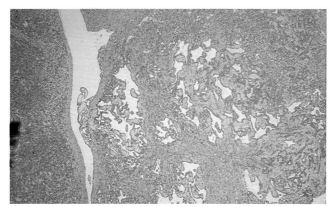

Figure 21.2: Histopathology of hemangioendothelioma type II

these lesions consists of the administration of corticosteroids (prednisolone, 4 to 5 mg/kg body weight per day for 28 days) in conjunction with diuresis and digitalis if CHF is present. Of lesions treated with steroids alone, 30 percent will not respond to therapy, 30 percent will resolve, and 40 percent will have a modified but unaltered course. The response is often noted within 1 to 2 weeks, but complete resolution requires approximately 5 months.[26] The mechanism of action of these steroids is unclear, but it has been postulated that they cause vasoconstriction of the lesion's vascular channels, which are lined by rapidly proliferating immature endothelial cells.[27] More recent studies have suggested treatment with α interferon[28] and γ interferon,[29] antiangiogenic agents that inhibit endothelial cell proliferation and migration, thus causing early regression of hemangioendotheliomas that have developed resistance to corticosteroids. Chemotherapy with cyclophosphamide[30] or doxorubicin[31] and radiation therapy[32,33] have also been used with variable degree of success. Secondary malignancy following radiation therapy has been reported.[34]

When medical treatment fails, the next step is angiography to determine the vascular supply of the lesion. The arterial supply may arise from collateral vessels?? from the superior mesenteric artery or from the intercostal, adrenal, or phrenic arteries; portal venous connection may also be present. Hepatic artery ligation is still controversial; several investigators have reported success in stabilizing the condition of infants with hemangioendothelioma by reducing arteriovenous shunting, thereby allowing time for tumor regression.[35] However, because the results have varied, some

investigators suggest that ligation should be avoided.[36] Hepatic artery embolization is an attractive alternative to hepatic artery ligation[25,37] because it is less invasive. However, percutaneous hepatic arterial embolization may be technically difficult in infants because they are small and because only a limited volume of contrast agent can be safely administered. Therefore, 2 or 3 embolization sessions may be required. Tumor regression may occur months to years after embolization. Two-thirds of embolization procedures are expected to be successful. Because the effect may be only temporary, this intervention is sometimes used to stabilize a patient's condition before transplantation can be performed or until other therapies such as a interferon can be effective. In cases of extensive collateralization and significant portal contribution, hepatic artery embolization should be avoided because it can result in hepatic necrosis, disseminated intravascular coagulopathy, and death.[38]

Surgical intervention for the child with symptomatic hemangioendothelioma is usually indicated only when all medical treatments have failed.[39] If possible, partial liver resection may be undertaken, but because symptomatic lesions are usually distributed throughout the liver, orthotopic liver transplantation is often required. A combination of medical management, embolization, and surgery has resulted in a survival rate of more than 70 percent for infants with severe symptoms.[19]

HEMANGIOMA

Hemangioma is the most common benign liver tumor in adults; the overall incidence at the time of autopsy is approximately 7 percent.[40] In children, however, hemangiomas are usually incidental findings in patients without symptoms. The lesions consist of blood-filled, nonanastomotic vascular spaces lined with flat endothelial cells and supported by fibrous tissue (Fig. 21.3). Most hemangiomas are small and may be multiple. Bleeding, thrombosis, necrosis, or calcification can occur in large hemangiomas, causing abdominal pain. The risk of spontaneous rupture and hemorrhage is exceedingly low.

Small hemangiomas appear on ultrasound images as well-defined, hyperechoic, homogeneous masses with mild posterior enhancement. CT with delayed imaging shows filling of a hypodense mass from the periphery to the center with globular pooling of the contrast agent in the periphery. Unless hepatomegaly is causing pain or disability, no treatment is recommended. When large hemangiomas are associated with pain or other clinical symptoms, surgical resection is the only effective treatment.

ARTERIOVENOUS MALFORMATION (AVM)

An AVM may occur within the liver parenchyma or outside the liver between the hepatic artery and the portal venous system. Like hemangioendothelioma, AVM is usually diagnosed when patients are less than 6 months of age; symptoms include hepatomegaly, CHF, and a bruit over the liver. Angiography is diagnostic, and embolization is therapeutic in some patients. Those whose condition cannot be managed successfully with embolization require arterial ligation, hepatic resection, or liver transplantation for cure.

MESENCHYMAL HAMARTOMA

Mesenchymal hamartomas of the liver are the second most common benign liver tumor of childhood,[41] usually presenting as a painless abdominal mass in a child younger than 2 years. The lesion consists of a mixture of mesenchymal tissue and bile ducts and is considered a developmental anomaly that arises from a mesenchymal rest that becomes isolated from the normal architecture of the portal triad. A mesenchymal hamartoma is not a true neoplasm but is differentiated independently.[2] The lesion grows along bile ducts and may incorporate normal liver tissue. Because the blood vessels and bile ducts are components of the mesenchymal rest, the biologic behavior of the tumor varies with the relative predominance of these tissues within the loose connective-tissue stroma that surrounds them. The tumor may then be a predominantly cystic structure or a predominantly vascular structure associated with CHF. Serum AFP concentrations are usually normal but can be mildly elevated. On imaging studies, the lesion appears as a large, multilocular, cystic mass with thin internal septation, usually without calcification (Fig. 21.4). Occasionally, the solid component of the lesion can be more predominant with multiple smaller cysts, giving the lesion a Swiss cheese appearance.[13]

Management of these lesions consists of complete surgical resection whenever possible. With huge lesions that involve both lobes of the liver, unroofing and marsupialization of the cyst are preferred, although the lesion can recur after incomplete removal. Malignant transformation into hepatic undifferentiated (embryonal) sarcoma has been reported.[42]

HEPATOCELLULAR ADENOMA

Hepatocellular adenoma (HCA) occurs predominantly in women between the ages of 15 and 50. Although uncommon in the general pediatric population, HCA occurs with increased frequency in patients with

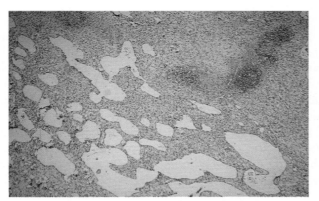

Figure 21.3: Hemangioma: histopathology showing vascular channel

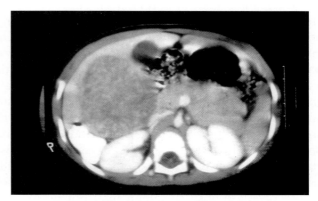

Figure 21.4: CT scan of mesenchymal hamartoma

predisposing disease or in teenagers who are taking birth control pills. Conditions predisposing pediatric patients to HCA include Fanconi's anemia, glycogen storage disease type 1, and the use of anabolic corticosteroids and estrogen. In association with Fanconi's anemia, HCA may develop after the use of androgen therapy to stimulate erythropoiesis or as the result of chronic iron overload caused by multiple blood transfusions.[5] Several mechanisms have been proposed for the development of HCA in patients with glycogen storage disease type 1, including an imbalance in the metabolism of insulin and glucagon.[6] These hormones are important in the regulation of hepatocyte proliferation and regeneration. Either response to glycogen overload or the presence of an oncogene may also play a role. In patients with these predisposing conditions, HCAs are most commonly multiple and variable in size. Hepatic adenomatosis, defined as the presence of more than 4 adenomas, rarely occurs in patients without predisposing factors.[43]

In pediatric patients, HCA is usually an asymptomatic mass. The results of liver function tests may be normal or abnormal, but the serum AFP concentration is not elevated. On imaging studies, the appearance of adenomas is nonspecific. Sonography shows a variable degree of echogenicity and may show heterogeneous hyperechoic tumor. The lesions tend to appear hypodense on CT scans performed without the administration of contrast agent, but they can appear as hyperdense areas of hemorrhage before contrast is administered and as low-density areas of necrosis after contrast has been administered. MR imaging shows hyperintense areas of hemorrhage or necrosis on T2-weighted images, but the signal may be variable according to the degree of fibrofatty change, hemorrhage, and hemosiderin deposition. Injection with the contrast agent gadolinium enhances the tumor.[13] Radionuclide imaging may show less uptake of Ga-67 in the adenoma than in normal liver, negative colloid (Tc-99m phytate) uptake in the adenoma, and early uptake and subsequent retention of Tc-99m PMT.[18] On microscopic examination, HCA is characterized by a hepatocellular proliferation intermingled with sinusoids without biliary structures; the tumor is often encapsulated. The cells have glycogen-filled cytoplasm and small nuclei without mitotic activity. Adjacent liver and vessels are compressed but not invaded. Pediatric patients usually do not have coexistent cirrhosis. Histologic findings are similar to those associated with well-differentiated hepatocellular carcinoma; studies of a core needle-biopsy specimen may not be able to

differentiate the two lesions. Development of hepatocellular carcinoma within an unresected HCA has been reported.[44]

HCA is unique in its tendency to rupture spontaneously, thus causing intraperitoneal hemorrhage. In adults, pregnancy and estrogen intake increase the risk of rupture. Regression of adenomas has been observed after discontinuation of oral contraceptives, but progressive enlargement is also possible.[45] In patients with glycogen storage disease, tumor regression may occur when the metabolic disturbance has been corrected.

Liver resection for HCA has been proved safe and is indicated even for asymptomatic HCA because of the risk of rupture and the association with malignancy. If resection cannot be accomplished without substantial risk, observation of the lesion and monitoring the serum AFP concentration may be appropriate. If the AFP concentration begins to rise or the lesion causes substantial symptoms and the risk of resection is unacceptably high, liver transplantation is a valid alternative. If the HCA ruptures, preoperative hepatic artery embolization can be used to stabilize the patient's condition and minimize intraoperative blood loss.[46]

FOCAL NODULAR HYPERPLASIA

Focal nodular hyperplasia (FNH) in pediatric patients is first seen as an irregularly shaped, nontender mass that is usually asymptomatic and may be found incidentally by radiographic study or laparotomy performed for other conditions. More than 80 percent of cases of FNH occur in female patients.[40] The results of liver function tests are elevated in fewer than 20 percent of cases, and the serum AFP concentration is normal. FNH is occasionally seen with vascular malformations and hemangiomas in the liver and probably develops as a result of a vascular malformation with unusual hyperplastic response to injury or ischemia; therefore, FNH is characterized by a hypervascular central scar.

Ultrasonography shows a well-defined lesion that may be isoechoic, hypoechoic, or hyperechoic in comparison with normal liver parenchyma. A central hyperechoic area is sometimes visible, and duplex Doppler ultrasound may show a hypervascular center. Multiple lesions are found in 10 to 15 percent of patients. Figure 21.5 depicts the imaging finding in a case of FNH. After the injection of a contrast agent, delayed CT images show the typical appearance of a hypervascular lesion with a dense stellate central scar. MR imaging shows isointensity on T1-weighted and T2-weighted images

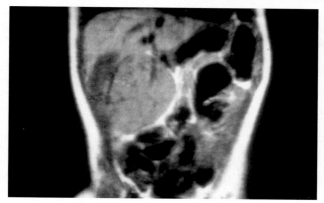

Figure 21.5: Focal nodular hyperplasia (FNH): appearance on CT scan

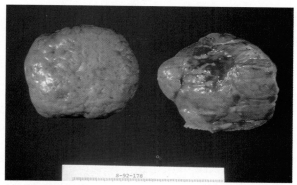

with a hyperintense central scar on T2-weighted images. After the injection of the contrast agent gadolinium, early enhancement is seen in the mass and late enhancement is seen within the scar.[13] Arteriography shows a hypervascular mass with feeding arteries entering the lesion and converging in the central portion of the tumor. Fibrolamellar hepatocellular carcinoma is radiographically indistinguishable from FNH on imaging studies; biopsy should be performed for accurate diagnosis.

Grossly, FNH appears as a lobulated, well-circumscribed, firm, unencapsulated lesion, occasionally pedunculated (Figs 21.6A to C). When the lesion is peripheral and more than 5 cm in diameter, it is often an umbilicated lesion on the liver surface. Microscopic examination shows proliferation of hepatocytes and bile ducts and the pathognomonic central fibrosis. Because the natural history of FNH is characterized by the absence of complications, expectant therapy is appropriate. When FNH is symptomatic, is diagnosed in a boy, or has other atypical features, or when the diagnosis of fibrolamellar hepatocellular carcinoma is entertained, a histologic diagnosis is mandatory.

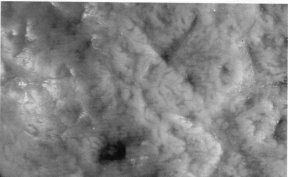

Figures 21.6B and C: Gross specimen of FNH

TERATOMA

Intrahepatic teratoma is a rare lesion that may contain calcification (Fig. 21.7). The serum AFP concentration may be mildly elevated. Resection is the treatment of choice because the lesion has the potential for malignancy when it contains immature elements.

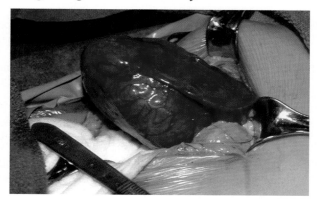

Figure 21.6A: Intraoperative picture of FNH

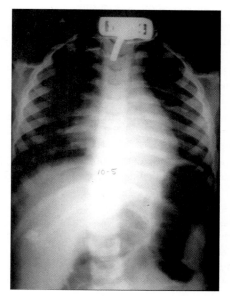

Figure 21.7: Plain radiograph of patient with hepatic teratoma with calcification in right upper quadrant of the abdomen

REFERENCES

1. Baggenstoss AH. Pathology of tumors of liver in infancy and childhood. RRCR 1970;26:240-5.

2. Edmonson HA. Differential diagnosis of tumors and tumor like lesions of liver in infancy and childhood. Am J Dis Child 1956;91:168-70.

3. Helmberger TK, Ros PR, Mergo PJ, et al. Pediatric liver neoplasms: a radiologic-pathologic correlation. Eur Radiol 1999;9(7):1339-47.

4. Ishak KG. Primary hepatic tumors in childhood. In Popper H, Schaffner F (Eds): Progress in Liver Diseases 1976;5:636-45.

5. Chandra RS, et al. Benign hepatocellular tumor in the young. Arch Pathol Lab Med 1984; 108:168-71.

6. Bianchi L. Glycogen storage disease I and hepatocellular tumors, Eu J Pediatr 1993;152:S63-70.

7. Jozwiak S, et al. Incidence of hepatic hamartomas in tuberous sclerosis. Arch Dis Child 1992;67:1363-5.

8. Kasabach HH, Meritt KK. Capillary hemangioma with extensive purpura. Report of a case. Am J Dis Child 1940;59:1063-70.

9. Fellows KE, et al. Multiple collateral to hepatic infantile hemangioendothelioma and arteriovenous malformation: effect on embolization. Radiology 1991;181:813-8.

10. Smith WL, Ballantine TVN, Gonzalez-Crussi F. Hepatic mesenchymal hamartoma causing heart failure in the neonate. J Pediatr Surg 1978;13:183-5.

11. Robinson D, Hambleton G. Cutaneous and hepatic hemangiomata. Arch Dis Child 1977;52:155-7.

12. Wu JT, Book L, Sudar K. Serum alphafetoprotein (AFP) levels in normal infants. Pediatr Res 1981;15:50-52.

13. Donnelly LF, Bisset GS. Pediatric hepatic imaging. Radiol Clin North Am 1998;36:413-27.

14. Thomas BL, et al. Use of intraoperative ultrasound during hepatic resection on pediatirc patients. J Pediatr Surg 1989;24:690-3.

15. Boechat MI, Kangarloo H, Ortega J, et al. Primary liver tumor in children: comparison of CT and MR imaging. Radiology 1988;169:727-32.

16. Weinreb JC, Cohen JM, Armstrong E, et al. Imaging of the pediatric liver: MRI and CT. AJR Am J Roentgenol 1986;147:785-90.

17. Horton KM, Bluemke DA, Hruban RH, et al. CT and MR imaging of benign hepatic and biliary tumors Radiographics 1999;19(2):431-51.

18. Kume N, Suga K, Nishigauchi K, et al. Characterization of hepatic sdenoma with atypical appearance on CT and MRI by radionuclide imaging. Clin Nuclear Med 1997; 22(12):825-31.

19. Selby DM, Stocker JT, Waclawiw VA. Infantile hemangioendothelioma of the liver. Hepatology 1994;20:39-45.

20. Dachman AH, Lichtenstein JE, Friedman AC, et al. Infantile hemangioendothelioma of the liver: a radiologic-pathologic-clinical correlation. AJR Am J Roentgenol 1983;140:1091-6.

21. Daller JA, Bueno J, Gutiarrez, et al. Hepatic hemagioendothelioma: clinical experience and management stategy.J Pediatr Surg 1999;34:98-106.

22. Jackson C, Greene HL, O'Neill JA, et al. Hepatichemagio-endothelioma. Am J Dis Child 1977; 132:74-7.

23. Pobeil RS, Bisset GS 3rd. Pictorail essay: imaging of liver tumors in the infant and child. Pediatr Radiol 1995;25:495-506.

24. Dehner LP, Ishak KG. Vascular tumors of the liver in infants and Children: a study of 30 cases and review of the literature. Arch Pathol 1971;92:101-11.

25. Burrows PE, Rosenberg HC, Chuang HS. Diffuse hepatic heamngiomas: percutaneous transcatheter embolization with detachable silicone balloons. Radiology 1985;156:85-8.

26. Touloukian RJ. Hemangioendothelioma during infancy: pathology, diagnosis and treatment with prednisolone. Pediatrics 1970;45:71-6.

27. Rocchini AP, Rosenthal A, Issenberg HJ, et al. Hepatic hemangioendothelioma: hemodynamic observations and treatment. Pediatrics 1976;57:131-5.

28. Ergowitz RAB, Mulliken JB, Folkman J. Interferon Alpha 2: a therapy for life threatening hemangiomas in infancy. N Eng J Med 1992;336:1456-63.

29. Friesel R, Komoriya A, Mackay T. Inhibition of endothelial cell proliferation by gamma interferon. J Cell Biol 1987;104:689-99.

30. Manglani M, Chari G, Sharma U, et al. Successful treatment with cyclophosphamide in a large hepatichemangioendo-thelioma. Indian Pediatr 1994;31:875-7.

31. Holcomb GW, O'Neill JA, Mahboubi S, et al. Experience woth hepatic hemangioendothelioma in infancy and childhood. J Pediatr Surg 1988;23:661-6.

32. Corbella F, Arico M, Podesta AF. Infantile hepatic hemangioendothelioma treated by radiotherapy. Pediatr Radiol 1983;13:297-300.

33. Kornfalt S, Norgren A, Henrikson H. Hepatic hemangioendothelioma treated by irradiation. Z Kinderchir 1975;16:37-40.

34. Haselow R, nesbit M, Dehner L, et al. Second neoplasm following megavoltage radiation in a pediatric population. Cancer 1978;42:1185-91.

35. Moazam F, Rodgers BM, Talbert JL. Hepatic artery ligation for hepatic hemangiomatosis of infancy. J Pediatr Surg 1983;18:120-33.

36. Nguyen L, Shandling B, Ein S, et al. Hepatic hemangioma in childhood: medical management or surgical management? J Pediatr Surg 1982;17:576-9.

37. Fellow KE, Hoffer FA, Markowitz RI. Multiple collaterals to hepatic infantile hemangio-endotheliomas and arteriovenous malformations: effect on embolization. Radiology 1991; 181:813-8.

38. Burke DR, Verstandig A, Edwards O, et al. Infantile hemangioendothelioma: angiographic features and factors

determining efficacy of hepatic artery embolization. Cardiovasc Intervent Radiol 1986; 9:154-7.

39. Samuel M, Spitz L. Infantile hepatic hemangioendo-thelioma: the role of surgery. J Pediatr Surg 1995;30: 1425-9.

40. Vauthey JN. Liver imaging: a surgeon's perspective. Radiol Clin North Am 1998;36:445-58.

41. Murray JD, Ricketts RR. Mesenchymal hamartoma of the liver. Am Surg 1998;64:1097-1103.

42. Lauwers GY, Grant LD, Donnelly WH, et al. Hepatic indifferentiated (embryonal) sarcoma arising in a mesenchymal hamartoma. Am J Surg Pathol 1997;21: 1248-54.

43. Brummett D, Burton EM, Sabio H. Hepatic denomatosis: rapid sequence MR imaging following gadolinium enhancement: a case report. Pediatr Radiol 1999;29:231-4.

44. Janes CH, et al. Liver cell adenoma at the age of 3 years and transplantation 19 years later after development of carcinoma: a case report. Hepatology 1993;17:583-5.

45. Nagorney DM. Benign hepatic tumors: focal nodular hyperplasia and hepatocellular adenoma. World J Surg 1995;19:13-8.

46. Leese T, Frages O, Bismuth H. Live cell adenomas. A 12-years surgical experience from a specialist Hepato Biliary Unit. Ann Surg 1988;2208:558-64.

CHAPTER 22

Kenneth W Gow
Chan Hon Chui
Sani Molagool
Bhaskar Rao

Malignant Liver Tumors in Children and Adolescents

HISTORY

In 1898, Misick gave the earliest description of a hepatoblastoma, which he termed a "teratoma hepatis".[1] The patient was a 3-week-old boy with a mass on the right side of his abdomen; respiratory symptoms developed, and the infant died at the age of 1 month. Autopsy findings showed that the right lobe of the liver was replaced by a multilobulated gray-yellow mass with prominent fibrous septa, smooth-walled cysts, and foci of bone and cartilage. The tumor had also invaded the hepatic veins. Microscopic examination identified embryonic-appearing hepatocytes, a spindle cell sarcomatous stroma, gland-like spaces, osteoid with osteoblasts, and squamous epithelium. The mass was considered a teratoma because it appeared to contain tissue representative of all three embryonic germ cell layers. However, we now recognize this type of tumor as a mixed epithelial mesenchymal variant of hepatoblastoma.

In 1962, Willis[2] proposed that "all embryonic tumors containing hepatic epithelial parenchyma" should be classified as hepatoblastomas. However, even during this period, the distinction was not often made in pediatric patients between hepatoblastoma and hepatocellular carcinoma. It was not until 1967 that Ishak and Glunz[3] set forth the morphologic criteria for differentiating hepatoblastoma from hepatocellular carcinoma.

EMBRYOLOGY

During the fourth week of gestation, the liver and biliary tract develop from the ventral bud arising from the caudal part of the endodermal lining of the foregut.[4] The hepatic diverticulum extends into the mesodermal tissue of the septum transversum, which lies between the pericardial cavity and the yolk stalk. The proliferating endodermal cells from the foregut give rise to interlacing cords of liver cells and to the epithelial lining of the intrahepatic portion of the biliary apparatus. The splanchnic mesenchyme of the septum transversum gives rise to connective tissue cells, Kupffer cells, and hematopoietic cells. Intrahepatic ducts develop in a centrifugal progression from the hilum outward. The mesenchymal tissue that accompanies portal veins growing into the parenchyma induces a transformation of hepatocytes into ductal tissue.

SURGICAL ANATOMY

Knowledge of the hepatic anatomy is an important factor guiding the surgeon to the limits of resection. However, subtle differences in terminology between anatomic and functional anatomy have confused some students. We will clarify these differences in terms as they arise.

The liver is suspended from the abdominal wall and the diaphragm by three ligaments: the falciform ligament, the coronary ligament, and the round ligament. On the left, the two leaves of the coronary ligament approach and join to form the left triangular ligament; on the right, their apposition forms the right triangular ligament. These ligaments must often be divided before the liver can be adequately exposed for resection. Anteriorly, the anterior layer of the coronary ligament forms a fold that extends over the superior surface of the liver, which is also known as the falciform ligament. Between the two layers of the fold, the remnant of the embryonic left umbilical vein forms the round ligament (ligamentum teres). The falciform and round ligaments extend into the liver to form the obvious fissure that separates the two segments of the left lobe.

The liver has both a right and left lobe, approximately equal in size. It is important to remember that the hepatic veins do not follow this division. On the visceral surface of the liver, the plane separating the right and left lobes passes through the bed of the gallbladder below and the fossa of the inferior vena cava (IVC) above. On the diaphragmatic surface, there is no visible external mark. The line of separation is an imaginary line that passes from the notch of the gallbladder anteriorly, parallel to the fissure of the round ligament, to the IVC above. The true left lobe thus consists of a left medial segment and a left lateral segment. The latter is the apparent left "lobe" of the older anatomists. Each of these segments may be divided into superior and inferior subsegments. The right lobe may be similarly divided into anterior and posterior segments by imaginary lines. The intersegmental fissure, when present, indicates this separation. Each of these segments may be divided again into superior and inferior subsegments. Therefore, the liver may be thought of as having four segments; right posterior, right anterior, left medial, and left lateral segments which is the basis of the terminology for resection (Fig. 22.1).

However, recently, with the introduction of the Couinaud's nomenclature, there has been confusion of the term "segment". What anatomists previously called segments is now referred to as sectors. What was previously called subsegments are now referred to as segments.

While imaginary lines may define the hepatic segments, the true segmental divisions can be observed only in cast specimens in which the hepatic artery, portal vein, and bile ducts have been injected. These casts have produced a "functional" anatomy that permits a description of hepatic segmentation based on the distribution of portal pedicles and the location of hepatic veins. This functional division of the liver is based on Couinaud's nomenclature and is shown in Figure 22.2. The liver is divided into two lobes by the portal scissura in which the middle hepatic vein courses. Each lobe has two sectors. In turn, each sector can be divided into two segments. The division of the sectors and segments is based on first-order and second-order branching of the

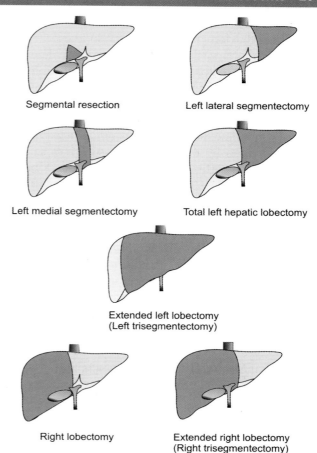

Figure 22.1: Summary of terminology used for extent of resection based on the anatomic segments

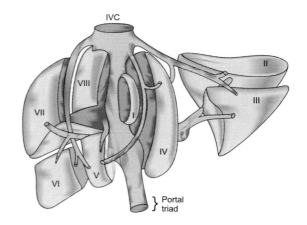

Figure 22.2: Couinaud's nomenclature with hepatic segmentation based on the distribution of portal pedicles and the location of hepatic veins. Sectors of the liver are depicted including sectors I through VIII

portal vein, the hepatic artery, and the bile ducts. The right lobe is divided into two "sectors" by the right portal scissura containing the right hepatic vein. The right posterolateral "sector" contains segment VI anteriorly and segment VII posteriorly. The right anterolateral "sector" contains segment V anteriorly and segment VIII posteriorly. The left lobe is divided by the left portal scissura containing the left hepatic vein. The left anterior sector is divided by the umbilical fissure into segment IV, the anterior part of which is the quadrate lobe, the segment III, which is the anterior part of the left lobe. The posterior sector is segment II. The caudate lobe (segment I) is unique and can be considered separate from the rest of the liver because it obtains its supply of blood directly from the right and left main branches of the portal vein and the hepatic artery, and drains bile directly into the bile duct. Its short, independent hepatic veins also provide hepatic venous drainage directly into the retrohepatic cava.

EPIDEMIOLOGY

The liver is the most common site of epithelial neoplasms in pediatric patients. Overall, hepatic malignancies are the tenth most common childhood tumor, representing 0.5 to 2 percent of all pediatric tumors[5,6] (Table 22.1). The annual incidence of malignant hepatic tumors in the United States is 1.6 per million children; hepatoblastoma (HB) is slightly more common, with an incidence of 0.9 per million, whereas the incidence of hepatocellular carcinoma (HCC) is 0.7 per million. Both tumors occur more often in boys than in girls (HB, 2:1 ratio; HCC, 1.4:1 ratio). The median age of patients at the time of diagnosis of HB is 1 year; most tumors occur during the patient's first 1.5 years of life. The median age of patients at the time of diagnosis of HCC is 12 years; most tumors occur when patients are 10 to 15 years of age.

Hepatoblastoma has been reported in association with maternal use of oral contraceptives[7,8] or gonadotropins[9] and in association with fetal alcohol syndrome.[10] The Children's Cancer Group (CCG) conducted a retrospective case-control study of risk factors for the development of HB; the study included 75 of a cohort of 120 pediatric patients.[11] The findings of the study showed that HB was more likely to occur after maternal exposure to metals (odds ratio [OR], 8.0), petroleum products (OR, 3.7), or paints or pigments (OR, 3.7) during pregnancy or during the year before pregnancy and after paternal exposure to metals,

Table 22.1: Classification of primary hepatic malignant tumors
Epithelial neoplasms
Hepatoblastoma
Hepatocellular carcinoma
Mesenchymal neoplasms
Undifferentiated embryonal sarcoma
Embryonal rhabdomyosarcoma
Epithelioid hemangioendothelioma
Germ cell tumors
Yolk sac tumor
Teratomas

especially lead (OR 3.0). The association between the occurrence of HB and parental exposure to hydrocarbons was of borderline significance. An association between development of poor-prognosis HB and low birth weight (less than 1500 grams) was recently reported by Ikeda et al,[12] but the exact mechanism of this association is unclear. Unlike HCC, HB has not been associated with any racial group.[13]

Environmental exposure to chemical carcinogens, such as aflatoxin and nitrosamines,[14] may induce HCC. Aflatoxins, the toxic metabolites of certain spoilage molds, are potent liver carcinogens in experimental animals and frequently contaminate human diets.[15] Interestingly, the frequency of HCC is related to geographic area in which patients live. The incidence of HCC is higher in Asia and Africa than in other areas of the world. In fact, HCC is so prevalent in some areas, such as Taiwan and Southern China, that it is three times as likely to occur as HB.[16] This prevalence is believed to be due to the close association between HCC and the hepatitis B virus (HBV); in one study, the serum of nearly 100 percent of pediatric patients with HCC tested positive for the hepatitis B surface antigen (HBsAg).[17] Mother-to-child transmission appears to be the primary route by which HBV is transmitted to pediatric patients with HCC. In an attempt to reduce the incidence of HCC in Taiwan, a nationwide hepatitis B vaccination program was launched in 1984. According to Chang et al,[18] this program reduced the average annual incidence of HCC in pediatric patients aged 6 to 14 years from 0.70 per 100,000 between 1981 and 1986 to 0.57 per 100,000 between 1986 and 1990. A further reduction to 0.36 per 100,000 was observed between 1990 and 1994. The corresponding rates of mortality due to HCC also decreased. The authors not only demonstrated the presumed connection between HCC and HBV but also showed that vaccination can effectively reduce the incidence of malignancy and mortality. Other nations such as India and Gambia are discussing[19] or beginning similar vaccination programs.[5,20] Finally, although the hepatitis C virus (HCV) is an important agent in the pathogenesis of HCC in adults, particularly in Japan, Southern Europe, the United States, South Africa, and other areas, it has not been related to the incidence of HCC in pediatric patients.[21]

GENETICS AND BIOLOGY

Hepatoblastoma

Beckwith-Wiedemann Syndrome

Congenital anomalies are frequently associated with HB. The most interesting association is that between the Beckwith-Wiedemann syndrome (BWS) and HB.[22] BWS is an autosomal-dominant syndrome consisting of macrosomia, macroglossia, abdominal wall defects, visceromegaly, neonatal hypoglycemia, and occasional hemihypertrophy. BWS is also associated with an elevated risk of Wilms' tumor, another embryonal neoplasm. Investigators have proposed that, in embryonal tumors, a developmental disturbance occurring during organogenesis permits inappropriate continuation of proliferation, thus resulting in a mass of immature tissue recognized as an embryonal tumor. In the case of Wilms' tumor, the homozygous expression of two different recessive mutant alleles, one at band 11p13 (*WT-1*)[23] and the other at band 11p15.5 (*WT-2*),[24] has been shown in tumor cells but not in cells from the surrounding normal kidney. This phenomenon, termed loss of heterozygosity (LOH), provides indirect molecular evidence of the presence of one or more tumor-suppressor genes.[25] Albrecht et al[26] detected this LOH on arm 11p in six of 18 HB specimens. The common region of overlap was restricted to the telomeric portion of arm 11p (band 11p15.5) and therefore excluded the *WT-1* tumor-suppressor gene at band 11p13. Maternal origin of the lost allele was determined in all six cases. The authors concluded that a tumor-suppressor gene at band 11p15.5 is involved in the pathogenesis of hepatoblastoma, and they also suggested that this chromosomal region is imprinted. Two notable genes are present on this portion of the chromosome: *H19* and *IGFII*. The precise role of the imprinting of these genes in carcinogenesis is unclear at this time.[27,28]

Cytogenetics

Other consistent clonal abnormalities in HB tissue have also been reported. Nagata et al[29] reviewed the chromosomal abnormalities in published cases of HB and in their own cases (a total of 38 detailed cases). The most consistently described chromosomal abnormalities were trisomy 1 or 1q (15 of 38 cases, 39.5%), trisomy 2 or 2q (17 of 38 cases, 44.7%), trisomy 20 (18 of 38 cases, 65.8%), and extracopies of chromosome 8 or 8q (15 of 38 cases, 39.5%). Further review of these chromosomal alterations demonstrated and noted that the most common breakages involved 1q (20/103 points, 19%), 2q (17/103 points, 17%), and 4q (15/103 points, 15%). Hu et al[30] recently studied 10 HB samples by using comparative genomic hybridization. This technique can screen the entire genome for genetic gains and losses without the need for growth in tissue culture, thereby removing the possibility of selection with cell suspensions. These authors reported that the most common recurrent abnormalities were gain of the long arm of chromosome 1 (6 of 10 tumors); gain of chromosomes 2 (7 of 10 tumors), 17 (4 of 10 tumors), and 20 (3 of 10 tumors); and loss of chromosomes 4 and 11 (2 tumors each). Four samples showed restricted regions of high-level gain at 1q32 or 2q24, regions that have previously been reported to be amplified in other tumors but not in HB. However, no specific amplified gene was identified in their study.

Familial Adenomatous Polyposis

Hepatoblastoma is also more prevalent in association with familial adenomatous polyposis coli (FAP).[31] The risk of the development of HB in a family with FAP was 0.42 percent in an international survey of FAP registries.[31] FAP, an autosomal-dominant disorder, is characterized by the development of numerous adenomatous colorectal polyps and colorectal carcinomas and is caused by germline mutations of the APC (adenomatous polyposis coli) gene located on band 5p21.[32,33] The APC gene product normally regulates the cytoplasmic level of β-catenin by targeting it for degradation.[34] Therefore, mutations of the *APC* gene will result in accumulation of β-catenin, which has been shown to induce malignant transformation. A variety of malignancies other than colorectal tumors occur in association with FAP. So far, more than 30 cases of HB have been reported in families with FAP.[35] Giardiello et al[36] identified a mutation at the end of the *APC* gene in eight children from FAP families. Wei et al[37] studied the levels of β-catenin in 11 HB samples. Using immunohistochemistry, they found that β-catenin accumulates in the nucleus and cytoplasm and suggested that activation of β-catenin may be an obligatory step in the pathogenesis of HB. They speculated that β-catenin may interfere with developmental signals that specify different tissue types at early stages of hepatic differentiation. Further evidence of the importance of β-catenin has been provided by Koch et al,[38] who reviewed 52 biopsy specimens and three cell lines from sporadic HB for mutations in β-catenin genes. These authors found that 48 percent of specimens had mutations affecting exon 3, which encodes the degradation targeting box of β-catenin; these mutations lead to accumulation of intracytoplasmic and nuclear β-catenin protein. This level of mutation is even larger than that seen in colorectal carcinomas (usually fewer than 25% of specimens are affected).[38] In view of the association between FAP and HB, Giardiello et al have suggested that it may be prudent to evaluate infants and young children from FAP families by screening for α-fetoprotein (AFP) concentrations and possibly by performing computed tomography (CT) scans of the abdomen.[39]

DNA Content

Flow cytometry (FC) is used to determine both the DNA content and the degree of proliferation of cells. DNA ploidy has been strongly associated with the prognosis of pediatric patients with acute lymphoblastic leukemia (ALL),[40] neuroblastoma,[41] and rhabdomyosarcoma (RMS).[42] FC may also be used to assess the percentage distribution of neoplastic cells in the various phases of the cell cycle. Such an assessment can provide an estimate of the proportion of neoplastic cells in the S, G2, and M phases of the cell cycle (i.e. the proliferative activity [PA]), which usually corresponds with the aggressiveness of the tumor.[43] The PA can also be semiquantitatively evaluated by microscopic count of cells exhibiting nuclear immunoreactivity for proliferating cell nuclear antigen (PCNA). PCNA is a nonhistone nuclear protein expressed in the G1, S, and G2 phases of the cell cycle and is easily detectable by immunohistochemical analysis. In the case of HB, studies[44,45] have shown a strong association between embryonal histology and aneuploidy and between fetal histology and diploidy. Furthermore, Rugge et al[45] have shown that embryonal HB is associated with a higher PA than is fetal HB. These authors suggest that the increased proliferation may make embryonal HB more susceptible to chemotherapy.

Hepatocellular Carcinoma

Tumor-suppressor Gene

Evidence suggests that a tumor-suppressor gene may be responsible for HCC oncogenesis. LOH has been frequently shown for many chromosomal regions in HCC cells, including arms 1p, 4q, 5q, 10q, 11p, 13q, and 17p. Nishida et al[46] examined 56 samples of HCC for LOH at 13 loci on five chromosomes. Allelic losses were most commonly detected on chromosome arms 13q (47%), 16q (40%), and 17p (64%). Losses on chromosome arms 4p and 11p were observed in fewer than 22 percent of samples. Interestingly, these chromosomal losses were more frequently associated with portal vein thrombosis, intrahepatic metastasis, increased tumor size, a poorly differentiated phenotype, and, most important, advanced clinical stage. Similarly, losses of arms 13q, 16q, and 17p were significantly more common in patients with clinical stage IV disease or histologically poorly differentiated tumors.

Metabolic and Genetic Diseases

Several diseases are associated with the development of HCC, including hereditary tyrosinemia, α-1-antitrypsin deficiency, porphyria cutanea tarda, Wilson's disease, hemochromatosis, and glycogen storage disease type I. The incidence of HCC is high in children with the chronic form of hereditary tyrosinemia who survive beyond the age of 2 years. In a series of 43 patients, HCC developed in 16 pediatric patients who survived beyond the age of two years.[47] Dietary avoidance of aromatic amino acids and methionine may not prevent liver diseases or the development of HCC in pediatric patients with tyrosinemia.[21] Although the other diseases listed above are associated with an increased incidence of HCC, the malignancy usually does not occur until patients reach adulthood. Finally, HCC has also been reported in 6 children with FAP.[48]

Cirrhosis

Cirrhosis occurs less frequently in pediatric patients with HCC than in adults with the disease. Regardless of cause, cirrhosis secondary to extrahepatic biliary atresia, neonatal hepatitis, or total parenteral nutrition is probably a precancerous state.[21] Esquivel et al[49] studied the explanted livers of 72 pediatric patients who underwent liver transplantation for end-stage liver disease; five livers demonstrated occult features of HCC and three demonstrated liver cell dysplasia, considered by some to be a preneoplastic condition. Chronic cholestasis without cirrhosis does not predispose patients to HCC, nor does biliary cirrhosis in the adult have a significant association with HCC. Thus, specific metabolic contributions to oncogenesis may be present in childhood hepatic tumors that develop in association with biliary cirrhosis.

CLINICAL PRESENTATION

Hepatoblastoma

In young children, HB is usually an asymptomatic abdominal mass detected by physical examination (Table 22.2) (Figs 22.3A and B). Systemic symptoms such as weight loss, anorexia, and weakness are less common. Jaundice is uncommon. Features of BWS, hemihypertrophy, or isosexual precocity can also be seen. Precocious puberty arises because the tumor produces β-human chorionic gonadotropin (β-hCG).[50] Severe osteopenia, with back pain, refusal to walk, and pathologic fractures of weight-bearing bones, may be seen at the time of presentation. Multiple vertebral compression fractures may be visible on radiographs. Some degree of osteopenia is present in one fourth of children with HB but usually resolves with tumor resection.

Hepatocellular Carcinoma

HCC usually remains asymptomatic until the tumor becomes very large. A palpable abdominal mass and

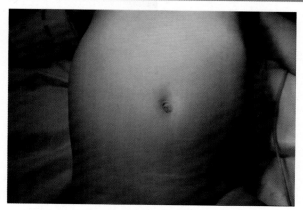

Figure 22.3A: Abdominal exam demons-trating hepatomegaly in a one-month-old infant with hepatoblastoma involving the left lobe of the liver

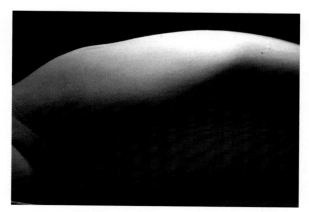

Figure 22.3B: Lateral view of hepatomegaly

abdominal distension are the most common symptoms of HCC in pediatric patients[51] (Table 22.3). Because of the relatively low incidence of HCC in pediatric patients, such a diagnosis is not usually considered at the time of presentation; thus, HCC is commonly diagnosed late in its course. Systemic manifestations such as anorexia, weight loss, and fever are more common with HCC than with HB. Jaundice is also more common with HCC than with HB and occurs in about 10 percent of patients. Splenomegaly may be present when the patient has coexisting cirrhosis, as may other features of chronic liver disease. Portal vein thrombosis is also common in pediatric patients with HCC.

HISTOLOGIC TYPES

Histologically, hepatoblastomas have been classified into six patterns with two main subtypes: epithelial and mixed (Table 22.4).[4] The epithelial subtype accounts for approximately 56 percent of cases, including pure fetal (31%), embryonal (19%), macrotrabecular (3%), and

Tabele 22.2: Presenting signs and symptoms of patients with hepatoblastoma	
Signs or symptoms	Frequency (%)
Upper abdominal mass	75
Weight loss	26
Anorexia	25
Abdominal enlargement	23
Pain	22
Vomiting	12
Jaundice	5
Weakness	Rare
Lethargy	Rare
Irritability	Rare
Diarrhea	Rare
Pruritus	Rare
Fever	Rare
Precocious puberty	Rare

Data from Exelby PR, Filler RM, Grosfeld JL. Liver tumors in children in the particular reference to hepatoblastoma and hepatocellular carcinoma: American Academy of Pediatrics Surgical Section Survey—1974. J Pediatr Surg 1975;10:329-37.[51]

Tabele 22.3: Presenting signs and symptoms of patients with hepatocellular carcinoma

Signs or symptoms	Frequency (%)
Upper abdominal mass	59
Abdominal enlargement	35
Anorexia	21
Weight loss	19
Pain	15
Vomiting	10
Jaundice	10
Fever	7

Data from Exelby PR, Filler RM, Grosfeld JL. Liver tumors in children in the particular reference to hepatoblastoma and hepatocellular carcinoma: American Academy of Pediatrics Surgical Section Survey—1974. J Pediatr Surg 1975;10:329-37.[51]

Table 22.4: Histologic classification of hepatoblastoma

Epithelial subtype
  Fetal pattern
  Embryonal and fetal pattern
  Macrotrabecular pattern
  Small-cell undifferentiated or anaplastic pattern

Mixed epithelial and mesenchymal subtype
  With teratoid features
  Without teratoid features

After JT Stocker. Hepatoblastoma, Sem Diagnost Pathol 1994; 11:136-43.[4]

small-cell undifferentiated patterns (3%). The mixed subtype consisting of epithelial and mesenchymal components, accounts for the remaining 44 percent of cases: 10 percent exhibit teratoid features such as striated muscle, bone, and squamous epithelium, and the remaining 34 percent do not exhibit such features.

Tumors of the fetal pattern of HB most closely resemble embryonal liver tissue. This pattern consists of uniform trabeculae of small, round to cuboidal cells with abundant cytoplasm and distinct cytoplasmic membranes (Fig. 22.4). The trabeculae are two to three cells thick and are arranged in alternating light and dark areas according to the amount of glycogen and lipid. Foci of extramedullary hematopoietic cells are found throughout the sinusoids in the lesion. Unlike other histologic patterns, however, tumors of the fetal pattern do not contain bile ducts and ductules.

Tumors of the embryonal pattern of HB display a more primitive histologic appearance than those of the

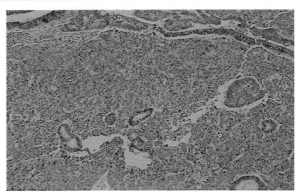

Figure 22.4: Photomicrograph of fetal type hepato-blastoma demonstrating uniform trabeculae of small, round to cuboidal cells with abundant cytoplasm and distinct cytoplasmic membranes

fetal pattern. This pattern consists of well-defined areas of fetal epithelial cells along with sheets and clusters of irregular, angulated cells with a high nucleocytoplasmic ratio, increased nuclear chromatin, and indistinct cytoplasmic membranes. The cells are loosely arrayed and display pseudorosette and acinar formations.

Tumors of the macrotrabecular pattern contain trabeculae that are at least 10 cells thick as part of a repetitive pattern. The tumor also contains cells of the fetal epithelial and embryonal patterns (Fig. 22.5).

Tumors of the small-cell undifferentiated or anaplastic pattern consist of cells that appear very much like neuroblastoma cells because of their typical scanty cytoplasm and hyperchromatic nuclei. These cells grow in sheets but lack cohesiveness and do not produce glycogen, fat droplets, or bile pigment. Incompletely formed bile ductules may be seen, but electron microscopic or immunohistochemical investigations are often necessary to confirm the diagnosis.

Tumors of the mixed subtype of HB consist of cells typical of both the fetal epithelial and embryonal patterns admixed with primitive mesenchyme and various mesenchymally derived tissues (Fig. 22.6). A constant aspect of this subtype of HB is the presence of osteoid-like material. The cells demonstrate a pale acellular matrix surrounding lacunar-like structures containing nuclei and cytoplasm with staining characteristics similar to those of the surrounding matrix. The cells typically resemble osteoblasts. A subset of this group contains a variety of teratoid features admixed with the epithelial, fibrous, and osteoid-like material.

Some studies suggest that the prognosis for patients with HB may be predicted on the basis of histologic

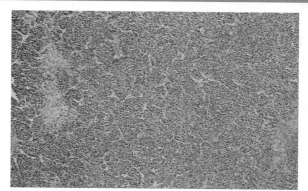

Figure 22.5: Photomicrograph of macrotrabecular hepatoblastoma demonstrating trabeculae that are at least 10 cells thick as part of a repetitive pattern

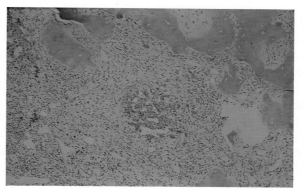

Figure 22.6: Photomicrograph of mixed hepato-blastoma demonstrating cells typical of both the fetal epithelial and embryonal patterns admixed with primitive mesenchyme and various mesenchymally derived tissues

features. In the series reported by Kasai and Watanabe,[52] a dominant fetal pattern in an infant less than 1 year of age was associated with the best prognosis (25% 2-year survival). Subsequent reports by Gonzales-Crussi et al[53] and Lack et al[54] also indicated that patients with a fetal pattern have a better outcome than patients with other histologic patterns of HB. In the latter study, 7 of the 13 pediatric patients with predominantly fetal tumors survived. The two patients with mixed HB who survived had tumors of a predominantly fetal pattern. None of the five patients with small-cell undifferentiated HB survived. Weinberg and Finegold[6] reported that six of eight patients with the fetal pattern of HB were long-term survivors. These authors also pointed out that classifying epithelial components in terms of predominant cell type may be less useful than ascertaining whether any embryonal or undifferentiated tissues are present, because the presence of such tissues indicates a poor prognosis. More recently, Haas et al[55] reported the outcome of 168 patients with HB who were enrolled in CCG and Pediatric Oncology Group (POG) studies. In cases of stage I disease (complete resection), patients a purely fetal pattern of HB fared substantially better than those with one of the other histologic patterns; however, the influence of histologic type on prognosis was not apparent beyond stage I. Similarly, in a 1992 series of 105 patients with HB reported by Conran et al,[56] the survival rate for patients with completely resected fetal HB was 93 percent, whereas that for patients with higher stages of disease was 11 percent. Although these studies suggest a more favorable outcome for patients with the fetal pattern of HB, this finding has not been universal,[57] and most studies have refrained from calling the fetal pattern a "favorable" histologic indicator.[58]

Hepatocellular carcinoma in pediatric patients is histologically similar to that in adults. It is distinguished from HB by the presence of tumor cells larger than normal hepatocytes in adjacent liver, broad cellular trabeculae, considerable nuclear prominence, and, frequently, giant cells (Fig. 22.7).[55] Fibrolamellar carcinoma (FLC) is a distinctive subtype of HCC that is characterized by broad fibrous septa and often by conspicuous hyaline or eosinophilic cytoplasm (Fig. 22.8). Several studies suggest that as many as 56 percent of patients with FLC survive[59,60] and that FLC is more resectable than typical HCC.[5,59] These superior survival rates have been disputed by Haas et al.[55] Recent findings suggest that FLC may not be a distinct entity but rather only a form of well-differentiated HCC; these studies indicate that the relatively good prognosis for patients with this type of tumor stems from its resectability in most cases, its tendency to occur in younger patients, and the absence of associated liver disease. A study of

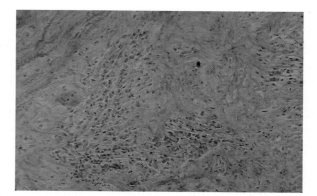

Figure 22.7: Photomicrograph of hepato-cellular carcinoma demonstrating tumor cells larger than normal hepatocytes in adjacent liver, broad cellular trabeculae, considerable nuclear prominence, and, frequently, giant cells

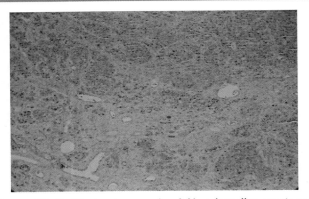

Figure 22.8: Photomicrograph of fibro-lamellar carcinoma characterized by broad fibrous septa and conspicuous hyaline or eosinophilic cytoplasm

low-grade HCC without fibrolamellar features in young patients who did not have cirrhosis showed that the prognosis was similar to that for patients with FLC.[61]

DIFFERENTIAL DIAGNOSIS

Approximately two-thirds of abdominal hepatic masses in pediatric patients are malignant. Of the primary malignancies, HB is the most common, followed by HCC. Other, less common hepatic malignancies include sarcomas (undifferentiated embryonal sarcoma, RMS, leiomyosarcoma, and angiosarcoma), lymphomas, malignant teratoma, and endocrine tumors. Most of the benign tumors are hemangiomas; other benign lesions include mesenchymal hamartoma, focal nodular hyperplasia, and adenoma.

Hepatoblastoma is often not difficult to diagnose if adequate tissue is available for review but can pose difficulties if the sample is small or shows only one type of differentiation, or if the entire tumor is of the fetal or macrotrabecular pattern.[62] Fetal HB must be differentiated from hepatic adenoma or normal infantile liver. Fortunately, adenoma is generally considered to be virtually nonexistent in children under the age of 10. Although macrotrabecular HB may be mistaken for trabecular HCC, it is important to note that, in pediatric patients, HCC essentially occurs only in conjunction with pre-established cirrhosis or a known metabolic disorder and is extremely rare in children under 3 years of age.[62]

Small nodules of well-differentiated HCC occurring in the cirrhotic liver usually pose a diagnostic problem because they can be difficult to distinguish from a regenerative, macroregenerative, or borderline (dysplastic) nodule. When well-differentiated HCC occurs in the noncirrhotic liver, other diagnoses that must be considered are adenoma and angiomyolipoma.[62]

INVESTIGATIONS

A complete blood count usually reveals a mild normochromic normocytic anemia, although polycythemia is sometimes seen in patients with HCC. Thrombocytosis in excess of 1×10^9/L may be seen in patients with either HB or HCC and is probably due to circulating thrombopoietin.[63] The activity of liver enzymes and alkaline phosphatase may be slightly elevated in patients with either disease, but elevation is more likely with HCC.

The most valuable laboratory test for both diagnosing and monitoring hepatic tumors is determination of the serum concentration of AFP. This fetal protein is a single-chain sialated glycoprotein with a molecular weight of 67.5 kD. It is initially synthesized in the yolk sac and the liver at 28 days of fetal life, but by 11 weeks' gestation it is made exclusively in the liver. Peak concentrations are reached at 14 weeks' gestation, at which time AFP is the dominant serum protein. After this point, the concentration rapidly declines until birth and continues to decline until the child reaches the age of 1 year, when it reaches adult levels. The serum concentration is 20 to 400 ng/ml at 2 months of age, 30 ng/ml at 6 months, and 3 to 15 ng/ml at 1 year. The normal serum half-life is five to seven days. AFP concentrations are elevated in 70 to 90 percent of patients with HB and in at least 50 percent of pediatric patients with HCC. Therefore, AFP is an excellent marker of hepatic malignancy, although it is not specific for hepatic tumors because an elevated AFP concentration is also associated with germ cell tumors. AFP can also serve as a useful marker for assessing the effects of treatment and for monitoring patients during follow-up. After resection, AFP concentrations may be monitored for a rising value, or the actual half-life may be calculated. Han et al[64] showed information about the recurrence of AFP-producing tumors can be obtained earlier by calculating the clearance of AFP than by waiting for an increase in the concentration of AFP. These authors found that the average half-life of AFP in patients who had undergone complete resection was 4 days, whereas that in patients who had undergone incomplete resection or had tumor recurrence was 25 days. A CCG study[65] showed that the strongest independent predictor of poor outcome in pediatric patients with unresectable or metastatic HB was the absence of decline in the AFP concentration by more than 2 logs before the second surgery.

Another potentially useful serum marker is the concentration of vitamin B_{12}–binding protein, which is often increased in patients with the fibrolamellar variant of HCC.[66] The concentration of this marker also correlates positively with disease progression.[67]

Diagnostic Imaging

Imaging is an essential part of the work-up of any intra-abdominal mass, especially a potentially malignant liver mass. The initial role of diagnostic imaging is to establish the location of the tumor, to determine whether the lesion is benign or malignant, and to suggest a diagnosis should the mass demonstrate typical features. Should the lesion appear to be malignant, diagnostic imaging may be able to suggest the extent of involvement and thereby be useful in staging the malignancy and guiding therapy. The sequence of investigation usually entails an initial ultrasound examination followed by CT scanning, magnetic resonance (MR) imaging, or both, depending on local resources and physician preference. The overall appearances are summarized in Table 22.5.

Ultrasound

The ultrasonographic appearance of HB is highly variable because of the various histologic types of the disease. Usually, hepatoblastomas are well delineated, multilobulated, and septated. The epithelial subtype is seen as a homogeneous, hypoechoic mass, whereas the mixed subtype is seen as a heterogeneous mass with hyperechoic foci resulting from calcifications and hypo- or anechoic areas resulting from liquefactive necrosis.[68]

Ultrasound shows HCC as predominately hypoechoic and sometimes isoechoic, with a thin hypoechoic halo corresponding to the tumor capsule. In diffuse HCC, there is subtle disruption of the normal echo pattern with anechoic areas resulting from necrosis.[68]

Computed Tomography

On nonenhanced CT images, the epithelial subtype of HB appears as a homogenous hypodense mass, and the mixed subtype appears as a more heterogeneous mass. Calcifications, which are present in half of cases,[69] can be detected in either subtype of HB; they are small and delicate in epithelial HB and coarse and extensive in mixed HB. After injection of a contrast agent, enhancement of a thick peripheral rim, corresponding to viable tumor or of septa, is seen in the early arterial phase (Fig. 22.9).

HCC is seen as a solitary, often well-defined mass with slightly lower attenuation than the normal liver, or

Tumor	Ultrasound	Computed tomography	Magnetic resonance imaging	Angiography
Hepato-blastoma	Well-delineated, septa, hetero-geneous, hypo-echoic (cysts, necrosis), calcifications	Epithelial subtype, homo-genous; mixed subtype, heterogenous, peripheral rim enhancement, septa, calcification	Epithelial subtype, hypointense on T1-weighted images and hypointense on T2-weighted images; mixed subtype, hyperintense on T1- and T2-weighted images	Malignant neo-vascularization, spokewheel wheel-spoke? pattern, vascular invasion
Hepato-cellular carcinoma	Hypoechoic, halo sign, diffuse: dis-organization of normal pattern	Hypodense, calcification, hemorrhage, fatty meta-morphosis, peripheral enhancement	Hypointense to hyper-intense on T1-weighted images because of nec-rosis, hemorrhage, septa, fat; hyperintense on T2-weighted images	Malignant neo-vascularization, vascular invas-ion (e.g. tumor thrombus in veins)
Undifferen-tiated em-bryonal sarcoma	Cystic-multi-septated, heterogeneous, calcification	Hypodense, septa, calci-fication, peripheral rim enhancement	Hypointense on T1-weighted images; hyperintense on T2-weighted images; hemorrhage, peripheral rim, and septa hypo-intense on both T1- and T2-weighted images	Nonspecific, mostly hypo-vascular, mass effect

Table 22.5: Radiologic findings associated with pediatric liver tumors

After Helmberger TK, et al. Pediatric liver neoplasms: a radiologic-pathologic correlation. Eur Radiol 1999;9:1339-47.[68]

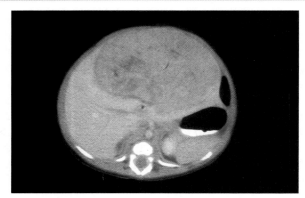

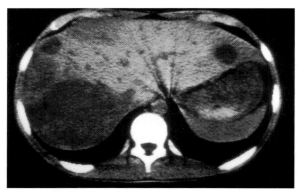

Figure 22.9: CT scan of the abdomen demonstrating hepatoblastoma in the left lobe of the liver in a one-month-old male infant. The lesion is noted to be replacing the left lateral segment and extends into the left medial segment

Figure 22.10: CT scan of the abdomen in a 15-year-old male demonstrating multifocal hepatocellular carcinoma involving the right and left lobe of the liver

as multiple, confluent masses that occupy large areas of the liver. Occasionally, CT may detect diffuse tumor infiltration as represented by a diffusely hypodense liver. Addition of a contrast agent improves the delineation of the lesion and may demonstrate a peripheral rim representing the tumor capsule (Fig. 22.10).

Magnetic Resonance Imaging

MR imaging is especially useful for the evaluation and characterization of pediatric liver lesions. It provides exquisite resolution, superb delineation of vascular structures, and multiple imaging planes, and it does not use ionizing radiation.[69] Compared with CT scanning, MR imaging and magnetic resonance angiography (MRA) offer several advantages. First, MRA clearly delineates hepatic arterial, portal venous, hepatic venous, and caval involvement by tumor.[70] Also, MR imaging can define the tumor margin and help determine the potential for resection.[71,72]

T1-weighted sequences provide excellent anatomic detail and superb contrast differentiation between fat and soft tissues. Furthermore, because these procedures use a short scanning time, they are effective in reducing artifact. T2-weighted images provide excellent contrast differentiation, especially between normal and abnormal soft tissues, and improved sensitivity for the detection of lesions, but they require longer imaging times than T1-weighted sequences and hence are subject to motion artifacts.[73]

On MR images, the epithelial subtype of HB is seen as a homogenous mass, hypointense on T1-weighted images and hyperintense on T2-weighted images. The mixed subtype presents a more heterogeneous appearance with hemorrhage seen as increased signal intensity set in a hypointense tumor on T1-weighted images (Fig. 22.11).[74]

On T1-weighted images, HCC is frequently seen as a mass with signal intensity lower than that of normal liver; however, variable signal intensity is possible.[68] On T2-weighted images, HCC is seen as a mass with mild hyperintensity relative to normal liver; increased signal intensity is seen in areas of necrosis[74,69] (Figs 22.12A and B).

Undifferentiated embryonal sarcoma has a heterogenous appearance on MRI but mostly hypointense on T1-weighted images, becoming hyperintense on T2-weighted images, corresponding with the predominately cystic nature of the lesions.[68] Typically, this entity is described as having paradoxical findings with ultrasound appearance of being solid but appearing cystic or necrotic on CT and MRI (Fig. 22.13).[75]

Selective Celiac or Hepatic Angiography

In patients with hepatoblastoma, angiography reveals the hypervascular nature of the tumor, which occasionally has a spoke-wheel pattern. Angiography allows visualization of malignant neovascularization, stretching of vessels, pooling of contrast media, and invasion or encasement of branches of the portal vein or the hepatic artery and vein.[68] In the case of HCC, angiography reveals malignant neovascularization with enlarged feeding arteries, tortuous vessels, early draining veins, pooling of contrast material, arteriovenous shunting, marked tumor blush, encasement of artery walls, and tumor thrombus in major veins.

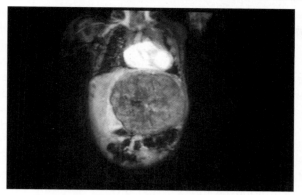

Figure 22.11: Gradient recalled echo post-contrast coronal MR of the abdomen demonstrating a large hepatoblastoma in a one-month-old infant involving the left lobe of the liver, pushing the right side over

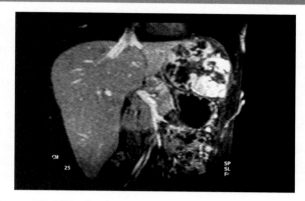

Figure 22.12B: Gradient recalled echo post- contrast coronal MR further demonstrating the extent of the lesion

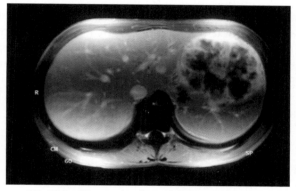

Figure 22.12A: T1 weighted axial MR of the abdomen in a 16-year-old male demonstrating a large necrotic fibrolamellar variant of hepatocellular carcinoma in the left lobe of the liver measuring 10 cm

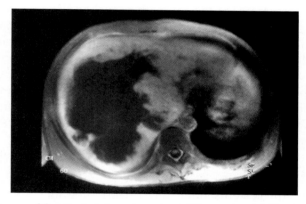

Figure 22.13: Axial post-contrast T1 weighted MR of the abdomen in a 12-year-old male demonstrating a large undifferentiated embryonal sarcoma of the right lobe of the liver. The center has the typical cyst-like or necrotic appearance while the rim appears solid and enhances

The role of angiography is now in question. Although some authors argue that angiography is useful for diagnostic purposes, such as determining resectability, caval involvement, and patency of the portal vein,[76] most investigators believe that MR imaging or MRA has superseded angiography for diagnostic purposes. Angiography may play an important role in certain therapeutic procedures, such as transarterial chemoembolization (TACE, discussed below).

Liver Biopsy

Two techniques may be used to establish the diagnosis of a malignant liver tumor: fine-needle aspiration (FNA) cytology or percutaneous core biopsy. FNA cytology is used to diagnosis of various mass lesions, but its use in pediatric patients has been limited. Perez et al[77] reviewed the use of this technique in 6 children with HB. In all

cases, the diagnosis was easily established. Furthermore, the specific histologic type could be narrowed to either undifferentiated small-cell or embryonic patterns or differentiated (fetal or macrotrabecular patterns). However, FNA is limited because the needle may miss the tumor, not enough tissue may be collected to allow a diagnosis, or both.

Core biopsies may provide more tissue with which to make a more definitive diagnosis. Hoffer[70] describes the safe and effective use of percutaneous biopsy for 22 patients at St. Jude Children's Research Hospital. The biopsies were performed under sonographic guidance; normal liver tissue was traversed before the mass was entered to minimize peritoneal spillage of tumor. Furthermore, when the biopsy path was selected, the portion of the liver that would probably be preserved in any future resections was avoided, thereby minimizing tumor seeding into other segments of the liver. An 18

G spring-loaded core biopsy needle was used; a median of three passes were performed for each patient. When the specimens had been acquired, 0.5 to 1.0 ml of an Avitene slurry, created by mixing 1 g of Avitene in 10 ml of normal saline, was injected into the sheath needle as it was withdrawn. This technique was used to minimize bleeding along the track of the biopsy needle.

The role of laparoscopic-guided biopsy of intra-abdominal masses has also been investigated. Alaish and Stylainos[78] point out that the ability to visualize very small lesions makes laparoscopy a better tool for diagnosing metastatic disease than CT or ultrasonography. Laparoscopy can also better reveal areas of decreased vascularity and areas that are believed to be representative of the mass, thus enabling the surgeon to obtain biopsy samples from these areas. Furthermore, with laparoscopy instruments the surgeon can obtain adequate specimens for all necessary pathologic investigations.[79] The long-term advantage of laparoscopy may be that it decreases the formation of adhesions [80]. This advantage is magnified if patients can avoid multiple laparotomies for initial biopsy, resection, and second-look surgery.[79]

STAGING

Several systems have been used to stage hepatic malignancies; unfortunately, no single system has yet been accepted. The best known is the adapted system proposed by the CCG and the Southwest Oncology Group (SWOG) (Table 22.6). A study using this classification system, which is based on operative findings, found good correlation between stage and outcome.[81]

The TNM (Tumor, Node, Metastasis) system was proposed for liver carcinoma by the International Union Against Cancer (UICC). von Schweinitz et al[82] reviewed several potential prognostic factors and found that extent of residual tumor, extent of liver involvement, focality of tumor, vessel involvement, and extrahepatic spread were significant prognostic variables. Because each variable forms the basis of the TNM system, this study supports the use of this staging system for future studies.

Recently, the SIOPEL I study group proposed a prechemotherapy and presurgery system called the Pre-Treatment Extension of Disease (PRETEXT) System (Fig. 22.14). This staging system, which has recently gained favor among all major study groups, is based on the anatomic segments and uses information obtained by diagnostic imaging. The liver is divided into four sectors; the left lobe of the liver consists of a lateral sector (segments II and III) and a medial sector (segment IV), and the right lobe consists of an anterior sector (segments V and VIII) and a posterior sector (segments VI and VII). On the basis of the affected sector(s), the tumor is classified into one of four groups.–Extrahepatic growth is indicated by adding one or more letters to the

Table 22.6: CCG and SWOG staging system for pediatric liver tumors	
Designation	Criteria
Stage I	Compete resection
Stage II	Microscopic residual disease, negative nodal involvement, no spilled tumor
Stage III	Grossly residual disease or nodal involvement or spilled tumor
	Primary tumor completely resected, but nodes positive, tumor spill, or both
	Primary tumor not completely resected and nodes positive, tumor spill, or both
Stage IV	Metastasis

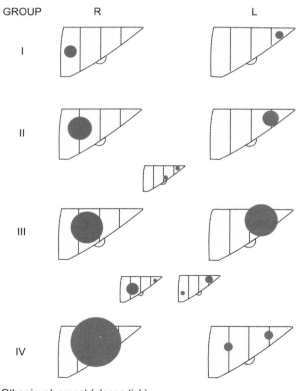

GROUP   R   L

I

II

III

IV

Other involvoment (please tick)
V hepatic vein ☐ P portal vein ☐ E extrahepatic ☐ M metastases ☐

Figure 22.14: The International Society of Pediatric Oncology pretreatment staging system

classification: V if the tumor extends into the vena cava, all three hepatic veins, or all of these structures; P if the main branch, both the left and right branches, or all of these branches of the portal vein are involved by tumor; E if there is evidence of extrahepatic intra-abdominal disease; and M if distant metastasis is present. As the name suggests, this system is used preoperatively and after chemotherapy to predict tumor response and resectability.

MANAGEMENT

The past three decades have seen remarkable advances in the treatment of pediatric patients with HB or HCC. In 1975, a survey of the Surgical Section of the American Academy of Pediatrics reviewed clinical data from 227 pediatric patients with HB and HCC.[51] Of these pediatric patients, 118 (52%) had undergone resection for cure, and 23 of these (19%) had died during the perioperative period. The overall survival rate for patients with HB was 35 percent; that for patients with HCC was 13 percent. An important finding was that there were no long-term survivors among patients who underwent incomplete resection of the malignant lesion. For those who underwent complete resection, the cure rate was 60 percent for HB and 33 percent for HCC.[51] This study pointed out two very important points for overall management. First, complete resection was mandatory if cure was to be achieved. Second, despite complete resection, a survival rate of 60 percent suggested that much could still be done to improve survival rates.

Surgical Management

With the assistance of diagnostic imaging, a plan for resection can usually be made before surgery. As much as 85 percent of the liver may be safely resected in pediatric patients, provided that the remaining liver is healthy. Both the extent of liver resection and the vascular anatomy should be known before resection. Standard anatomic resections based on the segmental distributions can be planned. If the lesion is small and limited, a segmental resection can be achieved. However, a more formal or extensive resection is usually required. Left lateral segmentectomy includes the liver substance to the left of the falciform ligament (segments II and III). Left medial segmentectomy consists of resection of liver parenchyma lateral to the falciform ligament and medial to the right lobe (segment IV). Left and right lobectomies consist of removal of the liver

tissue on either side of the anatomic plane that runs from the gallbladder bed to the suprahepatic vena cava. An extended right lobectomy (right trisegmentectomy) consists of the complete removal of the right lobe (segments V to VIII) plus the medial segment of the left lobe (segment IV). An extended left lobectomy (left trisegmentectomy) is the complete removal of the left lobe (segments II to IV) plus the anterior segment of the right lobe (segments V and VIII) [83]. Wheatley and LaQuaglia[84] point out that HB usually expands without breaching the umbilical fissure. Therefore, although tumors may be large, successful extended resection may still be possible. In contrast, HCC usually lacks such a capsule. The tumor commonly spreads diffusely through the liver, and the umbilical fissure does not constitute a barrier to spread; therefore, HCC is not commonly resectable.

Resection (Figs 22.15A to G) may be performed from either a standard transabdominal chevron incision or a thoracoabdominal incision. After initial visualization of the tumor, the vascular inflow and outflow are exposed for vascular control. Control of these structures is vital because the inability to manage hemorrhage resulting from damage to them is more life-threatening than any other aspect of the procedure.[84] The liver is mobilized by taking down the diaphragmatic ligamentous attachments, thereby exposing the suprahepatic vena cava. The porta hepatis is then dissected, and the vessels and bile ducts to the involved lobe are ligated and divided. Placing the patient into a slight Trendelenburg's position maintains a low central venous pressure during this portion of the procedure and helps to minimize blood loss. The liver capsule is then incised in an area demarcated by division of the hepatic artery and the portal vein. The use of intraoperative ultrasonography may assist complete resection and guide the operator to the exact location of vascular structures whose location may be distorted by the tumor.[85] The liver parenchyma may be dissected by finger fracture, suction knife, ultrasonic dissector, harmonic scalpel, or laser. These techniques are designed to quickly but carefully expose the bridging vessels so that they can be ligated or clipped to limit hemorrhage. After dissection through the liver substance, the hepatic veins must be ligated. In pediatric patients, these veins are quite short; therefore, to achieve adequate exposure for ligation, the vessel(s) may be dissected through the liver substance. After removal of the affected lobe, hemostasis must be achieved. The use of argon beam

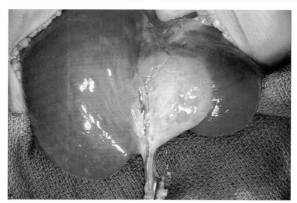

Figure 22.15A: Large left sided hepatoblastoma demonstrated after taking down the ligaments

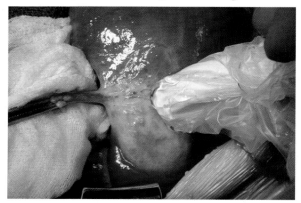

Figure 22.15B: Intraoperative ultrasound may be utilized to assess the extent of the lesion for planning the resection

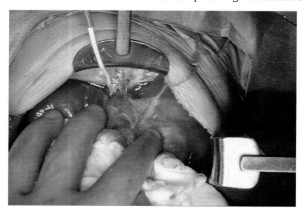

Figure 22.15C: The suprahepatic vena cava is dissected and the branches isolated

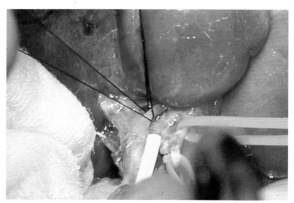

Figure 22.15D: The porta hepatis is dissected and the vessels and bile ducts isolated

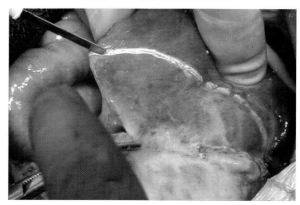

Figure 22.15E: The extent of resection is marked with electrocautery

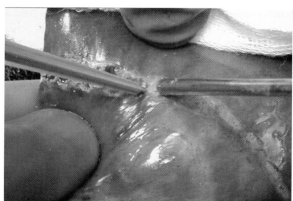

Figure 22.15F: The hepatic parenchyma is divided with ultrasonic dissector

coagulation is helpful for cauterizing the large raw surface that sometimes results after extensive resections. Finally, a drain is placed because of the risk of unrecognized biliary leaks from the transected surface.

Various techniques may assist the surgeon in reducing complications and facilitating resection. Such techniques have been shown to reduce both intraoperative blood loss and the risk of air embolism. Normothermic total vascular exclusion of the liver, although used in the adult population, has not been commonly used to treat pediatric patients.[86] Total vascular exclusion is most useful for central lesions involving the hepatic veins or IVC.

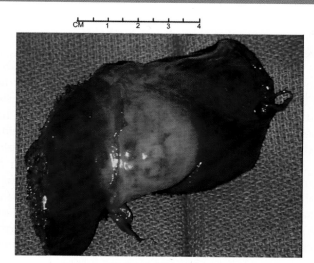

Figure 22.15G: The final resection specimen is sent to pathology

Ein et al[87] described the use of profound hypothermia and circulatory arrest (PH-CA) to achieve a bloodless operative field and minimize blood loss. However, the use of PH-CA may prolong operative times, and the coagulopathy that may develop as the result of hypothermia may in fact increase the likelihood of hemorrhage. Alternatively, standard cardiopulmonary bypass may be quicker and does not cause the coagulopathy that is associated with hypothermia.[88]

The tumor specimen should be submitted to the pathology laboratory in the intact, fresh, and unfixed state. Ideally, the pathologist should be asked to see the tumor in situ in the operating room. However, if this is not practical, the surgeon should carefully indicate the exact location and extent of the tumor. In general, it is recommended that one section should be taken for microscopic study for each centimeter of the largest tumor diameter, e.g. 12 sections for a tumor that measures $12.5 \times 6.3 \times 5.0$ cm.[89] In addition to sections taken for the examination of the resection margins, sections may be taken of the junction of the tumor with normal liver, areas that differ grossly, vessels near the edge of the tumor, and the liver at some distance from the tumor to detect the presence of preexisting liver disease.

Complications

Complications may be intraoperative or postoperative.[51] The most common intraoperative complication is hemorrhage. Other complications include air embolism, tumor embolus, hyperkalemia resulting from tumor lysis,

and primary or secondary (ischemic) bile duct injury. Postoperative complications include bile leak (caused by parenchymal transection and resolving spontaneously with drainage), subphrenic abscesses, pulmonary complications, adhesive bowel obstruction, and wound problems. Post-hepatectomy liver failure is unusual except for patients with cirrhosis. Surgical mortality rates have been reported to be 0 to 3 percent.[86]

Chemotherapy

Hepatoblastoma

In early clinical trials, childhood "hepatomas" were noted to be responsive to adriamycin (doxorubicin; ADR).[90] Later studies by Andrassy et al[91] and Weinblatt et al[92] showed that ADR was effective in combination with other agents given preoperatively to pediatric patients with HB. Cisplatin (CDDP) has emerged as an important agent in the treatment of HB; reports showed that it has therapeutic efficacy when used in combination with ADR[93] or vincristine (VCR) and 5-fluorouracil (5-FU).[94,95] Even when used as a single agent, high-dose CDDP brought about a significant tumor response in seven patients with advanced disease.[96] However, although the results of these studies were encouraging, the studies were limited to single institutions, and multi-institutional cooperative studies were needed to evaluate the role of chemotherapy.

Adjuvant Chemotherapy

In 1982, Evans et al[81] reported the results of two sequential prospective therapeutic trials sponsored by the CCG and SWOG. The first study (1972-1976) enrolled 40 patients; no adjuvant chemotherapy was given if the primary tumor was completely resected. Pediatric patients with residual disease were treated with radiation and chemotherapy using actinomycin D (AMD), VCR, and cyclophosphamide (CPM). Only seven patients who underwent gross total resection of the primary tumor were long-term survivors (18%). Seven of the 11 patients (63%) who underwent initial complete resections but no subsequent chemotherapy developed recurrent disease; this finding indicated the need for some form of effective adjuvant therapy. Because none of the patients who received chemotherapy alone survived, the cytotoxic agents were believed to be relatively ineffective, and the use of new agents was recommended. Evans et al[81] enrolled 62 pediatric patients in a follow-up study (1972-1978); these pediatric patients were treated with a combination of VCR, CPM, ADR, and 5-FU. All patients received chemotherapy, and those with residual or metastatic disease continued to receive radiotherapy. This study demonstrated a marked increase in the survival rates patients who underwent complete resection: 20 of 24 patients (83%) survived for two years with the addition of adjuvant chemotherapy. Responses to chemotherapy were seen in 12 of 37 patients (32%) with measurable disease (stages III and IV). However, the outcome for pediatric patients with incompletely resected tumors was discouraging; only 12 percent were alive after two years.

In the mid-1980s, both POG and the CCG developed treatment protocols based primarily on the use of CDDP. The CCG demonstrated that a regimen using CDDP and a continuous infusion of ADR achieved a measurable tumor response in 25 of 33 pediatric patients (75%) with initially unresectable HB. This response allowed gross tumor excision in 20 of the 25 patients, and 19 of these 29 remained free of disease treatment.[97] POG researchers used CDDP combined with VCR and 5-FU in a pilot study for patients with all stages of HB. The disease-free survival rate for patients who underwent initial tumor excision (stages I and II) followed by four courses of adjuvant chemotherapy was 90 percent. A partial response to chemotherapy was seen in 36 of 39 patients (92%) with advanced disease; 24 of 31 patients with stage III disease underwent complete excision of tumor after chemotherapy. Patients with stage IV disease did poorly; only 1 of 8 experienced long-term disease-free survival.[98]

From 1989 through 1992, the CDDP/VCR/5-FU regimen (regimen A) and the CDDP/ADR regimen (regimen B) were compared in a randomized intergroup protocol (CCG 8881/POG 8945) that enrolled 182 pediatric patients with HB.[99] After initial surgery (complete or gross total resections in stage I or II; biopsies in stage III or IV disease), patients were randomly assigned to receive either regimen. The 5-year event-free survival (EFS) estimate for patients on regimen A was 57 percent; that for patients on regimen B was 69 percent. Regimen B more commonly caused toxic effects, including cardiotoxicity and neutropenia. For regimen B, the 5-year EFS estimates were 91 percent for patients with stage I disease, 100 percent for patients with stage II disease, 64 percent for patients with stage III disease, and 25 percent for patients with stage IV disease. Outcome was similar for either regimen within disease stages. However, in view of the toxic effects of regimen B, regimen A was considered safer overall. Notably, 9

patients with stage I disease and the fetal pattern of HB were treated with four cycles of ADR alone; all survived free of tumor.

The German Cooperative Pediatric Liver Tumor Study evaluated the use of a combination of ifosfamide (IFOS), ADR, and CDDP to treat 37 pediatric patients with advanced or metastatic HB. Response to chemotherapy was seen in 35 of the 37 patients, with a disease-free survival rate of 73 percent at a median of 36 months' follow-up.[100] This study also defined a number of important prognostic criteria. The most unfavorable features appear to be incomplete initial resection, extensive primary tumor (i.e. multifocal or bilobar involvement), and vascular invasion.[82] The most recent study by the German Cooperative Pediatric Liver Tumor group used carboplatin and etoposide (VP-16) in combination with radical surgery to treat advanced and recurrent HB.[101] This treatment brought about cure in 7 of 14 patients (50%).

Neoadjuvant Chemotherapy

The routine use of preoperative chemotherapy has been the source of many debates. Those who believe that preoperative chemotherapy should not be used in all cases cite the following problems:[102] (i) diagnosis may be inaccurate if made on the basis of imaging studies alone; (ii) diagnostic imaging studies do not provide a completely accurate assessment of resectability; (iii) the likelihood of the development of drug resistance is increased; (iv) the use of chemotherapy automatically upstages tumors from a potential stage I lesion to a stage III lesion in most protocols; and (v) treatment with chemotherapy, with its inherent morbidity and mortality rates, is prolonged. Other researchers, however, cite several potential advantages of the use of preoperative chemotherapy:[103] (i) chemotherapy may make the tumor smaller and increase its demarcation from healthy liver parenchyma, thus increasing the likelihood of complete resection; (ii) the tumor may be made less vascular and more solid so that less bleeding occurs during surgery; (iii) effective therapy can begin without the delay that sometimes occurs before laparotomy can be performed; (iv) chemotherapy may limit intraoperative tumor spillage; (v) chemotherapy limits the number of laparotomies required and therefore may decrease the development of adhesions.

Over the last two decades, successive reports have described the use of various chemotherapy regimens to treat HB that has been considered unresectable; the aim of these regimens is to convert the tumors to resectable lesions (Figs 22.16A and B).[91,104-108] Results have steadily improved; in the first study, three of six patients survived;[91] more recently, fourteen of fifteen patients survived.[108] All authors have reported marked responses in most patients, with a significant reduction in the size of the tumor and a significant decrease in AFP. However, these reports have been limited in number, and chemotherapy was used because surgical therapy could not be initially offered. In contrast, the International Society for Pediatric Oncology (SIOP) recommends the use of preoperative chemotherapy as the initial treatment for all patients with a planned delayed resection. Pritchard et al[109] reports the most recent summary of findings from 154 patients with HB treated in this manner. After biopsy and assessment of pretreatment extent of disease, all patients were treated with a continuous 24-hour intravenous infusion of 80 mg/m^2 CPPD followed by 60 mg/m^2 ADR over a period of 48 hours. After four courses of treatment, patients

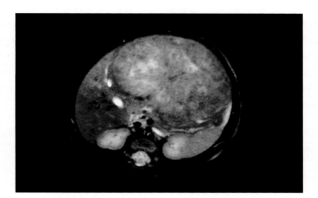

Figure 22.16A: T2 weighted axial MR of the abdomen demonstrating a large hepato-blastoma within the left lobe of the liver of a one-month-old infant

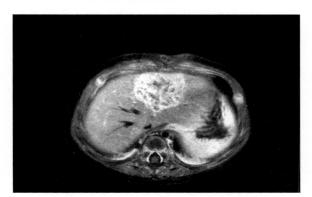

Figure 22.16B: Post-contrast T1 weighted axial MR of the abdomen now 12 weeks after chemotherapy demonstrating marked reduction in the size of the hepatoblastoma

were reassessed. When possible, the primary tumor was resected, and treatment was completed with two more courses of chemotherapy. Of the 154 patients registered, 138 received preoperative chemotherapy. A partial response, with tumor shrinkage and serial decrease in AFP, occurred in 113 patients (82%); 115 underwent delayed surgery; and 106 underwent complete resection of the primary tumor. The five-year EFS was 66 percent, and the overall survival was 75 percent. These authors noted that complete necrosis of the tumor occurred in 29 percent of cases, with no recognizable viable HB cells in the resected specimen. More than 50 percent necrosis was detected in most of the other specimens.

Hepatocellular Carcinoma

Chemotherapy plays a more limited role in the treatment of HCC than in the treatment of HB.[110] ADR, VP-16, and 5-FU have been reported to result in partial but short-lived remission in 18 to 28 percent of cases.[111,112] Also, because of the multicentric origin of HCC, preoperative chemotherapy is less likely to contribute significantly to subsequent successful resection. The most recent SIOP study of preoperative treatment of 40 patients with CPDD and ADR[113] found that partial response to chemotherapy occurred in only 43 percent of patients; 12 patients subsequently underwent complete resection. The overall 2-year survival rate was 40 percent.

Liver Transplantation

Orthotopic liver transplantation (OLTx) has gained favor for the treatment of a variety of liver diseases in pediatric patients. Originally, OLTx was used to treat patients with nonmalignant end-stage liver disease. On the basis of surgical and postoperative experience and with the introduction of new immunosuppressive regimens, overall survival rates have been excellent.[114-116] Because of the early experience with benign lesions, many surgeons questioned the use of OLTx to treat extensive but localized liver malignancies in pediatric patients. The advantage of OLTx is the ability to obtain complete resection of otherwise unresectable tumors, with the possibility of cure. The potential disadvantage is that patients with malignancies would require the administration of immunosuppressive agents, which may lead to tumor spread.

Because malignant liver lesions are not common in pediatric patients and because OLTx has only recently been used to treat these patients, the worldwide experience is somewhat limited. Only 2 percent of all liver transplants in pediatric patients are performed to treat malignancy.[115] However, several centers have reviewed their recent experiences, and these results may provide insight into the use of OLTx to treat pediatric hepatic malignancy (Table 22.7). Early results were mixed. Koneru et al[117] summarized the US experience up to 1990. Of 12 pediatric patients with HB treated with OLTx, 6 died of recurrence or graft failure. However, during this early era, chemotherapy had not yet been standardized. Since that time, the results of OLTx have steadily improved. Table 22.6 summarizes the results of OLTx for several recent reports documenting patients with stage III HB. Overall, approximately 75 percent of patients were alive with no evidence of disease at the time of publication.[118] Perhaps the most important factor in successful OLTx for HB is complete resection with no evidence of extrahepatic spread of tumor.[119,120]

OLTx has been less successful for pediatric patients with HCC; only 5 of 14 (36%) patients were alive 1 to 5 years after transplantation.[121-124] The largest single institutional study[125] reports a more favorable outcome. These authors reported the use of OLTx to treat 12 patients with HB and 19 with HCC. The survival rates after OLTx for HB were 92 percent at 1 year, 92 percent at 3 years, and 83 percent at 5 years. These authors

also showed that intravenous invasion, positive hilar lymph nodes, and contiguous spread had no significant adverse effect on outcome. The survival rates after OLTx for HCC were 79 percent at 1 year, 68 percent at 3 years, and 63 percent at 5 years. Vascular invasion, distant metastasis, lymph node involvement, tumor size, and male sex were significant risk factors for recurrence.

As OLTx becomes a more common treatment for pediatric liver malignancies, the supply of organs will be an issue, just as it is for other indications for transplantation. The size of the donor liver is an important issue, because size-matched organs are very rare. Therefore, reduced-size graft transplantation techniques will become more important. Techniques such as ex vivo reduction of larger whole organs to right lobe grafts, extended right lobe grafts, left lobe grafts, or left lateral lobe grafts with interposing vascular grafts have been recently developed.[118] Furthermore, split-liver grafting is becoming more common; in this procedure, a donor liver is divided into right and left lobes, and the two parts are transplanted into two recipients. Finally, because of the difficulty in obtaining cadaveric organs, many surgeons have turned to living-related donors to obtain split livers for transplantation. Notwithstanding the ethical issues involved, such transplant procedures have been undertaken with favorable results.

Table 22.7: Outcome of patients with stage III hepatoblastoma treated by orthotopic liver transplantation			
Reference	*Number of patients*	*Number of survivors*	*Duration*
Reyes et al, 2000[125]	1	1	More than 10 years
Al-Qabandi et al, 1999[120]	8	5	2-8 months
Laine et al, 1999[119]	5	5	0.5-8 years
Ringe et al, 1998[183]	2	1	More than 6 years
Bilik and Superina, 1997[184]	3	3	1-5 years
Ehrlich et al, 1997[107]	1	1	43 months
Achilleos et al, 1996[122]	2	2	25 and 37 months
Von Schweinitz et al, 1995[100]	1	1	More than 9 months
Stringer et al, 1995[185]	1	1	16 months
Pichlmayr et al, 1994[186]	1	1	11 years
Douglass et al, 1993[98]	3	2	More than 2 years
Tagge et al, 1992[123]	6	5	1.3 ± 0.9 years
Ninane et al, 1991[187]	1	1	7 months
Koneru et al, 1991[117]	12	6	24-73 months
Olthoff et al, 1990[121]	1	1	67 months
Total	48	36	

Adapted from Dower NA, Smith LJ. Liver transplantation for malignant liver tumors in children. Med Pediatr Oncol 2000;34:136-40.[118]

Pulmonary Metastases

Approximately 10 percent of patients have metastatic pulmonary lesions at the time of diagnosis of primary liver malignancies. Several investigators[126,127] argue for aggressive management, calling for resection for cure even if multiple thoracotomies are required. The results appear to justify this approach. Feusner et al[127] showed that pulmonary metastatectomy led to long-term survival for three of six pediatric patients with HB. Similarly, Black et al[126] reported long-term survival of four of five patients (four with HB and one with HCC) after aggressive treatment. These authors further pointed out that results are better if the primary tumor is completely excised and if the metastatic lesions develop more than six months after diagnosis; such late development implies that the tumor is less proliferative with longer doubling times.

Radiation Therapy

Radiotherapy plays a limited role in the treatment of liver malignancies in pediatric patients. Habrand et al[128] reviewed the role of radiotherapy in the treatment of fifteen pediatric patients with HB and HCC. In those difficult cases in which microscopic or gross residual tumor is left behind at the margin of resection or adjacent to important vascular structures, intraoperative radiation or brachytherapy may be considered. Furthermore, lung irradiation appears to play no role in the treatment of pulmonary metastases, nor does radiotherapy play a role in the treatment of HCC. There is a concern that, like chemotherapy, radiation therapy given immediately after resection limits liver regeneration. Indeed, doses sufficient to bring about cure would probably lead to overt toxicity to normal hepatocytes.[128]

FUTURE THERAPIES

The standard approaches of surgery, chemotherapy, and radiotherapy continue to be improved. However, novel approaches are being developed which may improve results in the future. These approaches have generally been investigated in adults, and no clear indications for their use in pediatric patients have yet been developed.

Chemoembolization

Arterial cannulization may be useful for local delivery of effective chemotherapeutic agents.[129-133] Several investigators have described small series of patients with various malignant pediatric liver tumors treated with transarterial chemoembolization (TACE) with cisplatin and doxorubicin. The studies describe remarkable shrinkage of tumors that were initially considered unresectable; on average, tumor diameter decreased by 31 percent and tumor volume by 69 percent.[130] Along with this, there was a marked drop in the serum concentration of AFP.[129-131] TACE appears to be effective for both HB and HCC but not for undifferentiated embryonal sarcoma.[129] Seki et al[132] used a combination of TACE and percutaneous microwave coagulation therapy to treat HCC. TACE reduces the vascularity of the tumor, thus increasing the effectiveness of microwave coagulation because normal blood flow removes the heat generated by the microwaves.

Portal Vein Embolization

A newly developed technique, portal venous embolization, obstructs the portal venous inflow of the segment involved with malignancy. This procedure is performed preoperatively to divert blood flow away from the segment that will eventually be resected. The anticipated result is hypertrophy of the future remnant liver. This procedure minimizes postoperative liver dysfunction and prevents postoperative liver failure, which is considered one of the most serious complications of hepatectomy. Various agents have been used as the embolic substance, including fibrin glue,[134] cyanoacrylate, gelfoam, coils,[135] and ethanol.[136]

Somatostatin Analog

Several reports have suggested that octreotide, a long-acting analog of somatostatin, may play a role in altering the growth of HCC tumors. Schindel and Grosfeld[137] studied a rat model of partial hepatectomy; hepatomas were introduced into the liver and subcutaneously. These authors found that, although the liver regeneration of animals treated with subcutaneously administered octreotide was reduced by 15 percent, a 90 percent reduction in tumor growth was also demonstrated. Kouroumalis et al[138] reported the results of the first study to demonstrate that patients with advanced HCC who were treated with octreotide had a survival advantage over untreated control patients. At this time, the exact mechanism by which octreotide functions is unclear, but it is possible that it may cause receptor augmentation or induction of apoptosis.[139]

Hormonal Therapy

The fact that HCC is consistently more common in male patients suggests that steroid hormones may play an important role in tumor formation.[140] Furthermore, the fact that the liver has been shown to be responsive to estrogen has lead many researchers to investigate the use of hormonal manipulation to treat HCC. Early reports suggested that use of the antiestrogen, tamoxifen was effective in palliation[141] and in prolonging the survival[142-144] of patients with advanced HCC. However, the exact mechanism by which tamoxifen functions is unclear; reports have shown no correlation between effectiveness and estrogen receptor status.[145] Indeed, most studies suggest function through estrogen receptor-independent mechanisms.[146-148] Recently, larger studies have challenged the effectiveness of tamoxifen in treating HCC.[149-152] Even further, there is some concern that tamoxifen may predispose patients to the development of HCC.[153] Certainly, the role of tamoxifen must to be clarified before a clear statement of its effectiveness can be made.

Interferon-alpha and Hepatitis C

The sequential development of cirrhosis and HCC in patients with transfusion-associated hepatitis was a clue leading to the identification of HCV as a risk factor for HCC in adults. It is thought that HCV may promote cancer by causing cirrhosis or possibly by interacting with cellular genes that regulate cell growth and differentiation.[154] Interferon-alpha is the only agent known to be effective against HCV infection. Recently, interferon-alpha was also shown to reduce the incidence of HCC.[155-162] However, not all patients are able to tolerate interferon-alpha,[163] and many patients with HCV infection may still develop HCC even after interferon therapy.[164]

Radiofrequency Ablation

Recently, percutaneous devices have been used to deliver focused radiofrequency waves to cause interstitial thermal ablation. Such treatment has been used as a definitive or palliative procedure for patients with extensive HCC.[165] Authors have reported its use to treat patients with HCC involving one lobe[166] or two lobes.[167] The advantage of this technique is that it provides a focused area of ablation and can be performed percutaneously, intraoperatively, or laparoscopically;[165] a single treatment is usually effective. However, when tumors are located near blood vessels, blood flow can create a heat sink by effectively removing the heat generated by the radiofrequency waves, thus limiting the volume of tumor treated.

Cryosurgery

Cryosurgical ablation of hepatic tumors relies on nonspecific tissue necrosis due to freezing and on microvascular thrombosis.[168] This technique has been used to treat patients with HCC for whom cirrhosis poses an excessive surgical risk. Cryosurgical ablation has been used as the sole procedure to eradicate the tumor,[168] to shrink the tumor to allow resection,[169] and to treat recurrent disease that cannot be re-resected.[170] It has also been used as a palliative procedure.[171]

Ethanol Injection

The percutaneous injection of absolute ethanol into HCC has been used as an alternative to surgical resection for patients with cirrhosis and prohibitive operative risks. Several large studies have reported adequate shrinkage of tumor and prolongation of survival for patients with small single lesions,[172] large single lesions,[173-174] or multiple lesions.[175] However, although this procedure causes tumor shrinkage, it is considered palliative and should not be performed with curative intent.[176]

RECOMMENDATIONS

The optimal approach to the management of HB and HCC is still being refined. The current recommendations consist of an initial attempt at complete resection should the findings of diagnostic imaging studies show no signs of extrahepatic spread. The role of preoperative chemotherapy is controversial, but we suggest that such treatment should be limited to those patients with unresectable tumors or extrahepatic spread. The currently recommended treatment is combination chemotherapy with the CDDP/VCR/5-FU regimen, which provides excellent results with relatively low toxicity. If this regimen achieves shrinkage of the tumor, a second-look laparotomy with the goal of complete resection should be performed. If the chemotherapy has no significant effect, alternative combinations may be attempted, or OLTx may be considered. Pulmonary metastasis should be treated aggressively with a realistic hope for cure if complete resection is possible.

RESULTS

When the approach described above is used to treat HB, one may hope to achieve 90 percent resectability; the most current 5-year EFS estimates are 91 percent for stage I disease, 100 percent for stage II disease, 64 percent for stage III disease, and 25 percent for stage IV disease.[99] The overall 5-year EFS estimate is approximately 60 percent.

For patients with HCC, the prognosis is generally poor. Complete resection is the only hope for cure but is possible in only about 10 to 33 percent of cases.[110,51] As a result, the overall 5-year survival is only 9 to 18 percent.[51,5,177,21]

OTHER TUMORS

Undifferentiated embryonal sarcoma (UES) has been referred to by various other terms, including malignant mesenchymoma, RMS of the liver, fibromyxosarcoma, undifferentiated sarcoma, and embryonal sarcoma.[178] It is considered the third most common malignant liver tumor, accounting for 13 percent of malignant liver tumors and 6 percent of all liver tumors in pediatric patients. UES is usually seen during late childhood (in patients 6 to 10 years of age) as a rapidly growing abdominal mass that may be associated with pain.[179] Typically, the imaging findings associated with this tumor are paradoxical: on ultrasound images the tumor appears solid, but on CT and MR images it appears cystic or necrotic (Table 22.5).[75] The best chance for cure lies in complete surgical resection. However, because the tumors are typically large, surgical resection may be difficult, and preoperative chemotherapy may be necessary. In either case, chemotherapy plays an important role because without the use of systemic therapy tumors often recur even after apparently compete resection.[178] Recent reports indicate that effective agents include VCR, IFOS, and ADR.[180]

Rhabdomyosarcoma of the biliary tract is rare: only 25 cases were reported in studies by the Intergroup Rhabdomyosarcoma Study Group (IRSG) between 1972 and 1998.[181] Diagnostic imaging is used to assess the extent of the tumor within the liver, regional spread, and distant metastases.[182] A careful search for extrahepatic disease is required because distant metastatic lesions suggest a poor outcome. The outcome has, however, improved over time with the introduction of better chemotherapeutic agents; with the exception of patients with metastatic lesions at the time of diagnosis, most pediatric patients with biliary RMS now become long-term survivors. Gross total resection of biliary RMS is rarely possible despite aggressive surgery, and outcome is good despite the presence of residual disease after surgery. Therefore, surgical exploration is recommended only for diagnosis and determination of extent of regional disease. Relief of biliary obstruction may be achieved with either endoscopic stent placement or systemic chemotherapy, but external biliary drains should be avoided because of the high risk of infectious complications.

Other malignant mesenchymal tumors of pediatric patients include angiosarcoma, liposarcoma, and leiomyosarcoma. Furthermore, malignant germ cell tumors and lymphoma can arise in the liver.

REFERENCES

1. Misick O. A case of teratoma hepatis. J Pathol Bacteriol 1898;5:128-37.
2. Willis RA. The pathology of the tumours of children. In Cameron R, Wright GP, (Eds): Pathological Monographs, London: Oliver and Boyd, 1962;57-61.
3. Ishak K, Glunz P. Hepatoblastoma and hepatocarcinoma. Cancer 1967;20:396-422.
4. Stocker JT. Hepatoblastoma. Sem Diag Pathol 1994;11(2):136-43.
5. Moore SW, Hesseling PB, Wessels G, Schneider JW. Hepatocellular carcinoma in children. Pediatr Surg Int 1997;12:266-70.
6. Weinberg AG, Finegold MJ. Primary hepatic tumors of childhood. Hum Pathol 1983;14:512-37.
7. Meyer P, LiVolse V, Cornog J. Hepatoblastoma associated with an oral contraceptive. Lancet 1974;2:1387.
8. Otten J, Smets R, Jager RD, Gerard A, Maurus R. Hepatoblastoma in an infant after contraceptive intake during pregnancy. N Engl J Med 1977;297:222.
9. Melamed I, Bujanover Y, Hammer J, Spirer Z. Hepatoblastoma in an infant born to a mother after hormonal treatment for sterility. N Engl J Med 1982;307:820.
10. Khan A, Bader J, Hoy G, Sinks L. Hepatoblastoma in child with fetal alcohol syndrome. Lancet 1979;1:1403-4.
11. Buckley J, Sather H, Ruccione K, et al. A case-control study of risk factors for hepatoblastoma. Cancer 1989;64:1169-76.
12. Ikeda H, Hachitanda Y, Tanimura M, Maruyama K, Koizumi T, Tsuchida Y. Development of unfavorable hepatoblas-toma in children of cery low birth weight. Cancer 1998;82:1789-96.
13. Mann JR, Kasthuri N, Raafat F, et al. Malignant hepatic tumours in children: incidence, clinical features and aetiology. Paediatr Perinat Epidemiol 1990;4:276-89.
14. Adamson R. Induction of hepatocellular carcinoma in nonhuman primates by chemical carcinogens. Cancer Detect Prev 1989;14:215-9.
15. Wogan GN. Impacts of chemicals on liver cancer risk. Sem Cancer Biol 2000;10:201-10.
16. Chen W, Lee J, Hung W. Primary malignant tumor of liver in infants and childhood in Taiwan. J Pediatr Surg 1988;23:457-61.
17. Chang M, Chen D, Hsu H, Hsu H, Lee C. Maternal transmission of hepatitis B virus in childhood hepatocellular carcinoma. Cancer 1989;64:23377-80.

18. Chang M.H, Chen CJ, Lai MS, et al. Universal hepatitis B vaccination in Taiwan and the incidence of hepatocellular carcinoma in children. N Engl J Med 1997;336:1855-9.

19. Karthikeyan G. Immunization for hepatocellular carcinoma. Indian Pediatr 1997;34:1141-3.

20. Gambia Hepatitis Study Group. Hepatitis B vaccine in the expanded programme of immunization: The Gambian experience. Lancet 1989;1:1057-60.

21. Chang MH. Hepatocellular carcinoma in children. Acta Paed Sin 1998;39:366-70.

22. Byrne J, Simms L, Little M, Algar E, Smith P. Three non-overlapping regions of chromosome arm 11p allele loss identified in infantile tumors of adrenal and liver. Genes Chromosomes Cancer 1993;8:104-11.

23. Koufos A, Hansen M, Lampkin B, et al. Loss of alleles at loci on human chromosome 11 during genesis of Wilms' tumour. Nature 1984; 309:170-2.

24. Koufos A, Grundy P, Morgan K, et al. Familial Wiedemann-Beckwith syndrome and a second Wilms' tumour locus both map to 11p15.5. Am J Hum Genet 1989;44:711-9.

25. Montagna M, Menin C, Chieco-Bianchi L, D'Andrea E. Occasional loss of constitutive heterozygosity at 11p15.5 and imprinting relaxation of the IFGII maternal allele in hepatoblastoma. J Cancer Res Clin Oncol 1994;120:732-6.

26. Albrecht S, Schweinitz DV, Waha A, Kraus JA, Deimling AV, Pietsch T. Loss of maternal alleles on chromosome arm 11p in hepatoblastoma. Cancer Res 1994;54:5041-4.

27. Ross JA, Radloff GA, Davies SM. H19 and IGF-2 allele-specific expression in hepatoblastoma. Br J Cancer 2000;82(4):753-6.

28. Rainier S, Dobry CJ, Feinberg AP. Loss of imprinting in hepatoblastoma. Cancer Res 1995;55: 1836-8.

29. Nagata T, Mugishima H, Shichino H, et al. Karyotypic analysis of hepatoblastoma: report of two cases and review of the literature suggesting chromosomal loci responsible for the pathogenesis of this disease. Cancer Genet Cytogenet 1999;114:42-50.

30. Hu J, Wills M, Baker BA, Perlman EJ. Comparative genomic hybridization analysis of hepatoblastomas. Genes Chromosomes Cancer 2000;27:196-201.

31. Hughes L, Michels V. Risk of hepatoblastoma in familial adenomatous polyposis. Am J Med Genet 1992;43:1023-5.

32. Nishisho I, Nakamura Y, Miyoshi Y, et al. Mutations of chromosome 5q21 gene in FAP and colorectal cancer patients. Science 1991;253:665-9.

33. Kinzler K, Nilbert M, Su L, et al. Identification of FAP locus genes from chromosome 5q21. Science 1991;253:661-5.

34. Orford K, Crockett C, Jensen J, Weissman A, Byers S. Serine phosphorylation-regulated ubiquitination and degradation of β-catenin. J Biol Chem 1997;272:24735-8.

35. Ding S-F, Michail NE, Habib NA. Genetic changes in hepatoblastoma. J Hepatol 1994;20:672-5.

36. Giardiello FM, Petersen GM, Brensinger JD, et al. Hepatoblastoma and APC gene mutation in familial adenomatous polyposis. Gut 1996;39:867-9.

37. Wei Y, Fabre M, Branchereau S, Gauthier F, Perilongo G, Buendia MA. Activation of β-catenin in epithelial and mesenchymal hepatoblastomas. Oncogene 2000;19:498-504.

38. Koch A, Denkhaus D, Albrecht S, Leuschner I, Schweinitz DV, Pietsch T. Childhood hepatoblastomas frequently xarry a mutated degradation targeting box of the β-catenin gene. Cancer Res 1999;59:269-73.

39. Giardiello F, Offerhaus G, Krush A, et al. Risk of hepatoblastoma in familial adenomatous polyposis. J Pediatr 1991;119:766-8.

40. Look A, Roberston P, Williams D, et al. Prognostic importance of blast cell DNA content in childhood acute lymphoblastic leukemia. Blood 1985;65:1079-86.

41. Tailor S, Locker J. A comparative analysis of nuclear DNA content and N-myc gene amplification in neuroblastoma. Cancer 1990;65:1360-66.

42. Shapiro D, Parham D, Douglass E, et al. Relationship of tumor-cell ploidy to histologic subtype and treatment outcome in children and adolescents with unresectable rhabdomyosarcoma. J Clin Oncol 1991;9:159-66.

43. Dressler L, Bartow M. DNA flow cytometry in solid tumors: practical aspects and clinical applications. Semin Diagn Pathol 1989;6:55-82.

44. Zerbini MCN, Sredni ST, Grier H, et al. Primary malignant epithelial tumors of the liver in children: a study of DNA content and oncogene expression. Pediatr Develop Pathol 1998;1: 270-80.

45. Rugge M, Sonego F, Pollice L, et al. Hepatoblastoma: DNA nuclear content, proliferative indices, and pathology. Liver 1998;18:128-33.

46. Nishida N, Fukuda Y, Kokurya H, et al. Accumulation of allelic loss on arms of chromosomes 13q, 16q, and 17p in the advanced stages of human hepatocellular carcinoma. Int J Cancer 1992;51:862-8.

47. Weinberg A, Mize C, Worthen H. The occurrence of hepatoma in the chronic form of hereditary tyrosinemia. J Pediatr 1976;88(3):434-8.

48. Gruner BA, DeNapoli TS, Andrews W, Tomlinson G, Bowman L, Weitman SD. Hepatocellular carcinoma in children associated with Gardner syndrome or familial adenomatous polyposis. J Pediatr Hematol Oncol 1998;20(3):274-8.

49. Esquivel CO, Gutierrez C, Cox KL, Garcia-Kennedy R, Berquist W, Concepcion W. Hepatocellular carcinoma and liver cell dysplasia in children with chronic liver disease. J Pediatr Surg 1994;29(11):1465-9.

50. Nakagawara A, Ikeda K, Tsuneyoshi M, et al. Hepatoblastoma producing both alpha-fetoprotein and human chorionic gonadotropin. Cancer 1985;56:1636-42.

51. Exelby PR, Filler RM, Grosfeld JL. Liver tumors in children in the particular reference to hepatoblastoma and hepatocellular carcinoma: American Academy of Pediatrics Surgical Section Survey—1974. J Pediatr Surg 1975;10(13):329-37.

52. Kasai M, Watanabe I. Histologic classification of liver cell carcinoma in infancy and childhood and its clinical evaluation: A study of 70 cases collected in Japan. Cancer 1970;25:551-63.

53. Gonzalez-Crussi F, Upton M, Maurer H. Hepatoblastoma: Attempt at characterization of histologic subtypes. Am J Surg Pathol 1982;6:599-612.

54. Lack E, Neave C, Vawter G. Hepatoblastoma. A clinical and pathologic study of 54 cases. Am J Surg Pathol 1982;6:693-705.

55. Haas JE, Muczynski KA, Krailo M, et al. Histopathology and prognosis in childhood hepatoblastoma and hepatocarcinoma. Cancer 1989;64:1082-95.

56. Conran R, Hitchcock C, et al. Hepatoblastoma. The prognostic significance of histologic type. Pediatr Pathol 1992;12:167-83.

57. Heifetz SA, French M, Correa M, Grosfeld JL. Hepatoblastoma: The Indiana experience with preoperative chemotherapy for inoperable tumors; clinicopathological considerations. Pediatr Pathol Laboratory Med 1997;17:857-74.

58. Dehner LP, Manivel JC. Hepatoblastoma: an analysis of the relationship between morphologic subtypes and prognosis. Am J Pediatr Hematol Oncol 1988;10(4):301-7.

59. Craig J, Peters R, Edmondson H, Omata M. Fibrolamellar carcinoma of the liver. Cancer 1980;46:372-279.

60. Farhi D, Shikes R, Silverberg S. Hepatocellular carcinoma in young people. Cancer 1983;52:1516-25.

61. Nagomey D, Adson M, Weiland L, Knight CD Jr., Smalley S, Zinsmeister A. Fibrolamellar hepatoma. Am J Surg 1985;149:113-9.

62. Ferrell L. Malignant liver tumors that mimic benign lesions: analysis of five distinct lesions. Semin Diagn Pathol 1995;12(1):64-76.

63. Naitoh-Komura E, Matsumura T, Sawada T, et al. Thrombopoietin in patients with hepatoblastoma. Proc Annu Meet Am Soc Clin Oncol 1997;16:A401.

64. Han SJ, Yoo SY, Choi SH, Hwang EH. Actual half-life of alpha-fetoprotein as a prognostic tool in pediatric malignant tumors. Pediatr Surg Int 1997:599-602.

65. Tornout JMV, Buckely JD, Quinn JJ, et al. Timing and magnitude of decline in alpha-fetoprotein levels in treated children with unresectable or metastatic hepatoblastoma are predictors of outcome: a report from the children's cancer group. J Clin Oncol 1997;15(3):1190-97.

66. Paradinas F, Melia W, Wilkinson M, et al. High serum vitamin B_{12} binding capacity as a marker of the fibrolamellar variant of hepatocellular carcinoma. Br Med J 1982;285:840-42.

67. Waxman S, Gilbert H. A tumor-related vitamin B_{12} binding protein in adolescent hepatoma. N Engl J Med 1973;289:1053-6.

68. Helmberger TK, Ros PR, Mergo PJ, Tomczak R, Reiser MF. Pediatric liver neoplasms: a radiologic-pathologic correlation. Eur Radiol 1999;9:1339-47.

69. Buetow PC, Rao P, Marshall WH. Imaging of pediatric liver tumors. MRI Clin Nor Am 1997; 5(2):397-413.

70. Hoffer FA. Liver biopsy methods for pediatric oncology patients. Pediatr Radiol 2000;30:481-8.

71. Finn JP, Hall-Craggs MA, Dicks-Mireaux C, Spitz L, Pritchard ERHJ, Vergani GM. Primary malignant liver tumors in childhood: assessment of resectability with high-field MR and comparison with CT. Pediatr Radiol 1990;21:34-8.

72. Boechat MI, Karngarloo H, Ortega J, et al. Primary liver tumors in children: comparison of CT and MR imaging. Radiol 1988;169:727-32.

73. Siegel MJ, Luker GD. MR Imaging of the liver in children. MRI Clin Nor Am 1996;4(4):637-56.

74. Powers C, Ros PR, Stoupis C, Johnson WK, Segel KH. Primary liver neoplasms: MR imaging with pathologic correlation. Radiographics 1994;14:459-82.

75. Buetow P, Buck J, Pantongrag-Brown L, et al. Undifferentiated (Embryonal) sarcoma of the liver: pathologic basis of imaging findings in 28 Cases. Radiol 1997;203:779-83.

76. Tonkin ILD, Jr. ELW, Hollabaugh RS. The continued value of angiography in planning surgical resection of benign and malignant hepatic tumors in children. Pediatr Radiol 1988;18:35-44.

77. Perez JS, Perez-Guillermo M, Bernal AB, Mercader JM. Hepatoblastoma: an attempt to apply histologic classification to aspirates obtained by fine needle aspiration cytology. Acta Cytol 1994;38:175-82.

78. Alaish SM, Stylianos S. Diagnostic laparoscopy. Curr Opin Pediatr 1998;10:323-7.

79. Saenz NC, Conlon KCP, Aronson DC, LaQuaglia MP. The application of minimal access procedures in infants, children, and young adults with pediatric malignancies. J Laparoendosc Advanced Surgical Techniques 1997;7(5):289-94.

80. Moore R, Kavoussi L, Bloom D, et al. Postoperative adhesion formation after urological laparoscopy in the pediatric population. J Urol 1995;16:792-5.

81. Evans A, Land V, Newton W, et al. Combination chemotherapy (vincristine, adriamycin, cyclophosphamide, and 5-fluorouracil) in the treatment of children with malignant hepatoma. Cancer 1982;50:821-6.

82. Schweinitz DV, Wischmeyer P, Leuschner I, et al. Clinico-pathological criteria with prognostic relevance in hepatoblastoma. Eur J Cancer 1994;30A(8):1052-8.

83. Glick RD, Nadler EP, Blumgart LH, Quaglia MPL. Extended left hepatectomy (Left Hepatic Trisegmentectomy) in Childhood. J Pediatr Surg 2000;35(2):303-8.

84. Wheatley JM, LaQuaglia MP. Management of hepatic epithelial malignancy in childhood and adolescence. Semin Surg Oncol 1993;9:532-40.

85. Thomas BL, Krummel TM, Parker GA, et al. Use of intraoperative ultrasound during hepatic resection in pediatric patients. J Pediatr Surg 1989;24(7):690-3.

86. Geiger JD. Surgery for hepatoblastoma in children. Curr Opion Pediatr 1996;8:276-82.

87. Ein S, Shandling B, Williams W, et al. Major hepatic tumor resection using profound hypothermia and circulatory arrest. J Pediatr Surg 1981;16:339-42.

88. Murakami T, Myojin K, Matano J, Kamikubo Y, Hatta E, Matsuzaki K. Resection of hepatoblastoma with right atrial extension using cardiopulmonary bypass. J Cardiovasc Surg 1995;36:455-7.

89. Stocker JT. An approach to handling pediatric liver tumors. Am J Clin Pathol 1998;109(Suppl 1):S67-S72.

90. Tan C, Rosen G, Ghavimi F, et al. Adriamycin (NSC-123127) in pediatric malignancies. Cancer Chemother Rep 1975;6:259-66.

91. Andrassy RJ, Brennan LP, Siegel MM, et al. Preoperative chemotherapy for hepatoblastoma in children: report of six cases. J Pediatr Surg 1980;15(4):517-22.

92. Weinblatt M, Siegel S, Siegel M, et al. Preoperative chemotherapy for unresectable primary hepatic malignancies in children. Cancer 1982;50:11061-4.

93. Quinn J, Altman A, Robinson H, et al. Adriamycin and cisplatin for hepatoblastoma. Cancer 1985;56:1926-9.

94. Douglass E, Green A, Wrenn E, et al. Effective cisplatin (DDP) based chemotherapy in the treatment of hepatoblastoma. Med Pediatr Oncol 1985;13:187-90.

95. Douglass E, Green A, Priest J, et al. Effective therapy for metastatic/unresectable hepatoblastoma (HB). Proc Am Soc Clin Oncol 1987;6:214.

96. Black CT, Cangir A, Choroszy M, Andrassy RJ. Marked response to preoperative high-dose cisplatinum in children with unresectable hepatoblastoma. J Pediatr Surg 1991;26(9):1070-3.

97. Ortega JA, Krailo MD, Haas JE, et al. Effective treatment of unresectable or metastatic hepatoblastoma with cisplatin and continuous infusion doxorubicin chemotherapy: a report from the childrens cancer study group. J Clin Oncol 1991;9(12):2167-76.

98. Douglass EC, Reynolds M, Finegold M, Cantor AB, Glicksman A. Cisplatin, vincristine, and fluorouracil therapy for hepatoblastoma: a pediatric oncology group study. J Clin Oncol 1993;11:96-9.

99. Ortega JA, Douglass EC, Feusner JH, et al. Randomized comparison of cisplatin/vincristine/fluorouracil and cisplatin/continuous infusion doxorubicin for treatment of pediatric hepatoblastoma: a report from the children's cancer group and the pediatric oncology group. J Clin Oncol 2000;18(4):2665-75.

100. Schweinitz DV, Hecker H, Harms D, et al. Complete resection before development of drug resistance is essential for survival from advanced hepatoblastoma - a report from the German

cooperative pediatric liver tumor study HB-89. J Pediatr Surg 1995;30:845-52.

101. Fuchs J, Bode U, Schweinitz DV, et al. Analysis of treatment efficiency of carboplatin and etoposide in combination with radical surgery in advanced and recurrent childhood hepatoblastoma: a report of the German cooperative pediatric liver tumor study HB 89 and HB 94. Klin Pediatr 1999;211:305-9.

102. Schweinitz DV, Burger D, Mildenberger H. Is Laparotomy the first step in treatment of childhood liver tumors? - The experience from the German cooperative pediatric liver tumor study HB-89. Eur J Pediatr Surg 1993;4:82-6.

103. Perilongo G, Shafford EA. Paediatric update: liver tumours. Eur J Cancer 1999;35(6):953-9.

104. Pierro A, Langevin AM, Filler RM, Liu P, Phillips MJ, Greenberg ML. Preoperative chemotherapy in "unresectable" hepatoblastoma. J Pediatr Surg 1989;24(1): 24-9.

105. King DR, Ortega J, Campbell J, et al. The surgical management of children with incompletely resected hepatic cancer is facilitated by intensive chemotherapy. J Pediatr Surg 1991;26(9):1074-81.

106. Reynolds M, Douglass EC, Finegold M, Cantor A, Glicksman A. Chemotherapy can convert unresectable hepatoblastoma. J Pediatr Surg 1992;27(8):1080-4.

107. Ehrlich PF, Greenberg ML, Filler RM. Improved long-term survival with preoperative chemotherapy for hepatoblastoma. J Pediatr Surg 1997;32(7):999-1003.

108. Seo T, Ando H, Watanabe Y, et al. Treatment of hepatoblastoma: Less extensive hepatectomy after effective preoperative chemotherapy with cisplatin and Adriamycin. Surgery 1998;123:407-14.

109. Pritchard J, Brown J, Shafford E, et al. Cisplatin, doxorubicin, and delayed surgery for childhood hepatoblastoma: a successful approach—results of the first prospective study of the international society of pediatric oncology. J Clin Oncol 2000;18(22):3819-28.

110. Chen JC, Chen CC, Chen WJ, Lai HS, Hung WT, Lee PH. Hepatocellular carcinoma in children: clinical review and comparison with adult cases. J Pediatr Surg 1998;33(9): 1350-4.

111. Chlebowski R, Brzechwa-Adjukiewcz A, Cowden A, Block J, Tong M, Chan K, Doxorubicin (75 mg/m2) for hepatocellular carcinoma: clinical and pharmacokinetic results. Cancer Treat Rep 1984;68:487-91.

112. Melia W, Johnson P, Williams R. Induction of remission in hepatocellular carcinoma: a comparison of VP 16 with Adriamycin. Cancer 1983;51:206-10.

113. Plashkes J, Perilongo G, Shafford E, et al. Response of hepatocellular carcinoma (HCC) to preoperative chemotherapy—cisplatin (CPDD) doxorubicin (DOXO) plado in the international society of paediatric oncology (SIOP) liver tumour study. Proc Annu Meet Am Soc Clin Oncol 1995;14: A1457.

114. Colombani PM, Lau H, Prabhakaran K, et al. Cumulative experience with pediatric living related liver transplantation. J Pediatr Surg 2000;35(1):9-12.

115. Reyes J, Marariegos G. Pediatric transplantation. Surg Clin North Am 1999;79:163-89.

116. Andrews W, Sommerauer J, Roden J, et al. 10-years of pediatric liver transplantation. J Pediatr Surg 1996;31:619-24.

117. Koneru B, Flye MW, Busuttil RW, et al. Liver transplantation for hepatoblastoma: the American experience. Ann Surg 1990;213(2):118-21.

118. Dower NA, Smith LJ. Liver transplantation for malignant tumors in children. Med Pediatr Oncol 2000;34:136-40.

119. Laine J, Jalanko H, Saarinen-Pihkala UM, et al. Successful liver transplantation after induction chemotherapy in children with inoperable, multifocal primary hepatic malignancy. Transplantation 1999;67(10):1369-72.

120. Al-Qabandi W, Jenkinson HC, Buckels JA, et al. Orthotopic liver transplantation for unresectable hepatoblastoma: A Single Center's Experience. J Pediatr Surg 1999; 34(8):1261-64.

121. Olthoff KM, Millis JM, Rosove JH, et al. Is liver transplantation justified for the treatment of hepatic malignancies. Arch Surg 1990;125:1261-8.

122. Achilleos O, Bruist L, Kelly D, et al. Unresectable hepatic tumors in childhood and the role of liver transplantation. J Pediatr Surg 1996;1996:1563-7.

123. Tagge E, Tagge D, Reyes J, et al. Resection, including transplantation for hepatoblastoma and hepatocellular carcinoma: impact on survival. J Pediatr Surg 1992;21:292-7.

124. Otte JB, Aronson D, Vraux H, et al. Preoperative chemotherapy, major liver resection, and transplantation for primary malignancies in children. Transplant Proceed 1996;28(4):2393-4.

125. Reyes JD, Carr B, Dvorchik I, et al. Liver transplantation and chemotherapy for hepatoblastoma and hepatocellular cancer in childhood and adolescence. J Pediatr 2000;136:795-804.

126. Black CT, Luck SR, Musemeche CA, Andrassy RJ. Aggressive excision of pulmonary metastases Is Warranted in the management of childhood hepatic tumors. J Pediatr Surg 1991;26(9):1082-6.

127. Feusner JH, Krailo MD, Haas JE, Campbell JR, Lloyd DA, Ablin AR. Treatment of pulmonary metastases of initial stage I hepatoblastoma in childhood: report from the childrens cancer group. Cancer 1993;71:859-64.

128. Habrand JL, Nehme D, Kalifa C, et al. Is there a place for radiation therapy in the management of hepatoblastomas and hepatocellular carcinomas in children? Int J Radiat Oncol 1992;23(3): 525-31.

129. Malogolowkin MH, Stanley P, Steele DA, Ortega JA. Feasibility and toxicity of chemoembolization for children with liver tumors. J Clin Oncol 2000;18(6):1279-84.

130. Han YM, Park HH, Lee JM, et al. Effectiveness of preoperative transarterial chemoembolization in presumed inoperable hepatoblastoma. J Vascul Intervent Radiol 1999;10:1275-80.

131. Oue T, Fukuzawa M, Kusafuka T, Kohmoto Y, Okada A, Imura K. Transcatheter arterial chemoembolization in the treatment of hepatoblastoma. J Pediatr Surg 1998;22(12):1771-5.

132. Seki T, Tamai T, Nakagawa T, et al. Combination therapy with transcatheter arterial chemoembolization and percutaneous microwave coagulation therapy for hepatocellular carcinoma. Cancer 2000;89:1245-51.

133. Ogita S, Tokiwa K, Taniguchi H, Takahashi T. Intrarterial chemotherapy with lipid contrast medium for hepatic Malignancies in infants. Cancer 1987;60:2886-90.

134. Nagino M, Nimura Y, Kamiya J, Kondo S, Kanai M. Selective percutaneous transhepatic embolization of the portal vein in preparation for extensive liver resection: the ipsilateral approach. Radiology 1996;200:559-63.

135. Baere Td, Roche A, Elias D, Lasser P, Lagrange C, Bousson V. Preoperative portal vein embolization for extension of hepatectomy indications. Hepatology 1996;24(6):1386-91.

136. Ogasawara K, Uchino J, Une Y, Fujioka Y. Selective portal vein embolization with absolute ethanol induces hepatic hypertrophy and makes more extensive hepatectomy possible. Hepatology 1996; 23(2):338-45.

137. Schindel DT, Grosfeld JL. Hepatic resection enhances growth of residual intrahepatic and subcutaneous hepatoma, which is inhibited by octreotide. J Pediatr Surg 1997;32(7):995-8.

138. Kouroumalis F, Skordilis P, Thermos K, Vasilaki A, Mochandrea J, Manousos O. Treatment of hepatocellular carcinoma with octreotide: a randomised controlled study. Gut 1998;42:442-7.

139. Raderer M, Hejna M, Muller C, et al. Treatment of hepatocellular cancer with the long acting somatostatin analog lanreotide in vitro and in vivo. Int J Oncol 2000;16(6):1197-1201.

140. Lui W, P'eng F, Liu T, Chi C. Hormonal therapy for hepatocellular carcinoma. Med Hypotheses 1991; 36(2):162-5.

141. Farinati F, Salvagnini M, Maria ND, et al. Unresectable hepatocellular carcinoma: a prospective controlled trial with tamoxifen. J Hepatol 1990;11(3):297-301.

142. Elba S, Giannuzzi V, Misciagna G, Manghisi O. Randomized controlled trial of tamoxifen versus placebo in inoperable hepatocellular carcinoma. Ital J Gastroenterol 1994; 26(2):66-8.

143. Cerezo FM, Tomas A, Donoso L, et al. Controlled trial of tamoxifen in patients with advanced hepatocellular carcinoma. J Hepatol 1994;20(6):702-6.

144. Manesis E, Giannoulis G, Zoumboulis P, Vafiadou I, Hadziyannis S. Treatment of hepatocellular carcinoma with combined suppression and inhibition of sex hormones: a randomized, controlled trial. Hepatol 1995;21(6):1535-42.

145. Jonas S, Bechstein WO, Heinze T, et al. Female sex hormone receptor status in advanced hepatocellular carcinoma and outcome after surgical resection. Surgery 1997;121(4):456-61.

146. Boix L, Bruix J, Castells A, et al. Sex hormone receptors in hepatocellular carcinoma. Is there a rationale for hormonal treatment? J Hepatol 1993;17(2):187-91.

147. Jiang S, Shyu R, Yeh M, Jordan V. Tamoxifen inhibits hepatoma cell growth through an estrogen receptor independent mechanism. J Hepatol 1995;23(6):712-9.

148. Tan C, Chow P, Findlay M, Wong C, Machin D. Use of tamoxifen in hepatocellular carcinoma: a review and paradigm shift. J Gastroenterol Hepatol 2000;15(7):725-9.

149. Castells A, Bruix J, Bru C, et al. Treatment of hepatocellular carcinoma with tamoxifen: a double-blind placebo-controlled trial in 120 patients. Gastroenterol 1995;109(3):917-22.

150. Liu C, Fan S, Ng I, Lo C, Poon R, Wong J. Treatment of advanced hepatocellular carcinoma with tamoxifen and the correlation with expression of hormone receptors: a prospective randomized study. Am J Gastroenterol 2000; 95(1):218-22.

151. Schachschal G, Lochs H, Plauth M. Controlled clinical trial of doxorubicin and tamoxifen versus tamoxifen monotherapy in hepatocellular carcinoma. Eur J Gastroenterol Hepatol 2000;12(3): 281-4.

152. Group C. Tamoxifen in treatment of hepatocellular carcinoma: a randomised controlled trial. Lancet 1998;352:17-20.

153. Moffat D, Oien K, Dickson J, Habeshaw T, McLellan D. Hepatocellular carcinoma after long-term tamoxifen therapy. Ann Oncol 2000;11:1195-6.

154. Colombo M. Hepatitis C virus and hepatocellular carcinoma. Baillieres Best Pract Res Clin Gastroenterol 1999;13(4):519-28.

155. Nishiguchi S, Kuroki T, Nakatani S, et al. Randomised trial of effects of interferon-alpha on incidence of hepatocellular carcinoma in chronic active hepatitis C with cirrhosis. Lancet 1995; 346(8982):1051-5.

156. Mazzella G, Accogli E, Sottili S, et al. Alpha interferon treatment may prevent hepatocellular carcinoma in HCV-related liver cirrhosis. J Hepatol 1996;24(2):141-7.

157. Imai Y, Kawata S, Tamura S, et al. Relation of interferon therapy and hepatocellular carcinoma in patients with chronic hepatitis C. Osaka Hepatocellular Carcinoma Prevention Study Group. Ann Intern Med 1998;15:94-9.

158. Yoshida H, Shiratori Y, Moriyama M, et al. Interferon therapy reduces the risk for hepatocellular carcinoma: National surveillance program of cirrhotic and noncirrhotic patients with chronic hepatitis C in Japan. Ann Intern Med 1999;131:174-81.

159. Toyoda H, Kumada T, Nakano S, et al. The effect of retreatment with Interferon-α on the incidence of hepatocellular carcinoma in patients with chronic hepatitis C. Cancer 2000;88:58-65.

160. Yabuuchi I, Imai Y, Kawata S, et al. Long-term responders without eradication of hepatitis C virus after interferon therapy: characterization of clinical profiles and incidence of hepatocellular carcinoma. Liver 2000;20(4):290-95.

161. Tanaka H, Tsukuma H, Kasahara A, et al. Effect of interferon therapy on the incidence of hepatocellular carcinoma and mortality of patients with chronic hepatitis C: a retrospective cohort study of 738 patients. Int J Cancer 2000;87(5):741-9.

162. Inoue A, Tsukuma H, Oshima A, et al. Effectiveness of interferon therapy for reducing the incidence of hepatocellular carcinoma among patients with type C chronic hepatitis. J Epidemiol 2000;10(4):234-240.

163. Llovet J, Sala M, Castells L, et al. Randomized controlled trial of interferon treatment for advanced hepatocellular carcinoma. Hepatol 2000;31:54-8.

164. Kubo S, Nishiguchi S, Tamori A, et al. Resected cases of hepatocellular carcinoma detected after interferon therapy for chronic hepatitis C. Hepatogastroenterology 2000;47(34):1100-02.

165. Curley S, Izzo F, Ellis L, Vauthey JN, Vallone P. Radiofrequency ablation of hepatocellular cancer in 110 patients with cirrhosis. Ann Surg 2000;232(3):381-91.

166. Rossi S, Stasi MD, Buscarini E, et al. Percutaneous radiofrequency interstitial thermal ablation in the treatment of small hepatocellular carcinoma. Cancer J Sci Am 1995;1(1):73.

167. Jiao L, Hansen P, Havlik R, Mitry R, Pignatelli M, Habib N. Clinical short-term results of radiofrequency ablation in primary and secondary liver tumors. Am J Surg 1999;17(4):303-6.

168. Crews K, Kuhn J, McCarty T, Fisher T, Goldstein R, Preskitt J. Cryosurgical ablation of hepatic tumors. Am J Surg 1997;174(6):614-7.

169. Adam R, Akpinar E, Johann M, Kunstlinger F, Majno P, Bismuth H. Place of cryosurgery in the treatment of malignant liver tumors. Ann Surg 1997;225(1):39-48.

170. Lam C, Yuen W, Fan S. Hepatic cryosurgery for recurrent hepatocellular carcinoma after hepatectomy: a preliminary report. J Surg Oncol 1998;68(2):104-6.

171. Wren S, Coburn M, Tan M, et al. Is cryosurgical ablation appropriate for treating hepatocellular cancer? Arch Surg 1997;132(6):599-603.

172. Bartolozzi C, Lencioni R. Ethanol injection for the treatment of hepatic tumours. Eur Radiol 1996; 6(5):682-96.

173. Livraghi T, Benedini V, Lazzaroni S, Meloni F, Torzilli G, Vettori C. Long-term results of single session percutaneous ethanol injection in patients with large hepatocellular carcinoma. Cancer 1998;83(1):48-57.

174. Lin S, Lin D, Lin C. Percutaneous ethanol injection therapy in 47 cirrhotic patients with hepatocellular carcinoma 5 cm or less: a long-term result. Int J Clin Pract 1999; 53(4):257-62.

175. Giorgio A, Tarantino L, Stefano GD, et al. Ultrasound-guided percutaneous ethanol injection under general anesthesia for the treatment of hepatocellular carcinoma on cirrhosis: long-term results in 268 patients. Eur J Ultrasound 2000;12(2):145-54.

176. Orlando A, D'Antoni A, Camma C, et al. Treatment of small hepatocellular carcinoma with percutaneous ethanol injection: a validated prognostic model. Am J Gastroenterol 2000;95(10):2921-7.

177. Lack E, Neave C, Vawter G. Hepatocellular carcinoma: review of 32 cases in childhood and adolescence. Cancer 1983;52:1510-15.

178. Webber EM, Morrison KB, Pritchard SL, Sorensen PHB. Undifferentiated embryonal sarcoma of the liver: results of clinical management in one center. J Pediatr Surg 1999;34(11):1641-4.

179. Stocker J, Ishak K. Undifferentiated (embryonal) sarcoma of the liver: report of 31 cases. Cancer 1978;42:336-48.

180. Douglass EC. Hepatic malignancies in childhood and adolescence (hepatoblastoma, hepatocellular carcinoma, and embryonal sarcoma). In Walterhouse DO, Cohn SI (Eds): Diagnostic and therapeutic advances in pediatric oncology. Boston: Kluwer Academic Publishers, 1997;201-12.

181. Spunt SL, Lobe TE, Pappo AS, et al. Aggressive surgery is unwarranted for biliary tract rhabdomyosarcoma. J Pediatr Surg 2000;35(2):309-16.

182. Roebuck DJ, Yang WT, Lam WWM, Stanley P. Hepatobiliary rhabdomyosarcoma in children: diagnostic radiology. Pediatr Radiol 1998;28:101-8.

183. Ringe B, Wittekind C, Bechstein W, et al. The role of liver transplantation in hepatobiliary malignancy. A retrospective analysis of 95 patients with particular regard to tumor stage and recurrence. Ann Surg 1988;209:88-9.

184. Bilik R, Superina R. Transplantation for unresectable liver tumors in children. Transplant Proceed 1997;29:2834-5.

185. Stringer MD, Hennayake S, Howard ER, et al. Improved outcome for children with hepatoblastoma. Br J Surg 1995;82:386-91.

186. Pichlmayr R, Weimann A, Ringe B. Indications for liver transplantation in hepatobiliary malignancy. Hepatology 1994;20:33S-40S.

187. Ninane J, Perilongo G, Stalens J-P, et al. Effectiveness and toxicity of cisplatin and doxorubicin (PLADO) in childhood hepatoblastoma and hepatocellular carcinoma: a SIOP pilot study. Med Pediatr Oncol 1991;19:199-203.

CHAPTER 23

Piotr Czauderna

Hepatocellular Carcinoma

INCIDENCE, EPIDEMIOLOGY AND ETIOLOGY

Hepatocellular carcinoma (HCC) is the fifth cancer worldwide but the second one regarding mortality statistics. In many western countries frequency of HCC has increased in recent years. However, still 80 percent of HCC occur in developing countries. HCC is more common in males than in females with 3:1 preponderance. Major reasons for HCC development worldwide are liver cirrhosis (due to various reasons including alcohol intake), viral hepatitis B and C, as well as oral intake of aflatoxines included in contaminated food. Due to above mentioned factors HCC is most common in Sub-Saharan Africa and South-east Asia, where its frequency may reach 90 to 100/100,000 of population. Incidence of HCC increases with age peaking at 45 years of age and then rising even further.

Only about 0.5 to 1 percent of HCC cases occur before 20 years of age, however in children it is the second liver neoplasm after hepatoblastoma. It is very unique below the age of five. Association of HCC with hepatic B antigen is common and varies greatly (from 10-70%) in different social classes, urban/rural areas, as well as geographical regions. In young children with HCC vertical perinatal transmission of the hepatitis B virus from the mother has been postulated. Due to aggressive introduction of HBV vaccination program in several endemic areas, like Taiwan or Saudi Arabia, frequency of HCC among children has decreased recently.[1] Pediatric HCC cases can also develop in association with congenital hepatic disorders such as biliary atresia, familial cholestatic cirrhosis, Alagille syndrome, glycogene storage diseases, hemo-chromatosis, alpha1-antitrypsin deficiency and in about half of all tyrosinemia cases.[2] It is well known that ongoing cycle of hepatocytes necrosis and regeneration in liver cirrhosis leads to carcinogenesis and HCC development. This effect may be potentiated by incorporation of elements of viral HBV/HCV genetic material into the cell's genome.[3] However, all above-mentioned reasons are true mainly in endemic HCC areas. On the contrary in Europe only about 30 percent of HCCs are linked to pre-existing liver disease and/or cirrhosis; others being *de novo* cases.[4] This experience is different from adult data, in which HCC constitutes the most common liver cancer and 85 percent of cases arise on the background of the liver cirrhosis.[2]

CLINICAL PRESENTATION

Main HCC symptoms are palpable hepatic mass, abdominal pain and in advanced cases cachexia and jaundice. Symptoms and signs of liver insufficiency can be present. Tumor can be unifocal or multifocal. Peritoneal implants and lymph nodes involvement at *porta hepatis* are common. Main metastatic sites are lungs.

HCC is frequently associated with elevated alpha-fetoprotein levels (AFP) which occurs in about 50 to 70 percent of cases.[4,5]

DIAGNOSTIC EVALUATION

Radiology

Imaging methods used in HCC are similar to those for hepatoblastoma. The typical sonographic HCC appearance is that of large or multifocal, heterogenous and predominantly hyperechoic mass but occasionally tumors may be hypoechoic or isoechoic.[6] Difficulties arise when HCC is formed in cirrhotic liver containing several regenerative nodules. In such cases contrast media (especially the second generation ones) can be of great help as they increase a difference between the tumor and surrounding liver. They also help to assess dynamic changes in arterial/portal and equilibrium phase.

In CT scan HCC appears as a low attenuation mass with calcifications in about 25 percent of cases (Fig. 23.1).[6] Triphasic CT scan is presently considered a golden standard to detect HCC foci in the cirrhotic liver. In fibrolamellar HCC a central scar seen in CT images have been reported in 70 percent of cases.[6]

In MRI hepatocellular carcinoma is hypointense in T1-weighted images, although high signal areas may be present due to steatosis or hemorrhage. On T2-weighted images it is usually slightly hyperintense in comparison with normal liver while regenerating nodules in cirrhotic liver usually remain hypointense. Early arterial enhancement with rapid washout my be present both in CT and MRI investigations.[6] Central scar associated with fibrolamellar HCC is hypointense in both T1- and T2-weighted images which helps to distinguish it from central scar observed in focal nodular hyperplasia.[6] There are also liver-specific MRI contrasts, like Ferumoxides or Mangafodipir, which may increase rate of HCC detection within cirrhotic liver even further.

Staging

There is no uniformly accepted staging system for HCC, especially that in cases of patients with liver cirrhosis

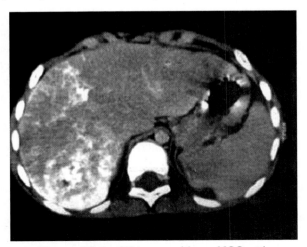

Figure 23.1: CT image of large HCC with visible calcifications (own material)

not only tumor itself but also patient's factors, i.e. Child-Pugh class (degree of liver compensation, hyperbilirubinemia, presence of ascites, hypoalbuminemia, etc.) have to be taken into account. Classical TNM system, although the oldest, does not seem to be particularly well suited to HCC. Most adult groups use Okuda system, Barcelona score (BCLC) or CLIPP scale.[7] In children with non-cirrhotic HCC traditional hepatoblastoma-type staging systems are used (i.e. PRETEXT) (Table 23.1).

Pathology

HCC is a malignant tumor derived from hepatocytes. It is histologically classified into: trabecular (plate-like) pattern, pseudoglandular and acinar pattern, compact pattern and scirrhous pattern. It has the following cytological variants: pleomorphic cell, clear cell, sarcomatous change and others. Pathologically HCC is formed by large, pleomorphic polynucleated cells. The morphology of childhood HCC is similar to that observed in adult patients.

Adult-type HCC occurring in cirrhotic livers may be associated with a distinctive spectrum of hepatocyte dysplasia and/or precursor lesions: liver cell dysplasia (LCD) = large cell (large cell dysplasia), liver cell dysplasia (LCD) = small cell (small cell dysplasia), dysplastic focus, dysplastic nodule.

A distinct variant is fibrolamellar HCC chiefly occurring in adolescents and young adults and accounting for 30 percent of the HCC presenting before 20 years of age. This tumor is histologically characterised by nests and cords of large and eosinophilic cells separated by hypocellular parallel bands of collagen-rich tissue (fibrolamellar structures).

Recently a a novel group of so called transitional liver cell tumors (TCLT) developing in older children and adolescents has been reported. These lesions are characterized by usually large hepatic masses, a very high serum AFP, an aggressive clinical course, histology intermediate between HCC and hepatoblastoma, and a distinctive beta-catenin expression pattern.[8]

Molecular Biology

The hypothesis on difference between adult and pediatric HCC could be supported by some molecular findings, too. For example, mutation of c-met gene was found only in children with HCC.[9] Also levels of cyclin D1 (regulatory protein of G1 phase cycle) expression are significantly lower in childhood HCC, while

Table 23.1: 2005 PRETEXT system: additional criteria

C

Caudate lobe involvement

C1   Tumor involving the caudate lobe

C0   All other patients

All **C1** *patients are at least PRETEXT II*

E

Extrahepatic abdominal disease

E0   No evidence of tumor spread in the abdomen (except M or N)

E1   Direct extension of tumor into adjacent organs or diaphragm

E2   Peritoneal nodules

Add suffix "a" if ascites is present, e.g. **E0a**

F

Tumor focality

F0   Patient with solitary tumor

F1   Patient with two or more discrete tumors

H

Tumor rupture or intraperitoneal hemorrhage

H1   Imaging and clinical findings of intraperitoneal hemorrhage

H0   All other patients

M

Distant metastases

M0   No metastases

M1   Any metastasis (except E and N)

Add suffix or suffixes to indicate location (see text)

N

Lymph node metastases

N0   No nodal metastases

N1   Abdominal lymph node metastases only

N2   Extra-abdominal lymph node metastases (with or without abdominal lymph node metastases)

P

Portal vein involvement

P0   No involvement of the portal vein or its left or right branches

P1   Involvement of either the left or the right branch of the portal vein

P2   Involvement of the main portal vein

See text for definition of involvement

Add suffix "a" if intravascular tumor is present, e.g. **P1a**

V

Involvement of the IVC and/or hepatic veins

V0   No involvement of the hepatic veins or inferior vena cava (IVC)

V1   Involvement of one hepatic vein but not the IVC

V2   Involvement of two hepatic veins but not the IVC

V3   Involvement of all three hepatic veins and/or the IVC

See text for definition of involvement

Add suffix "a" if intravascular tumor is present, e.g. **V3a**

frequency of loss of heterozygosity (LOH) on chromosomal arm 13q is much higher.[9] The exact meaning of these findings is not clear at the moment.

TREATMENT

Surgery

Biopsy

The aim of the biopsy in HCC is to obtain sufficient tissue to allow an accurate diagnosis, whilst avoiding complications. The most important potential immediate complication is hemorrhage. There is also the possibility of seeding tumor cells into an uninvolved segment of the liver, the abdominal wall, or peritoneal cavity. These risks can be minimized by using a percutaneous coaxial technique or (in case of laparoscopic approach) using protecting needle to guide tru-cut biopsies.

Obviously in a resectable tumor representing most probably case of HCC (i.e. older child or young adult with predisposing condition) primary resection should be undertaken without any attempt of biopsy. In clear HCC cases arising on the basis of liver cirrhosis diagnosis can be made on clinical ground providing tumor is more than 2 cm of diameter and it is associated with unequivocal rise in AFP and imaging results (US + helical CT and/or MRI). However, one has to keep in mind that in cirrhotic patients AFP may be permanently elevated due to ongoing liver regeneration process.

Tumor Resection

All the present studies have confirmed the importance of complete tumor resection for obtaining cure. However, only less than 20 percent of patients are amenable to initial surgical resection. Nevertheless, the ultimate goal of hepatocellular carcinoma treatment is to achieve complete tumor removal either in a primary or delayed setting. Standard hepatic resection techniques should be recommended: segmentectomies, hemihepatectomies and extended hemihepatectomies in advanced cases. As emphasised earlier, only complete (curative) tumor resection gives realistic hope of cure for patients with HCC. This implies that all options should be explored before declaring a tumour unresectable. In this regard, intraoperative US examination might be very useful, indeed, and it becomes a must when segmental hepatic resection is planned. Sampling of lymph nodes from hepato-dudodenal ligament should be performed in *every* case as their involvement has a significant impact on prognosis.

In fact even more extensive lymphadenectomy of the hepatic pedicle should be recommended.

Orthotopic Liver Transplantation (OLT)

Role of liver transplantattion in HCC remains still somewhat controversial. Generally, OLT should be favored in HCC with underlying cirrhosis on that condition that special tumor criteria are met. A clear advantage of OLT is that it also treats the basic pathologic process in the liver that is cirrhosis. Majority of transplantation centers do not accept patients with a single tumor larger than 5 cm or more than 3 tumors, especially when any of them exceeds 3 cm or their combined diameter is > 8 cm (Milano criteria). With such selection about 70 percent overall survival is achievable.[10-13] However, in cases of initially incomplete surgery 5-year survival after salvage transplant would be much lower in comparison with that for primary OLT (23 vs. 52%)—according to L.Wong estimates.[14]

There have been no prospective randomized, studies comparing outcome of liver resection with transplantation for HCC in the particular setting of non-cirrhotic livers. Actually these two options are difficult to compare fully as they deal with different groups of patients and are associated with completely different postoperative complications. Recurrence rates after standard surgery are 19 to 65 percent in comparison with 0 to 43 percent for transplantation.[15]

Pediatric liver transplantation experience in HCC is quite limited (only a few small series published and some of them are rather old).[16] There is only one fairly big pediatric series of transplanted HCCs (19 cases) from Pittsburgh, which confirms negative influence of tumor size and vascular invasion on prognosis—very much like in adults.[17] Two other, earlier reports: one by Tagge (from 1992) and one by Iwatsuki (early Pittsburgh series - from 1991) show low survival - in the range of 29 to 35 percent in patients with unresectable tumors.[18,19]

Because some data indicate possible difference in biology between pediatric and adult HCC it is not known whether adult lessons can be fully transposed to children. Very little is known on the role of OLT in patients with "de novo" HCC cases. Also some recent experience shows that the present cut off point of 5 cm of the tumor diameter may be somewhat extended without compromising patients' survival, even though such results are all retrospective and not collected in a pediatric population.[20,21]

Chemotherapy

Recently Katzenstein and Czauderna reported on the results of children and adolescents with hepatocellular carcinoma treated on the recently completed North American Intergroup Hepatoma study (INT-0098) and the first International Society of Pediatric Oncology liver tumor study (SIOPEL-1).[4,5] Both studies utilized preoperative chemotherapy in an attempt to increase surgical resectability since this is the foundation for curative therapy for liver tumors.

Forty-six patients were entered onto the North American Intergroup Hepatoma study. After initial surgery or biopsy all patients, 8 with stage I (completely resected tumors), 25 with stage III (unresectable tumor) and 13 with stage IV (metastatic disease) were randomized to receive cisplatin with either doxorubicin or 5-fluorouracil and vincristine. There was no difference regarding response, or survival rates between the two treatment regimens.

Seven of the eight patients (88%) with complete tumor excision at time of diagnosis (stage I) followed by adjuvant cisplatin-based chemotherapy survived. This is a significant improvement when compared with only 12 of 33 patients (36%) treated before the consistent use of adjuvant chemotherapy. This result suggests that adjuvant chemotherapy may be of benefit for patients with completely resected hepatocellular carcinoma. However, since some of these initially resected patients have faired well without any additional chemotherapy, this question will only be answered in a randomized trial. In contrast, outcome was uniformly poor for patients with advanced-stage disease. Five-year event-free survival for stage III and IV patients was 23 percent +/- 9 percent and 10 percent +/- 9 percent, respectively. Tumor resection after neoadjuvant chemotherapy was only feasible in 2 patients, and although they did have a prolonged survival they eventually died of recurrent disease.

Thirty-nine patients were entered onto the SIOPEL-1 study. Of these, 2 had complete resection of the tumor at diagnosis followed by chemotherapy, and 37 had preoperative chemotherapy with cisplatin and doxorubicin. Tumor extent determined based on radiologic findings, and classified according to a Pretreatment Extent of Disease System (PRETEXT). Disease was often advanced at time of diagnosis, 24 of 39 patients (62%) were classified as PRETEXT III and IV. Metastases were identified in 31 percent of the patients and extrahepatic tumor extension, vascular invasion or both in 39 percent. The tumor was multifocal in 56 percent of the patients. Although partial tumor response to therapy was observed in 49 percent (18/37) of the patients, complete tumor resection was achieved in only 36 percent (14/39) of the patients. Results of this study were also unsatisfactory with a 5-year event-free survival of 17 percent (Fig. 23.2). Presence of metastases was the most potent adverse prognostic factor (Fig. 23.3). PRETEXT category was able to discriminate patients' survival (Fig. 23.4). All long-term survivors had complete surgical excision of their tumor.

In the SIOPEL 2 study 21 patients with HCC were registered and their treatment intensity was increased, compared with the SIOPEL 1, by rapidly alternating the administration of cisplatin (every 14 days) with carboplatin and doxorubicin. Despite this intensification of standard systemic chemotherapy no improvement in EFS and OS has been achieved (unpublished data).

When we compare the results of these studies with three North American studies conducted between 1973 and 1984 (Haas) the outcome for patients with hepatocellular carcinoma has shown no significant improvement, despite of the improvements observed in surgical techniques, chemotherapy delivery and patient support. It seems obvious that a completely new treatment approach is needed to increase HCC cure rate.

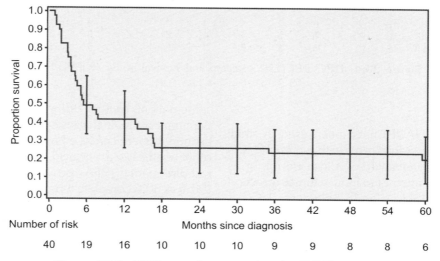

Figure 23.2: HCC event-free-survival in the SIOPEL 1 study

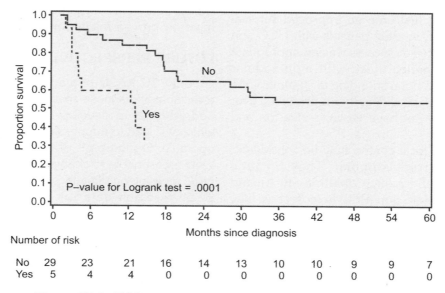

Figure 23.3: HCC: metastases and prognosis in the SIOPEL 1 study

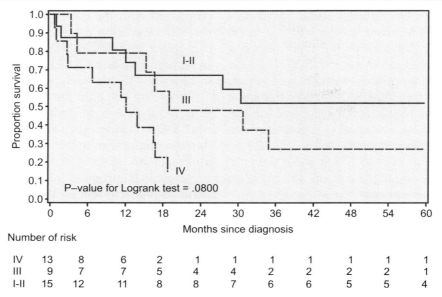

Figure 23.4: HCC: PRETEXT category and survival in the SIOPEL 1 study

Other Therapies

Chemoembolization (HACE) have been used in small number of children and adolescents with recurrent HCC while waiting for the availability of a liver donor, or as adjuvant therapy in an attempt to induce tumor resection (Fig. 23.5).[22] Since children and adolescents HCC is rarely associated with liver cirrhosis, a major limiting factor for the success of chemoembolization in adults, this therapeutic approach may be useful for these patients and further studies are warranted for this patient's population. Also recently Llovet et al. have demonstrated for the first time an improved survival associated with HACE in adult patients with HCC and liver cirrhosis.[23] The key to success was an appropriate patients' selection; hence those with multinodular tumors or large tumors not responding to systemic CHT are the best candidates providing ther is preserved liver function and they do not have vascular invasion and extrahepatic spread.

Other methods of local control may be considered, especially in recurrent tumors. They include percutaneous radiofrequency ablation (RFA) and percutaneous ethanol injection (PEI). In most cases they have palliative character and are suitable for smaller size tumors only: generally below 3-4 cm of diameter. However, these techniques are of low risk, are repeatable and do not damage non-neoplastic tissue which is especially important in cirrhotic patients. Additionally a combination of these techniques can be applied in the same patient. Neither PEI, nor RFA can be used, at least percutaneously, if the lesion is not recognizable in US examination. Recently, ethanol has been substituted with other agents like acetic acid. Tumor thermoablation with radiofrequency (RFA) provides better effect than PEI (90% vs 80% complete tumor necrosis) with less sessions (1.2 vs 4.8).[24] It is also associated with less side effects, thus in many centers RFA is preferred over PEI nowadays. However, it has to be mentioned that these techniques have not been well studied in children.

Other therapies like estrogens or androgens use, as well as treatment with sandostatin, have been shown to have no proven antitumoral effect.[7,24]

FUTURE PERSPECTIVES

As only 10 to 20 percent of pediatric HCCs are resectable at diagnosis specific issue, which needs to be addressed, is to develop a novel treatment strategy, which will lead to tumors shrinkage and rendering them operable. On the basis of several experimental data it seems reasonable to change the treatment approach in HCC focusing on targeting vascular supply of the tumor. Basic research data on HCC indicate that active angiogenesis takes place in HCC, especially in big and multifocal tumors, and that HCC gains hypervascularity during dedifferentiation and progression.[25-31] Elevated markers of angiogenesis (VEGF and bFGF) correlate with poor prognosis and a high chance for recurrence, as well as with vascular invasion, which is a major factor

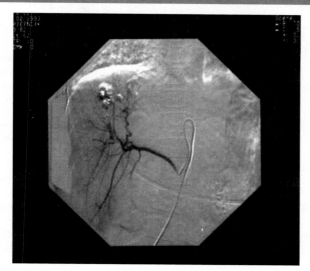

Figure 23.5: Example of chemoembolization in advanced HCC (own material)

associated with tumor recurrence and treatment failure.[29,30,32-34] Angiostatic treatment has several potential advantages: broad spectrum of activity, decreased resistance (as endothelial cells are genetically stable), improved drug access to targets, more tolerable side effects.[35] Activated tumor endothelium is a more specific target than tumor cells and inhibition of small number of tumoral vessels may affect the growth of many tumor cells. Recently, it has been proven that a combination of different angiostatic agents, which have several points of action, is superior to angiostatic monotherapy.[36,37] This results from the fact that different populations of tumor endothelial cells may relay on different angiogenic factors, which can also undergo change during the course of therapy. For optimal effect antiangiogenic treatment has to be given at frequent intervals to avoid recovery of endothelial cells from therapy insult. However, optimal dosing of angiostatic therapy is difficult to find as, on the contrary to chemotherapy, ideal dose is not necessarily maximum tolerated dose (MTD). It has also been known from several recent literature reports that angiostatic agents should not be used alone as they exert purely cytostatic action and most trials run that way led to disease stabilization only, thus they should be combined with cytotoxic therapy for maximum effect.[36,37] Thus it seems to be well justified in future HCC trials to combine systemic chemotherapy with angiostatic therapy in order to potentiate its antitumoral action.

REFERENCES

1. Chang, MH. Decreasing incidence of hepatocellular carcinoma among children following universal hepatitis B immunization. Liver Int 2003;23:309-14.
2. Czauderna P. Adult vs. childhood hepatocellular carcinoma—are they the same or different lesions? Biology, natural history, prognosis and treatment. Med Pediatr Oncol 2002;39:519-23.
3. Ganem D, Prince AM. Hepatitis B virus infection—natural history and clinical consequences. N Engl J Med 2004;350:1118-29.
4. Czauderna P, Mackinlay G, Perilongo G. et al. Hepatocellular carcinoma in children—results of the first prospective study of the International Society of Paediatric Oncology. J Clin Oncol 2002;20:2798-2804.
5. Katzenstein HM, et al. Hepatocellular carcinoma in children and adolescents: results from the Pediatric Oncology Group and the Children's Cancer Group Intergroup Study. J Clin Oncol 2002;20:2789-97.
6. Siegel MJ. Pediatric liver imaging. Semin Liver Dis 2001;21:251-69.
7. Llovet JM, Burroughs A, Bruix J. Hepatocellular carcinoma. Lancet 2003;362:1907-17.
8. Prokurat A, et al. Transitional liver cell tumors (TLCT) in older children and adolescents: a novel group of aggressive hepatic tumors expressing beta-catenin. Med Pediatr Oncol 2000;39:510-18.
9. Kim H, Lee MJ, Kim MR, et al. Expression of cyclin D1, cyclin E, cdk4 and loss of heterozygosity of 8p, 13q, 17p in hepatocellular carcinoma: comparison study of childhood and adult hepatocellular carcinoma. Liver 2000;20:173-8.
10. Hemming AW, et al. Liver transplantation for hepatocellular carcinoma. Ann Surg 2001;233: 652-9.
11. Klintmalm GB. Liver transplantation for hepatocellular carcinoma: a registry report of the impact of tumor characteristics on outcome. Ann Surg 1998;228:479-90.
12. Colombo M, Sangiovanni A. The European approach to hepatocellular carcinoma. Hepato-gastroenterol 2002;49:12-6.
13. Pons-Renedo F, Llovet J. Hepatocellular carcinoma: a clinical update. Medscape General Medicine 2003;5(3).
14. Wong LW. Current status of liver transplantation for hepatocellular cancer. Am J Surg 2002;183: 309-16.
15. Yeh CN, et al. Prognostic factors of hepatic resection for hepatocellular carcinoma with cirrhosis: univariate and multivariate analysis. J Surg Oncol 2002;81:195-202.
16. Achilleos O, et al. Unresectable hepatic tumors in children and the role of liver transplantation. J Pediatr Surg 1996;31:1563-7.
17. Reyes JD, et al. Liver transplantation and chemotherapy for hepatoblastoma and hepatocellular cancer in childhood and adolescence. J Pediatr 2000;136:795-804.
18. Tagge EP, et al. Resection, including transplantation, for hepatoblastoma and hepatocellular carcinoma: impact on survival. J Pediatr Surg 1992;27:292-7.
19. Iwatsuki S, et al. Hepatic resection vs. transplantation for hepatocellular carcinoma. Ann Surg 1991;214:221-9.
20. Roayaie S, et al. Long-term results with multimodal adjuvant therapy and liver transplantation for the treatment of hepatocellular carcinomas larger than 5 centimeters. Ann Surg 2002;235: 533-9.
21. Yao FY, et al. Liver transplantation for hepatocellular carcinoma: expansion of the tumor size limits does not adversely impact survival. Hepatology 2001;33:1394-403.

22. Arcement CM, Towbin RB, Meza MP, et al. Intrahepatic chemoembolization in unresectable pediatric liver malignancies. Pediatr Radiol 2000;30:779-85.

23. Llovet JM, Bruix J. Systematic review of randomized trials for unresectable hepatocellular carcinoma: chemo-embolization improves survival. Hepatology 2003;37:429-42.

24. Venook AP. Treatment of hepatocellular carcinoma: too many options? J Clin Oncol 1994;12: 1323-34.

25. Tang ZY, et al. Surgical treatment of hepatocellular carcinoma and related basic research with special reference to recurrence and metastases. Chin Med J 1999;112:887-91.

26. Ma J, et al. Clinicopathologic study of angiogenesis in human hepatocellular carcinoma. Zhonghua Bing Li Xue Za Zhi 2000;29:248-51.

27. Torimura T, et al. Increased expression of vascular endothelial growth factor is associated with tumor progression in hepatocellular carcinoma. Hum Pathol 1998;29:986-91.

28. Park YN, et al. Increased expression of vascular endothelial growth factor and angiogenesis in the early step of multistep hepatocarcinogenesis. Arch Pathol Lab Med 2000;124:1061-5.

29. Poon Rt, et al. Correlation of serum basic fibroblast growth factor levels with clinicopathologic features and postoperative recurrence in hepatocellular carcinoma. Am J Surg 2001;182:298-304.

30. Poon RT, et al. Serum vascular endothelial growth factor predicts venous invasion in hepatocellular carcinoma: a prospective study. Ann Surg 2001;233:227-35.

31. Tang ZY. Hepatocellular carcinoma—cause, treatment and metastasis. World J Gastroenterol 2001;7:445-54.

32. Li XM, et al. Serum vascular endothelial growth factor is a predictor of invasion and metastasis in hepatocellular carcinoma. J Exp Clin Cancer Res 1999;18:511-7.

33. Dhar DK, et al. Requisite role of VEGF receptors in angiogenesis of hepatocellular carcinoma: a comparison with Angiopoietin/ Tie pathway. Anticancer Res 2002;22:379-86.

34. Sugimachi K, et al. The mechanisms of angiogenesis in hepatocellular carcinoma: angiogenic switch during tumor progression. Surgery 2002;131:S135-41.

35. Liekens S, et al. Angiogenesis: regulators and clinical applications. Biochem Pharmacol 2001;61: 253-70.

36. Kerbel RS. Clinical trials of antiangiogenic drugs: opportunities, problems and assessment of initial results. J Clin Oncol 2001;18s:45s-51s.

37. Scappaticci F. Mechanisms and future directions for angiogenesis-based cancer therapies. J Clin Oncol 2002;18:3906-27.

Chan Hon Chui
Bhaskar Rao
Sani Molagool
Kenneth W Gow

CHAPTER **24**

Tumors of the Adrenal Gland (Other than Neuroblastoma)

Although neuroblastoma is the most common tumor of the adrenal gland in pediatric patients, other less common tumors should be considered in the differential diagnosis, such as the adrenocortical tumors (adrenocortical adenomas and carcinomas), pheochromocytomas, stromal tumors, metastatic adrenal gland malignancies, adrenal cysts, and adrenal hemorrhages. This chapter will discuss adrenocortical tumors and pheochromocytomas. Stromal tumors of the adrenal glands (fibroma, lipoma, hamartoma, neurofibroma, osteoma, hemangioma, lymphangioma, melanoma, and sarcoma) are very rare and usually do not cause symptoms. Nevertheless, these tumors should be excised because it is difficult to distinguish them from neuroblastoma and other malignant neoplasms.[1] Small hemorrhagic cysts of the fetal adrenal cortex are relatively common, are frequently bilateral, and are absorbed spontaneously.[1,2] Large cysts may be difficult to differentiate from solid tumors and may occasionally be malignant.[1] In newborns, adrenal hemorrhage due to fetal anoxia or difficult labor may produce adrenal insufficiency with shock and sepsis; this condition may be fatal if not treated promptly with replacement of adrenal cortical hormone.

ADRENOCORTICAL TUMORS

Introduction

Adrenocortical tumors (ACTs) are rare in children, accounting for only 2 to 12 percent of all childhood cancers.[3] The worldwide incidence of ACTs is 0.3 to 0.38 cases per million persons under the age of 15 years.[4]

Southern Brazil has reported a higher incidence of 3.4 to 4.2 cases per million persons in the same age group; this difference in incidence has not yet been accounted for. Unlike adults with ACTs, who generally have either abdominal masses or incidentalomas at the time of diagnosis, pediatric patients with ACTs usually have one of the clinical endocrine syndromes. Although ACTs are classified as either benign or malignant, it is often difficult to determine a histologic distinction between adrenocortical carcinoma and adenoma, and it is even more difficult to determine a difference in the prognosis of patients with these lesions. Total surgical resection of the tumor remains the mainstay of treatment.

Cause, Molecular Biology and Pathogenesis

Although the precise cause of ACTs is unknown, some researchers have suggested neoplastic transformation of adrenocortical tissue by chronic stimulation with adrenocorticotrophic hormone (ACTH) in cases of congenital adrenal hyperplasia.[5] ACTs can also occur independently of other disease.[6]

Approximately 50 percent of children with ACTs have genetic factors that predispose them to tumor development. Li-Fraumeni syndrome (LFS) and Beckwith-Wiedemann syndrome (BWS) are clearly associated with ACT. The associations of multiple endocrine neoplasia type I (MEN I) and Carney's complex with ACTs have been described in the adult population and may provide insight into other genetic factors that may cause ACTs.[6]

LFS is associated with alterations of the tumor-suppressor gene p53 on chromosome arm 17p.[7,8] The syndrome is a rare autosomal dominant condition with incomplete penetrance that causes many different types of tumors in affected family members. LFS is diagnosed when one family member is found to have sarcoma before the age of 45 years, a first-degree relative (parent, sibling, or offspring) is found to have cancer of any kind before the age of 45 years, and another first- or second-degree relative in the same lineage (grandparent, grandchild, or first cousin) is found to have any cancer before the age of 45 years or sarcoma at any age. Members of these families are at increased risk of leukemia, brain tumors, osteosarcomas, and ACTs; in fact, their risk of ACTs is 100 times higher than that of the general population.

Beckwith-Wiedemann syndrome (BWS) is another rare genetic disorder associated with a higher-than-expected incidence of ACTs. Symptoms of BWS include congenital umbilical hernia, macroglossia, and gigantism, but a wide phenotypic expression has been reported. Familial BWS is associated with abnormalities at chromosome band 11p15,[6] to which genes for insulin-like growth factor II (IGF-II) and H19 (a putative IGF repressor) have been mapped. These genes are important regulators of fetal adrenal growth. The loss of imprinting of these genes may cause their overexpression, thereby leading to oncogenesis. IGF II encodes an adrenal growth factor that is overexpressed in mRNA and protein in 84 percent of adrenal carcinomas but in only 6 percent of adenomas.[9] IGF-II has been shown to control the production of dehydroepiandrosterone sulfate (DHEAS) by the human fetal adrenal gland.[10]

Congenital hemihypertrophy, congenital deficiency of steroidogenic enzymes, and ACTH-dependent Cushing's syndrome have been associated with ACTs.[11,12] However, the causative genetic factor has not yet been identified because pediatric adrenocortical carcinomas are often associated with complex hyperdiploid karyotypes, involving multiple gains and losses of chromosomes and p53 mutations. We suspect that multiple hits are required for the formation of such tumors.

Environmental factors have been postulated as causes of ACTs, but proof is lacking. Reported associations between environmental factors and ACTs include fetal alcohol syndrome and maternal ingestion of hydroxy progesterone hexanoate or 75-selenomethionine during pregnancy. Carcinogenesis has been reported in animals receiving receiving diets low in linoleic acid.[3]

Pathology

It is difficult to distinguish benign ACTs from malignant ACTs solely on the basis of histopathological features, unless patients have obvious signs of malignancy such as metastatic disease or local invasion. The clinicopathologic studies of Hough and Weiss[13,14] attempted to distinguish benign lesions from malignant lesions in adults; however, many ACTs display both benign and malignant morphological characteristics. It is therefore not surprising to see local recurrences and late metastatic lesions in association with histologically benign lesions or to find lesions with malignant features that do not appear to be associated with an ominous prognosis. In general, the behavior of the tumor is inconsistent with the histological findings. Many pathologists consider other variables, such as tumor size, age of the patient, and presence of metastatic lesions, when making a final diagnosis of benign or malignant ACT.

Adrenocortical carcinomas are grossly larger than adenomas: adenomas tend to weigh less than 100 g, whereas carcinomas rarely weigh less than 200 g and frequently weigh more than 500 g. Because a solid mass weighing 100 g has a diameter of at least 6 cm, tumor diameter has been used as a guide for intervention in cases of adult nonfunctional adrenal tumors. Adrenocortical carcinomas appear lobulated, and their cut surface is variegated in color, ranging from tan-yellow to reddish-brown. The tumors may be encapsulated with zones of necrosis, hemorrhage, and calcification. Microscopic features include architectural disarray, frequent mitosis (including mitotic features), broad fibrous bands, marked cellular pleomorphism, nuclear atypia, hyperchromasia, necrosis, hemorrhage, calcification, and vascular invasion.

Adrenocortical adenomas are well encapsulated and more uniform in color than adrenocortical carcinomas; they are usually yellowish or, less commonly, reddish brown or brown. Their cut surface is uniform, and zones of necrosis, hemorrhage, and calcification are usually absent. Microscopic features include a well-preserved architecture with minimal mitotic activity and less variation in cell size and less nuclear pleomorphism than is seen in adrenocortical carcinomas. Necrosis, hemorrhage, and calcification are rare, and there is usually no evidence of invasion of the tumor capsule or blood vessels.

Clinical Features

The distribution of ACTs according to patient age is bimodal; these tumors usually occur in patients in the first and fifth decades of life. In the pediatric population, the median age of occurrence tends to be approximately 3 years. The female-male ratio is 2.3:1; this difference may represent sex-specific changes in the adrenal glands which are currently not understood. Twenty-five percent of ACTs are adenomas; the rest are carcinomas.[3,6]

Unlike adult ACTs, which commonly cause abdominal masses, most pediatric ACTs are hormonally active; only 10 percent of pediatric ACTs are nonfunctional. Thus, the symptoms they cause, such as virilization, feminization, and Cushing's and Conn's syndromes, depend largely on the specific adrenocortical hormones that the tumors secrete. ACTs may also secrete several different hormones and in such cases may cause signs and symptoms of multiple syndromes (mixed forms).

Virilization is the most common symptom of ACTs in pediatric patients, occurring in 80 percent of cases. More than 50 percent of ACTs secrete increased amounts of androgens; the rest secrete other hormones. Symptoms include deepening of the voice, acne, hirsutism, increase of muscle mass, and proliferation of sebaceous glands and their secretions, with a characteristic adult odor. Sex-specific changes in females include clitoral enlargement, facial and pubic hair with male escutcheon, amenorrhea, and occasional temporal balding. In males, penile enlargement and precocious isosexual pseudo-puberty may occur.

One third of patients with ACTs exhibit Cushing's syndrome. Only 8 percent of these exhibit isolated hyperadrenocorticalism, because most also exhibit virilization. Moon facies, weight gain, centripetal distribution of fat, plethora, hypertension, and striae are usually present.

Conn's syndrome is the manifestation of primary aldosteronism; in most cases, the associated pathological disorder is bilateral cortical hyperplasia. Aldosterone-producing adenoma is extremely rare in pediatric patients, occurring in only 1.6 percent of cases. Symptoms may include headaches, weak proximal muscles, polyuria, tachycardia, hypocalcemia, and hypertension.

Hypertension is associated with approximately 50 percent of ACTs. This symptom could be explained by an excess of glucocorticoids or mineralocorticoids or by the activation of the renin-angiotensin system because of compression of the renal vascular system by the tumor. Some patients exhibit hypertensive crises that are difficult to manage. However, hypertension usually improves after removal of the tumor.

Nonfunctional ACTs are uncommon in pediatric patients, accounting for only 5 percent of childhood ACTs. Because these tumors do not demonstrate endocrine hyperactivity, they usually cause symptoms of abdominal pain or fullness only after they have become quite large or have metastasized. The metastatic lesions frequently occur in the liver and lungs and are less common in the regional lymph nodes and bone.[6]

In many cases, the diagnosis of nonfunctional ACTs is delayed because of increased somatic growth, a generally healthy appearance, and the lack of palpability of the abdominal mass. The delay may range from 3 days to 61 months (median, 10 months).[3] Clinicians should maintain a high index of suspicion. Any child younger than 4 years with pubarche should be considered to have an ACT until proven otherwise. The presence of acne in an infant can be considered pathognomonic of an adrenocortical lesion.[15] Cushing's syndrome in children younger than 10 years should be considered highly indicative of ACT.[16]

Diagnosis

Because most pediatric ACTs are functional tumors, biochemical studies should be performed promptly. Testosterone and its precursors may be produced in significant amounts and may result in virilization. Evaluation should be directed toward the detection of androgens, including the plasma concentration of testosterone, the urinary and plasma concentrations of DHEA and DHEAS, and the urinary concentration of 17-ketosteroid (17-KS), a nonspecific measure of androgenic metabolites. The most specific assessment of adrenal androgen production is the plasma concentration of DHEAS; an elevation of the urinary concentration of 17-KS almost always indicates adrenal hyperactivity. Moreover, the concentration of 17-KS is usually markedly elevated in the case of malignancy but less so in the case of benign adrenal lesions.[17]

Patients with Cushing's syndrome exhibit hypercortisolism and the loss of diurnal variation. These symptoms are confirmed by detection of elevations in the plasma concentration of cortisol, the urinary concentration of 17-hydroxycorticosteroids, and the urinary concentration of free cortisol. It is interesting to note that the elevations in the concentrations of 17-hydroxycorticosteroid and plasma cortisol caused by adrenal malignancies are generally much larger than those caused by benign disease. In addition, determination of plasma ACTH activity and provocative tests using dexamethasone and metyrapone suggest the causes of Cushing's syndrome. Nevertheless, it is impossible to use biochemical tests to differentiate adrenal adenomas from carcinomas.[6,17]

When patients have with nonfunctional adrenocortical tumors that do not produce excessive amounts of active hormones, steroid precursors such as metabolites of pregnenolone may be produced in abundance.[18] In such cases, these urinary metabolites may serve as markers of tumor recurrence.

Imaging studies are as important as biochemical confirmation of adrenocortical overactivity in the diagnosis of ACTs. These studies localize and stage the tumor to facilitate surgical intervention.

In the evaluation of adrenal tumors in pediatric patients, ultrasound offers the advantages of being noninvasive and radiation-free. Lesions 3 cm or larger in diameter are readily delineated, and smaller tumors may be identified with realtime scanning. Color Doppler ultrasonography is considered reasonably accurate in the detection of tumor thrombus in the adrenal or renal vein or in the inferior vena cava (IVC). It is also ideal for the postoperative assessment of recurrence. Unfortunately, it cannot reliably identify smaller lesions as accurately as computed tomography (CT) and is operator dependent.

CT can detect adrenal gland tumors as small as 0.5 cm in diameter and can reliably detect lesions larger than 1 cm in diameter. In the pediatric population, the lack of retroperitoneal fat may pose some difficulty in the detection of ACTs. However, CT can be used to determine whether tumor thrombus is present in the adrenal or renal vein, the IVC, or the contralateral adrenal gland. CT can also be used to ensure contralateral renal function should ipsilateral nephrectomy be necessary. Only the presence of regional invasion or distant metastatic lesions (liver, lung, or brain) can reliably differentiate benign lesions from malignant tumors on CT images.

The role of magnetic resonance (MR) imaging in the evaluation of adrenal lesions is constantly expanding. (Fig. 24.1) The accuracy of MR imaging is comparable to that of CT in detecting adrenal masses larger than 1 or 2 cm in diameter. MR imaging has the advantage of

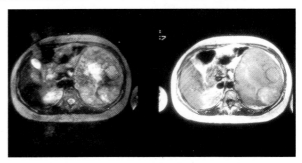

Figure 24.1: MR imaging of adrenocortical carcinoma

producing coronal slices, which can identify a 1 cm adrenal mass that is not visualized by a sector CT image. The various MR imaging techniques have been reported to be helpful in differentiating malignant from benign lesions. Using gradient and spin-echo images, MR imaging can accurately delineate the presence and extent of venous thrombus.

Arteriography and adrenal venography are generally unnecessary and dangerously invasive for pediatric patients. However, in special cases selective arteriography may be required for localization or angioembolization of a tumor before to surgery or to halt hemorrhage. Although venous blood sampling from the various levels of the IVC may be useful in aiding diagnosis, this procedure is associated with potential morbidity.

Adrenal scintigraphy using various iodocholesterol-labeled analogs has shown promise in diagnosing and differentiating functional adrenal lesions. This technique takes advantage of the uptake of radiocholesterol by adrenal cortical tissues. The current agent of choice is ^{131}I-6-beta-iodomethyl-19-norcholesterol (NP-59), which has provided functional information about the secretion of adrenal corticoids, mineralocorticoids, and androgen. With a documented glucocorticoid excess, symmetric uptake of NP-59 on bilateral images indicates adrenal hyperplasia. Unilateral uptake of the agent suggests adenoma, whereas bilateral nonvisualization suggests carcinoma. The use of this technique in pediatric patients is limited because of the long-term sequelae of radiation exposure. Whereas CT and MR imaging are quite effective in identifying abnormal adrenal anatomy, radiocholesterol scintigraphy can complement both biochemical and radiologic imaging data to identify abnormal adrenal function in adenomas and can suggest the presence of adrenal carcinoma or delineate the functional status of adrenal masses identified by CT or MR imaging.[6, 19,20]

Staging and Prognostic Factors

Because adrenocortical tumors are rare, risk-stratification and staging are difficult. Many researchers have attempted to formulate working systems for risk-stratification. It is hoped that the risks associated with each tumor can be better defined with the discovery of more molecular biological factors and with the currently known clinical and pathological features.

In general, the prognosis is very poor for patients with metastatic disease or gross residual tumor and very good for patients whose tumors can be completely resected and are small or have histologic features of adenoma. Sandrini et al proposed a staging system[21] based on the results of a review of 40 cases; this system, which is highly predictive of outcome for patients with either stage I or stage IV disease, takes into consideration tumor volume (< or > 200 cm^3), residual tumor (none, microscopic residual or gross residual) and hormonal levels after resection. Sandrini et al reported long-term survival for at least 90 percent of patients with stage I disease but for virtually none of those with stage IV disease (median follow-up time, 6.2 years; range, 1.4 to 13.7 years). Of the patients with stage II disease, 52 percent were alive and free of disease at the time of the report (median follow-up, 6.3 years; range, 0.1 to 17.8 years). Only 4 patients in the study had stage III disease; one of them was alive and had been free of disease for 6 years at the time of the report.[3,21]

Treatment

Complete surgical excision offers the best chance of cure for pediatric patients with stage I or II disease (Fig. 24.2). Invasion of the IVC by tumor should be considered tumor extension rather than metastatic disease. The surgical procedure should be aggressive in an attempt to remove completely the intravascular extension. The indications for total or near-total tumor excision in patients with stage III or IV disease remain controversial.

With new surgical techniques and better understanding of the perioperative care required for these patients, morbidity and mortality rates have markedly diminished.[6] Pediatric patients with ACTs tend to have endocrine syndromes that require preplanning and careful management. Because all patients with functional tumors are assumed to have contralateral suppression of adrenal function, replacement therapy should be started promptly. Electrolyte imbalance, hypertension, problems with surgical wound care, and infectious complications may arise as a result of the endocrine syndromes.

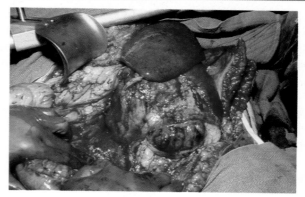

Figure 24.2: Left adrenocortical carcinoma and its adjacent spleen

An anterior transabdominal approach via a bilateral subcostal incision is preferred for optimal exposure. This approach affords the best opportunity to assess the extent of local invasion and lymph node involvement and to detect metastatic or contralateral disease. If the intrahepatic or intracardiac veins are involved, the cardiac surgery team should participate in the procedure.

Laparoscopic adrenalectomy has been widely used to treat adult adrenal neoplasms. The procedure is as effective as an open procedure, but the length of hospitalization and convalescence is markedly reduced.[22,23] Because adrenal neoplasms are uncommon in pediatric patients, laparoscopic experience with these tumors is lacking. Nevertheless, this minimally invasive surgical technique is a promising option for the treatment of pediatric adrenocortical carcinoma.

The use of chemotherapy in adrenocortical carcinoma has not been established. Mitotane [1,1-dichloro-2-(o-chlorophenyl)-2-(p-chlorophenyl)ethane, or o,p'-DDD], an insecticide derivative that produces adrenocortical necrosis, has been used extensively to treat adult patients with a high risk of relapse. However, preliminary results indicate that the rate of relapse has not been modified. The toxic effects of mitotane include nausea, vomiting, diarrhea, abdominal pain, somnolence, lethargy, ataxic gait, depression, and vertigo. Mitotane alters the metabolism of steroid hormone, and this alteration causes changes in the concentrations of steroids in blood and urine, rendering these biochemical markers inaccurate for the detection of disease recurrence. The use of mitotane to treat pediatric patients is still experimental. Other chemotherapeutic agents that have been used to treat pediatric patients with ACTs include cisplatin with etoposide; 5-fluorouracil (5-FU) with leucovorin; and ifosfamide, carboplatin with etoposide. Suramin, which is a polysulfated naphthylurea, and Gossypol, a biphenolic derivative extracted from cotton seeds, have demonstrated antitumor activity in vitro and have been used with some success to treat metastatic adrenal carcinoma in adults.

Adjuvant radiotherapy has not been shown to be effective in the treatment of adrenocortical carcinoma. However, it has been used as palliative care for patients with bone involvement.

Outcome

In his study of the natural history of untreated adrenocortical carcinoma, MacFarlane reported that the mean length of survival for 35 patients was 2.9 months.[24] The mortality rates in adult series are high: in one series, the mortality rate approached 90 percent;[25] in another, 50 percent of the patients died within 2 years after the onset of symptoms, and the 3-year survival rate was less than 25 percent.[26] Curitiba reported a series of 54 pediatric patients, 56 percent of whom were disease-free after initial treatment.[3] The time to tumor recurrence after surgery ranged from 1 to 48 months (median, 6 months). Recurrences were rapidly fatal; in nearly all cases, patients died within 11 months. Michalkiewics et al reported 20 pediatric patients with small, surgically resected adrenocortical tumors; the overall survival rate was 90 percent with a median follow-up time of 2.3 years.[27] As more data accumulate, the true prognosis for children with adrenocortical carcinoma will become clearer.

PHEOCHROMOCYTOMA

Introduction

Only 10 percent of all pheochromocytomas occur in pediatric patients.[28] The tumor is responsible for more than 1 percent of cases of childhood nonessential hypertension.[29] Although pheochromocytomas are usually found in the adrenal medulla, they may occur at extra-adrenal sites such as the organ of Zuckerkandl. The tumors are composed of chromaffin cells and secrete epinephrine, norepinephrine, or both; in some cases, they also secrete dopamine. They typically give rise to endocrine symptoms such as hypertension, palpitations, and hyperglycemia.

Epidemiology

Pediatric pheochromocytomas occur in patients between the ages of 6 and 14 years and are slightly more common in boys. Six percent of the tumors are malignant;[30] this diagnosis is more reliably determined by the presence of metastatic lesions than by microscopic features of the tumor. Approximately 70 to 80 percent of childhood primary pheochromo-cytomas arise in the adrenal medulla.[30-33] Approximately 30 percent of childhood pheochromocytomas are extra-adrenal, an incidence nearly twice as high as that in adults. These extra-adrenal tumors may occur in the paraganglia, the organs of Zuckerkandl, or the bladder. Simultaneous adrenal and extra-adrenal pheochromocytomas are rare. Nearly all childhood pheochromocytomas are functional. Although only 7 percent of adult pheochromocytomas are bilateral, as many as 70 percent of childhood pheo-chromocytomas are bilateral, as determined by studies of children who were followed up for many years.[29,31]

Genetics

Most pheochromocytomas occur sporadically; some are inherited. Some of the inherited tumors may occur alone, whereas others occur in combination with other endocrine tumors such as C-cell hyperplasia or medullary carcinoma of the thyroid in cases of MEN IIa or MEN IIb. Pheochromocytomas also occur with pancreatic cysts and islet cell tumors in patients with von Hippel-Lindau syndrome; in such cases they are also associated with retinal angiomatosis, cystic cerebellar hemangio-blastoma, and renal cell carcinoma.

Neurofibromatosis (NF), tuberous sclerosis, and Sturge-Weber disease are often associated with pheochromocytomas and other neuroendocrine tumors. The genetic transmission follows the pattern of an autosomal dominant gene with incomplete penetrance.[34]

The molecular pathogenesis of these tumors is difficult to define. Mutations in oncogenes, in tumor-suppressor genes, or in regulators of cell growth or proliferation and adhesion have been reported, especially in familial syndromes. Only a few of these genetic abnormalities have been found in sporadic cases; thus, it is difficult to identify any consistent or recurrent abnormalities.

The *RET* proto-oncogene is upregulated in pheochromocytoma cell lines and in tumor tissue from patients with MEN syndromes. Tumor cells from patients with MEN II a were found to have mutations in exons 10 and 11 of the *RET* proto-oncogene, which is located on chromosome 10. Mutations are found elsewhere in the same gene in tumor cells from patients with MEN IIb. Only 2 percent of sporadic pheochromocytomas exhibit mutations of the *RET* proto-oncogene.[34]

Mutations of the *VHL* (von Hippel-Lindau disease) tumor-suppressor gene on chromosome arm 3p cause pheochromocytomas in patients with VHL type 2.[35] Other identified mutations are not associated with pheochromocytomas (in particular, type 1). Defects in the neurofibromin and swannomin found in NF have not been found to be associated with pheochromocytomas, but they have been expressed in other neuro-endocrine tissues. Sturge-Weber syndrome has been postulated to arise from mutations in genes involved in angiogenesis and control of cellular adhesion.[34]

Pathology

Pheochromocytomas originate from chromaffin cells; these cells produce catecholamine and are precursors of the sympathetic paraganglia, the adrenal medulla, and the extra- and intra-adrenal paraganglia. These usually migrate along the aorta and its major bifurcation from the cervical region to the pelvis. Approximately 70 percent of pheo-chromocytomas in children occur in the adrenal medulla;[1,34] only about 5 percent occur extra-abdominally. Multicentricity has been reported in as many as one third of the cases. Children with familial syndromes are more likely to have bilateral tumors. Bilateral occurrence has been recognized in approximately 25 to 50 percent of pediatric patients but in only 10 percent of adults.[36]

Grossly, pheochromocytomas are often well-circumscribed, yellow-brown tumors that average 3 cm to 6 cm in diameter and weigh less than 100 g. They are vascular and may contain cystic and hemorrhagic areas. Their microscopic appearance is often variable, demonstrating islands of large cells containing typical catecholamine storage granules. Mitoses and multiple or pleomorphic nuclei may be found. The tumor may extend into the capsule or vessels.

The presence of metastatic lesions is an absolute indicator of malignancy. Relative indicators of malignant behavior include degree of necrosis, nuclear pleomorphism, mitotic rate, capsular invasion, and vascular invasion, but none of these indicators is completely reliable.[33] Malignant pheochromocytomas are rare and occur in only 6 to 10 percent of pediatric patients with pheochromocytomas, an incidence less than half that in adults. Possible areas of metastasis include liver, lung, lymph nodes, brain, and bone. Metastatic lesions should be distinguished from synchronous or metachronous lesions and occur in areas from which chromaffin derivatives are usually absent.

Clinical Manifestations

Nearly all pheochromocytomas cause endocrine symptoms. Arterial hypertension is the cardinal sign and is present in 70 to 80 percent of cases. Typically, the hypertension is refractory to conventional antihypertensive therapy. The symptoms are paroxysmal, are present most of the time, and may vary in intensity. The paroxysms include throbbing headaches, sweating, palpitations, anxiety, tremors, nausea, vomiting, abdominal and chest pain, and visual disturbances. Fatigue and exhaustion usually follow a paroxysmal attack. Between paroxysms, patients may experience orthostatic hypotension, increased sweatiness, cold hands and feet, weight loss, constipation, and low-grade fever. These symptoms occasionally lead to congestive heart failure, encephalopathy, and even death. Hyperglycemia is present with symptoms of polyuria and polydipsia.

Physical examination reveals the signs of hypertension, which include cardiomegaly and retinopathy. Episodes of tachycardia, systolic hypertension, and arrhythmia reflect the β-receptor effects of epinephrine secretion, whereas bradycardia and diastolic hypertension are evidence of the increased peripheral vasoconstriction by the α-adrenergic receptors in response to circulating norepinephrine. Contraction of the vascular system leads to decreased plasma volume and reduced erythrocyte mass, and inadequately functioning neurovascular reflexes may occasionally lead to orthostatic hypotension. Ectopic production of vasoactive intestinal peptide is present with symptoms of hypercalcemia, carbohydrate intolerance, watery diarrhea, hypokalemia, achlorhydria, and Verner-Morrison syndrome. If the tumor produces ACTH, Cushing syndrome may occur.

Diagnosis

Assays for catecholamines and their metabolites provide a biochemical diagnosis of pheochromocytomas. Patients with continuous hypertension or symptoms will require assays of the concentrations of catecholamines and metabolites (metanephrine [MN] and vanillylmandelic acid [VMA]) in plasma and 24-hour urine collections; these concentrations are increased when pheochromocytoma is present. Assays for concentrations of urinary free catecholamines and VMA yield false-negative results in approximately 25 percent of cases, whereas such results occur in only 4 percent of MN determinations.

Measurement of plasma catecholamine concentrations by radioenzyme assay may be more effective than determinations of either 24-hour urinary VMA or MN concentrations.[37] Malignant pheochromocytomas secrete large amounts of dopamine, and its metabolite, homovanillic acid (HVA), is excreted in the urine.[1] Patients with neuroblastoma characteristically secrete high levels of dopamine metabolites. During sampling, it is vital that patients avoid drugs and foods that may stimulate catecholamine secretion.

Once the diagnosis of pheochromocytoma or paraganglioma has been confirmed by chemical analysis, the tumor should be localized to facilitate surgical removal. Abdominal ultrasonography and CT are useful imaging methods; CT identifies approximately 95 percent of pheochromocytomas (Fig. 24.3). However, small lesions, extra-adrenal tumors, adrenal hyperplasia, and residual or recurrent tumors may be missed. MR imaging is more accurate than CT or ultrasonography in the diagnosis of pheochromocytoma and other adrenal tumors and is the method of choice for definitive evaluation of adrenal tumors in pediatric patients.[38] Radioisotopic studies with ^{131}I-labeled meta-iodobenzyl guanidine (MIBG) have been very useful in localizing abnormal medullary tissue in pheochromocytomas. After intravenous MIBG has been administered, a small fraction is concentrated by the tumor as determined by serial scintigraphy. Specificity has been reported to be 98 percent; sensitivity, 85 percent.[39] Not all pheochromocytomas produce detectable images. With advanced imaging techniques, angiographic procedures such as arteriography and venography are rarely required. When further studies are necessary, catecholamine concentrations are measured in blood samples obtained by percutaneous venous catheterization at various points along the IVC. Patients who require such studies must be given α-blocking agents before the procedure.

The histamine provocative test and other tests that increase catecholamine secretion have largely been abandoned because of risks associated with these tests in patients who are already hypertensive. The phentolamine test is useful only for patients with sustained hypertension and should rarely be used. The results are positive when pressure declines 5 to 10 minutes after intravenous injection of phentolamine (5 mg).

Treatment

Surgical removal is the mainstay of the treatment of pheochromocytoma. Careful presurgical preparation is required to reduce the risks of anesthesia and of the procedure itself; such preparation includes the administration of adrenergic antagonists (phentolamine, phenoxybenzamine, prazosin) that help reduce symptoms and blood pressure, ameliorate paroxysms, and expand the vascular bed and blood volume.

Phentolamine and phenoxybenzamine block the α-adrenergic receptors of epinephrine and norepinephrine. Because of the potential danger of hypertensive paroxysms, the patient should be given α-adrenergic blocking agents as soon as the diagnosis of pheochromocytoma has been confirmed and for at least 3 to 7 days before the surgical procedure.[40] Preoperative resolution of symptoms and normalization of blood pressure are the most reliable predictors of an uncomplicated postsurgical outcome. Normalization of MN concentrations is one of the best indicators that the patient's hypertensive paroxysms are adequately controlled. Phentolamine can be used for rapid alpha-adrenergic blockade, whereas phenoxybenzamine therapy for 1 to 2 weeks can be used when surgical intervention is not urgent.

Nitroprusside has occasionally been used before and during the surgical procedure to treat patients with crescendo symptoms or those whose disease has become refractory to oral and intravenous α-adrenergic blocking agents. Drugs that decrease catecholamine synthesis, such as α-methylpara tyrosine (AMPT), have been recommended as an alternative preoperative regimen. Patients with pheochromocytomas tend to exhibit hypovolemia, with an average 15 percent reduction of normal plasma volume. Carefully monitored preoperative re-expansion of the vascular system helps minimize the occurrence of fluctuations in blood pressure and intractable arrhythmias during the procedure. Anesthesia

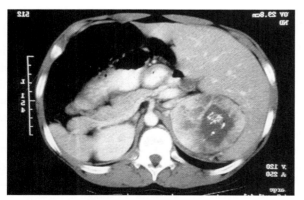

Figure 24.3: CT scan of a pheochromocytoma in the right adrenal gland

should be meticulously managed intraoperatively; invasive monitoring should be used, and antihypertensive and antiarrhythmic drugs should be readily available so that blood pressure can be maintained. Anesthetic drugs must be carefully chosen. Halothane is not used because it tends to sensitize the myocardium to the arrhythmic activity of catecholamines. Pancuronium bromide is preferable to succinylcholine or curare. After the tumor has been removed, hypotension can be controlled with transfusions and the administration of either norepinephrine or angiotensin II.

Pheochromocytomas are usually excised through a transabdominal approach, which allows exploration of adrenal glands and the periaortic sympathetic ganglia, the small intestinal mesentery, and the pelvis. The tumor should be gently dissected and manipulated only minimally, and venous drainage should be controlled early to avoid flooding the circulation with an excess of catecholamines (Fig. 24.4). The entire adrenal gland should be removed. Exploration of the contralateral adrenal gland is mandatory in all pediatric patients because of the high incidence of bilateral tumors. If bilateral adrenal tumors are present, both glands should be removed; glucocorticoid and mineralocorticoid replacement will be necessary. The prognosis is usually excellent after surgery, with 100 percent survival rates for patients with benign lesions.

Recent reports indicate that laparoscopic adrenalectomy can be performed when lesions are unilateral and less than 10 cm in diameter. This method lessens postoperative analgesic requirements and shortens hospital stay, although operative time is lengthened.[41]

Children who undergo resection of a pheochromocytoma should be examined at least twice annually for several years, and these examinations should include measurement of blood pressure and assays of urinary catecholamine concentrations. The risk of tumor recurrence is much higher in familial cases, particularly for patients with MEN II. The progeny and siblings of patients with pheochromocytoma also should be periodically evaluated for hypertension because of the high familial incidence of this tumor.

Unresectable malignant tumors or metastatic lesions are usually managed medically for long periods with phenoxybenzamine or alpha-methyltyrosine. Long-term survival has been reported for these patients. Metastatic lesions in bone respond well to radiotherapy. Chemotherapy regimens are similar to those used to treat neuroblastoma; chemotherapy may be used in

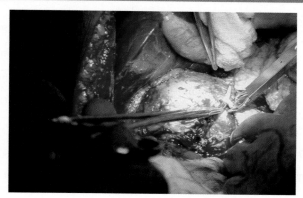

Figure 24.4: Early venous control in an adrenalectomy of a right pheochromocytoma

combination with radiotherapy. MIBG in higher doses has been used for radioablation of metastatic deposits.[42]

REFERENCES

1. Fonkalsrud EW, Dunn J. Adrenal glands, Pediatric Surgery 5th edition, Mosby – Year Book, Inc. Edited by O'Neill JA, Rowe MI, Grosfeld JL, Fonkalsrud EW, Coran AG. 1998;1558-73.
2. Wander JV, Das Gupta TK. Neurofibromatosis. Curr Probl Surg 1977;14:1-81.
3. Ribeiro RC, Michalkiewics EL. Adrenocortical tumors in children. Textbook of Uncommon Cancer 2nd edition, John Wiley & Sons Ltd, Edited by Raghavan D, Brecher ML, Johnson DH,Meropol NJ, Moots PL, Thigpen JT; 1999;611-20.
4. Young JLJ, Ries LG, Silverberg E, Horm JW, Miller RW. Cancer incidence, survival, and mortality for children younger than age 15 years. Cancer 1986;58(2suppl):598-602.
5. Nogeire C, Fukushima DK, Hellman L, Boyar RM. Virilizing adrenal cortical carcinoma. Cancer 1977;40:307-13.
6. Liou LS, Kay R. Adrenocortical carcinoma in children. Review and recent innovations. Urol Clin North Am 2000;27(3):403-21.
7. Li FP, Fraumeni JF Jr. Rhabdomyosarcoma in children: epidemiologic study and identification of a familial cancer syndrome. J Natl Cancer Inst 1969;43:1365-73.
8. Li FP, Fraumeni JF Jr. Prospective study of a family cancer syndrome. JAMA 1982;247:2692-4.
9. Ilvesmaki V, Kahri AI, Miettinen PJ, Voutilainen R. Insulin-like growth factors (IGFs) and their receptors in adrenal tumors: high IGF-II expression in functional adrenocortical carcinomas. J Clin Endocrinol Metab 1993;77:852-8.
10. Mesiano S, Jaffe RB. Interaction of insulin-like growth factor-II and estradiol directs steroidogenesis in the human fetal adrenal toward dehydroepiandrosterone sulfate production. J Clin Endocrinol Metab 1993;77:754-8.
11. Benson PF, Vulliamy DG, Taubman HO. Congenital hemihypertrophy and malignancy. Lancet 1963;1:468.
12. van Seters AP, van Aalderen W, Moolenaar AJ, Gorsiro MC, van Roon F, Backer ET. Adrenocortical tumor in untreated congenital adrenocortical hyperplasia associated with inadequate ACTH suppressibility. Clin Endocrinol 1981;14:325-34.
13. Hough AJ, Hollifield JW, Page DL, Hartmann WH. Prognostic factors in adrenal cortical tumors: a mathematical analysis of clinical and morphologic data. Am J Clin Pathol 1979;72:390-9.

14. Weiss LM, Medeiros LJ, Vickery AL Jr. Pathologic features of prognostic significance in adrenocortical carcinoma. Am J Surg Pathol 1989;13:202-6.

15. Stewart DR, Jones PH, Jolleys A. Carcinoma of the adrenal gland in children. J Pediatr Surg 1974;9:59-67.

16. Gilbert MG, Cleveland WW. Cushing's syndrome in infancy. Pediatrics 1970;46:217-29.

17. Chudler RM, Kay R. Adrenocortical carcinoma in children. Urol Clin North Am 1989;16:469-79.

18. Richie JP, Gittes RF. Carcinoma of the adrenal cortex. Cancer 1980;45:1957-64.

19. Ribeiro J, Ribeiro RC, Fletcher BD. Imaging findings in pediatric adrenocortical carcinoma. Pediatr Radiol 2000;30:45-51.

20. Wajchenberg BL, Albengaria Pereira MA, Medonca BB, et al. Adrenocortical carcinoma: clinical and laboratory observations. Cancer 2000;88(4):711-36.

21. Sadrini R, Ribeiro RC, Lacerda L. Extensive personal experience—childhood adrenocortical tumors. J Clin Endocrinol Metab 1997;82:2027

22. Aldrighetti L, Giacomelli M, Calori G, Pagnelli M, Ferla G. Impact of minimally invasive surgery on adrenalectomy for incidental tumors: comparison with laparotomy technique. Int Surg 1997;82:160-4.

23. Bornstein SR, Stratakis CA, Chrousos GP. Adrenocortical tumors: recent advances in basic concepts and clinical management. Ann Intern Med 1999;130:759-71.

24. MacFarlane DA. Cancer of the adrenal cortex: the natural history, prognosis and treatment in a study of fifty-five cases. Ann R Coll Surg Engl 1958;23:155-65.

25. Sullivan M, Boileau M, Hodges CV. Adrenal cortical carcinoma. J Urol 1978;120:660-5.

26. Lipsett MB, Hertz R, Ross GT. Clinical and pathological aspects of adrenocortical carcinoma. Am J Med 1963;35:374-83.

27. Michalkiewics EL, Sandrini R, Bugg MF, et al. Clinical characteristics of small functioning adrenocortical tumors in children. Med Pediatr Oncol 1997;28:175-8.

28. Kvale WF et al. Present day diagnosis and treatment of pheochromocytoma, JAMA 1957;164:854.

29. Bloom DA, Fonkalsrud EW. Surgical management of pheochromocytoma in children. J Pediatr Surg 1974;9:179-84.

30. Remine WH, Chong GC, van Heerden JA, Sheps SB, Harrison EG Jr. Current management of pheochromocytoma. Ann Surg 1974;179:740-8.

31. Stringel G, Ein SH, Creighton R, Daneman D, Howard N, Filler RM. Pheochromocytoma in children—an update. J Pediatr Surg 1980;15:496-500.

32. Stackpole RH, Melican MM, Uson AC. Pheochromocytoma in children: report of 9 cases and review of first 100 published cases with follow-up studies. J Pediatr 1963;63:315-30.

33. Ein SH, Weitzman S, Thorner P, Seagram CG, Filler RM. Pediatric malignant pheochromocytoma. J Pediatr Surg 1994;29(9):1197-1201.

34. Stratakis CA, Chrousos GP. Adrenal medulla and adrenergic ganglia tumors. Principles and Practice of Pediatric Oncology, 3rd edition, Lippincott William, Edited by Pizzo PA, Poplack DG. 1997;35:963-4.

35. Linehan WM, Lerman MI, Zbar B. Identification of the von Hippel-Lindau (VHL) gene. Its role in renal cancer. JAMA 1995;273:564-70.

36. Caty MG, Coran AG, Geagen M, Thompson NW. Current diagnosis and treatment of pheochromocytoma in children. Experience with 22 consecutive tumors in 14 patients. Arch Surg 1990;125:978-81.

37. Bravo EL, Tarazi RC, Gifford RW, Steward BH. Circulating and urinary catecholamines in pheochromocytoma. Diagnostic and pathophysiologic implications. N Engl J Med 1979;301:682-6.

38. Petrus LV, Hall TR, Boechat MI, et al. The pediatric patient with suspected adrenal neoplasm: which radiological test to use? Med Pediatr Oncol 1992;20:53-7.

39. Shapiro B, Copp JE, Sisson JC, Eyre PL, Wallis J, Beierwaltes WH. Iodine-131 metaio-dobenzylguanidine for the locating of suspected pheochromocytoma: experience in 400 cases. J Nucl Med 1985;26:576-85.

40. Heikkinen ES, Akerblom HK. Diagnostic and operative problems in multiple pheochromo-cytomas. J Pediatr Surg 1977;12:157-63.

41. Prinz RA. A comparison of laparoscopic and open adrenalectomies. Arch Surg 1995;130:489-92.

42. Sisson JC, Shapiro B, Beierwaltes WH, et al. Radio-pharmaceutical treatment of malignant pheochromocytoma. J Nucl Med 1984;25:197-206.

CHAPTER 25

Sandeep Agarwala
Devendra K Gupta

Rhabdomyosarcoma in Children

A malignant tumor of mesenchymal cell origin is called a sacroma. Mesenchymal cells normally mature into skeletal muscle, smooth muscle, fat, fibrous tissue, bone and cartilage. Tumors arising from these soft tissues are uncommon in children, and account for only 6 percent of all the childhood malignancies. More than half (53%) of the soft tissue sarcomas (STS) originate from the striated muscles and are called rhabdomyosarcomas (RMS). The remaining group (47%) consists of a heterogenous collection of subtypes referred to as non-rhabdomyosarcoma soft tissue sarcomas (NRSTS). Pediatric STS shows a striking difference in the incidence as compared to their adult counterparts. RMS, by far the commonest STS in children, is rare in adults. Also, pediatric RMS is commonly of the embryonal histology as compared to pleomorphic variety in adults. Similarly among the NRSTS, malignant fibrous histiocytoma (MFH) comprises the most common histology in adults, but is exceedingly rare in children. Of the MFH also, only the angiomatoid variety, a low-grade lesion of borderline behavior, occurs in children.

Rhabdomyosarcoma (RMS) is thought to arise from immature mesenchymal cells that are committed to skeletal muscle lineage,[1] but these tumors are also known to arise in tissues in which striated muscle is not normally found, such as urinary bladder. Rhabdomyosarcoma was first described by Weber in 1854[2] and is the most common soft tissue sarcoma in children, comprising more than 50 percent of all soft tissue sarcomas.[3] RMS is 7th in frequency, amongst childhood malignancy, after leukemia, central nervous system tumors, lymphomas, neuroblastoma, Wilms' tumor and bone tumors.[4,5]

Among the extracranial solid tumors of childhood, RMS is the third most common neoplasm after neuroblastoma and Wilms' tumor, comprising 15 percent of all solid tumors. Almost two-thirds of cases of RMS are diagnosed in children less than 6 years of age although there is another mid-adolescence peak. It is slightly more common in males than in females (1.3-1.4 : 1).[6] It is ubiquitous occurring almost everywhere but most commonly in the head and neck and the genitourinary areas. There are certain distinctive clusters of features regarding age at diagnosis, site of primary and histology. The head and neck tumors are most common in children younger than 8 years of age and if arising in the orbit, are almost always of embryonal histology. On the other hand the extremity tumors are more commonly seen in adolescents and are more frequently of alveolar histology. Vast majority of cases of RMS occur sporadically but the development of some cases of RMS has been associated with certain familial syndromes, such as neurofibromatosis and Li-Fraumani syndrome.[7]

The tumor spreads locally to invade adjacent structures and may also spread distantly via lymphatics and hematogenous routes. The most frequent sites of distant metastases are regional lymph nodes, lungs, bone marrow, bones, CNS, heart, liver and the breast.[8] Before the onset of combined treatment modalities, surgical extirpation of the primary was the treatment of choice but this often involved radical resections, such as amputations, orbital/pelvic exenterations or radical head and neck dissections.[7] Though these were mutilating surgeries with a lot of morbidity, it had resulted in an overall survival rates of 7 to 14 percent for head and neck tumors, 22 percent for trunk and approximately 70 percent for tumors of the bladder.[9] Radiation therapy had been used for RMS from 1950 onwards,[10] but it became a standard only after 1972.[11] Initially a variety of chemotherapeutic agents were tried as single agents and then combination chemotherapy came into practice from 1961.[12]

In 1972 members of the Children's Cancer Study Group (CCSG) and Pediatric Division of the Southwest Oncology Group, and the Cancer and Acute Leukemia Group B came together to form Intergroup Rhabdomyosarcoma Study (IRS). Till date 4 studies of this group have been conducted: IRS-I (1972-78; 686 patients), IRS-II (1978-84; 999 patients), IRS-III (1984-91; 1062 patients) and IRS-IV (1991-96). IRS-V is in the pilot stages. Pooled data from IRS-I, II and III[13-15] showed that the median age at diagnosis for RMS is 5-years and that almost two-thirds of the cases are diagnosed before 10 years of age. It also showed that the head and neck region was the commonest area involved (Table 25.1) comprising 35 percent of all RMS (parameningeal 16%, orbit 9%, and nonorbital nonparameningeal sites 10%) while the genitourinary was the second commonest site of involvement (26%) and the extremity tumors comprising 19 percent. This combined data showed that almost 45 percent of the cases were in clinical group (CG) III, 14 percent in CG-IV, 21 percent in CG-II, and 20 percent in CG-I.[13-16]

Currently approximately 70 percent of the patients survive for 5 years or more and are probably cured.[3,17] This is credited to the use of multi-modal, risk adapted therapy, refinements in tumor grouping and better supportive care which has emerged out of cooperative studies like IRS. In all likelihood, the molecular analysis of RMS will further refine current classification schemes, and knowledge of genetic features of the tumors will significantly improve the ability of investigators to identify patients at lower or higher risk of treatment failures, thus paving the way for advances in risk-based therapy.

TUMOR BIOLOGY

Chromosomes of this tumor contain both numerical and structural abnormalities.[18,19] In addition embryonal tumors are often hyperploid while the near tetraploid group has strong association with alveolar histology.[20] The tumor cell ploidy is believed by some to have a prognostic significance, with the hyperploidy conferring the best prognosis and diploidy the worst. This may be because the diploid tumors are made up of indolent, slowly growing tumor cells, which respond poorly to cytotoxic drugs. The prognostic implications of ploidy in embryonal and alveolar forms of RMS are controversial, so abnormalities of chromosome numbers have not widely been incorporated into clinical management. Structural chromosomal changes can further distinguish embryonal and alveolar tumors. The embryonal histology is rarely associated with translocations, while the alveolar type is chatacterized by a rearrangement of chromosome 2 and 13, the t(2;13)(q35;q14),[21,22] in which the PAX 3 gene within band 2q35 is fused with the FKHR gene within band 13q14.[23] This chimeric structure functions as an oncoprotein by inappropriately activating PAX 3 transcriptional targets, resulting in dysregulation of cell growth and transformation. The reverse transcriptase polymerase chain reaction (RT-PCR) can detect chimeric mRNA molecules in tumors bearing the t(2;13) rearrangement.[24] Alternatively, fluoroscence *in situ* hybridization (FISH) can be used to detect this.[25,26] Both

Table 25.1: The site of primary tumor with clinical group (CG) distribution in IRS-III[16]					
Site	*Total*	*CG-I*	*CG-II*	*CG-III*	*CG-IV*
Total	1062	213 (20%)	221 (21%)	478 (45%)	150 (14%)
All Head/neck	375(35%)	31(8%)	94(25%)	222(59%)	28(8%)
Orbit	109(10%)	3	46	58	2
Superficial	111(10%)	24	39	43	5
Parameningeal	155(15%)	4	9	121	21
GU (not BP)	167(16%)	89	36	33	9
GU-BP	110(10%)	9	7	88	6
Extremity	202(19%)	64	53	39	46
Others	208(20%)	20	31	96	61

BP = bladder/prostate

these techniques are methods of improved detection of alveolar cells that will aid in the diagnosis and staging. Even though the embryonal tumors lack tumor-specific translocations, they may undergo inactivation of one or more tumor suppressor genes, as indicated by the consistent loss of heterozygosity (LOH) for multiple closely linked loci at chromosome 11p15.5.[8,19,27] It has been shown that this LOH involves the loss of maternal genetic information with duplication of paternal genetic material at this locus.[28] This is also the region where IGF II gene resides. IGF II has been demonstrated to be imprinted with only the paternal allele being transcriptionally active.[29,30] Both alveolar and embryonal RMS appear to over produce IGF II, a growth factor that has been shown to stimulate the unregulated growth of these tumor cells.[31]

PATHOLOGY

Rhabdomyosarcomas are grossly firm, nodular, and of variable size and consistency. They are well circumscribed but not encapsulated, and often tend to infiltrate extensively into adjacent tissues. Sarcoma botryoides subtype has characteristic grape-like appearance with its grape-like clusters of tumors arising from a mucosa lined area. Histologically RMS falls into the broad category of small blue round cell tumor. The standard classification is still the one proposed by Horn and Enterline in 1958[32] which divided the tumor into four subgroups: embryonal, alveolar, botryoid and pleomorphic and noted that botryoid was actually a subtype of embryonal. The histologic distribution of the tumor in IRS-III is shown in Table 25.2. Since there was no overall agreement among the pathologists using the conventional classification therefore an international classification system for childhood RMS was proposed. This international classification system for childhood RMS being used in all new IRS studies beginning IRS-IV (Table 25.3).[33]

The differentiation of tumor type is made by a combination of light microscopy, immunohistochemical techniques, electron microscopy (EM) and molecular genetic techniques; the characteristic feature being the identification of myogenic lineage. This on light microscopy is the identification of cross-striations, characteristic of skeletal muscle, or characteristic rhabdomyoblasts.[35] Cross-striations are seen in 50 to 60 percent of the cases. Histologically *embryonal rhabdomyosarcoma* is composed of rhabdomyoblasts and small round cells. Rhabdomyoblast, the more

mature of the embryonal component, is characterized by bright eosinophilic cytoplasm and may appear in a variety of unusual shapes, termed "tadpole", "racquet" or "strap cells".[15,33] The embryonal type is commoner in children less than 8 years of age and comprise of 70 percent of the head and neck and the genitourinary rhabdomyosarcomas. *Sarcoma botryoides* is a morphologic variant of the embryonal RMS and often found in mucosa lined organs of the nasopharynx, auditory canal, genitourinary tract and the gastrointestinal regions, especially in the cavitatory structures. The polypoidal mass is composed of a subepithelial arrangement of tumor cells known as cambium layer.[15,33] This layer of small round cells surrounding a loose myxoid stroma and a central zone of round and spindle shaped cells more typical of the embryonal type. This subtype typically occurs under 4 years of age and is associated with the best outcome. Another subtype of embryonal RMS, the *spindle cell variant or the liomyomatous variant* is seen in the cases of paratesticular RMS predominantly and is also associated with a favorable outcome. This spindle cell variant may occasionally be seen in the orbit and the extremities.[36]

Alveolar RMS consists of rhabdomyoblasts mixed with a larger round cells with prominent eosinophilic cytoplasm. The tumor grows in cords and produces cleft-like spaces, namely alveoli. These fibrovascular spaces

Table 25.2: Histologic distribution in IRS-III[16]	
Histologic type	*Percentage*
Embryonal	59.4%
Alveolar	18.5%
Pleomorphic	0.5%
Undifferentiated	0.5%
RMS, type undetermined	13%
Extraosseous Ewing's sarcoma*	3.6%

RMS = rhabdomyosarcoma
* No longer defined as rhabdomyosarcoma

Table 25.3: International classification system for childhood rhabdomyosarcomas[34]	
I	Superior prognosis
	a) Botryoid
	b) Spindle cell
II	Intermediate prognosis
	a) Embryonal
III	Poor prognosis
	a) Alveolar
	b) Undifferentiated sarcomas

contain free floating monomorphous round malignant cells with abundant eosinophilic cytoplasm.[15,33] Even the presence of scattered foci of this alveolar pattern is adequate to exert an adverse influence on the clinical outcome and is considered sufficient to warrant it being classified as alveolar tumor. The alveolar histology is second in frequency and occurs more commonly in the extremities, trunk and the perineal areas. This type and the undifferentiated type have poor prognosis. Tumors, which have similar features as the alveolar type but lack classical clefts, are termed as *a solid variant* of alveolar RMS and have been associated with poorer prognosis.[36] This solid variant has been recently recognized on the basis of a storiform growth pattern with low cellularity and a paucity of round rhabdomyoblasts. The importance of the solid variant is that it can be easily mistaken for embryonal histology. The *pleomorphic RMS*, which is extremely rare in children show anaplastic cells present in large aggregates or as diffuse sheets.[37] It occurs in the extermities and the trunk.

Electron microscopy and immunohistochemical analysis of tumors are now useful tools for demonstrating characteristics of RMS, especially when light microscopy is inconclusive. The diagnostic EM features of RMS include visible z-bands, z-bands with or without insertion of thick and thin filaments, thick and thin filaments in hexagonal array, and an "Indian file" arrangement of the ribosome/myosin complexes.[15,38] Skeletal muscle or muscle-specific proteins, like antidesmin, muscle-specific actin and Myo D can be identified by immuno-histochemical staining. Monoclonal antibodies, like those to desmin, muscle-specific actin, sarcomeric actin and myoglogin have also been used to confirm the myogenic lineage with very good specificity and sensitivity.[15] Monoclonal antibodies against Myo D can be used in frozen section analysis also.[39]

Pooled data of IRS I, II, and III show that the 5-year survival is related to the histology with 95 percent survival for sarcoma botryoides, 75 percent for pleomorphic sarcoma, 66 percent for embryonal, 54 percent for alveolar and 40 percent for undifferentiated sarcomas.[3,14,17,33] There is conflicting evidence concerning the prognostic significance of histology and the importance of establishing the histologic subtypes. This is because analysis of large numbers of patients suggests that site, which is associated with histologic subtype, is an independent prognostic factor and histology is a prognostic factor only because of its association with site and other risk factors. The IRS-IV report on non-metastatic RMS showed a 3-year failure free survival rates of 83 percent for embryonal RMS,

66 percent for alveolar, 55 percent for undifferentiated and 66 percent for other sarcomas.[4]

STAGING

It is critical to assess the extent of tumor in every patient as the therapy and prognosis depends on the degree to which the mass has spread beyond the primary site. Several surgico-pathologic staging systems have been used historically,[40,41] but the clinical group staging system, developed by IRS in 1972 has been most widely used (Table 25.4).[3]

This recognizes four major categories of disease based on the amount of tumor remaining after initial surgery and the degree of tumor dissemination at the time of diagnosis.[3] This surgical staging may vary with operation techniques, and it excludes other important prognostic factors such as tumor size and site, IRS committee has now adopted a modification of the so-called TNM system.[7,42,43] This system (Table 25.5), modified for site of origin, is now the current system used in IRS-IV, which opened in 1992. The attractiveness of this approach is that it is less dependent on potentially subjective factors, such as the skill or aggressiveness of the operating surgeon, and is more reflective of the intrinsic biologic properties of the tumor. Most contemporary studies of RMS have relied on both the IRS clinical grouping system and the modified TNM staging (Table 25.5) to assign therapy and evaluate outcome.

Table 25.4: Clinical grouping system used by the IRS-I through III[3]

Group I: *Localized disease, completely resected*
    A Confined to the organ or muscle of origin
    B Infiltration outside organ or muscle of origin; regional nodes not involved

Group II: *Total gross resection with evidence of regional spread*
    A Grossly resected tumors with "microscopic" residual tumor
    B Regional disease completely resected with regional nodes involved, tumor extension into adjacent organs or both

Group III: *Incomplete resection or biopsy with gross residual disease remaining*
    A Localized or locally extensive tumor, gross residual disease after biopsy only
    B Localized or locally extensive tumor, gross residual disease after "major" resection (> 50% debulking)

Group IV: *Any size primary tumor, with or without regional lymph node involvement, with distant metastases, irrespective of surgical approach to the primary tumor*

Table 25.5: TNM pretreatment staging classification[7]

Staging prior to treatment requires thorough clinical examination and laboratory and imaging examinations. Biopsy is required to establish the histologic diagnosis. Pretreatment size is determined by external measurement or MRI or CT, depending upon the anatomic location. For less accessible primary sites, CT is employed as a means of lymphnode assessment as well. Metastatic sites require some form of imaging (but not histologic confirmation, except for bone marrow examination) confirmation

Stage	Sites	T	Size	N	M
1	Favorable	T_1 or T_2	a or b	N_0 or N_1 or N_x	M_0
2	Unfavorable	T_1 or T_2	a	N_0 or N_x	M_0
3	Unfavorable	T_1 or T_2	a	N_1	M_0
			b	N_0 or N_1 or N_x	M_0
4	Either	T_1 or T_2	a or b	N_0 or N_1	M_1

Definitions:
Site:
Favorable sites are orbit, head and neck (excluding parameningeal) or genitourinary (excluding bladder/prostate)
Unfavorable sites are bladder/prostate, parameningeal, extrimities, trunk and all others
Tumor:
T_1 = Tumor confined to anatomic site of origin
    a) Less than or equal to 5 cm in diameter
    b) Greater than 5 cm in diameter
T_2 = Extension and/or fixation to surrounding tissues
    a) Less than or equal to 5 cm in diameter
    b) Greater than 5 cm in diameter
Regional nodes:
N_0 = Regional nodes not clinically involved
N_1 = Regional nodes clinically involved by tumor
N_x = Clinical status of regional nodes unknown (specially sites which preclude
    lymph node evaluation)
Metastasis:
M_0 = No distant metastases
M_1 = Metastases present

In this system for localized tumors, the site and size (widest diameter) of the tumor are of primary importance, as is the presence or absence of macroscopic invasion into the adjacent structures. Therefore larger tumors (>5 cm) arising at unfavorable sites are upstaged to stage 3 (independent of LN status). Clinical involvement of LN results in upstaging (i.e. from stage 2 to 3) of small (< 5 cm) localized tumors arising in unfavorable sites (extremities, trunk, retroperitoneum, bladder/prostate and parameningeal) but does not affect the staging of tumors arising in favorable locations (orbit, non-parameningeal head and neck, paratesticular, vulva, vagina-uterus). This site based TNM staging is highly predictive of outcome,[13,42,44] and so the histologic subtype is no longer a factor considered in the staging. The IRS-IV report on non-metastatic RMS showed that 51 percent of the tumors were locally invasive (T_2), 51 percent were more than 5 cm in size (b), 80 percent were N_0, 15 percent N_1 and 5 percent N_x.[4]

The clinical work-up is a vital part of the overall management of rhabdomyosarcoma. The primary site, tumor size, and extent of disease must all be accurately determined, and adequate tissue must be provided for histologic, histochemical, electron microscopic and genetic studies. Diagnostic imaging should include both PA and lateral chest X-rays and CT scan and MRI of the primary tumor. Bone marrow examinations are also essential as are complete blood chemistries and blood counts to evaluate organ failure.

PATTERNS OF SPREAD

Fewer than 25 percent of the newly diagnosed patients have distant metastases, and almost half of those have only a single site of involvement (mostly one or more pulmonary metastases). The lung is the most frequent site of metastases (40-50%) (Fig. 25.1); Less common sites, either isolated or in conjunction with multi-

Table 25.7: Outline of the pulse VAC regimen for chemotherapy of RMS[7]

1. Vincristine- 2 mg/m^2 , IV weekly for 13 doses (covering 12 weeks), starting Day 0 (maximum dose = 2 mg), followed by a dose at week 16
2. Actinomycin D- 0.015 mg/kg/day, IV, weekly for 5 days, starting Day 0, Day 84 (week-12), Day 112 (week-16) (maximun dose = 0.5 mg)
3. Cyclophosphamide- 10 mg/kg/day, IV for 3 days starting Day 0, Day 84 (week-12), and Day 112 (week-16). Also one dose of 20 mg/kg*,IV, is given on Days 21,42, and 63 (weeks-3,6,9). Cyclophosphamide should be omitted on Days 42 and 63 in children who have the urinary bladder included in the radiation portal, or who will have large volumes or bone marrow irradiated, such as irradiation to the whole abdomen, including the pelvic bones
4. Radiotherapy is given to the tumor bed as well as to any sites of metastasis starting Day 42 (week-6)
5. Starting week-20, the following course is repeated every 4 weeks through week 104:
   Vincristine- 2mg/m^2, IV on Days 0 and 4 (max. single dose = 2mg)
   Actinomycin D- 0.015mg/kg/day, IV for 5 days starting Day 0 (max dose = 0.5 mg).
   Cyclophosphamide- 10 mg/kg/day,IV for 3 days, starting Day 0*

- *In IRS-IV, the dose of cyclophsophamide is 2.2 gm/m^2 per course given as an infusion. Mesna 450 mg/m^2, IV is given before and then every 3 hours for three doses following the cyclophosphamide dose*
- *Drug doses are reduced 50 percent in children < 1 year of age. If the drugs are tolerated, the doses are increased to 75 percent and then to 100 percent*

Table 25.8: Five-year survival rates as reported by IRS-III[7]

Site	CG-I/II/III	CG-IV
Orbit	95%	50%
Parameningel	74%	43%
Superficial (non-parameningeal Head and neck)	78%	40%
GU-non BP	89%	56%
GU- BP	81%	33%
Extremity	74%	28%
Others	67%	22%

CG—clinical grouping; GU—genitourinary; BP—bladder/prostate

The goal of identifying additional active agents is to be able to incorporate as many active agents as possible, without overlapping toxicities, to avoid the development of multidrug resistance. Additional agents like cisplatin, etoposide (VP-16) and dacarbazine (DTIC) have also been shown to be effective.[43] Trials with (i) carboplatin+ ADR+ ifosfamide +ACD or (ii) Ifosfamide+ ACD+ VCR have also been conducted for patients with advanced disease.[61,64] In IRS-IV stage 4 patients were to receive one of the three drug pairs (ADR+ ifosfamide or VCR+ melphlan or ifosfamide+ etoposide) before standard VAC regime was given.[65] Among the most promising new agents for treatment of RMS are Topotecan and Paclitaxel. For non-metastasic RMS, IRS-IV concluded that VAC+surgery+C-RT was the gold standard therapy.[4]

With the availability of combinations of hemopoietic growth factors, such as recombinant human granulocyte colony-stimulating factor (G-CSF) and the recently cloned "thromboprotein" to ameliorate myelotoxicity, an increased intensity of chemotherapy dose is feasible.

CLINICAL PRESENTATIONS AND MANAGEMENT FOR SPECIFIC SITES

The clinically evident signs and symptoms of RMS are in two main ways: The appearance of a mass lesion and disturbance of a normal body function by an unsuspected, critically located enlarging mass.

Head and Neck

The head and neck tumors are further divided into those that arise in the paramengeal region (50%) (Figs 25.2A and B), orbit (25%) (Fig. 25.3) and head and neck

kg/day for 3 days). One of the main questions that IRS-IV was attempting to answer in patients with non-metastatic RMS, is the comparasion of VAC vs VAI (VCR+ ACD+ ifosfamide) vs VIE (VCR+ ifosfamide+ etoposide). This randomization should permit direct comparison of efficacy of equitoxic doses of cyclophosphamide and ifosfamide in ACD containing regimes as well as ifosfamide-etoposide in the ifosfamide-ACD regimen. For non-metastatic RMS, the IRS-IV study[4] concluded that 3 year estimated failure free survival rates for VAC, VAI and VIE were 75, 77, and 77 percent respectively which was not significantly different. The overall survival rates for VAC, VAI and VIE were 84, 84 and 88 percent which was also not significant (p= 0.63). The result of treatment according to the site of primary and CG as reported by IRS-III is shown in Table 25.8.

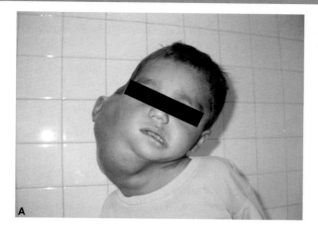

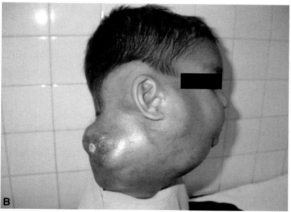

Figures 25.2A and B: Head and neck (parameningeal) RMS involving the mastoid region with intracranial extension and extension into the external auditory canal

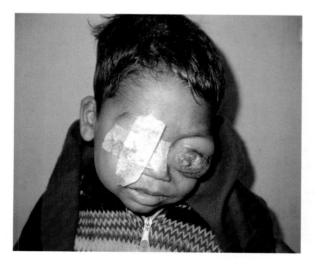

Figures 25.3: Head and neck (orbital) RMS

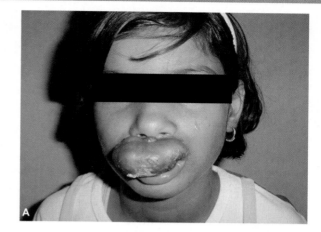

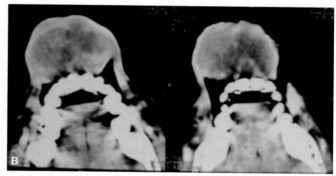

Figures 25.4A and B: (A) Head and neck (superficial) RMS involving the upper lip, **(B)** CECT scan of the same patient showing extensive involvement of the upper lip

superficial (Figs 25.4A and B), i.e. non-parameningeal (25%) (Table 25.9).[60]

Orbital RMS produces proptosis, chemosis, eyelid or conjunctival mass, opthalmoplegia and rarely blindness. These are usually diagnosed early before distant dissemination has occurred. Distant dissemination is late in orbital RMS because of tumor confinement by the bony orbit and the paucity of lymphatics. Parameningeal tumors usually cause nasal, aural or sinus obstruction. These are often associated with cranial bone erosions that can manifest as cranial nerve palsies. Erosion of contiguous bone at the cranial base and intracranial extension may lead to headache, vomiting, and systemic hypertension.[53,66] Nasophranygeal tumors can cause voice changes, airway obstruction, dysphagia and epistaxis while sinus tumor can be painful in addition to be having persistent nasal discharge and occasion epistaxis. Tumors of the middle ear or mastoid can present as a polypoidal growth from the ear, otitis media or facial palsy. Laryngeal tumors can present with hoarseness. Regional lymph node metastases to cervical

Table 25.9: Head and neck sites of rhabdomyosarcomas[60]

Category	Frequency	Specific sites
Parameningeal	50%	Nasopharynx, paranasal sinuses, middle ear, mastoid, pterygoid-infratemporal sites
Orbit	25%	Orbit and eyelid
Head and neck Superficial (non-parameningeal)	25%	Scalp, external ear, parotid, face, buccal mucosa, pharynx, larynx, tonsils, neck

lymph nodes may be present in up to 20 percent cases depending on the site. Distant metastasis is primarily to the lungs or the bones.[67] While the orbital tumors have very good prognosis, the parameningeal tumors have the poorest prognosis.

For orbital tumors non-excisional therapy is standard. Initial biopsy followed by chemotherapy and radiation leads to survival rates of > 90 percent (see Table. 25.8). IRS-IV study reported 3 year estimated failure free survival rates of 89 percent and overall survival rate of 100 percent for CG-I and II orbital and eyelid RMS.[4] Routine lymph node sampling is not indicated, as incidence of nodal spread is only 3 percent. Orbital exenteration is now recommended only for recurrent disease. Non-orbital, non-parameningeal tumors head and neck tumors (superficial) are mostly unresectable. These patients are best managed by an incisional biopsy followed by chemotherapy appropriate for their group.[16] Cervical lymph node dissection is not warranted, however, the clinically suspicious nodes must be biopsied, and if histologically positive they must be included in the RT portal. The 5-year survival rates are approximately 80 percent (see Table 25.8). Parameningeal tumors are at high risk for direct intracranial extension and may require RT right at the onset (Day 0), especially if there is bony erosion, cranial nerve palsy, or intracranial extension at presentation. These patients are treated with systemic chemotherapy and RT according to the group. RT is also necessary for the spinal cord if CSF is +ve for tumor cells. In addition, these patients with CSF +ve also need to be given intra-thecal chemotherapy (triple agent).[68] The 5-year survival rate is almost 70 percent for non-metastatic disease, but only 43 percent for metastatic disease (see Table 25.8).

Genitourinary Tract (GU)

These tumors arise in the bladder (Figs 25.5A and B), prostate, vagina, uterus, vulva (Fig. 25.6), paratesticular regions, and rarely the kidneys and ureter and constitute nearly 26 percent of all RMS cases (see Table 25.1). The embryonal histology is the commonest in this region and the most frequent of the GU RMS are those of the bladder/prostate (see Table 25.1). Within this category of genitourinary rhabdomyosarcomas are tumors with good prognosis, namely vulva, vagina and paratesticular and those with poorer prognosis, namely bladder and prostate. The bladder tumors usually grow intra-

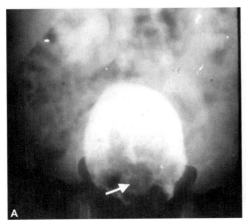
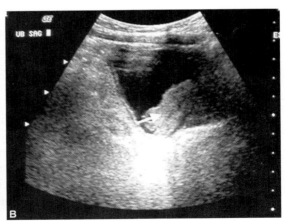

Figures 25.5A and B: (A) Micturating cystourethrogram showing RMS involving the bladder base, **(B)** Ultrasound of a patient with RMS of the bladder base and prostate

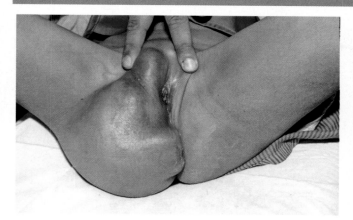

Figure 25.6: Genitourinary RMS involving the vulva in a girl

luminally, in the region of the trigone, and have a polypoidal appearance on gross or endoscopic examination. Tumors arising from the dome of the bladder (Figs 25.7A to C) are uncommon as compared to those from the trigone (Figs 25.8A to D and 25.9A to C), but the dome tumors have a better outcome. Children with bladder RMS are usually under four years of age and may present with hematuria, urinary obstruction, and rarely extrusion of tumor tissue. Prostatic tumors can occur in relatively older children and usually present as large pelvic masses with or without urethral strangury and/or constipation. Bladder tumors tend to remain localized while the prostatic tumors often disseminate early to lungs, bones and bone marrow.[69,70]

In the IRS-I the treatment used to be radical surgical removal (pelvic exenteration and total cystectomy) for bladder/prostate tumors. This gave excellent rates of local control but the morbidity of these operations was unacceptable and therefore now a conservative surgical approach in addition to adjuvant chemotherapy and RT is used.[71-74] IRS-IV recommends (Table 25.10) initial endoscopic, perineal or suprapubic diagnostic biopsy followed by intensive chemotherapy and early RT.[42] Initial complete resection is done only for those patients who have a tumor of the dome of the bladder and in whom the preservation of bladder and urethral function can be assured (Fig. 25.7). Anterior pelvic exenteration and total cystectomy is reserved for patients who do not achieve local control after chemotherapy and RT. Currently, 60 percent of the patients retain a functional bladder and the overall survival rate exceeds 85 percent (see Table 25.8).[73,74]

Paratesticular RMS arises in the distal area of the spermatic cord and may invade the testis and the surrounding tissues. These usually present as a unilateral painless scrotal swelling or a mass above the testis in pre or post-pubertal boys. Almost 30 percent of the paratesticular tumors are of the spindle cell variety which has an excellent prognosis.[7] Preoperative evaluation should include CT scan of the abdomen and pelvis to evaluate RPLN. Initial inguinal orchiectomy with the removal of the entire spermatic cord should be done. Scrotal voilation or trans-scrotal biopsy should be

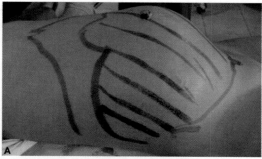

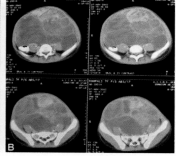

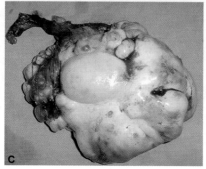

Figures 25.7A to C: A patient with RMS involving the fundus of the urinary bladder presenting as a large hypogastric mass **(A)** CECT scan of the same patient showing a large mass with variable attenuation and areas of necrosis **(B),** The gross specimen of the same patient after excision of the mass with a small portion of the dome of the bladder **(C)**

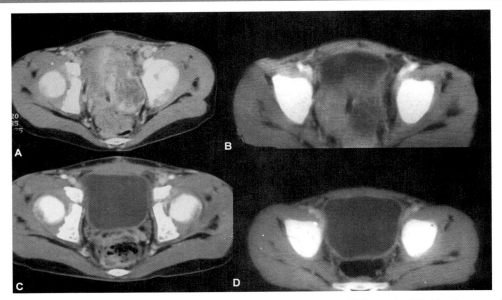

Figures 25.8A to D: (A and B) CECT scan of a patient showing RMS of the bladder base and the prostate [white arrow marking the compressed bladder neck and urethra], (**C** and **D**) the CECT scan of the same patient showing complete resolution following the chemotherapy and radiotherapy

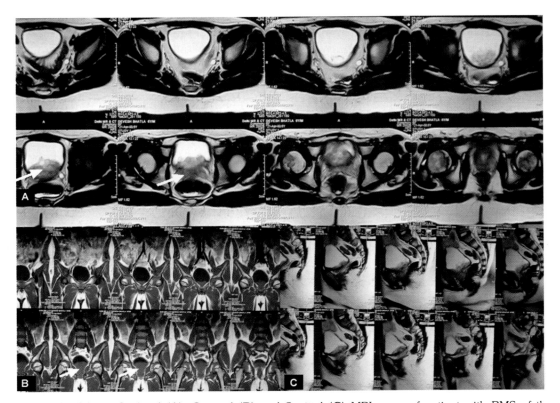

Figures 25.9A to C: Axial (**A**), Coronal (**B**) and Sagittal (**C**) MRI scans of patient with RMS of the bladder base and the prostate

Table 25.10: IRS-IV recommendation for treatment of RMS in childhood

Site	TNM	CG	Radiation therapy	Chemotherapy	Surgical
Orbit	1	I	None	VA × 32 weeks	Biopsy only
		II	4140 cGy CFI (starting week 9)	VA	
		III	5040 cGy HFI vs 5940 cGy HFI (starting week 9)	VAC × 52 weeks vs VAI × 52 weeks	
Non-parameningeal	1	I	None	VAC vs VAI vs VIE	Wide excision if possible, LN biopsy if clinically +ve
		II	4140 cGy CFI		
		III	5040 cGy CFI vs 5040 cGY HFI		
Paratesticular	1	I	None	VA	Inguinal orchidectomy
		II	4140 cGY CFI	VAC vs VAI vs VIE	
		III	5040 cGY CFI vs 5940 cGY HFI		
Vulua and vagina	1	I	None	VAC vs VAI vs VIE	Biopsy initially then 2nd look at week 9 and RT if +ve
		II	4140 cGY CFI		
		III	5040 cGY CFI		
Uterus	1	I	None	VAC vs VAI vs VIE	
		II	4140 cGY CFI		
		III	5040 cGY CFI vs 5940 cGY HFI		
Parameningeal/extremity/GU-BP/chest wall/trunk/retroperitoneum/others	2/3	I	None of TNM stage 2 4140 cGY CFI for Stage 3	VAC vs VAI vs VIE	Resection rarely feasible, begin RT Day 0 or week 9[1]
		II	4140 cGY CFI		
		III	5040 cGY CFI vs 5940 cGY HFI		
Any site	4	I	4140 cGY CFI	Trial combinations	See text
		II	4140 cGY CFI		
		III	5040 cGY CFI		

V—Vincristine; A—Actinomycin D; C—Cyclophosphamide; E—Etoposide; I—Ifosfamide; CFI—Conventional fractionation; HFI—Hyperfractionation

avoided to prevent scrotal contamination. In case there is scrotal voilation then hemiscrotectomy should be done to prevent metastases to the inguinal nodes (which are considered distant metastases and not local). Dissemination to retroperitoneal lymph nodes (RPLN) from paratesticular tumors is clinically (and on CT scan)

seen in 17 percent cases and pathologically in 27 percent.[7] Because of this it is advisable to do ipsilateral RPLN sampling in all cases of paratesticular tumors. Now, because of the availability of sensitive imaging techniques like spiral CT and MRI, IRS-IV does not recommend routine RPLN dissection for patients with completely resected localized tumors and negative imaging studies. The survival rates are now around 90 percent with adjuvant chemotherapy and RT directed to known nodal or residual disease.[75,76] In IRS-III the 5-year survival rate was 91 percent.[76] IRS-IV reaported a 3 year estimated failure free survival rate of 81 percent and 3 year survival rate of 90 percent for CG-I paratesticular RMS.[4]

Vaginal tumors present at a younger age than those of the uterine (mean age 2 years vs 14 years). Vaginal RMS is usually of the botryoid variety and present as mucosanguinous discharge, bleeding or a prolapsing polypoidal mass. Cervical and uterine sarcomas are diagnosed in older children who present with a mass and history of vaginal discharge. At present the IRS approach (see Table 25.9) is biopsy, to confirm diagnosis, cystoscopy, and CT scan of the pelvis to rule out local spread. Chemotherapy is followed by repeat vaginal examinations and biopsy without resectional surgery. Persistent disease is managed by local limited resection or partial vaginectomy. Uterine tumors are also initially treated with chemotherapy and second look surgery and radical resection (hysterectomy + proximal vaginectomy) is required only for gross residual disease who have failed to achieve a complete radiographic response within 6 months of induction chemotherapy and RT, or those who have early progression.[43]

Extremities

RMS involving the extremities comprises 19 percent of all RMS (see Table 25.1) and are characterized by a swelling in the affected body part (Figs 25.10A and B). They involve the lower extremity more than the upper and distal limb involvement is more common than proximal. Pain, tenderness and redness may occur and almost 45 percent of these are of alveolar histology.[77] Limb sparing, wide resection of the tumor is recommended whenever feasible and without loss of function since excision results in improved results.[78] Amputation should be avoided. Since more than one-fourth of these patients have metastases to the regional lymph nodes therefore IRS-IV recommends routine LN sampling, even if clinically negative. Positive lymph nodes warrant their inclusion in the RT portal. Involvement of ipsilateral supraclavicular LN for upper extremity tumors and of the iliac or para-aortic nodes for lower extremity tumors is considered distant metastases (stage-4). If surgical margins are microscopically positive the re-excision should be done prior to chemotherapy and RT.[56] Postoperatively all patients get chemotherapy and radiotherapy. The survival rate was 80 percent when lymph nodes were not involved as compared to 46 percent when involved.[78] There is also an increased rate of distant metastases when regional LN was involved.[79]

Retroperitoneum

Retroperitoneal (RP) tumors, excluding the genitourinary tract, account for 11 percent of cases, and can be either embryonal or alveolar. Complete resection of these tumors is often impossible for technical reasons and regional LN are often involved and distant metastases present at the time of diagnosis. Treatment includes chemotherapy and RT according to the clinical grouping. Patients with RP-RMS have the worst prognosis with a 5-year survival rate, of non-metastatic tumor, being only 50 percent.

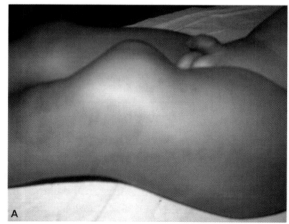 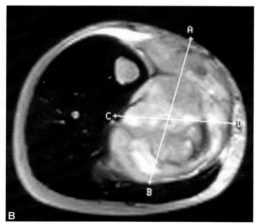

Figure 25.10A and B: (A) RMS (Extremity) involving the left quadriceps, **(B)** MRI scan of a child with undifferentiated RMS (extremity) involving the posterior compartment muscles of the calf

Trunk

These sites include tumors of the chest wall, paraspinal region (Figs 25.11A and B) and the abdominal wall in decreasing order of frequency and constitute 10 percent of all cases of RMS. Most of these are of alveolar histology and less than 30 percent are amenable to complete resection at diagnosis.[7] Whenever excised they have a tendency to local recurrence. Treatment includes chemotherapy and RT according to the clinical grouping.

COMPLICATIONS OF THERAPY

These include residual effects of operative management, radiotherapy, and chemotherapy. As the extent of surgical resection has a bearing on functional outcome, more and more conservative surgical approaches are being tried. Amputations, extensive lymph node dissections, and exenterations are now rarely resorted to. Infants tend to develop more chemotherapy related toxicities, like infections, anemia and bleeding, than older children. Combined therapy with drugs and irradiation can produce severe fibrosis and limitation of function in the irradiated sites. For example nearly 25 percent of those children with RMS of bladder prostate who do retain their bladders suffer from significant bladder dysfunction in the form of incontinence, frequency and nocturnal enuresis. All these patients are also at risk for hematuria, structural renal abnormalities and delayed growth and pubertal development requiring sex hormone replacement therapy. The incidence of hematuria after cyclophosphamide therapy can increase as much as four-fold if pelvic irradiation is used. The current use of Mesna has nearly eliminated this life-threatening complication. Infertility can result from effects of cyclophosphamide, radiotherapy, or the surgical intervention in the pelvic area. Ifosfamide is well known for nephrotoxicity with an overall incidence of 14 percent. The commonest is renal tubular dysfunction with aminoaciduria, glycosuria, cation leakage, increased serum creatinine, and acidosis and growth failure.

The most dreaded long-term complication is the development of second malignancy. These are usually bone sarcoma, leukemia or myelodysplastic syndrome.

FUTURE DEVELOPMENTS

The recent advances in understanding the biologic and genetic features of RMS as well as better scheduling of drugs have improved the survival of these children with RMS. The newly developed hemopoietic growth factors allow for further dose intensification that is likely to improve the outcome for metastatic and recurrent disease. The development of risk-based therapies is probably the most important strategy to minimize the late treatment related complications. While the children with low risk tumors are being treated with lesser drugs, the children with adverse prognostic factors are being treated with more and more intensive and complex therapies. Recently recognized translocation specific gene product (PAX 3-FKHR and PAX 7-FKHR) in alveolar RMS may provide molecular targets for future therapies. A relatively new approach in the treatment of many solid tumors is the use of angiogenic inhibitors. Many such compounds are currently being developed. Compounds like irinotecan and topotecan are being tried clinically and have demonstrated to have significant anti-angiogenic activity.

The ultimate goal of all these therapeutic maneuvers is the identification of better treatments, i.e. those that achieve maximum long-term survival with minimum short and long-term morbidity.

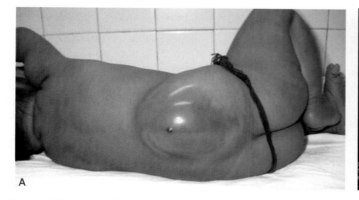 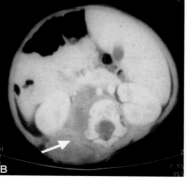

Figure 25.11A and B: (A) An infant with RMS (truncal) involving the left erector spinae muscles, **(B)** CECT scan of a child with alveolar RMS (truncal) involving the right erector spinae muscles

REFERENCES

1. Ruymann FB. Rhabdomyosarcoma in children and adolescents: a review. Hematol Oncol Clin North Am 1987;1:621.
2. Weber CO. Anatomische Unterschung einer zunge Nebst Bemerkungen 3 Uber de Neubildung quergestreiter Muskelfasern. Virchows Acrh Pathol Anat 1854;7:115.
3. Maurer HM, Beltangady M, Gehan EA, Crist W, Hammond D, Hays D, et al. The Intergroup Rhabdomyosarcoma Study-I: A final report. Cancer 1988;61:209-20.
4. Crist WM, Anderson JR, Meza JL, Freyer C, Raney RB, Ruymann FB, et al. Intergroup rhabdomyosarcoma study-IV: Results for patients with non-metastatic disease. J Clin Oncol 2001;19:3091-102.
5. Young JL, Miller RW. Incidence of malignant tumors in US children. J Pediatr 1975;86:254.
6. Maurer HM, Moon T, Donaldson M, Fernandez C, Gehan EA, Hammond D, et al. The Intergroup rhabdomyosarcoma Study: a preliminary report. Cancer 1977;40:2015.
7. Maurer HM, Donaldson SS, Wiener ES. Rhabdomyosarcoma in children. In Holland JF, Bast RC (Jr), Morton DL, et al (Eds): Cancer Medicine 4th edition, Wilams and Wilkins, Baltimore 1997;3023-34.
8. Ruymann FB, Newton WA, Ragab A, Donaldson MH, Foulkes M. Bone marrow metastasis at diagnosis in children and adolescents with rhabdomyosarcoma: a report from the Intergroup Rhabdomyosarcoma Study. Cancer 1984;53:368.
9. Green DM, Jaffe N. Progress and controversy in the treatment of childhood rhabdomyosarcoma. Cancer Treat Rev 1978;5:7.
10. Stobbe GC, Dragoon HW. Embryonal rhabdomyosarcoma of the head and neck in children and adolescents. Cancer 1950;3:826.
11. Sagerman RH, Tretter P, Ellsworth RM. The treatment of orbital rhabdomyosarcoma of children with primary radiation therapy. Am J Roentgenol Rad Ther Nucl Med 1972;114:31.
12. Pinkel D, Pickren J. Rhabdomyosarcoma in children. JAMA 1961;175:293.
13. Rodary C, Gehan EA, Flamant F, et al. Prognostic factors in 951 non-metastatic rhabdomyosarcoma in children: a report of the Intergroup Rhabdomyosarcoma Workshop. Med Pediatr Oncol 1991;19:89.
14. Newton WA, Soule EH, Hamoudi AB, Reiman HM, Shimada H, Beltangady M, Maurer HM. Histopathology of childhood sarcomas, Intergroup Rhabdomyosarcoma Studies I and II: clinicopathologic correlation. J Clin Oncol 1988;6:67.
15. Tsokos M. The diagnosis and classification of childhood rhabdomyosarcoma. Semin Diagn Pathol 1994;11:26-38.
16. Crist W, Gehan EA, Ragab AH, et al. The third Intergroup Rhabdomyosarcoma Study (IRS-III). J Clin Oncol 1995;13:610.
17. Maurer HM, Gehan EA, Beltangady M, Crist W, Dickman PS, Donaldson S, et al. The Intergroup Rhabdomyosarcoma Study II. Cancer 1993;71:1904-22.
18. Pappo AS, Crist WM, Kuttesch J, et al. Tumor cell DNA content predicts outcome in children and adolescents with clinical group III embryonal rhabdomyosarcoma. J Clin Oncol 1993;11:1901-5.
19. Scrable H, Witte D, Shimada H, et al. Molecular differential pathology of rhabdomyosarcoma. Genes Chromosomes Cancer 1989;1:23-35.
20. Shapiro DN, Parham DM, Douglass EC, Ashourn R, Webber BL, Newton WA Jr, et al. Relationship of tumor cell ploidy to histologic subtype and treatment outcome in children and adolescents with unresectable rhabdomyosarcoma. J Clin Oncol 1991;9:159.
21. Douglass EC, Rowe ST, Valentine M, et al. Variant translocations of chromosome 13 in alveolar rhabdomyosarcoma. Genes Chromosomes Cancer 1991;3:480.
22. Douglass EC, Valentine M, Etcubanas E, Parham D, Webber BL, Houghton PJ, et al. A specific chromosomal abnormality in rhabdomyosarcoma. Cytogenet Cell Genet 1987;45:148.
23. Shapiro DN, Sublett JE, Li B, et al. Fusion of PAX3 to a member of the forkhead family of transcription factors in human alveolar rhabdomyosarcoma. Cancer Res 1998;53:5108-12.
24. Downing JR, Khanderkar A, Shurltleff SA, et al. A multiplex RT-PCR assay for the differential diagnosis of alveolar rhabdomyosarcoma versus Ewing's sarcoma. Am J Pathol 1995;146:626-34.
25. Downing JR, Head DR, Parham DM, et al. Detection of the (11;22)(q24;q12) translocation of Ewing's sarcoma and peripheral neuroectodermal tumor by reverse transcription polymerase chain reaction. Am J Pathol 1993;143:1294-300.
26. Barr FG, Galili N, Holick J, et al. Rearrangement of PAX3 paired box gene in the pediatric solid tumor alveolar rhabdomyosarcoma. Nat Genet 1993;3:113-7.
27. Koufos A, Hansen MF, Copeland NG, Jenkins NA, Lampkin BC, Cavanee WK. Loss of heterozygosity in three embryonal tumors suggest a common pathogenetic mechanism. Nature 1985;316:330.
28. Scrable H, Cavanee W, Ghavimi F, et al. Molecular differential pathology of rhabdomyosarcoma tumorigenesis that involves genome imprinting. Proc Natl Acad Sci. USA 1989;86:7480.
29. Rainier S, Johnson LA, Dorby CJ, et al. Relaxation of imprinted genes in human cancer. Nature 1993;362:747.
30. Ogawa O, Eccles MR, Szeto J, et al. Relaxation of insulin like growth factor II gene imprinting implicated in Wilms' tumor. Nature 1993;362:749.
31. El-Bardy OM, Minniti C, Kohn EC, et al. Insulin-like growth factor II acts as an autocrine growth and motility factor in human rhabdomyosarcoma tumors. Cell Growth Differ 1990;1:325.
32. Horn RC, Enterline HT. Rhabdomyosarcoma: a clinicopathologic study and classification of 39 cases. Cancer 1958;11:181-99.
33. Newton WA, Gehan EA, Webber EL, et al. Classification of rhabdomyosarcoma and related sarcomas. Pathologic aspects and proposal for a new classification. An Intergroup Rhabdomyosarcoma Study. Cancer 1995;76:1073-84.
34. Asmar L, et al. Agreement among and within groups of pathologists in the classification of rhabdomyosarcoma and related childhood sarcomas: a report of an international study of four pathology classifications. Cancer 1994;74:2579.
35. Wexler LH, Helman LJ. Pediatric soft tissue sarcomas. CA Cancer J Clin 1994;44:211-47.
36. Leuschner I, Newton WA Jr, Schmidt D, et al. Spindle cell variant of embryonal rhabdo-myosarcoma in the paratesticular region: a report of the Intergroup Rhabdomyosarcoma Study. Am J Surg Pathol 1993;17:221-30.
37. Kodet R, Newton WA, Hamoudi AB, et al. Childhood rhabdomyosarcoma with anaplastic (pleomorphic) features: a report of the Intergroup Rhabdomyosarcoma Study. Am J Surg Pathol 1993;17:443-53.
38. Schmidt D, Harms D, Pilin VA. Small cell pediatric tumors: Histology, immunohistchemistry, and electron microscopy. Clin Lab Med 1987;7:63-89.
39. Dias P, Parham DM, Shapiro Dn, et al. Myogenic regulatory protein (Myo D1) expression in childhood solid tumors: Diagnostic utility in rhabdomyosarcoma. Am J Pathol 1990;137:1283-91.
40. Donaldson SS, Belli JA. A rational clinical staging for childhood rhabdomyosarcoma. J Clin Oncol 1984;2:135.

41. Maurer HM. The Intergroup Rhabdomyosarcoma Study (IRS): Objectives and clinical staging classification . J Pediatr Surg 1975;10:977.

42. Lawrence WJ, Gehan EA, Hays DM, et al. Prognostic significance of staging factors of the UICC staging system in childhood rhabdomyosarcoma: a report of the Intergroup Rhabdomyosarcoma Study (IRS-II). J Clin Oncol 1987;5:46-54.

43. Wexler LH, Helman LJ. Rhabdomyosarcoma and the undifferentiated sarcomas. In Pizzo PA, Poplack DG, (Eds): Principles and practice of pediatric oncology, 3rd edition. Lippincott-Raven Publishers, Philadelphia, 1997; 799-829.

44. Pedrick TJ, Donaldson SS, Cox RS. Rhabdomyosarcoma: the Stanford experience using a TNM staging system. J Clin Oncol 1986;4:370.

45. Raney RB Jr., Tefft M, Maurer HM, et al. Disease patterns and sruvival rate in children with metastatic soft-tissue sarcomas. Cancer 1988;62:1257.

46. Koscielniak E, Rodary C, Flamant F, et al. Metastatic rhabdomyosarcoma and histologically similar tumors in childhood: a retrospective European multicenter analysis. Med Pediatr Oncol 1992;20:209.

47. Lawrence W Jr. Hays DM, Heyn R, et al. Lymphatic metastases with childhood rhabdo-myosarcoma. Cancer 1977;39:556.

48. Shimada H, Newton WA Jr. Soule EH, et al. Pathology of fatal rhabdomyosarcoma. Report from Intergroup Rhabdomyosarcoma Study (IRS-I and IRS-II) Cancer 1987;59:459.

49. Gehan EA, Glover FN, Maurer HM, et al. Prognostic factors in children with rhabdomyosarcoma. Monogr Natl Cancer Inst 1981;56:83.

50. Okamura J, Sutow WW, Moon TE. Prognosis in children with metastatic sarcoma. Med Pediatr Oncol 1977;3:243.

51. LaQuaglia MP, Heller G, Ghavimi E, et al. The effect of age at diagnosis on outcome in rhabdomyosarcoma. Camcer 1994;73:109.

52. Weiner ES, Lawrence W, Hays D, et al. Retroperitoneal node biopsy in paratesticular rhabdomyosarcoma. J Pediatr Surg 1994;29:171.

53. Mandell LR, Massey V, Ghavani F. The influence of extensive bone erosion on local control in nonorbital rhabdomyosarcoma of the head and neck. Int J Ratiat Oncol Biol Phys 1989;17:649.

54. Niggli FK, Powell JE, Parkes SE, et al. DNA ploidy and proliferative activity (S-phase) in childhood soft-tissue sarcomas: their value as prognostic indicators. Br J Cancer 1994;69:1106.

55. Wijnaendts LCD, van der Linden JC, van Diest PJ, et al. Prognostic importance of DNA flow cytometric variables in rhabdomyosarcoma. J Clin Pathol 1993;46:948.

56. Hays DM, et al. Primary re-excision for patients with "microscopic residual" following initial excision of sarcomas of the trunk and extremity sites. J Pediatr Surg 1989;24:5.

57. Donaldson SS. Rhabdomyosarcoma: contemporary status and future directions. Arch Surg 1989;124:1015.

58. Mandell LR. Ongoing progress in the treatment of childhood rhabdomyosarcoma. Oncology 1993;7:71.

59. Teffts M. Radiation therapy guidelines in rhabdomyosarcoma: results of the Intergroup Rhabdomyosarcoma Studies. In Maurer HM, Ruymann FB, Pochedly C, (Eds): Rhabdo-myosarcoma and related tumors in children and adolescents, Boca Raton, Fla., CRC press 1991.

60. Wiener ES. Rhabdomypsarcoma. In O'Neill JA, Rowe MI, Grosfeld JL, Fonkalsrud EW, Coran AG (Eds) Pediatric Surgery 5th edition, Mosby, St Louis 1998; 431-45.

61. Kinsella TJ. Treatment of high risk sarcomas in children and young adults: analysis of local control using intensive combined modality therapy. Natl Cancer Inst Monogr 1988;6:291.

62. Teffts M, Lindberg R, Gehan E. Radiation therapy combined with systemic chemotherapy of rhabdomyosarcoma in children: local control in patients enrolled into the Intergroup Rhabdomyosarcoma Study. Natl Cancer Inst Monogr 1981;56:75.

63. Wilbur JR. Combination chemotherapy for embryonal rhabdomyosarcoma. Cancer Chemother Rep 1974;30:1632.

64. Ortega J, et al. A feasibility, toxicity, and efficacy study of ifosfamide, actinomycin D, and vincristine for the treatment of childhood rhabdomyosarcoma. A Report from Intergroup Rhabdomyosarcoma Study-IV pilot study. Am J Pediatr Hematol Oncol 1993;15:15.

65. Raney RB, Crist WM, Donaldson SS, Gehan EA, Maurer HM. A pilot study of ifosfamide/mesna and doxorubicin (IFOS/DOX) followed by vincristine, antinomycin D, cyclophosphamide (VAC) and hyperfractionated irradiation (HFRT) in children with metastatic soft-tissue sarcoma: a report from Intergroup Rhabdomyosarcoma Study (IRS) (abstract) Proc Am Soc Clin Oncol 1991;10:313.

66. Raney RB. Spinal cord "drop metastases" from head and neck rhabdomyosarcoma: proceedings of the Tumor Board of Children's Hospital of Philadelphia. Med Pediatr Oncol 1978;4:3.

67. Raney RB Jr, Tefft M, Newton WA, et al. Improved prognosis with intensive treatment of children with cranial soft tissue sarcomas arising in nonorbital parameningeal sites: a report from Intergroup Rhabdomyosarcoma Study Cancer 1987;59:147.

68. Ortega JA, Fryer C, Gehan E, Morris-Jones P, Raney B, Webber W, et al. Efficacy of reducing tissue volume irradiation in children with cranial parameningeal rhabdomyosarcoma. A report of the intergroup rhabdo-myosarcoma III. Proc Am Soc Clin Oncol 1990;9:296.

69. Hays DM, Raney RB Jr., Lawrence W Jr., Soule EH, Gehan EA, Tefft M. Bladder and prostatic tumors in the Intergroup Rhabdomyosarcoma Study (IRS-I) Cancer 1982;50:1472.

70. LaQuaglia MP, Ghavini F, Herr H, et al. Prognostic factors in bladder and bladder-prostate rhabdomyosarcoma. J Pediatr Surg 1990;25:1066.

71. Hays DM, Lawrence W Jr., Crist WM, et al. Partial cystectomy in the management of rhabdomyosarcoma of the bladder: a report from Intergroup Rhabdomyosarcoma Study. J Pediatr Surg 1990;25:719.

72. Hays DM, Raney RB, Wharam MD, et al. Children with vesical rhabdomyosarcoma (RMS) treated by partial cystectomy with neoadjuvant or adjuvant chemotherapy, with or without radiotherapy. J Pediatr Hematol Oncol 1995;17:46.

73. Hays DM. Bladder/prostate rhabdomyosarcoma: results of multi-institutional trials of the Intergroup Rhabdomyo-sarcoma Study. Semin Surg Oncol 1993;9:520.

74. Fryer CJH. Pelvic rhabdomyosarcoma: paying the price of bladder preservation. (editorial) Lancet 1995;345:141.

75. Raney RB Jr, et al. Paratesticular sarcomas in childhood and adolescence: a report from intreigroup rhabdo-myosarcoma studies I and II, 1973-1983. Cancer 1987; 60:2337.

76. Wiener ES, et al. Retroperitoneal node biopsy in para-testicular rhabdomyosarcoma. J Pediatr Surg 1994;29:171.

77. Hays DM, Soule EH, Lawrence W Jr, et al. Extremity lesions in the Intergroup Rhabdomyosarcoma Study (IRS-I): a preliminary report. Cancer 1982;49:1.

78. Lawrence W, Hays D, Heyn R, Beltangady M, Maurer HM. Surgical lesions from the intergroup rhabdomyosarcoma study pertaining to extremity tumors. World J Surg 1988;12:676.

79. Mandell R, et al. Prognostic significance of regional lymph node involvement in childhood extermity rhabdo-myosarcoma. Med Pediatr Oncol 1990;18:466.

CHAPTER 26

Sandeep Agarwala
Devendra K Gupta

Non-rhabdomyosarcoma Soft Tissue Sarcomas in Children

This heterogenous group of tumors of mesenchymal origin accounts for approximately 5 percent of all cancers in children less than 20 years of age. While RMS accounts for 60 percent of all STS in children less than 5 years of age, non-rhabdomyosarcoma soft tissue sarcomas (NRSTS) constitutes more than 75 percent of all STS in children 15 to 20 years of age. NRSTS, like RMS can arise in any part of the body, but the most common sites are extremities, trunk, abdomen and pelvis.[1] Extremities and trunk account for more than 50 percent of all NRSTS in children (Table 26.1).[2-5] Most NRSTS

present as painless asymptomatic masses. Sometimes symptoms may be due to local invasion of adjacent structures. Tumors like malignant peripheral nerve sheath tumor (MPNST) arise in a peripheral nerve and may show both motor and sensory involvement.

The incidence of occurrence of the varied histologic types of NRSTS depends on the age and the site (Tables 26.1 and 26.2). The most frequent histologic types are synovial sarcoma, neurofibrosarcoma and fibrosarcoma. In the extremities the tumor occurs mostly in the lower limbs. While most of the extremity NRSTS in children

Table 26.1: Common sites and age of onset of NRSTS in children		
Tumor type	*Most common sites*	*Usual age of onset*
Congenital fibrosarcoma	Extremity (70%), trunk (30%)	Most < 2 year
Adult form of fibrosarcoma	Extremity	15 years
Neurofibrosarcoma	Extremity(40%), RP (25%), Trunk (20%)	Younger in patients with neurofibromatosis-I
Malignant fibrous histiocytoma, angiomatoid form	Extremity	Young children
Synovial sarcoma	Extremity (lower more often than upper)	31% off in < 20 years age group
Hemangiopericytoma, infantile form	Extremity, trunk	< 1 year
Hemangiopericytoma, adult form	Extremity, RP, head and neck	10-20 years
Alveolar soft part sarcoma	Extremity, head and neck	15-20 years
Leiomyosarcoma	GI tract, vascular tissue,	Any age
Leiomyosarcoma, epithelioid form	Stomach	Younger girls
Liposarcoma	Extremity, RP	Two peaks, 0-2 years and second decade

Table 26.2: Distribution of histologic subtypes of NRSTS among children[2-5]

Tumor	Resected clinical group I and II	Unresectable clinical group III and IV
Synovial sarcoma	32%	14%
Malignant fibrous histiocytoma	14%	7%
Malignant peripheral nerve sheath tumor	10%	19%
Fibrosarcoma	10%	-
Leiomyosarcoma	10%	-
Alveolar soft part sarcoma	4%	14%
Others	20%	46%

Table 26.3: POG schema for grading of NRSTS in children

Grade 1
- Myxoid well differentiated liposarcoma
- Deep seated dermatofibrosarcoma protuberans
- Well differentiated or infantile (age < 5 years) fibrosarcoma
- Well differentiated or infantile (age < 5 years) hemangiopericytoma
- Well differentiated malignant peripheral nerve sheath tumor
- Angiomatoid malignant fibrous histiocytoma

Grade 2
- Sarcomas not specifically included in grade 1 or 3; < 15 percent of tumor showing geographic necrosis or the mitotic index is < 5 per 10 high power fields

Grade 3
- Pleomorphic or round cell liposarcoma
- Mesenchymal chondrosarcoma
- Extra-skeletal osteosarcoma
- Malignant triton tumor
- Alveolar soft part sarcoma

are synovial sarcomas, tumors of the trunk are predominantly malignant fibrous histiocytomas (MFH) or neurogenic in origin. Among the NRSTS, fibrosarcoma predominate in children younger than 1 year, whereas synovial sarcoma and malignant peripheral nerve sheath tumors are more common in children older than 10 years. The rarity and histologic heterogenecity of NRSTS in children preclude careful study of their natural history and response to therapy.

HISTIOLOGY AND GRADING OF NRSTS

Because of the inconsistencies in predicted behavior, a grading scheme for pediatric NRSTS is used, which takes into account the cytohistiologic features that are used for adult sarcomas, but with caveats of the childhood lesions (Table 26.3). This system is not used for RMS or for primitive neuroectodermal lesions, which are always considered high-grade tumors. The histologic grading system identifies three different grades of tumors based

on histopathologic subtypes: amount of necrosis, number of mitosis, and cellular pleomorphism. This histologic grading is highly predictive of clinical outcome (Table 26.4) and is therefore commonly used clinically.

PROGNOSTIC FACTORS AND OUTCOME FOR NRSTS

Overall clinical outcome for children with completely resected NRSTS is excellent but more than 20 percent of these will eventually develop disease recurrence and die of disease. Therefor the identification of risk factors for increased chances of recurrences in children with completely resected NRSTS is important so that these children can be put on adjuvant trials. The risk factors for local recurrence differ from those for metastatic recurrence. The most important risk factor for distant metastatic recurrence is high histologic grade, tumor size and invasiveness.[3] The factors associated with increased risk for local recurrence are:[2]

Table 26.4: Outcome for localized pediatric NRSTS according to histopathologic grading system proposed by Pediatric Oncology Group[2,3]

Grade	5-year survival (%)	5-year progression free survival (%)
1,2	99	84-93
3	73	52-67

- Microscopically positive margins
- Intra-abdominal primary tumors
- No radiotherapy
- Tumor size > 5 cm.
  Factors associated with decreased survival are:
- Microscopic positive margins
- Tumor size > 5 cm
- High histologic grade
- Intra-abdominal primary tumors.

Metastatic disease at the time of presentation occurs in about 15 percent of children with NRSTS,[4] and lungs is the commonest site of distant metastasis, although metastasis to bone, liver and mesentry have also been reported. Though lymphatic metastasis is rare for most NRSTS, it is commonly associated with high grade lesions like synovial sarcoma, angiosarcoma and epitheliod sarcoma.

In a review of 154 children with NRSTS treated at a single institution,[1] 31 percent of those with grade 1 or 2 lesions had treatment failures, while 73 percent of the children with grade 3 disease developed recurrent disease.

CLINICAL EVALUATION AND STAGING OF NRSTS

In all children suspected to have NRSTS the clinical evaluation should include routine hemograms, renal and liver function tests, bone scans and bone marrow examination. MRI scan is considered the imaging modality of choice for the evaluation of local and regional disease, particularly in the extremities, the pelvis and head and neck regions. The staging system currently used for NRSTS is the same as the modified TNM staging system used for RMS. The optimal method for obtaining tissue for diagnosis in patients with NRSTS is again datable. Although fine needle aspiration cytology (FNAC) is a useful diagnostic tool in the initial evaluation of NRSTS or a possible metastatic lesion, needle core biopsy (NCB) is better for providing enough tissue to permit accurate histological subtyping of a sarcoma. Excisional biopsy rarely should be used in the initial evaluation of these tumors. Simple excision of the tumor

violates the tissue planes and results in dissemination of the tumor cells throughout the operative field. Subsequent surgery in the region is thereby compromised. An excisional biopsy is undertaken only in those instances when the tumor is small (< 2.5 cm) or situated so that an eventual wide local resection can be done without risk or functional deformity. When an incisional biopsy is done it should be properly planned. For an extremity lesion, the incision should be planned longitudinally or parallel to the neurovascular bundle. At the time of biopsy, flaps should not be considered as they contaminate multiple compartments. Based on the plane of dissection there are four possible margins:

1. *Intralesional margin:* Dissection plane violating the pseudocapsule and only a portion of tumor is removed with obvious macroscopic residue.
2. *Marginal margin:* Pseudocapsule is the plane of dissection. Local recurrence rates in these cases are around 60 to 70 percent.
3. *Wide resection:* This includes the pseudocapsule and a margin of normal tissue removed en-bloc. There are no quantitative measurements in centimeters in the definition of wide margin. Recurrence rates are 5 to 10 percent.
4. *Radical margins:* Radical margin is defined as an extra-compartmental resection of the whole soft tissue compartment. Recurrence rates are less than 5 percent.

There are a number of staging systems used for pediatric NRSTS and these differ from their adult counterparts. Traditionally pediatric NRSTS have been staged according to the Intergroup RMS clinicopathologic staging system (clinical groups) (See Table 25.4 in chapter on RMS) and International Union against cancer staging system (TNM) (See Table 25.5 in chapter on RMS).

TREATMENT AND OUTCOME OF NRSTS (TABLES 26.5 AND 26.6)

During the past few years the surgical management of these tumors has undergone a considerable evolution with the realization that multimodal therapy provides

Table 26.5: Outcome of NRSTS in children according to the clinical groups[2,3,6]

Clinical group	5-year event free survival (%)	5-year survival (%)
I	72.83	84-90
II	65.72	84-88
III	-	35-54
IV	15 (2 year)	34 (2 year)

Table 26.6: Outcome for localized pediatric NRSTS according to International Union against Cancer staging system (TNM)[2]

Stage	5-year survival (%)	5-year progression free survival (%)
T_1	96	87
T_2	70	51
A	97	92
B	77	55

the best chance for survival. Unlike that for RMS, which is a highly chemosensitive tumor, the mainstay of treatment of NRSTS is complete surgical resection with or without adjuvant radiotherapy to prevent local recurrence.[7-9] Several prospective adult trials have failed to document survival benefit of adjuvant chemotherapy.[10] For pediatric NRSTS, some centers prefer to give pre-excision RT followed by surgery and then completion RT using external beam irradiation.[9,11] In some other centers, pre-excision chemotherapy is first used to reduce the size of local tumor and provide systemic therapy. This neoadjuvant chemotherapy is then followed by surgical excision; irradiation being used only if margins are positive. The only prospective pediatric trial addressing the value of adjuvant chemotherapy in patients with NRSTS was conducted by the Pediatric Oncology Group (POG). In this trial, 75 children with completely resected NRSTS lesions were assigned to receive observation vs adjuvant chemotherapy with VAC and doxorubicin. The 3-year disease free survival rate for the two groups did not differ (74% vs 76%). Sub-group analysis disclosed that patients with grade 3 lesions fared significantly worse than those with grade 1 and 2 lesions (3-year EFS, 75% vs 91%; p= 0,018). Distant relapses accounted for more than 80 percent of the failures in the high grade group. The outcome for children with metastatic NRSTS continues to be poor; fewer than 20 percent of the patients are disease free at 3-year.[10] The most active drugs against NRSTS include ifosfamide and doxorubicin. Currently POG is investigating the clinical activity of some combination chemotherapies for unresectable or metastatic NRSTS. If these prospective trials identify some beneficial outcomes then these active agents may be also tried as adjuvant chemotherapy in children with completely resected high grade NRSTS. There are some important differences from adults in the treatment of pediatric NRSTS:

- Biology of childhood NRSTS is significantly different.
- RT in rapidly growing child has much more morbidity than in adults.
- Successful limb sparing procedures in young growing child is much more difficult.
- Long-term consequences of irradiation and chemotherapy are a greater concern.

This is why wide local excision or en-bloc resection should be the primary form of treatment in children with NRSTS. All attempts should be made to obtain negative margins. What consists of an adequate margin of tissue is still debated. In some areas such as head and neck, mediastinum and retroperitoneum, wide local excision with clear margins may be impossible to achieve[12] without mutilating resections. The finding of microscopic involvement of surgical margins is highly predictive for local disease recurrence, distant disease recurrence and diminished overall survival.[13,14] This is why primary re-excision should have priority over any adjuvant therapy.[15] In a retrospective review from St. Jude's Children's Research Hospital the estimated 5-year survival was 89 percent with 12.8 percent of patients developing local recurrences and 11.8 percent a distant failure.[2] In contrast, only 50 percent of those with unresected disease and 34 percent of those with metastatic disease were alive at 5 year and 2 year respectively. Adjuvant RT is recommended in all cases of NRSTS in adults as these tumors respond to RT. This is not the case in childhood NRSTS. RT has been used sparingly in children because of its long-term effects.[16] Current recommendations for children are to avoid RT for grade 1 and 2 completely reseted tumors, however, incompletely reseted tumors require additional therapy for local control.

CONGENITAL FIBROSARCOMA

Fibrosarcomas are one of the commonest NRSTS in children and adults and it is one of the most common soft tissue sarcomas in children less than 1 year of age.[17] In the pediatric age group there are two peak incidences; one in infants and children less than 5 years of age and the other in 10-15 years age-group. According to the histological grading of NRSTS these are classified as grade I tumors and though it can have local recurrences, it usually does not metastasize with a metastatic rate of less than 10 percent.[17] Genetic studies have clearly documented a recurring t(12;15) translocation in fibrosarcomas. Histologically these tumors are composed of uniform population of fibroblasts or myofibroblasts, with little stroma of poorly formed collagen. Presentation is usually of a localized mass with no systemic symptoms and the commonest site being the extremities and the trunk. Retroperitoneal and head and neck tumors are uncommon and fare worse than the extremity lesions. Surgical removal by wide local excision, aimed at maintaining as much function as possible and avoiding amputation is the treatment of choice. The role of adjuvant chemotherapy is not established. Pre-excision chemotherapy or radiotherapy is advocated only if surgical removal is not feasible. In such cases pre-excision chemotherapy with VAC or VAI or VA have a good response in decreasing the size and making surgical excision feasible. The local recurrence rate for extremity and axial lesions are same at around 33 percent, but the metastatic rate of axial lesions is 26 percent which is much higher than the 10 percent for extremity lesions.[18,19]

FIBROSARCOMA

Conventional fibrosarcoma, nearly always occurs in post-pubertal adolescents and is a full fledged malignancy with a potential to metastasize as compared to congenital fibrosarcomas. Histologically it is a spindle cell tumor composed of characteristic "herring-bone" pattern of tumor cells; which are densely packed into interweaving fascicles of parallel arrays. The main differential diagnoses are aggressive fibromatosis, nodular fascitis, myositis ossificans, and inflammatory pseudotumor among the benign conditions and neurofibrosarcoma, malignant peripheral nerve sheath tumor, poorly differentiated embryonal rhabdomyosarcoma and spindle cell synovial sarcoma among the malignant lesions. Fibrosarcoma commonly occurs in the extremities and is treated according the protocol for other NRSTS and the 5-year survival rate is around 60 percent.

MALIGNANT PERIPHERAL NERVE SHEATH TUMOR (MPNST)

Malignant peripheral nerve sheath tumors (MPNST) (Fig. 26.1) accounts for around 5-10 percent of all NRSTS in children.[20,21] It has a known association with neurofibromatosis type -I with around two-thirds of children with MPNST having neurofibromatosis. About 15 percent of NF-I patients develop MPNST. Histologically there may be a variety of appearances and these must be differentiated from fibrosarcoma. In MPNST the cells are more variable in size and the characteristic "herring bone" pattern seen in fibrosarcoma is absent. There may be a myxoid stroma with palisading nuclei occasionally arranged in arrays, the so-called Verocay bodies.[22] Electron microscopy is useful in establishing a specific diagnosis. Alternatively immunohistochemistry with S-100 antibodies is often positive.[23] The most common presentation is of a

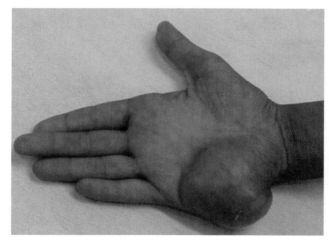

Figure 26.1: Malignant peripheral nerve sheath tumor involving the hypothenar aspect of right hand of a child

painless mass with occasional motor and/or sensory nerve involvement. The commonest primary sites are extremities (42%), retroperitoneum (25%) and the trunk (21%). Complete surgical excision plays a key role in the treatment of these children. Most children in whom the tumor is completely excised will live as compared to almost all children with incomplete tumor removal who die. Studies have shown that excision with a wide margin fares as well as grossly complete excision with local irradiation to microscopic residue.[24,25] The role of adjuvant chemotherapy is not well established though chemotherapy with VAC or VDC (vincristin, doxorubicin and cyclophosphamide) can produce tumor regression in patients with unresectable and metastatic disease.

MALIGNANT FIBROUS HISTIOCYTOMA (MFH)

Malignant fibrous histiocytosis (MFH) is less common in children than in adults, consisting of only 8-10 percent of all NRSTS as reported by the St Jude's and the SIOP series.[26,27] It is one of the most common radiation induced sarcomas. The typical microscopic appearance resembles that of fibrosarcoma but is distinct by the absence of "herring bone" pattern, presence of marked cellular pleomorphism, and multiple cell types (especially lipid laden tumor cells), and an overall more malignant appearance. The common type of MFH occurring in children less than 15 years of age is angiomatoid MFH, which has a very favorable prognosis. Grossly the tumor is very nodular like myofibroblastic tumor. Only 1 percent of MFH are reported to metastasize, the lungs being the commonest site, though metastasis to brain have also been reported. MFH can occur anywhere in the trunk and extremities and also the scalp. The initial management is by wide local excision as for other NRSTS and the outcome is usually favorable in children. MFH is a chemoresponsive tumor and in children with unresectable tumors it responds well to VAC with or without doxorubicin.[28] Responses with combination of ifosfamide and etoposide combinations have also been reported.[29]

SYNOVIAL SARCOMA

Synovial sarcoma is the most common NRSTS in adolescents and young adults (Fig. 26.2). The reported incidence varies between 17 percent of all NRSTS as per the SIOP report[27] to 26 percent as in the POG study report.[3] Overall synovial sarcoma is predominantly seen in the third decade with about 31 percent of patients

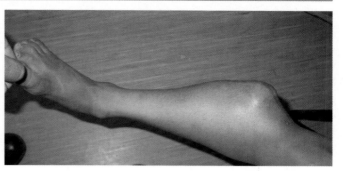

Figure 26.2: Synovial sarcoma of the lower limb

being younger than 20 years and in this pediatric population the median age is 13 years. Sixty percent of the tumors occur in the lower extremities with the upper extremity being the next most common site. It has been reported as the most common histology of soft tissue sarcoma occuring in the foot.[30] Ninety four percent of the metastatic disease is to the lungs and unlike other NRSTS, synovial sarcoma has a propensity to metastasize to the lymph nodes, though this is not so common in the pediatric population. Pathologically synovial sarcoma is unique for its propensity to differentiate into two distinct elements: a spindle cell fibrous stroma virtually indistinguishable from fibrosarcoma, and a distinct glandular component with absolute epithelial differentiation. In the absence of this glandular epithelial component it may be extremely difficult to diagnose synovial sarcoma unless immunohistochemistry with keratin antibodies is used. The spindle cells in synovial sarcoma are positive, unlike those in fibrosarcoma or any other STS.[31] Wide local excision is the treatment of choice with radiotherapy to the tumor bed to control microscopic disease. Although synovial sarcoma is a very chemosensitive tumor, the role of adjuvant chemotherapy is still not well established. These tumors respond well to ifosfamide or doxorubicin based regimes although combination of ifosfamide-etoposide has also been reported to be very effective.[29] The overall long-term survival rates reported by SIOP MMT 84 trial was 68 percent.[32] The survival rates reported by the St. Jude's Children Research Hospital was 80 percent for group I/II disease and 17 percent for group III/IV disease.[33]

ALVEOLAR SOFT PART SARCOMA (ASPS)

This is a very rare sarcoma even in adults comprising of less than 1 percent of all sarcomas in adults. In children it is even rarer. It is usually a slow growing indolent mass and the orbit and head and neck are the commonest site of primary disease in children. The most distinctive feature on histology is the presence of periodic acid-Schiff positive diastase resistant inclusions in the cytoplasm. The initial treatment is usually complete local excision with radiotherapy and chemotherapy reserved for recurrent disease. Most patients eventually relapse and subsequently die of the disease, sometimes as long as 20 years after the diagnosis.

HEMANGIOPERICYTOMA

Hemangiopericytoma are rare tumors and account for approximately 3 percent of all soft tissue sarcoma in children.[34-37] Cytogenetic abnormalities in the form of simple translocations t(12;19)(q13;13.3) and t(13;22)(q22;q11) have been reported in some of these tumors. Hemangiopericytoma occur more commonly in infants. As compared to adults the prognosis is good in these infants, though they can be more aggressive with higher incidence of metastatic disease in older children.[38,39] The tumor cells are thought to be derived from vascular pericytes, the first layer of support cells adjacent to the endothelial cells in normal vessels, but evidence to this origin is not well established. Histologically there is a pattern of uniform tumor with staghorn vascular pattern and reticulin positivity around each tumor cell that characterizes the diagnosis. The most common primary site of the tumor is lower extremity followed by retroperitoneum, head and neck and trunk. In infants the commonest sites are the tongue and the sub-lingual region. The most common sites of distant metastasis are the lungs and bone. Some of these children are reported to present with hypoglycemia or hypophosphatemic rickets that resolves with excision of the tumor.[40,41] The recommended primary treatment is wide local excision with radiotherapy being reserved for residual disease.[7] The role of adjuvant chemotherapy is not well established, however, the tumor is known to be responsive to vincristin, cyclophosphamide, doxorubicin, actinomycin D, methotrexate, mitoxantrone and other alkylating agents.

LEIOMYOSARCOMA

Leiomyosarcoma is a rare NRSTS in children accounting for less than 2 percent of cases.[42] There have been many reports of leiomyosarcoma in the skin, subcutaneous tissues and soft tissues after irradiation[43] suggesting irradiation as a predisposing factor. Recent reports have also suggested an increased incidence of leiomyosarcoma in adults and children infected with HIV.[44-46] These tumors have also been reported after treatment for acute lymphocytic leukemia[47] and during immunosuppression in transplant recipients.[48] Histologically the tumor cells are elongated with cigar shaped nuclei brightly eosinophilic cytoplasm (because of content of myofilaments) and these cells are arranged in closely packed parallel arrays. The most common primary site in children is the gastrointestinal tract, specially the stomach.[49] Less frequently it has been reported in retroperitoneum, peripheral soft tissues and the genitourinary tract.

The primary modality of treatment is wide local excision and the role of chemotherapy and radiotherapy are not yet known. The outcome is favorable for tumors outside the gastrointestinal tract, but GI lesions have a poorer outcome.[42,50]

LIPOSARCOMA

Liposarcomas are one of the most common soft tissue sarcomas in adults but in the pediatric population it is relatively uncommon. In children it usually occurs in the early part of the second decade of life[51] and rarely affects infants and young children. Consistent cytogenetic abnormalitiy of t(12;16)(q13;p11) translocation helps in differentiating from benign lipoblastoma and lipoblastomatosis. Histologically liposarcoma are of four types: myxoid, round cell, well differentiated and pleomorphic. The myxoid subtype is most common in children.[52] In this histologic variant most cells are fibroblastic with occasional cells showing conspicuous lipoblastic differentiation. The most common primary sites for liposarcoma in children are the lower extremities and trunk. Although metastasis is uncommon, the most common site of metastasis is the lung. As the tumor rarely metastasizes but can be locally invasive, the treatment of choice is wide local excision. Local recurrence with extension of tumor into adjacent vital structures is the usual cause of death. Radiotherapy is effective in the control of residual microscopic disease[7] and is strongly recommended for retroperitoneal tumors in children as in this location getting a wide margin is impossible. The role of adjuvant chemotherapy in liposarcoma in children has not yet been defined.

REFERENCES

1. Rao BN. Non-rhabdomyosarcoma in children: prognostic factors influencing survival. Semin Surg Oncol 1993;9:524-31.
2. Spunt SL, Popquette CA, Hurt YS, et al. Prognostic factors for children and adolescents with surgically resected non-rhabdomyosarcoma soft tissue sarcoma: an analysis of 121 patients treated at St. Jude's Children Research Hospital. J Clin Oncol 1999;17:3697-705.
3. Pratt CB, Pappo AS, Gieser P, et al. Role of adjuvant chemotherapy in the treatment of surgically resected pediatric NRSTS: a Pediatric Oncology Group study. J Clin Oncol 1999;17:1219.
4. Pappo AS, Rao BN, Jenkins JJ, et al. Metastatic non-rhabdomyosarcoma in children and adolescents: the St. Jude's Children Research Hospital experience. Med Pediatr Oncol 1999;33:76-82.
5. Spunt SL, Hill DA, Motosue AM, et al. Clinical features and outcome of children with unresected non-rhabdomyosarcoma soft tissue sarcoma. Med Pediatr Oncol 2000;35:279.
6. Pratt C, Maurer H, Gieser P, et al. Treatment of unresectable or metastatic pediatric soft tissue sarcoma with surgery, irradiation and chemotherapy: a Pediatric Oncology Group study. Med Pediatr Oncol 1998;30:201-9.
7. Potter DA, Kinsella TJ, Glatstein E, et al. High grade soft tissue sarcomas of the extremities. Cancer 1986;58:190.
8. Rosenberg SA, Tepper J, Glatstein E, et al. Prospective randomized evaluation of adjuvant chemotherapy in adults with soft tissue sarcomas of the extremities. Cancer 1983;52:424.
9. Bryant MH, Schray MF, Martinez AM, et al. Pre and/or postoperative adjuvant irradiation combined with limb sparing surgery for soft tissue sarcoma of extremities. Seventh annual meeting of European Society for Therapeutic Radiology and Oncology 1988;203.
10. Pappo AS, Parham DM, Rao BN, Lobe TE. Soft tissue sarcomas in children. Semin Surg Oncol 1999;16:121-43.
11. Schray MF, Gunderson LL, Sim FH, et al. Soft tissue sarcomas: integration of brachytherapy, resection and external beam irradiation Cancer 1990;66:451.
12. Pappo As, Shapiro DN, Crist WM. Rhabdomyosarcoma: biology and treatment(review). Pediatr Clin North Am 1997;44:953-72.
13. Andrassy RJ, Corporn CA, Hay D, et al. Extremity sarcomas. An analysis of prognostic factors from Intergroup Rhabdomyosarcoma Study III. J Pediatr Surg 1996;31:191-6.
14. Lawrence W Jr, Anderson JR, Gehan EA, Maurer H. Pretreatment TNM staging of childhood rhabdomyosarcoma: a report of Intergroup Rhabdomyosarcoma Study Group. Cancer 1997;80:1165-70.
15. Crist WM, Garnsey L, Beltangady MS, et al. Prognosis in children with rhabdomyosarcoma: a report of Intergroup Rhabdomyosarcoma Studies I and II. J Clin Oncol 1992;8:443-52.
16. Pinkel D, Piekren J. Rhabdomyosarcoma in children. JAMA 1962;175:293-8.
17. Soule EH, Prichard DJ. Fibrosarcoma in infants and children: a review of 110 cases. Cancer 1997;40:1711.
18. Blocker S, Koenig J, Ternberg J. Congenital fibrosarcoma. J Pediatr Surg 1987;22:665.
19. Ninane J, Gosseye S, Pantion E, et al. Congenital fibrosarcoma. Cancer 1986;58:1400.
20. D'Agostino AN, Soule EH, Miller RH. Primary malignant neoplasms of nerves (malignant neurilemomas) in patients without manifestations of multiple neurofibromatosis (von Recklinghausen's disease). Cancer 1963;16:1003.
21. Prichard DJ, Soule EH, Taylor WF, et al. Fibrosarcoma: a clinicopathologic and statistical study of 199 tumors of soft tissue of the extremities and trunk. Cancer 1994;33:888.
22. Enzinger FM, Weiss SW. Malignant schwannomas. In: Enzinger FM, Weiss SW (Eds): Soft tissue tumors. St. Louis: CV Mosby, 1995;889.
23. Weiss Sw, Langloss JM, Enzinger FM. Value of s-100 protein in the diagnosis of soft tissue tumors with particular reference to benign and malignant Schwann cell tumors. Lab Invest 1983;49:299.
24. Raney RB, Schnaufer I, Zeigler M, et al. Treatment of children with neurogenic sarcoma. Cancer 1987;59:1.
25. Treuner J, Gross U, Maas E, et al. Results of treatment of malignant schwannoma: a report from German soft tissue group (CWS). Med Pediatr Oncol 1991;19:399.
26. Marsden HB, VanUnnik AJM, Terrier-Lancombe MJ. Non-rhabdomyosarcoma tumors in the SIOP mesenchymal malignancy trials. Med Pediatr Oncol 1991;19:379.
27. Sonmelet-Olive D, Oberlin O, Flamant F, et al. Non-rhabdomyosarcoma malignant mesenchymal tumors in children: results of SIOP MMT 84 and 89 protocols. Proc Am soc Clin Oncol 1995;14:446.
28. Raney RB, Allen A, O'Neill J, et al. Malignant fibrous histiocytoma of soft tissue in childhood. Cancer 1986;57:2198.
29. Mieser JS, Kinsella TJ, Triche TJ, et al. Treatment of recurrent childhood sarcomas and primitive neural tumors with ifosfamide, etoposide and mesna. J Clin Oncol 1987;5:1191.
30. Gross E, Rao BN, Bowman L, et al. Outcome of treatment for pediatric sarcoma of the foot: a retrospective review over a 20-year period. J Pediatr surg 1997;32:1181-4.
31. Krall RA, Kostlanovsky M, Patchefsky AS. Synovial sarcoma: a clinical, pathologic and ultrastructural study of 226 cases supporting the recognition of the monophasic variant Am J Pathol 1983;5:136.
32. Sommelet D, Flamant F, Rodary C. A series of 100 soft tissue satcomas (STS) in childhood excluding embryonal rhabdomyosarcoma and schwannomas. Med Pediatr Oncol 1991;19:390.
33. Pappo AS, Fontanesi J, Luo K, et al. Synovial sarcoma in children and adolescents: the St Jude's Children's Research Hospital experience. J Clin Oncol 1994;12:2360.
34. Horowitz MD, Pratt CB, Webber BI, et al. Therapy of childhood soft tissue sarcoma other than rhabdomyosarcoma: a review of 62 cases treated at a single institution. J Clin Oncol 1986;4:559.
35. Salloum E, Flamant F, Calliaud JM, et al. Diagnostic and therapeutic problems of soft tissue tumors other than rhabdomyosarcoma in infants under 1 year of age: a clinicopathologic study of 34 cases treated at Institut Gustave Roussy. Med Pediatr Oncol 1990;18:37.
36. Skene AI, Barr L, Robinson M, et al. Adult type (non-embryonal) soft tissue sarcoma in childhood. Med Pediatr Oncol 1993;21:645.
37. Dillon P, Maurer H, Jenkins J, et al. A prospective study of non-rhabdomyosarcoma soft tissue sarcoma in pediatric age group. J Pediatr Surg 1992;27:241.
38. Atkinson JB, Mahour GH, Isacas H Jr, et al. Hemangiopericytoma in infants and children: a report of six patients. Am J surg 1984;148:372.
39. Virden CP, Lynch FP. Infantile hemangiopericytoma: a rare case of a soft tissue mass. J Pediatr Surg 1993;28:741.
40. Pratt CB. Clinical manifestation and treatment of soft tissue sarcomas other than rhabdomyosarcoma. In: Maurer HM, Ruymann FB, Podechly C, (Eds): Rhabdomyosarcoma and related tumors in children and adolescents. Boca Raton, FL: CRC 1991;421.

41. Hanukoghu A, Chalew SA, Sun CJ, et al. Surgically curable hypophosphatemic rickets: diagnosis and management. Clin Pediatr 1989;28:321.

42. Bolting AJ. Alveolar soft part sarcoma. Med Pediatr Oncol 1996;26:81-310.

43. Folberg R, Cleasby G, Flanagan JA, et al. Orbital leiomyosarcoma after radiation therapy for bilateral retinoblastom. Arch Ophthal 1983;101:1562.

44. Chadwick EG, Connor EJ, Hanson JC, et al. Tumors of smooth muscle origin in HIV infected children. JAMA 1990;263:3182.

45. Mc Loughlin LC, Nord KS, Joshi V, et al. Disseminated leiomyosarcoma in a child with acquired immunodeficiency syndrome. Cancer 1991;67:2618.

46. Mc Cain KL, Leach CT, Jensen HB, et al. Association of Epstein-Barr virus with leiomyosarcoma in children with AIDS. N Engl J Med 1995;332:12.

47. Shen SC, Yunis EJ. Leiomyosarcoma developing in a child during remission of leukemia. J Pediatr 1976;89:780.

48. Swanson PE, Denher LP. Pathology of soft tissue sarcoma. In: Maurer HM, Ruymann FB, Podechly C, (Eds): Rhabdomyosarcoma and related tumors in children and adolescents. Boca Raton, FL: CRC 1991;386.

49. Johnson H, Hatter JJ, Papanus SH. Leiomyosarcoma of the stomach: results of surgery and chemotherapy in an eleven-year-old girl with metastasis. Med Pediatr Oncol 1980;8:137.

50. Ranchod M, Kempson RL. Smooth muscle tumors of gastrointestinal tract and retroperitoneum: a pathological analysis of 100 cases. Cancer 1997;39:255.

51. Castleberry RP, Kelly DR, Wilson ER, et al. Childhood liposarcoma: report of a case and review of the literature. Cancer 1984;54:579.

52. LaQuaglia MP, Spiro SA, Ghavimi F, et al. Liposarcoma in patients younger than or equal to 22 years of age. Cancer 1998;72:3114.

CHAPTER 27

Hitoshi Ikeda
Yoshiaki Tsuchida

Germ Cell Tumors

Germ cell tumors in children are a disparate group of tumors comprising mature and immature teratomas, germinomas, embryonal carcinomas, yolk sac tumors, and choriocarcinomas. These germ cell tumors arise in the gonads or in extragonadal sites including the brain, face, neck, mediastinum, retroperitoneum, and sacrococcygeal region. The origin of extragonadal germ cell tumors is considered to be due to primordial germ cells that have aberrantly migrated.[1] Although a number of classifications for germ cell tumors and non-germ cell tumors of the gonads exist, that based on the WHO classification is widely accepted (Table 27.1).[2] Currently these classifications are highly influenced by Teilum's concept of the genesis of embryonic and extra-embryonic germ cell tumors with inclusion of the term "endodermal sinus tumor" or "yolk sac tumor" (Table 27.2).[3] In this chapter, the various germ cell tumors are discussed below.

TERATOMA

In 1869, Virchow described a tumor originating in the sacrococcygeal region using the term "teratoma," derived from the Greek "teraton" meaning "a monster".[4] Currently, teratomas are defined as neoplasms composed of one or more of the three embryonic germ cell layers: endoderm; mesoderm; and ectoderm. Tumors are often gonadal in origin but may be found anywhere in the body along the midline. Histologically, teratomas are classified into three types: mature

Table 27.1: Histological classification of germ cell tumors and non-germ cell tumors of the gonads

A. Germ cell tumors
 1. Pure form
  a. Dysgerminoma/germinoma/seminoma
  b. Embryonal carcinoma
  c. Yolk sac tumor/infantile embryonal carcinoma
  d. Choriocarcinoma
  e. Polyembryoma
  f. Teratomas
   • Mature teratoma
   • Immature teratoma
 2. Combined form
  a. Embryonal carcinoma + teratoma (teratocarcinoma)
  b. Embryonal carcinoma + yolk sac tumor
  c. Others
B. Sex-cord stromal tumors
 1. Granulosa cell tumor (common type, juvenile type)
 2. Sertoli cell tumor
 3. Leydig cell tumors
 4. Combined form
C. Tumor-like lesions
 1. Gonadoblastoma
 2. Others

Table 27.2: Histological classification of germ cell tumors according to Teilum[3]

• Embryonic structure [Teratoma]
• Tumor of totipotential cell [Embryonal carcinoma]
• Extraembryonic structure [Choriocarcinoma] [yolk sac tumor]
• Germ cell [Dysgerminoma/germinoma/seminoma]

teratoma; immature teratoma; and teratoma with malignant elements. Mature teratoma comprises only mature elements such as the skin, hair, fat tissue, cartilage, bone, glands, etc. Immature teratoma contains immature elements such as neuroepithelial tissue and immature mesenchyme. The presence of microscopic foci of yolk sac tumor, rather than the histological grade of immaturity, is a valid predictor of recurrence, and grading of immature teratoma is unnecessary in children.[5] In rare instances, mature teratoma also recurs as a malignancy, but a careful review of the original tumor usually reveals occult malignant elements.[6] The biological behavior of teratomas with malignant elements (yolk sac tumor, choriocarcinoma, seminoma, and dysgerminoma) is determined by the most malignant element in the tumor. Elevations of serum alpha-fetoprotein (AFP) levels usually indicate the presence of foci of yolk sac tumor somewhere in the tumor (Table 27.3). Therefore, when the serum AFP is high, the tumor should be extensively sampled and carefully examined before the patients' postoperative treatment is determined. The majority of children with teratoma, however, usually do well with surgery alone regardless of primary tumor location, and salvage chemotherapy is successful in the few instances of malignant recurrence.[7]

Mature Teratomas

These are usually multicystic tumors that may have bone, cartilage, teeth, and hair. The cysts have thick clear, mucoid, viscid or yellow material with intervening gray-tan tissues.[7] While those in the gonads are well encapsulated, the extragonadal one do not have a capsule. Histologically they have representative tissues from all the three germ cell layers, namely the ectoderm,

mesoderm and endoderm. Structures most commonly found are skin and its appendages, adipose tissue, brain, intestinal epithelium and cystic structures lined with squamous, cuboidal or flattened epithelium. In addition the mediastinal teratomas frequently contain hematopoietic, pancreatic or pituitary tissue.[8] In infants and young children, mature teratomas always behaves in a benign fashion. Many ovarian mature teratomas are associated with nodules of mature glial tissue implanted throughout the peritoneum- gliomatous peritonei,[9] or in the lymph nodes.[10] These mature glial implants do not alter the stage or prognosis but the same can not be said when there are implants of immature tissues.

Immature Teratomas

These are grossly and histologically similar to the mature teratomas, but in addition they have various immature tissues derived from the ectoderm, mesoderm or the endoderm. The grading of immature elements is done using the Dehner's modification[11] of the Thurlbeck and Scully system[12] (Table 27.4), on slide with the largest amount of aggregated immature tissue. This grading system basically uses the number of low power fields of primitive neuroepithelium per slide.[13] In children the immature teratomas are usually benign and are known to behave in a malignant fashion only if foci of malignant

Table 27.3: Normal ranges of serum AFP in infants

Age	Mean ± SD (hg/mL)
Premature	134,734 ± 41,444
Newborn	48,406 ± 34,718
0-2 weeks	33,113 ± 32,503
2 week-1mth	9,452 ± 12,610
2 month	323 ± 278
3 month	88 ± 87
4 month	74 ± 56
5 month	46.5 ± 19
6 month	12.5 ± 9.8
7 month	9.7 ± 7.1
8 month	8.5 ± 5.5

Table 27.4: Histologic grading system of ovarian immature teratomas (Dehner's)

Grade	Microscopic appearance
0	Mature tissue only
1	Mainly mature tissue, but some immature also
	Neuroepithelium or other immature tissue
	Limited to 1 low power field per slide
2	Moderate amount of immature tissue present
	Neuroepithelium or other immature tissue
	Occupies 1 to 3 low power field per slide
3	Abundant immature tissue
	Neuroepithelium or other immature tissue
	Occupies more than 4 low power field per slide.

germ cell element is present in which case the tumor is actually a mixed malignant germ cell tumor. The malignant element is usually endodermal sinus (EST or yolk cell tumor-YST) or rarely neuroblastoma or meduloblastoma. The malignant germ cell element can easily be missed histologically as they are small and are associated with immature neural elements and frequently do not stain positive for AFP. In a recent report from the POG/CCG in 1998,[5] it was noted 55.6 percent of the immature teratomas registered in this combined study of 135 immature teratomas were actually mixed tumors and all of these had yolk sac component with a few having additional malignant components as well. The remaining 44.4 percent were pure immature teratomas. Though 47 percent of the immature teratomas were of grade 3, but it was reported that the grade did not correlate with the age or the outcome. In this study[5] it was noted that there was significant correlation between the stage and the presence of foci of EST (YST) and that of grade and the presence of a foci of EST (YST). The study concluded that the presence of microscopic foci of EST rather than the grade of immature teratoma, was the only valid predictor of recurrences[5].

Malignant Teratomas

The teratomas containing yolk sac element grossly appear as mature teratomas but may be more solid depending on the quantity of malignant component tissue present. Microscopically the foci of yolk sac tumor in the teratomas appear as small glandular or reticular structures with large, vesicular nuclei within loose myxoid background. These yolk sac tumor elements do not stain positive for AFP.

Teratomas are described below according to their original sites.

SACROCOCCYGEAL TERATOMA

Sacrococcygeal teratoma is a tumor that frequently occurs in neonates and infants and affects predominantly female children.[15,16] Classically, tumors are classified into four types:[15] Altman type I (46.7%), the most common type are tumors that are predominantly external with a minimal presacral component; type II (43.7%) tumors are external but have a significant intrapelvic component; type III (8.8%) tumors are external but pelvic and extend significantly into the abdomen; and type IV (9.8%) tumors are entirely presacral.

Sacrococcygeal teratoma is a troublesome condition if the tumor is diagnosed after delivery has started. Dystocia at delivery and rupture of the tumor are often fatal to the infant. Recently an increasing number of sacrococcygeal teratomas have been detected by antenatal ultrasonographic (US) examination of the fetus.[17] Prenatal US and magnetic resonance imaging (MRI) are useful in making a differential diagnosis between sacrococcygeal teratoma, myelomeningocele, and other tumors. They also provide some information on the extent of the tumor extension into the pelvis and the presence or absence of polyhydramnios, fetal hydrops, and intratumoral hemorrhage. Massive hemorrhage into the tumor may occur spontaneously in utero and cause anemia and hypoproteinemia followed by fetal hydrops. Fetuses with sacrococcygeal teratoma that are mainly solid in appearance and are highly vascularized have a higher risk of developing hydrops, and the presence of a solid tumor is a significant negative prognostic factor.[17,18] High-output cardiac insufficiency as a result of vascular shunting through the tumor is another cause of fetal death. It is generally agreed that a fetus with a large sacrococcygeal teratoma (usually more than 5 cm in diameter) detected prenatally should be delivered by cesarean section to prevent death from tumor rupture or hemorrhage.[16] Since spontaneous intratumoral hemorrhage may result in fetal death, it is recommended that elective cesarean section be performed at a high-risk obstetric center at 32 to 34 weeks of gestation when fetal maturity is deemed adequate for neonatal survival.[16]

Primary treatment of sacrococcygeal teratoma is complete removal of the tumor along with the coccyx. Although emergency removal of the tumor is sometimes performed in a case with prenatally diagnosed sacrococcygeal teratoma, the removal can be delayed until the neonate's general condition becomes stabilized. During that time, the extent of the tumor is examined by MRI or computed tomography (CT), and the serum levels of AFP and beta-human chorionic gonadotropin (β-hCG) should be examined (Fig. 27.1). Tumor resection is usually carried out in the prone position and is performed using a chevron skin incision. When tumors extend extensively into the pelvis, initial dissection through the abdomen is necessary before the presacral dissection. The proximal extent of the tumor can be defined by rectal examination or by barium enema, and the tumor should be dissected close to its capsule so

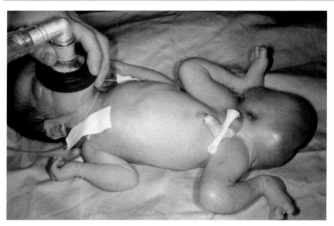

Figure 27.1: Appearance of a sacrococcygeal teratoma

that the retrorectal muscles and nervous network around the rectum can be preserved. Because failure to remove the coccyx is considered to be associated with a high recurrence rate, the coccyx should be removed with the tumor. The dissection between the coccyx and the sacrum makes it easier to dissect the tumor cranially into the retrorectal space. A significant proportion of patients who have undergone resection of sacrococcygeal teratoma are reported to have deficient anorectal function and urinary incontinence (neurogenic bladder).[19,20] These impairments are associated with surgical dissection, and therefore, careful and meticulous surgical techniques are required, especially when the tumor extends deeply into the pelvis and retroperitoneum.

Most tumors in the sacrococcygeal region are mature or immature teratomas, and less commonly yolk sac tumors. A retrospective survey by the Children's Cancer Group showed that 69 percent of sacrococcygeal teratomas were mature teratomas, 20 percent immature teratomas, and 11 percent yolk sac tumors at presentation.[21] The rate of malignancy increases with age at diagnosis, which is presumably caused by a delay in diagnosis of the less apparent lesions. Recurrent disease develops in 7 to 11 percent of sacrococcygeal teratomas within 3 years after resection.[21,22] The recurrent diseases usually are yolk sac tumors and are accompanied by an increase in serum AFP. In these instances in which a mature teratoma recurs as a malignancy, an occult focus of malignancy might have been overlooked when the original tumor was resected.[6] Studies suggest that patients should be carefully followed up for at least 3 years after the resection of benign

teratomas. Sacrococcygeal teratomas with malignant components and those with recurrent tumors as malignancy are treated according to the treatment protocol for malignant germ cell tumors. The staging for these malignant sacrococcygeal teratomas is done as for any extragonadal malignant germ cell tumor (Table 27.5).

OVARIAN TERATOMA

The majority of ovarian tumors in children and adolescents occur between ages 10 and 19 years, but they may occur at any age during infancy and childhood (Fig. 27.2). The most common of these tumors is benign cystic teratoma. These tumors usually present as an asymptomatic mass but may cause acute abdomen due to torsion of the ovary and the fallopian tube. Ovary-preserving tumor extirpation is the usual procedure for ovarian teratoma. Maintaining gonadal function and fertility is a concern, in particular when a teratoma develops in the bilateral ovaries, which occurs synchronously or metachronously in 4 to 7 percent of patients.[23,24] Minilaparotomy or laparoscopy-assisted cystectomy as minimally invasive surgery is an alternative to traditional laparotomy in patients with ovarian teratoma.[25] Salpingo-oophorectomy is necessary when ischemia of the ovary due to torsion is irreversible or when foci of malignant tumor are found by microscopic examination of the extirpated specimen.

Ovarian teratomas are sometimes associated with peritoneal implants that contain only mature glial tissues. Since the presence of gliomatosis peritonei does not alter patient prognosis, additional surgical approaches other than sampling or biopsy are usually unnecessary.[26] In patients with ovarian immature teratoma, surgery alone is also curative even if the serum AFP level is elevated.[27] Even when microscopic examination reveals small foci of yolk sac tumor, chemotherapy may be reserved until a recurrent tumor develops.[27] In such cases with relapse salvage is feasible with conventional chemotherapy.

Cystic ovarian tumors that are sometimes seen in newborns are usually not teratomas, but follicular cysts. They most often resolve spontaneously, but sometimes cause torsion, especially when they larger than 6 cm in diameter and 48 cm^3 in volume.[28] We have found that MRI is more useful than US in detecting hemorrhage and for determining indications for surgery in neonatal ovarian cysts.[28]

Table 27.5: Chemotherapy regimens for germ cell tumors in children

1. PVB (Ref.78)

Week	1	2	3
CDDP	↓		
VB	↓		
BL	↓	↓	↓

   CDDP (Cisplatin); 100 mg/m^2 on day 1, VB (Vinblastine); 0.15 mg/kg on day 2, BL (Bleomycin); 15 mg/m^2 on days 2, 9 and 16.

2. Modified PVB (Ref.130)

Week	1	2	3
CDDP	↓		
VB	↓		
BL	↓		

   CDDP (Cisplatin); 100 mg/m^2 on day 1, VB (Vinblastine); 0.15 mg/kg on day 2, BL (Bleomycin); 15 mg/m^2 on day 2.

3. BEP (Ref.39)

Week	1	2	3
CDDP	↓		
VP16	↓↓↓		
BL	↓		

   CDDP (Cisplatin); 100 mg/m^2 on day 1, VP16 (Etoposide); 120 mg/m^2 on days 1, 2 and3, BL (Bleomycin); 15 mg/m^2 on day 2.

4. JEB (Ref.130)

Week	1	2	3
Carbo.	↓		
VP16	↓↓↓		
BL	↓	↓	↓

   Carbo. (Carboplatin); dosage calculated from the EDTA glomerular filtration rate (approximately 600 mg/m^2 on day 1, VP16 (Etoposide); 120 mg/m^2 on days 1, 2 and 3, BL (Bleomycin); 15 mg/m^2 on days 2, 9 and 16.

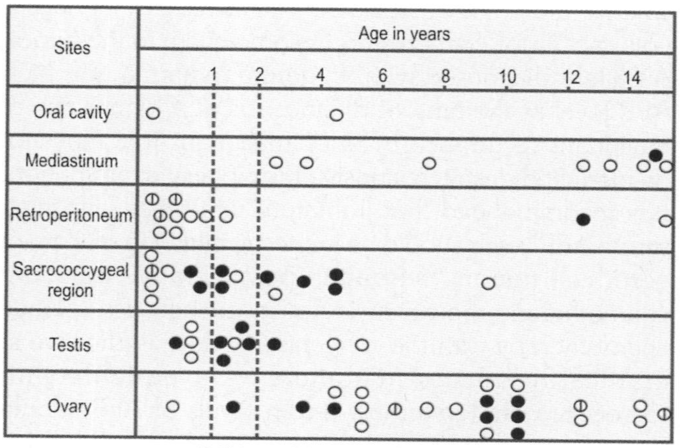

Figure 27.2: Age distribution of teratomas and malignant germ cell tumors according to the site of origin is shown. Cases are from a series at the Department of Pediatric Surgery, University of Tokyo

TESTICULAR TERATOMA

Testicular teratomas present as a painless scrotal mass in infants and children younger than two years of age and are sometimes found at birth.[29,30] Prepubertal teratomas of the testis may be associated with high serum AFP levels, but the clinical course of patients is equally uneventful with radical orchiectomy.[29,30] Because of the favorable characteristics of the disease, testis-sparing surgery or tumor enucleation is attempted in patients whose testicular parenchyme appears to be preserved.[31]

MEDIASTINAL TERATOMA

The mediastinum is the second most frequent site of extragonadal teratomas. Mediastinal teratomas occur in newborns to adolescents, and arise predominantly in the anterior mediastinum, occasionally in the posterior mediastinum, and rarely in the pericardial and intracardiac region.[32] Mediastinal teratomas typically manifest on CT as a heterogeneous mass containing soft tissue, fluid, fat, or calcification.[33] Some patients are asymptomatic and diagnosis is made incidentally by chest X-ray. However, affected children usually manifest symptoms such as dyspnea, cough, or chest pain. When the tumor causes severe respiratory distress in neonates mimicking congenital diaphragmatic hernia, emergency surgery to relieve lung compression and postoperative care supporting respiration are required.[32,34] Surgical approaches to mediastinal teratomas are either unilateral thoracotomy or median sternotomy, and the latter is necessary in some patients with large, bilaterally invasive lesions.

CERVICOFACIAL TERATOMA

Cervicofacial teratomas, arising in the oral cavity, nasopharynx, orbit, and anterior neck, are rare and usually noted at birth. A form of cervicofacial teratoma that arises from the palate or pharynx in the region of the basisphenoid (Rathke's pouch) is called epignathus.[35] Tumors may be diagnosed prenatally by US that is indicated for maternal polyhydramnios.[36] Polyhydramnios is caused by fetal inability to swallow the amniotic fluid. Life-threatening airway obstruction may occur at birth and require urgent resuscitation including bronchoscopy-assisted intubation or tracheostomy.[36] When an airway-obstructing mass is diagnosed prenatally, delivery by elective cesarean section is recommended, and the airway should be secured while the maternal-fetal placental circulation is maintained. Differential diagnosis includes cervical lymphangioma (hygroma), which should always be kept in mind. Careful examination and, if necessary, CT or MRI enable differential diagnosis between cervical teratoma and lymphangioma. Once the diagnosis of airway-obstructing teratoma is made, early resection after stabilization of the patient is the choice of treatment because it is the most effective method to control the airway.[35,36] The operative mortality rate is low, but significant morbidity such as recurrent nerve injury, hypothyroidism, or hypoparathyroidism may occur. The functional and cosmetic outcome of surgical treatment is generally excellent.

Others

Other sites of teratoma are the retroperitoneum, stomach, and intracranial region. Gastric teratomas account for only 1 percent of all teratomas in children and occur predominantly in boys.[37] A partial gastrectomy is required to remove the tumor.

TUMOR MARKERS FOR GERM CELL TUMORS

The clinical markers are useful in predicting response or indicating the presence of residual or progressive disease.[38] The markers are categorized as follows:
1. Oncofetoproteins – AFP and β-hCG
2. Cellular enzymes – LDH and placental alkaline phosphatase (PLAP).
3. Cytogenetic and molecular markers.

When a tumor of germ cell origin is among differential diagnoses, serum levels of AFP and β-hCG should be measured.

AFP

Serum AFP levels are elevated in patients with yolk sac tumors and correlate well with the clinical course. However, when the patient is younger than 10 months of age, serum AFP is physiologically elevated, and the normal ranges of AFP[39] should always be taken into account. Immunohistochemical staining demonstrates whether tumor cells are positive for AFP[40,41] (Figs 27.3A and B). After surgical excision of a yolk sac tumor, serum AFP levels decrease to normal with a half-life of approximately 5 days. Re-elevation of AFP levels in the serum indicates the presence of metastatic or recurrent disease.

Serum levels of AFP may be increased when there are foci of yolk sac tumors in teratomas. Conversely, when teratomas are associated with increased AFP levels, yolk sac tumor elements occur somewhere in the tumor. A patient diagnosed with immature teratoma and high AFP level at the time of diagnosis is at a higher risk of malignant recurrence.[42] Since malignant foci may not be identified despite extensive histological examination, it is recommended that immature teratomas with high serum AFP levels should be treated similarly to malignant germ cell tumors.[42] Routine postoperative adjuvant chemotherapy, however, is not given because salvage chemotherapy with the conventional dose is effective in eradicating recurrent tumors.[27] In patients with sacrococcygeal teratomas, serum levels of AFP should be measured during the postoperative follow-up, because yolk sac tumors recur in 7 to 11 percent of patients and almost all recurrences are accompanied by an increase in serum AFP level.[21,22] Only in a small number of patients with a huge immature teratoma does

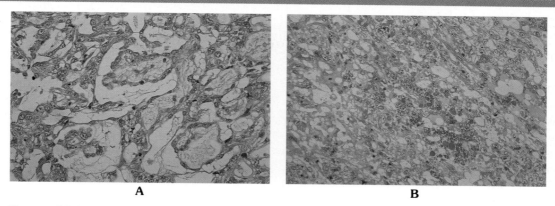

Figures 27.3A and B: (A) Histologically, yolk sac tumor is characterized by the formation of Schiller-Duval bodies, and **(B)** The presence of periodic acid Schiff (PAS)-positive eosinophilic hyaline globules

a moderate increase in serum AFP occur due to the gastrointestinal epithelia involved in the tumor.[43]

Analysis of the AFP subfraction profile is useful to distinguish germ cell tumor derived-AFP and that derived from hepatic tumors.[44-46] In germ cell tumors the fucosylation index, defined as the percentage of AFP of which the sugar chain is fucosylated and specifically binds to *Lens culinaris* agglutinin in total AFP, is 99 percent ±2 percent.[47] The glucosaminylation index, defined as the percentage of concanavalin A-nonreactive AFP in total AFP, is 45 percent ±20 percent. Both indices are significantly higher than those of AFP from hepatic tumors and benign liver disease (Figs 27.4A and B).[44,47] These

indices can also be used to differentiate AFP produced in yolk sac tumors from physiologically elevated AFP in early infancy.[39,44] Particularly, determination of the glucosaminylation index is sufficient to differentiate between AFP from yolk sac tumors and that from other sources.[44,45]

β-hCG

Choriocarcinomas secrete hCG, and β-hCG is measured to monitor the serum levels of hCG. Because the β subunit of hCG is identical in amino acid sequence to β subunits of pituitary hormones, radioimmunoassay with antibodies to β-hCG is used to measure serum levels

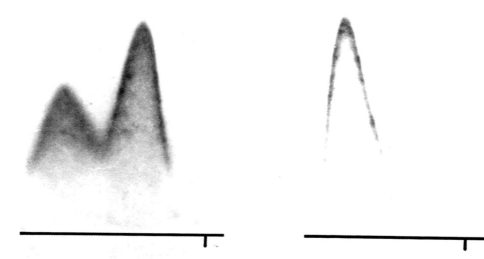

Figures 27.4A and B: Subfractionation of serum AFP was carried out using concanavalin A (Con A) affinity immuno-electrphoresis. In a patient with malignant yolk sac tumor, two peaks (Con A binding and Con A non-binding) appear **(A)**, whereas only one peak of Con A binding peak will appear in serum AFP from hepatoblastoma **(B)** and benign hepatic conditions such as biliary atresia[34]

of hCG. hCG is produced by one of the two components of choriocarcinoma, syncytiotrophoblasts, and serum β-hCG is a useful marker to monitor the disease course.

In addition to choriocarcinoma, some dysgerminomas contain reduced numbers of syncytiotrophoblasts in tumors, and are associated with slightly elevated serum levels of β-hCG. Elevation of serum β-hCG levels in dysgerminomas is limited compared with that in choriocarcinoma, but RIA for β-hCG is sensitive, and monitoring with β-hCG is sometimes useful in monitoring clinical course of patients with dysgerminoma.

Other Markers for Germ Cell Tumors

CA 125, an antigen defined by a monoclonal antibody, is related to a high molecular-weight glycoprotein that is expressed in coelomic epithelium during embryonic development.[48] In adults the normal values for CA 125 in serum are less than 35 U/ml, and the levels are increased in patients with epithelial ovarian cancer. On the other hand, little is known about the oncologic significance of the marker in children. An increase in serum CA 125 is observed in patients with yolk sac tumor and embryonal carcinoma.[49] Although the significance of CA 125 in childhood germ cell tumors is not yet fully understood, the measurement of serum levels may sometimes be useful in monitoring the disease.

Lactate dehydrogenase isoenzyme-1 (LDH-1) increases in the sera of patients with germ cell tumors including yolk sac tumor, dysgerminoma, and choriocarcinoma. Both total serum LDH activity and LDH-1 activity are increased in patients with yolk sac tumor.[50] The percentages of LDH-1 isoenzyme range from 60 to 88 percent in these patients and are higher than the normal value of 46 percent.

Cytogenetic Markers

Inspite of histologic heterogeneity, adolescent testicular germ cell tumors appear to be relatively genetically homogenous.[51] They have an aneuploid DNA content.[7,52] The characteristic cytogenetic finding is the presence of two copies of 12p of uniparental origin, with retention of 12q heterozygosity, i.e. i(12p).[51] Germ cell tumors associated with more than 3 copies of i(12p) are associated with poor prognosis.[53] The ovarian mature teratomas are cytogenetically normal in 95 percent cases,[54] while 60 percent of the immature teratomas show chromosomal abnormalities although the i(12p) has not been reported in them.[55,56] The histologic grade

of immature ovarian teratomas and their DNA content have been reported to be related; grade 1 and 2 tumors are diploid and grade 3 aneuploid.[57] It has also been observed that diploid grade 3 immature teratomas have a better prognosis than aneuploid grade-3 immature teratomas.[56] i(12p) which is absent in pure immature teratomas has been reported in the those immature teratomas containing endodermal sinus tumor component. Most malignant ovarian germ cell tumors are aneuploid and contain the i(12p).[58,59] In children less than 4 years of age, the histology and behavior of GCT derived from the gonadal or extragonadal sites are similar. Majority of these are teratomas, and regardless of the immaturity and site all are diploid tumors of normal karyotype and behave in a benign fashion if they can be resected.[60,61] Malignant GCT in this age group are almost exclusively yolk sac tumors which are often diploid or tetraploid.[57,62] The cytogenetic analyses of these malignant germ cell tumors in children less than 4 years of age has shown recurrent abnormalities involving chromosome 1,3, and 6 but have not shown the presence of i(12p).[62]

MALIGNANT GERM CELL TUMORS

Endodermal Sinus Tumor (Yolk Sac Tumors)

Endodermal sinus tumor (EST) are the commonest pure malignant germ cell tumor in children and the commonest germ cell tumor, benign or malignant, of testes in children.[63] It has been described in the testes, ovary, sacrococcygeal region and less frequently in the vagina, retroperitoneum, mediastinum and the pineal gland. They can metastasize to the lymph nodes, lungs, liver and bone. In the sacrococcygeal teratoma this is the only malignant form described,[64-66] and in most other extragonadal sites it occurs as a component of mixed malignant germ cell tumor.[8,67,68] Grossly they are pale gray to gray yellow tumors that are friable and have varying amounts of mucoid tissue, hemorrhage and necrosis. Microscopically the individual cell may be small, with pale scanty cytoplasm, round to oval nuclei, an inapparent nucleoli, or they may be medium to large sized cells with clear vesicular nuclei and prominent nucleoli.[69,70] Mitosis may be present. There are four basic histologic patterns of yolk sac tumors described, namely pseudopapillary or festoon pattern, microcystic or reticular pattern, solid pattern, and polyvesicular vitelline pattern.

Pseudopapillary or festoon pattern: This form has the classic Schiller-Duval bodies, which are basically composed of small central blood vessel closely surrounded by two layers of tumor cells, giving the appearance of a primitive glomeruli.

Microcystic or reticular pattern: This in addition to the Schiller-Duval bodies have many eosinophilic, hyalinized intra and extracytoplasmic globules and strands. The globules are positive for periodic acid-Schiff (PAS) and are diastase resistant and occasionally also stain for AFP and α-1 antitrypsin.The strands are also PAS positive and diastase resistant and also stain for laminin.[51]

Solid pattern: This pattern resembles embryonal carcinoma but the cells are smaller and less pleomorphic and have less prominent nucleoli than those of embryonal carcinoma. Hepatoid form, a variant of solid pattern, closely resembles fetal liver and stains for AFP, α-1 antitrypsin, albumin, and third and fourth components of complement.[71]

Polyvesicular vitelline pattern: This is characterized by small empty cystic structures, lined by single layer of malignant cells that are cuboidal to flat, in a loose myxoid stroma. This pattern is said to be associated with a better prognosis.[72]

There are two other distinct patterns described, namely enteric pattern[70] resembling fetal human gut, and the mesenchyme like pattern.[71]

Germinoma

The term germinoma was previously used for extragonadal malignant germ cell tumors which had the same histology as the dysgerminoma of the ovary and the seminoma of the testes.[73] Now the term germinoma is used for all these tumors regardless of the anatomic location.[74] In children germinomas are most commonly found in the ovary, anterior mediastinum and the pineal region. They account for 15 percent of all germ cell tumors.[75] They are the commonest malignant germ cell tumor of the ovary and the central nervous system.[7,66,67] Seminoma, though the commonest malignant germ cell tumor of the adult testis, is almost never found in the testes of infants and young boys, and rarely in adolescent testes.[63] Grossly these are solid, pinkish tumors with a rubbery consistency and have small areas of hemorrhage and necrosis. Microscopically the cells are large round, oval or polygonal, with clear cytoplasm, a distinct cell membrane, large nuclei with one or two prominent nucleoli. They are arranged in nests separated by bands of fibrous tissue with variable amount of lymphocytes. The tumor also has foreign body or Langhans giant cells

and granulomas.[51] Antiferritin antibody and placental alkaline phosphatase (PLAP) are positive in germinomas from all sites and are useful markers for this tumor.[76]

Gonadoblastoma

These are neoplasms found in dysgenetic gonads or are sometimes associated with malignant germinomas.[77] They are usually small, soft to firm, gray or brown with a lobulated surface. Multifocal calcification is present making the cut surface gritty. Histologically they are a mixture of immature germ cells and gonadal sex cord cells (granulosa or Sertoli cells).

Embryonal Carcinoma

In the pediatric age group pure embryonal carcinomas are rare, as they are usually a component of mixed malignant germ cell tumors of the testes or mediastinum. Microscopically they are composed of large cells with large overlapping nuclei and prominent nucleoli. There are three main patterns described, namely epithelial, pseudotubular and papillary. Epithelial form is composed of large nests of cells with varying amounts of central necrosis. The pseudotubular and papillary patterns may be mistaken for yolk sac tumor but the cells of this tumor stain negative for AFP and these tumors lack strands and the hyaline globules of yolk sac tumors.

Choriocarcinoma

In the pediatric age group this tumor is also usually a part of the mixed malignant germ cell tumors.[63,64] Choriocarcinoma has two distinct forms, gestational and non-gestational,[78] and these differ in biologic behavior and response to therapy.[74] The gestational form is one which arises from the placenta while the non-gestational form arises from extra-placental tissues in non-gravid individuals. They are very friable, hemorrhagic and necrotic. Microscopically they are composed of two types of cells, namely cytotrophoblasts and syncytio-trophoblasts. The cytotrophoblasts are closely packed nests of uniform, medium sized cells with clear PAS positive cytoplasm and a vesicular nuclei. The syncytiotrophoblasts tend to develop syncytia and cover the nests of cytotrophoblasts and stain positive for β-hCG. The placental form may be seen in very young infancys who present with disseminated metastases and elevated β-hCG. This is actually a metastatic lesion from the placental primary in the mother which has invaded the villous vessels and entered the umbilical vein and fetal blood.

Mixed Germ Cell Tumors

Mixed germ cell tumors are those germ cell tumors that contain multiple histologic types in at least 10 percent of the specimen. The prognosis for mixed germ cell tumors is worse than that for yolk sac tumors.[79]

TREATMENT OF GERM CELL TUMORS

Principles of Surgical Treatment

Surgery is the treatment of choice for all benign tumors like teratomas and also for malignant germ cell tumors, if feasible. In cases of malignant tumors the resection should not involve any vital structures as effective chemotherapy is available which can substantially reduce the bulk of the tumor and make resection less morbid. In such cases initial debulking or biopsy only is advisable followed by chemotherapy and a second look surgery.

Principles of Chemotherapy for Malignant Germ Cell Tumors

Since malignant germ cell tumors are relatively uncommon in the pediatric age group, most of the chemotherapies have been borrowed from the adult experience and they have been found to be equally effective. The common drugs found to be active against malignant germ cell tumors are Dactinomycin (A), vinblastine (V), bleomycin (B), doxorubicin (ADR), cisplatin (P), carboplatin (J) and etoposide (E). As single agents their response rates varies from 28 to 100 percent.[80-85] Synergistically active combinations of drugs have now been increasingly used and have been found

to be less toxic and at the same time more effective than single or dual agents. The addition of cisplatinum and carboplatin has further improved the results of these regimens. The commonly used pediatric combination are cisplatinum + vinblastine + bleomycin (PVB),[86] cisplatinum + etoposide + bleomycin (PEB)[87] and carboplatin + etoposide + bleomycin (JEB).[88] Currently PEB is the standard regimen being used in both POG and CCG trials of malignant germ cell tumors. In these trials there is randomization of the treatment of high risk tumors with standard PEB and high-dose cisplatinum + etoposide + bleomycin regimens. For salvage of relapsed or refractory patients, marrow ablative doses of carboplatin and etoposide followed by autologous marrow reinfusion is being tried.[89] Generally the low risk, stage-1 testicular and ovarian malignant germ cell tumors require no chemotherapy. Moderate risk tumors or those with progressive disease or tumor recurrences are managed with 3 to 4 courses of platinum based regimens. For higher risk tumors (higher stage testicular or ovarian tumors or extragonadal tumors) 6 months of platinum based regimen is indicated. Some of the common chemotherapeutic regimen are shown in Table 27.6.

Clinical Presentation, Staging and Treatment of Ovarian Germ Cell Tumors

Ovarian tumors constitute only 1 percent of all childhood malignancies[90] and are more common toward the end of the first decade. Two thirds (67%) of pediatric ovarian tumors are germ cell tumors and the most common of these being benign teratoma, 17 percent

Table 27.6: POG/CCG staging system for ovarian germ cell tumors[98]	
Stage	Extent of disease
I	• Limited to ovary/ovaries; peritoneal washings negative for malignant cells • No clinical, radiological or histological evidence of disease beyond Ovaries • Tumor markers negative after appropriate postoperative half-life • Gliomatosis peritonei does not upstage the tumor
II	• Microscopic residual or +ve LN (£ 2cm as measured by pathologist) • Peritoneal washings negative for malignant cells • Tumor markers +ve or –ve • Gliomatosis peritonei does not upstage the tumor
III	• LN with malignant metastatic nodule > 2 cm as measured by pathologist • Gross residual or biopsy only • Contiguous visceral involvement (omentum, intestine, bladder) • Peritoneal washings +ve for malignant cells • Tumor markers +ve or –ve.
IV	• Disseminated metastases including liver

are epithelial tumors and 12 percent sex cord-stromal tumors.[91] Two-thirds of the malignant ovarian tumors are germ cell tumors[92] and amongst the malignant germ cell tumors are, in the order of frequency, dysgerminoma, endodermal sinus tumors, immature teratoma, malignant mixed germ cell tumors and embryonal carcinoma.[11,52,90] Among the non-germ cell tumors are the epithelial tumors which are usually mucinous or serous cystadenomas and rarely cystadenocarcinoma.[93] Pseudomyxoma peritonei with tumor implantation on the peritoneal surfaces occurs mostly with mucinous cystadenomas.[94] Sex cord–stromal tumors are usually granulosa cell tumors which present as precocious pseudopuberty. The other sex cord-stromal tumors, namely, thecoma-fibroma and Sertoli-Leydig cell tumors (androblastoma, arrhenoblastoma) are rare. Most of the sex cord-stromal tumors should receive three courses of a cisplatinum based chemotherapy to enhance treatment results.[95]

The ovarian germ cell tumors can present as an asymptomatic abdominal or pelvic mass or with abdominal pain, which can be acute because of torsion of the pedicle. In addition there may be abdominal distension, constipation, enuresis, precocious puberty, vaginal bleeding or amenorrhea depending on the size of the tumor and secretion of various hormones. The initial investigation is an ultrasound of the abdomen and pelvis to localize the mass to the adnexa, to determine whether the mass is solid or cystic and to determine the presence of calcification.[96,97] Abdominal and pelvic CT scan will further help in defining the site of origin, extent and presence of other metastatic lesions. Since secondaries may appear in the thoracic lymph nodes, lung parenchyma or rarely bone,[51] it is essential to include a plain chest X-ray (PA and lateral), CT scan of the chest, skeletal survey and a radionucleide bone scan in the routine work up of these patients. The currently used surgico-pathological staging system for pediatric ovarian germ cell tumors is the one advocated by POG and CCG (Table 27.6). This four stage system is a refinement over the commonly used FIGO system (in adults) by accounting for:

- Higher risk of recurrence in patients with +ve peritoneal fluid washings (which leads to upstaging of the tumors).
- Utility of the tumor markers for prediction of outcome.
- Lack of negative prognostic impact of gliomatosis peritonei if only mature glial tissue is present.

Operative management is the mainstay of treatment of pediatric germ cell tumors but it is imperative to use reproductive sparing techniques. The basic steps[98] are the same as for adult ovarian tumors, namely:

- Collection of ascitic fluid of peritoneal washings for cytology,
- Examination of the entire peritoneal surface and liver and biopsy of any suspicious lesions,
- Unilateral oopherectomy or salpingo-oophrectomy,
- Wedge biopsy of any suspicious lesions of the contralateral ovary. Bilateral involvement is present in 10 to 15 percent of dysgerminoma, but is extremely rare with other histological types of GCT,
- Omentectomy,
- Bilateral retroperitoneal lymph node sampling including the internal iliac, common iliac, low paraaortic and perirenal lymph nodes.

VAC regimes were commonly used for malignant germ cell tumors of adults in the 1960s and 1970s and had led to improvement in survival rates but were associated with high relapse rates of nearly 46 percent.[99] When the same regimens were used in children[100] it that all stage I and II, 86 percent of stage III and 20 percent of stage IV children survived. Einhorn and Donohue in 1977[101] reported increased survival with PVB regimen in testicular malignant germ cell tumors and subsequently the same was reported for malignant ovarian germ cell tumors.[102-104] The currently used PEB regimens are expected to have survival rates of better than 90 percent with localized disease. The PEB regimen and it modification with high-dose cisplatinum has extensively tried by POG and CCG and their results are awaited. The currently used treatment protocol in the POG and CCG trials is shown in Table 27.5.

Endodermal sinus tumors (yolk sac tumors) (EST) of the ovary: EST is among the commoner malignant ovarian germ cell tumors[102] and are invariably associated with an elevated serum AFP level. The degree of elevation of aFP neither correlates with stage nor with the ultimate prognosis.[105] The tumor is so friable that tumor rupture has been reported in up to 33 percent of cases.[106] Though most of these are stage I tumors but surgery alone is inadequate as when surgery is the only modality used the survival rate is only 19 percent.[107] Therefore postoperative treatment with a platinum based regime is a must in all the cases to achieve a disease free survival rate of higher than 89 percent.[51] Also it is well known that EST is a radioresistant tumor[100] and so radiation therapy has no role in the treatment of EST.

Dysgerminoma of the ovary: Dysgerminoma is the commonest malignant germ cell tumor of the ovary in children and adolescents.[7,12] They usually occur in the genotypic females but can also occur in dysgenetic gonads and have an average age of presentation of about 16 years. These are usually large tumors and 10-15 percent of them are known to be bilateral. Majority of patients are developmentally normal but some are known to be associated with precocious sexual development.[100,108] Stage I patients have a high recurrence rate when treated with surgery alone,[109] and so they all must be treated with adjuvant chemotherapy with PEB, postoperatively.[110,111] There are some workers[115] who still recommend that stage I may be treated with oophrectomy or salpingo-oophrectomy alone and the patient followed up without further treatment unless they develop recurrence. These are very radiosensitive tumors and were extensively treated in the past with post-operative radiation therapy with extremely good results. Now, with the availability of effective chemotherapy and also with the awareness about the long-term morbidity following radiation therapy in young girls, specially with respect to reproductive functions, radiation treatment has more or less been given up.

Embryonal carcinoma of the ovary: This is a rare ovarian tumor comprising of only 6 percent of all ovarian malignant neoplasms.[75,112] These are the least differentiated form of germ cell tumors and are usually found admixed with other germ cell components such as mature cystic teratoma, EST or dysgerminoma.[112] By itself the embryonal carcinoma is hormonally inert but the presence of trophoblastic elements within the tumor may be manifested as precocious puberty, vaginal bleeding, amenorrhea, hirsuitism and a positive pregnancy test.[94,113,114] Only 50 percent of patients with stage I embryonal carcinoma of the ovary survive when surgery is the only treatment given and, therefore, postoperative chemotherapy is advocated for all patients and the approach is similar as for ovarian EST.[113-115]

Malignant mixed germ cell tumors of the ovary: These constitute 8 percent of the ovarian germ cell tumors and are usually EST in a dysgerminoma or immature teratoma.[116] Isosexual precocious puberty is seen in 30 percent of the children with this tumor.[116] These are classified and managed according to the predominant histologic type.[116]

Choriocarcinoma of the ovary: Non-gestational pure choriocarcinoma of the ovary is very rare in children

and comprises of 0.6 percent of all ovarian germ cell tumors. It is more often a part of a mixed ovarian germ cell tumor and manifests clinically as premature thelarche, pubarche and/or vaginal bleeding. This is a highly malignant tumor with early local, lymphatic and hematogenous spread.[108] Because of its malignant nature adjuvant chemotherapy is recommended for all patients irrespective of the stage of disease.

Polyembryoma of the ovary: There are only 12 reports of this extremely rare tumor in the literature and most of these are in association with other tumors.[117-120] This is again an exteremely malignant neoplasm which is not radiosensitive but responds well to chemotherapy with PEB.

Clinical Presentation, Staging and Treatment of Testicular Germ Cell Tumors

Pediatric testicular tumors are rare in prepubertal boys and account for 2 percent of solid malignant neoplasms in boys.[121,122] Seventy-five percent of these childhood neoplasms are germ cell in origin and two-thirds of the germ cell tumors are endodermal sinus tumors (EST) and lesser numbers are teratomas. The testicular tumors usually present as an asymptomatic scrotal mass. Nearly 85 percent of the testicular EST have elevated levels of AFP at presentation and rarely β-hCG is elevated. Ninety percent of the malignant testicular tumors are localized at presentation and metastatic disease, if present, is typically to the draining lymph nodes or the chest. Preopeartive assessment includes a scrotal ultrasound, ultrasound and CT scan of the pelvis, abdomen and chest, skeletal survey, radionucleide bone scan and evaluation of serum markers, namely, AFP and β-hCG. These are important for proper staging and patient monitoring. The surgical approach mandates an inguinal incision with occlusion of the cord structures by a vascular clamp. The testis is then mobilized into the operative field and a radical orchiectomy performed with ligation of all cord structures at the level of the internal ring (high ligation of the cord). The currently used POG staging system for testicular germ cell tumors is shown in Table 27.7. Boys with stage I or II tumors with normal or unknown markers, persistently elevated markers (after orchiectomy) or microscopic residual tumor in the cord structures should undergo an ipsilateral retroperitoneal lymph node (RPLN) sampling. This approach of RPLN sampling is controversial and some workers[123,124] have questioned its utility in stage I disease.

Stage	Extent of disease
I	• Limited to testis, completely resected by high inguinal orchiectomy or transscrotal orchiectomy with no spill
	• No clinical, radiographic, or evidence of disease beyond testes
	• Tumor markers normal after appropriate post-operative half life; patients with normal or unknown markers at diagnosis must have negative ipsilateral retroperitoneal node sampling to confirm stage I
II	• Transscrotal orchiectomy with gross spill of tumor
	• Microscopic residue present in scrotum or in spermatic cord (< 5 cm from proximal end)
	• Retroperitoneal LN involved (< 2 cm)
III	• Retroperitoneal LN involved (> 2 cm)
	• No visceral or extraabdominal involvement
IV	• Distant metastases, including liver

Table 27.7: POG/CCG staging of testicular tumors[98]

Known RPLN enlargement (stage II to IV disease) must be confirmed histologically by sampling.

In children 80 to 85 percent of the testicular germ cell tumors present as stage I disease.[98] As an adjuvant therapy most centers use PEB regimen for all testicular germ cell tumors more than stage I at presentation. For stage I disease surgery alone results in survival rates of 85 to 100 percent[125-128] and most of the others who relapse can be effectively treated with salvage chemotherapy with PEB.[109] The currently used protocol (POG and CCG) is shown in Table 27.5.

Testicular endodermal sinus tumors: These tumors are localized (stage I) in up to 85 percent of the cases and has an overall survival rate of about 70 percent.[79,126] For stage I tumors only surgery is recommended with a prolonged follow-up. While for stage II or III disease surgery should include high ligation and orchiectomy + RPLN sampling followed by chemotherapy with platinum based regime, namely PEB or JEB.

Clinical Presentation and Treatment of Extragonadal Malignant Germ cell tumors

Extragonadal germ cell tumors account for nearly two-thirds of all pediatric germ cell tumors.[62] The most common sites of extragonadal germ cell tumors in children are sacrococcygeal region, anterior mediastinum, pineal, and rarely the retroperitoneum, neck, stomach and vagina. Most of the extragonadal germ cell tumors are benign but when malignant these are very aggressive tumors and therefore adjuvant chemotherapy with PEB or JEB is recommended for all malignant extragonadal germ cell tumors, irrespective

Table 27.8: Staging of malignant extragonadal germ cell tumors (POG/CCG)[98]

Stage I	:	Complete resection at any site; coccygectomy for sacrococcygeal site; negative tumor margins; tumor markers positive or negative
Stage II	:	Microscopic residual; lymph nodes negative; tumor markers positive or negative.
Stage III	:	Gross residual or biopsy only; retroperitoneal nodes negative or positive; tumor markers positive or negative.
Stage IV	:	Distant metastases including liver

of the stage. The POG/CCG staging of extragonadal germ cell tumors is depicted in Table 27.8.

REFERENCES

1. Chaganti RSK, Rodriguez E, Mathew S. Origin of adult male mediastinal germ-cell tumors. Lancet 1994;343:1130–2.
2. Hata J. Germ cell tumors. In Shimizu K, Misugi K, Kobayashi Y, Hata J, Sasaki Y, Hamazaki M, (Eds): Pediatric Surgical Pathology. Tokyo, Bunko-do, 1995;48–56.
3. Teilum G: Special Tumors of the Ovary and Testis: Comparative Pathology and Histological Identification. Copenhagen, Munksgaard 1971.
4. Hawkins EP, Perlman EJ. Germ cell tumors. In Parham DM, (Ed.): Pediatric Neoplasia. Lippincott- Raven Publishers, Philadelphia, 1996,297–330.
5. Heifetz SA, Cushing B, Giller R, Shuster JJ, Stolar CJH, Vinocur CD, Hawkins EP. Immature teratomas in children: pathologic considerations: a report from the combined Pediatric Oncology Group/Children's Cancer Group. Am J Surg Pathol 1998;22:1115–24.

6. Hawkins E, Issacs H, Cushing B, Rogers P. Occult malignancy in neonatal sacrococcygeal teratomas: a report from a combined Pediatric Oncology Group and Children's Cancer Group study. Am J Pediatr Hematol Oncol 1993;15:406–09.

7. Talerman A. Germ cell tumors of the ovary. In: Kumarn RJ (Ed.): Blaustein's Pathology of the Female Genital Tract, 3rd ed New York: Springer-Verlag, 1987;659.

8. Dehner LP. Germ cell tumors of the mediastinum. Semin Diag Pathol 1990;7:266.

9. Harms D, Janig U, Gobel U. Gliomatosis peritonei in childhood and adolescence: clinicopathologic study of 13 cases including immunohistochemical findings. Pathol Res Pract 1989;184:422.

10. Shafie M, Furay RW, Chablani LV. Ovarian teratoma with peritoneal and lymph node metastases of mature glial tissue: a benign condition. J Surg Oncol 1984;27:18.

11. Dehner LP. Gonadal and extragonadal germ cell neoplasms: teratomas in childhood. In Finegold MJ, Bennington J (Eds): Pathology of neoplasia in children and adolescents. Philadelphia: WB Saunders, 1986;282.

12. Thurbeck WW, Scully RE. Solid teratoma of the ovary: a clinicopathologic analysis of nine cases. Cancer 1960;13:804

13. Norris HJ, Zirkin HJ, Benson WL. Immature (malignant) teratoma of the ovary: a clinical and pathological study of 58 cases. Cancer 1976;37:2359-72.

14. Heifetz SA, Cushing B, Giller R, Shuster JJ, Stolar CJ, Vinocur CD, Hawkins EP. Immature teratomas in children: pathologic considerations: a report from the combined Pediatric Oncology Group/Children's Cancer Group. Am J Surg Pathol 1998;22:1115-24.

15. Altman RP, Randolph JG, Lilly JR. Sacrococcygeal teratoma: American Academy of Pediatrics Surgical Section survey. J Pediatr Surg 1974;9:389–98.

16. Ikeda H, Okumura H, Nagashima K, Shinozaki K, Nagamachi Y, Fukaishi T, Ebara H, Sakaguchi M. The management of prenatally diagnosed sacrococcygeal teratoma. Pediatr Surg Int 1900;5:192–4.

17. Holterman A, Filiatrault D, Lallier M, Youssef S. The natural history of sacrococcygeal teratomas diagnosed through routine obstetric sonogram: a single institution experience. J Pediatr Surg 1998;33:899–903.

18. Westerburg B, Feldstein VA, Sandberg PL, Lopoo JB, Harrison MR, Albanese CT. Sonographic prognostic factors in fetuses with sacrococcygeal teratoma. J Pediatr Surg 2000;35:322–6.

19. Rintala R, Lahdenne P, Lindahl H, Siimes M, Heikinheimo M. Anorectal function in adults operated for a benign sacrococcygeal teratoma. J Pediatr Surg 1993;28:1165–7.

20. Uchiyama M, Iwafuchi M, Naitoh M, Yagi M, Iinuma Y, Kanada S, Takeda M. Sacrococcygeal teratoma: a series of 19 cases with long-term follow-up. Eur J Pediatr Surg 1999;9:158–62.

21. Rescorla FJ, Sawin RS, Coran AG, Dillon PW, Azizkhan RG. Long-term outcome for infants and children with sacrococcygeal teratoma: a report from the Childrens Cancer Group. J Pediatr Surg 1998;33:171–6.

22. Bilik R, Shandling B, Pope M, Thorner P, Weitzman S, Ein SH. Malignant benign neonatal sacrococcygeal teratoma. J Pediatr Surg 1993;28:1158–60.

23. Tapper D, Lack EE. Teratomas in infancy and childhood: a 54-year experience at the Children's Hospital Medical Center. Ann Surg 1983;198:398–410.

24. Ehren IM, Mahour GH, Isaacs H. Benign and malignant ovarian tumors in children and adolescents: a review of 63 cases. Am J Surg 1984;147:339–344.

25. Silva PD, Ripple J. Outpatient minilaparotomy ovarian cystectomy for benign teratomas in teenagers. J Pediatr Surg 1996;31:1383–6.

26. Nielsen SN, Scheithauer BW, Gaffey TA. Gliomatosis peritonei. Cancer 1985;56:2499–503.

27. Cushing B, Giller R, Ablin A, Cohen L, Cullen J, Hawkins E, Heifetz SA, Krailo M, Lauer SJ, Marina N, Rao PV, Rescorla F, Vinocur CD, Weetman RM, Castleberry RP. Surgical resection alone is effective treatment for ovarian immature teratoma in children and adolescents: a report of the Pediatric Oncology Group and the Children's Cancer Group. Am J Obstet Gynecol 1999;181:353–358.

28. Kuroiwa M, Suzuki N, Hatakeyama S, Takahashi A, Ikeda H, Tsuchida Y. Determination of indications of surgery with reference to magnetic resonance imaging (MRI) and ultrasound (US) studies. Pediatr Radiol (submitted)

29. Grady RW, Ross JH, Kay R. Epidemiological features of testicular teratoma in a prepubertal population. J Urol 1997;158:1191–2.

30. Gupta DK, Kataria R, Sharma MC. Prepubertal testicular teratomas. Eur J Pediatr Surg 1999;9:173–176.

31. Rushton HG, Belman AB, Sesterhenn I, Patterson K, Mostofi FK. Testicular sparing surgery for prepubertal teratoma of the testis: a clinical and pathological study. J Urol 1990;144:726–30.

32. Lakhoo K, Boyle M, Drake DP. Mediastinal teratomas: review of 15 pediatric cases. J Pediatr Surg 1993;28:1161–4.

33. Moeller KH, Rosado-de-Christenson ML, Templeton PA. Mediastinal mature teratoma: imaging features. Am J Roentgenol 1997;169:985-90.

34. Kuroiwa M, Suzuki N, Takahashi A, Ikeda H, Hatakeyama S, Matsuyama S, Tsuchida Y. Life-threatening mediastinal teratoma in a neonate. Pediatr Surg Int (in press)

35. Oliveira-Filho AG, Carvalho MH, Bustorff-Silva JM, Sbragia-Neto L, Miyabara S, Oliveira ER. Epignathus: report of a case with successful outcome. J Pediatr Surg 1998;33:520–1.

36. Azizkhan RG, Haase GM, Applebaum H, Dillon PW, Coran AG, King PA, King DR, Hodge DS. Diagnosis, management, and outcome of cervicofacial teratomas in neonates: a Children's Cancer Group study. J Pediatr Surg 1995;30:312–6.

37. Gengler JS, Ashcraft KW, Slattery P. Gastric teratoma: the sixth reported case in a female infant. J Pediatr Surg 1995;30:889–90.

38. Bale PM. Sacrococcygeal developmantal abnormalities and tumor in children. Perspect Pediatr Pathol 1984;1:9.

39. Tsuchida Y, Endo Y, Saito S, Kaneko M, Shiraki K, Ohmi K. Evaluation of alpha-fetoprotein in early infancy. J Pediatr Surg 1978;13:155–6.

40. Teilum G, Albrechtsen R, Norgaard-Pedersen B. Immunofluorescent localization of alpha-fetoprotein synthesis in endodermal sinus tumor (yolk sac tumor). Acta Pathol Microbiol Scand Sect A 1974;82:586–8.

41. Scully RE. Endodermal sinus tumor. In Tumors of the Ovary and Maldeveloped Gonads. Armed Forces Institute of Pathology, Washington, D.C., 1977;233–41.

42. Malogolowkin MH, Ortega JA, Krailo M, Gonzalez O, Mahour GH, Landing BH, et al. Immature teratomas: identification of patients at risk for malignant recurrence. J Natl Cancer Inst 1989;81:870–4.

43. Tsuchida Y, Hasegawa H. The diagnostic value of alpha-fetoprotein in infants and children with teratomas: a questionnaire survey in Japan. J Pediatr Surg 1983;18:152–5.

44. Tsuchida Y, Terada M, Honna T, Kitano Y, Obana K, Leibundgut K, Ishiguro T. The role of subfractionation of alpha-fetoprotein in the treatment of pediatric surgical patients. J Pediatr Surg 1997;32:514–17.

45. Ishiguro T, Tsuchida Y. Clinical significance of serum alpha-fetoprotein subfractionation in pediatric diseases. Acta Paediatr 1994;83:709–13.

46. Tsuchida Y, Honna T, Fukui M, Sakaguchi H, Ishiguro T. The ratio of fucosylation of alpha-fetoprotein in hepatoblastoma. Cancer 1989;63:2174–6.

47. Aoyagi Y, Suzuki Y, Igarashi K, Yokota T, Mori S, Suda T, et al. Highly enhanced fucosylation of -fetoprotein in patients with germ cell tumor. Cancer 1993;72:615–8.

48. Bast RC, Klug TL, St. John E, Jenison E, Niloff JM, Lazarus H, et al. A radioimmunoassay using a monoclonal antibody to monitor the course of epithelial ovarian cancer. N Engl J Med 1983;309:883–87.

49. Lahdenne P, Pitkänen S, Rajantie J, Kuusela P, Siimes MA, Lanning M, et al. Tumor markers CA 125 and CA 19-9 in cord blood and during infancy: developmental changes and use in pediatric germ cell tumors. Pediatr Res 1995;38:797–801.

50. Kinumaki H, Takeuchi H, Nakamura K, Ohmi K, Bessho F, Kobayashi N. Serum lactate dehydrogenase isoenzyme-1 in children with yolk sac tumor. Cancer 1985;56:178–81.

51. Castleberry RP, Cushing B, Perlman E, Hawkins EP. Germ cell tumors. In: Pizzo PA, Poplack DG (Eds): Principles and practice of pediatric oncology, Lippincott-Raven Publishers, Philadelphia, 1997:921-945

52. Hawkins EP. Pathology of germ cell tumors in childhood. Crit Rev Oncol Hematol 1990;10:165

53. Bosl GJ, Dmitrovsky E, Reuter VE, et al. Isochromosome of chromosome 12: clinically useful marker for male germ cell tuomrs. J Natl Cancer Inst 1989;81:1874

54. Surti U, Hoffner L, Chakravarti A, Ferrell RE. Genetics and biology of human ovarian teratomas:I. Cytogenetic analysis and mechanism of origin. AM J Hum Genet 1990;47:635

55. Ohama K, Nomura K, Okamoto E, Fukuda Y, Ihara T, Fujiwara A. Origin of immature teratoma of the ovary. Am J Obstet Gynacol 1985;152:895

56. King ME, DiGiovanni LM, Yung J, Clarke-Pearson DL. Immature teratoma of the ovary grade 3, with karyotype analysis. In J Gynecol Pathol 1990;9:178

57. Silver SA, Wiely JM, Perlman EJ. DNA ploidy analysis of pediatric germ cell tumors. Mod Pathol 1994;7:951

58. Speleman F, DePotter C, Dal Cin P, et al. i(12p) in malignant ovarian tumor. Cancer Genet Cytogenet 1990;45:49

59. Hoffner L, Shen-Schwartz S, Deka R, Chakravarti A. Genetics and biology of human ovarian teratoma: III. Cytogenetics and origins of malignant ovarian germ cell tumors. Cancer Genet Cytogenet 1992;62:58

60. Hoffner L, Deka R, Chakravarti A. Cytogenetics and origin of pediatric germ cell tumors. Cancer Genet Cytogenet 1994;74:54

61. Kashiwagi A, Nagamori S, Toyota K, Maeno K, Koyanagi T. DNA ploidy of testicular germ cell tumors in childhood: difference from adult testicular tumors. Nippon Hinyokika Gakkai Zasshi 1993;84:1655

62. Perlman EJ, Cushing B, Hawkins E, Griffin CA. Cytogenetic analysis of childhood endodermal sinus tumors: Pediatric Oncology Group study. Pediatr Pathol 1994;14:695

63. Young RH, Scully RE. Germ cell tumors: nonseminomatous tumors, occult tumors, effects of chemotherapy in testicular tumors. Chicago: ASCP Press, 1990:37

64. Hawkins EP, Perlman EJ. Germ cell tumors in childhood, morphology and biology. In Parham DM (Ed.): Pediatric Neoplasia: morphology and biology. New York: Raven Press 1996;297

65. Harms D, Janig U. Germ cell tumors of childhood: report of 170 cases including 59 pure and partial yolk sac tumors. Virchows Arch A Pathol Anat Histopathol 1986;409:233

66. Schropp K, Lobe T, Rao B, et al. Sacrococcygeal teratomas: experience of four decades. J Pediatr Surg 1992;27:1075

67. Felix I, Becker L. Intracranial germ cell tumors in children: an immunohistochemical and electron microscopic study. Pediatr Neurosurg 1990;16:156

68. Ho DM, Liu H. Primary intracranial germ cell tumor. Cancer 1992;70:1577

69. Ulbright T, Roth L, Brodhecker BS. Yolk Sac differentiation in germ cell tumors, a morphologic study of 50 cases with emphasis on hepatic, enteric and parietal yolk sac features. Am J Surg Pathol 1986;10:151

70. Ulbright T, Roth l. Recent developments in pathology of germ cell tumors. Semin Diagn Pathol 1987;4:304

71. Nakashima N, Fukatsu T, Nagasaka T, Sobue M, Takeuchi J. The frequency and histology of hepatic tissue in germ cell tumors. Am J Surg Pathol 1987;11:682

72. Nogales FF, Mantila a, Nogales-Ortiz F. Yolk sac tumors with pure and mixed polyvesicular vitelline patterns. Hum Pathol 1978;9:553.

73. Anderson T et al. Testicular germ cell neoplasm: recent advances in diagnosis and therapy. Ann Intern Med 1979;90:373

74. Albin A, Issac H. Germ cell tumors. In: Pizzo PA, Poplack DG (eds) Principles and practice of pediatric oncology, 2nd ed, Philadelphia, 1993, JB lippincott.

75. Dehner LP. Pediatric surgical pathology, 2nd ed, Baltimore, Williams and Wilkins, 1987:721

76. Witzelben Cl, Bruniya G. Infantile choriocarcinoma: a characteristic syndrome. J Pediatr 1968;73:374.

77. Scully RE. Gonadoblastoma: a review of 74 cases. Cancer 1970;25:1340.

78. Tapper D, Swain R. Teratomas and other germ cell tumors. In O'Neill JA, Rowe MI, Grosfeld JL, Fonkalsrud EW, Coran AG (Eds): Pediatric Surgery, Mosby, St. Louis, 1998:447-60.

79. Mann JR, Pearson D, Barrett A. Results of the United Kingdom Children's Cancer Study Group's malignant germ cell tumor studies. Cancer 1989;63:1657.

80. Merrin CE, Murphy GP. Metastatic testicular carcinoma: single agent chemotherapy (actinomycin d) in treatment. NY State J Med 1974;74:654.

81. Ameuls ML, Howe CD. Vinblastine in the management of testicular cancer. Cancer 1970;25:1009

82. Blum RH, Careter SS, Agre K. A clinical review of bleomycin: a new antineoplastic agent. Cancer 1973; 31:903.

83. Wollner N, Exelby PR, Woodruff JM, et al. VP-16-213 salvage therapy for refractory germinal neoplasms. Cancer 1980;96:2154.

84. Koshida K, Nishino A, Yamamoto H, et al. The role of alkaline phosphatase isoenzymes as tumor markers in testicular germ cell tumors. J Urol 1991;146:57.

85. Williams SD, Einhorn LH, Greco FA, et al. VP-16-213 salvage therapy for refractory germinal neoplasms. Cancer 1980;96:2154.

86. Einhorn LH, Williams SD, Troner M, et al. The role of maintenance therapy in disseminated testicular cancer. N Engl J Med 1981;305:727.

87. Hawkins EP, Finegold MJ, Hawkins HK, Kirscher JP, Starling KA, Weinberg A. Nongerminomatous malignant germ cell tumors in children: a review of 89 cases from the Pediatric Oncology Group, 1971-1984. Cancer 1986;58:2579.

88. Pinkerton CR, Broadbent V, Hoewich A, et al. "JEB": a carboplatin based regimen for malignant germ cell tumors in children. Br J Cancer 1990;62:257.

89. Nicholas CR, Anderson J, Lazarus HM, et al. High dose carboplatin and etoposide with autologous bone marrow transplantation in refractory germ cell cancer: an Eastern

Cooperative Oncology Group protocol. J Clin Oncol 1992;10;558.

90. Young Jl, Ries LJ, Silverberg E, et al. Cancer incidence, survival, and mortality for children younger than 15 years of age. Cancer 1986;58:598.

91. Breen JL, Maxson WS. Ovarian tumors in children and adolescents. Clin Obstet Gynecol 1977;20:607-23.

92. Lazar EL, Stolar CJ. Evaluation and management of pediatric solid ovarian tumors. Semin Pediatr Surg 1998;7:29-34.

93. Gribbon M, Ein SH, Mancer K. Pediatric malignant ovarian tumors: a 43 year review. J Pediatr Surg 1992;27:480-84.

94. Lack EE, Young RH, Scully RE. Pathology of ovarian neoplasms in childhood and adolescence. Pathol Ann 1992;27:281-356.

95. Calaminus G, Wessalowski R, Harms D, Gobel U. Juvenile granulosa cell tumors of the ovary in children and adolescents: results from 33 patients registered in a prospective cooperative study. Gynecol Oncol 1997; 65:447-52.

96. Sisler CL, Siegel MJ. Ovarian teratomas: a comparison of sonographic appearance in prebubertal and post-pubertal girls. Am J Roentgenol 1990;154:139.

97. Brown DL, Frates MC, Laing FC, et al. Ovarian masses: can benign and malignant lesions be differentiated with color Doppler US? Radiology 1994;190:333.

98. Rescorla FJ. Germ cell tumors. Semin Pediatr Surg 1997;6:29-37.

99. Slayton RE, Park RC, Silvergerg SG et al. Vincristine, dactinomycin, and cyclophosphamide in the treatment of malignant germ cell tumors of the ovary: a gynecologic oncology group study (a final report). Cancer 1985; 56:243-8.

100. Cangir A, Smith J, van Eys J, et al. Improved prognosis in children with ovarian cancers following modified VAC (vincristine sulfate, dactinomycin, and cyclophosphamide) chemotherapy. Cancer 1978;42:1234-8.

101. Einhorn LH, Donohue J. Cis-diamminedichloroplatinum, vinblastine, and bleomycin combination chemotherapy in disseminated testicular cancer. Ann Intern Med 1977;87:293-8.

102. Albin AR, Krailo MD, Ramsay NK, et al. Results of treatment of malignant germ cell tumors in 93 children: a report from the children's cancer group. J Clin Oncol 1991;9:1782-92.

103. Carlson RW, Sikie BI, Turbow MM, et al. Combination cisplatin, vinblastin and bleomycin chemotherapy (PVB) for malignant germ cell tumors of the ovary. J Clin Oncol 1983;1:645-51.

104. Jacob AJ, Harris M, Deppe G, et al. Treatment of recurrent and persistent germ cell tumors with cisplatin, vinblastin, and bleomycin. Obstet Gynecol 1982;59:129-32.

105. Kawai M, Kano T, Furuhasi Y, et al. Prognostic factors in yolk sac tumors of the ovary. A clinicopathologic analysis of 29 cases. Cancer 1991;67:184-92.

106. Copeland LJ. Malignant gynecologic tumors. In Sutow WW, Fernbach GJ, Vitte TJ (Eds): Clinical Pediatric Oncology. St Louis, MO, Mosby, 1984,744-60.

107. Kumaran RJ, Norris HJ. Endodermal sinus tumor of the ovary. Cancer 1976;38:2404-19.

108. Abell MR, Johnson VJ, Holtz F. Ovarian neoplasms in childhood and adolescence: part I. Tumors of germ cell origin. Am J Obstet Gynecol 1965;92:1059.

109. Gordon A, Lipton D, Woodruff D. Dysgerminoma: a review of 158 cases from Emil Novak ovarian tumor registry. Obstet Gynecol 1981,58:579-89.

110. Gershenson DM, Morris M, Cnagir A, et al. Treatment of malignant germ cell tumors of the ovary with bleomycin, etoposide and cisplatin. J Clin Oncol 1009;8:715-20.

111. Williams SD, Blessing J, Hatch K, et al. Chemotherapy of advanced ovarian dysgerminomas: trials of the Gynecologic Oncology Group. Proc Am Soc Clin Oncol 1991;9:155 (abstr).

112. Hawkins E, Perlman E. Germ cell tumors in childhood, morphology and biology. In Parham DM (Ed.): Pediatric neoplasia: morphology and biology. New York: Raven Press 1996;297.

113. Kumaran RJ, Norris HJ. Embryonal carcinoma of the ovary: a clinicopathologic entity distinct from endodermal sinus tumor resembling embryonal carcinoma of adult testis. Cancer 1976;38:2420.

114. Neubecker RD, Breen JL. Embryonal carcinoma of the ovary. Cancer 1962;15:546.

115. Greshenson DM. Update on malignant ovarian germ cell tumors. Cancer 1993;71:1582.

116. Kumaran RJ, Norris HJ. Malignant mixed germ cell tumors of the ovary: a clinical and pathological analysis of 30 cases. Obstet Gynecol 1976;48:579-89.

117. Beck JS, Fulmer HF, Lee ST. Solid malignant ovarian teratoma with "embryoid bodies" and trophoblstic differentiation. J Pathol 1969;99:67.

118. King ME, Hubbell MJ, Talerman A. Mixed germ cell tumor of the ovary with prominent polyembryoma component. Int J Gynecol Pathol 1991;10:88.

119. Takeda A, Ishizuka T, Goto T, et al. Polyembryoma of the ovary producing alpha-fetoprotein and HCG: immunoperoxidase and electron microscopic study. Cancer 1982;49:1878.

120. Simard LC, Polyembryonic embryoma of the ovary of parthenogenetic origin. Cancer 1957;10:215.

121. Brosman SA. Testicular tumors in prepubertal children. Urology 1979;13:581.

122. Pritchard J, Mitchell CD. Testicular tumors in children. In Broecker BH, Klein FA (Eds): Pediatric tumors of genitourinary tract. New York: Alan R Liss, 1988;187.

123. Filler RM, Hardy BE. Testicular tumors in children. World J Surg 1980;4:63-70.

124. Bracken RB, Johnson DE, Cangir A, et al. Regional lymph nodes in infants with embryonal carcinoma of testis. Urology 1978;11:376-79.

125. Peckham MJ, Barrett A, Husband JE, et al. Orchiectomy alone in testicular stage I non-seminomatous germ cell tumors. Lancet 1982;11:678-80.

126. Carroll WL, Kempson RL, Govan DE, et al. Conservative management of testicular endodermal sinus tumor in childhood. J Urol 1985;133:1011-4.

127. Kaplan GW, Gromie WC, Kelalis PP, et al. Prepubertal yolk sac tumors- report of testicular registry. J Urol 1988; 140:1109-12.

128. Huddart SN, Mann JR, Gornall P, et al. The UK Children's Cancer Study Group: testicular malignant germ cell tumors 1979-1988. J Pediatr Surg 1990;25:406-10.

129. Ikeda H, Matsuyama S, Suzuki N, Takahashi A, Kuroiwa M, Nagashima K, Hirato J. Treatment of a stage I testicular yolk sac tumor with vascular invasion. Acta Paediatr Jpn 1995;37:537-40.

130. Pinkerton CR, Broadbent V, Horwich A, Levitt J, McElwain TJ, Meller ST, Mott M, Oakhill A, Pritchard J. 'JEB'- a carboplatin based regimen for malignant germ cell tumors in children. Br J Cancer 1990;62:257–62.

CHAPTER 28

Andrew Pinter

Testicular Tumors

INTRODUCTION

Testicular tumors in childhood and adolescent boys represent approximately 1 percent of childhood malignancies, ranking seventh in order of malignant tumors.[1] Because of the low incidence of testicular tumors in boys, there is paucity of information. regarding appropriate management. A thorough literature review and experience gained by several national and international registries, like the UK Children's Cancer Study Group,[2] Paediatric Oncology Group or the Prepubertal Testis Tumor Registry established in 1980 by the Section of Urology of the American Academy of Pediatrics, help to elucidate the natural history, risk factors and optimal treatment of these rare tumors.

Because of the small series in prepubertal age, the experience with adult testicular tumors was extrapolated to infants and children. Time was needed to understand that distinct differences exist between natural history of the disease process in children and that in adult. In comparison with adults, childhood tumors are much more likely to be benign.

EMBRYOLOGY

Teilum initially proposed the germ cell origin of gonadal tumors.[3]

The process of differentiation of germ cell tumors is listed in Figure 28.1.[4] Seminoma or dysgerminoma is a primitive germ cell neoplasm that lacks the ability for further differentiation. Embryonal carcinoma is a tumor comprised of multipotential cells capable of further differentiation into embryonic (mature or immature teratoma) or extraembryonic (yolk sac or choriocarcinoma) tumors.[4]

This chapter, on the basis of the literature and of own experience, will try to provide an up-to date review of malignant and non-malignant testicular tumors in prepubertal boys.

NOMENCLATURE AND CLASSIFICATION

The initial lack of a worldwide-accepted classification of testicular tumors in children has resulted in some difficulty interpreting the data on the distribution and incidence of childhood testicular tumors of various histological types. Nomenclature and classification system formalized by the World Health Organization (WHO) divided the testis tumors into germ cell tumors and non-germ cell tumors,[5] however it was not easy to use in prepubertal boys, because certain carcinomas are almost never encountered in children, and yolk sac tumors are so common, the adult classification is not entirely accurate for infants and children.

Therefore, classification of prepubertal testicular tumors, based on histological appearance and combined with clinical and pathologic staging has been developed with the help of Mostofi and Sobin[5] and has been ratified by the Section of Urology of the American Academy of Pediatrics.[6] This classification includes germ cell tumors, gonadal stromal tumors, gonadoblastomas, tumor-like lesions, tumors of the adnexa, secondary tumors, lymphomas and leukemias (Table 28.1).

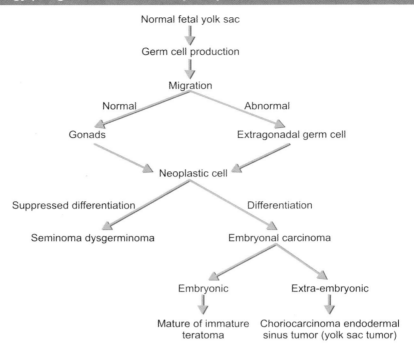

Figure 28.1: Classification system for development of germ cell tumors (Rescorla FJ. Sem in Ped. Surg 1997;6:29-37)

<table>
<tr><th colspan="2">Table 28.1: Classification of prepubertal testicular tumors</th></tr>
</table>

Germ cell tumors
- Yolk sac tumor
- Teratoma
- Seminoma
- Mixed germ cell tumor

Gonadal stromal tumors
- Leydig cell tumor
- Sertoli cell tumor
- Granulosa cell tumor
- Mixed gondal stromal tumor

Gonadoblastoma

Tumor-like lesions
- Epidermoid cyst
- Hyperblastic nodule secondary to congenital adrenal hyperplasia
- Simple cyst

Tumors of the adnexa
- Rhabdomyosarcoma, fibroma, fibrosarcoma, leiomyoma,
- leiomyosarcoma, hemangioma, lipoma

Secondary tumors
- Lymphoma and leukemia

DIAGNOSIS AND DIFFERENTIAL DIAGNOSIS

A prepubertal testicular tumor usually presents as a painless scrotal mass, noticed by the parents or the physician. The mass is firm and non-transilluminating, but it may associate with a reactive hydrocele. Some children may be misdiagnosed as having a hydrocele only. Less frequently presenting symptoms are trauma and swelling. With hormonally active tumors, scrotal examination may be unrevealing and the diagnosis is considered because of precocious puberty.

The duration of symptoms prior to the beginning of treatment averages 3 to 6 months in germ cell tumors but up to 2 months in non-germ cell neoplasms.[7,8]

The differential diagnosis includes: hydrocele, testicular trauma or infarct, torsion, mumps, orchitis, epididymo-orchitis.

To arrive at a decision on the appropriate management, the tumor extent needs to be assessed. Preoperatively, a scrotal ultrasound is beneficial and non-invasive means of detecting the characteristics of the mass. It is useful in the evaluation of local tumor extent, examination the contralateral testis and in prevention of an incorrect diagnosis (a simple hydrocele being mistaken for a coexisting hydrocele and tumor). Subsequently, the retroperitoneal lymph nodes, lungs, and liver need to be analysed for the presence of metastases. Besides abdominal and supraclavicular palpation and ultrasonography, computered tomographic examination of the abdomen and pelvis, skeletal X-ray survey and/ or bone scan are the most important staging measures to detect the possible metastases.

Biochemical tumor markers play an important role in the evaluation of children with testis tumors. Traditionally, both α-fetoprotein (AFP), produced by 90 percent of the yolk sac tumors, and the β subunit of humane chorionic gonadotropin (β-hCG), produced by trophoblastic elements, are two useful markers of germ cell tumors.

AFP made by the yolk sac cells of the embryo. The fetal levels are high and remain elevated after birth, declining to normal level at 9 months of age. The mean value for AFP for a newborn ~50.000 mg/ml, at 2 weeks of age ~10.000 mg/ml, at 1 months of age ~2.500 mg/ml, at 3 months of age ~90 mg/ml, and after 6 month of age < 15 mg/ml.[7] The half-life of AFP is prolonged in early infancy. By 8 months of age it drops to 5 days.[9]

Most yolk sac tumor have an elevation of AFP and in general may be extremely high. It has been estimated that as many as 10 percent of boys with yolk sac carcinoma do not have elevated AFP values.

β-hCG is produced by tumors with trophoblastic elements. Level of β-hCG is rarely elevated in yolk sac tumor in children but in germ cell tumors containing trophoblastic elements such as choriocarcinomas can produce elevation in β-hCG. The value of routinely measuring β-hCG in children with testicular tumors should be reassessed, since it is only elevated in a small number of patients.[2,8]

AFP and β-hCG can be obtained prior to or immediately after surgery for all suspicious testicular pathology. If elevated, these serum biological markers can be used as a baseline to monitor response to treatment or the occurrence of relapse.

Certain functional testicular tumors such as Leydig cell tumor produce increased hormonal (androgen) level arising from the gonadal cell tumors.

In general, all testicular masses should be explored for histological studies and definitive diagnosis. The surgical approach to a solid tumors mandates an inguinal incision to avoid contamination of the scrotum and its lymphatic drainage. The cord should be clamped with atraumatic clamp and the scrotal content and the intact tunica vaginalis delivered to the wound. If the mass involves a part of the testis and the gross appearance do not indicate a malignant process only, a biopsy or enucleation may be performed for frozen section histological diagnosis. If frozen section discloses a teratoma or other benign lesions enucleation is probably sufficient and the blood supply is restored and the testis is placed back into the scrotum. If a malignancy is confirmed, a radical orchiectomy is performed, with ligation of all cord structures at the level of the internal ring. Postoperatively, clinical staging and management vary by tumor and will be specified under the discussion of each individual tumor.

An overview of the diagnostic features of the most common testicular and paratesticular tumors in children taken from Coppes and coworkers[10] is presented in Table 28.2.

STAGING

Apart from a classification according to the histopathologic cell type (see Table 28.1), childhood testicular tumors can be classified according to their extend by the TNM staging classification. This classification takes into account the size of the primary tumor (T), regional lymph node involvement (N), and the occurrence of distant metastases (M).

TNM classification is based on evidence acquired from pathologic examination following surgical intervention; however, in most cases, routine lymph node dissection is not recommended anymore for staging purpose. In addition, a system for evaluating extent of disease has specifically been designed for testicular tumors by the Section of Urology, American Academy of Pediatrics (Table 28.3).

SURGICAL CONSIDERATIONS

Compared to adults, childhood testicular tumors are characterized by a higher percentage of benign clinical cause and much lower incidence of metastases. This has led to recommendations for an overall less aggressive cytostatic treatment and surgical approach to the management of testicular tumors in children.[11-13]

For appropriate therapy, the tumor extent must be known. The main diagnostic target organs are the retroperitoneal lymph nodes, lungs, liver and bone. Besides abdominal and supraclavicular palpation,

Table 28.2: Diagnostic features of the most common testicular and paratesticular tumors in children

Type	Age at diagnosis	Symptoms	Markers
Yolk sac tumor	Any age (most < 3 yrs)	Painless mass	Serum AFP elevated
Teratoma	Any age (most < 4 yrs)	Painless mass	
Leydig cell tumor	5-9 yrs	Precocious puberty	
TTAGS[a]	Most 0-9 yrs	Bilateral masses, symptoms of AGS[b]	ACTH low, 21-hydroxylase deficiency
Sertoli cell tumor	Any age	Painless mass	
Gonadoblastoma	Most after puberty	Virilization if phenotypic females, bilateral in 30 percent of cases	Phenotypic female with 46XY karyotype
Lymphoma/leukemia	Any age (most < 7 yrs)	Painless mass (can be occult)	Blasts in peripheral Blood/bone marrow
Rhabdomyosarcoma	Any age (most < 7 yrs)	Painless mass	

[a]TTAGS = Testicular tumor of the adrenogenital syndrome
[b]AGS = Adrenogenital syndrome

Table 28.3: Grouping of testicular tumors in children

Group I	:	Tumor confined to the testis, AFP levels normal within 1-2 months after orchiectomy, imaging of retroperitoneum and chest normal
Group II	:	Similar to group I, but retroperitoneal lymph node dissection reveals unsuspected nodal metastases
Group III	:	Retroperitoneal lymph node metastases demonstrated on imaging studies, serum AFP levels persistently elevated
Group IV	:	Demonstrable metastases beyond the retroperitoneum (bone, liver, lung)

sonography, X-ray and computer tomographic (CT) examination of the abdomen, pelvis and chest X-ray are the most important staging measures.

Tumor spread, contrary to the course of disease in adults, occurs more frequently by hematogenic metastases than by lymphogenic ones.

Inguinal orchiectomy allows an accurate histological differentation of the tumor and provides information on the local extension of the primary tumor. At the same time, it is in itself a sufficient therapy for most testicular tumors in stage I. Almost 75 percent of such children are cured by this method. It is essential to obtain histological confirmation of clear resection margins and presence or absence of vascular, lymphatic, tunica and cord infiltration.

The potential morbidity associated with paraaortic lymph node biopsy (intraoperative injuries, late bowel obstruction secondary to adhesions and potential ejaculatory dysfunction), especially if bilateral, is not considered to be justified by the information obtained.[14] A scrotal biopsy or orchiectomy can contaminate the surgical field, conceivably alter lymphatic drainage, may alter the histological stage and promote metastasis and lead to chemotherapy that would not have been otherwise necessary. Therefore, when a scrotal biopsy has been performed, a hemiscrotectomy should be done. The use of chemotherapy before orchiectomy or before thoracotomy in patients with bulky testicular tumors or lung metastases, appears to improve survival.

Theoretical concern related to testicular sparing procedures (enucleation) of prepubertal testicular tumors (teratoma, Leydig cell tumor) include the possibility of tumor seeding or spillage, incorrect diagnosis, sampling error or residual multifocal microscopic disease.

GERM CELL TUMORS

Germ cell tumors arising from the primitive germ cells or totipotent embryonal cells, may occur in any part of the reproductive tract. Germ cell tumors account for 2 to 3 percent of all childhood malignancies. The process of differentiation of germ cell tumor is listed in Figure 28.1.[4] Seminoma (or dysgerminoma) is a primitive germ cell neoplasm that lacks the ability for further differentiation. Embryonal carcinoma is a tumor comprised of multipotential cells capable of further differentiation into embryonic (mature or immature teratoma) or extraembryonic (yolk sac or chorio-carcinoma) tumor. The morphologic type and the biologic characteristics of each type of germ cell tumors vary depending on site of origin and age of patient. Mature cancers are managed by observation alone, whereas all other tumors require chemotherapy.

Yolk Sac Tumor

Yolk sac tumors which account for three quarters of malignant testicular tumors are the most common form of malignant tumor of the testis in infants and in children. In a detailed review of 556 prepubertal patients with testis tumors Brosman found 336 cases (60 percent) of yolk sac tumor.[8] They are clinically and histologically distinct neoplasms of the testis that occurs primarily in children < 2 years old. Almost all affected patients have an elevated serum AFP level.

This neoplasm has been referred to by many alternative names, including orchioblastoma, clear cell adenocarcinoma, juvenile embryonal carcinoma, embryonal cell carcinoma, archenteronoma, and infantile endodermal sinus tumor, however yolk sac is the preferred term, since the histology resembles that of the yolk sac.

Their clinical findings are of a painless and firm enlargement of the testis, often accompanied by a reactive hydrocele.

The initial staging should include determination of serum AFP, and adequate imaging of the chest, abdomen and pelvis. Preoperative high serum AFP levels do not necessarily predict metastases or poor prognosis. Review of the literature shows that nearly 60 to 90 percent of children present with elevated AFP levels and that approximately half are without metastases.[7,14]

Intraoperatively the yolk sac tumors present as solid pinkish-gray to yellow swellings; however, multicystic, necrotic or hemorrhagic lesion car also be seen.

Microscopically, yolk sac tumors have certain characteristics as distinguished from all other germ cell tumors. They are composed of epithelium and mesenchymal elements. The distinctive feature is the perivascular Schiller-Duval bodies. This is an arrangement of cells that form glomerulus-like structures.

In most children with yolk sac tumor, radical inguinal orchiectomy alone is curative. Scrotal orchiectomy is insufficient treatment and because of the high incidence of local or inguinal metastases after scrotal orchiectomy, it should be followed by radical orchiectomy and hemiscrotectomy. Nevertheless, the management of yolk sac tumor in children remains controversial, in particular the need for retroperitoneal lymph node dissections. In contrast to all adult testis tumors, which primarily metastasize via the lymphatic system to the retroperitoneum, data from the Prepubertal Testis Tumor Registry suggest that yolk sac tumor in children has a tendency to metastasize by hematogenous routes (lungs, liver, brain). Among 32 patients with metastatic disease at initial diagnosis, 11 had hematogenous spread (7 to the lung only, 4 to lungs and additional sites), 9 with metastases to the retropetineum only, and 6 patients had retroperitoneal metastases combined with hematogenous sites (lung in 4, vena cava in 1, and kidney in 1). These data suggest that particularly in young children, the treatment of Stage I. yolk sac tumor can be restricted to radical orchiectomy with close surveillance of the serum AFP levels, chest X-rays, and abdominal ultrasonography. In children, the risks of complications following retroperitoneal dissection (intraoperative injuries, late bowel obstruction secondary to adhesions, and potential for ejaculatory dysfunction) do not warrant its routine use in the surgical management of this neoplasm. A review of the disease-free survival of all reported testicular yolk sac tumors between boys undergoing orchiectomy alone or in combination with unilateral or bilateral retroperitoneal lymph node dissection showed no significant differences in survival. The complications combined with the incidence of lymphatic spread suggest that the risk of routine retroperitoneal lymph node dissection outweighs the benefit in clinical Stage I disease. For patients with Stage III disease, retroperitoneal lymph node sampling might be considered.

Following surgery, serum AFP levels must be monitored, monthly for a year and every two months in the second year. If AFP levels postorchiectomy do not return to normal within the expected length of time determined by half-life decay, metastatic disease must be suspected. The role of routine use for chest X-ray and abdominal ultrasonography and computerized axial tomography in patients in whom the AFP level has returned to a normal value is in question.

Chemotherapeutic agents effective in yolk sac tumor include vincristine, vinblastine, cisplatinium, actinomycin D, bleomycin, doxorubicin and' cyclophosphamide.[2,10,15,16] The optimum length of time for administration of the cytostatic drugs has not been clearly defined.

A recent Children's Cancer Group (POG) clinical trial evaluated surgery followed by observation for boys with Stage I testicular tumors. This strategy resulted in a 3-year event-free survival of 80 percent.[17] Most patients who developed recurrent disease following surgical resection of a testicular tumor were salvageable with standard cisplatin, etoposide and bleomycin (PEB), and the 3-year survival for these patients is 100 percent.[17] Thus, for young boys with Stage I disease, surgical resection by radical inguinal orchiectomy followed by close observation is the standard treatment approach. A cooperative study of 197 testicular germ cell tumors in childhood conducted by the German Society of Paediatric Oncology also demonstrated that in AFP producing Stage I tumors chemotherapy alone following radical orchiectomy reveals excellent result and radiotherapy or primarly lymphadenectomy can be omitted.[13]

In the same CCG/POG study described in the previous paragraph, boys with Stage II and III through IV testicular tumors treated with surgical resection followed by 4 courses of standard PEB therapy had event-free survival rates of 100 and 90 percent respectively.[17,18] Thus, for boys with state II through IV testicular germ cell tumors, surgical resection followed by 4 courses of standard PEB is the appropriate treatement approach.

Children with bulky disease should undergo cytoreductive chemotherapy" prior to the radical surgical intervention.

If residual or metastatic disease appears, aggressive chemotherapy combined with additional radiotherapy or an operation can result in salvage of approximately two- thirds of those patients with metastases.

Teratoma (Figs 28.2A to C)

The testicle is an uncommon site of teratomas in infancy and childhood, accounting for 2 to 7 percent of all teratomas.[19] The relative frequency of teratoma among testicular germ cell tumors in children varies from approximately 13 to 60 percent".[20] Of the 229 germ cell tumors included in the Prepubertal Testicular Tumor Registry 19 percent were classified as teratoma.[21] Their mean age at presentation was 18 months in this series, but they may be seen in the neonatal period. The tumor is derived from embryonic tissues and is composed of all three germ layers: ectoderm, mesoderm and endoderm although one layer may predominate. These tissues can show various stages of differentiation ranging from primitive structures to well matured tissues, such as teeth, cartilage, bony matrix. Macroscopically they present predominantly as multicystic structures of different size, colour, and consistency, often containing

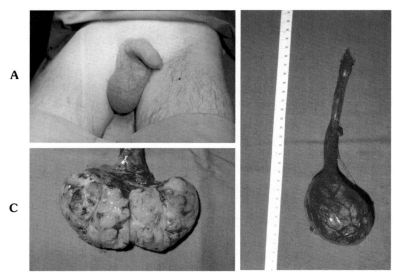

Figures 28.2A to C: Germ cell tumor- teratoma (**A**) Right-sided scrotal enlargement, (**B**) High orchiectomy -operative specimen, (**C**) Cut surface of the testis -tumor occupies the whole testis

gelationous fluid. Almost all prepubertal testicular tumors are of pure histological type. Of 353 childhood testis tumor in the American Testicular Tumor Registry, only 2 prepubertal patients had tumor containing yolk sac and teratomatosus elements, representing 0.85 of prepubertal boys with germ cell tumors.[22]

Although the final diagnosis can only be established by histopathologic examination, one can suspect this tumor in a prepubertal boy presenting with a testicular mass who does not have endocrine disturbances or an elevated serum APP. This suspicion will be confirmed by the presence of a circumscribed, partly cystic intratesticular mass on ultrasonography. Testicular teratoma in children is characterized by sonolucent areas with intervening septa and solid areas.[20] This finding contrast with other childhood intratesticular tumors, except for the rare cystic granulosa cell tumor.

Pure testicular teratomas have never been reported to be associated with elevated levels of serum AFP. However, testicular teratomas rarely containing yolk sac tumor component, can have elevated level of serum AFP.

As there have been no reports of metastatic teratoma in prepubertal boys, orchiectomy used to be the a curative procedure.[20,23] This is in contrast to the unpredictable outcome of testicular teratoma in adults.

However, surgical treatment for this condition has evolved over the last 3 decades, with the increasing recognition of their benign behavior, despite the presence of immature elements on histology. Favorable prognosis has been observed in the prepubertal age group not only for the mature and immature teratomas, but also for teratomas with malignant components.

This benign behavior of this neoplasm in all childhood has led to the recommendation of enucleation of the usually encapsulated tumors, which is a testicular sparing procedure (Fig. 28.3). In the 1990s there are increasing reports of testicular sparing, even enucleation when feasible, for prepubertal testicular teratomas.[20,23] This approach that has potential psychological cosmetic, and functional advantages for the developing child, is recommended unless the preoperative serum AFP or β-hCG levels are elevated. It is currently unclear whether or not biopsies need to be performed on the remaining ipsilateral testis to ensure that there is no carcinoma *in situ* or other germinal abnormalities.[20,23]

For testicular sparing procedure (enucleation or partial resection) an inguinal incision must be used and the cord clamped with an atraumatic clamp prior to handling the testis. Gross appearance and palpation should not indicate a malignant process and a biopsy or enucleation for frozen section histological diagnosis must be performed. In addition, the adjacent normal testicular tissue should also be biopsied to rule out pubertal changes and carcinoma in situ. Pathologic study of 17 orchiectomy specimens from the American Testicular Tumor Registry containing prepubertal teratomas did not reveal any instance of multifocal tumor, and all germ cells in the adjacent seminiferous tubules were negative for placental alkaline phosphatase, a highly sensitive marker for intratubular germ cell neoplasia.[20]

Seminoma

Seminoma, a malignancy related to spermatogenesis, is the most common testicular tumor in adult but is rarely seen in prepubertal boys. Because seminoma is related to spermatogenesis, it is questioned whether seminoma tumor could exist in prepubertal boys. Therefore uncertainity exists on how to best treat this neoplasm. Therefore, until clinical evidence suggests an alternative management, it is recommended to employ the same treatment used for adult patients: radical orchiectomy, proper staging and radiation therapy or chemotherapy for advanced stages. The recommended treatment according to the stages is the following: orchiectomy for stage I, orchiectomy (and retroperitoneal lymp node dissection) followed by chemotherapy or radiation therapy for stage II disease, and preoperative chemotherapy followed by surgery (and retroperitoneal lymph node dissection), radiation therapy, and eventually additional chemotherapy for stage III disease.

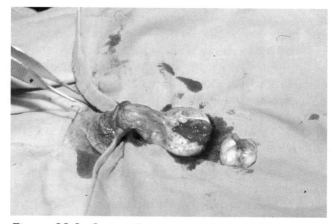

Figure 28.3: Germ cell tumor—teratoma, testicles sparing procedure (encapsulation)

Mixed Germ Cell Tumor

Tumors composed of more than one histological type of germ cell neoplasm occur in the central nervous system, anterior mediastinum, ovary and testis. The three most frequent combinations are teratoma with yolk sac, teratoma plus embryonal carcinoma and choriocarcinoma, and teratoma plus embryonal carcinoma.[24] In prepubertal boys with a mixed germ cell neoplasm, probably the most often encountered malignancy is teratoma with yolk sac.

Teratocarcinomas, which are composed of tissue of extraembryonal yolk sac tumor and of embryonal teratomatous tissue, belong to mixed germ cell tumors. Clinically they present like yolk sac tumors but in addition to AFP they may produce β-hCG. In contrast to the typical pulmonary metastasis of the yolk sac tumor, teratocarcinomas tend to metastasize in the lymphatic system. Therapy does not differ from that of yolk sac tumor, however the prognbstic marker is more often β-hCG, and the prognosis is worse.

β-hCG is elevated in those patients with histology other than yolk sac tumor. These tumors contain of choriocarcinoma and teratocarcinoma.

Treatment of these tumors is dictated by the most malignant component of the tumor.

Germ Cell Tumor – Late Effects

Survival for children with the most common types of germ cell tumors, which was only 10 to 20 percent before the development of effective chemotherapy, now approaches 70 percent with current treatment modalities.[12]

Systematic treatment used in the late 1970s to late 1980s resulted in large proportion of long-term sequelae, most frequently involving the musculoskeletal and endocrine systems. Children treated with combined modality therapy, including chemotherapy and radiotherapy were more likely to experience multisystem sequela compared to those who received either modality alone.[12]

GONADAL STROMAL TUMORS

The term of gonadal tumor refers to tumors of specialised gonadal stromal, neoplasms that contain cells resembling Sertoli, Leydig, and granulosa cells in varying combinations and degrees of differentiation.[25] Thus, we recognize tumors of Leydig, Sertoli and granulosa cells

or a mixture of these. These tumors account for 4 to 6 percent of all testicular neoplasms. Pathological recognition of these tumors is not easy and they sometimes are confused with germ cell tumors or sarcomas. The diagnosis of malignancy also is defined less clearly. The criteria of malignancies are hemorrhage and necrosis, polymorphism of cells, increased mitotic activity, vascular invasion and demonstration of metastasis.

Leydig Cell Tumor

Leydig cell tumors are the most common tumor of the gonadal stromas. They account for 1-4 percent of all testicular childhood neoplasm.[26] About 70 cases have been reported in children until 1991.[27]

Boys with Leydig cell tumor usually present between age 5 and 10 with a painless enlargement of the testis and signs of precocious puberty or other endocrine disturbances because the tumor secretes testosterone in abnormally high level. These signs include a growth spur, increased penile size, pubic hair, acne, deep voice, frequent erections without nocturnal emission, and variable psychosocial abnormalities. Ten to 15 percent of these patients present with gynecomastia, due to an imbalance between circulating androgen and estrogens.[27]

Children with Leydig cell tumors should be evaluated with an endocrinologic evaluation including serum testosterone levels, follicle stimulating hormone (FSH) levels, luteinizing hormone (LH) levels, and bone age. If ultrasonography confirms the presence of a small nonpalpable mass and the serum testosterone levels are elevated in the presence of low or normal FSH and LH levels, the presumed diagnosis is a Leydig cell tumor. Differential diagnosis includes all causes of precocious puberty, including poorly controlled congenital adrenal hyperplasia, adrenocortical carcinoma, and isosexual precocious puberty. Dexamethasone suppression of elevated plasma adrenocorticotropic hormone levels in congenital adrenal hyperplasia due to 21 or 11-hydroxylase deficiencies enables differentiation between these two disorders.[28] Occasionally, Leydig cell tumors have been reported in association with other genitourinary malformations (cryptorchidism and ambiguous genitalia) and Klinefelter syndrome.

To date, no malignant Leydig cell tumor has been reported in children,[29] therefore, simple tumor enucleation is a curative treatment for the disease.

Sertoli Cell Tumor

Sertoli cell tumor represents the second most common gonadal stromal tumor that account for less than 1 percent of testicular neoplasms. Approximately 15 percent of the reported cases occur in children. About 80 childhood cases have been reported in the literature.[30] Androblastoma, gondal stromal tumor and tubular adenoma are all considered Sertoli tumors.

Most of the patients present with a painless testicular mass. The majority of Sertoli cell tumors are benign, although in adults 10 to 20 percent metastasize primarily to the retroperitoneal nodes. In children few cases of malignant Sertoli cell tumors have been described, only one of which had metastasized. A variety of Sertoli cell tumors that tend to be bilateral and familiar, and are associated with precocious puberty, gynecomastia and atrial myxomas have been reported in the literature.[25]

The treatment of Sertoli cell tumor is inguinal orchiectomy but retroperitoneal extension must be ruled out by computer tomography or magnetic resonance imaging.

Granulosa Cell and Mixed Gonadal Stromal Tumors

Granulosa cell tumors account for approximately 15 percent of the gonadal stromal tumors[31] and they usually present before the patients are 6 months old. These tumors usually are cystic or mixed, or cystic and solid.[31] The juvenile type has been reported in undescended testis of infants with intersex disorders. The description of a patient with the Denys-Drash syndrome (Wilms' tumor, nephropathy and ambiguous genitalia) and a granulosa cell tumor in which WT-I was shown to be inactivated, suggest a possible role of this gene in the development of this malignancy.

GONADOBLASTOMA

Gonadoblastoma is a tumor that involves dysgenetic gonads, usually in patients with intersex anomalies. It more commonly appears after puberty but may rarely seen in the prepubertal child. They are usually small, 1 to 3 cm in diameter, soft to firm, gray-tan to brown, slightly lobulated tumors. Gonadoblastoma occurs almost exclusively in phenotypic females with 46 XY karyotype (male hermaphrodite) or 46 XY /45 XO (mosaicism) and intraabdominal testis. Only two cases were found in scrotal testis. Histological, the gonadoblastoma consists of three distinct elements; large germ cells similar to those of seminoma, sex-cord non-germinal elements (Sertoli or granulosa), and mesenchymal or stromal elements (Leydig).[27] Gonadoblastoma is usually benign and has never demonstrated malignant behavior. In most cases the patients present with an intraabdominal mass or signs of virilization or defeminisation.[32] Surgical removal of both gonads has been advocated because of the relatively high incidence of bilaterality.

TUMOR-LIKE LESIONS

Epidermoid Cyst

Epidermoid cysts account for less than 2 percent of childhood testicular tumors. They consist of stratified sqamous epithelium with keratinisation but without skin adnexal structures.[33]

Because they are intratesticular, it may be difficult to make the correct preoperative diagnosis. However, ultrasonography may demonstrate a complex heterogenous mass, which should suggest the possibility of an epidermoid cyst.

It is debated, whether should the lesion be regarded as a teratoma that is potentially malignant, or as a benign lesion amenable to conservative therapy. It is generally accepted that these tumors are benign, orchiectomy or enucleation are the recommended treatment of choice.[33,34] Ipsilateral testis biopsy is advocated if enucleation is performed, to rule out carcinoma *in situ*. However, to date carcinoma *in situ* has not been reported in prepubertal children with epidermoid cyst.

Hyperblastic Nodule Secondary to Congenital Adrenal Hyperplasia

It has been recognized that boys with congenital adrenal hyperplasia may develop testicular masses. In 1953, Prader demonstrated that the testicular masses in these patients are dependent on the elevated adreno-corticotrophic hormone (ACTH) level.[35] Most of these tumors are bilateral, although in some patients one testis is more enlarged than the contralateral side.[36] About two-thirds of tumors are larger than 2 cm in diameter and readily palpable. Rutgers and associated reviewed the literature and identified 40 patients with adrenogenital syndrome and testicular lesion, and only a few were children.[36]

These tumors decrease in size if the ACTH level is lowered by the administration of corticosteroids.[35] If the presence of the adrenogenital syndrome is not appreciated, the testicular mass is usually assumed to be neoplastic origin and an orchiectomy is performed. The presence of clinical features of the adrenogenital syndrome (vomiting, diarrhea, dehydratation, enlargement of genitalia, sexual precocity) will help to make the correct diagnosis, however, in some cases, careful endocrinologic testing is necessary to distinguish this disorder from the Leydig cell tumor to avoid unnecessary orchiectomies.

The treatment of choice is suppression of elevated ACTH levels (administration of corticosteroids). If the tumor does not response to corticosteroid suppression, one should consider a true neoplasm, in which case testis sparing surgery is indicated.

Simple Cysts

Preoperative ultrasound examination can suggest the benign lesion and enables the gondal preservation.[34] Altadona et al. described 2 cases of simple cysts of the testis in children treated by excision with gonadal preservation[37] (Figs 28.4A and B).

TUMORS OF THE ADNEXA

Although rhabdomyosarcoma is the most common neoplasm of the adnexa, some other tumors should also be considered. Paratesticular mesotheliomas, which may arise in the epididymis, tunica vaginalis or spermatic cord, usually occur after the age of 18 years and may be malignant. However, these tumors in children have a benign course. Paratesticular leiomyomas and leiomyosarcomas reported more frequently than their intratesticular counterparts.[38] Lipoma is another uncommon tumor, usually occurring in the spermatic cord.

Paratesticular Rhabdomyosarcoma (Figs 28.5A to C)

Any scrotal mass in a child is suspicious of a possible paratesticular rhabdomyosarcoma. About 10 percent of children with intrascrotal mass are discovered to have paratesticular rhabdomyosarcoma. Rhabdomyo-sarcoma arises from the distal spermatic cord and may invade the testis or surrounding tunics. The clinical presentation of rhabdomyosarcoma in the scrotum is a painless mass. Ultrasonography can distinguish a mass in the spermatic cord. AFP and β-hCG levels are normal. Rhabdomyosarcomas tend to spread by local invasion, lymphatic metastases occurring in approximately 30 to 40 percent of cases.[39]

The treatment of paratesticular rhabdomyosarcoma depends on the clinical and pathological staging advocated by the Intergroup Rhabdomyosarcoma Study (IRS). Initial treatment consists of a high inguinal orchiectomy and resection of the entire spermatic cord. If the scrotum has been violated by needle biopsy or a previous scrotal approach, a hemiscrotectomy should be performed.

Patients with paratesticular rhabdomyosarcomas like other rhabdomyosarcomas are classified into stages (I-IV). The current IRS protocol recommends not to perform ipsilateral retroperitoneal lymph node sampling in patients with stage I. Patients with higher stages are recommended to undergo lymph node sampling. All stages receive cytostatic treatment and advanced stages radiotherapy, too. The overall prognosis for patients with paratesticular rhabdomyosarcoma is good. The presence of unresectable retroperitoneal disease, the presence of distant metastases and age above 7 years are the three

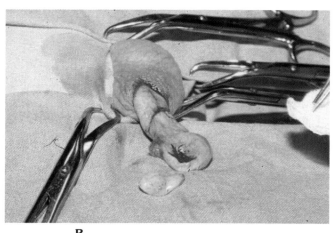

| A | B |

Figures 28.4A and B: Simple testicular cyst: (**A**) Preoperative ultrasound: fluid content circumscribed cyst, (**B**) Encapsulation of the cyst

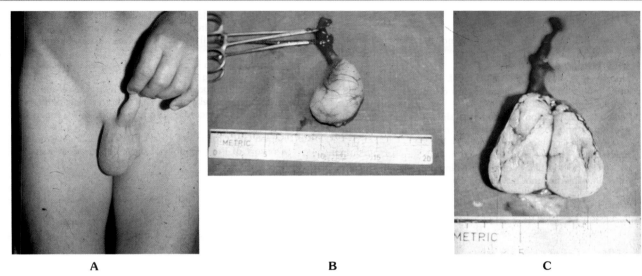

A **B** **C**

Figures 28.5A to C: Paratesticular rhabdomyosarcoma in a 12-year-old boy: (**A**) Right-sided scrotal enlargement, (**B**) High orchiectomy-operative specimen, (**C**) Cut surface of the tumor

major factors that may predict fatal outcome.[15,40] Rhabdomyosarcomas were found in 115 of 1431 patients (8%) in IRS II in 1987. This study demonstrated that the parastesticular rhabdomysarcoma had a mean age of presentation of 10 years and young age may be a favorable prognostic sign. Older children more often presented with more extensive and metastatic disease.

SECONDARY TUMORS

The testis is an uncommon site for metastatic spread. In adults, the most common primary sites of metastases to testis are prostate, lung malignant melanoma, colon, rectum and kidney. In children metastases to the testis can be found in patients with various neoplastic intraabadominal and retroperitoneal disorders, including neuroblastoma and Wilms' tumor.[41]

Lymphoma and Leukemia

Lymphoma and leukemia constitute 2 to 5 percent of all testicular tumors and account for most bilateral neoplasms. The testis represents a potential sanctuary site for tumor cells particularly in acute lymphoblastic leukemia (ALL). The incidence of testicular leukemia has increased with the improved survival in childhood ALL. Testicular involvement usually appears as a painless unilateral swelling.

It has been shown that occult testicular leukemia or leukemic testicular infiltration, in the presence of normal clinical examination of the testis at the cessation of therapy after 3 years of continued remission, has an incidence of approximately 11 percent and ranges from 0.9 to 40 percent.[42,43]

The high incidence of testicular involvement in ALL prompted a number of centres to advocate routine bilateral testicular biopsy either at some time during maintaince therapy or immediately prior to its cessation. Testicular biopsy, preferentially bilateral wedge biopsy is indicated to confirm the diagnosis. Optimal treatment of testicular relapse includes both administration of local radiotherapy to both testis and the use of chemotherapy.

Four cases of primary follicular lymphoma of the testis in young boys are reported.[44] Leonard and coworkers described a case of Burkitt's lymphoma involving the testis.[45]

CONCLUSIONS

Gonadal testicular germ cell tumors are infrequent in childhood, representing approximately 1 percent of cancers diagnosed in persons younger than 15 years of age. Until recently, the myriad of histological subtypes and sites:'of origin and the paucity of cases hindered the standardization of care for these children. The challenge presented by these neoplasms to the pediatric oncologist and pediatric surgeons is to control the tumor while maintaining future fertility. With the advent of effective chemotherapy and the recognition that many of these tumors are less malignant than it was thought before and respond in a similar manner, the management of testicular germ cell tumors is being clarified. However, because of the low incidence of these tumors, cooperative group studies will be necessary to extend future therapeutic advances.

Table 29.1: Classification of ovarian masses in girls (based on the WHO classification)

A.	Non-neoplastic cysts	
B.	Ovarian Tumors	
	1. Germ Cell tumors	(75-80%)
	a. Dysgerminoma	
	b. Teratoma	
	c. Yolk sac tumor	
	d. Gonadoblastoma	
	e. Other	
	2. Sex cord tumors	(5-10%)
	a. Granulosa-theca cell tumors	
	b. Sertoli-Leydig cell tumors	
	c. Other	
	3. Epithelial tumors	(5-10%)

(approximative frequence distribution of tumors is expressed in % [2-7])

fact, before the advent of ultrasonography, these masses rarely represented a clinical problem and it is likely that then and now they might resolve spontaneously in most instances.

These cystic ovarian masses are the result of stimulation of fetal follicular structures by maternal placental gonadotrophins. This explains their frequent postnatal resolution when transplacentally acquired hormone levels decrease. However, before or after birth the enlarged ovary may twist around its pedicle and then it undergoes edema, hemorrhage, ischemia and necrosis (Fig. 29.1). The size of the mass may reach 6 or more centimeters and it may become visible upon

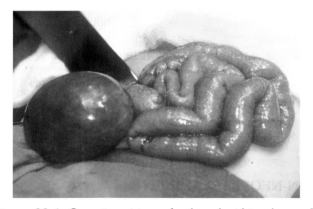

Figure 29.1: Operative picture of a 4-week girl in whom a 5-cm large cystic intra-abdominal mass was detected upon routine prenatal ultrasonography. The size of the mass did not change in the first month and we decided to excise it. A twisted, ischemic-hemorrhagic cystic ovary was found

fetal ultrasonography. Its ecographic structure is most often uniform, liquid, sometimes thick because of its bloody constituents and surrounded by a membrane or capsule that corresponds to the cortical of the ovary. The natural history is often autoamputation[8] and resorption but prenatal diagnosis raises the problem of inmediate prenatal or postnatal treatment measures.

These cysts, that often deserve the name of "chocolate cysts" due to their thick, brown content, are easily palpated in the newborn either because they have been seen upon prenatal ecography and are therefore looked for, or because they are detected upon careful abdominal palpation by the neonatologist. They can be huge but more often they are below 4 or 5 cm of diameter and can be manually moved around within the abdomen. It is suprising that sometimes they can be palpated in very high positions due to their elongated pedicle.[9] These masses are rarely painful mainly because upon diagnosis they have already a relatively long intrauterine life and are in fact in the process of spontaneous resolution. In rare opportunities they are associated with intestinal obstruction which leads to the diagnosis.[10-12] Fetal or neonatal ascites has been described as a rare symptom of ovarian cyst.[13]

Ultrasonography is the main diagnostic tool and very rarely other imaging procedures are necessary. The main concern is the presence of teratomatous tissue in one of these ovaries. This should be suspected when the ecographic pattern of the mass is uneven with liquid and solid components and when they have calcifications.[14] Both findings are really unusual at this age and some increase of blood levels of alpha-feto-protein is to be taken with caution because this is to be expected, to a certain extent, in newborns.

After a tendency to overzealous surgical indications developed in the past[15,16] there has been a trend towards more conservative therapeutic attitudes.[17-20] As we pointed out already, fetal and ovarian masses were practically unknown of before the advent of ultrasono-graphy but we are sure that they existed, evolved spontaneously and resolved by themselves most of the time without major clinical manifestations or untoward consequences. Only in very rare instances they caused intestinal obstruction, hemorrhage or severe pain. It is a general policy that only when they are very large or when they become symptomatic, they should be excised.[21] This is presently done laparoscopically in most cases[22-25] and any attempt at conservation of ovarian parenchyme is usually futile because the gonad and often the tube are twisted, necrotic, autoamputated or damaged to the point that they can be considered as already destroyed.

Cysts of similar nature can be observed in prepubertal or pubertal girls this time as a result of the onset of their own of hormonal secretion. In these cases the clinical picture is that of abdominal pain that is easily confused with appendicitis particularly when the right ovary is involved. Torsion can occur but it is certainly a quite rare event. In such cases the abdominal pain can be acute, anguishing and accompanied by nausea and vomiting, tenderness and guarding of the lower abdomen. Once again ultrasonography is of invaluable help in these cases and it allows detection of the cysts, assessment of the status of the ovary and blood flow within it, diagnosis of calcifications or solid components of a teratoma and inspection of the contralateral gonad.[26-28] Operative treatment in these cases should be restricted to the torsions, the teratomas and the very large cysts that can become twisted. All other cases can be treated under close observation with some rest and pain killers.[29] We must think that the presence of ovarian cysts is a normal event of the menstrual cycle and that their finding in a context of abdominal pain, except when they are large or when they are suggestive or torsion, might not be pathologic. It is therefore wise to restrict emergency operations for this reason to a minimum. In-hospital observation with additional imaging and hormonal tests may help to conserve some ovaries.[30]

OVARIAN TUMORS

The clinical picture accompanying the diagnosis of an ovarian tumor may orient the pathologic diagnosis but this does not happen all the time. These masses can produce acute or chronic **pain** related to size increase, hemorrhage, rupture or torsion. This pain is often abdominal rather than pelvic and it is generally difficult to relate it to the gonads. In some cases it acquires the features of acute abdomen making diagnosis with other conditions mandatory before adequate treatment. Another common presenting symptom is abdominal distension (Fig. 29.2). Right-sided tumors are particularly easy to be misdiagnosed as appendicitis for obvious reasons and it is customary to examine the right ovary when a non-inflamed appendix is found upon laparotomy in a girl. In cases of torsion the pain can be very upsetting and is accompanied by **nausea** and **vomiting** as well as by symptoms of visceral vascular compromise.

Tumors that secrete female hormones may manifest themselves by **isosexual precocious pseudopuberty** with early appearance of the secondary sexual characters (breast development, pubic and axillary hair, labial swelling and vaginal secretion or hemorrhage) in the absence of increased hypophyseal gonadotrophins. When this happens in a prepubertal girl the symptoms immediately draw the attention on the secreting organs and particularly on the ovary making diagnosis relatively easy. When the secretion from the tumor is androgenic, the **precocious pseudopuberty is heterosexual** with rapid somatic growth, bone age acceleration, muscle development, appearance of body hair and changes in the voice that are particularly striking in a girl. Overall, the proportion of hormone-secreting tumors in girls is low, and rarely above 10 percent.

In some cases an enlarged abdomen allows the diagnosis of the tumor. In some epithelial tumors, **ascitis** can be present when the neoplasm is extended and/or ruptured. In some large solid tumors or cysts the **mass** can be easily palpated upon physical examination.

The main diagnostic tool is, of course, ultrasonography, but other imaging procedures may help in establishing the diagnosis and particularly CT scanning and MRI (Figs 29.3A and B). The nature of hormonal secretions is also helpful to pinpoint preoperatively the histologic nature of the mass and the secretion of some tumor markers like alpha-feto-protein (yolk sac tumors, malignant teratoma), CA-125 (cystadenoma) or gonadotrophin (choriocarcinoma) may be extremely useful.

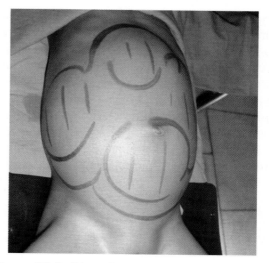

Figure 29.2: Bilateral ovarian tumors presenting as abdominal distension

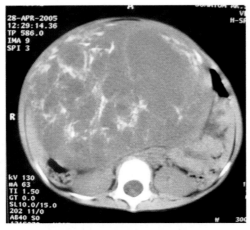

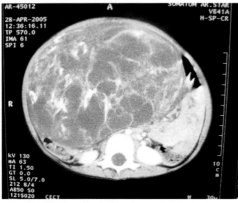

Figures 29.3A and B: CT scan abdomen in a case of ovarian tumor delineating the cystic nature of the tumor

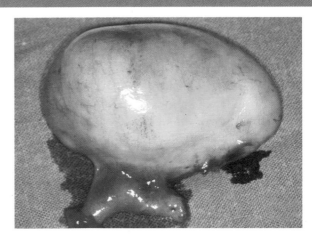

Figure 29.4: Ovarian dysgerminoma excised in a 23-month-old girl with mild signs of isosexual precocious puberty. The right tube was also excised and the bivalved biopsy of the remaining ovary did not show contralateral involvement. The patient did well after the operation

Although the treatment of ovarian tumors is far from being uniform, it is helpful to stage the malignant tumors in order to standardize the therapeutic protocols. The Children's Cancer Group-Pediatric Oncology group (CCG-POG) proposed four stages: I. Tumor limited to one ovary, totally resected with tumoral markers normal. II. Microscopic residual or positive lymph nodes (<2 cm) with markers +/−. III. Gross residual or biopsy alone. Lymph node or adjacent organ involvement or peritoneal washing positive. IV. Metastatic disease.

In the following paragraphs, we address the main features of the more common tumors of the ovary in girls.

Germ Cell Tumors

Tumors derived from the germ cells are by far the more frequent neoplasms of the female gonad in girls. The totipotent haploid germ cells that will give origin to the oocytes settle in the ovarian primordium after travelling from the extra-embryonic mesenchyme (the yolk sac or endodermal sinus) and they may undergo neoplastic changes in various directions: when they do not differentiate at all they evolve into **dysgerminomas** or **germinomas**. If differentiation into embryonal tissues takes place, they cause **teratoma** (benign or malignant) and if they differentiate into extraembryonal tissue they give rise to either **endodermal sinus-yolk sac tumors** or to **choriocarcinoma**. These germ-cell derivatives, except the undifferentiated ones, secrete alpha-feto-protein when they are immature or malignant and this is a very useful feature in terms of diagnosis and follow-up. Some tumors secrete β-hCG as well and this further helps to follow-up the course of the disease. Many germ cell tumors have cytogenetic anomalies that consist most often of isochromosome 1(12p) or 1p deletion.[31] Both anomalies have some prognostic significance because they bare associated with worse prognosis.

1. *Dysgerminomas:* This tumor is one of the most frequent in the ovary of prepubertal girls[7, 32] and it is histologically identical to seminoma of the testicle because its cells are totipotential undifferentiated germ cells. It is one of the varieties of tumor found in dysgenetic gonads. They are solid, white or yellowish firm tumors composed by lobules of large round cells with vesicle-rich nuclei and clear cytoplasm separated by conjunctive septa. A few of these tumors have some sincythiotrophoblastic elements than may secrete β-hCG. These masses can be huge at diagnosis (Fig. 29.4) and may cause symptoms of

compression and pain related to torsion, hemorrhage or rupture. Since they are not hormone-secreting masses, there cause no endocrine symptoms. In some mixed tumors in which there are components of sex cord cells, isosexual or heterosexual precocious puberty symptoms may occur.[33] The treatment is surgical and it should involve complete oophorectomy with salpyngectomy in unilateral Stage I cases. A considerable proportion of them (around 10%) are bilateral and this makes careful histologic staging of the contralateral gonad by bivalving biopsy mandatory. In any case, when the risk of local recurrence and the consequent mortality exists, it is indicated to complement this treatment with adequate chemotherapy including cisplatinum and bleomycin.

2. *Teratomas:* These tumors derive from the germinal cells differentiated in the direction of embryonal tissues that do not always pertain to the anatomical location of the mass. When they are mature they are composed by elements of the three blastodermic layers (ectoderm, mesoderm and endoderm) that may adopt an organoid pattern or eventually be shaped as a part of a normal organ. The three layers do not always participate in these tumors and this condition is not met in some of them in which components of only two of them are found. Teratomas may be seen almost everywhere in the body particularly along the migration route of the germ cells from their extra-embryonal origin in the endodermal sinus to their final destination in the gonads. They are more frequently observed in the sacrocoxigeal region and in the gonads. In the ovary they are bilateral in 10 percent of the cases approximately[34] and may be huge although this is not the rule. They are composed by mixtures of tissues like nervous system, gastrointestinal tract, cartilage, bone, teeth or glands. Very often they have cystic areas that, when internally lined by skin, may be filled by sebaceous secretion and hair.[35] In contrast with sacrocoxigeal teratomas which are present before birth, ovarian teratomas are rare in young girls and manifest themselves clinically near puberty or at adult age. Symptoms are related to the volume of the mass and usually consist of the perception of a space-occupying mass (Fig. 29.5) and pain due to twisting (Fig. 29.6), rupture or hemorrhage. Ultrasonographic and imaging diagnosis is not difficult because of their frequent cystic components, uneven ecographic consistence and frequent calcifications.[36,37] Treatment is always surgical and when the

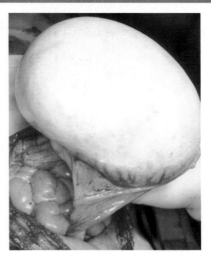

Figure 29.5: Huge right ovarian teratoma in a 12-year-old girl complaining of abdominal pain with rapid increase of abdominal girth. The ultrasonographic structure was uneven and there were several calcifications. The pedicle, which was intermittently twisted was very long since the mass was in fact located below the liver

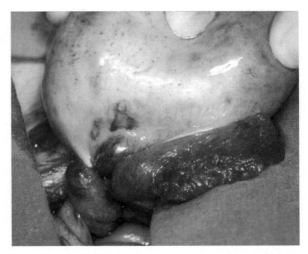

Figure 29.6: Twisted ovarian teratoma observed during laparotomy for acute abdomen in a 12-year-old girl

volume is not too large and/or when the cystic component is predominant, the laparoscopic approach is an atractive alternative to open surgery.[6] However, if this route is elected, the principles of treatment should be respected: the liquid contained in the cysts must not be spilled and the tumor should be excised trying to preserve some gonadal tissue for future hormonal secretion and reproduction. This can be feasible in unilateral cases but becomes a difficult issue in bilateral cases.

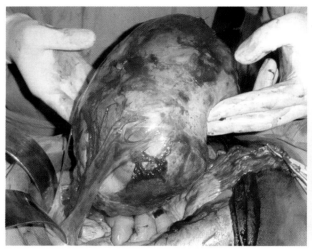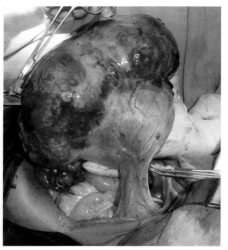

Figures 29.7A and B: Operative photograph of a yolk sac tumor
with cystic consistency and yellowish appearance

The other important problem is that these tumors are not always mature and that when some immature components are present the risks of recurrence and malignancy further impose strict surgical cleanliness during excision: The cystic components may contain undifferentiated cells able to implant themselves on the peritoneal surface to become immature or differentiated cells, frequently arranged as glial tissue (stage I tumors according to Thurlbeck and Scully[38]). The care to avoid any fluid spill during surgery must be exquisite and the laparoscopic approach should only be elected if clean aspiration and tumor bag removal are feasible.

When an immature teratoma has neuroepithelial or neuroectodermic components it becomes respectively a Thurlbeck y Scully Stage II or III tumor[38] with worse prognosis and adequate treatment is not possible without coadjuvant chemotherapy.

3. *Yolk sac (endodermal sinus) tumor:* When the germ cells undergo some differentiation towards extra-embryonic tissues they may give origin to this form of malignant neoplasm which grows very rapidly, is white or yellowish, it is sometimes cystic and often quite friable and in which uniform sheets of undifferentiated cells that sometimes group around the vessels in the form of Schiller-Duval bodies can be found (Figs 29.7A and B). This tumor secretes alpha-feto-protein (AFP) which is a very helpful tumor marker for diagnosis and follow-up. The symptoms are derived from the rapid growth of the mass and the diagnosis is usually easy by palpation, ecography and AFP measurements.[39] They are very sensitive to chemotherapy and they may even disappear with only this therapeutic modality.[4,40] Surgery is nevertheless attempted in almost every case at some point of treatment depending on the initial volume, the extension of the tumor and the involvement of adjacent organs[32] (Figs 29.8A and B).

4. *Gonadoblastomas:* These are tumors that appear generally in dysgenetic gonads of individuals with either XY karyotype or with mosaics in which Y chromosome elements are present (including Turner syndrome with SRY[41]). They consist of mixtures of sex cords and germ cell derivatives and are often combined with dysgerminoma elements. Sometimes they undergo partial calcification. Their malignant potential is one of the main reasons for castration in individuals with ambiguous genitalia and dysgenetic gonads with XY or Y-containing karyotypes. Their aspect is variable but they are often not very well delimited, with borders that cannot be separated from those of the gonad. This is often totally replaced by the tumor.

5. *Other tumors:* There are other rare ovarian tumos derived from the germ cells: **embryonal carcinomas**, related to the endodermal sinus tumors[4] are AFP and beta-HCG secreting masses that may cause isosexual precocious pseudopuberty. They require active chemotherapy coupled with extensive surgery.[2] **Choriocarcinoma** contains chorionic neoplastic tissue which is beta-HCG secretor and causes again isosexual precocious pseudopuberty. It

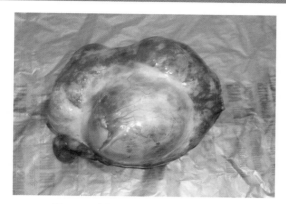

Figure 29.8A: Excised specimen of a yolk sac tumor

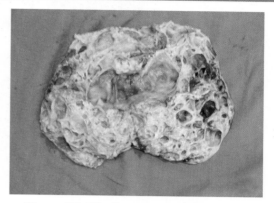

Figure 29.8B: Cut section of the excised specimen showing the cystic spaces

can be very huge, friable, hemorrhagic and extended to other organs.[42] Surgery can be very difficult and chemotherapy is always required for adequate treatment.

Sex Cord Tumors

Tumors derived from the sex cords are often secreting and since the differentiation of their cells can proceed in either direction, they can be accompanied by isosexual or heterosexual precocious pseudopuberty depending of their specialization (granulosa-theca cell tumors and Sertoli-Leydig cell tumors respectively).

1. *Granulosa-theca cell tumors:* The most frequent component is the granulosa cell and in these cases the tumor is almost constantly estrogen-secreting with normal gonadotrophin levels. Thelarche, axillary and pubic hair, vaginal hemorrhage and advanced somatic and bone growth are the main symptoms. The tumor is usually large and can be palpated or even seen upon abdominal inspection. Most children affected bear Stage I tumors and can be treated successfully with oophorectomy with salpyngectomy.[43,44] More extended cases have worse prognosis and require coadjuvant treatment based on modern chemotherapeutic protocols.[45,46]

2. *Sertoli-Leydig cell tumors:* This very rare tumor was formerly known as "arrhenoblastoma" or "andro-blastoma" and is androgen-secreting. Prepubertal patients may show heterosexual precocious pseudopuberty (accelerated somatic growth, hirsutism, voice changes, acne) and postpubertal girls may undergo loss of their feminine sexual characters followed by masculinization. These tumors occasionally secrete AFP that acts, together with androgens, as a tumor marker. Like the granulosa cell tumors, Sertoli-Leydig ones are treated with oophorectomy with salpingectomy when they are limited in extension[47] and with more extensive operations and chemotherapy in extended cases.

3. *Other sex-cord tumors:* Other rare neoplasm belonging to this category can be occasionally observed in girls: Fibromas,[48] Sex cord tumors with annular tubules, seen in association with the Peuts Jeghers syndrome[49] or sclerosing stromal tumors associated with the Chediak-Higashi syndrome in which there is albinism and a phagocytic disorder.

Epithelial Tumors

This variety of tumor, relatively frequent in adult women, is exceedingly rare in children and is practically only seen in adolescents.[4,50] They can be benign or malignant (the equivalent of ovarian carcinoma in adults). The tumors can be mucinous or serous[51] and are constituted by large cystic spaces sometimes lined by papillary tissue. They can extend into the other ovary or cause multiple implants on the omentum or on the peritoneal lining (Fig. 29.9). Some tumors secrete CA-125 which is another useful marker when positive.[52] Imaging procedures like MRI or CT-scan are useful for determining the extension of these masses. There is an intermediate form of low malignant potential in which the implants and the extension can be prominent but with little mytotic activity but this can only be determined upon histologic study.

These tumors are treated surgically and, when malignant, with chemotherapy. Surgery consists in total

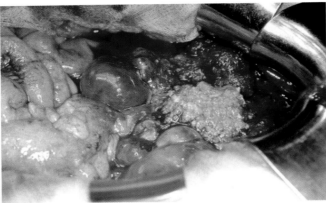

Figure 29.9: Operative picture of a 11-year-old patient with ascites, weight loss and a huge pelvic tumor. Bilateral ovarian involvement corresponding to a ruptured papillary cystadeno-carcinoma with epiploic involvement and numerous peritoneal implants was found. After large biopsy with omentectomy, adequate chemotherapy was instituted followed by bilateral salpingo-oophorectomy and hysterectomy. The patient is alive and well 9 years later

excision when possible including the ovary and the tube and it is doubtful for laparoscopy to be the more appropriate form of treatment in such cases because rupture of the cysts into the peritoneal cavity is to be avoided. In extended cases, surgery involves bilateral oophorectomy and histerectomy as well as omentectomy. Chemotherapy with cisplatinum and bleomycin are currently used for postoperative treatment in extended cases.[4] Cases with low malignant potential but advanced staging require very long follow-up because recurrences can be observed many years after the initial treatment.

REFERENCES

1. Larsen WJ. Human embryology. (2nd Ed.). New York, Churchill Livingstone, 1997.
2. Ehren IM, Mahour GH, Isaacs H, Jr. Benign and malignant ovarian tumors in children and adolescents. A review of 63 cases. Am J Surg, 1984;147:339-44.
3. Roth H, Daum R, Benz G, et al. Rare ovarian tumors in childhood. Eur J Pediatr Surg, 1991;1:210-5.
4. Gribbon M, Ein SH, Mancer K. Pediatric malignant ovarian tumors: a 43-year review. J Pediatr Surg, 1992;27:480-4.
5. Skinner MA, Schlatter MG, Heifetz SA, et al. Ovarian neoplasms in children. Arch Surg, 1993;128:849-53.
6. Templeman C, Fallat ME, Blinchevsky A, et al. Noninflammatory ovarian masses in girls and young women. Obstet Gynecol, 2000;96:229-33.
7. Terenziani M, Massimino M, Casanova M, et al. Childhood malignant ovarian germ cell tumors: a monoinstitutional experience. Gynecol Oncol, 2001;81:436-40.
8. Aslam A, Wong C, Haworth JM, et al. Autoamputation of ovarian cyst in an infant. J Pediatr Surg, 1995;30:1609-10.
9. Avni EF, Godart S, Israel C, et al. Ovarian torsion cyst presenting as a wandering tumor in a newborn: antenatal diagnosis and post natal assessment. Pediatr Radiol, 1983;13:169-71.
10. Ruiz Company S, Vilarino Mosquera A, Val F, et al. Síndrome Ovarico-intestinal. An Esp Pediatr, 1980;13:533-6.
11. Scholz PM, Key L, Filston HC. Large ovarian cyst causing cecal perforation in a newborn infant. J Pediatr Surg, 1982;17:91-2.
12. Koc E, Turkyilmaz C, Atalay Y, et al. Neonatal ovarian cyst associated with intestinal obstruction. Indian J Pediatr, 1997;64:555-7.
13. Vyas ID, Variend S, Dickson JA. Ruptured ovarian cyst as a cause of ascites in a newborn infant. Z Kinderchir, 1984;39:143-4.
14. Croitoru DP, Aaron LE, Laberge JM, et al. Management of complex ovarian cysts presenting in the first year of life. J Pediatr Surg, 1991;26:1366-8.
15. Zachariou Z, Roth H, Boos R, et al. Three years' experience with large ovarian cysts diagnosed in utero. J Pediatr Surg, 1989;24:478-82.
16. Bagolan P, Rivosecchi M, Giorlandino C, et al. Prenatal diagnosis and clinical outcome of ovarian cysts. J Pediatr Surg, 1992;27:879-81.
17. Widdowson DJ, Pilling DW, Cook RC. Neonatal ovarian cysts: therapeutic dilemma. Arch Dis Child, 1988;63:737-42.
18. Meizner I, Levy A, Katz M, et al. Fetal ovarian cysts: prenatal ultrasonographic detection and postnatal evaluation and treatment. Am J Obstet Gynecol, 1991;164:874-8.
19. Campbell BA, Garg RS, Garg K, et al. Perinatal ovarian cyst: a nonsurgical approach. J Pediatr Surg, 1992;27:1618-9.
20. Sapin E, Bargy F, Lewin F, et al. Management of ovarian cyst detected by prenatal ultrasounds. Eur J Pediatr Surg, 1994;4:137-40.
21. Dolgin SE. Ovarian masses in the newborn. Semin Pediatr Surg, 2000;9:121-7.
22. van der Zee DC, van Seumeren IG, Bax KM, et al. Laparoscopic approach to surgical management of ovarian cysts in the newborn. J Pediatr Surg, 1995;30:42-3.
23. Esposito C, Garipoli V, Di Matteo G, et al. Laparoscopic management of ovarian cysts in newborns. Surg Endosc, 1998;12:1152-4.
24. Jawad AJ, Zaghmout O, al-Muzrakchi AD, et al. Laparoscopic removal of an autoamputated ovarian cyst in an infant. Pediatr Surg Int, 1998;13:195-6.
25. Davies BW. An elegant method of reducing surgical trauma when dealing with a large simple neonatal ovarian cyst. J Pediatr Surg, 2002;37:143.
26. Brown MF, Hebra A, McGeehin K, et al. Ovarian masses in children: a review of 91 cases of malignant and benign masses. J Pediatr Surg, 1993;28:930-3.
27. Stark JE, Siegel MJ. Ovarian torsion in prepubertal and pubertal girls: sonographic findings. AJR Am J Roentgenol, 1994;163:1479-82.
28. Meyer JS, Harmon CM, Harty MP, et al. Ovarian torsion: clinical and imaging presentation in children. J Pediatr Surg, 1995;30:1433-6.
29. Liapi C, Evain-Brion D. Diagnosis of ovarian follicular cysts from birth to puberty: a report of twenty cases. Acta Paediatr Scand, 1987;76:91-6.
30. Piippo S, Mustaniemi L, Lenko H, et al. Surgery for ovarian masses during childhood and adolescence: a report of 79 cases. J Pediatr Adolesc Gynecol, 1999;12:223-7.
31. Bussey KJ, Lawce HJ, Olson SB, et al. Chromosome abnormalities of eighty-one pediatric germ cell tumors: sex,

age-, site-, and histopathology-related differences—a Children's Cancer Group study. Genes Chromosomes Cancer, 1999;25:134-46.

32. Cass DL, Hawkins E, Brandt ML, et al. Surgery for ovarian masses in infants, children, and adolescents: 102 consecutive patients treated in a 15-year period. J Pediatr Surg, 2001;36:693-9.

33. Lacson AG, Gillis DA, Shawwa A. Malignant mixed germ-cell-sex cord-stromal tumors of the ovary associated with isosexual precocious puberty. Cancer, 1988;61:2122-33.

34. Quint EH, Smith YR. Ovarian surgery in premenarchal girls. J Pediatr Adolesc Gynecol, 1999;12:27-9.

35. Masih K, Bhalla S. Gonadal teratomas: a study of 206 cases. Indian J Pathol Microbiol, 1993;36:495-8.

36. Kirks DR, Merten DF, Grossman H, et al. Diagnostic imaging of pediatric abdominal masses: an overview. Radiol Clin North Am, 1981;19:527-45.

37. Brammer HM, 3rd, Buck JL, Hayes WS, et al. From the archives of the AFIP. Malignant germ cell tumors of the ovary: radiologic-pathologic correlation. Radiographics, 1990;10:715-24.

38. Thurlbeck W, Scully RE. Solid teratoma of the ovary: a clinico-pathologic analysis of 9 cases. Cancer, 1960;13:801-5.

39. Levitin A, Haller KD, Cohen HL, et al. Endodermal sinus tumor of the ovary: imaging evaluation. AJR Am J Roentgenol, 1996;167:791-3.

40. Olsen L, Esscher T, Lundkvist K. Endodermal sinus tumour in girls—improved survival in metastatic disease. Z Kinderchir, 1989;44:83-5.

41. Krasna IH, Lee ML, Smilow P, et al. Risk of malignancy in bilateral streak gonads: the role of the Y chromosome. J Pediatr Surg, 1992;27:1376-80.

42. Szavay PO, Wermes C, Fuchs J, et al. Effective treatment of infantile choriocarcinoma in the liver with chemotherapy and surgical resection: a case report. J Pediatr Surg, 2000'35:1134-5.

43. Lack EE, Perez-Atayde AR, Murthy AS, et al. Granulosa theca cell tumors in premenarchal girls: a clinical and pathologic study of ten cases. Cancer, 1981;48:1846-54.

44. Zaloudek C, Norris HJ. Granulosa tumors of the ovary in children: a clinical and pathologic study of 32 cases. Am J Surg Pathol, 1982;6:503-12.

45. Vassal G, Flamant F, Caillaud JM, et al. Juvenile granulosa cell tumor of the ovary in children: a clinical study of 15 cases. J Clin Oncol, 1988;6:990-5.

46. Merras-Salmio L, Vettenranta K, Mottonen M, et al. Ovarian granulosa cell tumors in childhood. Pediatr Hematol Oncol, 2002;19:145-56.

47. Mann WJ, Chumas J, Rosenwaks Z, et al. Elevated serum alpha-fetoprotein associated with Sertoli-Leydig cell tumors of the ovary. Obstet Gynecol, 1986;67:141-4.

48. Bosch-Banyeras JM, Lucaya X, Bernet M, et al. Calcified ovarian fibromas in prepubertal girls. Eur J Pediatr, 1989;148:749-50.

49. Young RH, Dickersin GR, Scully RE. A distinctive ovarian sex cord-stromal tumor causing sexual precocity in the Peutz-Jeghers syndrome. Am J Surg Pathol, 1983;7:233-43.

50. Schwobel MG, Stauffer UG. Surgical treatment of ovarian tumors in childhood. Prog Pediatr Surg, 1991;26:112-23.

51. Deprest J, Moerman P, Corneillie P, et al. Ovarian borderline mucinous tumor in a premenarchal girl: review on ovarian epithelial cancer in young girls. Gynecol Oncol, 1992;45:219-24.

52. Magrina JF, Cornella JL. Office management of ovarian cysts. Mayo Clin Proc, 1997;72:653-6.

CHAPTER 30

Devendra K Gupta
Shilpa Sharma

Granulosa Cell Tumor of the Ovary

Granulosa cell tumors (GCT) comprising 2-3 percent of all ovarian neoplasms are rare tumors in the pediatric age group. They are the most common sex cord–stromal ovarian tumors in children consisting of granulosa cells, theca cells, and fibroblasts in varying degrees and combinations. Of the 17 children in one of the largest series of pediatric granulosa and theca cell tumors, 6 had juvenile granulosa cell tumors, 5 had adult-type granulosa cell tumors, 1 had luteinized granulosa cell tumor, 3 had gonadal stomal tumors, 1 had theca cell tumor and one had granulosa-theca cell tumor.[1]

Granulosa cell tumors commonly produce estrogen and are divided into adult (95%) and juvenile (5%) types based on histologic findings. Most juvenile GCTs develop in girls younger than 30 years and recur within the first 3 years.

ETIOLOGY

The etiology of GCT remains unknown. It is proposed that these neoplasms are derived either from the mesenchyme of the developing genital ridge or from precursors within the mesonephric and coelomic epithelium. Though no definite etiological factor has been identified, chromosomal anomalies and/or autocrine and endocrine signaling abnormalities along with a multifactorial etiology has been postulated.

CLINICAL SYMPTOMS

Seventy to 80 percent patients usually present with precocious pseudopuberty due to hormonal activity due to excess of estrogen and/or androgen (Figs 30.1 and

30.2). The patient may present with iso and heterosexual manifestations due to elevated testosterone and estradiol

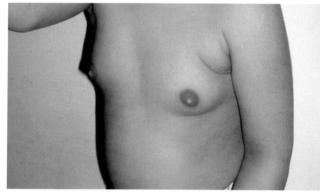

Figure 30.1: A 16-month-old child with granulosa cell tumor presented with thelarche

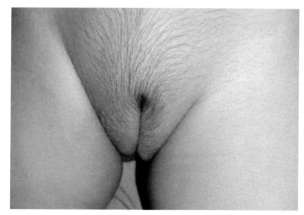

Figure 30.2: Signs of pseudoprecocious puberty visible as pubic hair growth in a 16-month-old child

levels.[2] Estrogen production by these tumors has been shown to cause endometrial hyperplasia. Most younger children present with precocious pseudopuberty while adolescents present with menstrual irregularities, secondary amenorrhea, virilization, abdominal swelling, and pain.[3,4] Rarely, a case of an 11-year-old girl presenting with galactorrhea and abdominal mass with increased prolactin and estradiol levels and decreased luteinizing hormone and follicle-stimulating hormone has been described.[5]

More than 90 percent of GCTs are diagnosed before spread occurs outside the ovary. Endorinological effects due to high estrogen levels usually regress after removal of the tumor. However, a small group of patients present with changes caused by androgen excess that may or may not only partially regress over time.

Most patients may have a palpable mass in the abdomen or pelvis felt per rectally that may lead to compressive symptoms like abdominal pain, dysuria, urinary frequency, and constipation. Acute onset of abdominal pain also can occur, although rarely due to adnexal torsion, rupture of a partially cystic GCT, or hemorrhage either within the tumor or into the peritoneum. Ascites may be associated occasionally in cases presenting late.[6]

Diagnosis based on a tumoral or acute abdomen has been associated with frequent intraperitoneal ruptures of the tumor in upto 50 percent and a risk of relapse.[4] These cases are usually diagnosed late despite previous endocrine signs.

Metastatic disease can involve any organ system, although tumor growth usually is confined to the abdomen and pelvis.

INVESTIGATIONS

Relevant investigations for reaching a diagnosis include serum estradiol, Müllerian-inhibiting substance, Inhibin, beta–human chorionic gonadotropin (β-hCG), alpha-fetoprotein (AFP), lactate dehydrogenase (LDH), and cancer antigen 125 (CA-125). The alpha subunit of Inhibin is confined largely to tumors in the sex cord–stromal group.

Müllerian-inhibiting substance, limited to tumors of ovarian origin has been shown to correlate with tumor presence in patients with GCTs. The tumor may be associated with raised serum oestradiol, androstenedione, inhibin and IGF-I.[7] Inhibin and estradiol may be elevated in a variety of other extraovarian disorders.

Ultrasonography can delineate presence of solid, complex, cystic components, bilateral involvement and free fluid in the peritoneal cavity.

GCTs have a heterogeneous appearance on both sonographic and CT imaging. Most commonly, they appear as round-to-ovoid masses that are multicystic, sometimes with solid components at the center or periphery.

Chest skiagram is useful to exclude pulmonary spread of malignant diseases of the ovary. Abdomino-pelvic CT scanning or MRI may help in diagnosing intraperitoneal spread or involvement of other organ systems prior to surgery or to confirm the presence of recurrent tumor identified after clinical examination (Fig. 30.3).

HISTOPATHOLOGY

Grossly, tumors can be cystic, solid, or a mixture of both (Fig. 30.4). On cut section, they usually are multicystic and may contain areas of hemorrhage (Fig. 30.5). Solid tumors appear grayish if they are nonsteroidogenic or yellow if they are steroid-producing neoplasms. Androgen-producing tumors more commonly are unilocular or solid in contrast to the multilocular tumors that make up most GCTs.

Microscopically, GCTs are composed of granulosa cells, theca cells, and fibroblasts in varying amounts and combinations (Fig. 30.6).

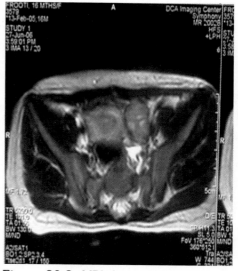

Figure 30.3: MRI depicting a left ovarian mass and bulky uterus in a girl who presented with vaginal bleeding

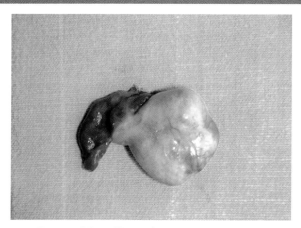

Figure 30.4: Excised specimen of a stage Ia ovarian tumor

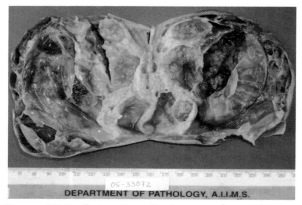

DEPARTMENT OF PATHOLOGY, A.I.I.M.S.

Figure 30.5: Cut section of a big granulosa cell tumor with cystic spaces

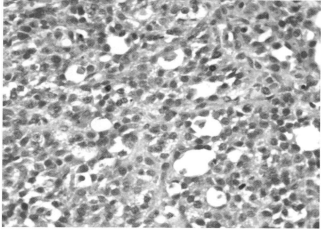

Figure 30.6: Photomicrograph of a granulosa cell tumor with HE staining

Adult GCTs have multiple histomorphologies, including well-differentiated microfollicular, macrofollicular, trabecular, and insular patterns and less well-differentiated types. Microfollicular is the most common subtype with characteristic Call-Exner bodies consisting of small rings of granulosa cells surrounding eosinophilic fluid and basement membrane material.

Rarely, mixed sex cord-stromal tumors that exhibit composite morphologic appearance histologically, including a combination of adult granulosa cell tumor, juvenile granulosa cell tumor (with areas of marked atypia), and Sertoli cell tumor have been reported in the pediatric age group.[8]

In adult GCTs, the nuclei usually are large pale ovoid or angular structures containing nuclear grooves that give them a "coffee-bean" appearance. Mitotic figures generally are few in number, and only mild nuclear atypia is found in most cases. Nuclear appearance and mitotic rate often are the key elements differentiating GCTs from other malignant tumors.

Histopathological evaluation substantially contributes to risk assessment and might be useful for therapy stratification in prospective therapeutic protocols. Compared with adult granulosa cell tumors, Juvenile GCT showed pronounced mitotic activity [mean 9.8 mitoses/10 high power field (HPF)], which was significantly higher than in other histological subtypes (2.7/10 HPF, P=0.001).[9] Immunohistochemical analysis revealed frequent coexpression of vimentin (positive in 52/52 examined tumors), cytokeratin (27/33), and inhibin (19/20). Mitotic rate was assessed by counting mitoses in at least 10 high-power fields (HPF) and was categorized as low, intermediate, or high when less than 10, 10 to 19, or more than 19 mitoses/10 HPF were found, respectively [10] (Fig. 30.7). The outcome has been found to significantly correlate with stage and mitotic activity (<20 versus > or =20 mitoses/10 HPF: event-free survival 1.0 versus 0.48 0.05, P=0.0001).[9]

Fortunately, majority of patients present at low tumor stage with excellent prognosis. Refractory tumors are characterized by high proliferative activity.

MANAGEMENT

Complete surgical staging should be performed and consists of pelvic washings, selective pelvic and periaortic lymph node sampling on the ipsilateral side, peritoneal biopsies, partial omentectomy, and biopsy of the contralateral ovary (only if it appears abnormal). If

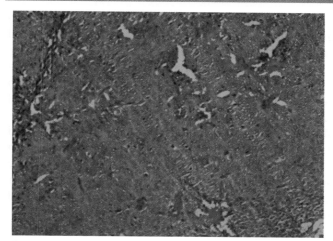

Figure 30.7: Photomicrograph of a granulosa cell tumor with a high mitotic index of 81 suggestive of poor prognosis

disease is identified outside the ovary, optimal debulking so that all remaining tumor nodules are smaller than 1 cm improves overall survival and decreases recurrences.

Previously, biopsy of the contralateral ovary was considered a routine part of the staging procedure but now is not required because only approximately 2 percent of tumors are bilateral.

Surgical treatment is considered first-line therapy for patients with GCTs. Unilateral salpingo-oophorectomy almost always provides sufficient treatment because most of these tumors are stage I. In Stage Ia, the tumor is limited to one ovary with an intact capsule, no tumor is present on the external surface of the capsule, and no ascites containing malignant cells are present. More widely spread tumors are difficult to treat and cause mortality.[3] Successful laparoscopic resection has also been done in a 6-year-old girl.[11]

Chemotherapy can be used as adjuvant therapy in patients with advanced or recurrent disease and has been effective for improving the disease-free survival. The rarity of this tumor has precluded randomized control trials; therefore, no prospective data are available regarding overall survival in high-risk patients, who receive adjuvant chemotherapy compared to those who have not.

The optimal chemotherapy regimen has been hard to identify given that the overall incidence of GCTs is relatively low. Various chemotherapy regimens have been used in patients with GCTs, with varying toxicity and response rates.

The BEP regimen is bleomycin at 20 U/m^2 (not to exceed 30 U) IV q3wk for 4 courses, etoposide at 75 mg/m^2 IV on days 1-5 q3wk for 4 courses, and cisplatin at 20 mg/m^2 IV on days 1-5 q3wk for 4 courses.

Older multidrug regimens included[1] cyclophosphamide, doxorubicin (Adriamycin), and cisplatin regimen, which includes cyclophosphamide at 500 mg/m^2 IV, Adriamycin at 40-50 mg/m^2 IV, and cisplatin at 40-50 mg/m^2 IV all given q4wk for 4-6 courses;[2] cisplatin and doxorubicin; and[3] cyclophosphamide, actinomycin, and 5-fluorouracil. These regimens have the benefit of fewer and less serious adverse effects. However, response rates often were poorer than for those of the newer cisplatin-based regimens.

Much less information is available for JGCTs with regard to treatment of advanced disease and recurrences. These tumors tend to behave more aggressively, with earlier recurrences and poorer responses to chemotherapeutic agents. High-stage tumors like natural stage IC tumors with preoperative rupture or malignant ascites can be effectively treated with adjuvant cisplatin-based chemotherapy, especially tumors with high mitotic activity. Advanced-stage tumors should be treated with at least four to six cycles of cisplatin-based chemotherapy.[10]

Case reports detailing complete responders can be found for patients treated with carboplatin and etoposide; methotrexate, actinomycin D, and chlorambucil; and methotrexate, actinomycin D, and cyclophosphamide. However, long-term survival rates in patients with JGCTs have been disappointing.

In the postoperative period, the elevated hormone levels return to normal values and the pseudopuberty reverts.[2] Postoperative serum MIS concentrations may be used to evaluate the completeness of tumor removal following initial surgery and serial MIS determinations may allow the detection of recurrences.[12] Two patients with high mitotic index in a series of 4 progressed and died after 10 and 14 months, and the others without high mitotic index obtained a complete remission for 25 and 32 months.[13] Thus, the prognosis is poor when patient has high mitotic index.[13] Cytoreductive surgery is the treatment of choice and combination chemotherapy may be helpful to improve the prognosis of JGCT.[13] In a series his among stage Ic patients with preoperative rupture, six tumors showed more than 20 mitoses/10 high-power fields, and four of these relapsed.[10]

Section Three

Leukemia

The Clinical Basis of Pediatric Medical Oncology

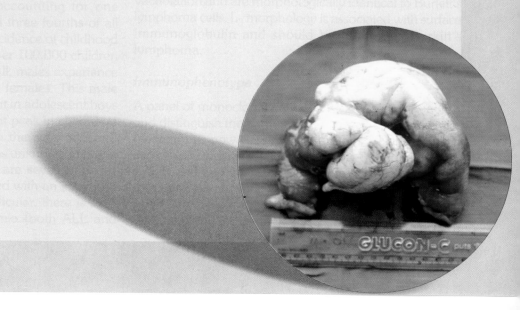

carry the immunophenotypes CD3, CD7, CD5 or CD2. The specific myeloid markers include CD13, CD14 and CD33. On the basis of immunophenotypic analysis a firm diagnosis can be made in 99 percent of cases.

Cytogenetics

Technological improvements now make it possible to demonstrate abnormalities in chromosomal number and/or structure in the majority of cases of ALL.[2,6] The presence of hyperdiploidy (chromosome number >50) is associated with a very good prognosis in contrast to the dramatic poor prognosis in patients with hypodiploidy (chromosome number <45 per cell).[7-9] Specific chromosomal translocations in ALL including the classical t(8;14) in B-cell ALL, t(4;11) in infant leukemia and t(9;22) translocation that forms the Philadelphia chromosome are associated with a poor prognosis.[10-12] The recognition of these abnormalities have contributed a lot to our understanding of the pathogenesis and prognosis of ALL patients.[13,14]

Prognostic Factors and Risk Assessment

Thirty-five years ago almost all children with acute lymphoblastic leukemia were dying with their disease and consequently all were considered as high risk. However, after introduction of chemotherapy and now, advances in cell biology and molecular genetics, the risk factors have been defined. Different study groups have defined different risk groups on the basis of clinical and biological features present at the time of diagnosis such as age at diagnosis, WBC count, sex, tumor load, CNS disease at diagnosis, immunophenotype, cytogenetics and DNA content and response to therapy. The two most important prognostic factors are age at diagnosis and the initial WBC count. Children less than one year of age have a very poor prognosis whereas children between the ages of 1 and 9 years do very well. A WBC count of more than $50,000/mm^3$ at diagnosis has a very bad prognosis.

Clinical Presentation

The clinical features of ALL are those of bone marrow infiltration with leukemic cells (bone marrow failure) and the extent of extramedullary disease spread. The most common symptoms and signs are usually manifestations of the underlying anemia, thrombocytopenia and neutropenia. Pallor, fatigue due to anemia, petechiae, purpura/bleeding due to thrombocytopenia and fever/ infections due to neutropenia are the usual presenting features. Lymphadenopathy, hepatomegaly and splenomegaly that are present in more than 60 percent of cases are the manifestations of extramedullary disease spread. Bone or joint pain which are present in about 25 percent of cases are due to leukemic involvement of the periosteum of bone or joint. Infants and young children may present with a limp or refusal to walk. Bone tenderness may be present. The incidence of central nervous system (CNS) involvement at diagnosis is about 4 to 5 percent of cases. The patient may present with signs or symptoms of raised intracranial pressure but most of the patients are asymptomatic. The diagnosis of CNS leukemia is made by examination of cerebrospinal fluid (CSF). Even a single blast in CSF is sufficient to diagnose CNS leukemia. Overt testicular leukemia may be seen in about 1 percent of cases at the time of diagnosis. It presents with firm, painless unilateral or bilateral swelling of the testes. The diagnosis should be confirmed by the testicular biopsy. Other rare sites of extramedullary involvement include heart, lungs, kidneys, ovaries, skin, eye or gastrointestinal tract. The duration of symptoms in a child with ALL may vary from days to weeks and in some cases few months. However, most of them present with 3 to 4 weeks history of presenting symptoms.

Investigations

a. Complete blood count including peripheral smear examination.
b. Bone marrow aspiration.
c. CSF for cytology.
d. Chest X-ray.
e. Uric acid.
f. Liver function tests.
g. Where facilities are available, investigations for membrane markers, cytogenetics and HLA typing of the patient with siblings should be undertaken.

Differential Diagnosis

These include infectious mononucleosis, acute infectious lymphocytosis, idiopathic thrombocytopenic purpura, pertussis and parapertussis and various viral infections like cytomegalovirus, EB virus and other viruses that result in leukemoid reactions and pancytopenia. ALL must also be differentiated from aplastic anemia which may present with pancytopenia. Some times when the child with ALL presents with fever, bone or joint complaint (limp, arthritis or arthralgia), pallor, splenomegaly and leukocytosis, the disease may be confused with juvenile rheumatoid arthritis. If there is some doubt about the diagnosis, the bone marrow aspirate should be done to exclude leukemia. ALL must also be distinguished from other pediatric cancers that may present with bone marrow involvement. They include neuroblastoma, non-Hodgkin's lymphoma (NHL), rhabdomyosarcoma, Ewing's sarcoma and retinoblastoma. Although there is usually evidence of a primary tumor in some other sites in these cases, a diagnosis of ALL must be confirmed by bone marrow examination. It should also be emphasized that leukemia may present as an acute emergency with life threatening complications such as infection, hemorrhage, organ dysfunction secondary to leukostasis or signs and symptoms of superior vena cava syndrome due to anterior mediastinal mass in cases of T-cell ALL.

Treatment

The treatment of ALL is divided into 4 stages (i) Induction (to attain remission) therapy, (ii) Intensification (consolidation), (iii) CNS prophylaxis or CNS preventive therapy and (iv) maintenance or continuation therapy. The average duration of treatment in ALL ranges between 2 and 2½ years and there is no advantage of treatment exceeding 3 years.[15,16] The two drugs regimen of vincristine and prednisolone induces remission in 80 to 95 percent of children with ALL. Since both the remission rate and duration of remission can be improved by the addition of a third or fourth drug (L-asparaginase and/or anthracycline) to vincristine and prednisolone, current induction regimens include vincristine, prednisolone, L-asparaginase and anthracycline. Currently a remission rate is achieved in 95 to 98 percent of cases;[17] the remission induction therapy lasts for 4 to 6 weeks.

CNS Preventive Therapy

The concept of CNS preventive therapy is based on the fact that most children with leukemia have subclinical CNS involvement at the time of diagnosis and central nervous system acts as a sanctuary site where leukemic cells are protected from systemic chemotherapy because of the blood brain barrier. The early institution of CNS prophylaxis is essential to eradicate leukemic cells that have passed the blood brain barrier. CNS prophylaxis has made a major contribution to the increased survival rates in leukemia. Most children receive a combination of intrathecal methotrexate and cranial irradiation.

Recent attention has been focussed on the long-term neurotoxicity and rarely development of brain tumor with this combination. The current goal is therefore to achieve effective CNS prophylaxis while minimizing neurotoxicity. Most centers use a low dose of cranial irradiation (1800 cGy) with intrathecal methotrexate. Other alternative regimens include the use of triple intrathecal therapy consisting of methotrexate, hydrocortisone and cytarabine without cranial irradiation.[18,19]

Intensification (Consolidation) Therapy

This is a period of intensified treatment administered shortly after remission induction. Some new chemotherapeutic agents are administered to tackle the problem of drug resistance. There is enough evidence to suggest that intensification of treatment has improved the long-term survival in all patients and it has become a common practice in many treatment protocols particularly for high-risk patients.

Maintenance (Continuing) Therapy

Once remission has been achieved, therapy is continued for an additional 2 to 2.5 years. Without maintenance or continuation therapy all patients, except those with B-cell ALL, relapse within 2 to 4 months. The main drugs used for maintenance therapy include 6-mercaptopurine daily and methotrexate once a week given orally with or without pulses of vincristine and prednisolone or other cytostatic drugs. It is imperative to carefully monitor children on maintenance therapy for both drug related toxicity and compliance.

Supportive Care

Aggressive supportive care like blood component therapy (red blood cell and platelet transfusion), detection and management of infectious complications, nutritional and metabolic needs and psychosocial support are important.

Treatment After Relapse

Despite the success of modern treatment, 25 to 30 percent of children with ALL still relapse. The most common site of relapse is in the bone marrow (20%), followed by CNS (5%) and testis (3%). The prognosis for a child with ALL who relapses depends on the site and time of relapse. Children with late relapse have a better prognosis than those with early relapse. Early bone marrow relapse before completing maintenance therapy has the worst prognosis with a long time survival of only 10 to 20 percent; late relapses occuring after cessation of maintenance therapy has a better prognosis. Relapse in extramedullary sites particularly testes compared with bone marrow relapse is more favorable in terms of survival. The treatment of relapse must be more aggressive than the first line therapy with induction of new drugs to overcome the problem of drug resistance. Bone marrow transplantation offers the better chance of cure than conventional chemotherapy particularly in early relapse. The overall survival after relapse is 20 to 40 percent in different series.

Late Effects of Treatment

Long-term effects of treatment that may take years to become apparent are issues of increasing concern today. Therefore, continued evaluation of an ALL survivor for prolonged periods is an essential part of follow-up. It is now clear that children who received cranial irradiation at a younger age are at increased risk of cognitive and intellectual impairement and development of CNS neoplasms. There is a risk of development of secondary acute myeloid leukemia after the intensive use of epipodophylotoxin (etoposide or tenoposide) therapy. Endocrine dysfunctions leading to short stature, obesity, precocious puberty, osteoporosis, thyroid dysfunction and growth retardation due to growth hormone deficiency are reported. The most worrying late effect of treatment is anthracycline induced cardiac toxicity.

Indian Scenario

There are ongoing Indo-US multicentric trials for characterization and treatment of ALL at Cancer Institute, Madras; Tata Memorial Hospital, Mumbai; All India Institute of Medical Sciences, New Delhi; and Kidwai Memorial Institute of Oncology, Bangalore. The five year survival of ALL patients from these centers is reported to be 45-55 percent.[20] The event free survival from our center is about 51 percent.[21] Various reasons have been attributed for the reduced survival rates of childhood malignancies including ALL in developing countries including India. Financial burden of treatment, often resulting in poor compliance and dropouts is a principal problem. The high incidence of infections among these immunocompromised patients, lack of availability of good supportive care and poor tolerance to chemotherapy in a largely malnourished group of patients contributes to a high mortality in our set up.

Over the years there has been a gradual improvement of outcome of ALL patients in our country and the future looks encouraging.

ACUTE MYELOID LEUKEMIA

Acute myeloid leukemia (AML) accounts for 15 to 20 percent of childhood leukemia. AML is a much more complex and resistant disease than the ALL.[22] With intensive myelosuppresive induction and further post remission therapy, however, about one-third of such patients can now achieve long-term survival and probably cure.

Epidemiology

The ratio of AML to ALL is approximately 1:4. AML can occur at any age but the incidence is slightly more during adolescence. Congenital leukemia (leukemia occuring during first 4 weeks of life) is mostly AML. Males and females are affected equally. The etiology is generally not known. However, an excess of AML is seen following ionizing radiation exposure. There are certain known congenital and acquired predisposing factors. Down syndrome (trisomy 21) is the most common genetic predisposing factor associated with a high risk of leukemia. Other predisposing factors are Fanconi's anemia, Bloom's syndrome, Kostmann syndrome and Diamond-Blackfan anemia. Certain drugs like alkylating agents and epipodophyllotoxins are well established predisposing factors for secondary AML.

Biology

AML can be divided into several subgroups according to the French-American-British (FAB) morphological classification system (M_0 to M_7). M_0 = immature, M_1 = Acute myeloblastic leukemia with minimal maturation, M_2 = Acute myeloblastic leukemia with maturation, M_3 = Acute promyelocytic leukemia, M_4 = Acute myelomonocytic leukemia, M_5 = Acute monoblastic leukemia, M_6 = erythroblastic leukemia, M_7 = Acute megakaryoblastic leukemia. About 30 to 40 percent of cases of AML are M_1 and M_2 and about same percentage is M_4 and M_5. M_3 type of AML constitutes about 5 to 10 percent. Specific chromosomal abnormalities have been found in various FAB subclasses.

Clinical Presentation

Most patients with AML presents with pallor, fatigue, bleeding or fever as manifestations of their underlying anemia, thrombocytopenia and neutropenia due to bone marrow failure. Unlike ALL, the bulky lymphadenopathy and massive hepatosplenomegaly is not very common in AML. However, infants and toddlers with AML may have more organomegaly, high WBC counts and CNS disease at diagnosis. Disseminated intravascular coagulation (DIC) may occur with any subgroup but is especially common in acute promyelocytic leukemia (M$_3$). Chloromas (also called granulocytic sarcoma) are localised collections of leukemic cells seen almost exclusively in patients with AML. They may occur at any site including CNS, bones (typically orbit) and skin. Gingival hypertrophy may be present. Diagnosis must be confirmed by bone marrow examination; the morphologic, cytochemical, immunophenotypic and genetic characteristics of the leukemic blast cells should be determined, if possible. Sometimes, the diagnosis of AML is preceded by a prolonged pre-leukemic phase lasting several weeks or months. Usually, this is characterized by a lack of one of the normal blood cell lineages, resulting in either a refractory anemia or a moderate degree of neutropenia or thrombocytopenia. The condition is often referred to as a myelodysplastic syndrome (MDS). Some children may be seen with hypoplastic marrow that may develop later into an acute leukemia.

Treatment

Compared to ALL, the cure rate is hampered by a lower remission rate, an increased relapse rate and a greater risk of death in remission due to infections and hemorrhage. Nevertheless, during the past two decades, the long-term survival for children with AML has increased from less than 10 percent to almost 40 percent. This is due to intensification of therapy along with improved supportive care including early use of empiric broad-spectrum antibiotics and prophylactic platelet transfusion. The main drugs used for induction therapy are combination of cytosine arabinoside (Ara-C) and an anthracycline (doxorubicin or daunorubicin). Some investigators have added other drugs like etoposide and thioguanine during induction therapy but without much significant success. With the current regimen, remission could be induced in about 70 to 80 percent of children with AML. However, without further therapy most children relapse within one year. Post-remission therapy (consolidation therapy) includes high dose chemotherapy utilizing Ara-C and etoposide or bone marrow transplantation. Most studies now suggest that bone marrow transplantation during early remission is superior to intensive chemotherapy alone.

The subset acute promyelocytic leukemia (M$_3$) that accounts for about 10 to 15 percent of children with AML should be treated separately. Probably, the best therapy is to induce remission by All-transretinoic acid (ATRA) as a single agent and then the remission is consolidated with post-remission intensive chemotherapy.

Because of severe myelosuppression following intensive chemotherapy in children with AML, these children require intensive blood component support including platelets and broad-spectrum antibiotics for control of severe infections. Therefore, these children should be treated by a pediatric oncologist in a tertiary care hospital where all the supportive care facilities are available.

ADULT VARIETY OF CHRONIC MYELOID LEUKEMIA (ACML)

Adult type of chronic myelogenous leukemia is a clonal panmyelopathy involving all the hemic lineages.[23] It is one of the commonest leukemias encountered in adults. However, it is quite rare in pediatric age group accounting for only 3 to 5 percent of all childhood leukemias. It is usually easily recognized because more than 95 percent of patients have a distinctive cytogenetic abnormality, the Philadelphia chromosomoe (ph^1).

Clinical Features

The onset of the disease is insidious. The presenting symptoms generally consist of mild fever, malaise and weight loss. Occasionally, patients present with more acute symptoms such as bone or joint pain or priapism. Splenomegaly is the most common physical finding and is usually massive. Mild hepatomegaly and lymphadenopathy may be present. Leukocytosis is present in all cases and 80 percent patients have a WBC count above 100,000/mm^3. The differential count shows all forms of myeloid cells from promyelocytes to polymorphonuclear leukocytes. Basophilia is common. Mild anemia is common but thrombocytopenia is rare. In contrast, thrombocytosis is relatively common. Bone marrow aspirate demonstrates a shift in the myeloid series to immature forms that increase in number as patients progress toward the blastic phase of the disease. Leukocyte alkaline phosphatase (LAP) activity is low. Philadelphia chromosome is positive in more than 90 percent of cases.

Treatment

The aim of treatment during chronic phase is to control the increasing white cell counts. This can usually be achieved by single agent chemotherapy with either busulfan or hydroxyurea. The blood counts returns to normal or near normal in almost all patients within 6 to 8 weeks. Spleen size also decreases. With this conventional treatment, the average survival is 3 to 4 years. Survival after development of accelerated phase is usually less than a year and after blastic transformation only a few months. The curative therapy is bone marrow transplantation when appropriate donors are available. Alpha-interferon may produce partial or complete remission in the chronic phase of CML.

JUVENILE CHRONIC MYELOID LEUKEMIA

Juvenile chronic myelogenous leukemia (JCML) is an uncommon hematological malignancy of childhood and accounts for less than 2 percent of all leukemias in children.[23] Compared to the adult variety of chronic myeloid leukemia (ACML), JCML is a disease of infancy and early childhood below the age of 5 years, has a more acute and severe course with relatively more frequent lymphadenopathy, anemia, hepatospleno-megaly, skin involvement, infection and thrombo-cytopenia.

Fetal hemoglobin values are elevated in most of the cases. Hematological features usually include a leukocytosis of less than $100,000/mm^3$. Monocytosis is a striking feature in the peripheral blood. Thrombo-cytopenia and anemia are common. Peripheral smear shows evidence of myeloid hyperplasia with the full spectrum of granulocytic precursors and increased normoblasts. The leukocyte alkaline phosphatase score is normal or low. Bone marrow aspirates show increased cellularity with predominance of granulocytic cells in all stages of maturation. Megakaryocytes are normal or decreased. Most of these patients have normal karyotypes or nonspecific chromosomal abnormalities. Philadelphia chromosome is always negative.

Treatment

JCML has a much more fulminant course. Chemotherapy has limited value. Drugs used for adult variety of CML like busulfan or hydroxyurea are of no value. Sequential subcutaneous cytosine arabinoside and oral 6-mercaptopurine are said to offer some systemic relief, but do not appear to prolong survival. Recently isotretinoin (13-cis-retinoic acid) has been used with some success. Allogeneic bone marrow transplantation is the only hope for these unfortunate children at the moment.

REFERENCES

1. Pui CH. Acute lymphoblastic leukemia. Pediatr Clin North Am 1997;4:831-46.
2. Pui CH, Evans WE. Acute lymphoblastic leukemia. N. Eng J Med 1998;339:605-15.
3. Gurney JG, Severson RK, Davis S, et al. Incidence of cancer in children in the United States. Cancer 1995;75:2186-95.
4. Young J, Gloeckler RL, Silverberg E, et al. Cancer incidence, survival and mortality for children younger than age 15 years. Cancer 1986;58:598-602.
5. Pui CH. Childhood leukemias. N Eng J Med 1995; 332: 1618-30.
6. Williams DL, Harber J, Murphy SB, et al. Chromosomal translocations play a unique role in influencing prognosis in acute lymphoblastic leukemia. Blood 1986;68:205-12.
7. Look AT, Roberson PK, Williams DL. Prognostic importance of Blast cell DNA content in childhood acute lymphoblastic leukemia, Blood 1985;65:1079-86.
8. Jackson JF, Boyett J, Pullen J, et al. Favourable prognosis associated with hyperdiploidy in children with acute lymphoblastic leukemia correlates with extra chromosome 6, a Pediatric Oncology Group Study. Cancer 1990; 66:1183-9.
9. Trueworthy R, Shuster J, Look T, et al. Ploidy of lymphoblasts is the strongest predictor of treatment outcome in B-progenitor cell acute lymphoblastic leukemia. J Clin Oncol 1992; 10:606-13.
10. Pui CH, Franket LS, Carroll AJ, et al. Clinical characteristics and treatment outcome of childhood acute lymphoblastic leukemia with the t (4; 11) (q21; q23): a collaborative study of 40 cases. Blood 1991;77:440-47.
11. Fletcher JA, Lynch EA, Kimball VM, et al. Translocation (9; 22) is associated with extremely poor prognosis in intensively treated children with acute lymphoblastic leukemia. Blood 1991;77: 435-9.
12. Pui CH, Crist WM. Biology and treatment of acute lymphoblastic leukemia. J Pediatr 1994; 124:491-503.
13. Pui CH, Behm FG, Downing JR, et al. 11 q 23/MLL rearrange-ment confers a poor prognosis in infants with acute lymphoblastic leukemia. J Clin Oncol 1994; 12:909-15.
14. Look AT. Oncogenic transcription factors in the human acute leukemias. Science 1997;278:1059-64.
15. Childhood ALL collaborative group. Duration and intensity of maintenance chemotherapy in acute lymphoblastic leukemia: overviews of 42 trials involving 12,000 randomized children. Lancet 1996;347:1783-8.
16. Nesbit MJ, Sather H, Robinson L, et al. Presymptomatic central nervous system therapy in previously untreated childhood acute lymphoblastic leukemia: comparision of 1800 rad and 2400 rad: a report for children cancer study group Lancet 1981;1:461-5.
17. Reiter A, Schrappe M, Ludwig WD, et al. Chemotherapy in 998 unselected childhood acute lymphoblastic leukemia patients. Results and conclusions of the multicenter trial ALL-BFM 86. Blood 1994;84:3122-33.
18. Pullan J, Boyett J, Shuster J, et al. Extended triple intrathecal chemotherapy trial in prevention of CNS relapse in good-risk and poor-risk patients with B-progenitor acute lymphoblastic leukemia: a Pediatric Oncology group study. J Clin Oncol 1993;11:839-49.
19. Abromowitch M, Ochs JS, Pui CH, et al. High-dose methotrexate improves clinical outcome in children with acute lymphoblastic

leukemia. St. Jude total therapy study X. Med Pediatr Oncol 1988;16:297-303.

20. Advani S, Pai S, Venzon D, et al. Acute Lymphoblastic leukemia in India: An analysis of prognostic factors using single treatment regimen. Ann Oncol 1999; 10:167-76.

21. Arya LS Jain Y, Bhargava M, Gupta S, Tomar S. Acute lymphoblastic leukemia: results of an aggressive induction consolidation regimen in India. Med Pediatr Oncol (abstr) 1999;33:152.

22. Golub TR, Weinstein HJ, Grier HE. Acute Myelogenous Leukemia. In: Pizzo PA, Poplack DG, (Eds): Principles and Practice of Pediatric Oncology. Philadelphia: Lippincott-Raven, 1997;1025-49.

23. Altman AJ: Chronic Leukemias of Childhood. In: Pizzo PA, Poplack DG, (Eds): Principles and Practice of Pediatric Oncology. Philadelphia: Lippincott-Raven, 1997;483-507.

CHAPTER 32

Sameer Bakhshi

Lymphoma

NON-HODGKIN'S LYMPHOMA

Pediatric lymphomas are the third most common group of malignancies in children and adolescents accounting for about 12 percent of all newly diagnosed cancers in this age group. Lymphomas are uncommon below the age of 5 years and the relative incidence increases with increasing age. Pediatric non-Hodgkin's lymphomas (NHL) are quite different than lymphomas in adults. Low-grade lymphomas that are common in adults are rare in children. Pediatric lymphomas are high-grade lymphomas that are diffuse and aggressive lymphomas that have a propensity for wide spread dissemination. Unlike adults with NHL, who most often present with lymph node disease, children typically have extranodal disease involving the mediastinum (in 26 % of cases), abdomen (in 31 %), or head and neck (in 29 %).

Cellular Origin, Immunophenotype and Histopathology of Childhood NHL

Lymphomas efface the lymph node architecture although in the early stages, there may be preservation of the architecture in some areas of the lymph node. In non-lymphoid tissue, the lymphoma cells tend to infiltrate in between the normal cells, collagen, or muscle fibers of the involved tissue. The three main histological subtypes of NHL in childhood are:

1. *Lymphoblastic lymphoma:* These cells are indistinguishable from those of acute lymphoblastic leukemia. The distinction is arbitrarily based on bone marrow examination with blasts>30 percent being classified as leukemia. They may be of either B or T cell origin, and the few translocations that do occur frequently involve the T-cell receptor genes.

2. *Small non-cleaved cell lymphomas:* These cells have a high nuclear-cytoplasmic ratio; the cytoplasm is very basophilic and usually contains lipid vacuoles (staining positive with oil red O). These are sub-divided into:
   a. Burkitt's (cells uniform in size and shape)
   b. Non-Burkitt's (heterogeneous cells) lymphoma.

   They are of B-cell origin, and involve a chromosomal translocation of a protooncogene involved in cellular proliferation (c-myc on 8q24).

3. *Large cell lymphoma:* They may be of high or intermediate grade, and of either T or B cell origin, and may be classified diffuse, immunoblastic or anaplastic. Anaplastic large cell lymphoma is a new clinicopathologic variant of large cell lymphoma, CD30 positive, wherein the cells characteristically involve the lymph node sinus as well as extranodal sites (skin, bone and soft tissue) where the cells grow in a cohesive pattern, and contain frequent, large, bizarre cells, with abundant cytoplasm and irregular nuclei. The most frequently observed translocation is t(2;5)(p12;q35). It forms 10 percent of childhood lymphomas and roughly 30 to 40 percent of the pediatric large cell lymphomas.

Epidemiology

Childhood lymphomas occur throughout the world, although the relative frequency and incidence of NHL show significant geographic variations. In equatorial

Africa, for example, 50 percent of all cancers are lymphomas (Burkitt's lymphoma being predominant). In United States and Europe about one-third of childhood lymphomas are lymphoblastic, one half small, noncleaved cell lymphomas (Burkitt's and nonburkitt's or Burkitt like) and the rest are large cell lymphomas. In India probably lymphoblastic lymphoma is more common. There is no evidence that NHL is predisposed by radiation exposure. Patients with Hodgkin's disease treated with combined modality treatment (chemotherapy and radiation) are at increased risk of development of NHL (perhaps 4-5% over a 10-year period). Patients with immunodeficiency and DNA repair deficiency syndromes (eg. Wiskott-Aldrich syndrome, X-linked lymphoproliferative disorder and ataxia telangiectasia) and acquired immunodeficiency syndrome like human immunodeficiency virus (HIV) infection, following immunosuppressive therapy (e.g. Post-transplants) malaria and infection with Ebstein-Barr virus and malaria are believed to be risk factors for development of Burkitt's lymphoma in equatorial Africa.

Clinical Presentation

Patients with NHL usually present with clinical features that correlate with histologic subtype. Patients with lymphoblastic lymphoma most commonly present with an intrathoracic tumor, particularly a mediastinal mass (50-70% cases) and often have a pleural effusion. The presenting features may include dyspnea, dysphagia, chest pain or superior vena caval obstruction. Most often the lymphadenopathy is supradiaphragmatic, and the immunophenotype T cell type. Cutaneous lymphoblastic lymphomas are generally of the B-precursor type.

Small non-cleaved cell lymphomas manifest as abdominal pain, ascites, palpable abdominal mass, intestinal obstruction or intussusception. Presentation with a right iliac fossa mass is quite common and can be confused with appendicitis or appendicular inflammatory mass (Fig. 32.1). Lymphadenopathy is usually subdiaphragmatic. Jaw involvement is most frequent site in African Burkitt's lymphoma (70%) occurring particularly in young children younger than 5 years of age. Jaw involvement in non-African Burkitt's lymphoma occurs in 15 percent of patients at presentation, and is not age related (10-15%).

Large cell lymphomas occur at a variety of sites including mediastinum, abdomen, head and neck region; in unusual sites like bone and CNS, as well as in immunodeficiency associated lymphoma. Anaplastic large cell lymphomas typically involve the skin, bone and lymph node sinuses.

NHL are very rapidly growing tumors. Almost two thirds of the children have a widespread disease at the time of diagnosis that may involve the bone marrow, central nervous system or both. Further, because of their high turnover especially in case of Burkitt's lymphoma, there is high risk of tumor lysis. There may be obstruction to the renal outflow system by the abdominal mass or direct infiltration of the kidneys.

Diagnosis

NHL is a rapidly growing neoplasm, so rapid diagnosis is essential (Table 32.1). Selection of the appropriate node or mass for histological material is important. Histology remains the primary means for definitive diagnosis and should be supplemented if possible with immunophenotypic and cytogenetic studies. If the

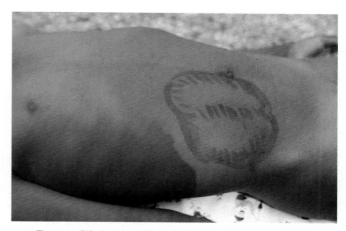

Figure 32.1: Non Hodgkin's lymphoma presenting as a mass in the right iliac fossa

Table 32.1: Evaluation of patient with non-Hodgkin's lymphoma
• History and physical examination
• Complete blood count
• Bone marrow aspirations and biopsy
• CSF examination (Cytology)
• Cytology from other body fluids if available like pleural, pericardial or peritoneal fluid
• LFT, renal function tests, serum electrolytes, LDH, uric acid
• Chest radiograph
• CT scan of chest and abdomen
• Bone scan

patients clinical condition is not suitable for biopsy particularly under general anesthesia due to large mediastinal mass causing superior vena cava syndrome, the diagnosis should be made with less invasive procedures like percutaneous needle aspiration of accessible lymph node, examination of body fluids or bone marrow. It must be remembered that in patients with large mediastinal mass, there may be acute deterioration after endotracheal intubation and general anesthesia because of edema in an already compromised airway. Further venous engorgement because of superior vena caval obstruction may result in profuse intraoperative bleeding.

Histopathology or FNAC reveals a round cell tumor that needs to be differentiated from other small round blue cell tumors in childhood such as neuroblastoma, peripheral neuroectodermal tumor and rhabdomyosarcoma using appropriate immunocytochemical stains.

Staging

The most widely used staging system is that of St. Jude (Table 32.2) which is applicable to all histological types of childhood lymphoma.

Prognostic Features

The tumor burden, reflected by both the stage of the disease and the serum lactate dehydrogenase concentration, is the single most important predictor of the outcome. Among patients with Burkitt's lymphoma, central nervous system disease at the time of diagnosis is associated with the greatest risk of treatment failure. In patients with large-cell lymphoma, bone marrow involvement and a T-cell or indeterminate immunophenotype appear to be associated with a poorer prognosis. Finally, the expression of CD30 may be a favorable prognostic feature in patients with large-cell lymphomas, although this finding is controversial. In lymphoblastic lymphoma as in acute lymphoblastic leukemia, T cell immunophenotype is more aggressive than B-precursor type.

Management

The dramatic improvement in the overall survival of patients with NHL is because of the development of highly effective, multiagent chemotherapy and supportive care. Surgery has very limited role in treatment other than for diagnostic purposes. Surgery

has very limited role in treatment other than for diagnostic purposes. Occasionally for small tumors, complete excision may be attempted (Fig. 32.2). Radiotherapy is also restricted to emergency situations like superior vena cava syndrome or spinal cord compression due to paraspinal disease. Thus systemic combination chemotherapy is the main treatment of NHL. Different chemotherapeutic regimens are used for treatment depending on the histology and stage of the disease.

Table 32.2: St. Jude's staging system for Non-Hodgkin's lymphoma
Stage I
• Single nodal or extranodal site excluding mediastinum and abdomen
Stage II
• Single extranodal site with regional node involvement
• Two or more nodal areas on the same side of the diaphragm
• Two single (extranodal) tumors with or without regional node involvement on the same side of the diaphragm
• Primary gastrointestinal tumor usually in the ileocecal area with or without involvement of associated mesenteric nodes (resectable)
Stage III
• Two extranodal sites on opposite sides of the diaphragm
• Two or more nodal areas above and below the diaphragm
• Primary intrathoracic tumors (mediastinal, pleural, thymic)
• Extensive intra-abdominal disease (not resectable)
• All paraspinal or epidural tumors
Stage IV
• CNS or bone marrow involvement

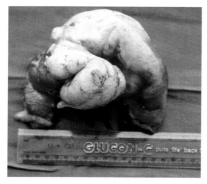

Figure 32.2: Resected specimen of intestine with non-Hodgkin's lymphoma presenting with intestinal obstruction

In non-lymphoblastic localized NHL (stages I and II) large cell as well as small noncleaved B-cell, a 9-week regimen of modest intensity—3 cycles of CHOP (cyclophosphamide, doxorubicin, vincristine and prednisone) without any irradiation may be sufficient therapy. However, most pediatric oncologists use chemotherapy regimens for lymphoblastic lymphoma that are based on protocols for ALL. These are intensive protocols that use combinations of 8 to 10 drugs over a prolonged duration of 1.5 to 2 years. Cranial irradiation or prophylactic intrathecal chemotherapy to prevent CNS relapse as in ALL, although the risk for CNS relapse is less than that for ALL. A short course therapy for early stage lymphoblastic lymphoma is generally not used because of the high recurrence rate in the following 1 to 2 years. The long-term survival in patients with lymphoblastic lymphoma with limited disease is excellent in the range of 80 to 90 percent and in advanced stage disease it is about 65 to 75 percent. Patients with lymphoblastic lymphoma who remain relapse free for 36 months after diagnosis are considered as cured.

The chemotherapeutic regimens for small non cleaved B-cell lymphoma (Burkitt's and non-Burkitt's) consist of short duration, intensive alkylating agent therapy (cyclophosphamide or ifosfamide) coupled with intermediate or high dose methotrexate, vincristine, anthracyclines, etoposide and cytarabine. CNS prophylaxis in the form of intrathecal chemotherapy is also given. Total duration of therapy is approximately 6 months for stage 3 and 4 disease. Long-term event-free survival is excellent—more than 90 percent in patients with limited disease and 75 to 85 percent in patients with extensive disease.

There is no consensus on the appropriate therapy for advanced-stage large cell lymphomas, perhaps because of the biologic heterogeneity of these tumors. The most recent data suggests that immunophenotype-directed treatment in large cell lymphoma may be more effective in improving survival. B-cell tumors respond well to a variety of treatments, including the short-term, intensive chemotherapeutic regimen used for Burkitt's lymphoma. Tumors of T-cell origin probably require more intensive or prolonged (perhaps lymphoblastic-specific) therapy. A possible exception is the CD30+ large-cell subtype, which may respond to the treatment used for Burkitt's lymphoma.

HODGKIN'S LYMPHOMA

Hodgkin's lymphoma (HL) is characterized by the progressive enlargement of lymph nodes. The disease is usually considered unicentric in origin and has a predictable pattern of spread by extension to contiguous nodes. While the etiology of HL still remains unknown, the biology of the disease confirms malignant behavior.

Epidemiology and Etiology

The annual incidence of HL is approximately 5 to 7 cases per million children younger than 15 years. The age specific incidence of HL exhibits a characteristic bimodal distribution. In the developed countries, the early peak occurs in the age group of 20 to 30 years and the second peak after the age of 50 years. In developing countries, however, the early peak occurs before adolescence. HL is rare before the age of five years. It is more common in males than in females. The exact cause of HL is not known. Epidemiologic studies suggest that a large proportion of patients with HL have high EBV antibody titers along with in situ hybridization evidence of EBV genomes in Reed-Sternberg cells. EBV positive tumor genomes are more frequently observed in children aged less than 10 years of age, Asian ethnicity especially in developing countries and histologically in the mixed cellularity subtype.

Pathology

HL is divided in main categories: classic Hodgkin's and nodular lymphocytic predominant Hodgkin's (NLPHL). Classic Hodgkin's in turn is divided into 4 subtypes: nodular sclerosis, mixed cellularity, lymphocyte-rich classic HL, and lymphocyte-depleted disease. The characteristic cells were termed as Hodgkin's and Reed-Sternberg cells in classic Hodgkin's lymphoma and lymphocytic and histiocytic cells in NLPHL.

NLPHL cells consistently express B cell markers like CD 20 and B cell receptor that are rarely expressed by other types of HL. Although identification of the characteristic Reed-Sternberg cell, a large multinucleated giant cell with abundant cytoplasm and either multiple or multilobed nuclei, facilitates the diagnosis of HL, it is not pathognomonic. Rarely, Reed-Sternberg cells can be seen in reactive lymphoid hyperplasia, NHL and non-lymphoid malignancies. Nodular sclerosing is the most common type in developed countries whereas in

CHAPTER 33

Tulika Seth

Histiocytosis

INTRODUCTION

The histiocytoses are a group of rare diseases that involve histiocytes, which are derived from bone-marrow stem cells. In 1953, these conditions were unified under the terminology-histiocytosis X. In 1987, the term Langerhans cell histiocytosis syndromes were adopted by the histiocyte society.[1] The two forms of histiocytosis most often encountered in children are Langerhans cell histiocytosis (LCH) and hemophagocytic lympho-histiocytosis, the first a disease of epidermal antigen-presenting dendritic cells called Langerhans cells (LCs), and the second of mononuclear phagocytes. In both conditions there may be accumulation of histiocytic cells in organs and tissues throughout the body.[2] This article will discuss Langerhans cell histiocytosis (LCH) in detail.

LCH in children is a very diverse disease. The overall mortality in LCH is 10-20 percent, however, many survivors suffer severe long-term consequences of the disease and subsets of patients continue to have progressive disease that is refractory to current therapies. LCH in children is very diverse. Approximately two-thirds of patients, present with single-system disease with the skeleton being the commonest site.[3] Many of these patients require minimal treatment or resolve spontaneously, but even in these patients there may be permanent, mainly orthopedic consequences.[4] At the other extreme most often in young infants, the presentation is multisystem with organ failure. Among patients who do not respond to treatment within the first few weeks, mortality may be as high as 20 percent irrespective of treatment.[5,6] Between these extremes lie patients with multisystem disease without organ failure in whom the disease runs a fluctuating course and may eventually 'burn out'; often leave serious residual disabilities.[7]

PATHOLOGY

Langerhans cells are the resident dendritic cells of the skin and are responsible for antigen uptake, processing and presentation. If inflammation occurs in the skin, the Langerhans cells become activated. The clinical signs and symptoms, as well as the morphology of LCH, indicate that disordered cytokine and chemokine production and responses are important in the pathogenesis of the disorder. In the LCH lesion, up to 80 percent of the T cells are memory helper T cells.[3,8] These T cells express CD40 ligand (CD40L);[9] a marker of activated T cells, whereas antigen-presenting cells express CD40. The CD40-CD40L interaction is known to activate T cells to produce cytokines. The interaction of CD40+ LCH cells and CD40L+ T cells in LCH potentiates the cytokine storm,[9] this term refers to both the high level and diversity of cytokines produced locally.[10,11] Higher than normal levels of granulocyte-macrophage colony stimulating factor (GM-CSF), tumor-necrosis factor-alpha (TNFα) and interleukin-3 (IL-3) are present in LCH. These cytokines function as chemo-attractants to recruit eosinophils, neutrophils, macrophages and CD34+ Langerhans cell precursors into the lesions.[12]

The cytokines provide an ideal microenvironment to prolong the viability of the interacting inflammatory cells by creating autocrine and paracrine loops. In LCH, cytokines known to influence osteo-clastogenesis, such as IL-1, IL-6, TNFα, receptor activator of nuclear factor-B ligand RANKL, GM-CSF and M-CSF, are highly expressed.[11,13] LCH cells, and the T cells in close proximity to them, express RANKL and M-CSF.[8] Aberrant production of M-CSF and RANKL-RANK interaction is therefore probably responsible for the large number of osteoclasts and the prominence of osteolysis in LCH.[8] The RANK- RANKL interaction provides a survival signal for these cells,[14-16] which perpetuates the survival of LCH cells. Chemokine and chemokine-receptor expression patterns, might explain the predilection of LCH for particular sites and the cellular composition of the lesions. Maturation of LCs is associated with the coordinated down regulation of receptors for inflammatory chemokines, for example CCR6 and CCL20. Dendritic cells found in LCH lesions retain many features of normal skin LCs, such as expression of CD1α antigen, langerin and Birbeck granules, they are equally clearly abnormal.[17,18] Normally, cytokine production by LCs is triggered by pathogen-associated molecular patterns,[19] while the trigger for cytokine production by LCH cells remains unknown. Furthermore, the lesional cytokine storm would be expected to induce differentiation from an antigen processing to an antigen-presenting cell and migration of LCs to the draining lymph nodes. This does not occur in LCH. Therefore, the failure of LCH cells to differentiate and migrate produces a self-sustaining lesion, providing a microenvironment in which many cell types survive and precursors might differentiate to inappropriate effector cells causing pathological damage.

DEFINITION

Langerhans cell histiocytosis (LCH) is an abnormal proliferation of Langerhans cells with expression of CD1α, S-100 protein and the presence of Birbeck granules by ultrastructural examination[20].

Synonyms and Historical Annotation

Previously described as Histiocytosis X, this disease was first described in clinical variants as Solitary Eosinophilia Granuloma, Hand Schuller Christian disease and Letterer-Siwe disease.

EPIDEMIOLOGY

Incidence is 5/100,00,00 with most cases presenting in childhood.[21] A male predominance is seen 3.7:1.[22] The peak age in children is 1 to 4 years. It may be associated with acute lymphoblastic leukemia and lymphoma.[23]

ETIOLOGY

The exact etiology is unknown. There is some evidence of viral infections, e.g. human herpes virus 6, Ebstein-Barr virus, herpes simplex, adeno virus, cytomegalo virus, T cell leukemia virus type 1 and 2 have been implicated.[23-25] History of exposure to neonatal infections, viral infections, lack of childhood vaccination and exposure to solvents has been described.[23]

Debate Malignancy vs Non-malignancy

Genetic studies of X-linked androgen receptor gene have revealed the monoclonal nature of proliferation of the Langerhans cell.[26] The association with clonal malignant diseases of early hematopoietic precursor cells indicates that there might be underlying genetic abnormalities in these cells in LCH, a finding that is in accord with the finding of a common immunoglobulin gene rearrangement in B cells and LCH cells.[27]

More recently, the arguments in favor of a non-neoplastic origin for LCH have been set out[28] Histologically, LCH lesions are granulomatous in character and do not have the cellular homogeneity of a malignant neoplasm. The uniform distribution of LCH lesions, indicating orderly recruitment of the cells to tissues, is unlike the haphazard spread of malignant neoplasms. Regression of LCH lesions is frequent but rare in true malignancies. So far, it has not been possible to culture 'LCH cells' and produce any cell lines.

CLINICAL FEATURES

Patients can present with:
1. Unifocal bone lesions of skull or diaphysis. They may present with a localized mass (Fig. 33.1) and radiologically a lytic lesion is seen with erosion of cortical bone and other extranodal sites (e.g. skin).
2. Multifocal unisystem disease presents mostly in young children with multiple destructive bone lesions, associated with adjacent soft tissue masses. The children may present with exophthalmos, diabetes insipidus, and tooth loss.

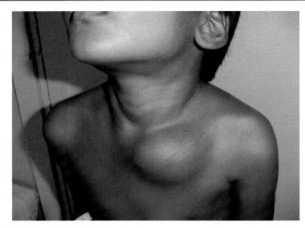

Figure 33.1: Histiocytosis may present as a mass lesion

3. Multifocal, multisystem disease presents with systemic symptoms of fever, pancytopenia, hepatospleno-megaly, lymphadenopathy, skin and bone lesions.[3]

SITES OF INVOLVEMENT

Bone

Painful bone lesions are common. They occur commonly in the skull as punched-out lytic lesions, without evidence of marginal sclerosis or periosteal reaction. Bone involvement of the mandible and maxilla and soft-tissue involvement of the gingiva may result in the loss of teeth. Involvement of vertebra can result in vertebral collapse (vertebra plana) and lesions of long bones may result in fractures. Radionuclide bone scan (99mTc-polyphosphate) may show localized increased uptake at the site of involvement. Magnetic resonance imaging (MRI) shows bone lesions not identifiable by either radiographic or radionuclide scans. The differential diagnoses are osteomyelitis, malignant bone tumors, and bony cysts.[29]

Skin

Cutaneous eruptions consist of:
1. Diffuse papular scaling lesions, resembling seborrheic eczema (most common)
2. Petechiae and purpura
3. Granulomatous ulcerative lesions
4. Xanthomatous lesions
5. Bronzing of the skin

Lungs

Lung involvement may result in pulmonary dysfunction with tachypnea and/or dyspnea, cyanosis, cough, pneumothorax or pleural effusion. Radiographic densities or infiltrates consisting of diffuse cystic changes, nodular infiltrations, or extensive fibrosis can occur. The radiographic appearance may resemble military tuberculosis.

Liver

Hepatomegaly may be present, liver dysfunction may consist of hypoproteinemia (total protein less than 5.5 g/dl and/or albumin less than 2.5 g/dl), edema, ascites, and/or hyperbilirubinemia (greater than 1.5 mg/dl, not attributable to hemolysis). A baseline liver biopsy may reveal portal triditis and rarely fibrohistiocytic infiltrate may be seen. Patients with fibrohistiocytic infiltrates are more likely have progressive liver disease and develop cirrhotic changes.

Hematopoietic System

Hematopoietic system dysfunction may consist of:
1. Anemia (hemoglobin level less than 10 g/dl, not due to iron deficiency or superimposed infection), leukopenia (neutrophils less than 1500/mm[3]), or thrombocytopenia (less than 100,000/mm[3]). If abnormal hemogram report then a bone marrow evaluation is mandatory. An excessive number of histiocytes in the marrow aspirate alone, are not considered evidence of dysfunction. It must be demonstrated that they are abnormal histiocytes.

Lymph Nodes

Occasionally, massive lymph nodes enlargement of cervical nodes occurs without other evidence of histiocytosis.

Central Nervous System

Clinically, four groups of patients can be distinguished:
1. Patients with a disorder of the hypothalamic pituitary system.
2. Patients with symptoms of space-occupying lesions such as headache and seizures.
3. Patients with neurological dysfunction — ataxia, tremor, intellectual impairment or dysarthria with variable progression to severe CNS deterioration.
4. Patients who present with an overlap of the above symptoms.
   Patients who develop CNS disease are more likely to have multisystem disease and skull lesions with skull and temporal bone lesions, orbital involvement, diabetes insipidus and endocrinopathies.[29,31]

Hypothalamic Pituitary Involvement

Signs and symptoms: Hypothalamic involvement: disturbances in social behavior, appetite, temperature regulation, sleep pattern.

Posterior pituitary involvement: diabetes insipidus (DI), polyuria and polydypsia.

Anterior pituitary involvement: growth failure, precocious or delayed puberty, amenorrhea, and hypothyroidism.

Of all these presentations, DI is the most common manifestation. The incidence of this complication ranges from 5 to 50 percent. DI is more likely to develop within 5 years of diagnosis and it may manifest before any extracranial manifestations of LCH. DI is commonly associated with multisystem LCH.

Laboratory studies for the diagnosis of DI include:
1. Water deprivation test.
2. Measurement of urinary arginine vasopressin (ADH).

It is important to perform these tests to discriminate partial from complete DI. Partial DI fluctuates spontaneously. Gadolinium-enhanced MRI studies show thickening of the hypothalamic pituitary stalk (>2.5 mm) and absence of a posterior pituitary "bright" signal in T1 weighted images. These lesions are caused by the infiltration of LCH cells.

There is no convincing evidence that established DI can be reversed by any treatment modality. However, there is some evidence that early radiotherapy for incipient DI may be useful. Replacement therapy with desmopressin (DDAVP) is recommended for patients with DI. The rapid institution of systemic chemotherapy for disseminated disease seems to prevent the occurrence of DI and might be responsible for the low frequency of DI.

Space Occupying Central Nervous System Lesions

These lesions may arise from adjacent bone lesions, brain meninges, or choroid plexus. They usually give rise to signs and symptoms of increased intracranial pressure. They are also site specific and size dependent. Such symptoms include headaches, vomiting, papilledema, optic atrophy, seizures, and other focal symptoms. Even diffuse meningitis-like manifestations can occur. These lesions may occur without any other evidence of LCH. Mass lesions respond well to treatment, leaving minimal or even no residual defects.[29] Treatment options are:
- Surgical excision, (depending on the site and the relationship of the lesion to the vascular and neural structures)

- Systemic chemotherapy
- Local radiotherapy
- Steroids.

Cerebellar Syndrome/Neurologic Degeneration

The cerebellum is the second most common site of LCH CNS involvement. The symptoms mainly follow the pontine-cerebellar pattern, beginning as a discrete reflex abnormality or gait disturbance, and/or nystagmus. They can progress to disabling ataxia. Pontine symptoms include dysarthria, dysphagia, and other cranial nerve deficits, ultimately leading to fatal CNS degeneration. On MRI, lesions in the pons, basal ganglion, and cerebellar peduncles show white matter lesions without enhancement. MRI of the cerebrum may show white-matter lesions in the periventricular area. There is no effective treatment available and prognosis is poor. However, early intervention with etoposide therapy may merit consideration.

In addition to the above lesions, therapy-related CNS changes should also be taken into consideration in the differential diagnosis of LCH CNS lesions.[29-33]

DIAGNOSIS (TABLE 33.1)

The key feature for diagnosis is the demonstration of Langerhans[3] cells. Langerhans cells are 10 to 15 μ in size, with grooved, folded and indented nuclei, fine chromatin and inconspicuous nucleoli and a thin nuclear membrane. Cytoplasm is moderately abundant and is slightly eosinophilic. Variable number eosinophils, histiocytes, neutrophils and small lymphocytes are present.[2,29]

Table 33.1: Diagnosis of Langerhans' cell histiocytosis
1. Presumptive diagnosis: light morphologic characteristics
2. Designated diagnosis a. Light morphologic features plus b. Two or more supplemental positive stains for • Adenosine triphosphatase • S100 protein • α-D-Mannosidase • Peanut lectin • Positive by flow for vimentin, HLA- DR, CD45, CD68, lysozyme
3. Definitive diagnosis a. Light morphologic characteristics plus b. Birbeck granules in the lesional cell with electron microscopy and/or c. Positive staining for CD1α antigen on the lesional cell ± Langerin

Ultrastructure

The hallmark of LCH is the presence of cytoplasmic Birbeck granules. They are tennis racket shaped, 200 to 400 nanometer long and 33 nanometer wide. Variable numbers may be present in the LCH lesions. Earlier lesions may have more granules.

Cytochemistry

LCH lesions express CD1α, S100 protein (2,20) and are weakly positive for vimentin, HLA-DR and placental alkaline phosphatase. The LCH immunophenotype is usually negative for B-cell and T-cell markers (except CD4). May be weakly positive for CD45, CD68 and lysozyme. They are negative for CD30, MPO, CD34, and negative for dendritic cell markers like CD21 and CD35. Ki 67 may stain in 10 percent of LCH cases.[22] CD1α is a surface antigen, which is useful, but not specific. CD1α can be expressed on Rosai-Dorfman disease and deep-seated juvenile xantho granulomatosis.[34]

Langerin is a recently identified lectin, which can be used as immuno-histochemical marker of Langerhans[9] cells (LCs). Langerin on epidermal LCs has a coarsely granular cell membrane and a cytoplasmic staining pattern that is always associated with CD1α expression. In a study all 24 cases of LCH were Langerin (+)/CD1α (+). Lymph node sinuses and hepatic sinusoids show Langerin (+)/CD1α (-) cells, indicating that, when used alone to confirm LCH infiltration, it should be used with caution. At other sites, its diagnostic accuracy is similar to that of CD1α.[35]

Genetics

The immunoglobulin heavy chain genes and b,d,g chain genes of T-cell receptors are in a germline state.[36] No numeric or structural karyotype abnormality has been seen in LCH.

Workup

CXR and Skeletal survey
Complete hemogram
Liver function test
Coagulation profile
Urine osmolality and overnight water deprivation test
See Table 33.2.

Staging

Group A: Patients with multifocal bone disease – lesions in multiple bones or more than two lesions in one bone.

Group B: Patients with soft tissue involvement, with or without bone lesions, but without signs of organ dysfunction $\geq$ patients with single bone lesion and a biopsy proven contiguous soft tissue mass, regional lymph node involvement, or endocrinologic disabilities (e.g., diabetes insipidus, growth hormone deficiency).

Group C: Patients with dysfunction of any of the following organ systems: liver, lung, or hematopoietic system as defined as hemoglobin level of less than 9.0g/dl in infants and less than 10 g/dl in older children.[29]

	Table 33.2: Required laboratory and radiographic evaluation of new patients with Langerhans' cell histiocytosis		
	Follow-up test interval when organ system is:		
Tests	*Involved*	*Not involved*	*Single-bone lesion*
Hemoglobin	Monthly	6 months	None
White blood cell count and differential count	Monthly	6 months	None
Platelet count	Monthly	6 months	None
Liver function tests (SGOT, SGPT, Alkaline phosphatase, bilirubin, Total proteins, albumin)	Monthly	6 months	None
Coagulation studies (PT, PTT, fibrinogen)	Monthly	6 months	None
Chest radiograph (PA and lateral)	Monthly	6 months	None
Skeletal radiograph survey	6 months	None	Once, at 6 months
Urine osmolality measurement after overnight water deprivation	6 months	6 months	None

Treatment

In patients with localized disease, local therapy is recommended. Current knowledge suggests tailoring the therapy to the extent of disease. In single-system disease, treatment by excisional biopsy, low-dose radiotherapy, or mild chemotherapy and topical steroids for skin lesions is successful.[36] Multifocal disease can be life threatening and warrants an aggressive approach[4,5] Chronic disease, exacerbation and remission are seen. Thus a unique approach is needed to treat each patient.[39,40]

All Groups

Initial Treatment (first 6 weeks)

Prednisone: 40 mg/m²/day PO for 28 days followed by a two week steroid taper.
30 mg/m²/day PO for 7 days
20 mg/m²/day PO for 7 days
Vinblastine: 6 mg/m²/ IV bolus on days 1, 8, 15, 22, 29, and 36
Etoposide: 60 mg/m²/day, days 1-5
Etoposide: 150 mg/m²/day, days 18, 25, 32, 39

Continuation Treatment (starting week 9)

Group A
Prednisone: 40 mg/m²/day PO, days 1-5 of weeks 9, 12, 15, 18, 21 and 24,30,36,42
Vinblastine: 6 mg/m²/IV bolus, day 1 of weeks 9, 12, 15, 18, 21 and 24,20,36,42
6 mercaptopurine 50 mg/m²/day week 6-52

Group B
Etoposide: As above with addition of
150 mg/m²/day, day 18,25,32,36,42

Group C
Etoposide: As above with addition of
150 mg/m²/day, day 18,25,32,36,42
Methotrexate: 500 mg/m² IV day 1 of week 8,12,15,18,24,36,42 (with leukovorin rescue)

Group A: Patients with multifocal bone disease-lesions in multiple bones or more than two lesions in one bone.
Group B: Patients with soft tissue involvement, with or without bone lesions, but without signs of organ dysfunction ≥ patients with a single bone lesion and a biopsy proven contiguous soft tissue mass, regional lymph node involvement, or endocrinologic disabilities (e.g. diabetes insipidus, growth hormone deficiency).
Group C: Patients with dysfunction of any of the following organs systems: liver, lung or hematopoietic system as defined as hemoglobin level of less than 9.0 g/dl in infants and less than 10 g/dl in older children.

The above protocol is recommended for the following reasons:

High rate of resolution (Group A: 89%; Group B: 91%; Group C: 67%)

Low frequency of recurrence (Group A: 12%; Group B: 23%; Group C: 42%)

Low incidence of permanent complications (e.g. diabetes insipidus)

Low incidence of drug toxicity or late effects

Options for Multisystem Disease

2-chlorodeoxyadenosine (2CDA): A purine analogue exerts a toxic effect on monocytes. It has been reported to induce response in many patients with severe or refractory multisystem disease.[41]

Pamidronate has been used for multifocal bone pain unresponsive to chemotherapy, corticosteroids, anti-inflammatory and narcotic analgesics.[42]

Salvage Treatment for Refractory Patients

Cyclosporine A, antithymocyte globulin and prednisolone have been employed. If a matched sibling is available and the patient has unresponsive and progressive disease, allogeneic bone marrow transplant can be utilized after the administration of a conditioning regimen consisting of busulfan, etoposide, and cyclophosphamide.[43]

PROGNOSIS AND PREDICTIVE FACTORS

The clinical course depends on whether multisystem involvement is present of not. Certain organs like liver and lung are poor prognostic sites. Multiple bone lesions and absence of any other system involvement is a good prognostic factor. Only 10 percent of unifocal bone lesions may progress to multisystem disease. Unifocal disease patients have a greater than 95 percent overall survival (OS). When two organs are involved the OS is 75 percent liver and lung.

In the absence of frankly malignant cytological features, the presence of atypia or high mitotic index does not correlate with prognosis.[37] DAL-HX 83/90 &

LCH1 trials have found initial response to therapy can be used to identify patients most at risk for death.[4,5] Prognostic factors include:[29]

1. Initial response to therapy
2. Age at diagnosis (<24 months, 55-60% mortality)
3. Number of organs involved at diagnosis:

Number of organs	Mortality (%)
1-2	0
3-4	35
5-6	60
7-8	100

4. Organ dysfunction (e.g. lung, liver, bone marrow) at diagnosis:

Organ dysfunction	Mortality (%)
Present	66
Absent	4

5. Natural history on treatment:

Group	Description	Mortality (%)
A	No disease progression over 6-12 months	0
B	Progressive disease without organ dysfunction	20
C	Development of organ dysfunction during course of disease	100

SEQUELAE

Even inactive lesions may have late sequelae that significantly impact the quality of life of survivors of LCH. The risk of development of these complications must be considered in the planning of critical therapy.

Sequelae are common in patients with multisystem disease and include small stature because of growth-hormone deficiency, diabetes insipidus, cerebellar ataxia, deafness, orthodontic problems, lung fibrosis and liver cirrhosis.[6,7] Central nervous system (CNS) damage especially neuropsychological problems can be a major problem. Other sequelae include orthopedic problems, poor dentition, pulmonary fibrosis and hepatic cirrhosis.

Newer Options for Therapy of Langerhans' Cell Histiocytosis

a. Recent developments have resulted in more innovative forms of therapy, including the experimental testing of an antibody against CD1α for diagnostic immuno-localization and therapy of LCH. Radiolabelled monoclonal antibody to CD1α, localizes to active Langerhans cell histiocytosis lesions in the bones of the skull. This provides encouraging evidence that it may be a possible effective therapeutic target to LCH cells in patients.[44]

b. The humanized anti-CD52 monoclonal antibody, alemtuzumab (or Campath-1H), has been shown to potently deplete lymphocytes in human patients. CD52 is expressed on normal lymphocytes, monocytes, some dendritic cell subsets and normal Langerhans cells (LC) in the skin do not bind alemtuzumab. The pathologic LC of Langerhans' cell histiocytosis (LCH), express CD52 and can be targeted by this antibody.[45]

Tumor necrosis factor alpha (TNF-α) seems to play a key role in the pathogenesis of Langerhans' cell histiocytosis (LCH). Thalidomide is an immuno-modulating agent of inflammatory cytokines including TNF-alpha. Thalidomide has reportedly been used to treat disseminated LCH successfully.[46]

Novel treatments that can improve results and decrease sequelae are being tried. Imatinib mesylate has been tried for cerebral Langerhans' cell histiocytosis, which is associated with a dismal prognosis; further studies are required to assess its role.[47] Amifostine differentiating agent, is being studied in LCH cord blood and bone marrow cultures, however the results are preliminary.[48]

Further study of the etiopathogenesis and clinical trials by collaborative groups, and the research efforts of organizations like the Histiocytosis society and Nikolas symposia will help to improve treatment of LCH and related diseases, in the future.[42]

Special Situations

1. Patients with oral involvement-panoramic dental radiographs of the mandible and maxilla every 6 months.
2. Presence of malabsorption, unexplained chronic diarrhea, or failure to thrive requires endoscopic biopsy, upper gastrointestinal study with small-bowel follow-up, 72-hours stool fat.
3. Patients with neurologic or possible hormonal abnormalities- MRI scan or contrast-enhanced computed tomography (CT) scan of the brain and hypothalamic pituitary axis.
4. Patients with pulmonary symptoms, superior vena cava syndrome or significant mediastinal widening on chest X-ray—high-resolution CT of the lungs

5. Ear involvement—CT of temporal bones and ENT review
6. Hepatosplenomegaly—ultrasound of the abdomen
7. Soft-tissue tumors—MRI of involved.

Technetium-99m labeled scintography for bone lesions and routine radiographic skeletal examinations are complementary to each other, because radiography is more likely to detect older and quiescent lesions and scintography is more likely to detect newer aggressive lesions.

REFERENCES

1. Writing Group of the Histiocyte Society, et al. Histiocytosis syndromes in children. Lancet 1987;1:208-9.
2. Weiss LM, Grogan TM, Muller-Hermelink HK, Stein H, Dura T, Favera B, Paulli M, Feller AC. Langerhans cell Histiocytosis. Tumours of Haematopoietic and Lymphoid Tissues, edited by Elaine S Jaffe, Nancy Lee Harris, Harold Stein, James W. Vardiman. IARC 2001.
3. Peter C. L. Beverley, R. Maarten Egeler, Robert J. Arceci and Jon Pritchard The Nikolas Symposia and histiocytosis. Nature Cancer Reviews.
4. Titgemeyer C, et al. Pattern and course of single-system disease in Langerhans cell histiocytosis data from the DAL-HX 83- and 90-study. Med. Pediatr. Oncol 2001;37:108-14.
5. Minkov M, et al. Treatment of multisystem Langerhans cell histiocytosis. Results of the DAL-HX 83 and DAL-HX 90 studies. DAL-HX Study Group. Klin. Padiatr 2000;212:139-44.
6. Haupt R, et al. Permanent consequences in Langerhans cell histiocytosis patients: a pilot study from the Histiocyte Society-Late Effects Study Group. Pediatr. Blood Cancer 2004;42,438-44.
7. Willis B, Ablin A, Weinberg V, Zoger S, Wara WM, Matthay KK. Disease course and late sequelae of Langerhans' cell histiocytosis: 25-year experience at the University of California, San Francisco. J Clin Oncol 1996;14(7):2073-82.
8. Annels NE, et al. Aberrant chemokine receptor expression and chemokine production by langerhans cells underlies the pathogenesis of langerhans cell histiocytosis. J. Exp. Med. 2003; 197:1385-90.
9. Egeler RM, Favara BE, Laman JD, Claassen E. Abundant expression of CD40 and CD40-ligand (CD154) in paediatric Langerhans cell histiocytosis lesions. Eur. J. Can. 2000;36:2105-10.
10. de Graaf JH, Tamminga RYJ, Kamps WA, Timens W. Langerhans cell histiocytosis: expression of leukocyte cellular adhesion molecules suggests abnormal homing and differentiation. Am. J. Path. 1994;144:466-72.
11. Egeler M, Favara B, van Meurs M, Laman JD, Claassen E. Differential in situ cytokine profiles of Langerhans-like cells and T cells in Langerhans cell histiocytosis: abundant expression of cutokines relevant to disease and treatment. Blood 1999;94:4195-4201.
12. Caux C, Dezutter-Dambuyant C, Schmitt D, Banchereau J. GM-CSF and TNFα cooperate in the generation of dendritic Langerhans cells. Nature 1992;360:258-60.
13. da Costa CE, et al. Presence of osteoclast-like multinucleated giant cells in the bone and nonostotic lesions of Langerhans cell histiocytosis. J. Exp. Med. 2005;201:687-93.

14. Servet-Delprat C, et al. Flt3+ macrophage precursors commit sequentially to osteoclasts, dendritic cells and microglia. BMC Immunol 2002;3:15-25.
15. da Costa CE, et al. Presence of osteoclast-like multinucleated giant cells in the bone and nonostotic lesions of Langerhans cell histiocytosis. J. Exp. Med 2005;201:687-93.
16. Cremer I, et al. Long-lived immature dendritic cells mediated by TRANCE-RANK interaction. Blood 2002;100:3646-55.
17. Schouten B, et al. Expression of cell cycle-related gene products in Langerhans cell histiocytosis. J. Pediatr. Hematol. Oncol 2002;24:727-32.
18. Hage C, Willman CL, Favara BE, Isaacson PG. Langerhans' Cell Histiocytosis (Histiocytosis X): immunophenotype and growth fraction. Hum. Path 1993;24:840-5.
19. Medzhitov R, Janeway CA. Innate immunity: impact on the adaptive immune response. Curr. Op. Immunol 1997;9:4-10.
20. Krenacs L, Tiszalvicz L, Krenacs T, Boumsell L. Immunohistochemical detection of CD1A antigen in formalin-fixed and paraffin-embedded tissue sections with monoclonal antibody 010. J Pathol 1993;171:99-104.
21. Nicholson HS, Egeler RM, Nesbit ME. The epidemiology of Langerhans cell histiocytosis. Hematol Oncol Clin North Am 1998;12:379-84.
22. Pileri SA, Grogan TM, Harris NL, Banks P, Campo E, Chan JK, et al. Tumors of histiocytes and accessory dendritic cells. An immunohistochemical approach to classification from the International Lymphoma Study Group based on 61 cases. Histopathology 2002;41(1):1-29.
23. Neumann MP, Frizzera G. The coexistence of Langerhans' cell granulomatosis and malignant lymphoma may take different forms: report of seven cases with a review of the literature. Hum Pathol 1986;17:1060-65
24. McClain K, Jin H, Gresik V, Favara B. Langerhans cell histiocytosis: lack of a viral etiology. Am J Hematol 1994;47:16-20.
25. Egeler RM, et al. The relation of Langerhans cell Histiocytosis to acute leukaemia, lymphoma and other solid tumours. Hematol. Oncol. Clin. North Am. 1998;12:369-78.
26. Yu RC, Chu CE, Buluwela L, Chu AC. Langerhans cell histiocytosis: a clonal proliferation of langerhans cells. Lancet 1994;343:767-8.
27. Magni M, et al. Identical rearrangement of immunoglobulin heavy chain gene in neoplastic Langerhans cells and B-lymphocytes: evidence for a common precursor. Leuk. Res. 2002;26:1131-3.
28. Nezelof C, Basset F. An hypothesis Langerhans cell histiocytosis: the failure of the immune system to switch from an innate to an adaptive mode. Pediatr. Blood Cancer 2004;42:398-400.
29. Histiocytosis Syndromes. Manual of Pediatric Hematology Oncology. Academic Press, Third edition 1999. Philip Lanzkowsky.
30. Arico M, Egeler RM. Clinical aspects of Langerhans cell histiocytosis. Hematol Oncol Clin North Am. 1998;12(2):247-58.
31. Grosis N, Prayer D, Prosch H, Lassmann H. CNS LCH Co-operative Group. Neuropathology of CNS disease in Langerhans cell histiocytosis. Brain 2005;128(4):829-38.
32. Grois N, Potschger U, Prosch H, Minkov M, Arico M, Braier J, et al. Risk factors for diabetes insipidus in langerhans cell histiocytosis. Pediatr Blood Cancer. 2005 Jul 26; [Epub ahead of print].
33. Nanduri VR, et al. Cognitive outcome of long-term survivors of multi-system Langerhans cell Histiocytosis: a single institution cross-sectional study. J. Clin. Oncol 2003; 21: 2961-7.

34. Carbone A, Passannante A, Gloghini A, Devaney KO, Rinaldo A, Ferlito A. Review of sinus histiocytosis with massive lymphadenopathy (Rosai-Dorfman disease) of head and neck. Ann Oncol Rhinol Laryngol 1999;108:1095-104.

35. Chikwava K, Jaffe R. Langerin (CD207) staining in normal pediatric tissues, reactive lymph nodes, and childhood histiocytic disorders. Pediatr Dev Pathol 2004;7(6):607-14.

36. Yu RC, Chu AC. Lack of T-cell receptor gene rearrangements in cells involved in Langerhans cell histiocytosis. Cancer 1995;75:1162-6.

37. Risdall RJ, Dehner LP, Duray P, Kobrinsky N, Robinson L, Nesbit ME, Jr. Histiocytosis X (Langerhans' cell histiocytosis). Prognostic role of histopathology. Arch Pathol Lab Med 1983; 107:59-63.

38. Ladisch S. Langerhans cell Histiocytosis. Curr Opin Hematol 1998;5(1):54-8.

39. McLelland J, Broadbent V, Yeomans E, Malone M, Pritchard J. Langerhans cell histiocytosis: the case for conservative treatment. Arch Dis Child 1990;65(3):301-3.

40. Arceci RJ. Treatment options-commentary. Br J Cancer Suppl. 1994; 23:S58-60. Review.

41. Stine KC, Saylors RL, Saccente S, McClain KL, Becton DL. Efficacy of continuous infusion 2-CDA (Cladribine) in pediatric patients with Langerhans cell histiocytosis. Pediatr Blood Cancer. 2004;43(1):81-4.

42. Farran RP, Zaretski E, Egeler RM. Treatment of Langerhans cell histiocytosis with pamidronate. J Pediatr Hematol Oncol. 2001;23(1):54-6.

43. Morgan G. Myeloblative therapy and bone marrow transplantation for Langerhans' cell histiocytosis. Br J Cancer Suppl. 1994;23:S52-3.

44. Beverley PC, Egeler RM, Arceci RJ, Pritchard J. The Nikolas Symposia and histiocytosis. Nat Rev Cancer 2005;5(6):488-94.

45. Jordan MB, McClain KL, Yan X, Hicks J, Jaffe R. Anti-CD52 antibody, alemtuzumab, binds to Langerhans cell in Langerhans cell histiocytosis. Pediatr Blood Cancer 2005;44(3):251-4.

46. Mauro E, Fraulini C, Rigolin GM, Galeotti R, Spanedda R, Castoldi G. A case of disseminated Langerhans' cell histiocytosis treated with thalidomide. Eur J Haematol 2005;74(2):172-4.

47. Montella L, Insabato L, Palmieri G. Imatinib mesylate for cerebral Langerhans'cell histiocytosis. N Engl J Med 2004;351(10):1034-5.

48. Danilatou V, Dimitriou H, Stiakaki E, Kalmanti M. Amifostine as differentiating agent in cord blood and bone marrow cultures from children with hematological disorders. Pediatr Hematol Oncol 2004; 21(2):125-34.

Head and Neck Tumors

Pediatric Tumors and the Subspecialities

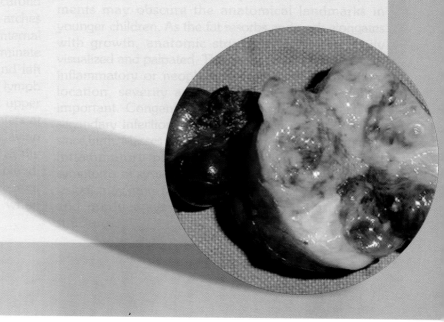

and may be candidates for bone marrow transplantation.

NEUROBLASTOMA

Neuroblastoma may occur primarily in the head and neck region in 2-4 percent of afflicted children. Metastatic disease from a distant site is much more common. Infants are more likely to present with tumors in the cervical region.

Patients with cervical neuroblastoma usually present in the first year of life with a firm mass in the lateral neck. Horner's syndrome may be seen. Cervical neuroblastoma may be confused with an infectious process and recognized only after attempted incision and drainage of the neck mass. Metastatic neuroblastoma to the orbits is more common than primary cervical neuroblastoma and may produce proptosis and periorbital ecchymosis (Fig. 34.1). Cervical neuroblastoma spreads by local invasion of surrounding tissue and shows a high propensity for regional lymph node metastases (Fig. 34.6) Distant disease, bone, and bone marrow involvement is common at presentation. Head and neck tumors are evaluated with CT or MRI of the head, neck and chest. Nearly all neuroblastomas produce catecholamines and their byproducts, homovanillic acid and vanillyllmandelic acid can be measured in the urine. Bone and bone marrow biopsies are performed in all cases.

For localized cervical neuroblastoma, surgical excision may be curative. Further therapy may be indicated for tumors with unfavorable prognostic features. Multiagent chemotherapy is used in patients with unresectable disease and advanced disease. Common regimens include cyclophosphamide, doxorubicin, with cisplatin and either teniposide or etoposide reserved for more resistant tumors. Traditionally, radiation has been used for incompletely resected cervical neuroblastoma. The role of radiation in these patients is being redefined because of the improved outcome following the use of multiagent chemotherapy.

Primary tumors of the head and neck and those occurring in infants are favorable prognostic features. The survival rate is greater than 90 percent in children of any age with localized disease that is completely resected. Localized unresectable disease treated with subtotal resection or biopsy followed by chemotherapy is associated with a 75-90 percent probability of long-term survival. Survival for regional neuroblastoma with positive lymph nodes is dependent on age. More than 80 percent of children under 1 year of age treated with surgery or chemotherapy are cured. Older children treated with more intensive therapy have a cure rate of 50 to 70 percent. Long-term survival in children over 1 year of age is 10-30 percent. Recurrent disease is usually widespread and prognosis is poor.

GERM CELL TUMORS

Approximately 5 percent of germ cell tumors arise in the extracranial head and neck region (Fig. 34.7). Though 25-35 percent of all germ cell tumors are malignant, malignant germ tumors of the head and neck are rare. The majority of cervical germ cell tumors are congenital and present at birth or in early infancy. The anterior lateral neck is the most common site of occurrence. These tumors have also been found in the pharynx, nasopharynx, paranasal sinuses and orbit.

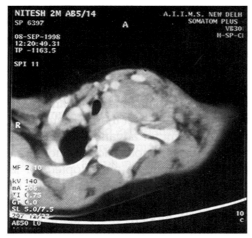

Figure 34.6: C T Scan delineating the extent of a cervicothoracic neuroblastoma

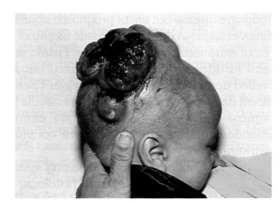

Figure 34.7: Germ cell tumor of the scalp with lobulated appearance

Large congenital lesions may obstruct the pharynx and produce maternal polyhydramnios or non-immune fetal hydrops. Following birth, obstructing tumors produce respiratory distress and dysphagia and may require intubation and emergency surgical decompression. Germ cell tumors arise from primitive germ cells and are characterized histologically by the presence of mature tissue from all three germ cell layers. The most common histologic features include skin and cutaneous appendages, adipose tissue, cystic structures and intestinal epithelium. Immature tissue elements are commonly seen in neonatal cervical teratomas. Although rare in the cervical region, pure yolk sac tumors (endodermal sinus tumors) or mixed tumors with yolk sac elements behave as malignant tumors and metastases from congenital teratomas have been reported.[8,9] To date, fewer than 20 cases of cervical endodermal sinus tumors have been reported in the literature.[10] Serum alpha-fetoprotein may be elevated in head and neck tumors with endodermal sinus elements. Excision of benign teratomas result in cure. Malignant lesions are treated with surgical resection whenever possible followed by a prolonged course of multidrug chemotherapy. Patients with unresectable tumors or residual disease may receive irradiation to the primary tumor site. Most patients initially respond to therapy and estimates of long-term disease free survival in children with unresectable germ cell tumors is around 50 percent.

OTHER SOFT TISSUE SARCOMAS

Soft tissue sarcomas other than rhabdomyoasarcoma in infants and small children primarily occur in the head and neck region and make up 3 percent of all tumors in children (Fig. 34.8). Soft tissue sarcomas in infants and younger children often have less aggressive behavior and an excellent prognosis with surgery. Sarcomas that present during adolescence behave more like tumors in the adult population. Most soft tissue sarcomas present as painless, asymptomatic masses in the neck unless there is compression or invasion of adjacent structures. Because of the rarity of these lesions in childhood, most of the available data for treatment comes from the adult population. In general, wide local excision is the treatment of choice. Because of the difficulty in obtaining wide negative margins in the head and neck, adjuvant therapy is often used in conjunction with surgical excision.

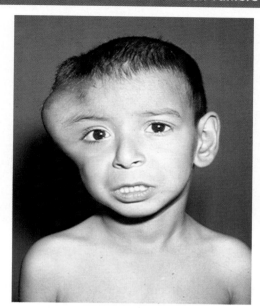

Figure 34.8: Soft tissue sarcoma of the temporal region

FIBROSARCOMA

Fibrosarcoma is the most common soft tissue sarcoma in infancy and most common soft tissue sarcoma after rhabdomyosarcoma in all children accounting for 15-20 percent occur in the head and neck. These tumors occur in two age periods: infants to 5 years and in older children aged 10-15 years. It is thought that tumors in infants tend to have a more benign course. Congenital fibrosarcomas possess non-random chromosomal changes that are not seen in adult fibrosarcoma. Histologically, fibrosarcoma tumors consist of spindle cells with a characteristic herringbone pattern. Fibrosarcomas in the first year of life rarely metastasize and can be treated with wide local excision. Radiation is indicated if complete excision is not possible. Fibrosarcoma tumors in adolescence are more aggressive and require multimodality therapy. Survival for non-metastatic tumors range from 83 to 92 percent in children under 5 years of age and 60 percent for those older than 5 years.

MALIGNANT PERIPHERAL NERVE SHEATH TUMOR

Malignant peripheral nerve sheath tumors arising from the cranial nerves, cervial plexus, or sympathetic chain account for 5 percent of all soft tissue sarcomas in

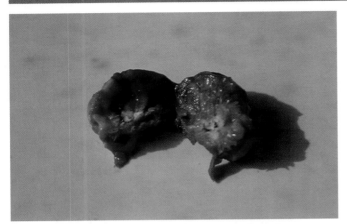

Figure 34.9: Excised neuroectodermal
tumor from the upper jaw

children and 10 percent occur in the head and neck region (Fig. 34.9). In contrast to other head and neck soft tissue sarcomas, MPNSTs commonly present with pain, paresthesias and muscle weakness. They are associated with neurofibromotosis type I which is characterized by café au lait spots, neurofibromas, skeletal dysplasia, and many neoplasms. They are similar in appearance to fibrosarcomas but are far more aggressive. The tumor cells of MPNST, in contrast to fibrosarcoma, are more variable in size and shape and lack a herringbone pattern. Because these tumors are very aggressive, wide surgical excision is advocated in all instances. Irradiation is used for local control and vincristine, actinomycin D, cyclophosphamide and doxorubicin are used in chemotherapy regimens. Survival is generally good for early stage tumors (50-75%) and poor for advanced disease (15-30%).

SYNOVIAL SARCOMA

Synovial sarcoma is rare in children. These tumors occur more commonly in older children and young adults and histologically differentiate into a spindle fibrous stroma similar to fibrosarcoma and a glandular component with epithelial differentiation. In contrast to other non-rhabdomyosarcoma soft tissue sarcomas, synovial sarcomas commonly present with both lymph node and lung metastases. Local disease is treated with local excision. Controversy exists as to the role of radiation and chemotherapy in these patients. Since vital structures in the neck preclude wide negative margins and these tumors are chemoresponsive, postoperative radiation and chemotherapy should be strongly considered. Patients with metastatic disease should receive

chemotherapy. The 5-year survival rates are greater than 50 percent.

HEMANGIOPERICYTOMA

Hemangiopericytoma accounts for 3 percent of all soft tissue sarcomas and occurs most commonly in the lower extremities and retroperitoneum. These tumors occur rarely in the nasal cavity, paranasal sinuses, orbital region, parotid gland and the neck. It is thought that hemangiopericytomas arise from vascular pericytes or alternatively from mesenchymal cells with pericytic differentiation. Multiple simple and complex genetic translocations have been demonstrated in these tumors. Wide local excision and postoperative chemotherapy is the recommended treatment. Irradiation is added for incompletely resected tumors. Hemangiopericytomas in infants are associated with a better prognosis than those occurring in older children and adults. The reported 5-year survival rates for these tumors are stage-dependent and range from 30 to 70 percent.

MALIGNANT FIBROUS HISTIOCYTOMA

These are rare sarcomas with multiple tissue elements commonly present in the head and neck region. They rarely occur during infancy. Ring chromosomes and 19p+ alterations have been observed in these tumors. Microscopically, MFH resembles fibrosarcoma but lacks a herringbone pattern. In addition, in MFH multiple cell types, marked cellular pleomorphism and a storiform pattern of tumor cells are seen. Treatment is with wide excision and local irradiation for residual tumor. These tumors are chemosensitive and advanced tumors have responded well to multidrug therapy. The 3-year survival for head and neck tumors is greater than 50 percent.

ALVEOLAR SOFT PART SARCOMA

Alveolar soft part sarcoma is rare in childhood, but when it occurs, it most commonly involves the head and neck. The precise cell of origin of these tumors is unknown and there is no known normal tissue counterpart. The diagnosis is made based on characteristic light and electron microscopic findings. The presence of adenosine triphosphatase in these tumors suggests a myogenic origin. In contrast, a neuroepithelial origin for these tumors is suggested by the presence of neurosecretory granules; although, these inclusions have also been seen in muscle. In addition, immunocytochemical studies overwhelmingly support a myogenic origin. These tumors are slow-growing and 80 percent of children are alive 2 years after diagnosis. Most patients, however, eventually die of the disease. Alveolar soft parts sarcoma in younger children and those arising in the head and neck have a better prognosis. Treatment is with wide local excision. Because these sarcomas are very slow growing tumors, radiation and chemotherapy are reserved for recurrent and distant disease.

LARYNGEAL TUMORS

A. *Benign:* juvenile papilloma is the commonest neoplasm of childhood. It arises due to benign overgrowth of epithelial tissues induced by human papilloma virus giving rise to hoarseness, dysphonia, and inspiratory stridor commonly from 1 to 7 years. It has tendency for spontaneous regression during puberty and also for local invasion and malignant degeneration. Laser excision offers best outcome. Other benign tumors include hemangioma, lymphangioma.

B. *Malignant:* rarely squamous carcinoma in teenage has been reported.the prime etiology is juvenile papilloma received radiotherapy. Presents with hoarseness, dyspnea, cough, aphonia, aspiration, stridor and cervical nodes. Surgery or radiotherapy or both offers good survival.

NASOPHARYNGEAL CARCINOMA

Nasopharyngeal carcinoma represents 1 percent of cases pediatric malignancy, is common in adolescents. It is also known as lymphoepithelioma, transitional cell carcinoma, and epidermoid carcinoma. There is a slight male predilection and a higher incidence in teenagers of African-American descent Its incidence is 1 case per 1,00,000 population world wide but highest in southeast Asia namely china, Hongkong where the incidence is 25 per 1,00,000 population, And 10 per 1,00,000 in Africa The proved causative factor is Epstein Barr virus (EBV). It arises from the fossa of Rossenmuller.

WHO classification of nasopharyngeal carcinoma consists of three types.

Type 1: Squamous cell carcinoma.

Type 2: Non keratinizing carcinoma

Type 3: Undifferentiated carcinoma.

Undifferentiated nasopharyngeal carcinoma, also known as lymphoepithelioma, is most common in children and is associated with EBV exposure

Type 2 and 3 are associated with inflammatory infiltrate of lymphocytes, plasma cells and hence the term lymphoepithelioma. It spreads locally to oropharynx, base of skull, cranial nerves, typically to upper deep cervical level II, posterior cervical level V nodes and distant metastasis to lungs, mediastinum, bone and liver. Most children have metastatic spread to cervical lymph nodes at the time of diagnosis.[11] The most common presenting symptoms include neck mass, hearing loss, otalgia, nasal obstruction and epistaxis. Other presenting symptoms include cervical node; otitis media, trismus and cranial nerve palsy. Paraneoplastic syndrome include osteoorthropathy, clubbing, and joint swelling. Children with ear symptoms often have a persistent middle ear effusion for many months prior to diagnosis of nasopharyngeal cancer. Cranial nerve palsies and head pain suggest invasion of the skull base.

Nasopharyngeal examination and biopsy and EBV serology is performed for diagnosis and CT scan and MRI are equally useful for staging nasopharyngeal carcinoma. TNM staging is used for staging In addition, CT of the chest and abdomen and radionuclide bone scanning should be performed to evaluate for metastatic disease. Surgery has fewer roles, as nasopharynx is difficult to approach and mostly advanced. Radiotherapy has dominant role but xerostomia, trismus is the problem. 5-FU, methotrexate, bleomycin, and ciplatinum has beneficiary role. Differential diagnosis includes rhabdomyosarcoma, Burkitt's lymphoma and angiofibroma. Undifferentiated nasopharyngeal carcinoma is radiosensitive and responds well to radiotherapy.[12] Chemotherapy is added for advanced stage disease. The overall 5-year survival of children with nasopharyngeal carcinoma approaches 40 percent.[12,13] Stage 1 and 2 has 54 percent survival; stage 4 has zero percentage 5 year survival

SALIVARY GLAND TUMORS

Benign and malignant tumors arise from the major and minor salivary glands. The benign tumors include hemangioma, lymphangioma or cystic hygroma, which are common in infancy and pleomorphic adenoma which arise from myoepithelial component are seen in adolescent age group. The lympho vascular benign tumors are soft, compressible with bluish skin cast. The lymphovascular swelling usually present with slow growing swelling and sometimes with sudden pain and rapid increase in size due to bleed inside. The classic benign tumor of the salivary gland tumor is pleomorphic tumors and Warthins tumor that are slow growing. Warthins tumor is extremely rare in childhood and show hot spot in technetium scan. Benign tumors may mimic sialadenitis and chronic parotitis. Malignant tumors do occur in salivary glands commonly in parotid. As a rule of thumb the neoplasm involving the parotid gland is that 50 percent are vascular, 50 percent are solid, and 50 percent of the solid tumors are malignant. Sixty percent of submandibular and 80 percent of minor salivary gland tumors are malignant Mucoepidermoid carcinoma is the commonest malignant tumor. Cylindroma has tendency to involve sub maxillary gland with perineural spread and pulmonary metastasis the risk is high in children received radiation to head and neck. Malignant tumors can spread to local organs; invade cranial nerves and neck vessels. Metastasis to lung and bone are seen in high grade tumors and anaplastic tumors. Lymphoma and metastatic involvement of the periparotid lymph node should be considered in differential diagnosis.

The common malignant tumors are:
- Mucoepidermoid carcinoma
- Acinar cell carcinoma
- Undifferentiated carcinoma
- Adenocarcinoma
- Undifferentiated sarcoma
- Adenoid cystic carcinoma
- Squamous cell carcinoma
- Lymphoma
- Rhabdomyosarcoma.

FNAC, CT scans, MRI and silogram help in diagnosis and staging. Silogram is replaced by CT scan with intravenous contrast. Surgical excision with radiotherapy is the mode of treatment. In the absence lymph node enlargement no need for lymph resection. Radiotherapy is reserved for high grade tumors. Long term follow up is required as late recurrence is reported.

About half of all epithelial salivary gland tumors are malignant. Malignant salivary gland tumors can occur at any age; however, most occur in older children and adolescents. Histologically, salivary neoplasms in children are similar to those seen in adults. The pleomorphic adenoma is the most common benign neoplasm and mucoepidermoid carcinoma the most common salivary gland malignancy.[14,15] Mucoepidermoid carcinoma contains dermoid and mucus-containing cells. Two-thirds of these tumors are low-grade and are associated with a low incidence of recurrence and cervical lymph node metastases. Low-grade acinic cell carcinoma, undifferentiated carcinoma, adenocarcinoma, adenoid cystic carcinoma and malignant mixed tumors occur less

commonly. In children the majority of salivary gland tumors involve the parotid gland. The presence of a firm preauricular mass is the most common finding.

Rapid growth, facial weakness or pain and associated cervical lymphadenopathy are suggestive of malignancy. A swelling of the parotid gland not suggestive of acute or recurrent inflammation should be investigated by ultrasound, sialogram and CT scan. Histological confirmation is essential. A simple hemangioma or lymphangioma only require surgical excision. A pleomorphic adenoma requires a superficial parotidectomy to avoid recurrence. Mucoepidermoid carcinoma requires a total parotidectomy since even well differentiated tumors extend beyond the resection margins. For the soft tissue sarcomas, frozen section allows surface markers, cytogenetic studies and electronmicroscopy and they are treated appropriately according to the sarcoma or lymphoma protocols.

All firm salivary gland masses should be biopsied.[16] While fine needle aspiration has been used with success in adults, its role in children has not been determined. Incisional biopsy of the parotid gland should be avoided due to the risk of injuring the facial nerve. The only indication for incisional biopsy is for histologic diagnosis of large, unresectable tumors. Superficial conservative parotidectomy in case of parotid and complete removal of the gland in case submandibular and sublingual gland are the main stay of treatment.

Superficial parotidectomy with preservation of the facial nerve or total excision of the submandibular gland should be the initial procedure. High grade malignancies and tumors in the deep lobe require total parotidectomy. The role of neck dissection in the management of salivary gland malignancies is controversial.

Many surgeons advocate neck dissection for high-grade malignancies or clinically palpable disease. Some centers routinely perform a conservative neck dissection for mucoepidermoid carcinoma which can be converted to a radical or modified neck dissection for grossly or histologically positive lymph nodes.[17,18] Adjuvant radiation can be used for local control of high-grade, high stage tumors. Most centers use radiation for adenoid cystic carcinoma, which often spreads along nerve sheaths and is difficult to eradicate by surgical resection. Chemotherapy is reserved for high-grade or unresectable lesions. Cyclophosphamide, doxorubicin and cisplatin are frequently employed. Survival largely depends on histopathology and tumor grade. The prognosis for low-grade mucoepidermoid carcinoma, acinic cell carcinoma and well-differentiated adenocarcinoma is good, whereas high grade mucoepidermoid carcinoma, poorly differentiated adenocarcinoma, and undifferentiated tumors do poorly. Overall, the 5-year survival in children with mucoepidermoid and acinic cell carcinomas is greater than 90 percent.[19]

REFERENCES

1. Derias NW, Chong WH, O'Connor AFF. Fine needle aspiration cytology of head and neck swelling in a child: a non-invasive approach to a diagnosis. J Laryngol Otol 1992;106:755-7.
2. Knight PJ, Hamoudi AB, Vassy LE. The diagnosis and treatment of midline neck masses in children. Surgery 1984;93:603-11.
3. Moussatos GH, Baffes TG. Cervical masses in infants and children. Pediatrics 1963;32:251-8.
4. Knight PJ, Mulne AF, Vassy LE. When is lymph node biopsy indicated in children with enlarged peripheral nodes? Pediatrics 1982;69:391-6.
5. McGill T. Rhabdomyosarcoma of the head and neck: an update. Otolaryngol Clin North Am 1989;22:631-6.
6. Ben-Yehuda D, Polliack A, Okon E, et al. Image-guided core-needle biopsy in malignant lymphoma: experience with 100 patients that suggests the technique is reliable. J Clin Oncol 1996;14:2431-4.
7. Hayes DM, Ternberg JL, Chen PT, et al. Post splenectomy sepsis and other complications following staging laparotomy for Hodgkin's disease in childhood. J Pediatr Surg 1986;21:328628-32.
8. Shoenfeld A, Ovadia J, Edelstein T, Liban E. Malignant cervical teratoma of the fetus. Acta Obstet Gynecol Scand 1982;61:7-12.
9. Pearl RM, Wisnicki J, Sinclair G. Metastatic cervical teratoma of infancy. Plast Reconstr Surg 1986;77:469-73.
10. Stephenson JA, Mayland DM, Kun LE, et al. Malignant germ cell tumors of the head and neck in childhood. Laryngoscope 1989;99:732-5.
11. Fernandez C, Cangir A, Samaan N, Rivera R. Nasopharyngeal carcinoma in children. Cancer 1976;37:2787-91.
12. Ahern V, Jenkin D, Banerjee D, et al. Nasopharyngeal carcinoma in the young. Clin Oncol 1994;6:24-30.
13. Baker S, McClatchey K. Carcinoma of the nasopharynx in childhood. Otolaryngol Head Neck Surg 1981;89:555-9.
14. Schuller D, McCabe B. Salivary gland neoplasms in children. Otolaryngol Clin North Am 1977;10:399-412.
15. Malone B, Baker S. Benign pleomorphic adenomas in children. Ann Otol Rhinol Laryngol 1984;93:210-4.
16. Baker S, Malone B. Salivary gland malignancies in children. Cancer 1985;55:1730-6.
17. Byers R, Piorkowski R, Luna M. Malignant parotid tumors in patients under 20 years of age. Arch Otolaryngol 1984;110:232-5.
18. Callender DL, Frankenthaler RA, Luna MA, et al. Salivary gland neoplasms in children. Arch Otolaryngol 1992;118:472-6.
19. Castro E, Huvos A, Strong E, Foote F. Tumors of the major salivary glands in children. Cancer 1972;29:312-7.

CHAPTER 35

Spencer W Beasley

Mediastinal Masses

INTRODUCTION

Most mediastinal masses are diagnosed incidentally in an asymptomatic child, but when they do produce symptoms, it is usually because of their space occupying effects, i.e. from compression of the airway, esophagus and lung. Sometimes they present with pain from infection or perforation of a cyst, or from invasion of the chest wall by a malignant tumor.[1] The symptoms tend to be nonspecific, and therefore generally are unhelpful in establishing a specific diagnosis.[2] In contrast, the location of the mass suggests its likely origin. For example, posterior mediastinal lesions are likely to be neurogenic tumors, whereas anterior tumors are more likely to be teratomas. Children) under six years of age are more likely to have benign lesions, whereas older children are more likely to have malignancies[3] Overall about 40 percent of mediastinal masses in children are malignant.

MEDIASTINAL COMPARTMENTS

The mediastinum is an anatomical region between the base of the neck and diaphragm that is limited by the sternum anteriorly, the spine posteriorly, and the lungs laterally.[4] For convenience it is divided into three compartments: anterior, posterior and visceral (or middle) (Fig. 35.1). The anterior compartment contains the thymus, lymph nodes and the lower pole of the thyroid. The posterior compartment contains the sympathetic chain with its ganglia and the lateral surface of the vertebral bodies. The visceral compartment includes the heart, pericardium, the great vessels, thoracic duct, lymph nodes and nerves (vagal and phrenic). Each compartment produces specific lesions

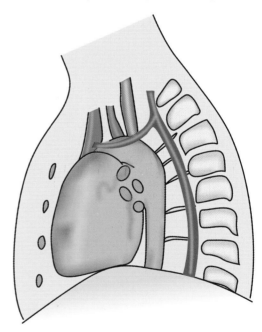

Figure 35.1: The superior mediastinum extends from the thoracic inlet to the upper border of the pericardial sac. The inferior mediastinum is divided into three compartments (a) Anterior: between the sternum and the pericardium, (b) Middle: between the anterior and posterior surfaces of the pericardium and (c) Posterior: from the back of the pericardium to the vertebral bodies. For practical purposes, the superior and anterior compartments are considered as one.

(Table 35.1) which is the reason that knowledge of the location of a mediastinal mass provides clues to its likely nature.

Masses in the anterior mediastinum tend to produce respiratory symptoms from tracheal compression, which is relevant in determining how and when tissue diagnosis and resection should be undertaken. Sudden respiratory collapse is a well-recognized hazard of general anesthesia in children with an anterior mediastinal mass.

Lesions of the visceral compartment include lymphomas and phaeochromocytomas.[4] Pericardial cysts tend to occur at the cardiophrenic angle.

Masses in the posterior mediastinum are usually neurogenic in origin; they may be glial (neuroblastoma, ganglioneuroma, ganglioneuroblastoma); neuronal (schwannoma, neurinoma, neurofibroma); or paraganglial (phaeochromocytoma).[4] Extralobar pulmonary sequestrations are found in the posterior mediastinum and usually have a direct arterial supply from the aorta. Bronchogenic cysts and esophageal duplications may arise either in the posterior or visceral mediastinum.[1]

The age of the child also provides clues to the likely diagnosis. For example, neural tumors, which predominate in the costovertebral sulcus (posterior mediastinum), occur in children younger than 3 years of age.[5] Lymphomas are the most common tumor in older children and adolescents. Thymomas, a common mediastinal tumor in adults, are extremely rare in children.[6,7]

CLINICAL MANIFESTATIONS

Mediastinal masses produce symptoms in two thirds of patients.[5] The remaining are diagnosed incidentally by skiagram chest or ultrasonography done for other reasons. Symptoms like cough, dyspnea and repeated respiratory infection tend to be nonspecific and may arise from airway obstruction. In the neonatal period and during infancy respiratory distress and cyanosis predominate. Symptoms of respiratory obstruction do not distinguish benign from malignant masses. Occasionally patients may present with paraneoplastic syndromes: for example, Cushing syndrome (thymoma), hypercalcemia (lymphoma), and gynecomastia (germ cell tumor). Several specific systemic syndromes are also recognised: opsoclonus-myoclonus (neuroblastoma); Horner syndrome (neuroblastoma involving the cervical sympathetic trunk); myasthenia gravis (thymoma); scleroderma (thymoma); and vertebral anomalies (intestinal duplications). Caval compression may produce superior vena cava syndrome.

INVESTIGATIONS

Laboratory Tests

There are a number of laboratory tests that assist in the diagnosis and follow-up of some tumors. Tumor markers like β-HCG and α-fetoprotein levels are often elevated in children with germ cell tumors, and can be used as tumor markers to detect recurrence following resection. Elevated levels of vanillylmandelic and homovanillic acid are seen in neuroblastoma.

CXR

A posteroanterior and lateral skiagram chest will detect a mediastinal lesion in over 90 percent[5] and usually enables lesions to be categorized to a specific mediastinal compartment. In combination with the age of the child, the location is predictive of the likely diagnosis.[2]

Ultrasonography

Ultrasonography is used to determine whether the mass is solid or cystic, and is particularly useful for small central lesions that may be difficult to see on plain radiology.[8,9] Ultrasonography is also used to assist with needle biopsies of mediastinal lesions.

Table 35.1: The differential diagnosis of mediastinal masses according to mediastinal compartment

Mediastinum	Likely Lesions
Superior	• Cardiothoracic cystic hygroma/lymphangioma • Thymoma or thymic cyst • Substernal thyroid
Anterior	• Teratoma • Lymphoma • Germ cell tumor
Middle	• Pericardial cyst • Bronchogenic cyst • Esophageal duplication • Lymphoma
Posterior	• Neurogenic tumor (especially neuroblastoma or ganglioneuroma) • Esophageal duplication/neurenteric canal • Bronchogenic cyst • Pulmonary sequestration

Occasionally, the tumors are "functioning", in that the symptoms reflect the hormone or enzyme that they secrete (ectopic gastric mucosa may cause massive hemoptysis and pancreatic islet tissue may cause hypoglycemia, or they may become infected.[28,29] There is an association between malignant thoracic teratomas, malignant histiocytosis and Klinefelter's syndrome and there are now many reports of the association of mediastinal germ cell malignant tumors with acute myelogenous leukemia.[30,31]

Investigation of GCT

A plain skiagram chest may reveal most of the tumors. A CT scan highlights the heterogeneous nature of the tumor, and identifies fat and calcification.[32] When the tumor is intrapericardial, angiography may be helpful to delineate its vascular anatomy.

Tumors with yolk sac (endodermal sinus) elements secrete alpha-fetoprotein (a-FP), and those with elements of choriocarcinoma secrete beta human chorionic gonadotropin (b-HCG). Consequently, serum alpha-fetoprotein (a-FP), carcinoembryonic antigen (CEA) and HCG levels should be measured, and if elevated, provide a useful marker of tumor activity following excision. Alpha-fetoprotein also is produced by the fetal liver and yolk sac, and has a half-life of 4 days, which means that the age of the infant affects true hermaphrodite interpretation of the level in the first year of life.[33]

Treatment of GCT

Mediastinal teratomas should be excised, but the surgical approach depends on the size and the location of the tumor. Often they are well encapsulated and easy to remove despite their large size, although the more posterior lesions (pericardial or posterior mediastinal) may have prominent vessels from the aorta. Left untreated, benign teratomas continue to grow and may cause death by compression of vital structures.[34] Malignant teratomas may be more difficult to resect and have a poorer prognosis.[24]

Outcome of GCT

The prognosis for resectable mediastinal mature cystic teratoma and seminoma is good.[18] Nonseminomatous malignant germ cell tumors of the mediastinum often present with advanced disease and do not respond well to chemotherapy. Nonetheless, it is important to

distinguish mediastinal germ cell tumors from other undifferentiated malignant tumors, especially thymic carcinoma, which has a poor prognosis.[18]

Malignant mediastinal germ cell tumors have been reported to have a 4-year survival rate of 48 percent, although the experience of Lakhoo[24] indicates a somewhat poorer outcome. The use of platinum-based chemotherapy in combination with bleomycin and etoposide offers survival rates of 55-70 percent.[35] Malignant mediastinal teratomas have a poor prognosis than those in gonadal sites hence long term follow-up is required for all children operated for a mediastinal teratoma.[3]

Lymphoma

The most common anterior and middle mediastinal masses in children are lymphomas.[36] Hodgkin's lymphomas often will have both cervical and mediastinal components. Non-Hodgkin lymphomas tend to be more disseminated and are usually lymphoblastic T cell in origin.[36] More than 50 percent of children with a lymphoblastic lymphoma present with an anterior mediastinal mass, and more than one third of patients with non-Hodgkin's lymphoma have their primary site in the mediastinum.[37]

Presentation

Hodgkin's disease usually presents with cervical or supraclavicular lymphadenopathy.[38] Night sweats, fever and weight loss occur in about 25 percent.[39] The symptoms produced by mediastinal lymphomas depend on their location, size and rate of growth: compression of adjacent structures may cause respiratory distress or superior vena cava syndrome.[36] Sometimes, a mediastinal lymphoma can appear as an incidental finding on chest X-ray. Airway obstruction results in symptoms, which range from a mild cough to severe dyspnoea and stridor particularly in non-Hodgkin's lymphoma.[40] Non-Hodgkin's lymphomas often grow rapidly and produce their symptoms within a short period, and pose specific risks under general anesthesia.

Investigations for Lymphomas

A mediastinal mass will be evident on a chest X-ray, and a pleural effusion is common. CT scan of the chest defines the exact location for the tumor and the degree of major airway compression. A CT scan of the abdomen and pelvis assess sub diaphragmatic disease. Staging laparotomy is now rarely performed, as it does not influence management.

Histological confirmation of the diagnosis is obtained by a tissue biopsy, usually of a regional lymph node, but may require thoracoscopy or thoracotomy.[37] A Sample of pleural effusion fluid or bone marrow aspirate may also be diagnostic. Fine needle aspiration of the mediastinal lesion is often unsatisfactory.

Treatment

The treatment of lymphomas does not involve surgery, apart from assistance in obtaining a tissue biopsy and insertion of a central venous line for chemotherapy. Biopsy of the mediastinal mass is required when there are no accessible peripheral lymph nodes.

Outcome

The 5 to 10 year disease-free survival rate for Hodgkin's disease is 70 to 90 percent[39] year survival rate of children with a mediastinal lymphoblastic lymphoma is 75 percent.[41]

Lymphangioma

Lymphangiomas are nonmalignant congenital abnormalities that can vary from predominantly cystic (e.g. cervicothoracic cystic hygroma) to predominantly vascular elements (Lymphangioma). Isolated mediastinal lymphangiomas (usually anterior) account for 1 percent of all lymphangiomas although large cervical lymphangiomas extend into the chest in up to 10 percent of cases[3]. Lymphatic lesions do not to involutes nor respond to drug therapy. They often require resection or sclerotherapy.[42]

Presentation

Cervical lymphangiomas are usually readily apparent at birth or within months thereafter and may cause airway obstruction -some of these extend into the posterior mediastinum as a cervicothoracic cystic hygroma. Isolated mediastinal lymphangiomas tend to present later as an incidental radiological finding or with symptoms of respiratory obstruction. Rapid enlargement of a lymphangioma may occur because of hemorrhage into the cystic spaces and lead to acute symptoms of obstruction or pain. They may also become infected. Increasingly, they are being diagnosed on antenatal ultrasonography: nuchal lesions appear as multiseptated cysts and are suggestive of Turner syndrome, Noonan syndrome or a fetal trisomy.

Investigation

The clinical appearance of the cervical component of a cystic hygroma is well known. On plain radiology, a mediastinal hemangioma looks homogenous. Ultrasonography shows its cystic nature, but the appearance may be complex and the cysts often contain debris. A CT scan shows the degree to which it involves other structures (Fig. 35.4).

Treatment

The optimal treatment is surgical excision with preservation of all important structures. In reality, it is not always possible to completely excise the lymphangioma safely without damage to key structures: consequently, alternative modalities may be required to deal with residual disease. Intralesional injection of bleomycin and OK432 have been employed with some success.[43,44] Other agents used include tetracycline, steroids, iodine and glucose.[3] Macrocystic lesions respond best to sclerotherapy. Microcystic lesions do not respond to sclerotherapy, and are difficult to resect surgically. Lymph accumulation after resection is common and may necessitate aspiration.

Thymic Tumors

Thymomas are extremely rare in children. Some patients may have myasthenia gravis.[45] Thymic carcinomas in

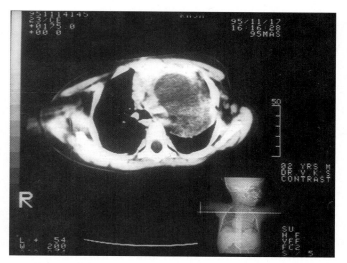

Figure 35.4: CT scan chest demarcating the extent of a lymphangioma left hemithorax

children are aggressive malignancies and may cause chest pain and shortness of breath.[23] Treatment involves surgical resection through a median sternotomy, followed by postoperative chemotherapy and radiotherapy. The longterm outcome is variable.[46-48]

Thymic cysts are thin-walled and may grow large with time. They contain clear fluid (unless hemorrhage has occurred) and may be uni- or multilocular. The surgical approach for excision depends on the degree to which they are cervical or intrathoracic. They should be distinguished from cystic nodular sclerosing Hodgkin's disease, seminoma and cystic teratoma.[47]

Bronchogenic Cysts

These are the main cystic lesions in the posterior mediastinum. Bronchogenic cysts are usually lined by respiratory epithelium.

Diagnosis

They may be diagnosed on plain radiology, although a bronchogenic cyst near the carina may be difficult to see on plain radiology. A barium swallow may demonstrate posterior compression or displacement of the esophagus. Their cystic nature is confirmed on ultrasonography. A CT scan or MRI may be required to differentiate them from other posterior mediastinal masses.

Treatment

They should be excised because they tend to slowly increase in size as they accumulate secretions, and may become infected or turn malignant.[1] Often, they can be resected through a thoracoscopic approach.

Neuroblastoma and Ganglioneuroma

Neurogenic tumors include a variety of tumor types that arise from neurogenic structures in the thoracic cavity. They represent the most common mediastinal lesions,[2] accounting for about 35-40 percent.[49] They are found primarily in the paravertebral sulcus where they arise from the sympathetic chain or one of their rami. The tumors of the sympathetic ganglia (ganglioneuroma, ganglioneuroblastoma and neuroblastoma) are derived from neural crest cells, and represent a biological continuum of maturation and differentiation.[50] Ganglioneuromas are fully differentiated and do not metastasize, but their growth through the vertebral foramina may produce symptoms from nerve root and spinal cord compression. Paragangliomas and neurofibromas are discussed separately below.

Presentation

Neuroblastoma and ganglioneuroma are frequently identified as asymptomatic lesions on a plain chest X-ray. Ganglioneuromas, in particular, can often reach a huge size before being discovered. Symptoms pertain to compression of the neural elements or other intrathoracic structures. Horner's syndrome may occur with apical tumors if the stellate ganglion is involved (Fig. 35.5).

Investigation

Once discovered on a chest X-ray, an MRI should be performed to identify any extension through the vertebral foramina or spinal compression.

Treatment

Ganglioneuromas normally require resection, and morbidity relates to surgical consideration of its location and size (Fig. 35.6). If there is uncertainty about the diagnosis (including assessment of the N-myc expression status) asymptomatic lesions can be left untreated.

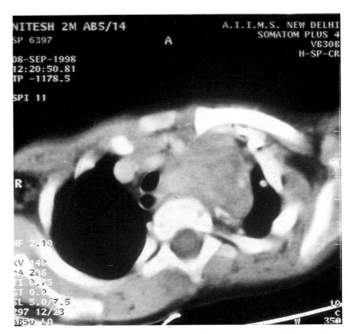

Figure 35.5: CT Scan image of a superior mediastinal neuroblastoma lifting the blood vessels

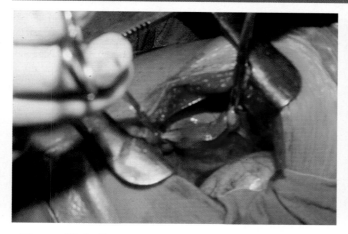

Figure 35.6: Extensive intrathoracic neuroblastoma with intraspinal extension

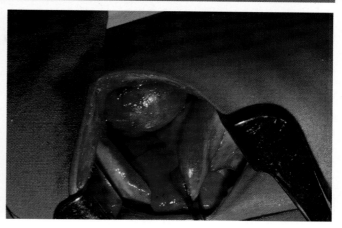

Figure 35.7: Operative photograph of a mediastinal neuroblastoma

For neuroblastomas, complete surgical excision by thoracotomy offers the best opportunity for cure (Fig. 35.7). The best surgical approach for tumors extending through the foramina is unresolved: some advocate a combined approach to the intraspinal (laminectomy) and intrathoracic components,[51] whereas others prefer to perform the laminectomy first because, excision of the mediastinal component alone may be complicated by hemorrhage and edema of the residual tumor in the spinal canal and lead to neurological sequelae.

Cystic neuroblastomas are extremely rare and are usually adrenal, but may occur in the mediastinum,[52] All cases have been diagnosed in children under the age of two years. They tend have a benign course and recurrence is unlikely after resection.

Outcome

Information about the likely biological behavior of the tumor comes from histological examination of the resected specimen and analysis of N-myc expression. Amplification of the proto-oncogene N-myc is indicative of rapid tumor progression and a poor prognosis Additional adverse prognostic features include: age greater than 12 months at diagnosis; primary tumor unresectable; distant metastases to bone, and bone marrow involvement, Various other biological parameters of poor outcome include: serum ferritin >142 ng/ml; serum lactate dehydrogenase level >1500 u/l; low TRK-A expression; and low VMA/HVA ratio in urine.[53-56]

Chemotherapy is used for Stage 4 tumors. It may be used also following initial biopsy of an unresectable "high-risk" tumor, following which the tumors often become resectable. Follow-up involves serial urinary catecholamine levels and regular imaging.

Paraganglionic Tumors

A phaeochromocytoma located outside the adrenal gland is called paraganglioma. In the posterior mediastinum these tumors are related to the thoracic sympathetic chain. They may be asymptomatic (incidental diagnosis) or produce headaches from excessive catecholamine secretion. The tumor may be located with a I^{131} MIBG scan, and further information is provided on MRI T2-weighted images. Those, which secrete catecholamines, require careful perioperative management with volume replacement, α adrenergic and β-blockade; otherwise a hypertensive crisis may occur during surgical handling of the tumor.

Neurofibroma

Neurofibromas are benign tumors that are similar in their presentation and behavior to schwannomas (neurilemmomas). These spherical homogenous nonencapsulated tumors are of interest in that they are a manifestation of the autosomal dominant disorder neurofibromatosis 1 (NF1), which affects 1: 2500 people. Other lesions include optic gliomas, peripheral (appear in adolescence) and plexiform neurofibromas (appear early) and phaeochromocytomas. Children with mediastinal neurofibromas and NF1 are at increased risk of malignant transformation of the tumor; they should be excised.

Hemangiomas

Vascular anomalies include a variety of hemangiomas and other vascular malformations, and are relatively rare, comprising only 3 to 6 percent of mediastinal masses in children[42]. Unlike most mediastinal masses, they may involve more than one compartment. They are often misdiagnosed and treated inappropriately.

Diagnosis

The correct diagnosis can be established from a combination of the history, external examination, associated anomalies, bronchoscopy and radiological studies. Red skin discoloration of those with a cervical component often becomes visible in the first few weeks of life and tends to be central or bilateral. About 10 percent will have multiple hemangiomas.

Treatment

Haemangiomas are benign tumors that involute spontaneously. Sometimes, however, they may cause tracheal compression and require anti-angiogenic therapy (e.g. Prednisone 2 mg/kg/day or interferon or bronchoscopic endoluminal laser ablation to maintain airway patency prior to involution. They may cause intrinsic or extrinsic compression of the trachea sometimes requiring a tracheostomy.

REFERENCES

1. Shamberger RC, Mediastinal masses. In: Rob and Smith Operative Surgery 5th Edn. Spitz L and Coran AG. (Eds) Chapman and Hall Medical, London 1995 pp 89-200.
2. Massie RJ, Van Asperen PP, Mellis CM. Review of open biopsy for mediastinal masses. J Pediatr and Child Health. 1997;33(3):230-3.
3. Rodgers BM, McGahren ED Mediastinum and pleura. In Surgery of Infants and Children scientific principles and practice Eds Oldham KT, Colombani PM, Foglia RP, Lippincott-Raven Publishers, Philadelphia 1997 pp 927-33.
4. Esposito C. Romeo Seminars. Surgical anatomy of the mediastinum. Sem Pediatr Surg 1999;8(2):50-3.
5. Esposito G. Diagnosis of mediastinal masses and principles of surgical tactics and techniques for their treatment. Sem Pediatr Surg 1999;8(2):54-60.
6. Azarow KS, Pearl RH, Zurcher R, et al. Primary mediastinal masses. A comparison of adult and pediatric populations. J Thorac Cardiovasc Surg 1993;106:67-72.
7. Spigland N, Di Lorenzo M, Hernandex R, et al. Malignant thymoma in children; a 20 year review. J Pediatr Surg 1990;25:1143-6.
8. Meza MP, Benson M, Slovis TL. Imaging of mediastinal masses in children. AJR 1992;158:825- 32.
9. Durand G, Bandain P, Pin I, et al. Usefulness of ultrasonography (US) in the diagnosis of a mediastinal opacity. Pediatr Pulmonol Suppl 1997;16:56-7.
10. Landwehr, P., Schulte O, Lackner, K. MR Imaging of the chest: mediastinum and chest wall European Radiology. 1999; 9(9):1737-44.
11. Ryckman FC, Rodgers BM. Thoracoscopy for intrathoracic neoplasia in children. J Pediatr Surg 1982;17:521-4.
12. Azizkhan RG, Dudgeon DL, Buck JR, et al. Life-threatening airway obstruction as a complication to the management of mediastinal masses in children. J Pediatr Surg 1985;20:816-22.
13. Neuman GG, Weingarten AE, Abramowitz RM, et al. The anaesthetic management of the patient with an anterior mediastinal mass. Anesthesiology 1984;60:144-7.
14. Jeffrey GM, Mead GM, Whitehouse JMA. Life threatening airway obstruction at the presentation of Hodgkin's disease, Cancer 1991;67:506-10.
15. Miller RD, Hyatt RE. Evaluation of obstructing lesions of the trachea and larynx by flow-volume loops. Am Rev Respir Dis 1973;108:475-81.
16. Ferrari LR, Bedford RF. General anesthesia prior to treatment of anterior mediastinal masses in pediatric cancer patients. Anesthesiology 1990;72:991.
17. Loeffler JS, Leopold KA, Retch A, et al. Emergency previously radiation for mediastinal masses. Impact on subsequent pathological diagnosis and outcome. J Clin Oncol 1986;4:716-21.
18. Weidner, N. Germ cell tumors of the mediastinum. Seminars in Diagnostic Pathology. 1999;16(1):42-50.
19. King M, Telander RL, Smithson WA, et al. Primary mediastinal tumors in children. J Pediatr Surg 1982;17:512-9.
20. Azarow KS, Pearl RH, Zurcher R, et al. Primary mediastinal masses. J Thorac Cardiovasc Surg 1993;106:67-72.
21. Grosfield JL, Skinner MA, Rescoria FJ, et al. Mediastinal tumors in children; experience with 196 cases. Ann Surg Onc 1994;1:121-7.
22. Massie RJH, Van Seperen PP, Mellis CM. A review of open biopsy for mediastinal masses. J. Pediatr Child Health 1997;33:230-3.
23. Billmire DF. Germ cell mesenchymal and thymic tumors of the mediastinum. Sem in Pediatr Surg 1999;8(2):85-91.
24. Lakhoo K, Boyle M, Drake DP. Mediastinal teratomas; review of 15 pediatric cases. J Pediatr Surg 1993;28:1161.
25. Kuller JA, Laifer SA, Martin JG, et al. Unusual presentations of fetal teratoma. J Perinatal 1991;40:294-6.
26. Deenadayalu RP, Tuuri D, Dewall RA, et al. Intrapericardial teratomas and bronchogenic cyst. J Thorac Cardiovasc Surg 1974;67:945-2.
27. Zerell JT, Halpe DCE. Intrapericardial teratoma-neonatal cardio-respiratory distress amenable to surgery. J Pediatr Surg 1980;15:961-3.
28. Robertson JM, Fee HJ, Mulder DG. Mediastinal teratoma causing life-threatening hemoptysis. Am J Dis Child 1981;135:148-50.
29. Honiky RE, dePapp EW. Mediastinal teratoma with endocrine function Am J Dis Child 1973;126:650-3.
30. Beasley SW, Tiedemann K, Howat AJ, Auldist AW, Werther G, Touhy P. Precocious puberty associated with malignant thoracic teratoma and malignant histiocytosis in a child with Klinefelter's Syndrome. Medical and Pediatr Oncology 1987;15:277-80.
31. Woodruff K, Wang N, May W, Androne E, Denny C, Feig SA. The clonal nature of mediastinal germ cell tumors and acute myelogenous leukemia. A case report and review of the literature. Cancer Genetics and Cytogenetics 1995;79:23-31.
32. Link KM, Samuels LJ, Reed JC, et al. Magnetic resonance imaging of the mediastinum. J Thorac Imaging 1993;8:34-53.

33. Tsuchida V, Endo V, Saito S, et al. Evaluation of alpha-fetoprotein in early infancy. J Pediatr Surg 1978;13:155-6.
34. Lack EE, Weinstein HJ, Welch KJ" Mediastinal germ cell tumors in childhood. J Thorac Cardiovasc Surg 1985;89:826-35.
35. Berkow RL, Kelly OR. Isolated CNS metastasis as the first site of recurrence in a child with germ cell tumor of the mediastinum. Med Pediatr Oncol 1995;24:36-9.
36. Mauch PM, Kalish LA, Kaden M, et al. Patterns of presentation of Hodgkin's disease: implications for etiology and pathogenesis. Cancer 1993;71:2062.
37. Glick RD, La Quaglia MP. Lymphomas of the anterior mediastinum. Sem Pediatr Surg 1999;8(2):69-97.
38. La Quaglia MP. Non-Hodgkin's lymphoma and Hodgkin's disease in childhood and adolescence in O'Neil JA Jr, Rowe MI, Grosfield, et al (eds): Pediatric Surgery (ed 5) St Louis, MO, Mosby Year Book 1998. pp461-481.
39. Hudson MM, Donaldson 88. Hodgkins disease. Pediatr Clin North Am 1997;44:891-906.
40. Shields TW. Primary Mediastinal Tumors and Cysts and Their Diagnostic Investigation, in Shield TW (ed): Mediastinal Surgery. Malvern PA, Lea and Febiger, 1991, pp 111-7.
41. Shepherd SF, A'Hern RP, Pinkerton CR. Childhood T-cell lymphoblastic lymphoma: Does early resolution of mediastinal mass predict for final outcome? The United Kingdome Children's Cancer Study Group (UKCCSG). Br J Cancer 1995;72:752-6.
42. Fishman SJ. Vascular anomalies of the mediastinum. Sem Pediatr Surgery. 1999;8(2):92-8.
43. Okada A, Kubota A, Fukuzawa M, et al. Injection of bleomycin as a primary therapy of cystic lymphangioma. J Pediatr Surg 1992;27:440.
44. Ogita S, Tsutot T, Deguchi E, et al. OK-432 therapy for unresectable lymphangiomas in children. J Pediatr Surg 1991;26:263-70.
45. Furman WL, Buckley PJ, Green M, et al. Thymoma and myasthenia gravis in a 4-year-old child Case report and review of the literature. Cancer 1985;56:2703-6.
46. Ramon y Cajal S, Suster S: Primary thymic epithelial neoplasms in children. Am J Surg Pathol 1991;15:466-74.
47. Lam WWM, Chan FL, Lau YL, et al. Pediatric thymoma: unusual recurrence in two siblings. Pediatr Radiol 1993;23:124-6.
48. Dehner LP, Martin SA, Sumner HW. Thymus related tumors and tumor like lesions in childhood with rapid clinical progression and death. Hum Pathol 1977;8:53-66.
49. Wychulis AR, Payne WS, Clagett OT, et al. Surgical treatment of mediastinal tumors; a 40 year experience. J Thorac Cardiovasc Surg 1971;62:379-92.
50. Saenz NC. Posterior mediastinal neurogenic tumors in infants and children. Sem in Pediatr Surg 1999;8(2):78-84.
51. Grillo HC, Ojemann RG, Scannell JF, et al. Combined approach to "dumbbell" intrathoracic and intraspinal neurogenic tumors. Ann Thorac Surg 1983;36:402-7.
52. Richards ML, Gundersen AE, Williams MS. Cystic neuroblastoma of infancy. J Pediatr Surg 1995; 30(9):1354-7.
53. Evans AE, D'Angio GJ, Propert K, Anderson J, et al. Prognostic factor in neuroblastoma. Cancer 1987;59:1853-9.
54. Shuster JJ, McWilliams NB, Castleberry R, et al. Serum lactate dehydrogenase in childhood neuroblastoma. A Pediatric Oncology Group recursive partitioning study. Am J Clin Oncol 1992;15:295-303.
55. Nakagawara A, Arima M, Azar CG, et al. Inverse relationship between trk expression and N-myc amplification in human neuroblastomas Cancer Res 52 1364-1368,1992
56. Laug WE, Siegel SE, Shaw KN, et al. Initial urinary catecholamine metabolite concentrations and prognosis in neuroblastoma Pediatrics 1978;62:77-83.

CHAPTER 36

Devendra K Gupta
Akshay Pratap

Tumors in
Intersex Disorders

Patients with intersex syndromes are rare in the general population. In addition to anatomic, endocrinologic, psychologic, and sexual identity issues, patients, families and physicians must consider the risks of tumor occurrence and tumor behavior in the various intersex syndromes at the time of diagnosis. Treating and consulting urologists must understand the risk of tumor development and tumor behavior when counseling intersex patients and their families. Although some syndromes share the occurrence of cryptorchidism, individual risks for tumor development are intrinsic to the specific syndrome.

ANDROGEN INSENSITIVITY SYNDROME

The most frequent cause of male pseudo-hermaphroditism is androgen insensitivity syndrome (AIS), which is encountered in infancy, adolescence adulthood, and middle to old age. At birth and in childhood, the phenotypic female may present clinically with inguinal hernias. At the time of herniorrhaphy, crypt orchid gonads may be found in the hernial sac. Biopsy will permit the recognition of prepubertal testes. Further clinical examination will confirm the diagnosis of androgen insensitivity syndrome. Malignant intratubular germ cells have been identified in infancy. These cells do not have an immediate risk of clinical malignancy but in the course of decades may evolve into a malignant germ cell tumor. It is generally recommended that the patient retain crypt orchid gonads through puberty to receive benefit from their hormone production and then have the gonads removed.

There is a risk for malignancy in androgen insensitivity syndrome gonads owing to the occurrence of germ cell tumors. The cumulative risk for a germ cell tumor is greater than 30 percent by 50 years of age.[1] Malignant intratubular germ cell neoplasia has been described in infancy, adolescence, and adulthood. This lesion cannot be seen grossly. Microscopically, it consists of malignant germ cells within seminiferous tubules. These cells contain large nuclei with irregular nuclear borders and prominent nuclei and are larger than spermatogonia. The diagnosis of malignant intratubular germ cells can be confirmed with immunoperoxidase stain for placental alkaline phosphatase in patients over 1 year of age. Other types of germ cell tumors resemble lesions in descended testes grossly and histologically. In patients with androgen insensitivity syndrome, all types of germ cell tumors have been reported and have the same prognosis as similar tumors in patients without androgen insensitivity syndrome.

Androgen insensitivity syndrome can also present at adolescence when the patient realizes that she has not experienced menarche. Investigations at this time indicate the diagnosis. If there is no clinical mass, the gonads should be removed after completion of puberty because of the risk for neoplasm. Androgen insensitivity syndrome can also be discovered in the course of an infertility evaluation, at which time the gonads should be removed. Androgen insensitivity syndrome is genetically determined and is occasionally discovered as a result of the diagnosis in a sibling. In post-pubertal patients, the gonads should be removed at the time of discovery because of the risk for germ cell tumors.

Other masses may occur in the crypt orchid testes and may be present at the diagnosis of androgen insensitivity syndrome. These so called Sertoli cell adenomas (SCA) are not neoplastic and have no malignant potential. The gonad is of a normal to slightly small size for the patient's age. Along the medial border, there may be a mass of benign smooth muscle thought to be of mullerian duct origin. On cut section, testicular parenchyma is tan to brown and may have none to multiple white nodules up to 25 mm in diameter. These nodules are SCA. Sertoli cell adenomas are seen grossly and consist of tissue demarcated from surrounding testicular parenchyma. The adenomas may or may not be encapsulated and are composed of multiple small tubules lined principally by prepubertal type Sertoli cells. Microscopically, the non-adenomatous testicular parenchyma is composed of seminiferous tubules, populated by post-pubertal and prepubertal-type Sertoli cells. Variable numbers of primary spermatocytes are present. In the interstitium, Leydig cells are prominent and increased in number. Variable amounts of cellular spindled connective tissue resembling ovarian stroma may course through the testicular parenchyma. Although these masses may become large and clinically evident, their cellular composition and the fact that Sertoli cell adenomas do not become malignant are consistent with the interpretation that they are benign and harmartomatous.

PERSISTENT MÜLLERIAN DUCT SYNDROME

At the time of diagnosis, patients with persistent mullerian duct syndrome usually have normal adult male external genitalia. Other findings are possible unilateral or bilateral cryptorchidism, normal Wolffian duct derivatives, and an infantile uterus, usually with one or two fallopian tubes, or within an inguinal hernia. Patients are usually diagnosed at the time of herniorrhaphy. Persistent mullerian duct syndrome is caused by a genetic mutation in the gene for antimullerian hormone (AMH), on chromosome 19 or possibly in the gene for the end organ receptor.[2]

Patients have an approximately 15 percent risk for associated germ cell neoplasm.[3] Any type of germ cell neoplasm may occur in these testes, including malignant intratubular germ cell neoplasia and bilateral mixed malignant germ cell neoplasms.[3,4] Eastham[3] and coworkers found 12 germ cell tumors in 84 patients. Malignancy in persistent müllerian duct syndrome presents in the cryptorchidism testes, and thus consideration should be given to removal of intraabdominal or inguinal testes. There is no known risk of malignancy of the müllerian duct derivatives,

fallopian tubes, and uterus; therefore, these organs can be left in place. Fertility may occur in patients with this syndrome.

GONADAL DYSGENESIS

Gonadal dysgenesis consists of a spectrum of disorders with ambiguous genitalia, persistent mullerian duct structures, Wolffian duct derivatives, karyotypes having a Y or marker chromosomes with or without molecular biologic evidence of a Y chromosome, and the potential for neoplastic transformation of the gonads. Entities within this spectrum include mixed gonadal dysgenesis, pure gonadal dysgenesis, and dysgenetic male pseudohermaphroditism (Fig. 36.1). Patients with bilateral streak gonads (Turner's syndrome) should also be considered to have the syndrome because of molecular biologic evidence showing a Y chromosome in some patients and because of the risk for gonadoblastoma and other germ cell tumors. Rutgers and Scully[1] reported tumors in 9 to 30 percent of patients with mixed gonadal dysgenesis. The most common tumors in these patients is a neoplasm composed of intimately admixed germ cells and sex cord cells circumscribed nests with focal or diffuse calcification. Hyaline basement membrane material is often present within these nests. Approximately 80 percent of patients with gonadoblastomas are phenotypic female, and 20 percent are males.[1] In about 50 percent of the patients tumor cells invade stroma and form a germinoma, term synonymous with seminoma. Approximately 17 percent of germinomas arising in gonadoblastoma are bilateral. Although gonadoblastomas do not metastasize, other types of germ cell tumors occurring in association with

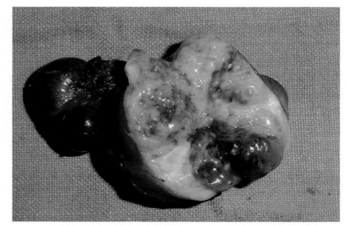

Figure 36.1: Gonadoblastoma in a case of mixed gonadal dysgenesis

them may metastasize. Some germ cell tumors occurring in dysgenetic gonads may not contain gonadoblastoma owing to overgrowth of the gonadoblastoma or origin of the germ cell tumor in malignant intratubular germ cell. In a study of 15 patients with gonadal dysgenesis, Wallace[5] et al found gonadal tumors in seven, all phenotypic females. These patients had five gonadoblastoma, four germinomas, and one malignant intratubular neoplasia. One patient had a gonadal stromal tumor. Because of the risk for malignant germ cell tumors in gonadoblastoma, the presence of a Y chromosome should be investigated with a karyotype analysis or molecular techniques. The gonads should be removed if the patient has a diagnosis of a mixed gonadal dysgenesis or gonadoblastoma with Y chromosome material. These gonads are not fertile. There is a small risk for endometerial adenocarcinoma, particularly if the patient is treated with unopposed estrogens.

Juvenile granulosa cell tumor has been described in patients with mixed gonadal dysgenesis. These tumors are associated with 45XO/46Y and 45,XO/46,X, iso (Yq), and other sex chromosomal mosaicism.[6,7] The tumors are usually found in descended testes, although they have been discovered in cryptorchidism and torsed testes. The tumor is unassociated with isosexual precocity but has been found in patients with intersex disorders. The testes harbouring such tumor are usually enlarged, solid or cystic. Tumors range in size from four microscopic lobules to 13 cm. Follicular structures of varying size are lined by one to multiple layers of cells and contain pale eosinophilic or basophilic material. The stroma is fibrous and contains groups of granulose cells that do not resemble the cells of adult granulose cell tumor. In the solid areas, the cells have round to oval nuclei and pale to eosinophilic cytoplasm. Tumor cells stain for vimentin, and some cells stain positively for keratin and S-100 protein. Immunohistochemistry has demonstrated universal tumor cell positivity for inhibin in juvenile granulosa cell tumor of the ovary. This finding is also expected to occur in the testes. Mitosis may be numerous. Tumor cells may be present in relationship to seminiferous tubules and have been described even within a seminiferous tubule.

Juvenile granulosa cell tumor of the ovary has a mortality rate of approximately 5 percent. In contrast, there is no indication that juvenile granulosa cell tumor of the testes recurs after orchiectomy. The differential diagnosis of juvenile granulosa cell tumor of the testes includes tumors developing in the neonatal period. Most

congenital testicular tumors and tumors discovered in the first four months of life are juvenile granulosa cell tumor rather than yolk sac tumors. Yolk sac tumors may be cystic or solid and may have micro-cystic or macrocystic areas, whereas definitive diagnostic areas of yolk sac tumors including Schiller-Duval bodies, hyaline droplets, and staining for alpha-fetoprotein are negative in juvenile granulosa cell tumor.

CONGENITAL ADRENAL HYPERPLASIA

Although congenital adrenal hyperplasia affects boys with the same frequency as girls, those with 21 hydroxylase and 11b hydroxylase deficiencies do not cause male pseudohermaphroditism. They do, however need to take cortisol to correct the metabolic defect, but are frequently not motivated to do so and are therefore poorly controlled. Continuing ACTH drive may result in Leydig cell adenomas, which usually present as bilateral testicular enlargement later in adolescence and young adulthood. In the study by Rutgers and co-workers,[8] masses occurred at an average of 22.5 years. Clinical recognition that the masses are a part of the congenital adrenal hyperplasia syndrome will obviate the need of orichiectomy. Ultrasound is useful in the diagnosis and follow up of intratesticular masses in congenital adrenal hyperplasia.[9] Grossly the Leydig cell adenomas appear as well-encapsulated lesions. Microscopically, sheets of cells with eosinophilic cytoplasm and round nuclei are present in the testes. The cytoplasm may have a fine brown granularity owing to lipochrome pigment. In no cases have Rinkes's crystals been reported. Although specimens observed in low and high power microscopic fields may be indistinguishable from Leydig cell tumors, the pathologist must recognize and communicate the fact that "the tumors of congenital adrenal hyperplasia" are nonneoplastic and consequently nonmalignant. Only one case in the literature describes a malignant Leydig cell tumor in a patient with congenital adrenal hyperplasia.[10]

TRUE HERMAPHRODITE

True hermaphrodite is a state in which there is a testes on one side and an ovary on the other or unilateral or bilateral ovotestes. The ovary is physiologically dominant and the testis usually undergoes atrophy and scarring. There is an increased incidence of germ cell neoplasia including gonadoblastoma (Fig. 36.2). Because patients with true hermaphrodite have a Y chromosome and

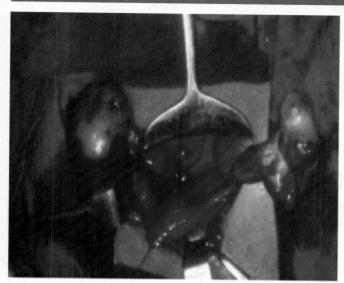

Figure 36.2: Gonadoblastoma in a case of true hermaphrodite

undescended gonads, ovotestes, and testes should be removed because of the risk for a germinal neoplasm.

CONCLUSION

A variety of intersex syndromes occur that have different clinical presentations. Gonads that are cryptorchid and have a Y chromosome or Y chromosome material detected by molecular techniques are at risk for germinal neoplasms. Gonads with dysgenesis are at risk for gonadoblastomas and other malignant germ cell tumors. Not all masses are malignant in patients with intersex syndromes. Masses in the testes and paratesticular tissues are almost benign in patients with congenital adrenal hyperplasia.

REFERENCES

1. Rutgers JL, Scully RE. Pathology of the testis in intersex disorders. Semin Diagn Pathol 1987;4:275-91.
2. Cohen-Haguenauer O, Picard JY, Mattei G, et al. Mapping of the gene for anti-mullerian hormone to the short arm of human chromosome 19. Cytogenet Cell Genet 1987;44:2.
3. Eastham JA, McEvoy K, Sullivan R, et al. A case of simultaneous bilateral nonseminomatous testicular tumors in persistant mullerian duct syndrome. J Urol 1992;148:407-8.
4. Williams JC, Merguerian PA, Schned AR, et al. Bilateral testicular carcinoma in situ in persistant mullerian duct syndrome: a case report and literature review. Urology 1994;44:595-8.
5. Wallace TM, Levin HS: Mixed gonadal dysgenesis. A review of 15 patients reporting single cases of malignant intratubular germ cell neoplasia of the testis, endometrial adenocarcinoma and a complex vascular anomaly. Arch Pathol Lab Med 1990;114:679-88.
6. Tanaka Y, Sasaki Y, Tachibana K, et al. Testicular juvenile granulosa cell tumor in an infant with X/XY mosaicism clinically diagnosed as true hermaphroditism. Am J Surg Pathol 1992;18:316-22.
7. Raju U, Fine G, Rajasekharan W, et al. Congenital testicular juvenile granulosa cell tumor in a neonate with X/XY mosaicism. Am J Surg Pathol 1986;10:577-83.
8. Rutgers JL, Young RH, Scully RE. The testicular "tumors" of the adrenogenital syndrome: a report of six cases and review of the literature on testicular masses in patients with adrenocortical disorders. Am J Surg Pathol 1988;12:503-13.
9. Vanzulli A, DelMaschio A, Paesano P, et al. Testicular masses in association with adrenogenital syndrome: US findings. Radiology 1992;183:425-9.
10. Davis JM, Woodroof J, Sadasivan R, et al. Case report: congenital adrenal hyperplasia and malignant Leydig cell tumor. Am J Med Sci 1995;309:63-5.

CHAPTER 37

Gauri Kapoor

Therapeutic Advances in Pediatric Malignant Bone Tumors

INCIDENCE

Osteosarcoma and Ewing's sarcoma are the two most common bone cancers in children. Based on the Surveillance, Epidemiology and End Results (SEER) report of the NCI, USA, malignancies of the bone comprise 6 percent of all cancers in children younger than 20 years of age. The incidence of osteosarcoma and Ewing's sarcoma are observed to be 56 and 34 percent respectively among all bone cancers.[1] The other bone cancers including chondrosarcoma and malignant fibrous histiocytoma are rare in children and are not dealt with here. For all bone malignancies there occurs a steady increase in incidence with age, the steepest rise coinciding with the adolescent growth spurt, the peak is higher in osteosarcoma as compared to Ewing's sarcoma. Figure 37.1 shows the age distribution of malignant bone tumors as per the tumor registry of the Rajiv Gandhi Cancer Institute and Research Centre and the peak incidence is between ages 15 to 24. The most frequent site of bone cancer is the long bones of the lower limbs, however it constitutes 78 percent of all sites in osteosarcoma and only 29 percent for the Ewing's sarcoma (central axis involvement is more common).

DIAGNOSTIC WORK-UP AND STAGING

Most patients with bone tumors present with pain and swelling in the involved region and often have symptoms for several months before a diagnosis is established.

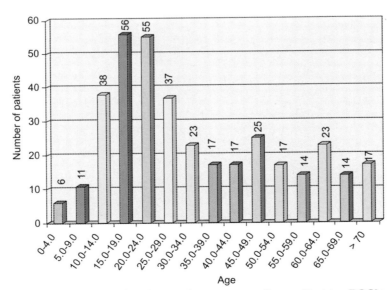

Figure 37.1: Age distribution of malignant bone tumors: Tumor Registry RGCI and RC 1996-2002

Ewing's sarcoma patients may in addition have constitutional symptoms, symptoms from metastatic disease and local signs of inflammation making infection an important differential diagnosis. In osteosarcoma the most common primary site is the metaphysis of long bones with 50 percent of tumors arising around the knee area and less than 10 percent occurring in the axial skeleton. Ewing's sarcoma equally involves the extremity (53%) and central axis (47%, pelvis, chest wall, spine, skull bones). Metastasis at diagnosis occurs in 15 to 20 percent of osteosarcoma patients, lung is the most common site and less commonly bone and other soft tissue. In Ewing's sarcoma 25 percent have metastasis at diagnosis, involving lung (35%), bone (3%) and bone marrow (11%).[2]

Hence diagnostic work-up is done to establish diagnosis and stage the disease. Although diagnosis of a bone cancer can often be predicted by radiographic appearance and location, a biopsy for pathologic confirmation is mandatory. Imaging is done to define local tumor extent and soft tissue involvement by CT scan or MRI as well as to detect metastatic disease by imaging of chest (plain radiograph or CT), radionucleide bone scan (for skip lesions or distant bony metastases) and in Ewing's sarcoma bone marrow aspirate and biopsy (to detect marrow involvement). These have an important bearing on management of the patient. Role of PET scan in these tumors is still evolving and has not proven to be very accurate for detecting pulmonary metastasis. However the most interesting aspect is its potential use in assessing tumor response after initial chemotherapy.

Staging

The surgical staging of osteosarcoma developed by Enneking is summarized below:[3]
- **Stage IA** (G1,T1,M0) low-grade and intra-compartmental (T1), no metastatsis.
- **Stage IB** (G1,T2,M0) low-grade type extra-compartmental (T1), no metastasis.
- **Stage IIA** (G2,T1,M0) high-grade, intra-compartmental (T1), no metastasis.
- **Stage IIB** (G2,T2,M0) high-grade extra-compartmental (T1), no metastasis.
- **Stage IIIA** (G1 or G2,T1,M1) any grade intra-compartmental (T1), with metastasis.
- **Stage IIIB** (G1 or G2,T2,M1) any grade extra-compartmental (T1), with metastasis.

Staging of Ewing's sarcoma, at present there is no formal staging system for Ewing's sarcoma. Most patients are grouped depending on whether cancer is restricted to only one site (*localised disease/limited stage disease*) or whether it has spread (*metastatic disease*).

WHO **histological classification** recognizes three major subtypes of conventional osteosarcoma osteoblastic, chondroblastic and fibroblastic osteosarcoma reflecting the predominant type of matrix[4] and two variants telangiectatic and small cell osteosarcoma. Low-grade intramedullary osteosarcoma and surface osteosarcoma (periosteal and parosteal) are very rare in children and therefore not included in this review. On the other hand Ewing's sarcoma is morphologically a blue round cell tumor characterized by immunoreactivity with MIC-2 and the typical t(11;21)(q24;q12) translocation (85% of cases).

Some of the common **cytogenetic** associations of bone cancers are:
1. Osteosarcoma
   - RB gene locus on chromosome 13q (60-75%)
   - Mutation of p53 gene on chromosome 17 (30-50%)
   - Increased risk in individuals with inherited abnormality of p53 (Li Fraumeni familial cancer syndrome)
   - Increased risk in individuals with inherited RB gene abnormality.
2. Ewing's sarcoma
   - Reciprocal t(11;22) translocation (90-95%)
   - Reciprocal t(21;22) translocation (5-10%)
   - Poor prognosis associated with: p53 alteration; deletion of INK4A (cell cycle regulator); gain of 1q chromosome aberration; loss of 16q associated with dissemination at diagnosis.

TREATMENT

The successful treatment of bone cancers requires the use of systemic chemotherapy in combination with local control with surgery alone in osteosarcoma and surgery and or radiotherapy in Ewing's sarcoma (Table 37.1). The goal of treatment is to cure the disease while preserving organ/limb function and minimizing long-term sequelae.

Table 37.1: Modern management of bone sarcomas has evolved mainly due to

a. Multi-agent chemotherapy
b. Better diagnostic imaging (CT scan. and MRI)
c. Improved surgical techniques
d. Supportive care (antibiotics, nutrition, anesthesia, biomedical engineering, rehabilitation)
e. Aggressive surgery of metastasis

Systemic Treatment

Prior to the advent of effective chemotherapy, most patients with bone cancers were treated with local control measures alone ie surgical resection and or radiotherapy and had 5yr DFS of 15-20 percent, implying thereby that most of these patients had microscopic metastases at diagnosis. Over the past 3 decades the role of systemic combination chemotherapy in treatment of both osteosarcomas and Ewing's sarcomas has been clearly established.

Osteosarcoma

The most active chemotherapeutic agents in osteosarcoma are cisplatin, doxorubicin, high dose methotrexate and now ifosphamide as well. Early trials with combination chemotherapy did reveal better outcomes,[5] but were not convincing because they were non-randomized trials. Two subsequent randomized studies by Link et al (1991) and Eilber et al (1987) clarified this controversy.[6,7] The former reported 6yr RFS of 66 percent for the group also treated with adjuvant chemotherapy as against 17 percent for surgery alone, Eilber et al reported similar results. It was Rosen et al (1979) who introduced the concept of administering chemotherapy prior to definitive surgery, now termed as neo-adjuvant chemotherapy.[8] It was initially started to provide time for preparing custom endoprosthesis for limb-salvage procedures. Subsequently it also provided the opportunity to examine the histologic response of the tumor to induction chemotherapy. Now we know that a strong correlation exists between degree of tumor necrosis grade and DFS, also confirmed by others.[9] Hence now there are three *histological grading systems* for osteosarcoma to assess *response to induction chemotherapy*. That developed by Huvos et al (1977) is used at the Memorial Sloane Kettering Cancer Centre, that developed by Salzer-Kuntshik (1983) and the one more commonly used by us is that developed by Picci et al (1985) at the Instituti Ortopedico Rizzoli in Bologna.[9-11] The latter have classified response into 4 categories: Total response (no viable tumor); Good response (90-99% necrosis); Fair response (60-89% necrosis); Poor response (< 60% necrosis). Most data now accept >90 percent necrosis as favorable prognosis. Attempts to modify or intensify induction chemotherapy upfront or in those with poor histologic response have not provided any survival advantage. The chemotherapy doses used by the Cooperative

Osteosarcoma Study Group before 1998 per course include doxorubicin 60-90 mg/m^2, cisplatin 90 to 150 mg/m^2, methotrexate 12 g/m^2 with leucovorin rescue, ifosphamide 6-9 g/m^2.[12] Actuarial 10-yr overall and event free survival were 59.8 percent and 48.9 percent. The favorable prognostic factors were younger age, limb lesions better than axial, non-metastatic disease and size less than one third of limb. Good histologic response to chemotherapy was associated with better survival (73 vs 47% in poor responders) and so was completeness of surgery (complete 65% vs incomplete 15%). However it is relevant to mention that the role of high dose methotrexate in primary non-metastatic osteosarcoma remains controversial and the European Osteosarcoma Intergroup still use the 2 drug combination of cisplatin and doxorubicin with good results.[13] The drug combination of bleomycin, cyclophosphamide, actinomycin D are no longer used nor has the intra-arterial chemotherapy added any advantage.

For metastatic and recurrent osteosarcoma ifosphamide, etoposide combination and high dose methotrexate are usually used additionally. Surgical resection of pulmonary lesions is usually attempted for metastatic as well as recurrent disease. Involvement of multiple bone sites is associated with a very grave outcome.

The Standard of Care for Osteosarcoma

Given the advantages in facilitating limb-salvage procedures and assessing chemotherapy response, the use of neoadjuvant chemotherapy (9 to 12 weeks) followed by surgery with adequate (wide or radical) margins has become the standard approach to treatment. The total duration of chemotherapy ranges from 24 to 28 weeks. At present there is no role for radiotherapy in primary treatment.

Ewing's Sarcoma

Ewing's sarcoma, unlike osteosarcoma, is a disease that is exquisitely sensitive to both chemotherapy and radiotherapy. The two most well studied chemotherapeutic agents in Ewing's sarcoma are cyclophosphamide and doxorubicin and were found to produce complete response as single agents in the 1960s and 1970s.[14,15] Subsequently Jaffe et al (1976) found vincristine and dactinomycin to be also effective.[16] The first IESS (Inter Ewing's sarcoma Study Group): 1973-1978, established the importance of using multiagent adjuvant chemotherapy, VACA regimen. The study clearly showed that addition of doxorubicin improved 5 yr DFS to 60 from 24 percent.[17] The second IESS, 1978-1982, established better outcome with high dose intermittent chemotherapy as against moderate or low dose frequent administration.[18] These studies also established certain poor prognostic factors like large size, pelvic location and poor histologic response to neo-adjuvant chemotherapy. At the same time the St Jude Children's Research Hospital (SJCRH) study ES 79: 1978-1986, reported 5 yr DFS for localized disease based on tumor size, <8 cm vs > 8 cm, to be 82 and 64 percent.[19] The CESS-81 (German Multi-Institutional Cooperative Ewing's Sarcoma Study) used VACA and reported 80 percent 5 yr DFS of 80 percent for tumor volume <100 ml vs 54 percent for tumor volume >100 ml.[20] In the early 1980s ifosphamide was tried for resistant sarcomas, subsequently CESS-86 used ifosphamide instead of cyclophosphamide in high risk Ewing's sarcoma patients and observed favorable results, later confirmed by the UK National Ewing's tumor study 2, ET-2 (5 yr DFS 62%).[21,22] Subsequently etoposide alone and then in combination with ifosphamide has emerged and the latter showed response rates as high as 90 percent. Hence the POG 8850/CCG7881 showed the benefit of multiagent combination chemotherapy, reporting 5 yr DFS of 69 percent in VACA+IE vs 54 percent in VACA alone.[23] Similarly the EICESS 92 randomized both standard and high risk patients to the above two arms and reported survival advantage in both the arms using VACA+ IE over VACA alone.[24]

Treatment for metastatic tumors of the Ewing's family may be one of the following:

1. Combination chemotherapy followed by radiation therapy to all sites of gross disease with possible selected surgical excision.
2. High-dose chemotherapy with or without radiation therapy plus additional stem cell support.
3. Clinical trials of intensive chemotherapy with multiple chemotherapy drug combinations and newer agents for recurrent tumors. For metastatic Ewing's sarcoma the overall cure rate is about 20 percent and results with VACA± IE are similar. For patients with progressive or recurrent disease the various chemotherapy combinations that may be tried include IE if not used earlier, cyclophosphamide and topotecan combination, or irinotecan and cisplatin combination.

Role of Stem cell transplant as consolidation for Ewing's sarcoma with high risk disease or metastatic disease has been tried using various conditioning regimens like melphalan+TBI, thiotepa+carboplatin, etc. However, so far no survival advantage has been observed. A randomized trial of post-surgical chemotherapy with or without stem cell transplant is ongoing. Role of allogenic BMT using *ex vivo* purging with antisense oligoneuclotide is in a trial phase and may hold promise for the future.

The Standard of Care for Ewing's Sarcoma

Hence the current standard of care for Ewing's sarcoma is neoadjuvant chemotherapy (VAC+IE) followed by local control with surgery and or radiotherapy followed by adjuvant chemotherapy.

Local Control

Optimum outcome in malignant bone tumors requires a multidisciplinary approach and close cooperation between members of the various teams, pediatric oncology, pediatric surgery, orthopedics and radiation oncology. Cure is possible only if both systemic chemotherapy as well as local control measures (surgery/radiotherapy) is employed. The timing and sequence of these therapies is also very crucial to outcome.

Surgery

The surgical management of bone cancers has evolved into a complex field. Importance of surgical margins in malignant osseous tumors cannot be undermined. Precise definition and classification of surgical margins is essential for planning of surgical procedures and include intralesional, marginal, wide and radical. The goal of surgery is to perform complete, enbloc removal of lesion with adequate margins. The use of neoadjuvant chemotherapy and advances in imaging techniques has now enabled the oncologic surgeon to obtain local control rates equivalent to amputation with limb salvage procedures. Hence limb salvage surgery has now become standard of care except in situations where it may compromise on oncologic outcome.

Two broad criteria must be fulfilled before considering limb salvage surgery, (i) satisfactory surgical margin must be possible so that the risk of local recurrence is low (less than or equal to that with amputation) and (ii) functional outcome should be greater than or equal to that achieved by amputation and prosthetic fitting.

Below are mentioned some of the options for limb sparing procedures.[25]

Limb sparing surgical options for children with extremity bone cancers:
1. Endoprosthetic replacement
2. Allograft
3. Sterilization and reimplantation of bone
4. Vascularized fibula graft
5. Vascularized graft combined with allograft
6. Bone distraction
7. Rotation plasty.

The overall goals of Limb sparing surgical options for children with extremity bone sarcomas are therefore to (1) Maintain adequate function, (2) Improve quality of life/preserve body image, (3) maintain low local recurrence/failure rates and (4) Maintain survival rates.

Osteosarcoma

The surgical options available to the patient include limb salvage surgery and amputation. Most advanced centers offer the latter to nearly 85 percent of the patients, however it cannot be at the cost of a good margin especially so in case of osteosarcoma. As mentioned above, surgery is the only curative local therapy available for osteosarcoma. Hence surgery must be done with wide margins. The balance between wide margin and limb preservation must be very finely balanced and tumor control is the ultimate goal. For patients with lung metastasis pulmonary metastatectomy is indicated. More than 85 percent o recurrences in osteosarcoma occur in the lung, and complete surgical resection with wide margins can be accomplished with relative ease (repeatedly). Complete surgical resection of all overt metastatic disease is a prerequisite for long-term salvage.

Ewing's Sarcoma

The management of local tumor site in Ewing's sarcoma is not only complex but also quite controversial. This is in part because both the options i.e. surgery and radiotherapy are available and effective. The selection of local modality is therefore dependent on relative efficacy and treatment related effects. Concerns regarding late effects including secondary malignancies and loss of growth often move oncologists to a primary surgical approach for local therapy. Non-randomized studies suggest superior outcome with local surgical therapy, although bias exists in selecting smaller more peripheral tumors for definitive surgical resection. Krasin et al (2005) reported 5yr EFS and local recurrence rate of 71.5 and 12.5 percent in 33 patients with localized Ewing's sarcoma treated with systemic chemotherapy and surgery alone at the SJCRH.[26] The same authors reported 30 percent local failure rates with radiation alone and 10.8 percent with combined surgery and radiotherapy as local control.[27,28]

Although the surgical principles applicable to the treatment of Ewing's sarcoma are similar to those followed in the treatment of osteosarcoma, three main differences characterize the approach to Ewing's sarcoma: (i) Ewing's sarcoma is radiosensitive, whereas osteosarcoma is not; (ii) Ewing's sarcoma tends to occur in a younger population than osteosarcoma; and (iii) Ewing's sarcoma tends to arise in the diaphysis of long bones, whereas osteosarcoma has a predilection for the metaphyseal area. Hence in Ewing's sarcoma the option of radiotherapy is available for cases with positive margins and here limb is preserved and amputations are rare if ever. The selection of a local control modality has evolved gradually over the past 25 years from primary irradiation to surgical resection with reconstruction if the morbidity is acceptable.

Role of Radiotherapy

Ewing's sarcoma are radiosensitive tumors and local cure can be achieved by definitive radiotherapy. In most prospective trials however surgery has yielded better local control rates and in all treatment protocols surgery is the local treatment option of first choice. Combined local therapy (surgery plus radiation therapy) has also provided excellent local control rates. Indications for post-operative radiotherapy are marginal resection, positive margins and poor histological response. Indications for radiotherapy as the only local control measure mainly include inoperable sites (e.g. pelvis) and large tumors requiring mutilating surgery. Recommended radiotherapy doses in this setting are 55 to 60 Gy; in postoperative setting with gross disease are 55.8 Gy; and microscopic disease requires 45 Gy. Doses would also be adjusted for tumor site and age of patient.

LATE EFFECTS

Late effects of chemotherapy must be monitored for and these include cisplatin-induced ototoxicity and electrolyte imbalance and doxorubicin related cardiomyopathy. It is therefore important to have baseline audiogram and ECHO for ejection fraction in these children. In addition sperm banking for males should be offered as chemotherapy for both bone cancers has the potential for producing sterility.

Second malignancies particularly t-AML/MDS do occur in about 2-8 percent of patients of Ewing's sarcoma and usually happen about 2-5 yrs from diagnosis.[29-31] Second solid tumors have a cumulative incidence of 5 to 10 percent at 15 to 20 years.

FUTURE CONSIDERATIONS

It is quite apparent that the survival of children with metastatic and recurrent bone cancers remains dismal. There is a clear need for newer and effective agents which could be used in clinical trials. Use of monoclonal antibodies such as Trastuzumab (Herceptin) that targets epidermal growth factor 2, is currently under investigation for osteosarcoma. Monoclonal antibodies specific for the ganglioside GD2, a cell surface antigen expressed by human neuroblastomas also recognize osteosarcomas and may be considered for therapy. Other biologic agents under investigation include use of inhaled GM-CSF and interferon-α; interleukin-12 and interferon-α; insulin-like growth factor I; use of radio pharmaceuticals for drug delivery; adenoviral gene therapy using selective promoters controlling a suicide gene (thymidine kinase) are also under study. Trimetrexate is a new agent under research investigation for osteosarcoma Bone seeking isotopes such as Sumariam have shown dramatic though transient initial responses in osteosarcoma.

The chimeric protein, EWS-FLI1 [t(11;22)] identified in most Ewing's sarcomas, is shown to be associated with tumorigenicity and is an important focus of targeted therapy for these tumors. As p21 expression is inhibited by EWS-FLI1, histone deacetylase inhibitors (known to upregulate p21) may show promise as cancer therapy. Ewing's tumor expresses kit and treatment with imatinib (KIT tyrosine kinase inhibitor), inhibits of KIT and increases sensitivity of tumor cells to doxorubicin and vincristine. This is a potential use for metastatic/recurrent disease.[32]

REFERENCES

1. Dahlin DC, Unni KK. Bone Tumors: General aspects and data on 8542 cases, 4th edn. Springfield,IL: Charles C. Thomas; 1986.
2. Ginsberg JP, et al. Ewing's sarcoma family of tumors: Ewing's sarcoma of bone and soft tissue and the PNETs. In: Pizzo PA, Poplack DG, (Eds): Principles and Practice of Pediatric Oncology, 4th edn. Lippincott William and Wilkins, 2002; 972-1016.
3. Enneking WF, Spanier SS, Goodman MA. A system for the surgical staging of musculoskeletal sarcoma. Clin Orthop 1980;153:106.
4. Raymond AK, Ayala AG, Knuutila S. Conventional osteosarcoma. In Kleihues P, Sobin L, Fletcher C, et al, (Eds): WHO Classification of Tumors: Pathology and Genetics of Tumors of Soft Tissue and Bone. Lyon, France: IARC Press, 2002;264-70.
5. Pratt C, Rivera G, Shanks E, et al. Combination chemotherapy for osteosarcoma. Cancer Treat Rep 1978;62:251-7.
6. Link MP, Goorin AM , Horowitz M, et al. Adjuvant chemotherapy of high-grade osteosarcoma of the extremity. Updated results of the multi-institutional osteosarcoma study. Clin Orthop 1991;(270):8-14.
7. Eilber F, Giuliano A, Eckardt J, et al. Adjuvant chemotherapy for osteosarcoma: a randomized prospective trial. J Clin Oncol 1987;5:21-6.
8. Rosen G, Marcove RC, Caparros B, et al. Primary osteogenic sarcoma: the rationale for preoperative chemotherapy and delayed surgery. Cancer 1979;43:2163-77.
9. Huvos AG, Rosen G, Marcove RC. Primary osteogenic sarcoma pathologic aspects in 20 patients after treatment with chemotherapy en-block resection and prosthetic bone replacement. Arch Pathol Lab Med 1977;101:14.
10. Salzer-Kuntshik M, Delling G, Beron G, Sigmund R. Morphological grades of regression in osteosarcoma after poly-chemotherapy-study COSS 80. J Cancer Res Clin Oncol 1983; 106(S):21.
11. Picci P, Bacci G, Campanacci M, et al. Histologic evaluation of necrosis in osteosarcoma induced by chemotherapy. Regional mapping of viable and nonviable tumor. Cancer 1985;56:1515.
12. Bielack SS, Kempf-Bielack B, Delling GG, et al. Prognostic factors in high-grade osteosarcoma of the extremities or trunk: an analysis of 1,702 patients treated on Neoadjuvant Cooperative Osteosarcoma Study Group protocols. J Clin Oncol 2002;20:776-90.
13. Lewis IJ, Nooij M, for the European Osteosarcoma Intergroup. Chemotherapy at standard doses or increased dose intensity in patients with operable osteosarcoma of the extremity: a randomized controlled trial conducted by the European Osteosarcoma Intergroup (ISRCTN 86294690) Proc Am Soc Clin Oncol 2003;22:816.
14. Haggard ME. Cyclophosphamide (NSC-26271) in the treatment of children with malignant neoplasms. Cancer Chemother Rep 1967;51:403-5.
15. Oldham RK, Pomeroy TC. Treatment of Ewing's sarcoma with adriamycin (NSC-123127). Cancer Chemother Rep 1972; 56:635-9.
16. Jaffe N, Paed D, Traggis D, et al. Improved outlook for Ewing's sarcoma with combination chemotherapy (vincristine, actinomycin D, and cyclophosphamide) and radiation therapy. Cancer 1976;38:1925-30.
17. Nesbit Jr ME, Gehan EA, Burgert Jr EO, et al. Multimodal therapy for the management of primary, non-metastatic Ewing's sarcoma of bone: a long-term follow-up of the first Intergroup study. J Clin Oncol 1990;8(10):1664-74.
18. Burgert Jr EO, Nesbit ME, Garsney LA, et al. Multimodal therapy for the management of nonpelvic, localized primary, Ewing's sarcoma of bone:Intergroup study IESS-II. J Clin Oncol 1990;8:1514-24.
19. Hayes FA, Thompson EI, Meyer WH, et al. Therapy for localized, Ewing's sarcoma of bone. J Clin Oncol 1989;7:208-13.
20. Jurgens H, Exener U, Gadner H, et al. Multidisciplinary treatment of Ewing's sarcoma of bone: a 6 yr experience of a European cooperative trial. Cancer 1988;61:23-32.
21. Paulussen M, Ahrens S, Dunst J, et al. Localized Ewing's sarcoma of bone: final results of the Cooperative Ewing's Sarcoma Study CESS86. J Clin Oncol 2001;19:1818-29.

22. Craft ACS, Malcolm A, et al. Ifosphamide containing chemotherapy in Ewing's sarcoma: The second UKCCSG and MRC Ewing's Tumor Study. J Clin Oncol 1998;16:3628-33.

23. Grier HE, Krailo MD, Tarbell NJ, et al. Addition of ifosphamide and etoposide to standard chemotherapy for Ewing's sarcoma and PNET of bone. N Engl J Med 2003;348(8):694-701.

24. Paulussen M, Ahrens S, Braun-Munzinger G, et al. EICESS 92 (European Intergroup Co-operative Ewing's sarcoma study – preliminary results. Klin Padiatr 1999;211(4):276-83.

25. Grimer RJ. Surgical options for children with osteosarcoma. Lancet Oncology 2005;6:85-92.

26. Krasin MJ, Davidoff AM. Rodriguez-Galindo C, et al. Cancer July 15, 2005/Volume 104/Number 2:367-73.

27. Krasin MJ, Rodriguez-Galindo C, Billups CA, et al. Int. J. Radiation Oncology Biol. Phys., 2004;Vol. 60, No. 3: 830-38.

28. Krasin MJ. Rodriguez-Galindo C, Davidoff AM, et al, Pediatr Blood Cancer 2004;43:229-36.

29. Carvajal R, Meyers P. Ewings sarcoma and primitive neuroectodermal family of tumors. Hematol Oncol Clin North Am. 2005;19(3);501-25.

30. Kushner BH, Heller G, Cheung NK, et al. High risk of leukemia after short-term dose intensive chemotherapy in young patients with solid tumors. J Clin Oncol 1998;16:3016-20.

31. Rodriguez-Galindo C, Poquette CA, Marina NM, et al. Hematologic abnormalities and acute myeloid leukemia in children and adolescents administered intensified chemotherapy for the ESFTs. J Pediatr Hematolo Oncol 2000;22:321-9.

32. Gonzalez I, Andreu EJ, Panizo A, et al. Imatinib inhibits proliferation of Ewing tumor cells mediated by the stem cell factor/KIT receptor pathway, and sensitizes cells to vincristine and doxorubicin-induced apoptosis. Clin Cancer Res. 2004;15;10(2):751-61.

CHAPTER 38

VS Mehta
PS Chandra

Cranial Tumors in Children

The management of brain tumors constitutes perhaps the single most important neurosurgical procedure after trauma in any large neurosurgical center. Treatment involves the very best of both technical skills and human interaction.

Historically in Hindu mythology, Jivaka, the personal physician of Gautama Budha was said to have had removed intracranial tumors using trephine holes.[1]

The treatment of brain tumors has expanded rapidly over the past decades. It was the discovery by Schleiden and Schwann in 1838 and 1839 and the description of neuroglia by Virchow in 1846 that formed the basis for neuropathology of tumors. Modern brain tumor surgery was made possible by three discoveries of the 19th century—anesthesia, asepsis and neurological localization of cerebral lesions.

Despite some earlier reports of surgical success, modern brain tumor surgery is generally thought to have commenced on 25th November 1884, when Rickman Godlee operated on a 25-year-old Scottish farmer named Henderson who had suffered from focal motor epilepsy and a progressive hemiparesis. It was Harvey Cushing who introduced methodical meticulous techniques of Halsted to the neurosurgical operations.[2,4] Dandy in 1921 advocated radical internal decompression.[5] The improvement in the treatment of patients with brain tumors has been related to advances in surgical techniques, the introduction of adjuvant therapies, the revolution in imaging brain tumors, and an improved understanding of the biology of these tumors. Stereotactic equipment has enabled a safer and more accurate approach to deep intracranial tumors.

Pediatric brain tumors are particularly challenging as these patient group are intolerant to hypovolumia, hypothermia and have a greater incidence of developing respiratory problems.

PATHOLOGY OF BRAIN TUMORS

Although the gross and microscopic features of the brain tumors in adults and pediatric age groups are same, the incidence of the types of pathologies vary widely. The most common tumors in adults include anaplastic astrocytoma, glioblastoma, meningiomas, metastatic tumors, pituitary tumors and acoustic tumors in that order.[6] In children, on the other hand, the astrocytic tumors tend to be histologically and biologically benign, meningiomas and pituitary tumors are rare and metastatic tumors are almost unheard of. At the same time, there are a number of tumors, which are very specific to the pediatric age group. These include pilocytic astrocytoma (typically located in cerebellum, diencephalon and the optic apparatus), brainstem gliomas, embryonal neuroepithelial tumors (commonly arising from the cerebellum), mixed neuronal—glial tumors, ependymomas and choroid plexus neoplasms, craniopharyngiomas, germ cell tumors, and atypical teratoid—rhabdoid tumors.

Another fundamental difference between adult and childhood CNS tumors involves the site of origin. The cerebrum is the favored location among adults, whereas the cerebrum and cerebellum each give rise to one-third of the primary CNS neoplasms among children. The following chapter focuses on the biology, gross and microscopic features of CNS tumors in infants and children below 18 years of age. Table 38.1 shows the distribution of various tumor types from a large series.[7-20] Table 38.2 shows the WHO classification of

Table 38.1: Biopsy diagnosis of CNS tumors in 1038 children aged 0-18 years (Values in parentheses are percentages[7])

	No. of patients
Gliomas	*435(41.9)*
Pilocytic	140(32.2)
Astrocytoma	136(31.3)
Anaplastic/ glioblastoma multiforme	59(13.6)
Mixed glioma	28(6.4)
Brainstem glioma	47(10.8)
Gliomatosis cerebri	8(1.8)
Oligodendroglioma	17(3.9)
Mixed neuronal-glial	*122(11.8)*
Ganglioglioma	93
Giant cell tumor of tuberous sclerosis	17
Pleomorphic astrocytoma	6
Desmoplastic astrocytoma/ ganglioglioma	6
Embryonal neuroepithelial tumors	*188(18.1)*
Primitive neuroectodermal tumor	163
Medulloepithelioma	8
Atypical teratoid-rhabdoid tumor	17
Ependymal-choroid plexus tumors	*94(9.1)*
Ependymoma	64
Choroid plexus papilloma	30
Craniopharyngioma	61(5.9)
Germ cell tumors	43(4.1
Meningioma	26(2.5)
Pineocytoma	6(0.6)
Miscellaneous	22(2.0
Cysts	19(1.8)
Lymphoma	9(0.9)
Pituitary adenoma	11(1.0)
Chemodectoma	1(0.1)
Olfactory neuroblastoma	1(0.1)

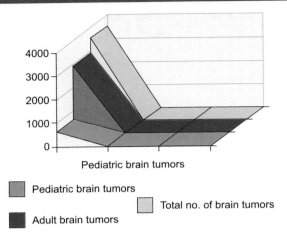

Pediatric brain tumors

■ Pediatric brain tumors

□ Total no. of brain tumors

■ Adult brain tumors

Figure 38.1: Incidence of pediatric brain tumors as seen in dept of neurosurgery, All India Institute of Medical Sciences (AIIMS, New Delhi). A total of 3545 tumors were operated and pathologically diagnosed over 10 years (1989-1999), of which 613 (17.3%) were in the pediatric age group ($\leq$ 15 years) Source: Prof Chitra Sarkar, dept of Neuropathology

course, whereas those within the substance of the pons pursue a more malignant course.[9] For the same reasons many authors recommend that for the final diagnosis of a tumor not only the histologic type is to be specified but the site is also to be designated.[7,8] A modification of revision of the World Health Organization Classification of Brain Tumors in Childhood is provided in Table 38.2. Histopathological features of some of the important childhood tumors are mentioned.

brain tumors. Figure 38.1 showing distribution of brain tumors reported at AIIMS.

BRAIN TUMOR CLASSIFICATION

The recent revision of World Health Organization (WHO) classification represents a consensus-compromise among representatives from 13 countries. However delineation of criteria to be used in making accurate diagnosis is often lacking, particularly to the large group of gliomas.[7] Unfortunately, vague imprecise terminology forms the basis of much of the problem.

Consideration of the specific tumor type must include not only histologic features but also location within the CNS, as it appears that local environment of a tumor influences its growth. For example, the biology of brainstem gliomas is quite different if the tumor arises in the midbrain and medulla rather than in the pons. In the former two they tend to exhibit an indolent

CEREBELLAR TUMORS IN CHILDREN

Cerebellar tumors are common lesions in children. About 54 to 70 percent of all childhood brain tumors originate in the posterior fossa proper. Most of western literature has reported the cystic cerebellar astrocytoma to be the most common tumor in the posterior fossa, accounting for about 12 to 28 percent of all pediatric brain tumors, and representing nearly one third of all posterior fossa tumors in children.[21] Although reported in older adults, the tumor almost exclusively occurs in children and older adults. The cerebellar primitive neuroectodermal tumors (PNET) is regarded as second to cerebellar astrocytoma in frequency of occurrence, constituting approximately 25 percent of all intracranial tumors of childhood.[12] Our own data from (Neurosciences dept, AIIMS) revealed a somewhat different picture. We analyzed a total of 3545 primary intracranial tumors (excluding pituitary adenomas) over 10 years (189-199). Posterior fossa tumors accounted for 48.3 percent (296/613) of all intracranial neoplasms in

Table 38.2: Modification of Revision of the World Health Organization Classification of brain tumors in childhood

I. Tumors of neuroepithelial tissue
A. Glial tumors
1. Astrocytic tumors
   a. Astrocytoma (fibrillary, protoplasmic, gemistocytic, pilocytic, gigantocellular)
   b. Anaplastic astrocytoma
2. Oligodenroglial tumors
   a. Oligodendroglioma
   b. Anaplastic oligodendroglioma
3. Ependymal tumors
   a. Ependymoma
   b. Anaplastic ependymoma
4. Choroid plxus tumors
   a. Choroid plexus papilloma
   b. Choroid plexus adenoma
   c. Choroid plexus carcinoma
5. Mixed gliomas
   a. Oligoastrocytoma
   b. Ependymoastrocytoma
   c. Oligoastroependymoma
   d. Gliofibroma
6. Gliomatous tumors
   a. Glioblastoma multiforme
   b. Giant cell glioblastoma
   c. Gliosarcoma
7. Gliomatosis cerebri
B. Mixed glial-neuronal tumors
1. Ganglioglioma
   a. Dysembryonic neuroepithelial tumor
2. Superficial cerebral astrocytoma/ desmoplastic infantile ganglioglioma
3. Pleomorphic xanthoastrocytoma
4. Subependymal giant cell tumor
5. Anaplastic ganglioglioma
C. Neuronal tumors
1. Gangliocytomas
2. Neurocytomas
D. Embryonal tumors
1. Primitive neuroectodermal tumors (PNET)
   a. PNET not otherwise specific
   b. PNET with glial differentiation
   c. PNET with ependymal differentiation
   d. PNET with neuronal differentiation
   e. PNET with retinal differentiation
   f. PNET with mesenchymal differentiation
   g. PNET with melanocytic differentiation
   h. PNET with differentiation along multiple lines

2. Medulloepithelioma
3. Atypical teratoid-rhabdoid tumor
E. Pineal cell tumors
II. Tumors with meningeal and related issues
A. Meningiomas
1. Epithelial meningiomas
2. Anaplastic meningiomas
B. Meningeal sarcoma
C. Melanocytic tumors
III. Tumors of nerve sheath cells
A. Neurilemmoma (schwannoma, neurinoma)
B. Neurofibroma
1. Neurofibrosarcoma
IV. Primary malignant lymphoma
V. Tumors of blood vessel origin
A. Hemangioblastoma
B. Hemangiopericytoma
C. Hemangiosarcoma
VI. Germ cell tumors
A. Germinoma
B. Embryonal carcinoma
C. Choriocarcinoma
D. Endodermal sinus tumor
E. Teratomous tumors
   1. Immature teratoma
   2. Mature teratoma
   3. Teratocarcinoma
F. Mixed
VII. Malformative tumors
A. Craniopharyngiomas
B. Rathke's cleft cyst
C. Epidermal cyst
D. Dermoid cyst
E. Colloid cyst of third ventricle
F. Enterogenous or bronchial cyst
G. Cyst , NOS
H. Lipoma
I. Granular cell tumor (choristoma)
J. Hamartoma
1. Neuronal
2. Glial
3. Neuroglial
4. Meningoangioneuromatosis
VIII. Tumors of neuroendocrine origin (pituitary adenomas, paragangliomas)
IX. Local extension from regional tumors
X. Metastatic tumors

children in contrast to a lower percent in adults (25%). About 38 percent of all childhood posterior fossa tumors were constituted by medulloblastomas. (courtesy- Prof Chitra Sarkar, Neuropathology). This is unlike the western literature, where cerebellar astrocytomas were reported to be the most common posterior fossa tumor. The other posterior fossa tumors seen in pediatric population in our series included ependymomas (8%), acoustic neurinomas (6%), meningiomas (1%), hemangioblastomas (1%) and other uncommon tumors constituting 7 percent.

CLINICAL APPROACH TO POSTERIOR FOSSA TUMORS IN CHILDREN

Posterior fossa tumors constitute a major chunk of neoplasms seen in pediatric age group, hence it is important that the referring or the treating physician has a proper perspective to localize them clinically. Following clinical examination it is important to ascertain: (i) whether it arises from the cerebellar or brainstem neuraxis, (ii) whether the tumor is situated cerebellar hemispheric region or in the midline. The clinical features of the brainstem neoplasms are described in the next section.

The clinical features of cerebellar tumors though give a fairly good localization but are not specific to point out the pathology. These are related to the symptomatology due to obstructive hydrocephalus, midline posterior fossa mass lesions and cerebellar hemispheric mass lesions. Obstructive hydrocephalus gives rise to headache, vomiting and lethargy, which occur early in the course of illness, usually not more than 2 months after its onset.[17] A typical symptom of raised intracranial pressure in children is constipation, which occurs as the child is reluctant to strain while passing stools. In some cases severe vomiting may present itself as marasmus/ chronic dehydration which is resistant to all forms of treatment. Ependymomas have been described to present with vomiting as one of its early symptoms due to its origin from the area postrema. The features of raised pressure on examination include papilledema, bilateral 6th nerve paresis and neck stiffness. Bilateral 6th cranial nerve paresis is a common sign of raised intracranial pressure ('false localizing sign') and occurs due to its long intracranial course and also due to its stretching over the petrous due to cranio-caudal herniation ("being pulled like the reins of a horse"). Neck stiffness occurs due to tonsillar herniation and some children may present with ophisthotonic posturing.

Midline cerebellar signs are difficult to detect in infants and children. Midline tumors include medulloblastomas, astrocytomas and more uncommonly ependymomas. An important finding is deterioration in motor milestones and refusal of the child to perform any motor activity. Most often a child with gait disturbance with cerebellar signs will often refuse to walk rather try to walk and then fall down. Other clinical features include a gaze-evoked nystagmus. Here the patient will develop a jerky nystagmus with fast and slow components. The slow component is in the direction of the gage with the fast corrective component in the opposite direction. Usually the nystagmus is horizontal but there may be an added rotational component if the vestibular nuclei are involved. Older children usually present with classical signs of gait ataxia, dysmetria, finger nose incoordination and dysdiadokinesia. Atypical presentations may be observed in some 10 percent of cases[17] of medulloblastomas and include only increasing head size in infants, meningeal signs due to subarachnoid seedling, presentation as a catastrophic intratumoral hemorrhage, or with features of spinal cord or cauda equina compression[27]

Cerebellar hemispheric tumors present with unilateral cerebellar signs consisting of dysmetria, dysdiadochokinesia, past pointing and rebound phenomenon involving the limbs. These features are more noticeable on the side of tumor involvement. When the tumor extends to the midline patients develop features of truncal ataxia, nystagmus and dysarthria. These features are once again seen in older children. Infants and younger children usually present with decreased spontaneous motor activity on the affected side. Astrocytomas are the commonest cerebellar hemispheric tumors. Uncommonly medulloblastomas may also occur in the cerebellar hemisphere (especially the desmoplastic variant). The clinical features of astrocytomas are usually characterized by an indolent picture with several months history of episodic headache and vomiting. Indeed, in most children the diagnosis is made usually 5 to 18 months after the onset of symptoms. In some cases the recognition of the tumor is made in older children and adolescents, who present with macrocrania, delayed milestones, late acquisition of standing ability and, uncertain gait. Often, these patients have been already evaluated by a number of physicians before being referred to a neurosurgeon. Classically, the patients are usually well preserved unlike the patients with medulloblastomas. They present with a long history of headaches and vomiting.

Following this appraisal of clinical features, each of the common posterior foassa tumors are discussed in terms of epidemiology, etiopathogenesis, pathology, neuroimaging and management. Lastly the surgical approaches are described in brief.

MEDULLOBLASTOMA

Medulloblastoma is a posterior fossa tumor composed of malignant embryonal tissue that occurs primarily in the childhood.[7] This has been described as a specific entity by Bailey and Cushing more than 70 years ago.[16] There have been significant advances during the past 20 years, and the average survival period has steadily increased.

Epidemiology and Etiology

Medulloblastoma is one of the common intracranial tumors of the childhood, accounting for 15 to 20 percent of central nervous system neoplasms and for about one-third of posterior fossa tumors in the pediatric population (< 15 years).[17] The incidence of this tumor is about six per million per year. Males are affected more than females. Seventy-five percent of the cases are observed in childhood, with median at diagnosis of 9 years. Analysis of our data on brain tumors (Neuroscience's center, AIIMS), over a 10 year period (n= 3545, 1989-1999) showed that medulloblastomas accounted for 5 percent (181/1030) of all intracranial tumors. They were the commonest posterior fossa tumor in the pediatric age group. About 38 percent (112/ 296, total no. of posterior fossa tumors in the pediatric age group=296) of all childhood posterior fossa tumors were constituted by medulloblastomas (Courtesy: Prof Chitra Sarkar, Neuropathology). This is in contrast to most of the western literature , where cerebellar astrocytomas were reported to be the most posterior fossa tumor.

Etiological Factors

These are not clearly understood, even though rare cases of tumors occurring within the same family or even in siblings have been described. Association of medulloblastoma with various congenital anomalies like ataxia telangectasia,[22] Rubinstein-Taybi syndrome,[23] and Gorlin syndrome[24] have been reported. Studies on genetic factors are under development. The most significant cytogenetic abnormality found to date is an isochromosome 17q in 30 percent of cases.[25] This anomaly has been associated with poor prognosis. Loss of function of the tumor suppressor gene p53 located on the short arm of the chromosome 17, which has been implicated in the genesis of several malignancies does not seem to occur in medulloblastomas.[26]

Pathology

Medulloblastomas are thought to develop from residual neuroectodermal cells of the median and posterior velum of the vermis or from the external granular layer of cerebellar cortex. In children the tumor almost always arises in the vermis and fills the fourth ventricle.[17] They are included in the group of primitive neuroectodermal tumors (PNET). *Macroscopically*, the tumor is frequently pink-gray in color, soft, homogenous, and sometimes cystic or hemorrhagic. *Microscopically* the tumor is by presence of densely cellular lesions that have a intense overall blue color on routine H and E staining. The classic appearance is characterized by dense population of small, round, deeply basophilic nuclei without much perceptible surrounding cytoplasm. Nuclear size and configuration may vary from small to medium. Mitotic activity is variable and cell necrosis is common. Homer Wright rosettes are commonly seen. The various histological patterns include desmoplastic variant, neuroblastic variant, PNET with ependymal rosettes, PNET with astrocytic differentiation, PNET with melanin bearing cells and PNET with striated or smooth muscle differentiation.[15]

Medulloepitheliomas are found exclusively in infants and children and said to be the most primitive of all CNS tumors. The tumor is highly cellular with very little stroma.[12] Both the biology and nosology is much debated but some authors have categorized it into the PNET group.

Neuroimaging

CT scan and MR imaging have radically changed the diagnosis and localization of posterior fossa tumors.

CT scan is the basic procedure for evaluation. It is still the single most investigation before surgical intervention particularly in our country where most of the patients cannot afford MR imaging. Typically, this shows a well defined, midline located tumor filling the fourth ventricle. Most frequently, the tumor is hyperdense and enhances markedly on contrast administration.[27, 28] Less frequently, the tumor is isodense on plain scans and enhances moderately on contrast. Sometimes a cap of CSF may be seen encircling the tumor ventrally indicating its intraventricular location. Atypical features include areas of hemorrhage, necrosis, and cystic changes.[29]

MR imaging has become the standard in the diagnosis of brain tumors. It provides much more superior anatomic features necessary for surgical procedures and can screen the spine as well for 'drop metastasis'. The image generally appears hypointense on T1-weighted images. On proton density images, the tumor becomes brilliant and homogenous[30] (Fig. 38.2). On contrast injection (gadolinium-diethylenetriame penta-acetic acid-DTPA), the tumor becomes brilliantly enhanced. Occasionally, they appear heterogeneous on MR imaging, with areas of cystic degeneration, and central necrosis. These features portend a poorer prognosis and may be present in 10 percent of cases.[30] Other 'atypical' features include calcification and eccentric location and lack of contrast enhancement. However, all these features are not specific to medulloblastomas.

Recently, magnetic resonance spectroscopy (MRS) has been used to give further information concerning some metabolites of cerebral tissue (choline, creatine, N-acetyl-aspartate). The ratios of these metabolites are disrupted in pediatric brain tumors, generally demonstrating a high choline peak. However, the accuracy of these techniques does exceed 80 percent.[31] Using neural networks, the accuracy of the diagnosis may further be increased to 96 percent.[32]

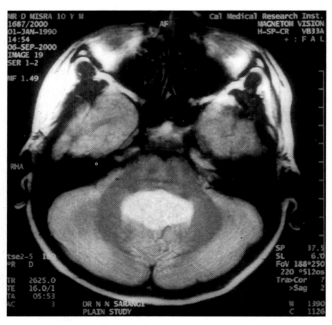

Figure 38.2: MR imaging T1 sequence showing a medulloblastoma

Surgical Management

To '*shunt or not to shunt*' remains a controversial factor in management of hydrocephalus in medulloblastomas. Abraham and Chandy[33] were the first to advocate a preoperative shunt operation for patients with posterior fossa tumors. Ever since there have been a number of papers dealing with the advantages and disadvantages of performing a shunt before definitive surgery.[34-38] The disadvantages of preoperative shunting however include shunt infection, caudo-cranial transtentorial herniation, subdural hematoma and trans shunt metastasis.[36-39] At the same time it is not usual to find patients in our country who present with severe hydrocephalus, in a compromised condition, with dehydration and a poor nutritional status. It may not be an unwise decision in such cases to perform a shunt first, and then subject the patient to tumor surgery once his general condition improves. More so, performing the surgery electively especially for large tumors, allows the surgeon to use all the advantages of an elective theatre like use of special instruments (ultrasonic aspirator, etc), preparing the blood bank for massive transfusions if necessary and performing the surgery with a more refreshed mind. Thus, the patients particularly in a developing country like ours are best managed by individual assessment.

Staging Procedure and Prognostic Factors

For children with medulloblastoma, careful and accurate staging is essential at diagnosis. The procedure includes an early postoperative contrast enhanced cranial CT scan or MR imaging, lumbar cerebrospinal fluid cytology (not later than 15 to 20 days after surgery), and spinal MRI. All this data allows the determination of individual prognostic factors and accordingly the patients may be assigned to '*low*' or '*high*' risk groups, and then treated appropriately.[17,26,37,39,40] Many prognostic factors have been proposed over a number of years. Presence of large tumor size (tumor filling the whole of the fourth ventricle and extending through the foramen of Luschka, Magendie and also through the aqueduct), subtotal or partial resection, presence of metastasis (either within the neuaxis or rarely outside the CNS) and age of presentation being less than 1 year are the classic adverse factors.[26,41-43] The size of the tumor is a relative adverse factor, being largely determined by the extent of surgical resection. During the last decade, biological factors have been proposed to determine the prognosis. These include ploidy,[44] isochromosome 17q,[45] amplification of the c-myc oncogene,[46] or neural cell adhesion molecule levels in cerebrospinal fluid.[47]

Adjuvant Therapy

Radiotherapy has moderate efficacy against medulloblastomas.[48] Postoperative craniospinal irradiation at a dose of 35 to 40 Gy with a posterior fossa boost up to 50 to 55 Gy, delivered in 1.8 Gy daily fractions, has become the standard treatment for more than four decades.[49] Before 1970s, the approximate survival for 5 years was 30 percent. With advancement in neuroimaging, microneurosurgical techniques and the adjuvant therapy, the 5-year survival has increased to the range of 50 to 70 percent.[50-52] Local control of the disease is dependent on the dose to the posterior fossa, which must be greater than 50 Gy.[49] Adverse late effects of neuraxis irradiation in children is a major problem. Neurointellectual sequel range from learning disabilities to severe neurocognitive handicaps in about two-thirds of patients who need either special institutional care.[53]

Endocrine dysfunctions are observed in more than half of the long-term survivors who develop various aspects of hypopituitarism. Growth impairment occurs as a result of growth hormone deficiency, and direct damage to vertebral cartilage occurs in about 60 percent of patients usually after 2 years of irradiation.[54] Other dysfunctions include precocious puberty, hypo-gonadism, hypothyroidism and hypocorticism though are less frequent have been reported.[55,56] Various authors have tried to avoid these complications by subjecting the patients to lesser amount of radiation (25-35 Gy) or by using fractionated therapy.[57] Radiosurgery for patients with medulloblastomas have been also reported but seems to be limited at the moment. It has been used as a technique for boosting sites of residual tumor, but it cannot be recommended as a single salvage procedure.[58]

Chemotherapy has been shown to be sensitive to medulloblastomas both *in vivo* and *in vitro*. In the middle 70's two large prospective multi-institutional studies undertaken (CCSG in United States[59] and SIOP I in Europe[60]) have shown an improvement in disease free survival rate in children with 'high-risk' disease, with use of vincristine and CCNU. Another study a further advantage by adding cisplatin to this regimen.[42] The role of use of chemotherapy for 'low-risk' disease is however still controversial.[42] A major advantage of chemotherapy that has been proposed is reduction of whole brain radiation either preceding or following radiotherapy. Some studies have shown a 70 percent disease-free survival rates at 5 years using this regimen.[61,62]

Outcome

The duration of survival of medulloblastomas has significantly improved over the past two decades. This has been mainly due to the dramatic improvement in the microneurosurgical techniques, improvement in neuroimaging, and introduction of newer adjuvant therapies. The 5-year survival has steadily improved from a dismal 0.5 percent in the early sixties[63] to a 60 to 70 percent survival presently.[50-52,61,62] Long-term survivals have been reported in isolated cases (Bailey-19 years,[64] Penfield-24 years[65]). We have had a case surviving without recurrence for more than 17 years (personal communication: Prof P.N. Tandon). A number of authors believe that *Collin's law*[66] is applicable to medulloblastomas. The rule states that the period of risk of recurrence is equal to the age at presentation plus 9 months of gestational age. Survival beyond this period of risk, represents a presumed curve. However, this rule is not infallible and recurrences have been reported beyond the period of risk.[67] Recurrence is usually at the original site or along the cerebrospinal pathways, frequently in the spinal subarachnoid space. A child operated for a medulloblastoma may present several years later, with back pain and radiculopathy. MR imaging will reveal 'drop' metastasis encasing the roots.[51]

CEREBELLAR ASTROCYTOMA

These tumors, among tumors of glial type, hold a special concern to the pediatric neurosurgeon. Nearly 90 percent of cerebellar astrocytoma are low-grade tumors which tend not recur when excised completely. About two-third of these tumors occur in children and adoloscents.[68] Thus in majority of the cases the surgical management is a highly rewarding experience.

The *incidence* of these tumors as stated in the literature, in children account for 5 to 6 percent of all,[69-72] 20 percent of all pediatric central nervous system tumors[69-72] and 30 to 40 percent of all tumors in the posterior fossa.[69-72] Our own analysis showed that of the 296 pediatric fossa tumors studied from 1989 to 1999, about 26 percent of these were pilocytic astrocytomas and 14 percent were grade II, III, or IV astrocytomas. This is in contrast to the adult posterior fossa tumors in adults (n = 1030) where only 11 percent were pilocytic astrocytomas and 6 percent were astrocytomas of other grades (Prof Chitra Sarkar, dept of Neuropathology, AIIMS).

These tumors occur predominantly in early life, but are rare in neonates infants. The peak incidence occurs between 6 and 9 years of age with a second peak in the young adulthood.[69,70] There is usually no sex preponderence.[70]

Pathological Features

Macroscopically, cerebellar astrocytomas are characterized by discrete, circumscribed and well demarcated masses. However, in spite of their gross appearance these tumors may extend into the surrounding white matter for some distance. The infiltrative capability of pilocytic astrocytomas is more limited than fibrillary variant, although they tend to extend more easily into the perivascular spaces. More than three-quarters of astrocytomas have a cystic component (usually the pilocytic type), which acquires a huge size in nearly half of cases. The fluid within the cystic component is yellow or brown in color due to its high protein content. Hemorrhages within the tumor is very rare. In some cases, there is a presence of mural nodule to one side. In such cases, this is the only neoplastic component that is left, and is characterized by easy bleeding due to abnormally high vascularity. In about one fifth of cases, the tumor is grossly solid (usually the fibrillary type), predominantly located in the midline and with less demarcated boundaries with the surrounding parenchyma.[12,21,73,74] The more malignant lesions are characterized by ill defined, ill demarcated lesions with associated edema. Histologically, the gliomas could pilocytic (juvenile), fibrillary, and less commonly anaplastic or malignant. The pilocytic variety ahs the best prognosis and are categorized as Grade I in the WHO classification, the fibrillary variety being in the Grade II.

Imaging

Findings on imaging are dependent on macroscopic appearance due to variable combination of solid and cystic components. Generally, for *pilocytic astrocytomas* three main patterns are recognized: (i) large cystic tumor with solid mural nodule; (ii) solid tumor with cystic areas; (iii) cystic tumor surrounded by thick neoplasm rim. The *fibrillary type* is generally characterized as ill- defined mass lesions. The anaplastic astrocytomas are ill-defined heterogeneous mass lesions with surrounding edema.

CT scan: The *pilocytic astrocytomas* are characterized by well defined lesions. The cystic areas are usually hypodense. The solid component is iso-hypodense. Calcifications are unusual. Following contrast injection, there is an intense homogenous enhancement of the solid tumor. Often, the pericystic area also enhances indicating neoplastic tissue. In the *fibrillary astrocytomas*, the tumor is characterized by an ill-defined homogenous enhancement which, usually does not enhance with contrast. Calcifications are seen in about 10 to 20 percent. In *anaplastic and malignant varieties*, the tumor is characterized by a greater degree of heterogeneity and edema.[75-77]

MR imaging: As in CT scan, the *pilocytic astrocytomas* are well defined masses. The cystic content exhibits a variable signal due to protein concentration ranging from iso to hyperintense (Fig. 38.3). Solid components are hypointense in T1 sequences, becoming hyperintense on T2 weighted sequences and shows homogenous enhancement after injection with gadolinium contrast. The *fibrillary type* ill-defined homogenous lesions, hypointense on T1 and hyperintense on T2, showing either no or patchy enhancement. The *anaplastic or malignant* variants have same picture as the fibrillary type, but show patchy enhancement and have marked perilesional edema, better seen on T2 weighted sequence.[77,78]

MR Spectroscopy are being used more recently. They have been performed more for pilocytic astrocytomas and exhibit decreased creatinine choline and N-acetylasparatate/ choline ratios and increased lactate.[31]

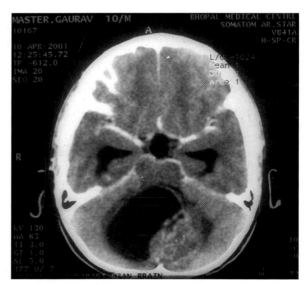

Figure 38.3: MR imaging, T1 sequence showing evidence of a cystic astrocytoma in the posterior fossa

Management

The ideal treatment of cerebellar astrocytomas is total microsurgical excision. In the cystic variety, the cyst wall should be excised completely, unless it is adherent to the brainstem. The solid tumors should also be excised completely. There is hardly any role for radiotherapy except for the uncommon malignant variety. The details of operative surgery will be dealt in detail in a separate section.

Prognosis

Patients who undergo total excision of a benign cerebellar astrocytoma can except long-term relapse-free survival in 80 to 100 percent[79,80] of cases. The prognosis of patients who undergo subtotal or partial tumor removal is more difficult to establish, as some authors emphasize the possibility of long-term survival in these cases, whereas others stress the high risk of recurrence and advocate reoperation or adjuvant therapy. Regular imaging is essential regularly (initially for every 6 months, later every year for 5 years) to look for any recurrence. In patients, who could not undergo total excision, it is preferable to perform a reoperation. However, some surgeons prefer to regularly follow-up these patients and subject them to surgery or adjuvant therapy only when there is radiological evidence of regrowth.[81,82] Malignant transformation of these tumors on long term follow-up though uncommon is a definite possibilty.[82]

EPENDYMOMAS

These uncommon tumors are derived from and have the appearance of differentiated ependymal cells. They arise from the ependymal cells lining the ventricles. They arise most commonly from the posterior fossa in the pediatric age. They have been described to occur in younger patients, with nearly 50 percent presenting in children less than 3 years of age.[83] However, our own study shown that a majority of the patients were in the older age group at about 4 years of age. Pediatric ependymomas constituted about 50 percent of all patients.[84] Our series have shown a higher male preponderance (1: 1.3), contrary to what described in the literature. *On gross inspection*, these tumors are multicystic, hemorrhagic and calcified; not surprisingly these features are typified on imaging.[83] The microscopic appearance is characterized by formation of typical pseudorosettes. Most often the cell processes attach themselves to the adventitia of the vessel. Nuclei tend to have a monotonous character and mitotic activity is variable.

CT scan or MR imaging usually corroborates with the above gross findings. CT will show a iso-hyperdense within the posterior fossa, with areas of calcification (seen in about 45% of the cases) enhancing heterogeneously on contrast. the tumor is intraventricular in location characterized by a cap of CSF on the posterior and the lateral aspects. MR imaging will show a tumor isointense on T1 becoming hyperintense on T2 sequence. Enhancement with contrast is almost always seen, though heterogeneously. The anatomic details are more clearly made out on MR imaging. The major point of distinction is that these tumors arising from the floor of the fourth ventricle, cannot be differentiated from it. Surgical approach is similar to medulloblastomas, however a thin lining of tumor tissue should be left along the floor of the floor ventricle to avoid damage to the brainstem.

We have studied about 33 intracranial ependymomas over a period of 5 years (1994-1998) of which 22 were infratentorial in location. Total excision of the tumor was performed in 25 (76%) patients and a subtotal excision was performed for other 8 cases. This was mainly due to the fact that the tumor was adherent to the floor of the brainstem and a thin rim of tumor was removed on the surface. This technique is better than to attempt a total excision, which may result in serious morbidity.[84]

Although radiotherapy has a significant impact on survival, controversy still exists on the dose and the extent. Generally 50 to 55 Gy over the primary site is recommended spaced over 5-6 weeks. Higher doses may be needed for patients with higher grade tumors. Chemotherapy (CCNU based) is especially indicated for infants and younger children.[85] Prophylactic craniospinal irradiation is usually not indicated except for anaplastic ependymomas and ependymoblastomas.[86-88]

The *outcome* depends on several factors, the most important being the extent of surgical excision and the adjuvant therapy given.[87] In addition our study showed that strong positivity with cell marker-proliferative cell nuclear antigen (PCNA) had a linear correlation with the duration of survival.[84] Sutton et al studied 80 patients with ependymomas and reported 51 percent, 5 year progression free survival (PFS), in patients who have had total excision as compared to 21 percent of PFS in patients with incomplete resection.[87] The five year survival in the literature has varied from 16 to 58 percent.[87,88] In our series follow-up data was available for 18 patients who were doing well at a mean follow-up of 34 months.[84]

Other posterior fossa tumors: Other posterior fossa tumors are uncommonly seen in children. In our study of the 296 patients of posterior fossa tumors studied in children, acoustic neurinomas were seen in about 6 percent of cases and meningioms and haemangioblastomas were seen in less than 1 percent of cases each. This is unlike in adults, where these are common tumors (Courtesy: Prof Chitra Sarkar, Neuropathology).

SURGICAL APPROACHES FOR POSTERIOR FOSSA TUMORS

Most cerebellar tumors may be approached through a prone position. This position minimizes the risk of air embolism seen more commonly in children, especially in sitting position.[89-92]

In patients who have associated hydrocephalus, an occipital burr hole for draining the ventricle. The skin incision is given starting from the inion to the midcervical region. The muscles are split in the midline along the white line. The occipital bone and the C1 spinous process is exposed. A craniectomy of size 5 cm × 5 cm is usually sufficient. Once the dura is opened the margins of the dura is hitched open with stitches. Brain swelling in the posterior fossa should be avoided at all costs. If the brain is tense before dural opening, then the CSF should drained from the ventricles through a parieto-occipital burr hole and also from the cerebellomedullary cisterns. This would make the brain more lax and aids in tumor dissection. The tumor is identified next. If it's a *midline tumor* like medulloblastoma or ependymoma the tumor may not be seen on the surface, but indirect evidence may be present in form of widening of the vermis, flattening of the sulci over its surface, and presence of 'yellowish' deposits over the surface of the brainstem. The tumor may be now approached in two ways, either through the foramen of magendie- "the trans-foraminal route" or splitting through the vermis—"the trans-vermian route." Most of the tumors, even the very large ones may be approached through the foramen of magendie (trans-foraminal route), the tonsils and the vermis may be just separated by self retaining retractors. It is rarely required to split the vermis, i.e. through the "trans-vermian route." In most of the cases, the tumor can be separated from the floor completely. In tumors like ependymomas, the tumor would be arising from the floor of the fourth ventricle, and it is preferable to remove a thin layer on the floor rather than to attempt total excision to prevent serious morbidity.

In hemispheric tumors like cerebellar astrocytomas, the tumor is usually visualized on the surface. If the tumor is deep seated, indirect evidence in form of widening of the gyri or obliteration of sulci may be found. A preoperative ultrasound may also be used to locate the tumor. The principles of tumor removal is same the same. In cystic tumors like pilocytic astrocytomas, the cytic is decompressed first. Following this the mural nodule is identified and then excised. This is often quite vascular and sometimes may be confused for the nodule of cystic hemangioblastoma, though it is quite uncommon in pediatric age group. It is also essential to excise the wall of the cavity as it often contains tumor tissue.[90-92]

BRAINSTEM GLIOMAS

Brainstem gliomas constitute about 1-4 percent of all intracranial gliomas.[93] They comprise about 10 to 20 percent of all intracranial procedures in children and comprise 25 to 30 percent of all posterior fossa tumors in the pediatric age group.[94-96] In our study they constituted 2.18 percent of all intracranial tumors (Jan 1983 to march 1997, Neurosurgery dept, AIIMS).[97] These are treacherous lesions, which, unfortunately involve the pediatric age group. Our study showed a maximum involvement between 6 and 10 years of age.[97] This is concordance with the figures quoted in the literature, though a second peak has been reported in the fourth decade of life.[97-100] These tumors were initially considered inoperable, but with advent of modern neuroimaging and microneurosurgical techniques there has been a dramatic change in the management of these tumors.

Pathologic Features

Most astrocytomas of the brainstem are infiltrative tumors fibrillary type, similar to diffuse cerebral astrocytomas. Macroscopically, they are usually characterized by a symmetrical enlargement of the pons (diffuse hypertrophy). The expanding structure encroaches posteriorly and superiorly upon the fourth ventricle. Occasionally, there may be anterior enlargement. The medulla is often spared. Sometimes, however it originates from medulla and may spread to the upper cervical region.[101] *Histologically,* there is a diffuse replacement of nervous tissue by small and large astrocytic cells, stellate, pilocytic, and gemistocytic either randomly dispersed or arranged in smaller or larger groups. These morphologic diversity reflects the cellular heterogeneity even in absence of anaplasia. In some cases there may frank features of anaplasia, necrosis and endothelial proliferation as seen in glioblastoma multiformes.[101]

Depending on the macroscopic appearance, the brain stem gliomas have been divided into the following categories:[98-100,102]

1. *Diffuse:* This is a 'stereotype' of brainstem tumors that have been recognized since the beginning of neurosurgery. These neoplasms present with a short history and present with multiple cranial nerve palsies along with involvement of long tracts. MR imaging is virtually diagnostic of these lesions. The tumor is invariably malignant and the only form of therapy advisable is radiotherapy or chemotherapy. Surgery is not indicated. Even stereotactic biopsy is not advised as the procedure may cause additional morbidity, and the biopsy may not contain representative tissue.

2. *Focal:* These more commonly involve the medulla and is often associated with a relatively long clinical history. Neurological usually reveal focal deficits, i.e. either a sixth or seventh nerve palsy. These neoplasms are commonly low-grade astrocytomas and are amenable for surgical excision.

3. *Cervicomedullary tumors:* These are invariably low-grade astrocytomas and gangliogliomas and amenable to radical excision.

4. *Cystic tumors:* These are usually low-grade pilocytic astrocytomas and highly amenable for surgical excision (Figs 38.4A and B).

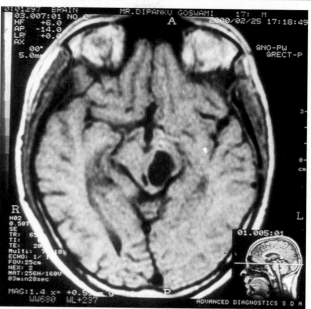

Figure 38.4B: After surgery. These lesions are completely amenable to surgery, but require the expertise of a surgeon who has enough experience in the field

5. *Exophytic tumors:* These tumors are characterized by exophytic growth either ventrally, laterally into the cerebellopontine angle or dorsally into the fourth ventricle. Of these, the dorsally exophytic tumors have the best prognosis, are amenable for radical excision and is associated with long-term neurological recovery (Fig. 38.5). The other variants have a poor prognosis.

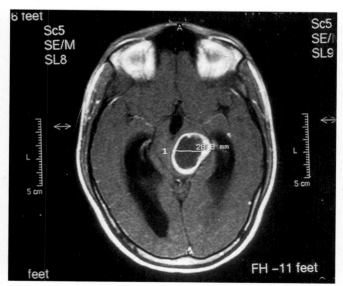

Figure 38.4A: MR imaging showing a focal cystic tumor in the midbrain, Fig. 38.4A Before surgery, note the intense enhancement of the wall with contrast

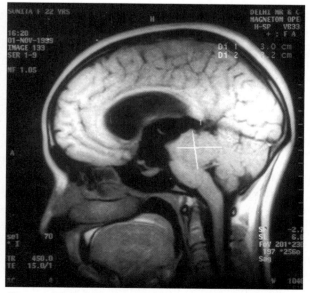

Figure 38.5: MR image, sagittal section, T1 sequence showing a dorsally exophytic brainstem tumor

6. *Tectal plate gliomas:* These are uncommon in the pediatric age group. The main presenting feature is hydrocephalus. These are diagnosed on MR imaging with gadolinium contrast and are managed by performing a ventriculoperitoneal shunt.[103] These may be simply followed up and if they increase in size may be subjected to radiotherapy. Radiosurgery has been also used recently. Endoscopic third ventriculostomy or aqueductal stenting may be a better alternative to a shunt surgery.

Clinical Features

These are characterized by an insidious onset, but a short course of illness. Vomiting is a common symptom and is usually due to involvement of area postrema and the other medullary nuclei by the tumor. Ataxia is usually due to involvement of cerebral peduncles. Motor weakness due to involvement of pyramidal tracts is common. Extra-occular movement palsy is characterized by squint usually noticed by parents or school teachers. Additional signs include nystagmus, skew deviation, and internuclear ophthalmoplegia.[97,98,100,102] The latter sign is a hallmark of intrinsic brainstem involvement characterized by failure to adduct the eye on the side of the lesion and presence of nystagmus on abducting the eye on the opposite side. This occurs due to the involvement of medial longitudinal fasciculus. Other signs of cranial nerve involvement include facial weakness, dysarthria, and swallowing difficulties. Features of raised intracranial pressure may occur due to obstruction of CSF pathways. Uncommonly, focal intrinsic tumors from the tectum can cause obstruction early in the course of illness.[103] The following features are characteristic of an intrinsic brainstem neoplasm: (i) Internuclear ophthalmoplegia; (ii) Horner's syndrome; (iii) cranial nerve involvement with crossed motor involvement, e.g. ipsilateral third nerve paresis with contralateral hemiparesis (Weber's syndrome); (iv) Combination of certain cranial nerve nuclei e.g. 6th and 7th cranial involvement on one side indicates an intrinsic pathology. This is because the 7th nerve fibres loop around the 6th nerve nuclei within the brain stem (internal genu); (v) Presence of nuclear type of third nerve paresis, i.e. bilateral superior rectus palsy, bilateral levator superioris palsy or a complete third nerve paresis on one side with one of or more of the previous findings in the other eye. This occurs due to complex and large size of the third nerve nuclei and involvement of only one of the components by the tumor. In our series[97] headache was the most common feature (78%), followed by cranial nerve paresis in 65 percent of cases. Other features include papilledema (46%), cerebellar signs (65%) and motor involvement in 68 percent of cases.

Neuroimaging

CT scans are uncommonly used for diagnosis. MR imaging is virtually diagnostic and is also useful for planning surgery. CT scan usually shows an hypodense areas within the brain-stem with expansion of the brain-stem. The lesion usually does not enhance or partly enhances with contrast. MR imaging is always essential not only for diagnosis, but also for planning surgery. In diffuse lesions, the entire brain-stem is found to be expanded and MR imaging is diagnostic. In focal lesions, there will be a discrete lesion in the brain-stem, usually hypo to isointense on T1 sequence and hyperintense on T2 sequence. The tumor usually enhances well with contrast. The cystic lesions do not take up contrast (Figs 38.4A and B). There are very few differential diagnosis, however arterio-venous malformations and cavernous malformations have to be kept in mind.[93,96-98,100,102]

Management

The diffuse tumors carry the worst prognosis and the survival is usually not more than 18 months after diagnosis. Parts of the tumor may start off as a fibrillary astrocytoma but by the time of death, usually the entire tumor is either a malignant astrocytoma or a glioblastoma multiforme. Thus a stereotactic biopsy is totally unreliable for diagnosis, while the imaging characteristics are almost diagnostic of this dreadful condition.[104] These patients may be directly subjected to radiotherapy. The type of radiotherapy is undergoing a change. The standard therapy has been 55 Gy to the tumor area with weekly dose of 800 to 1000 cGy. In hyper-fractionated therapy, higher doses up to 76 Gy may be tolerated and has improved short-term survival without obvious toxicity.[105]

The surgical indications for brain-stem gliomas include focal, cystic, dorsally exophytic, and cervico-medullary tumors. The focal solid tumors are managed by surgery alone, without radiotherapy, particularly when a complete excision has been performed.[104] The patient needs to be followed up with regular neuroimaging. The patients with focal cystic tumors may undergo decompression of the cyst, which is fairly an easy procedure. However, focal radiotherapy may be required to prevent recollection of the cyst. In patients with dorsally exophytic tumors, decompression may be carried out till the tumor is shaved off flush with the floor of fourth ventricle. It is advisable to remove a thin carpet of tumor on floor to prevent serious morbidity. A large number of patients with low-grade astrocytomas and gangliogliomas will have a good outcome.[102-104] The uncommon type of "tectal plate" gliomas may be managed by shunt alone with regular follow-up neuroimaging.[103-104] Recently, we have performed aqueductal endoscopic stenting and simultaneous biopsy of the lesion for this condition with satisfactory results (unpublished).

Surgical Approaches

Most of the brainstem gliomas may be approached through a midline suboccipital craniectomy as described for the posterior fossa tumors. Only the ventrally exophytic or laterally situated tumors will require an approach through the cerebellopontine angle. In these tumors, it is essential to have a good view of the floor of the fourth ventricle. The surgery is performed under the operating microscope. Once the tumor is identified, adequate biopsy should be obtained. Internal decompression should be performed before attempting excision.[106] Special instruments like micro-CUSA may be used to assist excision. Intraoperative brainstem evoked potentials may be used to monitor the patient intra-operatively.

PINEAL REGION TUMORS

Pineal region tumors represent 3 to 8 percent of all intracranial tumors in children.[106] These tumors are difficult to access due to the anatomic considerations, close proximity to the deep venous system, and the brain-stem. In our own series these tumors represented the entire range of posterior third ventricular tumors represented 0.8 percent of all intracranial tumors (a total of 50 tumors of 6300 intracranial tumors operated between May 1989- May1999). Of these 15 patients were in the pediatric age group.[107] The management of pineal region tumors has undergone several significant changes since Dandy's initial effort to approach them surgically. The high complication rates by the initial surgeries, lead many physicians to abandon surgery and subject the patients directly to surgery regardless of the histopathology of the tumors.[108]

Pathology

Histologic classification involves three major groups among the pineal region tumors: germ cell tumors, pineal cell tumors and nonspecific tumors.[11] *Primary germ cell tumors* of the nervous system appear mainly in the suprasellar and pineal regions. They represent 50 percent of all pineal tumors. There are five major subtypes: (i) Germinomas; (ii) Embryonal carcinomas, including yolk sac or endodermal sinus tumors, (iii) Choriocarcinomas; (iv) Teratomas: mature and immature; (v) Mixed germ cell tumors. *Germinomas* are the most common type of germ cell tumors. Histologically they contain a combination of large round cells with clear cell borders, eosinophilic cytoplasm and a central nucleus containing a prominent nucleolus along with lymphocytes and plasma cells. Histiocytes are also seen and may form granulomas. Mitotic activity is variable. Immunohistochemical studies may help in distinguishing subtypes of the germ cell tumors. Pure germinomas and mature teratomas have the best prognosis. The former respond to radiotherapy and the latter are best managed by surgical resection.[19,20]

The *pineal cell* tumors arise from the specific pineal cells and represent 20 percent of all pineal tumors. They constitute pinealocytomas or pinealoblastomas. They are further classified into pure pinealocytomas (malignant), astrocytic differentiated pinealocytomas (benign or malignant) and neuronal differentiated pinealocytomas (benign). The other nonspecific tumors represent 30 percent of all the tumors of pineal region which, include low-grade astrocytomas, ependymomas, oligodendrogliomas, and choroid plexus papillomas.[11,109]

Clinical Features

These often progress insidiously often over a period of 4 months. They depend on compression on neighboring structures or are due to obstructive hydrocephalus. The latter is the most common feature seen in about 85 percent of cases.[106] In our own series features of raised intracranial pressure was seen in about 80 percent of cases.[107] Neuro-ophthalmogic features are unique for these group of tumors, and these occur due to compression of the posterior white commissure and pretectal region. This results in *Perinaud's syndrome*, characterized by upward gaze paresis and less commonly others signs like convergence retraction nystagmus, spasm of convergence may also occur. As the tumor expands long tracts like pyramidal and sensory fibers may get affected. Neuroendocrine manifestations are observed frequently and justify a complete endocrine work-up for all the patients. Pre-operative diabetes insipidus is commonly associated with germinomas, and is due to seedling of the tumor to the anterior part of the third ventricle.

Precocious puberty may occur and is due to secretion of B-human chorionic gonadotrophin mainly seen in choriocacarcinomas. Less commonly hypopituitarism, thermoregulatory disorders, abnormal alimentary behavior and jet-lag syndrome may occur.[109-111]

Investigations

Neuroimaging: X-rays which initially played an significant role in diagnosis has now lost much of its importance. This may show 'pressure atrophy' of dorsum sella and posterior clinoids due to hydrocephalus. A pineal calcification of more than 10 mm size in a 10 year old may be highly suspicious of pineal tumor etiology. Similarly presence of pineal tumor calcification below the age of 10 years is highly suspicious of a pineal region tumor.[112]

CT scan with or without contrast makes usually makes the diagnosis. Generally, the tumor is characterized by a well lesion which is iso to hyperdense on plain scans located in the posterior part of the third ventricle. Tumors like germinomas usually enhance brilliantly with contrast. However Zimmermann[113] et al have reported that diagnosis of germ cell tumors on the basis of CT only is not reliable.

MR imaging is very advantageous to define the various characteristics of the tumor but still is ineffective to make an histological diagnosis. Further more with different sequences, three-dimensional MRI, and MR angiography one may evaluate the surgical approaches, extension of tumor and nature of tumor (infiltrative or limited). Germinomas are usually iso-intense on T1 sequences and iso-hyperintense on T2 weighted images, with small cystic areas and without calcification and enhance brilliantly with contrast. Calcification is more common in pineal parenchymal tumors. Similarly presence of hemorrhage may suggest a choriocarcinoma. Non-germinomatous tumors show a mixed signal intensity signals on both T1/T2 sequences.[114] *Digital angiography* or *MR angiography* usually is not necessary except in suspected meningiomas with vascular encasement, angiomas, or aneurysm of vein of Galen.

CSF cytology: This is a very important investigation. The characterization of clusters of two types of cells indicates the probability of germinomas. Analysis of CSF is also a good measure during the follow-up period.[115]

Tumor markers: Radioimmunologic analysis of tumor markers in blood and CSF and immunocytochemistry in tumor tissue are very important for diagnosis and prognosis. There are three essential types of markers: B-hCG for choriocarcinoma (trophoblastic secretion), alpha- fetoprotein (AFP) for endodermal sinus tumors,[115] and placental alkaline phosphatase (PAL) for germinomas[116]. The specific markers for pineal cells still remains in the field of research. Markers like hydroxy-indol-o-methyltransferase (HIOMT), antigen-S are under consideration.[117]

Management

Surgery

The first attempts to remove this tumor was performed by Horsley[118] in 1905. Since then many surgical approaches have been described.[119-123] Presently, only the superior and inferior transtentorial approaches are mostly used. Most of the patients with pineal region tumors have hydrocephalus, and this must be relieved either by a shunt or by third ventriculostomy before surgery. As an alternative an intraventricular drain may be placed before approaching the tumor. The *supracerebellar transtentorial approach* is preferably performed in a 'sitting-slouch' position, unless there are strong contraindications against this approach (age less than 2 years, severe degree of hydrocephalus). The patient should be monitored for air embolism, which include a Doppler probe, end-tidal PCO_2 evaluation and modest positive pressure ventilation. Here a midline suboccipital craniectomy is performed, the dura is opened and the cerebellum is retracted downwards. The surgeon then follows the inferior surface of the tentorium and approaches the posterior third ventricular area.[124-128] The *occipital trans-tentoria (Poppen's approach)l* approach is uncommonly used. Here, an occipital craniotomy is performed, the occipital lobe is then retracted and the falco-tentorial junction is then followed as a guide to reach the posterior third ventricular region.[126-128]

Adjuvant Therapy

The role of preoperative *radiotherapy* is controversial.[129] With the availability of tissue diagnosis, the treatment with radiotherapy will depend on the histological subtype of the tumor. Radiosensitivity is usually good, germinomas being highly radiosensitive. This is to the extent that if the diagnosis could be made on CSF cytology, then radiation may be given directly. They are known to melt like 'butter'. Whole brain radiation with 5500 rads to the area of the tumor is usually recommeded.[129,130] Chemotherapy is increasingly playing an important role in management of these tumors. This is especially so for non-germinomatous tumors. In germinomas which, are highly radiosensitive chemotherapy seems to have a role in recurrent and systemic disease.. Cisplatin seems to be the most effective drug.[131,132]

CRANIOPHARYNGIOMAS

These are benign tumors of epithelial origin that arise in the surprasellar area. Despite its benign histology, these are difficult lesions to treat and despite therapy, the disease may progress leading to progressive deterioration and patients may die of disease. On the other hand, most of these tumors may resected completely and patients may have complete cure. The surgical management remains controversial with some individuals opting for an aggressive approach, while others proposing a more conservative attitude utilizing radiotherapy.

Pathology

The well accepted hypothesis that craniopharyngiomas arise from embryonic squamous cell rests of an incompletely involuted hypophyseal-pharyngeal duct was first proposed by Erdheim. These squamous cell nests lie in the pituitary stalk extending from the tuber cinereum to the pituitary gland. For this reason this tumor is typically adherent to the tuber cinereum and can insinuate itself into the substance of hypothalamus. Elsewhere the tumor is covered with arachnoid, which is easily separable from the tumor along with blood vessels.. If the diaphragma sellae has a large opening, the tumor can invade the pituitary gland as well and enlarge the sella tursica. These tumors are typically cystic. The material in the cyst consists of cholesterol crystals formed from chronic bleeding from the cyst wall. The cyst also always contain calcium deposits which distinguish it from other suprasellar tumors. The cyst walls are composed of columnar or stratified squamous epithelium resting on a collagenous basement membrane which separate the tumor from the surrounding meninges. In the solid portion the epithelial elements are separated by loosely arranged stellate cells, giving rise to adamantinomatous pattern. Thus two morphologic variants rare observed: the adamantimatous and the papillary. Both are observed in adults, but in children the adamantinoma is nearly always present in children. Masses of keratin coalesce into large foci of calcification.[133]

Two theories for craniopharyngiomas have been debated:

1. that the tumor is developed from embryonic remnants of Rathke's pouch and
2. a metaplasia of the cells of adenohypophysis. Immunohistochemical studies have shown that glcoprotein P and human chorionic gonadotrophin are coexpressed.[134,135]

Clinical Features and Clinical Evaluation

Craniopharyngiomas by virtue of their location may produce a combination of neurologic and endocrine symptoms. The main presenting symptoms are visual disturbances. In 70 percent of patients, visual field deficits are present. An inferior temporal quadrantopia may be found in early tumors with compression of the optic chiasm from the superior aspect. This is a point of clinical difference from pituitary adenomas which produce compression over the inferior part of the optic chiasm and produce superior temporal quadrantopia.[135-137] In 50 percent of cases there are features of raised intracranial pressure and papilledema may be in up to 18 percent of patients. The frequency of endocrine manifestations ranges from 25 to 50 percent in pediatric age groups. It is higher in adults (75%). The endocrinopathy are usually those of growth retardation (33%), obesity (25%), diabetes insipidus (20%) and delayed puberty in about 50 percent of patients.[137, 138]

A complete endocrine work-up is mandatory for all patients with craniopharyngiomas. Endocrine deficits are reported as follows: growth hormone (GH): 60 percent, leteinizing hormone/ follicle-stimulating hormone (LH/FSH): 60 percent, adrenocorticotrophic hormone (ACTH): 30 percent, and thyroid hormone (TH) in 30 percent of cases.[137, 138]

Neuroimaging

CT scan and MR imaging are the standard neuroimaging tools. However, MR imaging is the prime imaging tool for imaging. *CT scan* generally a shows a well defined mass in the supra-sellar region. Larger masses would show lobulations with extensions into the lateral, anterior, or supra-sellar compartments. Some tumors may be entirely cystic, but most often there are mixed areas of cystic and solid components. Contrast enhancement is modest on CT scan. CT scan is useful in evaluating changes of bony structures in the skull base and also to detect tumor calcifications. *MR imaging* is presently the gold standard for evaluating the imaging characteristics of craniopharyngiomas. Generally, the tumor is iso-hypo intense on T1 sequences. Presence of fat may be hyperintense on T1 sequence. Fat suppression sequences should be performed in such cases. T2 weighted images show hyper intense images. Contrast administration is necessary, and this shows enhancement of solid component but not the cystic part. An additional advantage of MR imaging is that, it gives an idea about the condition of the surrounding vessels (Fig. 38.6). MR angiography may be also performed wherever necessary.[139-141] Conventional angiography is rarely necessary.

Management

There is abundant controversy among physicians dealing with this type of tumor concerning the choice of treatment for craniopharyngiomas. Most neurosurgeons prefer total excision as the treatment of choice, but in some cases when the tumor is densely adherent to the infundibulum, leaving some portion of tumor and treating the residual tumor with radiotherapy may not be an unwise decision. Other options that have been tried include stereotactic aspiration for cystic craniopharyngiomas with or without intra-cavitory instillation of beta-emitting isotopes or beomycin.[142] Hydrocephalus is a complicating factor found in 15 to 30 percent of craniopharyngioma patients.[143] Management of cases should be individualized. A preoperative shunt placement may be performed for large tumors or in cases where the surgeon is not sure of excising the tumor completely. On the other hand, a single stage tumor excision may treat the hydrocephalus as well.[135]

Surgical Approaches

The optimal approach to these tumors is to be decided by the operating surgeon. It would depend on the size, shape and the direction of projection of the tumor. The two most preferred approaches include the sub-frontal and the pterional approaches (Fig. 38.7). A trans-sphenoidal approach would be required in the occasional intra-sellar tumor. Other routes like trans-callosal/trans-cortical-transventricular[144] (for intra-ventricular tumors), subtemporal[145] (small retrochismatic tumors) and transpetrosal[145] (large retro-chiasmatic tumors with extension along the clivus) approaches are rarely indicated.[135,137,138]

Postoperative management: The most common postoperative complications are related to endocrine disturbances. Diabetes insipidus is common especially after radical excision and may occur in about 70 percent of cases. Most of them subside with treatment. A few cases may require life-long replacement. This may be managed by administration of injectable or nasal desmopressin (DDAVP). Oral carbamazepine is useful in controlling less severe cases. Other endocrine disturbances include GH (95%), TH(90%), ACTH(75%) and LH/FSH in 95 percent of cases. All of these should be treated with replacement therapies. Postoperative

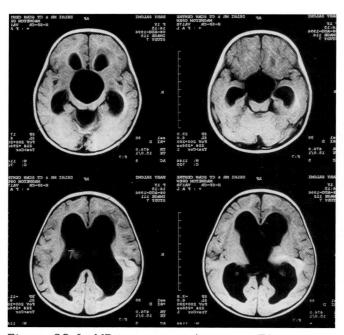

Figure 38.6: MR imaging, axial sections, T1 sequences showing a cystic craniopharyngioma with obstructive hydrocephalus

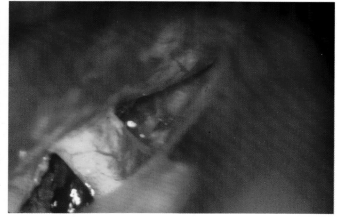

Figure 38.7: Craniopharyngioma as seen through the pterional route. Note the tumor seen lateral to the optic nerve (the white band like structure)

hypothalamic syndromes may occur and these include hypersomnia, temperature dysregulation, profound amnesia, electrolyte and caloric disturbances.[138,146,147]

Radiation Therapy

Radiotherapy has been demonstrated to have a destructive effect on craniopharyngiomas even though the brain parenchyma would be expected to be harmed by doses high to effect the tumor. Radiotherapy is effective for patients who have undergone a subtotal resection,[148] but this is not always true and sometimes these tumors may continue to grow relentlessly and also make any further surgery extremely difficult. Radiosurgery avoids complications of external beam radiation and is useful for small recurrences.[149]

Results

The overall 10-year post-treatment survival rate for craniopharyngiomas is 92.5 percent after total removal and 85.6 percent after subtotal removal. This increases to 90 percent if radiotherapy is combined with subtotal excision.[138]

The quality of life has become more important for these patients. Most of the patients have a worse endocrine status after surgery. About 70 percent of the patients have diabetes insipidus, but this subsides in most of the patients.[138] The figures of other endocrine dysfunction has been already quoted earlier. Neuropsychological abnormalities have been observed in 30 to 60 percent of patients.[138] In one study it has been seen that 88 percent of patients had a normal neuropsychological assessment as compared to 22 percent in cases who received radiotherapy.[150]

OPTIC PATHWAY TUMORS

Primary tumors of the optic pathways occur most commonly in the first two decades of life, peaking during the middle of the first decade. They represent from 0.5 to 5 percent of brain tumors and are not common. There seems to be a predominance of females over males.[151-154]

Pathology

These tumors arise from the astroglia of the optic nerve. Oligodendroglial elements are occasionally present, but neoplastic astrocytic cells are usually the predominant component. Most astrocytomas of the optic nerve are composed of highly elongated astrocytic cells with long,

fine fibrillary processes. Because of this feature they are often called pilocytic astrocytomas, juvenile astrocytomas or piloid astrocytomas. A more detailed description of these tumors has been provided in the earlier section on pathology.

There have been two patterns of growth observed in optic nerve gliomas. In one type the tumor growth has been restricted to the optic nerve with minimal involvement of leptomeninges. In other there is invasion of tumor into the subarachnoid space, often with a marked proliferative fibroblastic response and hyperplasia of meningothelial cells. It has been suggested that the latter type is associated with neurofibromatosis.[151]

Clinical Features and Biological Behavior

The most frequent complaint is visual symptoms and loss of acuity. Proptosis, nystagmus, strabismus, visual field defect, headache, diencephalic syndrome, and hemiparesis may also be observed. Examination usually reveals visual loss, and optic atrophy is common. Typical chiasmal visual field defects are uncommon. Various reports show that about 10-50 percent of patients have features of neurofibromatosis. It is now recognized that patients with neurofibromatosis have an higher incidence for harboring single (58%) or multicentric (100%) optic nerve astrocytomas, while there is a low incidence of neurofibromatosis (9%) in patients with chiasmal glioma.[152] The biological of these tumors has been highly variable especially with reference to the association with neurofibromatosis-I. Earlier reports were equivocal, but the more recent reports have demonstrated a protective effect of neurofibromatosis over optic nerve gliomas.[153] Some of the recent reports have even demonstrated spontaneous regression of these tumors in presence of neurofibromatosis.[154]

Neuroimaging

Skull roentgenography was extensively utilized in the past for the diagnosis. In a J-shaped sella (due to erosion of posterior margin of sphenoid plane) and alterations in the shape and size of optic foramina (size of optic foramen being more than 7 mm in any dimension or a difference of the two foramina being more than 20%) was considered pathognomic of optic pathway neoplasms.[112] CT scan and MR imaging are extremely helpful in diagnosis, however MRI with gadolinium contrast is superior to CT scanning. Saggital oblique MRI with fat suppression technique gives the entire definition of optic nerve from the globe to the chiasm. CT scanning is useful to delineate bone destruction. When the tumor is mainly intracranial CT scan images show a hypodense, less frequently an isodense mass which obliterates partially or completely the prechiasmatic cistern, and the anterior third ventricle. Presence of small cystic areas or specks of calcification, not as common as cranio-pharyngiomas may be seen. Contrast injection usually shows good enhancement, but heterogenously. MR imaging shows excellent anatomic details of the tumor with the surrounding structures. The optic chiasm may be seen thickened and is not seen separately from the tumor. The tumor appears hypo-intense on short TR/TE (T1) sequences, being iso-to-moderately hyper-intense on T2 sequences. Contrast enhancement is variable. The coronal cuts give the best appreciation of the tumor in optic canals, and its relation to optic chiasm and the hyothalamus.[155-157]

Management

The management of optic pathway gliomas reflects the same uncertainties that have been highlighted regarding pathogenesis and biologic behavior. Furthermore, the association of neurofibromatosis-I, which according to many authors should confer a protective effect is certainly another factor to be included when planning any therapeutic modality. In fact many of the tumors associated with NF-I are not treated by many surgeons and are just closely monitored by regular neuroradiologic investigations. However in children without neurofibro-matosis, histologic diagnosis is mandatory in order to ascertain the nature of suprasellar mass, and also because of reported possibility of tumor involution after partial excision or even biopsy.[154,158]

Radiation therapy has been long considered the main, if not the only therapeutic means for treating these tumors. However, there has been a growing criticism due to its deleterious side effects, despite of the fact that many of these tumors responding well to radiotherapy. Intellectual and endocrinologic sequelae have been reported after irradiation to the suprasellar region.[159-162] Chemotherapy, which is the emerging therapeutic modality, has not yet shown sufficient evidence of effectiveness to be proposed as the first choice of treatment.[158] On the above grounds, surgery is still the first choice of therapeutic modality, the adjuvant therapy being reserved when surgery fails to stabilize the tumor growth.

Surgical Management of Anterior Optic-pathway Gliomas

Gliomas limited to one optic nerve (either pure intraorbital, or intraorbital gliomas with intracranial extension, but not affecting the chiasm) are best treated by surgical excision. However, surgical intervention must be undertaken only when there has been complete loss of vision in that eye, and the major indications of surgery in these cases include unsightly proptosis, risk of losing ocular globe, and prevention of retrograde spread of tumor into the chiasm. In patients, where vision is preserved, especially in those with NF-I, a cautious 'wait and watch policy' is advised. Regular neuroimaging should be performed and an surgical intervention must be performed only when there is progressive loss of vision and/or growth in the size of the tumor. The tumor is usually approached through a lateral orbitotomy approach. Alternatively, an orbito-frontal craniotomy may be performed through a small eye-brow incision or a curvilinear incision over the hairline starting from the tragus to the midline. The anterior and posterior limits of the tumor is then exposed and the tumor along with the nerve is transected just behind the globe and just proximal to the annulus.[163-165]

Surgical Management of Chiasmatic-hypothalamic Gliomas

These lesions were not considered amenable for surgical resection and till recently only radiotherapy was advised as the only mode of therapy. However, the emergence of microneuro-surgical techniques has made significant changes in management of these tumors. The primary aim of surgery is debulking. In patients with stable vision, the surgical debulking should be, however, more conser-vative. In patients with blindness complete resection may be opted. Chemotherapy is the first adjuvant therapy of choice as most of the patients are children. Regular neuroimaging is mandatory. If there is any evidence of tumor growth, then radiotherapy may be given, other-wise only regular follow-up is required. If patients have hydrocephalus, then a shunt may be performed before surgery. However, due to the peculiar location of the tumor both the ventricles do not communicate, hence two separate ventricular ends may need to be inserted. Alternatively, an endoscopic septostomy along with a single side shunt may be performed. The surgical route is usually same as that for craniopharyn-giomas.[165,166]

Outcome

The remarkably different biologic behavior makes it difficult to define the prognosis. Despite these marked differences, overall survival rates at 5 years for patients submitted to partial resection or even biopsy followed by adjuvant therapy has ranged from 70-100 percent. These long term survival rates have been reported at 57-90 percent at 10 years and 50 percent at 13 years.[167-170] Presence of NF-I has been shown to confer a protective effect and some tumors have even shown spontaneous regression.[153,154]

SUPRATENTORIAL TUMORS

The infratentorial tumors have an higher incidence in the pediatric population, but supratentorial tumors are not rare. In most reported series they comprise about 30-40 percent of all cerebral neoplasms in children.[171] However, the incidence of supratentorial tumors was higher in our study. We have studied a total of 3545 primary intracranial tumors (excluding pituitary adenomas) over 10 years (1989-1999), and there were a total of 613 pediatric cases of which 317 (51.7%) had tumors in the supratentorial compartment. (courtesy-Prof Chitra Sarkar, Neuropathology).

A brief discussion of most of the common supratentorial tumors will be provided in the following section:

Astrocytoma

These are the commonest tumors of the cerebral hemispheres, and account for approximately 50 percent of all astrocytomas in children. There is no sex predilection and they occur at all ages with peak incidence between 8 and 12 years.[171,172] About half of them are benign and half malignant The majority of them (50-70%) are associated with a cyst and the cyst wall contains the tumor in most of the cases. The natural history of these tumors is variable. Even with benign histology, only 60-70 percent of children with low-grade tumors will have long term survival.[173] Glioblastomas have a dismal prognosis with a five-year survival of 5-15 percent and 20-40 percent survival for anaplastic tumors.[174,175] Surgical excision remains the primary option. Radiation therapy has continued to be the traditional adjuvant treatment for malignant or incompletely resected tumors. While there is a definitive advantage for malignant tumors, there remains a controversy for subtotally resected low-grade tumors. Chemotherapy has shown to increase the survival significantly in children with malignant astrocytomas. This is particularly important in children below 3 years of age, where radiation may have deleterious effects.[174-176]

Ependymomas

These constitute 8 to 10 percent of all intracranial tumors in pediatric age group.[11] About 30 to 50 percent are supratentoraial. Unlike the posterior fossa ependymomas, which are always located in the fourth ventricle, the supratentorial tumors arise from ectopic rests of ependymal cells adjacent to the ventricles.[177,178] Large cysts occur in 50 percent of supratentorial tumors, but this is not associated with benign histology. Even though most often they are histologically benign their biological behavior is often malignant, usually due to incomplete removal. The microscopic appearance is characterized by formation of typical pseudorosettes. Most often the cell processes attach themselves to the adventitia of the vessel. Nuclei tend to have a monotonous character and mitotic activity is variable.[10,12]

Calcification is found in about 50 percent of cases. Surgical excision with postoperative therapy is the optimal therapy of choice. The principles for surgery as same as that for astrocytomas.[177,178] The results of 5-year survival rate with surgery alone has been in the range of 17 to 27 percent. With radiotherapy, it improved to 40 to 87 percent.[179] Chemotherapy has been also used as an adjuvant but its role is controversial.

Oligodendrogliomas

These are rare in children accounting for 1 to 2 percent of hemispheric tumors, when they are pure and arise from oligodendrocyte cells alone. However, so-called 'mixed gliomas', containing astrocytes as well are more common (9-30%).[180] These tumors tend to be slow growing lesions with a peak incidence in children between 6 to 12 years, and there is a strong male dominance.[181,182]

These tumors have a gelatinous character and may or may not have a well defined borders on gross examination. They have a gritty component due to calcification, which is a very common feature present in about 90 percent of cases. Evidence of old hemorrhages may be seen on cut sections.[12] The microscopic appearance is characterized by sheets of cells with small, round nuclei surrounded by a clear zone bordered by a delicate membrane ('fried egg appearance') incompletely separated into lobules by a delicate fibrovascular stroma. The cells generally have a monotonous appearance although the malignant varieties are characterized by anaplastic nuclei and variable number of mitotic figures.[12,13]

Calcification is common and may be also seen on plain skull radiography. CT and MR imaging usually shows a irregularly defined lesion with patchy contrast enhancement, with cystic changes commonly seen. Surgical excision is the most effective treatment. Radiation therapy is of doubtful benefit for pure oligodendrogliomas but may improve outcome for mixed gliomas. Chemotherapy has been shown to be beneficial for malignant tumors or recurrent tumors. The 5-year survival rate for pure oligodendrogliomas ranges from 75 to 85 percent. There seems to be a role for repeat surgical resections.[180-183]

Gangliogliomas

This is a mixed tumor composed of neurons and astrocytes. They were first described by Courville in 1930 and they account for about 4 to 8 percent of childhood brain tumors.[183] Their histological grading is similar to astrocytomas. They may arise from any part of the brain but are more common in the medial temporal lobe and the floor of the third ventricle.

Radical surgical excision is the treatment of choice. In patients presenting with refractory seizures, the surrounding area needs to be also removed as it is epiletogenic. Radiotherapy is not indicated unless malignant changes are observed. The long-term disease-free survival following surgical excision is 75 to 90 percent.[184,185]

Other Uncommon Glial Tumors

Some of the examples include gliomatosis cerebri, subependymal giant cell astrocytoma, dysembryoplastic neuroepithelial tumors and hypothalamic hamartomas.

Gliomatosis cerebri produce diffuse enlargement of the brain with microscopic evidence of infiltrating gliomas cells along anatomic pathways throughout the central nervous system. The age ranges from 9 to 60 years. Obstructive hydrocephalus may occur and can be managed by shunting, otherwise there no treatment and the outcome is dismal.[186]

Subependymal giant cell astrocytoma: These occur in tuberous sclerosis, arising form subependymal nodules in the walls of the lateral ventricles. If asymptomatic, they require no treatment. They are very slow growing and malignant changes have not been reported.[187]

Dysembryoplastic neuroepithelial tumors: These were initially described by Daumas-Duport[188] et al in 1988. The age ranges from 1 to 19 years (mean 9 years), and there is a male preponderance. The tumors are located in the temporal lobe, but also may occur in other lobes as well. They usually present with seizures. The optimal treatment is surgical excision , if necessary under electro-cortcographic survey. Surgical excision will produce a complete cure and adjuvant therapy is not indicated.[188,189]

Hypothalamic hamartomas: These are uncommon and usually occur in the ventral hypothalamus and are either sessile or pedunculated. Most patients present with precocious puberty. They may be associated with other midline anomalies like agenesis of corpus callosum, optic malformations, and dysgenesis of cerebral hemispheres. Other clinical features like behavioral changes, gelastic epilepsy ('laughing fits') or intellectual deficits, visual disturbances, and autonomic disturbances (hyperphagia, hyperactivity, or somnolence) may occur. CT scan shows the tumor typically to be isodense with cerebral gray matter and does not enhance with contrast. MR imaging does not show nay contrast enhancement, and the tumor is usually of the same signal as the cerebrospinal fluid or the parenchyma. Histologically, the tumor consists of mature neurons, without evidence of neoplastic differentiation. Some neurons may contain neurosecretory granules. Based on these findings, it has been suggested that the tumor may cause precocious puberty either by its intrinsic secretory function or by compressing the inhibitory pathways from the hypothalamus to the pituitary gland. Treatment is controversial. Medical treatment with gonadotrophin-releasing analogs may be given for precocious puberty but is expensive. The role of surgery is doubtful. If at all, it may be carried out for pedunculated hamartomas. Sessile hamartomas need to be decompressed very conservatively. Most of the surgeons feel that surgical intervention should be kept in reserve particularly when it is associated with other anomalies and there is nor progression.[190-192]

INTRAVENTRICULAR TUMORS IN CHILDREN

These tumors have a peculiarity of remaining clinically silent until they attain a large size or produce hydrocephalus. In young infants they may present with macrocrania. The best known examples are Choroid plexus papillomas, subependymomas, and colloid cysts. Colloid cysts are very rare in infants and children.

Choroid plexus papillomas: are rare tumors of neuroectodermal origin with an incidence of 0.4 to 0.6 percent of all intracranial tumors, but the majority of them occur in the first 2 years of life. Histologically, most tumors are benign, but 10 percent show malignant changes (choroid plexus carcinoma). Choroid plexus papilloma is derived embryologically form the ependymal lining of the neural tube. These tumors may occur anywhere in the ventricular system, but are more frequent in the lateral ventricle in children, and in adults in the fourth ventricle. Tumors in the third ventricle are rare. Clinically they present with features of raised intracranial pressure due to hydrocephalus. Hydrocephalus in these tumors has been reported to be not only due to obstruction, but also due to micro-hemorrhages leading to defective absorption and increased secretion of the cerebrospinal fluid. CT scan usually shows a homogenous lobulated mass that shows marked contrast enhancement. A heterogeneous enhancement may suggest malignant changes. MR imaging is more sensitive and delineates a more detailed anatomy, showing the characteristic molding of the tumor within the ventricle, changes due to vascularity, calcification, and old hemorrhage. With high resolution, it may be also possible to identify the hypertrophied vessels. Usually the blood supply is from the anterior choroidal, posterior choroidal, or lateral striate vessels. Surgical excision is treatment of choice, however intraoperative hemorrhage is a common complication, which in young children with limited blood volume is critical. Outcome is good if total excision is achieved. Choroid plexus carcinoma have a bad prognosis and require radiotherapy/chemotherapy.[193-195]

The above section has dealt with most of the intracranial tumors found in the pediatric age group. The pathological, clinical and radiological aspects including the recent developments, have been dealt in a comprehensive manner. A brief overview of the surgical approaches has been also provided. It is important for the pediatric surgeon to diagnose a brain tumor in a child and have a knowledge of most of the common tumors found in children.

REFERENCES

1. Bhatia LS. A History of medicine with special reference to the Orient. Office of Medical Council of India, New Delhi, 1997.
2. AlRodhan NRF, Laws ER Jr. Meningioma: a historical study of the tumour and its surgical management. Neurosurgery 1990;26:832-47.
3. Cushing H. Intracranial tumours. Charles C Thomas, 1932.
4. Hitselberger WE, House WF. Surgical approaches to acoustic tumours, Arch Otolaryngol. 1966;84:286-91.
5. Salcman M. The morbidity and mortality of brain tumours. Neurol Clin 1985;3:229.
6. Rorke LB, Gilles FH, Davis RL, et al. Revision of the World Health Organisation classification of brain tumours for childhood brain tumours. Cancer 1985;56:1869-86.
7. Rorke LB. Pathology of brain and spinal cord tumours In, Choux M, Rocco DC, Hockley AD, Walker ML, (Eds): Pediatric Neurosurgery, Churchill Livingstone, London, 1999;395-426.
8. Albright AL, Wisoff JH, Zeltzer P, et al. Prognostic factors in children with supratentorial (nonpineal) primitive neuro-ectodermal tumours. Pediatric Neurosurg 1995;22:1-7.
9. Kernohan JW, Mahon RF, Svien HJ, et al. A simplified classification of gliomas. Proc Staff Meet Mayo Clinic 1949; 24:71-5.
10. Rubinstein LJ. Discussion on polar spongioblastomas. Acta Neurochir Suppl (Wein) 1964;10:132-40.
11. Russell DS, Rubinstein LJ. Pathology of Tumours of the Nervous System, 5th ed. Baltimore: Williams and Wilkins, 1989.
12. Dumas-Duport G, Scheithauer BW, O'Fallon J, Kelly P. Grading of astrocytomas: a simple and reproducible method. Cancer 1988; 62: 2152-65.
13. Becker LE. Primitive neuroectodermal tumours: views on a working classification. In: Fields WS, (Ed.): Primary Brain Tumours. A Review of Histological Classification. New York: Springer, 1989: 59-69.
14. Rorke LB. Primitive neuroectodermal tumours. In Nelson JS, Parisi JE, Schochet SS Jr, (Eds): Principle and Practice of Neuropathology. St Louis: CV Mobsy, 1993: 185-202.
15. Bailey P, Cushing H. Medulloblastoma cerebelli: a common type of midcerebellar glioma of childhood. Arch Neurol Psychiat 1925;14:192-224.
16. Choux M, Lena G. Le medulloblastome. Neurochirurgie 1982; 28(Suppl 1):11-23.
17. Rorke LB, Packer RJ, Biegel JA. Central nervous system atypical/rhabdoid tumours of infancy and childhood: definition of an entity. J Neurosurg 1996; 85: 56-65.
18. Rubinstein LJ. Justification for a cytogenetic scheme of embryonal central neuroepithelial tumours. In: Fields WS, (Ed.): Primary Brain m. A Review of Histological Classification. New York: Springer, 1989; 16-27.
19. Mostofi FK, Price EB Jr. Tumours of the Genital system. Washington DC: Armed Forces Institute of Pathology, 1973.
20. Sutton L, Schut L. Cerebellar astrocytomas, In McLaurin R, Scut L, Venes J, Epstein F, (Eds): Pediatric Neurosurgery: Surgery of the Developing Nervous System, Philadelphia, WB Sauders, 1989;338-46.
21. Shuster J, Hartz Z, Stimson CW, et al. Ataxia telangectasia with cerebellar tumour. Paediatrics 1986;37:776-86.
22. Miller RW, Rubinstein JH. Tumours in Rubinstein-Taybi syndrome. Am J Med Genet 1995;56:112-5.
23. Neblett CR, Waltz TA. Neurological involvement in the neuroid basal cell carcinoma syndrome. J Neurosurg 1971; 35: 577-84.
24. Beigel J, Rorke L, Packer R, et al. Isochromosome 17q in primitive neuroectodermal tumours of the central nervous system. Genes Chromosom Cancer 1989;1:139.
25. Allen J, Epstein F. Medulloblastoma and other primary CNS malignant neuroectod ermal tumours: the effect of age and extent of disease on prognosis. J Neurosurg 1982; 57: 446-51.
26. Park TS, Hoffman HJ, Hendrick EB, et al. Medulloblastoma, clinical presentation and management. Experience at the Hospital for Sick Children, Toronto, 1950-1980. J Neurosurg 1983; 58: 543-52.

27. Bilaniuk LP, Zimmerman RA, Schut L, et al. Computed neuroimaging of Pediatric infra-tentorial brain tumours. J Neuroradiol 1984;8:224-42.

28. Sandhu A, Kendall B. Computed tomography in management of medulloblastomas. Neuroradiology 1987;29:444.

29. Atlas S. Intraaxial brain tumours, In Magnetic Resonance Imaging of Brain and Spine. New York, Raven Press. 1991;273-326.

30. Sutton LN, Wehril SL, Gennarelli L, et al. High-resolution H-magnetic resonance spectroscopy of Pediatric posterior fossa tumours *in vitro*. J Neurosurg 1994;81:443-8.

31. Arle JE, Morris C, Wang ZJ, et al. Prediction of posterior fossa tumour type in children by means of magnetic resonance image properties, spectroscopy, and neural networks. J Neurosurg 1997;86:755-61.

32. Abraham J. Epidemiology of brain tumours. In Neuro-oncology. Deshpande DH, Vidyasagar C, Narayana Reddy GN, (Eds). NIMHANS, Eastern Press, 1981;57.

33. Bongartz EB, Bamberg M, Nau HF, et al. Optimal therapy in medulloblastoma. Acta Neurochir (Wein) 1979;50:117.

34. Hekmatpanah J, Mullan S. Ventriculaocaval shunt in the management of posterior fossa tumours. J Neurosurg 1967; 26:609.

35. Hoffman HJ, Hendrik EB, Humphreys RP. Metastasis via ventriculoperitoneal shunt in patients with medulloblastoma. J Neurosurg 1976; 44: 562.

36. Park TS, Hoffman HJ, Hendrick EB, et al. Medulloblastoma: Presentation and management. Experience at the hospital for children. Toronto 1950-1980. J Neurosurg 1983; 58: 543.

37. Lodha DC, Bhatia R, Tandon PN. Evaluation of ventriculoatrial shunts in posterior fossa tumours. Neurol India 1981; 29: 1.

38. Sharma BS, KAK VK, Banerjee AK, et al. The management of medulloblastomas in childhood (Chandigarh experience with review of literature). Neurol India 1989; 37: 97-102.

39. Chang CH, Housepian EM, Herbert C, et al. An operative staging system on megavoltage radiotherapeutic technique for cerebellar medulloblastoma. Radiology 1969;93:1351-9.

40. Laurent JP, Chang CH, Cohen ME. A classification system for primitive neuroectodermal tumours (medulloblastomas) of the posterior fossa. Cancer 1985;57:446-51.

41. Packer RJ, Sutton LN, Elterman R, et al. Outcome for children with medulloblastoma treated with radiation and cisplatic, CCNU, and vincristine chemotherapy. J Neurosurg 1994;81: 690-8.

42. Bouffet E, Gentet JC, Doz F et al. Metastatic medulloblastomas: the experience of the French Co-operative M Group. Eur J Cancer 1994;30A:1478-83.

43. Schofield DE, Yunis EJ, Greyer R, et al. DNA content and other prognostic features in childhood medulloblastoma. Cancer 1992; 69: 1307-14.

44. Batra SK, McLendon RE, Koo JS. Prognostic implications of chromosome 17p deletions in human medulloblastomas. J Neurooncol 1995;24:39-45.

45. Wasson JC, Saylors RI, Zeltzer P, et al. Oncogene amplification in Pediatric brain tumours. Cnacer Rexss 1990; 50: 2987-90.

46. Figarella-Branger D, Dubois C, Chauvin P, et al. Correlation between polysialic-neural cell adhesion molecule levels in CSF and medulloblastoma outcomes. J Clin Oncol 1996;14:2066-72.

47. Weichselbaum RR, Liszcsack Phillips JP, et al. Characterisation and radiobiologic parameters of medulloblastomas *in vitro*. Cancer 1977;40:1087-96.

48. Patterson E, Farr RF. Cerebellar medulloblastoma: treatment by irradiation of the whole central nervous system. Acta Radiol 1953; 39: 323-36.

49. Berry M, Jenkin R, Keen C, et al. Radiation therapy for medulloblastoma: a 21-year-old review. J Neurosurg 1981; 55: 43-51.

50. Silverman CL, Simpson JR. Cerebellar medulloblastoma: importance of posterior fossa dose to survival and pattern of failure. Int J Radiat Biol Phys 1982; 8: 1869-76.

51. Alken JC, Bloom J, Ertel I, et al. Brain tumours in children: current co-operative and institutional chemotherapy trials in newly diagnosed and recurrent disease. Semin Oncol 1986; 1: 110-22.

52. Hoppe-Hirsch E, Brunet L, Laroussinie F, et al. Intellectual outcome in children with malignant tumours of the posterior fossa: influence of the field of irradiation and quality of surgery. Childs Nerv Syst 1995;11:340-5.

53. Shalegt SM, Beardwell CG, Aarons BM, et al. Growth impairment in children treated for brain tumours. Arch Dis Chid 1978;53:491-4.

54. Rappaport R, Brauner R, Czernichow P, et al. Effect of hypothalamic and pituitary irradiation on pubertal development with cranial tumours. J Clin Endocrinol Metab 1982;54:1164-8.

55. Shalegt SM, Clayton PE, Price DA. Growth and pituitary function in children treated for brain tumours or acute lymphoblastic leukaemia. Horm Res 1988;30:53-61.

56. Allen JC, Donahue B, Da Rosso R, Nirenberg A. Hyper-fractionated craniospinal radiotherapy and adjuvant chemotherapy for children with newly diagnosed medulloblastoma and other primitive neuroectodermal tumours. Int J Radiat Oncol Biol Phys 1996;36:1155-61.

57. Patrice SJ, Tarbell NJ, Goumnerova LC, et al. Results of radiosurgery in the management of recurrent and residual medulloblastoma. Pediatr Neurosurg 1955;22:197-203.

58. Evans EA, Jenkins RDT, Sposto R et al. The treatment of medulloblastoma- results of a prospective randomised trial of radiation therapy with and without chloroethyl-cyclohexyl nitrosourea, vincristine and prednisolone. J Neurosurg 1990; 72: 572-82.

59. Tait DM, Thorton-Jones H, Bloom HJG, et al. Adjuvant chemotherapy for medulloblastoma: the first multicentre control trial of the International Society of Pediatric Oncology (SIOP). Eur J Cancer 1990;26:464-9.

60. Levin VA, Rodriguez LA, Edwards MSB, et al. Treatment of medulloblastoma with procarbazine, hydroxiurea, and reduced radiation dose to whole brain and spine. J Neurosurg 1988; 68:383-7.

61. Halberg FE, Wara WM, Fippin LF, et al. Low dose craniospinal radiation therapy for medulloblastoma. Int J Radiat Oncol Biol Phys 1991; 20: 651-4.

62. Cushing H. Experiences with cerebellar medulloblastomas. A critical review. Acta Pathol et Microbiol Scandinav 1930;7:1-7.

63. Ingraham FD, Bailey OT, Barker WF. Medulloblastoma cerebelli, diagnosis, treatment survivals, with report of fifty-six cases. N Eng J Med 1948;238:171.

64. Penfield WB, Feindel W. Medulloblastoma of the cerebellum with survival for seventeen years. Arch Neurol Psychiat 1947; 57: 481.

65. Quest DO, Brisman R, Antunes JL, et al. Period of risk for recurrence of medulloblastoma. J Neurosurg 1978;48:159.

66. King GA, Sagerman RH. Lobe recurrence in medulloblastoma. Am J Roent Rad Ther Nucl Med 1975;123:7-9.

67. Zulch KJ. Brain tumours. Berlin: Springer, 1986.

68. Schneider JH, Raffel C, McComb G. Benign cerebellar astrocytomas of childhood. Neurosurgery 1992;30:58-63.

69. Berger MS. Cerebellar astrocytomas. In Youmans JR, (Ed): Neurological Surgery. Vol IV. 4th ed. Philadelphia: Saunders, 1996; 2593-2602.

70. Ilgren EB, Stiller CA. Cerebellar astrocytomas. Clinical characteristics and prognosis indices. J Neurooncol 1987; 4: 293-308.

71. Sutton LN, Schut L. Cerebellar astrocytomas. In McLaurin RL, Schut L, Venes JL, et al, (Eds): Pediatric Neurosurgery. 2nd ed. Philadelphia: Saunders, 1989;338-46.

72. Mishra BK, Tandon PN, Banerji AK, et al. Intracranial tumours of infancy, childhood and adolescence. Ind J Cancer 1984; 21: 63-8.

73. Hayostek CJ, Shaw EG, Scheithauer B, et al. Astrocytomas of the cerebellum. A comparative clinicopathological study of pilocytic and diffuse astrocytomas. Cancer 1993; 72: 856-69.

74. Segall HD, Zee CS, Naidich TP, Ahmadi J, Becker TS. Computed tomography in neoplasms of the posterior fossa in children. Radiol Clin North Am 1982; 20: 237-53.

75. Segall HD, Batnitzky S, Zee CS, Ahmadi J, Bird CR, Cohen ME. Computed tomography in the diagnosis of intracranial neoplasms in children. Cancer 1985;56:1748-55.

76. Lee YY, Van Tassel P, Bruner JM, et al. Juvenile pilocytic astrocytomas: CT and MR characteristics. Am J Neuroradiol 1989;10:363-70.

77. Brant-Zawadski M, Kelly W. Brain tumours. In Brant-Zawadski M, Norman D, (Eds): Magnetic Resonance Imaging Of The Central Nervous System. New York: Raven Press, 1987:151-85.

78. Gjerris F, Klinken L. Long-term prognosis in children with benign cerebellar astrocytomas. J Neurosurg 1978;49:179-84.

79. Ilgren EB, Stiller CA. Cerebellar astrocytomas: clinical characteristics and prognostic indices. J Neurosurg 1987; 4: 293-308.

80. Klein DM, McCullough DC. Surgical staging of cerebellar astrocytomas in childhood. Cancer 1985;56:1810-1.

81. Budhka H. Partially resected and irradiated cerebellar astrocytoma of childhood. Malignant evolution after 28 years. Acta Neurochir (Wein) 1975;32:146-8.

82. Kline LE, Kovnar EH, Stanford RA. Ependymomas and ependymoblastomas in chidden. Pediatric Neurosci 1988;14: 57-63.

83. Naik AL, Chandra PS, Mehta VS. A retrospective analysis of ependymomas in 5 years (1994-1998): Thesis submitted to the dept of Neurosurgery, AIIMS, New Delhi. Jan 2000.

84. Fitz C, Rao K. Primary tumours in chidden, In Lee S, Rao K, (Eds): Cranial Computed Tomography and MRI. New York, McGraw-Hill, 1987; 365-412.

85. Heideman RL, Paeker RJ, Reaman GH. A phase II evaluation of thiotepa in Pediatric CNS malignancies. Cancer 1993;72: 271-5.

86. Sutton LN, Goldwein J, Perilongo G. Prognostic factors in childhood ependymomas. Ped Neurosurg 1990;16:57-65.

87. Dohrman G, Farwell J, Flannery J. Ependymomas and ependymoblastomas in children. J Neurosurg 1976;45:273-83.

88. Salazar OM, Castro-Vita H, VanHoutte P, et al. Improved survival in cases if intracranial ependymoma after radiation therapy. J Neurosurg 1983;59:652-9.

89. Matson D. Surgery of posterior fossa tumours in childhood. Clin Neurosurg 1968;15:247-64.

90. Tomita R, Raimondi A. Fourth ventricular tumours. In McLaurin R, Schut L, Venes J, Epstein F, (Eds): Pediatric Neurosurgery: Surgery of the developing nervous system. New York, Grune and Stratton, 1982; pp 383-93.

91. Petronio J, Walker ML. Surgical management of cerebellar tumours in children. In Schmidek HH, Sweet WH, (Eds): Operative Neurosurgical Techniques 3rd ed 1995, W.B. Saunders and Co, Philadelphia: pp 801-12.

92. Hoffman HJ, Becker L. A clinically and pathologically distinct group of benign brainstem gliomas. Neurosurg 1980; 7: 243-8.

93. Albright AL, Guthkelch AN. Prognostic factors in Pediatric brain-stem gliomas. J Neurosurg 1986;65:751-5.

94. Farwell JR, Dohrmann GJ. Central nervous system tumours in children. Cancer 1977;40:3123-32.

95. Koos WT, Miller MH. Intracranial Tumours In Infants And Children. Stuttgast: Thieme, 1971;346-50.

96. Kansal S, Jindal A, Mahapatra AK. Brain-stem gliomas: A study in 111 patients. Indian Journal of Cnacer 1999;36:99-108.

97. Tokuriki Y, Handa H. Brain-stem gliomas: An analysis of 85 cases. Acta Neurochirur 1986;79:67-73.

98. Mantravadi RVP, Phatak R. Brain-stem gliomas: An autopsy study of 25 cases. Cancer 1984;49:1294-6.

99. Vandertop WP, Hoffman HJ. Focal midbrain tumours in children. Neurosurgery. Neurosurg 1992;31:186-94.

100. Russell DS, Rubinstein LJ. Pathology of Tumours of the Nervous System. 4th ed. Baltimore: Williams and Wilkins, 1977; 181-3.

101. Epstein F, McLeary EL. Intrinsic brain-stem tumours of childhood: surgical indications. J Neurosurg 1986;64:11-5.

102. May PL, Blaser SI, Hoffman HJ, et al. Benign intrinsic tectal "tumours" in children. J Neurosurg 1991;74:867-71.

103. Hoffman HJ, Goumnerova L. Pediatric brain stem gliomas. In Wilkins H, Rengachary SS, (Eds): Neurosurgery 2nd ed. McGraw Hill, New York 1996; 1183-94

104. Pakisch B, Urban C, Slave I, et al. Hyperfractionated radiotherapy and polychemotherapy in brain-stem tumours in children. Childs Nerv Syst 1992; 8: 215-8.

105. Epstein FJ, Farmer JP. Intrinsic tumours of the brainstem. In Apuzzo MLJ (Ed.): Brain Surgery: complications avoidance and management. Churchill Livingstone, New York, 1992; 1835.

106. Sano K. Diagnosis and treatment of tumours in the pineal region. Acta Neurochir (Wein) 1976; 34: 153-7.

107. Arora T, Mehta VS, Singh VP, et al. A retrospective study of posterior third ventricular tumours over 10 years. Thesis submitted to the faculty of the dept of Neurosurgery, AIIMS, New Delhi 1999.

108. Cummins FM, Taveras JM, Schlesinger EB. Treatment of gliomas of the third ventricle and pinealomas with special reference to the value of radiotherapy. Neurology 1960; 10: 1031-6.

109. Asha T, Shankar SK, Das BS, et al. True pinelomas and germinomas- a clinicopathological appraisal. Neurol (India) 1990; 38: 31-42.

110. Keane JR. The pretectal syndrome- 206 patients. Neurology 1990; 40: 684-92.

111. Rout D. Sharma A. Radhakrishnan VV, et al. Exploration of the pineal region: observations and results. Surg Neurol 1984; 21: 135-42.

112. Taveras JM, Wood EH. Diagnostic Neuroradiology 2nd ed. Williams and Wilkins, Baltimore, 214-6.

113. Zimmerman RA. Pineal region masses; Radiology, In. Wilkins RH, Rengachary SS, Neurosurgery (Eds). McGraw-Hill, 1985; 680-92.

114. Chi Shing Zee, Seagull H, Apuzzo M, et al. MR imaging of pineal region neoplasms. J Comput Assist Tomog 1991; 15: 56-61.

115. Jeffrey C, Allen MD, Morton K, et al. Alpha-feto protein and human chorionic gonadotropin dissemination in CSF. Neurosurgery 1979; 51: 368-74.

116. Herrick MK. Pineal tumours: classification and pathology. In Wilkins RH, Rengachary SS, (Eds): Neurosurgery. New York: McGraw-Hill 1996: 995-1001.

117. Bruce JN, Stein BM. Pineal tumours. Neurosurg Clin N Am 1990; 1: 123-8.

118. Horsley V. Discussion. Proc R Soc Med 3 (Pt 2): 1910: 77.

119. Dandy WE. An operation for removal of pineal tumours. Surg Gynecol Obstet 1921; 33:113-8.

120. Van Wagenen WP. A surgical approach for the removal of certain pineal tumours. Report of a case. Surg Gynecol Obstet 1931; 53: 216-23.

121. Stein BM. The infratentorial supracerebellar approach to pineal lesions. J Neurosurg 1971; 35: 197-201.

122. Poppen JL. The right occipital approach to a pinealoma. J Neurosurg 1968; 28: 357-61.

123. Jamieson KG. Excision of pineal tumours. J Neurosurg 1971; 35: 550-62.

124. Suzuki J, Iwabuchi T. Surgical removal of pineal tumours (pinealomas and teratomas). J Neurosurg 1965; 23: 565-71.

125. Page LK. The infratentorial-supracerebellar exposure of the tumours in the pineal area. Neurosurgery 1977; 1: 36-40.

126. Stein BM, Bruce JN. Surgical management of pineal region tumours. Clin Neurosurg 1992; 39: 509-32.

127. Bruce JN, Stein BM. Infratentorial approach to pineal tumours, In Wilson CB (Ed): Neurosurgical Procedures: Personal approaches to classic operations. Baltimore, Williams and Wilkins, 1992; 63-76.

128. Bruce JN, Stein BM. Supracerebellar approaches in the pineal region, In Apuzzo MLZ, (Ed): Brain Surgery: Complication avoidance and management. New York, Churchill-Livingstone, 1993, pp 511-36.

129. Danoff B, Sheline GE. Radiotherapy of pineal tumours. In: Neuwelt EA. (Ed.): The diagnosis and Treatment of Pineal Region Tumours. Williams and Wilkins 1984;300-26.

130. Sano K, Matsutani M. Pinealoma (germinoma) treated by direct surgery and postoperative radiation. A long-term follow-up. Child's Brain 1981; 8: 81.

131. Sawaya R, Hawley DK, Tobler WD, et al. Pineal and third ventricular tumours. In (Ed). Youmans JR. Neurological Surgery WB Saunders Co, 1990, pp 3171-236.

132. Herrmann HD, Wincler D, Westpal M, Treatment of tumours of pineal region and posterior part of the third ventricle. Acta Neurochir (Wein) 1992; 116: 137.

133. Szeifert GT, Sipos L, Hovarth M, et al. Pathological characteristics of surgically removed craniopharyngiomas: analysis of 131 cases. Acta Neurochir (Wein) 1993; 124: 139-43.

134. Tachibana O, Yamashima T, Yamashita J, et al. Immmunohistochemical expression of human chorionic gonadotrophin and P glycoprotein in human pituitary glands and craniopharyngiomas. J Neurosurg 1994; 80: 79-84.

135. Sammi M, Bini W. Surgical treatment of craniopharyngiomas. Zentralblatt fur Neurochirurgie 1991; 52: 17-23.

136. Raimondi AJ. Pediatric Neurosurgery. Berlin, Springer-Verlag, 1987, 277-91.

137. Symon L. Experiences with radical excision of craniopharyngioma. In Samii M (Ed.): Surgery of the sellar region and paranasal sinuses. Berlin, Springer-Verlag, 1991, 373-80.

138. Choux M, Lena G, Genitoiri L. Le craniopharyngiome de L'enfant. Neurochirurgie 37 (Suppl): 1991: 1-174.

139. Bonneville JE, Cattin F. The role magnetic resonance imaging in the diagnosis of endocrine tumours of the sellar region in children. Horm Res 1995; 43(4): 151-3.

140. Donovan JL, Nesbit GM. Distinction of masses involving the sellar and suprasellar space: specificity of imaging features. AJR Am J Roentgenol 1996; 167(3): 597-603.

141. Adambaum C, Chaussain JL. Diagnostic strategies in Pediatric imaging. Horm Res 1996; 46(4-5): 165-69.

142. Broggi G, Giorgi C, Franzini D, et al. Preliminary results of intracavitory treatment of craniopharyngioma with bleomycin. J Neurosurg Sci 1989; 33: 145-48.

143. Banna M, Hoare RD, Stanley P, et al. Craniopharyngioma in children. J Pediatr 1973; 83:781-5.

144. Long DM, Leibrock L. The transcallosal approach to the anterior ventricular system and its application in the therapy of craniopharyngiomas. Clin Neurosurg 1980; 27: 160-8.

145. Ammirati M, Sammi M, Sephernia A, et al. Surgery of large retrochiasmatic craniopharyngiomas in children. Childs Nerv Syst 1990;6:13-7.

146. Tiupakoov AN, Mazerkina NA, Brook CG, et al. Growth in children with craniopharyngiomas following surgery. Clin Endocrinol (Oxf) 1998; 49(6): 733-8.

147. Lehmbecher T, Muller- Scholden J, Danhauser-Leister I, et al. Perioperative fluid and electrolyte management in children undergoing surgery for craniopharyngiomas: A 10-year experience in a single institution. Childs Nerv Syst 1998; 14(6): 276-9.

148. Bloom HJ. Tumours of the central nervous system. In Voute PA, et al, (Eds): Cancer in Children. 2nd ed. New York: Springer, 1986: 197-222.

149. Laws ER Jr, Vance ML. Radiosurgery for pituitary tumours and craniopharyngiomas. Neurosurg Clin N Am 1999;10(2):327-36.

150. Pierre-Khan A, Braunner R, Renier D, et al. Traitement des craniophryngiomes de l'enfant. Analyse retrospective de 50 observation. Arch Fr Pediatr 1988; 45: 163-7.

151. Stern J, Jakobiec FA, Housepian EM. The architecture of optic nerve gliomas with or without neurofibromatosis. Arch Ophthalmol 1980; 98: 505-11.

152. Housepian EM. Management and results in 114 cases of optic glioma. Neurosurgery 1977; 1: 67-68 (abstr).

153. Listermick R, Charrow J, Gutmann DH. Intracranial gliomas in neurofibraomatosis type I. Am J Med Genet 1999; 89(1): 38-44.

154. Perilongo G, Moras P, Carollo C, et al. Spontaneous partial regression of low-grade glioma in children with neurofibromatosis-I: a real possibility. J Chil Neurol 1999; 14(6): 352-6.

155. Davis PC, Hopkins KL. Imaging of the paediatric orbit and visual pathways.: computed tomography and magnetic resonance imaging. Neuroimaging Clin N Am 199; 9(1): 93-114.

156. Jakobiec FA, Depot MJ, Kennerdell JS, et al. Combined clinical and computed tomographic diagnosis of orbital glioma and meningioma. Ophthalmology 1984; 91: 137-55.

157. Brown EW, Riccardi VM. Mawad M, et al. MR imaging of optic pathways in patients with neurofibromatosis. Am J Neuroradiol 1987; 8: 1031-6.

158. Venes JL, Latack J, Kandt RS. Postoperative regression of optochiasmatic astrocytoma: a case for expectant therapy. Neurosurgery 1984; 15: 421-3.

159. Brand WN, Hoover SV. Optic glioma in children. Review of 16 cases given megavoltage radiation therapy. Childs Brain 1979; 5: 459-66.

160. Danoff BF, Kramer S, Thomson N. The radiotherapeutic management of optic nerve gliomas in children. Int J Radiat Oncol Biol Phys 1980; 6: 45-50.

161. Bataini JP, Delanian S, Povert D. Chiasmal gliomas: results of irradiation management in 57 patients and review of the literature. Int J Radiat Oncol Biol Phys 1991; 21: 615-23.

162. Mohadjer A, Etou A, Milios E, et al. Chiasmatic optic glioma. Neurochirurgica (Stuttg) 1991; 34: 90-3.

163. Housepian EM, Marquardt MD, Behrens M. Optic gliomas. In Wilkins RH, Rengachary SS, (Eds). Neurosurgery. 2nd ed. New York: Mc-Graw Hill, 1996: 1401-5.

164. Oxenhandler DC, Sayers MP. The dilemma of childhood optic gliomas. J Neurosurg 1978; 48: 34-41.

165. Hoffman HJ. Optic pathway and hypothalamic gliomas in children. In Youmans JR, (Ed.): Neurological Surgery. 5th ed. Philadelphia: WB Saunders, 1995; pp 2521-8.

166. Wisoff JH, Abott R, Epstein F. Surgical management of exophytic chiasmatic-hypothalamic tumours of childhood. J Neurosurg 1990; 73: 661-7.

167. Alvord EC, Lofton S. Gliomas of the optic nerve or chiasm. Outcome by patient's age, tumour site, and treatment. J Neurosurg 1988; 68: 85-98.

168. Flikinger JC, Torres C, Deutsch M. Management of low-grade gliomas of the optic nerve and chiasm. Cancer 1988; 61: 635-42.

169. Rodriguez LA, Edwards MSB, Levin VA. Management of hypothalamic gliomas in children: an analysis of 33 cases. Neurosurg 1990; 26: 242-7.

170. Tenny RT, Laws ER Jr, Younger BR, et al. The neurosurgical management of optic glioma. Results of 104 patients. J Neurosurg 1982; 57: 452-8.

171. Hoffman HJ. Supratentorial brain tumours in children. In Youmans JR, (Ed.): Neurological Surgery. Philadelphia: WB Saunders, 1982: 2702-32.

172. Dohrmann GI, Farwell JR, Flannery JT. Astrocytomas in childhood. A population based study. Surg Neurol 1985;23: 64-8.

173. Laws ER, Taylor WF, Clinton MR, et al. Neurosurgical management of low-grade astrocytomas. J Neurosurg 1984; 61: 665-73.

174. Farwell JR, Dohrmann GI, Flannery JT. Central nervous system tumours in children. Cancer 1977; 40: 3123-32.

175. Young JL Jr, Miller RW. Incidence of malignant tumours in US children. J Pediatr 1975; 86: 254-8.

176. Marchese MJ, Chang CH. Malignant astrocytic gliomas in children. Cancer 1990; 65: 2771-8.

177. Coulon RT, Till K. Intracranial ependymomas in children. A review of 43 cases. Childs Brain 1977; 3: 154.

178. Dohrmann GJ, Farwell JR, Flannery JT. Ependymomas and ependymoblastomas in children. J Neurosurg 1976;45:273-83.

179. Pollack IF, Gerszten PC, Julio Mertinez A, et al. Intracranial ependymomas of childhood. Long- term outcome and prognostic factors. Neurosurgery 1995; 37: 655-66.

180. Dohrmann GJ, Farwell JR, Flannery JT. Oligodendrogliomas in children. Surg Neurol 1978; 10: 21-25.

181. Favier J, Pizzolato GP, Berney J. Oligodendroglial tumours in childhood. Childs Nerv Syst 1985; 1: 33-8.

182. Warwick RE, Edwards MSB. Pediatric brain tumours. Curr Probl Pediatri 1991; 21: 129-32.

183. Courville CB. Ganglioglioma. Tumour of the central nervous system. Review of the literature and report of two cases. Arch Neurol Psychiatry 1930; 24: 434-7.

184. Sutton LN, Packer RJ, Rorke LB, et al. Cerebral gangliogliomas during childhood. Neurosurgery 1983; 13: 124-8.

185. Berger MS, Kincaid J, Ojemann GA, et al. Brain mapping techniques to maximise resection, safety, and seizure control on children with brain tumours. Neurosurgery 1989; 25: 786-92.

186. Cough JR, Weiss SA. Gliomatosis cerebri: report of four cases and review of literature. Neurology 1974; 24: 504-11.

187. Shepherd CW, Scheithauer BW, Gomez MR, et al. Subependymal giant cell astrocytoma. A clinical, pathological and flow cytometric study. Neurosurgery 1991; 28: 864-8.

188. Daumas-Duport C, Scheithauer BW, Chodkiewicz JP, et al. Dysembryoblastic neuro-epithelial tumor: a surgically curable tumor of young patients with intractable partial seizures. Neurosurgery 1988; 23: 545-56.

189. Kirkpatrick PJ, Honavar M, Janota I, et al. Control of temporal lobe epilepsy following en bloc resection of low-grade tumours. J Neurosurg 1993; 78: 19-25.

190. Le Marquand HS, Russell DS. A case of pubertas praecox (macrogenitosomia precox) in a boy associated with a tumor in the floor of third ventricle. Berkeley Hospital Report 1934;3:31.

191. Albright AL, Lee PA. Neurosurgical treatment of hypothalamic hamartomas causing precocious puberty. J Nuerosurg 1993; 78: 77-82.

192. Starceski PJ, Lee PA, Albright AL, et al. Hypothalamic hamartomas and sexual precocity. Evaluation of treatment options. Am J Dis Child 1990; 144: 225-8.

193. Ho DM, Wong T, Liu H. Choroid plexus tumours in childhood; histopathological study and clinico-pathological correlation. Childs Nerv Syst 1991; 7: 437-41.

194. Sahar A, Feisod M, Beller AJ. Choroid plexus papilloma: hydrocephalus and cerebrospinal fluid dynamics. Surg Neurol 1980; 13: 476-8.

195. Pillay PK, Humphreys RP, St Clair S, et al. Choroid plexus carcinomas in childhood. A note for preresection chemotherapy. AANS Annual Meeting, 1992: 484 (Abstract).

CHAPTER 39

Supriyo Ghose
Sanjeev Nainiwal
Mridula Mehta

Retinoblastoma

A typical "Cat's eye" reflex or leukocoria (Fig. 39.1) is a well-known feature of retinoblastoma.[1-4] However, many other congenital and acquired conditions may produce an identical pupillary reflex such as retinal dysplasia, retinal vascular folds, persistent hyperplastic primary vitreous (PHPV), retinal detachment, retained intraocular foreign body, endophthalmitis, cataract, uveitis, Coats' disease, and retrolental fibroplasia (RLF) or retinopathy of prematurity (ROP). Retinoblastoma is usually associated with neovascularization, high intraocular tension, features of bilateral involvement, optic nerve extension with distant metastases, and hereditary predisposition. Besides the pathognomic yellowish-white reflex, retinoblastoma may present with a squint, red eye, pain and secondary glaucoma and other atypical presentations. A number of atypical presentations like orbital cellulitis, endophthalmitis, phthisis bulbi, staophyloma, etc. have are also uncommonly seen.[5] These children should be immediately referred for further investigations and management, because delay may adversely affect survival. In spite of various imaging modalities, the differential diagnosis during the early stage may be difficult, and the exact diagnosis may be possible only after histopathological examination after enucleation of the eye. Earlier radical treatment modalities, as enucleation are giving way to eye salvaging procedures of cryotherapy, chemoreduction and lens-sparing techniques of modern radiotherapy.

Retinoblastoma (RB), as we all know, is the commonest intraocular malignancy in children. Though this is not a common condition, it is one of the few life-threatening conditions that present to an ophthalmologist. A timely diagnosis and early treatment could thus save the life of the child. Now, with the advent of newer therapeutic modalities like laser, chemotherapy and radiotherapy, an early diagnosis and the use of combination therapy can result in preservation of vision thus avoiding enucleation. The goal of RB therapy now is to **save the life *and* preserve the vision.**

HOW *NOT* TO MISS THE DIAGNOSIS OF RETINOBLASTOMA

The commonest presentation of retinoblastoma is leukocoria in a child aged 1 to 5 years. In a typical case it may not be so difficult to make the diagnosis. However, given the grave consequences of a missed or delayed diagnosis, it is prudent for ophthalmologists to maintain a high index of suspicion so as to pick up all the cases at the earliest. The clinical features together with the investigations can correctly establish the diagnosis in most cases.

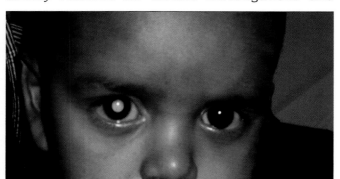

Figure 39.1: Full blown retinoblastoma presenting as leukocoria in right eye

Age: Though RB commonly presents between 18 and 24 months, in our country we often find children presenting at a later age. A word of caution: RB can present in neonates and also in older children (7-8 years) so one should be careful to rule it out in all cases of leukocoria. It has been diagnosed prenatally in fetus by ultrasonography on one hand, and rarely an adult with an intraocular mass may turn out to have retinoblastoma.

Family history and genetics: RB is said to be familial in 25 to 30 percent but in Indian conditions, we are not always able to elicit a positive family history. One should look for regressed lesions in the parents of bilateral cases and ask for a history of deaths in early childhood in the family. Also, screening of siblings (aged less than 5 years) of all cases should be done, whether unilateral or bilateral. Though the genetic abnormality is identifiable in some cases, chromosomal analysis may not be practical in our scenario since it is expensive and the results take a long time. The study of the effect of birth rank showed a significant association between sporadic retinoblastoma (bilateral and unilateral) and late para, indicating that fresh germline mutations must have taken place in some of the sporadic cases. Familial retinoblastoma is significantly associated with early para, suggesting early parental age, on the other hand, a high paternal age may be associated with sporadic bilateral (sporadic hereditary) retinoblastoma.[6]

Leukocoria: Leukocoria, unilateral or bilateral, is by far the commonest presentation of RB (Fig. 39.1). There may be overlying engorged vessels or calcification visible. There is a long list of differential diagnosis of leukocoria usually clubbed a 'pseudoglioma'. The ones likely to cause a diagnostic dilemma are PHPV, organized vitreous hemorrhage, endophthalmitits and Coats' disease in older children. The associated anterior segment findings may help, in the form of microcornea in PHPV and a low tension in endophthalmitis. Raised IOP, ectropion uveae, rubeosis and pseudohypopyon are all pointers to a tumor in the eye, which has reached an advanced stage.

Squint: Any squint in a child warrants a fundus examination with dilated pupils. A macular tumor causing the squint can be picked up even with a cursory indirect ophthalmoscopic examination, so there is no excuse for telling the parents to bring the child back for squint surgery later, without seeing the fundus.

Secondary glaucoma: If the parents miss the initial leukocoria, RB can present as secondary glaucoma with an opaque cornea. Therefore, one should rule out a tumor in these cases by examining the other eye and doing an ultrasound, if possible.

Proptosis: Unfortunately in India, there are still a large number of children presenting with proptosis. A history of leukocoria may sometimes be forthcoming. Though orbital cellulitis is still the commonest cause of proptosis in children, tumors like orbital RB and rhabdomyosarcoma should be kept in mind.

Pseudohypopyon and endophthalmitis: Though infections are rare in RB, it can present as pseudohypopyon in an inflamed eye and/or masquerading as endophthalmitis. One needs a high index of suspicion in these cases especially if seen in older children.[6]

Orbital cellulitis (pseudocellulitis): Sterile orbital cellulitis can be seen in tumors undergoing necrosis. Such inflammation is in response to inflammatory factors released during necrosis and is responsive to oral steroids. The case should be re-evaluated after inflammation has subsided for proper assessment of optic nerve involvement.

Phthisis bulbi: Such a presentation is usually preceded by massive inflammation and results from immune response against the tumour. Viable tumour cells may still be present in them.

HOW TO INVESTIGATE A CASE OF SUSPECTED RETINOBLASTOMA

Investigations are aimed at confirming the diagnosis and establishing extent of disease both for the prognosis and therapy decisions.

Examination under anesthesia: Complete evaluation of anterior and posterior segment, including corneal diameters, intraocular pressures, examination of vitreous and retina by indirect ophthalmoscopy (Figs 39.2A and B). Careful colored drawings of the tumor should preferably be made. Attention should also be paid to presence of low set and posteriorly rotated ears, simian crease in palms, broad thumb, telecanthus, hypertelorism and other minor congenital anomalies. These findings may suggest presence of 13q deletion syndrome.

Wide-angle retinal photography or RetCam 120 digital imaging: Extremely useful for documenting size and location of the tumour. It allows comparison of images on serial follow-up and pictures from it can be shown to family members to better understand the disease.

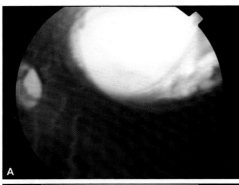
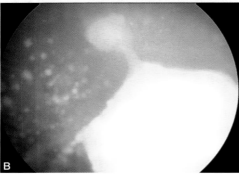

Figures 39.2A and B: (A) Intraocular retinoblastoma as a well defined mass lesion. (B) Intraocular retinoblastoma with vitreous seeds

Fluorescein angiography is also possible with this system for diagnosis and management of the tumor.

Ultrasonography: USG is an important tool in establishing the diagnosis of RB. RB is usually seen as a mass lesion of moderate to high internal reflectivity, arising from the retina.[2] There may be an overlying detachment visible. Calcification, characterized by spikes of 100 percent reflectivity, is seen in 90 percent cases and is diagnostic of RB. Optic nerve involvement and scleral infiltration may also be picked up. USG monitoring of tumor height is important when the patient is on chemoreduction. Recently, three-dimensional ultrasonography of retinoblastoma is available for better delineation of tumor form and volume.

CT Scan: On CT Scan, RB is seen as a moderately attenuating mass lesion with calcification. Extraocular spread in the form of optic nerve or scleral infiltration and/or intracranial extension is well demonstrated. CT Scan is required for radiotherapy planning as well.

MRI: MRI is not as useful in the diagnosis of RB except in cases where vitreous hemorrhage/exudative retinal detachment is suspected. Though calcification is not so well demonstrated, the soft tissue visualization is better especially in case of chiasmal involvement. A Gadolinium enhanced MRI with specific cuts directed through region of pineal gland is advisable to rule out possibility of trilateral retinoblastoma (Bilateral retinoblastoma and pineloblastoma).

Special Investigations

In most cases the diagnosis can be clinched with the above-mentioned clinical features and investigations. In certain cases where the diagnosis is difficult, like leucocoria without calcification, non-responsive uveites/vitritis in children older age groups etc., some special investigations may be indicated. One such investigation is Fine Needle Aspiration Biopsy (FNAB). FNAB done under indirect ophthalmoscopic guidance and with an experienced cytopathologist can be a useful diagnostic tool.

Investigations for Metastasis

The investigations for determining the spread of RB are CSF examination and bone marrow biopsy. Bone scanning may be done if metastasis is suspected.

STAGING OF RB

As in all cancers, staging of the disease is essential both for prognostication and for planning the treatment. The age-old Reese-Ellsworth classification, though still followed in a number of centers, may not be so relevant today. For one, it is only an intraocular classification and secondly, anterior lesions, which today can easily treated with cryotherapy, have been assigned a worse prognosis. Other classifications like the St. Jude's Hospital classification have included both extraocular and intraocular disease. The RPC-IRCH classification also lays the basis for combined modality (local therapy, radiotherapy and chemotherapy) treatment. Recently, International Classification of Retinoblastoma has come up that groups intraocular Rb and predicts response to chemoreduction and focal treatment.

MANAGEMENT OF RB

The emphasis in RB management has now shifted from enucleation to the use of combination therapy in an effort to preserve vision and salvage the globe. For this multi-modality therapy to work, good co-operation is ***essential*** between the ophthalmologists, pediatric oncologists and radio-therapists. The therapy of each child needs to be carefully planned with active involvement of the concerned doctors and family of the child if optimum results are to be obtained.

The therapeutic options available are:

1. Local treatment: Cryotherapy
                      Laser therapy
                      Transpupillary thermotherapy.
2. Surgical: Enucleation
                      Exenteration.
3. Chemotherapy: Chemoreduction with various drugs—Etopside, carboplatin, vincristine, cyclophosphamide
4. Radiotherapy: Brachytherapy with radioactive plaques—Iodine-125, ruthenium-106
                      External beam radiotherapy (EBRT)

Local Treatment

Local treatment is directed at small lesions away from the fovea and optic nerve that are accessible either with laser or cryotherapy. It may either be the primary therapy or used after chemoreduction—this has been described as serially aggressive local therapy (SALT). Cyrotherapy is done by elevating the lesion on a cryoprobe and applying the triple freeze-thaw technique . The endpoint of the cryo is when the ice ball reaches the surface of the tumor into the overlying vitreous. Patient should be reviewed after 2-3 weeks and cryo may be repeated if required. The lesion usually regresses to a flat scar. On subsequent follow-up the edges of the scar need to be carefully examined for recurrence. Laser treatment is suitable for small lesions (1-1.5 disc diameter with minimal elevation). Here contagious laser spots are applied around the lesion to cut off the vascular supply. These lesions then may regress completely without any scarring.

All patients treated with local modalities need to be carefully followed up at monthly intervals initially.

Indications of cryotherapy
- < 3.5 mm in diam
- < 2 mm in thickness
- Anterior to equator
- Residual or recurrent tumour after chemoreduction and EBRT.

Method

Retinal cryoprobe –70°C is used.

Tumor is elevated on tip and freezing is applied until the surrounding retina turns white and ice crystals appear in overlying vitreous requires 10 to15 sec, then it is allowed to thaw.

Three successive freeze and thaw applications are used may be repeated in 3 to 4 weeks if required. Successful if flat, pigmented, avascular scar results with no signs of viable tumor. The recurrence rate is 33 percent.

Surgical Treatment

Most children present with the eye full of tumor, leaving enucleation as the only option. During enucleation, one should take care to obtain a long stump of the optic nerve and also subject the globe to histopathological examination to confirm the diagnosis and determine the extent of infiltration of the intraocular structures; information that has a bearing on the overall prognosis. All attempts should be made to give a good cosmetic result in the form of an implant and a good fitting prosthesis. Presently integrated implants (Hydroxy-apatite, Porous polyethylene) are available on which the muscles can be attached and give better outcome in terms of motility and cosmesis.

Orbital retinoblastoma is treated with exenteration followed by radiotherapy. However, once the tumor breaches the sclera and extends to the orbit, the prognosis for life is very dismal.

Chemotherapy

The newer drugs with better ocular penetration like carboplatin and etoposide have ensured that chemotherapy now has an important role in RB management, that of chemoreduction (Fig. 39.3). In this, a few cycles of the chemotherapeutic drugs are given to shrink the tumors which are then treated with local therapy: cryotherapy/laser.[7]

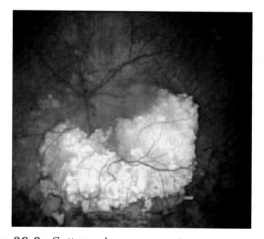

Figure 39.3: Cottage cheese regression pattern in retino-blastoma this may be after treatment or even spontaneous

vertically upwards and slightly backwards. It also gives off the zygomatic branch that runs obliquely upwards and forwards. The lower division splits off a buccal branch that runs horizontally forward in close proximity with the parotid duct. It then continues inferiorly and divides to give off a small cervical branch and a longer, slender mandibular branch that runs forward across the mandible. This branch has a variable course and may loop down low into the neck before ascending. It is the most frequently injured branch of the facial nerve and its loss is associated with the typical appearance of drooping of the corner of the mouth when the patient is asked to show his teeth.

Once each of the branches has been traced and clearly displayed, the whole of the parotid tissue lying superfical to this plane can be easily removed (Fig. 40.5). Bleeding is usually controlled by traction on the gland and use of the bipolar cautery. If a decision is made to do a total parotidectomy then the deep lobe needs to be removed as well. This is done in the same way by teasing apart the glandular tissue from the underlying muscle and fascia using the blunt tip of the haemostat. Each branch of the nerve is gently separated from the gland tissue that is then delivered upwards and removed from its attachments. The process is repeated with each of the branches until all the remaining glandular tissue has been elevated off from its bed. The use of nerve hooks or rubber slings to hold the branches of the facial nerve is not advisable as sudden traction may tear the delicate filaments. This part of the dissection is much like working through a lattice and is not difficult as the deep lobe in most cases is much smaller than the superficial lobe. The parotid duct is ligated as far forwards

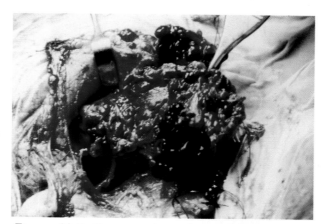

Figure 40.5: Cavernous type of parotid hemagnioma showing large vascular spaces with thrombus

as possible. Haemostasis is then secured using the bipolar cautery and the wound is closed in layers with drainage.

Complications of Parotidectomy

Facial nerve palsy, either temporary or permanent, remains the most important consideration in parotid gland surgery. The incidence of this complication depends on several factors including the disease pathology, extent of the lesion, the type of surgical resection and the experience of the operator. Retraction of the nerve or its branches, particulary the mandibular branch, may result in facial weakness but this will usually recover within a few weeks. Division of the nerve if recognised at the time of surgery should be dealt with by nerve grafting. Direct suture of the cut facial nerve should not be attempted, as the results are uniformly unsuccessful.

The other complication unique to parotid surgery is Frei's syndrome that is gustatory sweating over the hemiface. It is thought to be due to aberrant regeneration of nerve branches to sweat glands of the face. Several techniques have been described to prevent its occurrence by interposing tissues or implants between the parotid bed area and the overlying flaps.[21,22] When the syndrome is established and causes significant disability a recently described technique of injecting botulinum toxin intracutaneously into the affected area has been highly effective.[23,24]

LYMPHANGIOMATOUS MALFORMATIONS

Unlike hemangiomas, lymphangiomas seldom occur only within the parotid gland. They usually involve the parotid as part of a larger lesion in the head and neck region (Table 40.4).

Macroscopically, two types can be distinguished and they have very different outcomes:

1. Macrocystic lymphangioma (cystic hygroma) (Figs 40.6 and 40.7): This is the more common type, presenting with large cystic spaces filled with clear or straw-coloured fluid. Haemorrhage into the cysts may result in a sudden increase in size and sometimes cause airway obstruction (Figs 40.8 to 40.10). The natural history of these lesions is that they enlarge in size as the child grows and do not show any tendency towards spontaneous regression. However, the wall of these cysts can be clearly demarcated from

Table 40.4: Distribution of lymphangioma by anatomical region[30]

Anatomical Region	Percentage
Cervical	31.4%
Craniofacial	18.9%
Extremity	18.8%
Trunk	9.2%
Intraabdominal	9.2%
Cervicoaxillothoracic	4.9%
Multiple	3.8%
Total	193 cases

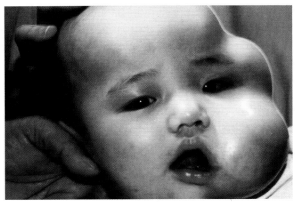

Figure 40.8: Sudden enlargement in cystic hygroma due to bleeding

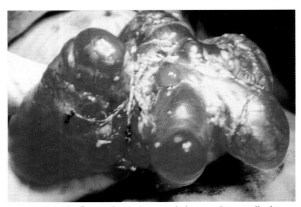

Figure 40.6: Cystic hygroma with large, thin-walled cysts easily separated from surrounding tissues. Note the facial nerve stretched across the cysts

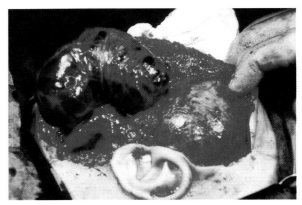

Figure 40.9: Operative findings showing massive hemorrhage into cysts

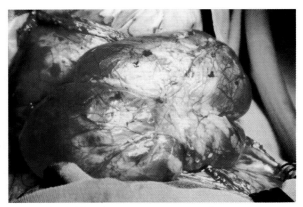

Figure 40.7: Very large cysts in cystic hygroma involving parotid and extending into neck

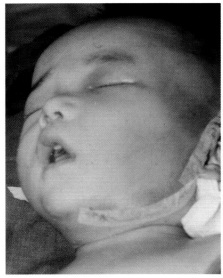

Figure 40.10: Appearance after complete excision. The facial nerve was preserved with all its branches

surrounding structures from which it can be easily separated (Fig. 40.11).

2. Microcystic lymphangioma (lymphangiomatous malformation): In this lesion multiple cysts of various sizes, usually small are intimately interspersed with normal tissues and no plane of separation can be

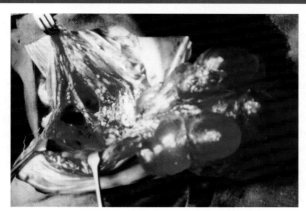

Figure 40.11: Mixed lesion with lymphangioma and hemangioma

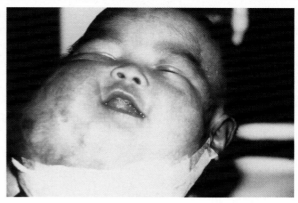

Figure 40.13: Hemorrhage and infection following attempted aspiration. Patient developed acute airway obstruction and needed tracheostomy

identified (Figs 40.12 and 40.13). Unlike cystic hygromas, no clearly defined wall can be recognised. These lesions tend to grow and infiltrate into surrounding structures (Fig. 40.14).

Clinically, lymphangiomas most commonly present as an asymptomatic neck mass.[25] Unlike hemangiomas, these lesions do not regress spontaneously but rather progressively increase in size as the child grows. The diagnosis is easily made on clinical examination. The lesions have a soft, cystic feel and are often brilliantly transilluminant.

Antenatal diagnosis with ultrasound examination can reveal the diagnosis and MRI may be helpful in evaluating the extent of the disease.[26] This may have implications in the decision to terminate pregnancy if the lesions are extensive and not amenable to treatment.

Ultrasound characteristics of lymphangiomas have been well described.[27] MRI gives excellent resolution

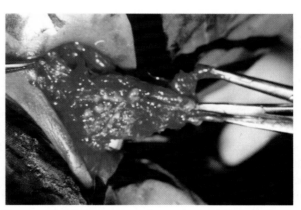

Figure 40.14: Resection of microcystic lymphangioma. Note the extensive infiltration into tissues

both in confirming the diagnosis and precisely localising the tissue characteristics.[28] Contrast-enhanced MRI is very helpful in differentiating hemangiomas from lymphangiomas.[29] All hemangiomas show enhancement following intravenous administration of contrast while lymphangiomas do not show this feature at all.

Management

Lymphangiomas are highly complex lesions and treatment can vary from simple excision to radical surgical procedures requiring major reconstruction of soft tissues. Both non-surgical and surgical therapies have been used with varying claims for success.

Needle Aspiration: Although some recent reports have referred to the use of this method the results are poor[25]. Lymphangiomas are composed of multiloculated cystic spaces and it is impossible to aspirate all the cysts.

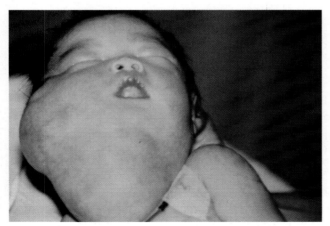

Figure 40.12: Typical appearance of microcystic lymphangioma

Furthermore, leaving the lining behind results in rapid re-accumulation of fluid in these cavities. A particularly dangerous complication is when infection occurs after aspiration. The whole mass becomes very tense and swollen with severe, spreading cellulitis.

Sclerotherapy: A number of different agents have been used to cause regression of lymphangiomas. These include the following:
1. The 50 percent dextrose[30]
2. Doxycycline[28]
3. Bleomycin[31]
4. α - Interferon[32]

The mechanism of action is uncertain and the results are unpredictable although in reported series cure rates over 80 percent have been claimed.[31]

Sclerotherapy received a significant boost with the introduction of OK-432 (picibanil) in Japan. This is an antigen derived from streptococcus pyogenes and it induces an inflammatory response that leads to sclerosis and resolution of the lesion. Ogita and his colleagues reported their experience in 64 patients over a 6-year period in both primary cases as well as those that recurred following incomplete surgical removal.[33] They noted good results with cystic lesions while cavernous types did poorly. Again, in secondary treatment after failure of surgery or bleomycin the results were not as good as in the primary cystic type lesions. Since then numerous other investigators have reported favorable results with the use of OK-432.[34,35,36,37,38] Overall, the experience with OK-432 suggests that the best response to this type of therapy occurs with macrocystic lymphangiomas of the infratemporal fossa or cervical region.

Surgical Excision: Complete surgical excision provides the only permanent cure for lymphangiomas. In a large series of 164 patients undergoing primary surgical therapy, the recurrence rate after total excision was 11.8 percent compared to 52.9 percent after partial excisions.[30] In the author's experience, complete excision for parotid lymphangiomas always requires parotidectomy, as it is impossible to separate the cysts from gandular tissue. The operation can be safely done without injury to the facial nerve but it requires considerable experience of parotid gland surgery.

Surgical removal of cystic hygromas should be done as early as possible as the ease of dissection is greatest when the infant is very young. The author carries out this operation as soon as the diagnosis is made even in the neonatal stage. The parotid part of the lesion will usually require total parotidectomy with sparing of the facial nerve.

Cavernous, microcystic lymphangiomas continue to pose a difficult surgical problem. Surgical removal can be extremely difficult owing to the extensive infiltration into tissues. Incomplete removal always results in rapid recurrence of the lesion. Although benign, these lesions can behave almost like malignant tumors. Complete surgical excision is necessary to cure this condition but this may require sacrifice of significant areas of normal tissue (Fig. 40.15). The resulting deformity will then need plastic surgical reconstruction.

SOLID NEOPLASMS OF THE PAROTID

In children these lesions are rare and generally the principles of treatment follow the same guidelines as for adults (Fig. 40.16).

Pleomorphic Adenoma

This is the most common benign solid tumor and usually occurs in older children between 10 and 15 years of age. It usually presents as a very slow growing, painless hard mass. The most common site of involvement is the superficial lobe. Occasionally, it may be confined solely to the deep lobe and it then presents as an intra-oral mass in the lateral wall of the pharynx where it may cause airway problems.

The tumor itself is composed of glandular and stromal elements and has a gritty, cartilage-like appearance. Although it appears well encapsulated there are always

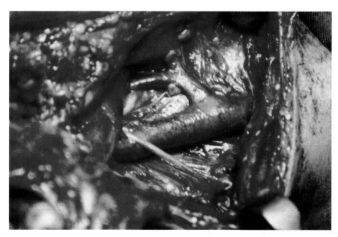

Figure 40.15: Completed resection of microcystic lymphangioma. The resection required radical excision of all involved tissues leaving a large soft-tissue defect

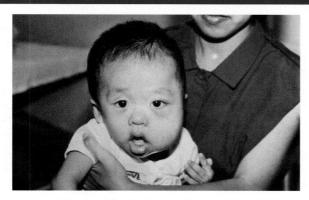

Figure 40.16: Neurofibromatosis
involving the parotid gland

numerous surface projections that extend out like feet into the surrounding parenchyma. For this reason, enucleation will not remove the tumor completely and recurrence is the rule.[39] The diagnosis is made on CT or MRI and surgical treatment is always indicated. The tumor is removed by excising the lobe in which it arises e.g. superficial parotidectomy for a lesion in the superficial lobe. It is essential to ensure complete removal as recurrences are liable to undergo malignant transformation. As the facial nerve is never involved it is always possible to carry out nerve-sparing surgery without endangering the adequacy of the resection.

Mucoepidermoid Carcinoma

This is the most common malignant neoplasm of the parotid gland in children but is rarely found under the age of 10 years.[40] Unlike the adult variety, those that occur in children tend to be less aggressive and are locally recurrent. Adequate resection with clearance of involved lymph nodes can give a good prognosis.

In malignant parotid gland tumors surgical resection may require the sacrifice of the facial nerve. If this is necessary immediate nerve grafting using the lesser occipital or transverse cervical branches to bridge the defect can be performed. The results are very good but functional recovery may take up to one year.

Other Parotid Tumors

The parotid gland may become involved in other malignancies that may be local or systemic. Rhabdomyosarcoma occurs most commonly in the head and neck region but rarely involves the parotid gland primarily.[41] It usually presents as a mass that may be mistaken for an inflammatory swelling. FNAC may sometimes be helpful especially if combined with immunohistochemical studies. Adjuvent chemotherapy can be effective in controlling the disease.

First branchial cleft cysts sometimes present as parotid tumors.[42] These cysts are derived from the first branchial cleft and histologically are composed of lympho-epithelial tissue.

Malignant parotid tumors may sometimes arise as second neoplasms in children who have been previously treated for primary childhood cancer.[43] In a series of 8 such cases 7 mucoepidermoid and 1 acinar cell carcinoma occurred in patients who had previously had acute leukemia (n = 7) or neuroblastoma (n = 1). The time of occurrence of the second tumor ranged from 4 to 16 years with a median of 9 years. Interestingly, 6 percent of second cancers involved the parotid gland whereas primary malignant salivary gland neoplasms constituted only 0.08 percent of all primary cancers diagnosed in the same period. With the increasing survival of children with primary malignancies it is important that patients be kept under careful followup for parotid gland neoplasms.

REFERENCES

1. Orvidas LJ, Kasperbauer JL, Lewis JE, et al. Pediatric parotid masses. Archives of Otolaryngology – Head and Neck Surgery 2000;126:177-84.
2. Al-Khafaji BM, Nestok BR, Katz RL. Fine-needle aspiration of 154 parotid masses with histologic correlation: ten-year experience at the University of Texas M. D. Anderson Cancer Center. Cancer 1998;84:153-9.
3. Filopoulos E, Angeli S, Daskalopoulou D, et al. Pre-operative evaluation of parotid tumors by fine needle biopsy. European Journal of Surgical Oncology 1998;24:180-3.
4. Liu KK, Lam WW. Parotid hemangioma in infancy: diagnosis with technetium 99m-labeled red blood cell pool imaging. Otolaryngology–Head and Neck Surgery 1995;112:780-1.
5. Carvalho MB, Soares JM, Rapoport A, et al. Perioperative frozen section examination in parotid gland tumors. Sao Paulo Medical Journal–Revista Paulista de Medicina 1998;117:233-7.
6. Horie Y. Kato M. Juvenile hemangioma (infantile hemangio-endothelioma) of the parotid gland associated with cyto-megalovirus infection. Pathology International 1999;49:668-71.
7. Sabatino G, Verrotti A, de Martino M, et al. Neonatal suppurative parotitis: a study of five cases. European Journal of Pediatrics 1999;158:312-4.
8. Wang SL, Jou ZJ, Yu SF et al. Recurrent swelling of parotid glands and Sjogren's syndrome. International Journal of Oral and Maxillofacial Surgery 1993;22:362-5.
9. Chiu CH, Lin TY: Clinical and microbiological analysis of six children with acute suppurative parotitis. Acta Paediatrica 1996;85:106-8.
10. Reid E, Douglas F, Crow Y, et al. Autosomal dominant juvenile recurrent parotitis. Journal of Medical Genetics 1998;35:417-9.
11. Chitre VV, Premchandra DJ. Recurrent parotitis. Archives of Disease in Childhood 1997;77:359-63.
12. Giglio MS, Landaeta M, Pinto ME. Microbiology of recurrent parotitis. Pediatric Infectious Disease Journal 1997;16:386-90.

13. Mandel L, Kaynar A. Recurrent parotitis in children. New York State Dental Journal 1995;61:22-5.

14. Wang S, Li J, Zhu X, et al. Gland atrophy following retrograde injection of methyl violet as a treatment in chronic obstructive parotitis. Oral Surgery, Oral Medicine, Oral Pathology, Oral Radiology, and Endodontics 1998;85:276-81.

15. Sadeghi N, Black MJ, Frenkiel S. Parotidectomy for the treatment of chronic recurrent parotitis. Journal of Otolaryngology 1996;25:305-7.

16. Bartunkova J, Sediva A, Vencovsky J, et al. Primary Sjogren's syndrome in children and adolescents: proposal for diagnostic criteria. Clinical and Experimental Rheumatology 1999;17: 381-6.

17. Carroll CM, Amin H. Non-tuberculous mycobacterial infection of the parotid gland. Irish Medical Journal 1997;90:152-4.

18. Dubois J, Garel L. Imaging and therapeutic approach of hemangiomas and vascular malformations in the pediatric age group. Pediatric Radiology 1999;29:879-93.

19. Horie Y, Kato M. Juvenile hemangioma (infantile hemangio-endothelioma) of the parotid gland assocaited with cyto-megalovirus infection. Pathology International 1999;49: 668-71.

20. Blei F, Isakoff M, Deb G. The response of parotid hemangiomas to the use of systemic interferon alfa-2a or corticosteroids. Archives of Otolaryngology – Head and Neck Surgery 1997;123:841-4.

21. Ahmed OA, Kolhe PS. Prevention of Frey's syndrome and volume deficit after parotidectomy using the superficial temporal artery fascial flap. British Journal of Plastic Surgery 1999;52:256-60.

22. Dulguerov P, quinodoz D, Cosendai G, et al. Prevention of Frey syndrome during parotidectomy. Archives of Otolaryngology – Head and Neck surgery 1999;125:833-9.

23. Laskawi R, Drobik C, Schonebeck C. Up-to-date report of botulinum toxin type A treatment in patients with gustatory sweating (Fey's syndrome). Laryngoscope 1998;108:381-4.

24. Laccourreye O, Muscatelo L, Naude C. Botulinum toxin type A for Frey's syndrome: a preliminary prospective study. Annals of Otology, Rhinology and Laryngology 1998;107:52-5.

25. Fageeh N, Manoukian J, Tewfik T, et al. Management of head and neck lymphatic malformations in children. Journal of Otlaryngology 1997;26:253-8.

26. Kaminopetros P, Jauniux E, Kane P, et al. Prenatal diagnosis of an extensive fetal lymphangioma using ultrasonography, magnetic resonance imaging and cytology. British Journal of Radiology 1997;70:750-3.

27. Kapoor R, Saha MM, Talwar S. Sonographic appearances of lymphangiomas. Indian Pediatrics 1994;31:1447-50.

28. Wimmershoff MB, Schreyer AG, Glaessl A, et al. Mixed capillary/lymphatic malformation with coexisting port-wine stain: treatment utilizing 3D MRI and CT-guided sclerotherapy. Dermatologic Surgery 2000;26:584-7.

29. Yonetsu K, Nakayama E, Kawazu T, et al. Value of contrast-enhanced magnetic resonance imaging in Oral Surgery, Oral medicine, Oral Pathology, Oral Radiology, and maxillofacial region. Endodontics 1999;88: 496-500.

30. Hancock BJ, St-Vil D, Luks FI, et al. Complications of lymphangiomas in children. Journal of Pediatric Surgery 1992; 27:220-4.

31. Zhong PQ, Zhi FX, Li R, et al. Long-term results of intratumorous bleomycin-A5 injection for head and neck lymphangioma. Oral Surgery, Oral Medicine, Oral Pathology, Oral Radiology, and Endodontics 1998;86:139-44.

32. Reinhardt MA, Nelson SC, Sencer SF, et al. Treatment of childhood lymphangiomas with interferon-alpha. Journal of Pediatric Hematology/Oncology 1997;19:232-6.

33. Ogita S, Tsuto T, Nakamura K, et al. OK-432 therapy in 64 patients with lymphangioma. Journal of Pediatric surgery 1994;29:784-5.

34. Brewis C, Pracy JP, Albert DM. Treatment of lymphangiomas of the head and neck in children by intralesional injection of OK-432 (Picibanil). Clinical Otolaryngology and Allied Sciences 2000:25:130-4.

35. Luzzatto C, Midrio P, Tchaprassian Z, et al. Sclerosing treatment of lymphangiomas with OK-32. Archives of Disease in childhood 2000;82:316-8.

36. Greinwald JH JR, Burke DK, Sato Y, et al. Treatment of lymphangiomas in children: an update of Picibanil (OK-432) sclerotherapy. Otolaryngology – Head and Neck Surgery 1999; 121:381-7.

37. Schmidt B, Schimpl G, Hollwarth ME. OK-432 therapy of lymphangiomas in children. European Journal of Pediatrics 1996;155:649-52.

38. Mikhail M, Kennedy R, Cramer B, et al. Sclerosing of recurrent lymphangioma using OK-432. Journal of Pediatric Surgery 1995;30:1159-60.

39. Laskawi R, Schott T, Schroder M. Recurrent pleomorphic adenomas of the parotid gland: clinical evaluation and long-term follow-up. British Journal of Oral and Maxillofacial surgery 1998;36:48-51.

40. Khadaroo RG, Walton JM, Ramsay JA, et al. Mucoepidermoid carcinoma of the parotid gland: a rare presentation in a young child. Journal of Pediatric Surgery 1998;33:893-5.

41. Salomao DR, Sigman JD, Greenebaum E, et al. Rhabdo-myosarcoma presenting as a parotid gland mass in pediatric patients: fine-needle aspiration biopsy findings. Cancer 1998; 84:245-51.

42. Baader WM, Lewis JM. First branchial cleft cysts presenting as parotid tumors. Annals of Plastic Surgery 1994;33:72-4.

43. Kaste SC, Hedlund G, Pratt CB. Malignant parotid tumors in patients previously treated for childhood cancer: clinical and imaging findings in eight cases. American Journal of Roentgeno-logy 1994;162:655-9.

RK Minkes
MA Skinner

Thyroid Tumors in Children

The thyroid gland develops as a diverticulum from the endoderm of the floor of the pharynx and descends along the thyroglossal tract to the level of the laryngeal primordium. Two pairs of parathyroid glands develop from separate pharyngeal pouches. The inferior parathyroid glands are derived from the third pharyneal pouch and descend with the thymus gland, which is also derived from the third pouch. The superior thyroid glands are derived from the fourth pharyngeal pouch and descend adherent to the posterior aspect of the thyroid capsule

Thyroid carcinoma accounts for 1 percent of all childhood malignancies and 7 percent of cancers arising in the head and neck. The incidence of clinically detectable thyroid cancer ranges from 0.2 to 5 per million children annually and is at least twice as common in females (Fig. 41.1).[1] The incidence increases with age

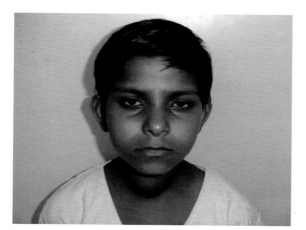

Figure 41.1: Midline thyroid swelling in a girl. Thyroid cancers are more common in females

and peaks during adolescence. Differentiated thyroid cancer is rare before the age of 3 years.

The role of radiation in the development of benign and malignant thyroid disease is well established and radiation doses exceeding 150 cGy increase the risk of thyroid cancer.[2] Historically, 80 percent of all new cases of thyroid cancer were related to neck irradiaton for benign infant disorders such as enlarged thymus, hypertrophied tonsils and adenoids, hemangiomas, nevi, eczema and cervical adenitis. Higher radiation doses, young age at radiation initiation and female sex are significant risk factors for the development of thyroid cancer following radiation exposure. The cessation of irradiation for benign conditions led to a decrease in the incidence of thyroid carcinoma. However, an increase in the number of childhood thyroid cancer cases has being reported following nuclear power station accidents. Most of these tumors are extremely aggressive and have occurred as soon as only 4 years following the disaster.

Another risk factor for thyroid cancer is the successful treatment of previous childhood malignancies. Up to 50 percent of children receiving irradiation and chemotherapy for Hodgkin's disease, leukemia and other head and neck malignancies develop elevated thyroid stimulating hormone (TSH) levels within 1 year of treatment.[3,4] Thyroid cancer may develop after a latency period of up to 25–30 years. Environmental factors are also thought to play a role in thyroid carcinoma. For example, follicular carcinomas are increased in areas with iodine deficiency and dramatic decreases are seen when iodinated salt is used in the diet. Finally, there are some genetic factors responsible for thyroid carcinoma such as in the multiple endocrine neoplasia (MEN) 2 syndromes. At least 30–50 percent of medullary thyroid carcinoma are related to these autosomal dominant familial syndromes.

HISTOLOGIC TYPES—FOLLICULAR OR PAPILLARY

Follicular adenoma is the most common cause of solitary thyroid nodules in the pediatric population.[5] Adenomas are solitary, are well circumscribed and well encapsulated, and are composed of glandular epithelium. Thyroid nodules occur in 4-7 percent of the general adult population and in only 1-2 percent of the pediatric population; however, solitary nodules in children reportedly have a 20-73 percent incidence of malignancy.[6] The incidence of malignancy is much higher in pediatric nodules. Five percent of nodules in adults are malignant while in the pediatric population, the percentage of malignant nodules is 33 percent.[7-9]

The histologic subtypes of thyroid cancer include:[10-14]

1. Papillary or mixed (70–80%)
2. Follicular (20%)
3. Medullary (5–10%)
4. Anaplastic (Rare)

Papillary tumors consist of epithelial cells arranged as papillae disseminated throughout the gland. Lymphocytic infiltrates and psammoma bodies are common. In follicular carcinoma, the malignant cells are adenomatous with follicle formation and are distinguished from benign adenomas only by the presence of nuclear abnormalities, capsular invasion or vascular invasion.

Follicular carcinoma lesions usually are encapsulated and have highly cellular follicles and microfollicles with compact dark-staining nuclei of fairly uniform size, shape, and location. Pathologic diagnosis can be made only when invasion of the capsule, adjacent glands, lymphatics, or blood vessels is seen. When a portion of the cells in the tumor is found to be oxyphilic (Hürthle cells), it is called a Hürthle cell tumor. These lesions tend to have a less favorable prognosis.

Follicular tumors with any papillary elements behave as papillary malignancies and are considered papillary tumors with follicular architecture. Medullary thyroid carcinoma (MTC) arises from the parafollicular C cells, which secrete calcitonin and derived from neural crest cells and ultimobranchial body. Hyperplasia of the C cells is thought to represent a precancerous state. These tumors appear as solid islets of regular, undifferentiated cells with abundant granular cytoplasm. The nuclei are hyperchromatic, and mitoses are common. The cells have a fusiform shape and may form a whorling pattern. The stroma contains fibrotic tissue, amyloid and may contain calcifications in 50 percent of these lesions.

PATHOGENESIS

The only established risk factor for differentiated thyroid cancer is ionizing radiation. Specific genetic mutations identified in recent years have helped to elucidate the pathogenesis of thyroid cancer. Activating mutations in the RAS proto-oncogene can be demonstrated in both benign follicular adenomas and 80 percent of follicular carcinomas.[15] The RAS mutation is present in only 20 percent of papillary tumors. A translocation involving the RET proto-oncogene is present in 35 percent of papillary carcinomas.[16,17] Mutations in the RET proto-oncogene are present in both sporadic and familial forms of MTC. Approximately 80 percent of children who undergo thyroidectomy based on the presence of the RET mutation have foci of MTC within the gland. Different mutations in the RET proto-oncogene identified in MEN2A and 2B may be responsible for the phenotypic variance seen in these syndromes.

In children MTC is usually familial, either associated with the MEN2 syndromes or the familial MTC (FMTC) syndrome. MEN2A is characterized by MTC, pheochromocytoma, and parathyroid hyperplasia. Children with MEN2B develop a more virulent form of MTC, pheochromocytomas, and multiple neuromas and have a characteristic phenotypic appearance; MTC is the first tumor to develop in MEN patients and is the most common cause of death in these patients. A history of Graves disease, hypothyroidism, or goiter can indicate benign thyroid disease.

CLINICAL PRESENTATION

Most pediatric thyroid nodules are asymptomatic and are detected by parents or by physicians on routine examination. Only about 50 percent of children with thyroid carcinoma present with nodular thyroid enlargement as the presenting symptom. A painless noninflammatory metastatic cervical mass is the presenting symptom for 40-60 percent of patients.[18] Malignant lesions most commonly are papillary and follicular carcinomas, and previous radiation therapy is a significant risk factor.

Pediatric thyroid carcinoma occurs more frequently in adolescents but has been reported in the neonatal period.[19]

Children commonly present with advanced disease. The lungs are the most common site of metastasis. Carcinoma of the thyroid gland presents as a painless thyroid mass, cervical adenopathy, or a combination of the two. Carcinoma in pediatric patients most commonly manifests as an asymptomatic neck mass incidentally noted by parents or patients or by physicians during routine physical examination. Palpable cervical adenopathy is present in up to two-thirds of cases and may be present without a palpable primary thyroid tumor.[13] Rarely, with advanced disease or anaplastic carcinoma, dysphonia and tracheal and esophageal compressive symptoms can occur. Hoarseness indicates compression or invasion of the recurrent laryngeal nerve. Up to 50 percent of patients with papillary tumors have metastases to local cervical or mediastinal lymph nodes and 6–20 percent have lung metastases at the time of diagnosis.[20] Local lymph node disease is less common in follicular variants but bone metastases are more common. Rapid growth rate may indicate a poorer prognosis. Pain is rarely associated with malignancy except transiently in association with hemorrhage into a nodule.

Tenderness suggests hemorrhage into a nodule, a cyst, or an inflammatory process. A soft compressible nodule is less likely to be malignant than a firm one. Fixation of the mass to surrounding tissues and vocal fold paralysis suggest malignancy. Lymphadenopathy further increases the likelihood of malignancy. Diffuse thyroid enlargement or multiple nodules are more suggestive of a benign process

Mucosal neuromas of the tongue, palpebral conjunctiva, and lips with marfanoid body habitus may suggest MEN syndrome with medullary carcinoma.

INVESTIGATIONS

The evaluation for a thyroid mass should begin with thyroid function tests, which are normal in the majority of cases (Fig. 41.2). Ultrasonography will determine whether the lesion is cystic or solid. Many investigators consider cystic lesions to be benign lesions that represent hemorrhage into or degeneration of an adenomatous nodular goiter. One of the most helpful capabilities of ultrasound is guidance of percutaneous needle biopsy. A solid nodule has a higher chance of being malignant; however, up to 50 percent of malignant lesions may

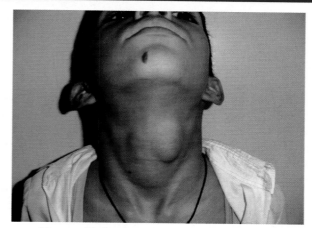

Figure 41.2: Left thyroid swelling in a boy

have a cystic component.[21] Approximately 8 percent of cystic lesions are malignant.[22] The incidence of malignancy in multinodular goiter is 1-7 percent and in solitary nodules is 10-25 percent.[7]

A thyroid scan with Tc 99m-pertechnetate will determine if the mass contains functioning thyroid tissue. Radionucleotide scan Thyroid scintiscans are most useful in evaluating tissue function in thyroglossal duct cysts, in evaluating the thyroid in a normal location, and in diagnosing ectopic thyroid; however, they have not proven very worthwhile in distinguishing malignant from benign disease.

Cold nodules are most often benign adenomas, although in children, carcinoma is identified in 30 percent of children who undergo surgical resection for cold nodules.

CT scans can be helpful in patients with substernal extension, local invasion, or lymph node metastasis.

The pathologic diagnosis is established by FNA cytology or frozen section at the time of surgery. The use of FNA to evaluate thyroid nodules is well established in adults and its use in adults has decreased the incidence of thyroidectomy for benign conditions and has increased the number of surgical patients with carcinoma. Limitations of FNA include an incidence of false negative cytology from 1 percent to 6 percent, which may result in a delay in diagnosis and treatment of carcinoma, availability of an experienced cytopathologist and an inability to differentiate benign from malignant follicular lesions. Results of FNA cytology indicate cancer, a benign lesion, or a lesion suspicious for cancer. In addition, it has been demonstrated, in adults, that benign nodules may be followed safely with serial physical and ultrasound examinations; the nodules are resected if growth is demonstrated during the observation period. Surgical resection is indicated for malignant or suspicious nodules. Aspirated cysts that collapse completely can be observed, but should be surgically removed if they recur.

The usefulness of FNAC in children is less well defined. A recent study of 57 children with thyroid nodules revealed malignancy in 18 percent.[23] There was one false negative FNAC, in which papillary carcinoma was diagnosed as a benign nodule; the malignancy was subseqently recognized and resected after clinical follow-up. Since the pattern of thyroid disease in children older than 13 years is similar to that in adults, it is likely that aspiration cytology is an acceptable way to evaluate thyroid nodules in adolescents.[24] In children younger than 13 years of age, aspiration is exceedingly more difficult to perform and the pattern of benign disease is different than in adults. The natural history of these lesions and the safety of a non-operative approach is unknown. Therefore, FNA should probably not be used in young children, and all children younger than 13 years of age should undergo surgical excision.

MEDICAL MANAGEMENT

Radioactive therapy with iodine 131 (^{131}I) is indicated to ablate residual normal thyroid and treat functioning metastases in differentiated thyroid tumors. Since pediatric patients are few and the prognosis is generally excellent, ^{131}I usually is recommended only for patients with extensive unresectable cervical nodal involvement, invasion of vital structures, or distant metastases. Very few instances of solid tumors or leukemia associated with ^{131}I treatment have been reported.[25]

SURGICAL MANAGEMENT

There are controversies on the specific type of initial surgical resection on the thyroid, the role of lymph node dissection, and the optimal treatment of recurrence. For differentiated thyroid carcinoma the surgical options include either total or subtotal thyroidectomy. Good long-term outcomes with mortality rates ranging from 0–17 percent up to 28 years after treatment are seen irrespective of which surgical procedure is performed. Thyroid lobectomy is the initial procedure of choice for most solitary thyroid lesions to adequately remove the pathology and to spare enough thyroid tissue to maintain a euthyroid state.[26] A completion total or subtotal thyroidectomy can be performed at a later date if final pathology proves carcinoma.. A near-total

thyroidectomy with radical lobectomy on the side of the primary lesion and subtotal removal of the contralateral lobe is recommended if the lesion is proven or suggestive of carcinoma.[18] The indolent nature of differentiated thyroid carcinoma and the increased risk of recurrent laryngeal nerve injury (0–24 percent) and hypoparathyroidism (6–27%) reported in the literature are arguments against performing total thyroidectomy.[13,27]

Proponents of total thyroidectomy argue that aggressive surgical resection with lymph node dissection of involved regional nodes is the best method for local control of the tumor. Some surgeons suggest that a thyroid lobectomy with isthmus resection is acceptable for 'minimal' differentiated carcinoma clearly isolated to one lobe. However, in one series 66 percent of patients had bilateral tumors and 81 percent of the tumors were multifocal.[14] Thus, most surgeons recommend total or near-total thyroidectomy for known cancer. When surgery is performed for a thyroid nodule without a histologic diagnosis, thyroid lobectomy and isthmus resection is indicated. If frozen section of the resected nodule reveals malignancy, then a total thyroidectomy should be completed. Although total thyroidectomy has not been proven to decrease recurrence, supporters of this method argue that remaining thyroid tissue may interfere with the use of radioactive iodine in the postoperative diagnostic scanning and in the treatment of microscopic regional and distant disease. Residual thyroid tissue also provides a source of thyroglobulin that may diminish the specificity of the test as a tumor marker postoperatively.[28]

Care should be taken to avoid injury to the recurrent laryngeal nerve. In particular, the nerve should be identified along its entire course and be seen entering the larynx. The right recurrent laryngeal nerve arises from the vagus nerve and passes around the posterior aspect of the first part of the subclavian artery. The right recurrent laryngeal nerve ascends lateral to the tracheal esophageal groove as it passes posterior to the inferior pole of the thyroid. The nerve then travels obliquely, closer toward the gland and crosses the inferior thyroid artery and ascends to enter the larynx. A non-recurrent right laryngeal nerve, which occurs 0.5–1 percent of the time, courses directly off the vagus nerve to enter the larynx. It does not cross the inferior thyroid artery. The left recurrent laryngeal nerve arises from the vagus and passes inferior and medial to the aorta and ascends to enter the larynx. The nerve usually travels in the tracheal–esophageal groove but may be more medial on the anterior aspect of the trachea.

Tumor involving the recurrent laryngeal nerve should be shaved off, thus preserving the nerve. The parathyroid glands should also be protected. If there is any question as to the viability of the parathyroid glands, they should be autotransplanted into the sternocleidomastoid muscle or non-dominant forearm.

Technique for Thyroidectomy

A curvilinear incision is made above the sternal notch in a skin crease. Dissection is carried down through the platysma muscle. Subplatysmal flaps are elevated superiorly to the thyroid notch and inferiorly to the sternal notch.

The strap muscles are separated in the midline to expose the thyroid gland. Crossing branches of the anterior jugular vein may need to be divided. There is no need to divide the strap muscles unless there is tumor invasion necessitating resection. The thyroid lobe with the nodule or known cancer is then mobilized. Exposure is obtained by dissecting the strap muscles laterally. There should be a relatively avascular plane that allows dissection past the posterior aspect of the thyroid gland. The middle thyroid veins arising on the anterolateral surface in the middle of the thyroid gland are encountered first and must be ligated to allow mobilization of the lobe. Many surgeons advocate identifying the recurrent laryngeal nerve prior to mobilizing the superior pole. The strap muscles are retracted laterally and the thyroid gland is grasped with a Babcock clamp and retracted anteromedially. The recurrent laryngeal nerve is identified by its relationship to the inferior thyroid artery. The nerve may pass over, under or branch around the artery. With the exception of a right non-recurrent laryngeal nerve there is always a crosspoint. The nerve should be traced along its anterior plane until it can be seen entering the larynx. The terminal portion of the recurrent laryngeal nerve passes posterior to a lateral extension of thyroid tissue.

This portion of the gland may be left in situ in a near-total thyroidectomy. If medial retraction limits exposure, the superior pole of the gland should be mobilized. The superior pole is approached by dividing the thin anterior suspensory muscle over the larynx. An avascular plane between the thyroid and cricothyroid muscle is entered and the branches of the superior thyroid vessels are divided close to the thyroid gland below the external branch of the superior thyroid nerve. Division of the upper pole pedicle between clamps, en mass, results in a high frequency of injury to this nerve and should be avoided. With the superior pole free the gland may be retracted medially.

The parathyroid glands are at risk during thyroidectomy primarily due to devascularization when dividing the inferior thyroid arteries, which supply both the superior and inferior parathyroid glands 80 percent of the time. Branches of the inferior thyroid artery should be divided individually distal to the end branches supplying the parathyroid glands. Division within the thyroid sheath may be necessary. The parathyroid glands are gently teased laterally away from the thyroid capsule. Following division of the inferior thyroid artery the inferior pole vessels are divided. The remaining posteromedial attachment of the thyroid, referred to as the ligament of Berry, is closely related to the recurrent laryngeal nerve. Complete dissection of the nerve allows safe division of the ligament and retraction of the thyroid medially away from the nerve. The thyroid lobe is dissected off the pretracheal fascia until the junction of the isthmus and the contralateral lobe is reached. A pyramidal lobe, if present should be included. The junction of the isthmus and opposite lobe is transected with electrocautery when performing a lobectomy and isthmusectomy. For a total thyroidectomy the isthmus is not transected and the contralateral lobe is mobilized as described. Suspicious regional lymph node chains should be included.

After hemostatis is assured, the strap muscles are approximated with interrupted absorbable sutures. A small drain may be placed below the strap muscles and brought out through a separate skin incision if the operative field is not completely hemostatic. The platysma muscle is closed with interrupted absorbable sutures and the skin closed using a running subcuticular stitch. Some surgeons advocate routine autotransplantation of one or two parathyroid glands into the sternocleidomastoid muscle or forearm muscle to prevent permanent hypoparathyroidism.[29] Autotransplantation is required when a parathyroid gland cannot be preserved or if there is a question about its viability. Intrathyroidal parathyroid glands occur 1 percent of the time and if recognized following thyroidectomy should be autotransplanted. The removed parathyroid glands are placed in a specimen cup of sterile saline submerged in sterile ice until the thyroidectomy is completed. For parathyroid autotransplantation, the excised parathyroid glands are minced into several small pieces. Small wells are made within the sternocleidomastoid muscle or forearm muscle by gently spreading with fine forceps. Two or more pieces of parathyroid tissue are placed in each well and marked with a silk suture.

Neck dissection in pediatric thyroid surgery is indicated for regional lymph node metastasis. Perform a unilateral selective neck dissection, inspecting lymph nodes in the paratracheal region, in the tracheo-esophageal groove, and laterally. Excise nodes that are suspicious for pathology.

Formal neck dissection has not been shown to improve outcome and has an increased risk of minor surgical complications.[30]

Postoperatively, the head of the patient's bed should be elevated 30 degrees. Clear oral liquids can be given the night of surgery. The drain is removed the following morning. Serum calcium levels are measured daily for the first 2-4 postoperative days in all patients who have undergone a total or subtotal thyroidectomy. A slight decrease in the calcium level (to ~7.0 mg/dl) usually occurs as the remaining parathyroid tissue recovers from surgical trauma. Mild hypocalcemia of this level requires treatment only if symptomatic. Mild symptoms include a positive Trousseau or Chvostek sign, mild cardiac arrhythmia, or perioral tingling. Treatment of these mild symptoms requires only oral calcium combined with vitamin D. Intravenous calcium gluconate is used for a more rapid replacement with severe arrhythmia or impending tetany.

Patients undergoing total parathyroidectomy with reimplantation often require calcium and vitamin D replacement until the autotransplanted tissue functions adequately. Thyroidectomy patients should be treated with exogenous thyroid hormone to suppress TSH-mediated stimulation of the gland. To detect distant metastases or residual disease, radioiodine 131I scanning should be performed 6 weeks following surgery and discontinuation of exogenous thyroid replacement. If residual thyroid cancer is detected, then therapeutic doses of 131I should be administered until all disease is erradicated. Diagnostic scans are then repeated yearly. Thyroglobulin levels should also be obtained yearly; an elevated level should raise the suspicion of recurrent thyroid carcinoma. The recurrance rate of differentiated thyroid carcinoma in children followed for 20 years is 30 percent and most recent series report greater than 90 percent long-term survival rates.[14]

The only effective treatment for MTC is surgical resection. Unfortunately, radioiodine, external beam radiation, and chemotherapy have not been found to be effective in treating MTC. Management of MTC in children from families with MEN2 relies on presymptomatic detection of the RET proto-oncogene mutation. Genetic screening is now possible for the MEN2 gene and prophylactic total thyroidectomy to prevent MTC at about age 5 is recommended for children with MEN2A and FMTC to prevent the occurrence of C-cell hyperplasia or carcinoma,[31,32] (Lallier, 1998 Because of the increased virulence of MTC in MEN2B, thyroidectomy is recommended in infancy.[33] These children require total thyroidectomy and removal of all lymph nodes in the central compartment of the neck, medial to the carotid sheaths and between the hyoid bone and the sternum. In patients with MEN2A, the lifetime risk of hyperparathyroidism is 30 percent.[34] Thus, to prevent the possibility of reoperating in the neck to remove residual hyperparathyroid tissue when hyperparathyroidism develops, strong consideration should be given to routine heterotopic auto-transplantation of the glands at the time of prophylactic thyroidectomy.[31]

RECURRENCE

Papillary thyroid carcinoma in children behaves in a different manner from adults. Children with advanced local disease, lymph node involvement, and distant metastases have better long-term morbidity and mortality than adults.

Papillary or papillary-follicular histology has been shown to be a major risk factor associated with recurrence after surgical resection with a recurrence rate of 35 percent to 45 percent in children. This rate of recurrence is substantially higher than the 5 percent to 20 percent rate in adults. Risk factors for disease recurrence include age younger than 10 years, male sex, palpable lymph nodes at initial presentation , multiple nodules at initial presentation and tenderness at presentation.

Meticulous regional lymph node dissection is an essential, indispensable part of treatment for children with a formal modified regional neck dissection removing the pretracheal, paratracheal, lower spinal accessory, upper, middle, and lower jugular lymph nodes and recurrent laryngeal nerve chain. This necessitates identification, exposure, and preservation, when possible, of the recurrent laryngeal nerve every single time. Papillary thyroid carcinoma in children has an excellent prognosis despite distant diseases.

Thyroid resection combined with selective use of radioactive iodine ablation is a safe and effective treatment for recurrent PTC in children. The best predictors of recurrent disease are lymph node involvement and multiple thyroid nodules at presentation. Either subtotal or total thyroid resection is an adequate initial therapy, but a formal neck dissection completely removing regional lymph nodes is an essential and key step in the treatment of children with PTC. This includes exposure and preservation, when possible, of the recurrent laryngeal nerve.

COMPLICATIONS

Surgical complications include recurrent laryngeal nerve injury, hypoparathyroidism, hypothyroidism, and wound infection. The most common complication of a total thyroidectomy in children is parathyroid gland injury in 6-15 percent of patients, resulting in permanent hypoparathyroidism.[30,32] Another importan complication is recurrent laryngeal nerve injury. Hypoparathyroidism may be prevented by exhaustive search for parathyroid glands during thyroidectomy with routine autotransplantation Hypothyroidism in all patients after total thyroidectomy is avoided by thyroid hormone replacement. Hypothyroidism occurs in 6.5-49 percent of patients who have had a subtotal thyroidectomy.

PROPHYLACTIC THYROIDECTOMY

In children with RET proto-oncogene mutation, curative treatment of medullary thyroid carcinoma is possible by prophylactic thyroidectomy. In 46 RET gene carriers, prophylactic thyroidectomy was carried out between the ages of 4 and 21 years and it was conclude that if prophylactic thyroidectomy is done at early ages, cure rate is high.[35] Timing and extent of prophylactic thyroidectomy can be modified by individual RET mutation.

PROGNOSIS

Pediatric patients seem to have higher local and distant recurrence rates than adults, but the prognosis for children is excellent, with mortality rates of less than 10 percent.[28] The overall 20-year survival rate is 92-100 percent. In adults, smokers have been found to have a worsened prognosis compared to nonsmokers.[36] A family history of thyroid cancer had a nonsignificant negative effect on survival.

FUTURE DEVELOPMENTS

Recent experience in the management of differentiated thyroid carcinoma in children, especially in the use of radioiodine after recombinant human thyroid stimulating hormone (rhTSH) stimulation has been reported.[37] The dosage of 131I ranged from 1.5 to 3.7 × 10(9) Bq. Radioiodine therapy under rhTSH was reported as an effective and safe adjuvant treatment.

REFERENCES

1. Anderson A. Bergdahl L, Boquist L. Thyroid carcinoma in children. Am J Surg 1977;43:159-63.
2. Favus M, Schneider A, Stachura M et al. Thyroid cancer occurring as a later consequence of head and neck irradiation: evaluation of 1056 patients. New Engl J Med 1976;294:1019-25.
3. Vane D, King D, Boles T Jr. Secondary thyroid neoplasms in pediatric cancer patients: increased risk with improved survival. J Pediatr Surg 1984;19:855-60.
4. Smith MB, Xue H, Strong L et al. Forty-year experience with second malignancies after treatment of childhood cancer: analysis of outcome following the development of second malignancy. J Pediatr Surg 1993;28:1342-8.
5. Festen C, Otten BJ, van de Kaa CA. Follicular adenoma of the thyroid gland in children. Eur J Pediatr Surg 1995;5: 262-4.
6. Schneider K. Sonographic imaging of the thyroid in children. Prog Pediatr Surg 1991; 26: 1-14.
7. Garcia CJ, Daneman A, Thorner P, Daneman D. Sonography of multinodular thyroid gland in children and adolescents. Am J Dis Child 1992;146:811-6.
8. Khurana KK, Labrador E, Izquierdo R, et al. The role of fine-needle aspiration biopsy in the management of thyroid nodules in children, adolescents, and young adults: a multi- institutional study. Thyroid 1999;9:383-6.
9. Lugo-Vicente H, Ortiz VN, Irizarry H, et al. Pediatric thyroid nodules: management in the era of fine needle aspiration. J Pediatr Surg 1998;33:1302-5.
10. Desjardins JG, Khan AH, Montupet P, et al. Management of thyroid nodules in children: a 20-year experience. J Pediatr Surg 1987;22:736.
11. Hung W, Anderson KD, Chandra RS, et al. Solitary nodules in 71 children and adolescents. J Pediatr Surg 1992;27:1407-9.
12. Samuel AM, Sharma SM. Differentiated thyroid carcinomas in children and adolescents. Cancer 1991;67:2186-90.
13. Harness JK, Thompson NW, McLeod MK, et al. Differentiated thyroid carcinoma in children and adolescents. World J Surg 1992;16:547-53.
14. Schlumberger M, DeVathaire F, Travagli JP, et al. Differentiated thyroid carcinoma in childhood: long term follow-up in 72 patients. J Clin Endocrinol Metab 1987;65:1088-94.
15. Lemoine NR, Mayall ES, Wyllie FS, et al. Activated ras mutations in human thyroid cancers. Cancer Res 1988;48:4459-63.
16. Bongarzone I, Butti MG, Coronelli S, et al. Frequent activation of ret protooncogene by fusion with a new activating gene in papillary thyroid carcinomas. Cancer Res 1994;54:2979–85.
17. Sozzi G, Bongarzone I, Miozzo M et al. A (t910;17) translocation creates the RET/PTC2 chimeric transforming sequence in papillary thyroid carcinoma. Genes Chrom Cancer 1994;9: 244-50.
18. Joppich I, Roher HD, Hecker WC, et al. Thyroid carcinoma in childhood. Prog Pediatr Surg 1983;16:23-8.
19. Estevao-Costa J, Gil-Da-Costa MJ, Medina AM, Sobrinho-Simoes M. Thyroid carcinoma in a newborn: clinical challenges in managing the first recorded case. Med Pediatr Oncol 2000;34: 290-2.
20. Exelby PE, Frazell EL. Carcinoma of the thyroid in children. Surg Clin North Am 1969;49:249-59.
21. Bajpai M, Ramaswamy S, Gupta DK, et al. Solitary thyroid nodule. Indian Pediatr 1992;29:116-8.
22. Yoskovitch A, Laberge JM, Rodd C, et al. Cystic thyroid lesions in children. J Pediatr Surg 1998; 33:866-70.

23. Raab SS, Silverman JF, Elsheikh TM, et al. Pediatric thyroid nodules: disease demographics and clinical management by fine needle aspiration biopsy Pediatrics 1995;95:46-9.

24. Yip FW, Reeve TS, Poole AG, et al. Thyroid nodules in childhood and adolescence. Aust N Z J Surg 1994;64:676-8.

25. Yeh SD, La Quaglia MP. 131I therapy for pediatric thyroid cancer. Semin Pediatr Surg 1997;6:128-33.

26. Bryarly RC, Shockley WW, Stucker FJ. The method and management of thyroid surgery in the pediatric patient. Laryngoscope 1985;95:1025-8.

27. Zimmerman D, Hay ID, Gough IR, et al. Papillary thyroid carcinoma in children and adults: long-term follow-up of 1039 patients conservatively treated at one institution during three decades. Surgery 1988;104:1157-66.

28. Alessandri AJ, Goddard KJ, Blair GK, et al. Age is the major determinant of recurrence in pediatric differentiated thyroid carcinoma. Med Pediatr Oncol 2000;35:41-6.

29. Wells SA Jr, Farndon JR, Dale JK, et al. Long term evaluation of patients with primary parathyroid hyperplasia managed by total parathyroidectomy and heterotopic autotransplantation. Ann Surg 1980;192:451-8.

30. La Quaglia MP, Telander RL. Differentiated and medullary thyroid cancer in childhood and adolescence. Semin Pediatr Surg 1997;6:42-9.

31. Wells SA Jr. Chi DD, Toshima K et al. Predictive testing and prophylactic thyroidectomy in patients at risk for multiple endocrine neoplasia type 2a. Ann Surg 1994;220:237–47.

32. Lallier M, St-Vil D, Giroux M, et al. Prophylactic thyroidectomy for medullary thyroid carcinoma in gene carriers of MEN2 syndrome. J Pediatr Surg 1998;33:846-8.

33. Samaan NA, Draznin MB, Halpin RE, et al. Multiple endocrine syndrome type IIb in early childhood. Cancer 1991;68:1832-4.

34. Howe JR, Norton JA, Wells SA Jr. Prevalence of pheochromocytoma and hyperparathyroidism in multiple endocrine neoplasia type 2A: Results of long-term follow-up. Surgery 1993;114:1070-7.

35. Frank-Raue K, Buhr H, Dralle H, Klar E, Senninger N, Weber T, Rondot S, Hoppner W, Raue F. Long-term outcome in 46 gene carriers of hereditary medullary thyroid carcinoma after prophylactic thyroidectomy: impact of individual RET genotype Eur J Endocrinol. 2006;155:229-36.

36. Ihre Lundgren C. Are possible risk factors for differentiated thyroid cancer of prognostic importance? Thyroid 2006;16:659-66.

37. Lau WF, Zacharin MR, Waters K, Wheeler G, Johnston V, Hicks RJ. Management of paediatric thyroid carcinoma: Recent experience with recombinant human thyroid stimulating hormone in preparation for radioiodine therapy Intern Med J. 2006;36:564-70.

CHAPTER 42

Devendra K Gupta
Shilpa Sharma

Pancreatic Tumors in Childhood

Tumors arising from the pancreas are not so common in children and adolescents. Malignant pancreatic tumors in children show a pattern different from that in Adults. Since these tumors are occasionally seen, they can pose a diagnostic dilemma and are therapeutic challenges. A high index of suspicion is required to get the proper array of investigations done and reach the proper diagnosis. Some of these tumors are mild in nature and can be easily cured if diagnosed in time while some have an aggressive course and high mortality. The major problem encountered is a lack of accepted therapeutic strategies.

There is no accepted etiology or recognized genetic syndromes associated with pancreatic tumors in children or adolescents, although endocrine tumors of the pancreas may be associated with other hormone-producing tumors. Congenital pancreatoblastoma has been found in association with the Beckwith-Wiedemann syndrome.

These tumors can arise at any site within the pancreas. Pancreatoblastomas and solid cystic tumors are mainly found in the head of the pancreas. Most pancreatic tumors do not secrete hormones; however few may be functional presenting with symptoms related to the secretion of hormones. Some tumors secrete insulin, which can lead to symptoms of weakness, fatigue, hypoglycemia, and coma. If the tumor interferes with the normal function of the islet cells, there may be symptoms of watery diarrhea or abnormalities of salt balance. Both carcinoma of the pancreas and pancreaticoblastoma can produce active hormones and can be associated with abdominal mass, clinically apparent wasting, and back pain. Obstruction of the duodenum and gastric outlet by tumors the head of the pancreas may be associated with jaundice and gastrointestinal bleeding.

Venous obstruction may be associated with varices, hemorrhage, and ascites. Tumors of the body or tail of the pancreas may erode into the stomach and cause hemorrhage. Ascites and hepatic failure may result with involvement of the liver and peritoneum. Progressive weight loss and anorexia may lead to fatal outcome.

The diagnosis of a pancreatic neoplasm is usually established by biopsy, using laparotomy or minimally invasive surgery. The differential diagnosis includes various benign neoplasms such as papillary-cystic tumors and hemagioma and other malignant lesions. Various serum markers, including carcinoembryonic antigen (CEA), α-fetoprotein, CA19-9, and pancreatic oncofetal antigen, amylase, lipase, alkaline phosphatase, lactate dehydrogenase, transaminase may be of value in the diagnosis and in follow up. Alpha-fetoprotein may be elevated in pancreatoblastoma.

Radiological studies include contrast studies of the upper gastrointestinal tract, abdominal ultrasonography and CT scan of the abdomen

Treatment includes various surgical procedures to remove the pancreas and duodenum or removal of part of the pancreas. Operative procedures include pancreaticoduodenectomy, total pancreatectomy, regional pancreatectomy, and distal pancreatectomy. Complete resection is usually possible and long-term survival is likely, although pancreatoblastoma has a high recurrence rate.[2]

For pediatric patients, the effectiveness of radiation therapy is not known. Chemotherapy may be useful for treatment of localized or metastatic pancreatic carcinoma. The combination of cisplatin and doxorubicin has produced responses in pancreatoblastoma prior to tumor resection. Other agents that may be of value include 5-fluorouracil, streptozotocin, mitomycin C, carboplatin, gemcitabine, and irinotecan. A complete resection of the primary tumor has been achieved in upto 82 percent, and most of the cases in the pediatric age group have good long-term survival.[1,2] However, the prognosis depends on the stage at the time of diagnosis, radio sensitivity and chemosensitivity of the tumor.

CLASSIFICATION OF MALIGNANT PANCREATIC TUMORS

The various malignant lesions of the pancreas are classified in Table 42.1. They may alos be classified according to cell of origin as; duct cell origin (e.g. adenocarcinoma, squamous cell carcinoma); acinic cell origin (e.g. acinic cell carcinoma); connective tissue origin (e.g. liposarcoma); lymphatic origin (e.g. lymphoma); uncertain origin (e.g. malignant papillary cystic carcinoma, pancreatoblastoma) and islet cell origin (e.g. malignant insulinoma, glucagonoma, and gastrinoma). In the pediatric age group, three types of pancreatic tumors are most commonly reported.[1-3] These include pancreatoblastomas, endocrine carcinomas of the pancreas and solid cystic tumors. The first two will be discussed in this chapter and the third in a separate chapter. Other pancreatic neoplasms are typically found in adults, such as ductal adenocarcinoma, acinar cell carcinoma, solid and papillary epithelial neoplasms and adenomas though they may be seen in adolescents. Rarely, secondary tumors of the pancreas can be associated with certain primary malignancies.[4]

Table 42.1: Classification of malignant lesions of the pancreas
1. Pancreaticoblastoma
2. Papillary-cystic carcinoma
3. Pancreatic neuroendocrine tumors (PNET).
4. Ductal Adenocarcinoma
5. Acinic cell carcinoma
6. Cystadenomas and cystadenocarcinomas
7. Squamous cell carcinoma
8. Liposarcoma
9. Lymphoma
10. Others—rhabdomyosarcoma, hemangioendothelioma

PANCREATOBLASTOMA

Pancreatoblastoma, originally known as infantile carcinoma of the pancreas, is a rare pancreatic neoplasm of childhood. Becker first reported it in 1957 though the earliest histopathologic description was published by Frable et al in 1971.[5,6] Its histologic resemblance to fetal pancreatic tissue at approximately 7 weeks gestation led Horie et al, in 1977, to propose that the original name be replaced with pancreatoblastoma.[7] Pancreatoblastoma is now the accepted term and is used interchangeably with pancreaticoblastoma.[8] The authors have seen and managed 3 cases though just over 50 cases have been reported in the literature.[9,10]

Pancreatoblastoma usually affects patients between 1 and 8 years of age though it has been reported in neonates and in the elderly also. The cystic congenital form is associated with Beckwith-Wiedemann syndrome. A male predominance has been found. All the 3 cases seen by the authors were males. Most of the cases have been reported in Asians.

Pancreatoblastoma is a heterogeneous, fairly well circumscribed tumor; its origin may be difficult to determine. It may appear to have a pancreatic or hepatic origin, clinically as well as radiologically. It has a tendency to behave aggressively, with evidence of local and distant spread. Pancreatoblastoma is slow growing and clinically occult tumor that is quite large at the time of diagnosis.[11]

Pancreatoblastoma should be considered in the differential diagnosis of an upper abdominal mass in a child, especially when the mass appears to arise from the pancreas or liver (Fig. 42.1). Symptoms are usually related to the mass effect and include epigastric fullness,

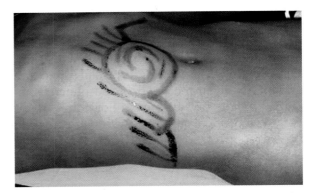

Figure 42.1: A mass in the right hypochondrium of an eleven-year-old boy with uncertain organ of origin. The mass was present since 1 year and associated with intermittent dull aching pain. It was 11×10 cm in size, firm in consistency and inseparable from the liver

vomiting, constipation, and pain. Rarely, pancreato-blastoma has also presented as chronic diarrhea with failure to thrive.[3]

The heterogeneous character of the tumor is well appreciable on contrast enhanced CT scan (Figs 42.2A and B). The tumor has low to intermediate signal intensity on T1-weighted MR images, high signal intensity on T2-weighted MR images, isointensity relative to the spleen on T1-weighted MR images, and slight hypointensity to the spleen on T2-weighted MR images.[9] Clustered tumor calcifications and rim calcifications have been noted (Fig. 42.3).

Pancreaticoblastoma may have exocrine and endocrine components associated with zymogen and neuroendocrine granules. Cushing's syndrome and the syndrome of inappropriate antidiuretic hormone secretion have been reported.[12] One of the patients in the authors' series also presented with features of Cushing's syndrome with raised ACTH levels (Fig. 42.4). These endocrine syndromes are postulated to be the

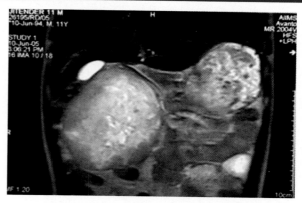

Figure 42.3: MRI scan delineating the focal calcification within the mass

result of adrenocorticotrophic hormone secretion by the tumor. Elevated serum levels of α-fetoprotein, α_1-antitrypsin, or lactate dehydrogenase have also been reported.[3,13,14] The liver is the most common site for metastasis.[15] Other sites include the lung, bone, and posterior mediastinum.

The organ of origin can become very difficult to determine; only half of the patients have radiologically identified pancreatic origins.[9] While approximately half of all pancreatoblastomas arise in the pancreatic head, obstructive symptoms are unusual, despite the large size of the tumor as the tumor has a soft, gelatinous consistency pathologically.[16]

Local spread to omentum, peritoneal cavity and adjacent portal and mesenteric vessels has been described. The tumor may appear malignant with lobulations (Fig. 42.5).

The tumor is a partially circumscribed, lobulated mass with variable consistency. Necrosis and calcification may be associated. Extension into the peripancreatic tissues with invasion of the duodenum and adjacent soft tissues

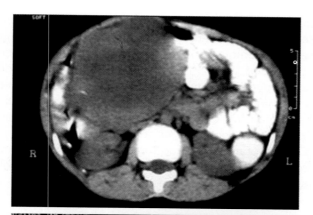

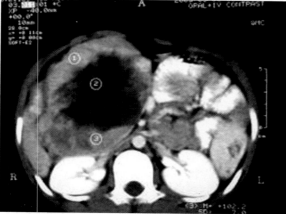

Figures 42.2A and B: CT scan depicting the hetero-geneous nature of the mass, adherent to the duodenum, liver and pancreas

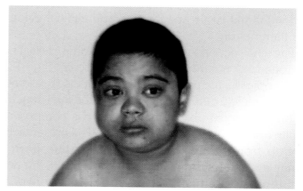

Figure 42.4: A patient with pancreatoblastoma presenting with Cushing's syndrome

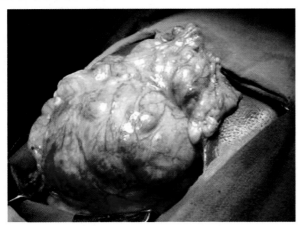

Figure 42.5: At laparotomy, pancreatoblastoma appears malignant. Note the visible lobulated appearance

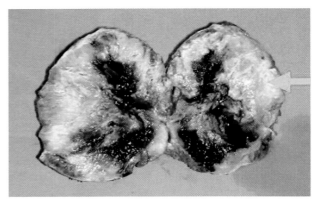

Figure 42.6: The cut section of pancreatoblastoma showing the central necrosis

may occur commonly. Portal and mesenteric vascular and perineural invasion has also been described. Ascites may be an indicator of tumor spread.

The differential diagnosis in a child includes any large abdominal mass, particularly when the tumor is large and when its origin is uncertain. This includes Neuroblastoma, Non-Hodgkin lymphoma, or Wilms' tumor. Neuroblastoma and American Burkitt lymphoma may secondarily involve the pancreas. When the tumor appears to arise from the liver, a pancreatoblastoma may resemble other primary hepatic neoplasms, such as hepatocellular carcinoma, hepatoblastoma, and mesenchymal hamartoma. The distinction of a pancreatoblastoma from hepatocellular carcinoma and hepatoblastoma may be difficult as all three tumors may occur with an elevated level of -fetoprotein and with heterogeneous hepatic masses with or without calcifications. When the tumor is clearly pancreatic in origin, the differential diagnosis includes pancreatic abscess, pseudocyst, and other pancreatic neoplasms. Abscess and pseudocysts are characterized by their predominantly cystic appearance and clinical evidence of inflammation.

The cut section of pancreatoblastoma depicts the heterogenous nature with central necrosis (Fig. 42.6). Microscopically, the pancreatoblastoma closely resembles the incompletely differentiated acini of the fetal pancreas. Although pancreatoblastoma primarily is composed of primitive acinar elements, islet cells may be present which develop from groups of cells that separate from the primitive ductal system and settle between the acini. Immunohistochemistry is essential to confirm the diagnosis. Pancreatoblastomas stains positive for epithelial membrane antigen, neuron specific enolase,

synaptophysin, pan-cytokeratin and carcinoembryonic antigen (Fig. 42.7).

Fibrotic capsules with rare, late metastases are characteristics of these tumors.[17] Thus, therapy consists of surgical resection of the localized tumor. The role of adjuvant chemotherapy for a resectable tumor is uncertain. Radiation therapy and chemotherapy are used to treat recurrent or metastatic disease. The drugs used for chemotherapy include adriamycin, ifosfamide, cisplatin and VP16.[17] Response to cyclophosphamide, dactinomycin, bleomycin, or vinblastine is variable. Surgical excision and radiation therapy are necessary after obtaining chemotherapy response to prevent regrowth of tumor in case of advanced disease.

The prognosis is good for patients with localized, surgically resectable disease. Patients with nonresectable disease have a poorer prognosis.

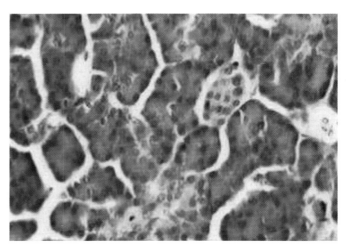

Figure 42.7: Histopathological picture of pancreatoblastoma

PANCREATIC DUCTAL ADENOCARCINOMA

Ductal adenocarcinoma is typically a small tumor that arises in the pancreatic head of elderly men, though few reports in children have been reported.[18] The male-to-female ratio is 2:1.

Several genetic, environmental, and disease-related risk factors have been identified including an increased association with cigarette smoking, high meat and fish consumption and exposure to amines. Certain diseases like chronic pancreatitis, diabetes mellitus, and hereditary cancer syndromes (e.g. familial adenomatous polyposis) are predisposing factors. Hereditary pancreatitis caused by mutation of the cationic trypsinogen gene is characterized by acute recurrent pancreatitis in childhood, which progresses to chronic pancreatitis and pancreatic cancer in early adulthood.

Sixty percent develop in the pancreatic head; 40 percent develop in the body and tail. Symptoms include progressive deep and boring epigastric pain, anorexia, weight loss, and jaundice associated with pruritis and steatorrhea. The patient is usually cachexic. An abdominal mass may be palpable along with ascites. The patient may have left cervical lymphadenopathy (Virchow's node). Unlike pancreatoblastoma, necrosis, hemorrhage, and calcifications are rare.

The diagnostic modality of choice is contrast-enhanced computed tomography (CT) with thin cuts through the pancreas.

MRI may improve differentiation of a pancreatic cancer from chronic pancreatitis in evaluating a pancreatic head mass, and offers simultaneous assessment of the pancreatic and bile ducts by heavily T2-weighted imaging (MR-cholangiopancreatography).

Endoscopic ultrasound is an accurate test for diagnosing and staging pancreatic ductal cancer and has the greatest role in the detection of small tumors missed by CT. It may offer a better assessment of local blood-vessel involvement, and allows fine needle aspiration of tumor and lymph nodes. Disadvantages include increased invasiveness, operator dependence, lack of widespread availability, and inability to detect distant metastasis.

ERCP is most useful for detecting small tumors not visualized by CT, palliating unresectable tumors causing biliary obstruction, and ruling out differential causes of pain or jaundice. It has more than 90 percent sensitivity. Suggestive features include an irregular, solitary pancreatic duct stenosis >1 cm long, abrupt cutoff of the main pancreatic duct, or an obstruction of both pancreatic and bile ducts. Brush cytology from the pancreatic duct has 70 percent sensitivity and good specificity for adenocarcinoma.

Tumor marker, CA19-9, in a concentration above 70 U/ml has 70 percent sensitivity for pancreatic cancer though it may be elevated in benign conditions such as choledocholithiasis and cholangitis. Specific genetic mutations of the K-ras oncogene, c-erb B-12 oncogene, and p16 tumor suppressor genes have been described and may have a role in screening high-risk individuals.

Biopsy of a pancreatic mass or metastasis may be obtained percutaneously under CT guidance or by endoscopic ultrasound guided FNAC. Current imaging tests may underestimate tumor, nodal, and metastatic staging. Staging laparoscopy with or without laparoscopic ultrasound improves accuracy through detection of small hepatic or peritoneal metastases, widespread sampling of regional lymph nodes, and direct visualization of the primary tumor and its relationship to peripancreatic vessels.

Surgical resection is the only hope for curative therapy. The tumor is resectable if it is confined to the pancreas without: (i) encasement of adjacent surrounding major vessels (superior mesenteric artery or vein, portosplenic confluence, celiac trunk or aorta); (ii) extensive peripancreatic lymph node involvement; or (iii) distant metastases. Unfortunately, due to late presentation and delay in diagnosis, only 20 percent cases present with resectable disease. The long-term prognosis is poor with a 5-year survival after resection with tumor-free margins being about 20 percent. The standard operation for adenocarcinoma in the pancreatic head is the pancreaticoduodenectomy, or Whipple operation with resection of the pancreatic head, duodenum, common bile duct, distal stomach, and gallbladder followed by pancreaticojejunostomy, hepatoicojejunostomy, and gastrojejunostomy. Complications include anastomotic leaks and ulcerations, dumping syndrome, and bile gastritis.

Chemotherapy and radiotherapy may help in shrinkage of the primary tumor, improvement of symptoms, and prolongation of survival. Single-agent gemcitabine and combined 5-fluorouracil-based chemotherapy with external beam radiation have been tried.

For locally advanced and metastatic disease, symptomatic therapy for pain (neural plexus invasion), jaundice (biliary obstruction), or vomiting (gastric outlet obstruction) may be provided. Surgical biliary bypass or percutaneous or endoscopic bile duct stenting may be offered for biliary obstruction. Gastric outlet obstruction may be managed by surgical gastro-jejunostomy or endoscopic stenting

ACINAR CELL CARCINOMA

It has been rarely reported to occur in the pediatric age group.[2] Acinar cell carcinoma, can be a soft, large, lobulated, well-demarcated tumor with areas of necrosis and with metastases to the liver and lymph nodes. The absence of calcifications and the propensity for lung metastases may help in distinguishing this tumor from pancreatoblastoma.

SOLID AND PAPILLARY EPITHELIAL NEOPLASMS

Solid and papillary epithelial neoplasms are found most frequently in African-American and Asian female patients aged 10 to 50 years. Approximately 30 percent of the cases occur in adolescents. These tumors, like pancreatoblastoma, are usually well demarcated, large, and often-heterogeneous masses that may contain peripheral calcifications. However, aggressive behavior in these tumors is rare. These are discussed in detail in another chapter in this book.

ADENOMAS

Adenomas are large, slow-growing tumors that occur in middle-aged and elderly women. Although cysts and calcifications are common, the presence of a central stellate scar at CT and the absence of aggressive features may help in distinguishing this tumor from pancreatoblastoma.

Hemangioendothelioma, and rhabdomyosarcoma involving the pancreas have also been reported in children.[18,19] Rhabdomyosarcoma has a poor prognosis if it is associated with progressive disease.[18]

PANCREATIC NEUROENDOCRINE TUMORS

Pancreatic neuroendocrine tumors, also known as islet-cell tumors, are rare tumors arising from endocrine cells within or near the pancreas. The incidence rate is 5 cases per million person years. They may occur sporadically or as part of the multiple endocrine neoplasia type 1.

Most of these primary tumors arise within the "gastrinoma triangle," composed of the joining of the cystic and common hepatic ducts, the joining of the second and third portions of the duodenum, and the border of the body and tail of the pancreas. Patients with functional endocrine tumors usually present with the secondary clinical features of hormone secretion (Table 42.2). Patients with insulinoma present with symptomatic hypoglycemia from hyperinsulinemia. Gastrinomas produce recalcitrant peptic ulcer disease resulting from hypergastrinemia (Zollinger-Ellison syndrome). Less commonly encountered tumors include glucagonoma, VIPoma (secreting vasoactive intestinal polypeptide), somatostatinoma, and PPoma (secreting pancreatic polypeptide).

Insulinoma is the most common endocrine tumor of the pancreas. Over 90 percent of the insulinomas are benign and single, and can be cured by simple excision. Insulinomas are evenly distributed between the head, body and tail of the pancreas.[20] The release of insulin leads to fasting hypoglycemia producing fatigue,

Table 42.2: Pancreatic neuroendocrine tumors		
Tumor type	*Clinical features*	*Symptomatic treatment*
Insulinoma	Hypoglycemia	Octreotide diazoxide
	Symptoms of catecholamine excess	
	Mostly benign	
Gastrinoma	Peptic ulcer disease	Proton pump inhibitor
	GERD secretory diarrhea	Octreotide
	Most common NET in MEN 1	
	Mostly malignant	
Glucagonoma	Glucose intolerance	Octreotide
	Migratory necrolytic erythema	Insulin
	Weight loss	Zinc supplement (rash)
	Mostly malignant	TPN
Somatostatinoma	Diabetes	Octreotide
	Gallstones	
	Secretory diarrhea	
VIPoma	Secretory diarrhea	Octreotide
	Hypokalemia	
	Hypochlorhydria	

restlessness, malaise followed by confusion, hypothermia, staggering gait, loss of consciousness, coma or convulsions. These symptoms may appear as intermittent attacks, most frequently in the early morning hours. The hypoglycemia in turn can induce the release of catecholamines producing tachycardia, trembling and diaphoresis. The Whipple's triad characteristically seen in adults includes symptoms of hypoglycemia, glucose level below 50 mg/dl and relief of symptoms by the administration of glucose Familial insulinoma has been described in a father and daughter.[21]

Carcinoid tumors are also included in this group but are rarely found in the pancreas. These tumors may be suspected based on symptoms related to the secretory product. Some patients develop watery diarrhea, hypokalemia, and achlorhydria (WDHA) due to overproduction of pancreatic polypeptide.

Nonfunctioning islet cell tumors are usually associated with recurrent multiple peptic ulcer disease involving abnormal sites like jejunum and ileum due to the elaboration of gastrin by the tumor. Nonfunctional tumors are occasionally detected on imaging tests done for other indications or for abdominal pain in patients with significant tumor growth. They are most often indolent but may demonstrate malignant behavior, including metastases. The prognosis for nonfunctional tumors may be poorer than functional ones due to a delay in diagnosis.

When suspected, imaging tests are vital to locate the primary tumor and determine the presence of metastases though they may be difficult to localize as they are usually very small and radiographically occult (Fig. 42.8). Contrast-enhanced CT and MRI may have a low yield for small tumors that may be picked up with

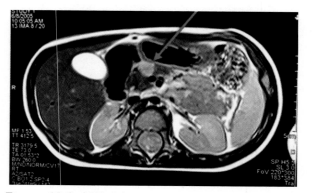

Figure 42.8: MRI delineating a space-occupying lesion in the pancreas (arrow) that was diagnosed as insulinoma in the setting of hyperinsulinemic hypoglycemia in a 22-month-old girl with symptoms of hypoglycemia

endoscopic ultrasound that may also allow simultaneous FNAC for tissue diagnosis. The disadvantages of endoscopic ultrasound include increased invasiveness, inability to consistently visualize the pancreatic tail, and lack of widespread availability. Functional tests may be helpful in localizing neuroendocrine tumors not detected on standard imaging tests. Nuclear imaging after administration of radiolabeled octreotide can aid in location of most neuroendocrine tumors. Insulinomas are not well visualized with octreotide scans because they do not possess high concentrations of somatostatin receptors.

Octreotide has been found to provide a reasonable addition or alternative to diazoxide in controlling symptoms of congenital hyperinsulinism.[22] The overall sensitivity of noninvasive methods like combined endoscopic ultrasonography and somatostatin receptor scintigraphy has been found as 89 percent for insulinoma and 93 percent for gastrinoma.[23] The diagnostic value of three simple functional tests, the inhibitory effect of insulin on ketogenesis and on glycogenolysis and the stimulatory effect of leucine on insulin secretion has also been found useful in absence of fasting hyperinsulinemia.[24] Provocation tests, for the diagnosis of insulinoma include tolbutamide, glucagon, glucose and arginine tests that have been found to cause increased levels in the maximal plasma insulin in 100, 91, 63, and 56 percent cases respectively.[25] Though intra-arterial calcium stimulation test with venous sampling has been described as the most sensitive preoperative test for regionalizing insulinoma by some authors, others have found intraoperative ultrasound more useful.[26-29] Catheterizing the splenic and portal vein through a branch of the splenic vein and serial sampling at 2 cm intervals along the portal and splenic veins for rapid determination of insulin levels by quick double-antibody radioimmunoassay have been used to localize pancreatic adenomas and to decide how much pancreas to remove in diffuse lesions avoiding "blind" pancreatectomies.[30]

Realtime intraoperative ultrasonography of the pancreas has been used to localize additional adenomas intraoperatively and allowed a 90 percent pancreatectomy with enucleation of small adenomas in the remaining head.[31] Manual palpation can be relied upon with a high positivity.[29] The authors could localize a tumor as small as 1.5 cm by manual palpation and then enucleate it from the normal looking surrounding pancreatic tissue (Figs 42.9 and 42.10). Multiple insulinomas may be missed on initial diagnosis so careful

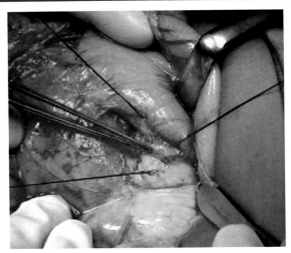

Figure 42.9: An insulinoma palpable at junction of head and body of pancreas that was successfully enucleated

palpation should be done for localization of any other tumor.[32]

Laparoscopic resection of pancreatic insulinoma is another alternative to surgical resection but has the disadvantage of not allowing manual palpation.[33]

Depending on the location, insulinomas can be enucleated, might require partial or distal pancreatectomy or pancreaticoduodenectomy.

Treatment consists of excision of the insulinoma or, if it is not possible to localize the tumor, subtotal or total pancreatectomy.[34] It is suggested that in the very young when there is no evidence of an insulinoma, resection at the initial operation should be up to 90 percent, than the previously recommended 75 percent.[35] When hyperinsulinemic hypoglycemia first manifests after 1 year of age, it is always caused by an islet cell adenoma, which is cured by enucleation.[36]

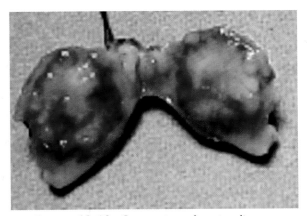

Figure 42.10: Cut section of an insulinoma showing homogeneous appearance

Tumors confined to the pancreas should be surgically resected, either through enucleation or more extensive resection of the head (Whipple procedure), body, or tail of the pancreas. Most insulinomas can be treated by enucleation.[18] Intraoperative ultrasound may be advantageous to localize the tumor. Before resection, symptoms of hormonal excess must be treated and controlled. Histopathology with immunohistochemistry along with clinical correlation form the mainstay for the diagnosis. Pancreatic neuroendocrine tumors stain positive for neuron specific enolase, chromogranin and synaptophysin (Fig. 42.11).

Malignant gastrinomas and malignant insulinomas should primarily be treated with radical surgery, including extensive lymph node dissection.[16] In case of distant metastases, local resection of the liver may be done.[16] Patients with metastatic disease can be managed medically with octreotide, chemotherapy (streptazocin in the case of malignant insulinomas), or radiographic embolization of the primary tumor and metastases. Debulking of primary and metastatic disease may also be considered for patients with debilitating symptoms related to tumor secretory products.

Aggressive surgical therapy is warranted in the management of pediatric pancreatic tumors as the long-term results have been reported to be encouraging.[1] Long-term follow-up of insulinoma should include prevention of metastasis or recurrence, and testing for multiple endocrine neoplasia type 1.[37] The patients should be closely followed up, as recurrence may develop up to 15 years after surgery.[21]

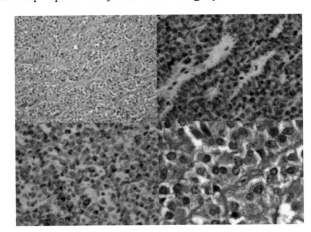

Figure 42.11: Microphotographs of the histopathology along with immunohistochemistry of a pancreatic tumor that was positive for neuron specific enolase, chromogranin and synaptophysin suggestive of neuroendocrine tumor

PANCREATIC CYSTIC NEOPLASMS

Most pancreatic cysts are inflammatory pseudocysts arising from acute or chronic pancreatitis. Other types of pancreatic cysts include simple cysts and cystic neoplasms. Cystic neoplasms are reported to account for less than 1 percent of pancreatic cancers. They are usually indolent tumors with varying malignant potential. Serous cystadenomas are composed of multiple small cysts (microcystadenoma) that are lined by glycogen-rich cells. Although serous tumors may be large and cause pain, they have a low potential for malignant transformation. Mucinous cystadenomas and cystadenocarcinomas are composed of one or a few large cysts, often with thickened and irregular walls. Mucinous cystadenomas have been reported in infants.[18] All mucinous neoplasms have malignant potential and should be resected when possible. Malignant recurrence following cyst excision and resulting in mortality has also been reported in the pediatric age group.[18] Intraductal papillary mucinous neoplasms arise from either the main pancreatic ductal epithelium or side-branches and consist of dilated ductal segments, often with papillary projections that secrete mucin with a high potential for malignant transformation.

The primary aim of diagnosis is to differentiate benign from malignant cysts.

In the absence of pancreatitis, radiographic features are poorly reliable in differentiating mucinous from other types of pancreatic cysts. If there is no history of pancreatitis to suggest a pseudocyst, cystic masses greater than 1 cm in size and producing symptoms should be resected. In asymptomatic patients, EUS allows improved characterization of cyst features and also simultaneous aspiration of cyst fluid for chemical analysis. Fluid may be analyzed for cytology, tumor markers (CEA, CA19-9, CA15-3), and amylase. A positive mucin stain of cyst fluid may also be helpful in ruling in a mucinous cystic neoplasm. The ERCP features of Intraductal papillary mucinous neoplasms include a gaping papilla with extrusion of mucin and global or segmental main-duct or side-branch dilation with papillary projections. Symptomatic or enlarging pancreatic pseudocysts may be drained surgically, endoscopically, or percutaneously. Resection should be considered for mucinous cystic neoplasms and symptomatic or enlarging serous cysts.

REFERENCES

1. Jaksic T, Yaman M, Thorner P, Wesson DK, Filler RM, Shandling B. A 20-year review of pediatric pancreatic tumors. J Pediatr Surg 1992;27:1315-7.
2. Shorter NA, Glick RD, Klimstra DS, Brennan MF, Laquaglia MP. Malignant pancreatic tumors in childhood and adolescence: The Memorial Sloan-Kettering experience, 1967 to present. J Pediatr Surg 2002;37:887-92.
3. Wang JS, Lee HC, Sheu JC, Chang PY, Liang DC, Chen BF.Pancreatic tumors in children: report of three cases. Acta Paediatr Taiwan 1999; 40:335-8.
4. Nijs E, Callahan MJ, Taylor GA. Disorders of the pediatric pancreas: imaging features. Pediatr Radiol. 2005; 35:358-73. Epub 2004 Nov 5.
5. Becker WF. Pancreatoduodenectomy for carcinoma of the pancreas in an infant. Ann Surg 1957;145:864-72.
6. Frable WJ, Still WJS, Kay S. Carcinoma of the pancreas, infantile type: a light and electron microscopic study. Cancer 1971; 27:667-73.
7. Horie A, Yano Y, Kotoo Y. Morphogenesis of pan-creato-blastoma, infantile carcinoma of the pancreas: report of two cases. Cancer 1977;39:247-54.
8. Cubilla AL, Fitzgerald PJ. Classification of pancreatic cancer (nonendocrine). Mayo Clin Proc 1979; 54:449-58.
9. Montemarano H, Lonergan GJ, Bulas DI, Selby DM Pancreatoblastoma: Imaging Findings in 10 Patients and Review of the Literature. Radiology 2000;214:476-82.
10. Chun Y, Kim W, Park K, Lee S, Jung S. Pancreatoblastoma. J Pediatr Surg 1997 Nov;32(11):1612-5.
11. Mergo PJ, Helmberger TK, Buetow PC, et al. Pancreatic neoplasms: MR imaging and pathologic correlation. Radio-Graphics 1997;17:281-301.
12. Passmore SJ, Berry PJ, Oakhill A. Recurrent pan-creatoblastoma with inappropriate adrenocorticotropic hormone secretion. Arch Dis Child 1988;63:1494-6.
13. Ohaki Y, Misugi K, Hirose M. Pancreatic carcinoma of childhood: report of an autopsy and review of the literature. Acta Pathol Jpn 1985;35:1543-54.
14. Willnow U, Willberg B, Schwamborn D, et al. Pancreato-blastoma in children: case report and review of the literature. Eur J Pediatr Surg 1996;6:369-72
15. Klimstra DS, Adair CF, Hefess CS. Pancreatoblastoma: a clinicopathologic study and review of the literature. Am J Surg Pathol 1987;11:855-65.
16. Kloppel G, Maillet B. Classification and staging of pancreatic nonendocrine tumors. Radiol Clin North Am 1989;27:105-19.
17. Vossen S, Goretzki PE, Goebel U, Willnow U Therapeutic management of rare malignant pancreatic tumors in children. World J Surg 1998; 22:879-82.
18. Grosfeld JL, Vane DW, Rescorla FJ, McGuire W, West KW. Pancreatic tumors in childhood: analysis of 13 cases. J Pediatr Surg 1990;25:1057-62.
19. Tunell WP. Hemangioendothelioma of the pancreas obstructing the common bile duct and duodenum. J Pediatr Surg 1976; 11:827-30.
20. Vazquez Quintana E. The surgical management of insulinoma. Bol Asoc Med PR 2004;96:33-8
21. Maioli M, Ciccarese M, Pacifico A, Tonolo G, Ganau A, Cossu S, et al. Familial insulinoma: description of two cases. Acta Diabetol 1992;29:38-40.
22. Barrons RW.Octreotide in hyperinsulinism. Ann Phar-macother 1997;31:239-41.

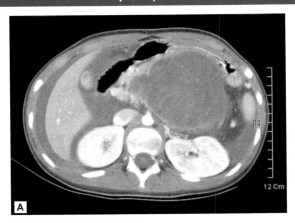

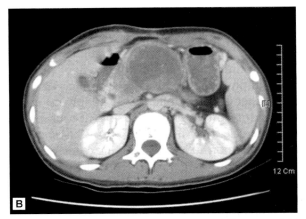

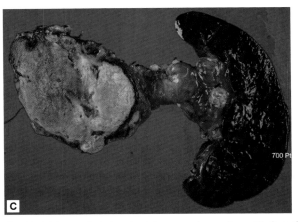

Figures 43.1A to C: (A) Initial abdominal CT scan of 12-year-old girl with history of abdominal trauma showed an 11.0 × 9.0 cm mass within the pancreatic body and tail with intraperitoneal fluid collection (case #23). No intra-abdominal metastatic lesion or lymphadenopathy. Laparotomy showed huge, unresectable intra-abdominal tumor originated from pancreas suggestive of pancreatic cancer. Tumor biopsy revealed SPT. **(B)** Abdominal CT scan shows decrease in size of the pancreatic mass (7.0 × 6.0 cm) after three-month course of chemotherapy. she received subtotal pancreatectomy with splenectomy **(C)** Resected specimen of pancreas and spleen)

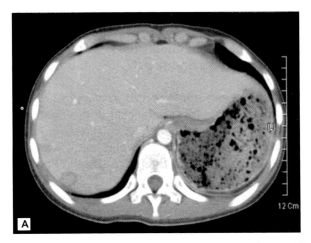

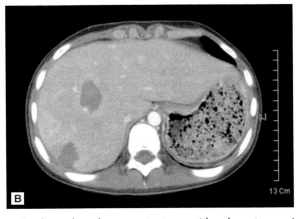

Figures 43.2A and B: (A) Abdominal CT scan (case #23) three month after subtotal pancreatectomy with splenectomy, single intra-hepatic metastatic lesion is noted in segment VII of the liver. **(B)** After Radiofrequency ablasion and chemotherapy, another metastatic lesion was found in segment VIII of the liver. This patient is now alive, under chemotherapy

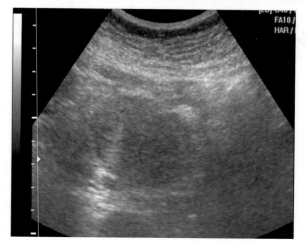

Figure 43.3: Ultrasonographic finding of SPT in the pancreatic head. A solid, well-demarcated, 3 cm sized hypoechoic round lesion in pancreas head portion. which is heterogeneous in echo texture, containing hypoechoic fluid-filled cystic areas

pancreatic leakage or pancreatitis increases when *solid pseudopapellary tumor of the pancreas 3*—the tissue-sparing surgery such as tumor enucleation or laparoscopic pancreatectomy is performed by an inexperienced surgeon. The decision for enucleation should be based on the histopathological results from frozen sections, the macroscopic appearance of the tumor especially size of the tumor, and location within pancreas (Figs 43.7A and B). But if preoperative radiologic finding is consistent with SPT, enucleation can be performed without confirming result of the frozen biopsy. Some surgeons regard this minimally invasive operation as an adequate approach for histology-proven SPT[21,23] whereas others recommend partial (pylorus-preserving) pancreaticoduodenectomy.[22] The latter is certainly an oncologically adequate intervention and is a safe procedure in terms of prognosis. Overall five-year survival is reported to be above 95 percent.[24] The

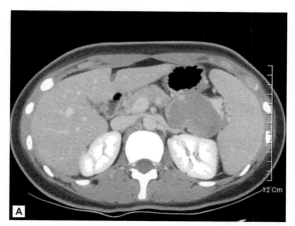

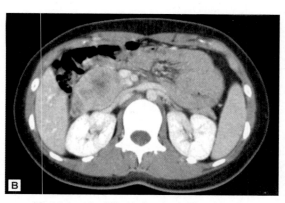

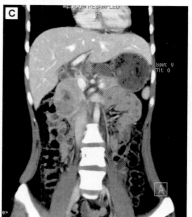

Figures 43.4A to C: (A) Abdominal CT scan of 13-year-old girl with SPT (case #16). 6 cm-sized spherical, cystic tumor located in the pancreas tail, she received distal pancreatectomy with splenectomy. (**B** and **C**) Abdominal CT scan of 14-year-old girl (case #20). 4.7 cm-sized relatively well-circumscribed mass (abutting portal vein) probably arising from pancreatic head suggestive of SPT. she underwent simple tumor enucleation

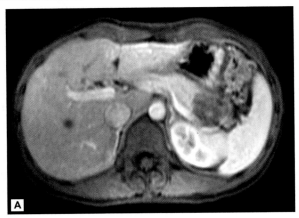
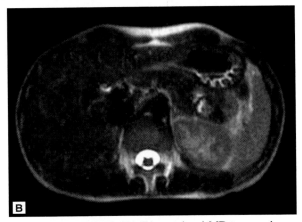

Figures 43.5A and B: 4.8 cm-sized mass within the pancreatic tail suggestive of SPT. **(A)** T1-weighted MR image shows high-signal areas, corresponding to hemorrhage, and often a relatively hypointense rim. **(B)** The signal intensity on T2-weighted MR image is usually heterogeneous, a low-signal rim is present

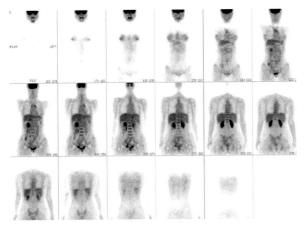

Figure 43.6: FDG-PET scan of 14-year-old girl (case #20). A mass of increased FDG uptake along the margin in pancreatic head. No other areas of abnormal uptake in the rest of the imaged body.

incidence of distant metastasis is reported in 12-15 percent of cases,[6,10,24] for the most part, synchronous metastasis. Survival of these patients is usually not quite poor even if surgical metastasectomy is not possible.[25]

Adjuvant therapy such as chemotherapy[1,26,27] or radiotherapy[28] has been anecdotally reported to be beneficial in several cases of SPT, but until now, there is no clear role of chemotherapy or radiotherapy. Strauss reported a 15 cm, unresectable SPT in the pancreatic head adhered to SMV reduced to 3.5 cm following six-month course of chemotherapy with cis-platin and leukovorin, Strauss could resect the tumor. Rebhandl reported a case of SPT in which serial meta-stasectomy(segmentectomy, omentectomy and splenectomy) and chemotherapy (ifosfamid, cis-platin and VP-16) completely cured the cancer. Fried et al reported a case in which an 18-year-old female patient was cured by six weeks of radiotherapy alone (4,000

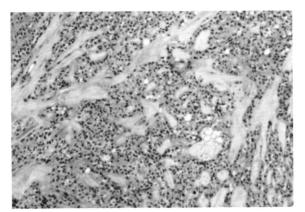
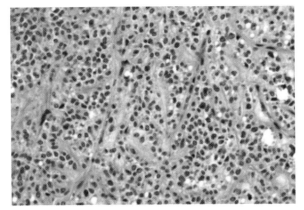

Figures 43.7A and B: Histopathology of SPT **(A)** Pseudopapillary pattern with one to two layers of tumor cells lining elongated fibrovascular stalks. Cells were stained with H and E and are magnified at 40X. **(B)** Solid pattern of sheets of polyhedral tumor cells. The nuclei are round or oval with dispersed chromatin and small nucleoli. Cells were stained with H and E and are magnified at 100X

cGy). Shorter et al reported a case in which an SPT with multiple liver metastases was treated with a short course of Tamoxifen.[28] The patient remained disease free for twelve year disease free. On the other hand, Alex reported a case in which a 15-year-old female patient had a 15 cm SPT in the pancreatic head as well as multiple liver metastases and periaortic lymph node invasion. The patient died despite a subtotal pancreatectomy and adjuvant chemoradiotherapy.

Until now, there has been no sufficient explanation for this diverse clinical course or prognostic markers for SPT. Nishihara et al[29] reported signals such as venous invasion, nuclear atypia, high mitotic index and the presence of necrobiotic cell nest to be good prognostic markers, however, these are not unanimously accepted.[30] Pasquiou et al[31] reported that factors such as: male gender, old age and tumor rupture(due to external trauma or tumor resection) are important in determining a poor prognosis. Other studies have also shown that tumor rupture and subsequent peritoneal seeding to be important prognostic factors in patient survival.

Recently, much research has been focused on the origin and pathogenetic mechanisms of SPT.[32-34] Until now, SPT is believed to be originated from pancreatic pluripotent stem cells, This is because immunohistochemical staining fails to show a clear-cut lineage. Chen found melanin pigment in SPT and suggested that SPT was originated from neural crest cells. Kosmahl[32] set up an interesting hypothesis that SPT was derived from genital ridge/4 pediatric oncology ovarian anlage tissue, which became attached to the dorsal portion of the pancreas during early embryogenesis.

Mutation in β-catenin, intranuclear accumulation of β-catenin and transcriptional activation of the oncogenes c-Myc and cyclin D1 have been accepted as pathogenetic mechanisms for tumorigenesis of SPT.[35-38] Another mechanism, in which β-catenin is stabilized, is constitutive activation of the Wnt/wingless signal transduction pathway. This could be affected by a mutation in APC, GSK-3 β-Axin.[39-40]

Previously, we microdissected SPT tumor cells from twenty patients including adults. We found that all patients showed strong intranuclear β-catenin immunostaining (Figs 43.8A to C). 80 percent (16/20) of patients showed a mutation at GSK-3

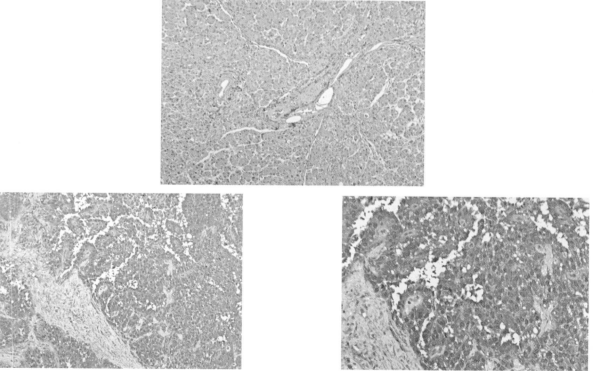

Figures 43.8A to C: Immunostaining for β-catenin (A) β-catenin immunostain in normal pancreatic tissue. Acinal cells, duct cells, and some islet cells in the nonneoplastic pancreatic parenchyma showed only weak or absent membranous staining. (B) β-catenin immunostain in solid (right bottom) and pseudopapillary (middle upper) areas of tumor. Almost all tumor cells show cytoplasmic and nuclear staining. Membranous staining is weak and discontinuous. Cells were counterstained with hematoxylin and magnified at 100X. (C) β-catenin immunostain in areas of tumor. Cells are counterstained with hematoxylin and magnified at 200X

β-phosphorylation sites in β-catenin exon 3 (codon 32,33,or 37). 56 percent (10/18) of patients showed an allelic loss in 5q22.1(APC gene locus). Abraham[37] suggested that mutations in β-catenin are good prognostic markers for SPT. Our previous study, however, included patients with no allelic loss at 5q22.1 or β-catenin mutations. In addition, all of these patients are still alive. Therefore, an alternate mechanism of β-catenin stabilization must exist.

Two recently-performed researches should be noticed. One is the research of Iwai. he found that in immunostaining of SCC cell line, there was also some β-catenin (function as cofactor bind E-cadherin and β-catenin) immunoreactivity in plasma membrane of cancer cell. He suggested that E-cadherin continuously function as an inhibitor of cancer cell dehiscence and metastasis. The other is the research of Morales.[41] Contrary to previous results, He found that estrogen receptor(ER- β) was constitutively expressed in SPT cells. ER- β) is known to be an inhibitor of overexpression of the oncogene cyclin D1[42], Taken together, these two results may help explain the slow growth and favorable prognosis characteristic of SPT.

REFERENCES

1. Rebhandl W, Felberbauer FX, Puig S, et al. Solid-pseudopapillary tumor of the pancreas (Frantz tumor) in children: Report of four cases and review of the literature. J Surg Oncol 2001;76:289-96.
2. Klimstra DS, Wenig BM, Heffess CS. Solid pseudopapillary tumor of the pancreas: a typically cystic carcinoma of low malignant potential. Semin Diagn Pathol 2000;17:66-80.
3. Matsunou H, Konishi F, Yamamichi N, et al. Solid, infiltrating variety of papillary cystic neoplasm of the pancreas. Cancer 1990;65:2747-57.
4. Potrc S, Kavalar R, Horvat M, et al. Urgent Whipple resection for solid pseudo papillary tumor of the pancreas. J Hepatobiliary Pancreas Surg 2003;10:386-9.
5. Franz VK. Papillary tumors of the pancreas: benign or malignant?, in Franz VK (Eds): Atlas of Tumor Pathology, Washington DC, US Armed Forces Institute of Pathology, 1959;pp32-33.
6. Wang KS, Albanese C, Dada F, et al. Papillary cystic neoplasm of the pancreas: A report of three pediatric cases and literature review. J Pediatr Surg 1998;33(6):842-5.
7. LH Tang, H Aydin, MF Brennan, DS Klimstra. Clinically Aggressive Solid Pseudopapillary Tumors of the Pancreas: A Report of Two Cases with Components of Undifferentiated Carcinoma and a Comparative Clinicopathologic Analysis of 34 Conventional Cases. Am J Surg Pathol 2005;29(4):512-19.
8. Lam KY, Lo CY, Fan ST. Pancreatic solid cystic papillary tumour: clinicopathologic features in eight patients from Hong Kong and review of the literature. World J Surg 1999;23:1045-50.
9. Zhou H, Cheng W, Lam KY, et al. Solid cystic papillary tumour of the pancreas in children. Pediatr Surg Int 2001;17:614-20.
10. Jung SE, Kim DY, Park KW, et al. Solid and papillary epithelial neoplasm of the pancreas in children. World J Surg 1999;23:233-6.
11. Sun CD, Lee WJ, Choi JS, et al. Solid Pseudopapillary tumors of the pancreas:14 years experience ANZ J Surg 2005;75:684-9.
12. Buetow PC, Buck JL, Pantongrag-Brown L, et al. Solid and papillary epithelial neoplasm of the pancreas: imaging-pathologic correlation in 56 cases. Radiology 1996; 199:707–11.
13. Wunsch LP, Flemming P, Werner U, et al. Diagnosis and treatment of papillary cystic tumor of the pancreas in children. Eur J Pediatr Surg 1997;7:45–7.
14. Poustchi-Amin M, Leonidas JC, Valderrama E, et al. Papillary-cystic neoplasm of the pancreas. Pediatr Radiol 1995;25:509–11.
15. Cantisani V, Mortele KJ, Levy A, et al. MR imaging features of solid pseudopapillary tumor of the pancreas in adult and pediatric patients. AJR 2003;181:395-401.
16. Lee, Jong-Kang MD *; Tyan, Yeu-Sheng MD. Detection of a Solid pseudopapillary Tumor of the Pancreas with F-18 FDG Positron Emission Tomography. Clinical Nuclear Medicine. 2005; 30(3):187-8.
17. Sperti, Cosimo, Pasquali, Claudio, Chierichetti, Franca, Liessi, Guido, Ferlin, Giorgio, Pedrazzoli, Sergio. FACS Value of 18-FDG-PET in the management of Patients with Cystic Tumors of the Pancreas. Annals of Surgery 2001;234(5):675-80.
18. Ashton J, Sutherland F, Nixon J, Nayak V. A case of solid-pseudopapillary tumor of the pancreas: preoperative cyst fluid analysis and treatment by enucleation. Hepato-gastroenterology. 2003 Nov-Dec; 50(54):2239-41.
19. Bektas AH, Werner AU, Kaaden AS, Philippou AS, Kloppel AG, Klempnauer AJ. Solidpseudopapillary tumor of the pancreas—a rare and frequently misdiagnosed neoplasm Langenbeck's Archives of Surgery 1999;384(1):39-43.
20. Murat ZEYTUNLU Ozgur FIRAT, Deniz NART, Ahmet COKER. Solid and cystic papillary neoplasms of the pancreas: Report of four cases Turk J Gastroenterol 2004;15(3):178-82.
21. Carricaburu E, Enezian G, Bonnard A, Berrebi D, Belarbi N, Huot O, Aigrain Y, de Lagausie P. Laparoscopic distal pancreatectomy for Frantz's tumor in a child. Surg Endosc 2003; 17(12):2028-31.
22. Kloppel G, Maurer R, Hofmann E, Oscarson J, Forsby N, Ihsel, Ljungberg O, Heitz PU. Solid cystic (papillary-cystic) tumors within and outside the pancreas in men: report of two patients. Virchows Arch A Pathol Anat Histopathol 1991;418:179-83.
23. Siech M, Merkle E, Mattfeldt T, Wiedmeier U, Brambs HJ, Beger HG. Solid-pseudopapillare Tumoren des Pankreas. Chirurg 1996;67:1012-5.
24. Akiyama H, Ono K, Takano M, et al. Solid pseudopapillary tumor of the pancreatic head causing marked distal atrophy. Int J Pancreatol 2002;32:47-52.
25. CM Vollmer Jr, E Dixon, DR Grant. Management of a solid pseudopapillary tumor of the pancreas with liver metastasis 2003;5(4):264-7.
26. Strauss JF, Hirsch VJ, Rubey CN, et al. Resection of a solid and papillary epithelial neoplasm of the pancreas following treatment with cis-platinum and 5-Fluorouracil: A case report. Med Pediatr Onc 1993;21:365-7.
27. Fried P, Cooper J, Balthazar E, et al. A role for radiotherapy in the treatment of solid and papillary neoplasms of the pancreas. Cancer 1985;56:2783-5.
28. Shorter NA, Glick RD, Klimstra DS, et al. Malignant pancreatic tumors in childhood and adolescence: The Memorial Sloan-

Kettering experience, 1967 to present. J Pediatr Surg 2002; 37(6):887-92.

29. Ky A, Shilyansky J, Gerstle J, et al. Experience with papillary and solid epithelial neoplasms of the pancreas in children. J Pediatric Surg 1998;33:42-44.

30. Nishihara K, Nagoshi M, Tsuneyoshi M, et al. Papillary cystic tumors of the pancreas. Assessment of their malignant potential. Cancer 1993;71:82-92.

31. Huang HL, Shih SC, Chang WH, et al. Solid-pseudo-papillary tumor of the pancreas: Clinical experience and literature review World J Gastroenterol 2005;11(9):1403-9.

32. Pasquiou C, Scoazec JY, Gentil-Perret A, Taniere P, Ranchere-Vince D, Partensky C, Barth X, et al. Solid pseudopapillary tumors of the pancreas. Pathology report of 13 cases Gastroenterol Clin Biol 1999;23(2):207-14.

33. Kosmahl M, Seada LS, Janig U, et al. Solid-pseudo-papillary tumor of the pancreas: its origin revisited. Virchows Arch 2000;436(5):473-80.

34. Nadler EP, Anna Novikov, Landzberg BR, et al. The use of endoscopic ultrasound in the diagnosis of solid pseudopapillary tumors of the pancreas in children. J Pediatric Surg 2002;37(9):1370-73.

35. Chen Chen, Wen Jing, Priya Gulati, et al. Melanocytic differentiation in a solid pseudopapillary tumor of the pancreas Case report J of Gastroenterol 2004;39(6):579-83.

36. Behrens J, Jerchow BA, Wurtele M, et al. Functional Interaction of an Axin Homolog, Conductin, with β-Catenin, APC, and GSK-3a. Science 1998;280:596-9.

37. Tanaka Y, Kato K, Notohara K, et al. Frequent β-catenin mutation and cytoplasmic or nuclear accumulation in pancreatic solid-pseudopapillary neoplasm. Cancer Res 2001;61(23): 8401-4.

38. Abraham SC, Klimstra DS, Wilentz RE, et al. Solid-Pseudopapillary Tumors of the Pancreas Are Genetically Distinct from Pancreatic Ductal Adenocarcinomas and Almost Always Harbor β-catenin Mutations Am J Pathol 2002;160(4):1361-9.

39. Tanaka Y, Notohara K, Kato K, et al. Usefulness of a-Catenin Immunostaining for the Differential Diagnosis of Solid-Pseudopapillary Neoplasm of the Pancreas. Am J Surg Pathol 2002;26(6):818-20.

40. Nakamura T, Hamada F, Ishidate T, et al Axin, an inhibitor of the Wnt signalling pathway, interacts with beta catenin, GSK-3 beta and APC and reduces the beta catenin level Genes Cells 1998;3:395-403.

41. Soichi Iwai, Wataru Katagiri, Chie Kong, Shigeki Amekawa Mutations of the APC, β-catenin, and axin-1 genes and cytoplasmic accumulation of β-catenin in oral squamous cell carcinoma J Cancer Res Clin Oncol 2005;131:773-82.

42. A Morales, A Duarte-Rojo, A Angeles. The beta Form of the Estrogen Receptor Is Predominantly Expressed in the Papillary Cystic Neoplasm of the Pancreas Pancreas 2003;26(3):258-63.

43. PA Hershberger, AC Vasquez, B Kanterewicz, et al. Opposing Action of Estrogen Receptors and on Cyclin D1 Gene Expression J Biol Chem 2002;277(27):24353-60.

have been reported.[6] Immunophenotype shows vimentin positivity with variable positivity with muscle markers. The differential diagnosis of this type is infantile fibrosarcoma. The tumor may recur locally if inadequately excised. The progression is unpredictable.

Extra-abdominal Fibromatosis

These occur most commonly on the back, chest wall, head and neck, or lower extremity (Figs 44.2A and B).They have a male predominance. Most patients complain of a painless mass of several months or years' duration.

Desmoplastic Fibroma

It is a benign intraosseous neoplasm recognized as the intraosseous counterpart of soft tissue fibromatosis. It has a propensity for locally aggressive behavior and local recurrence. Desmoplastic fibroma has been reported in sites like maxilla and mandible.[7,8] They usually present

as a rapidly expanding, painless mass and may be adequately treated surgically.

Desmoplastic fibromas of the pediatric skull are uncommon lesions with similarity to benign skull lesions though they are locally aggressive.[9] Local recurrence is common after curettage alone but complete resection appears to be curative.[9] Close follow up of incompletely resected lesions is essential.

Intra-abdominal Fibromatosis

Intra-abdominal fibromatosis is a rare benign neoplasm arising from the abdominal fibrous tissue, mostly in the mesentery. Rarely, it may occur in the retroperitoneum. It is characterized by a tendency to infiltrate the surrounding vessels and vital structures and recurrence after usually incomplete surgical removal. Thus, they are associated with considerable morbidity and mortality. Though they are rare in childhood, their high potential for local invasiveness and recurrence makes it vital to diagnose them in time. They usually present as a mass abdomen along with pressure symptoms like intermittent nausea and vomiting, abdominal fullness, constipation and urinary frequency. Although abdominal desmoids have an increased incidence in Gardner's syndrome, they are rarely found in isolated form. The authors have managed a rare case of retroperitoneal fibromatosis causing intestinal obstruction (Fig. 44.3). Although intraabdominal desmoids are usually detected as a

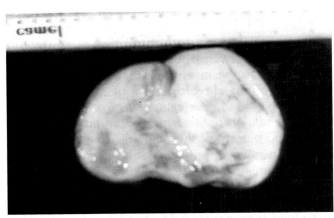

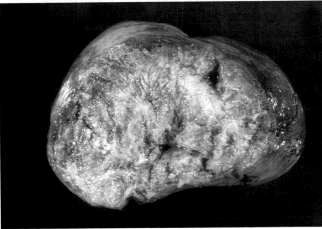

Figures 44.2A and B: Excised specimen of fibromatosis involving the chest wall

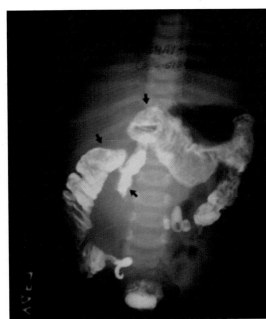

Figure 44.3: Barium enema in one-year-old child with retropeitoneal fibromatosis presenting with intestinal obstruction

solitary lesion, occassionally there may be multiple lesions Intestinal obstruction and invasion of colon wall have also been reported.[10]

Abdominal Fibromatosis (Desmoid Tumor)

Fibromatosis tumors of the anterior abdominal wall are much less common than extra-abdominal fibromatosis.

Desmoid tumor is a slow growing non-metastasizing locally aggressive tumor that arises from the rectus sheath or surgical scar tissue on the abdominal wall. Wide local excision with 2 cm margin offers good outcome. There is a high incidence of recurrence if a wide margin is not excised. For recurrent, aggressive and irresectable lesions tamoxifen, NSAID sulindac or combination has been used with anecdotal success.

Desmoid tumor may also involve the chest wall exclusively or both the chest wall and adjacent structures.[11] Positive margins at resection, reoperation and postoperative radiation are associated with a high risk of local recurrence.[11]

INVESTIGATIONS

Skiagram (AP and lateral) may be helpful to delineate the extent of a superficial lesion (Fig. 44.4). Ultrasonographic examination may be useful for the initial diagnoses which may be supplemented with other investigations like computed tomography and magnetic resonance imaging [MRI] for delineating the exact extent of the lesion. Barium studies may be helpful in intra abdominal fibromatosis presenting with bowel symptoms.

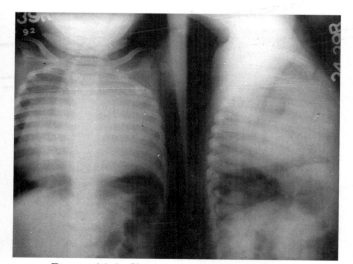

Figure 44.4: Skiagram chest (AP and lateral) outlining a chest wall fibromatosis

Most lesions were ovoid (52%) or infiltrative (34.5%) in outline with an irregular or lobulated contour (76%) on MRI.[4] The lesions may cross major fascial boundaries in upto 30 percent cases.[4] Accurate diagnosis and staging of aggressive fibromatosis by MRI have important treatment and prognostic implications Homogeneous isointensity or mild hyperintensity on T1-weighted images and heterogenous high signal on T2-weighted or STIR images are seen on MRI. All lesions usually enhance avidly after IV gadolinium. The MRI findings cannot predict recurrence.[4]

DIFFERENTIAL DIAGNOSIS

Fibroma: A case of oral giant cell fibroma has been reported in a 3-year-old boy was successfully excised by electro surgery without any recurrence.[12]

Fibrous hamartoma (FH) of infancy is a benign mesenchymal tumor, occurring as a superficial mass. Complete excision is curative. A nonradical excision has also been found to be curative in some cases so an aggressive approach may be avoided, as the overall prognosis is excellent.[13] Chemotherapy has been required for a synchronous desmoid fibromatosis so follow up with histopathology is important.[13]

Fibrolipomas: These benign tumors are more frequent in males than in females, built mostly of fibrous connective tissue. Their surface is shiny, pink and plain. They are well separated from the surrounding tissues. The treatment of fibrolipomas is only surgical. Fibrolipomas occur usually in adults and are extremely rare in children.[14] The asymptomatic course, allows them to grow for many years. Treatment is sought for cosmetic reasons. The final diagnosis must always be confirmed by histological examination.

Prepubertal vulval fibroma: It is a mesenchymal tumor that arises in the vulvar region in the prepubertal years. Most cases arise from the labia majora. The median age at presentation is 8 years.[15] The differential diagnoses include hemangioma, lipoma, lymphangioma and Bartholin cyst.

The tumors are usually unilateral, ill defined, located in the submucosa or subcutaneous tissue, and range from 2.0 to 8.0 cm in size in maximum dimension. Microscopically, they are poorly marginated, hypocellular neoplasms composed of bland spindle-shaped cells in a variably collagenous to edematous or myxoid stroma, diffusely infiltrating between preexisting normal vascular, adipose, and neural tissues. The tumor cells are immunoreactive for CD34 but not for smooth muscle actin, desmin, and S-100 protein.[15] Treatment is by local excision. There is a tendency for local recurrence.

Chondromyxoid fibroma: An extensive chondromyxoid fibroma invading the lamina of the second thoracic vertebra has been described in a 7-year-old child causing extensive cord compression and progressive neurological deterioration.[16] This is an extremely rare bone tumor with only 25 such cases of spinal involvement being reported.[16]

PATHOLOGY

These tumors are not encapsulated tumor and thus have the potential for local reccurence. Macroscopically, cut surface is usually pale, whorled and fibrous with irregular margin. The histology shows that the tumour is composed of a proliferation of sheets of uniform, bland spindle cells within a dense collegenous stroma. Microscopically, there is proliferation of palely eosinophilic fibroblasts and myofibroblasts. There is an infiltrative pattern with presence of abundant collagen between the tumour cells and absence of cytological features of malignancy.

Cellularity and mitotic activity are extremely variable. Other light microscopic features include thick-walled blood vessels sharply outlined from surrounding tissue, perivascular lymphocytic infiltrate at the advancing edge of the tumour and rarely metaplastic ossification or cartilage formation. The immunohistochemistry is positive with vimentin, variably positivity for SMA, CD117 and desmin and negative for CD34. Staining correlates with the cellularity. Ultrastructural study confirms fibroblastic and myofibroblastic features with presence of intracytoplasmic collagen formation.

The histologic features do not vary with the MRI signal characteristics of the lesion and are not helpful in predicting recurrence.[4]

Fibromatosis may be confirmed by the presence of vimentin and absence of other biological cell markers.[17]

Sharma V et al tried to determine the impact of prognostic variables on local control in patients with aggressive fibromatosis treated with or without radiation.[18] It was found that on univariate analysis, age, sex, positive margins, primary or recurrent presentation, site of involvement and initial treatment did not affect local control significantly.[18]

TREATMENT

General recommendations for the clinical management of pediatric patients with aggressive fibromatosis remain undetermined.

Surgical Excision

Surgical excision is the usually recommended treatment of pediatric fibromatosis (Figs 44.5A and B). However the invading nature of this tumor is responsible for recurrences leading to mutilating surgery and eventually to death despite the histologically benign appearance. The primary treatment of fibromatosis is local surgical excision with a wide local excision or muscle group resection if possible (Fig. 44.6). Negative surgical margins is the most vital factor determining the success of primary treatment Outcome of the tumor depends on early

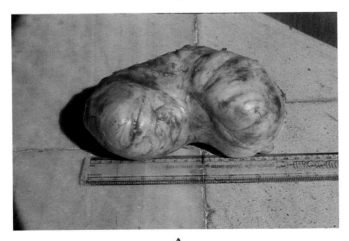

A

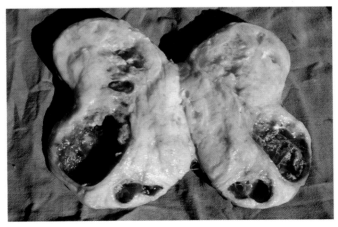

B

Figures 44.5A and B: (A) Excised specimen of a retroperitoneal fibromatosis, **(B)** cut section of the specimen

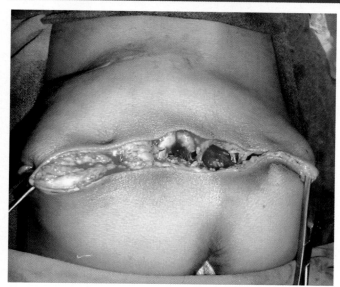

Figure 44.6: Surgical excision of an extensive recurrent fibromatosis. Note the scar of the previous incision site superior to the incision

diagnosis and complete tumor resection, and, if indicated, timely employment of neo/adjuvant chemotherapy. Incomplete resection with positive margins is the most important determinant for disease recurrence.[19]

Chemotherapy

Patients with fibromatosis not amenable to surgery may suffer from high morbidity. Various chemotherapeutic regimens have been tried in these patients with limited success as the results of chemotherapy have been variable without consistency.

A chemotherapy trial with vincristin and methotrexate proved to be effective in reducing the tumor burden and improving the general condition of a boy who presented with a large intraabdominal fibromatosis at the age of 5 years and had undergone 4 subsequent abdominal explorations for diagnosis, tumor reduction, and intestinal obstructions.[17]

Preoperative chemotherapy and adjuvant treatment following incomplete resection with combined vincristine, actinomycin-D, and cyclophosphamide (VAC) has been found to be useful by some.[19] On the other hand a combination of ifosfamide, vincristine and actinomycin was found to be ineffective in one series.[20]

Intensive chemotherapy with Actinomycin 750-1,500 microgram/m^2 at Day 1 and vincristine 1.5 mg/m^2 at Day 1 and Day 8 repeated every four weeks has been found to be effective in extensive fibromatosis.[20]

The tumor has been found to decrease slowly but constantly. A mild treatment but for a long time, 10-17 months has been reported to succeed in cases where more intensive courses have failed.[20] The tumor biopsy after the course of chemotherapy may confirm the nonprogressive nature of the residual fibromatosis or reveal a scar without progressive fibromatosis.

Pegylated liposomal doxorubicin has been used as a therapeutic option in patients with progressive unresectable fibromatosis in unfavorable localizations heavily pretreated with various chemotherapeutic agents without results[21] 3-weekly cycles liposomal doxorubicin were given in a dose range of 20-50 mg/m^2 /day.

Radiotherapy

Local radiotherapy with a total dose of 5000 rads has been found to be useful for incompletely resected tumors in some cases. However, the addition of radiation therapy to surgery was found to have no impact on local control by others.[18]

The morbidity of radiation treatment is considerable and adjuvant radiation therapy should therefore be considered only in situations where the risk of recurrence and the morbidity of re-excision are high.[18] Fourty two percent cases receiving radiation have been reported to develop severe moist desquamation following treatment with doses of 60 Gy or more.[18]

Radiotherapy must be thus be considered in life-threatening conditions as the last resort in a growing child.[17]

FOLLOW UP

Regular follow up is essential as there is a high incidence of recurrence. Also, there is a risk of malignant conversion. The development of a fibrosarcoma of the thigh has been reported as long as 28 years after excision of fibromatosis.[22]

REFERENCES

1. Dehner LP. Mesenchymal neoplasms in childhood. Insights of Arthur Purdy Stout and where they have taken us. Am J Surg Pathol 1986;10Suppl1:32-42.
2. Hicks J, Mierau G. The spectrum of pediatric fibroblastic and myofibroblastic tumors. Ultrastruct Pathol 2004;28:265-81.
3. Chung EB, Enzinger FM. Infantile myofibromatosis. Cancer 1981;48:1807-18.
4. Lee JC, Thomas JM, Phillips S, Fisher C, Moskovic E. Aggressive fibromatosis: MRI features with pathologic correlation AJR Am J Roentgenol 2006;186:247-54.
5. Fetsch JF, Laskin WB, Miettinen M. Palmar-plantar fibromatosis in children and preadolescents: a clinicopathologic study of 56

cases with newly recognized demographics and extended follow-up information. Am J Surg Pathol 2005;29:1095-105.

6. Desai SR, Dombale VD, Janugade HB. Infantile fibromatosis (desmoid type)—a case report. Indian J Pathol Microbiol 2005;48:379-80.

7. Ogunsalu C, Barclay S. Aggressive infantile (desmoid-type) fibromatosis of the maxilla: a case report and new classification. West Indian Med J 2005;54(5):337-40.

8. Said-Al-Naief N, Fernandes R, Louis P, Bell W, Siegal GP. Desmoplastic fibroma of the jaw: a case report and review of literature. Oral Surg Oral Med Oral Pathol Oral Radiol Endod 2006;101:82-94.

9. Wolfe SQ, Cervantes L, Olavarria G, Brathwaite C, Ragheb J, Morrison G. Desmoplastic fibroma of the pediatric skull. Report of three cases. J Neurosurg 2005;103:362-5.

10. Eren S. A sporadic abdominal desmoid tumour case presenting with intermittent intestinal obstruction. Eur J Pediatr Surg 2005;15:196-9.

11. Abbas AE, Deschamps C, Cassivi SD, Nichols FC. 3rd, Allen MS, Schleck CD, Pairolero PC Chest-wall desmoid tumors: results of surgical intervention. Ann Thorac Surg 2004;78:1219-23;discussion1219-23.

12. Braga MM, Carvalho AL, Vasconcelos MC, Braz-Silva PH, Pinheiro SL Giant cell fibroma: A case report. J Clin Pediatr Dent 2006;30:261-4.

13. Carretto E, Dall'Igna P, Alaggio R, Siracusa F, Granata C, Ferrari A, Cecchetto G. Fibrous hamartoma of infancy: an Italian multi-institutional experience. J Am Acad Dermatol. 2006;54:800-3.

14. Janas A, Grzesiak-Janas G.The rare occurence of fibrolipomas Otolaryngol Pol 2005;59:895-8.

15. Iwasa Y, Fletcher CD. Distinctive prepubertal vulval fibroma: a hitherto unrecognized mesenchymal tumor of prepubertal girls: analysis of 11 cases. Am J Surg Pathol 2004;28:1601-08.

16. Meredith CC, Kepes JJ, Johnson P, Sebastian CT, McMahon JK, Arnold PM. Chondromyxoid fibroma of the upper thoracic spine in a 7-year-old patient. A case report and review of the literature Pediatr Neurosurg 2004;40:190-5

17. Alebouyeh M, Moussavi F, Tabari AK, Vossough P. Aggressive intra-abdominal fibromatosis in children and response to chemotherapy. Pediatr Hematol Oncol 2005;22:447-51.

18. Sharma V, Chetty DN, Donde B, Mohiuddin M, Giraud A, Nayler S. Aggressive fibromatosis—impact of prognostic variables on management. S Afr J Surg 2006;44:6-8,10-1.

19. Buitendijk S, van de Ven CP, Dumans TG, den Hollander JC, Nowak PJ, Tissing WJ, Pieters R. van den Heuvel-Eibrink MM Pediatric aggressive fibromatosis: a retrospective analysis of 13 patients and review of literature. Cancer. 2005;104:1090-9.

20. Mitrofanoff P, Vannier JP, Bachy B, Hemet J, Boillot B, Borde J. Fibromatosis in children: regression with prolonged chemotherapy. Apropos of 2 cases Chir Pediatr 1988;29:325-9.

21. Wehl G, Rossler J, Otten JE, Boehm N, Uhl M, Kontny U, Niemeyer C. Response of progressive fibromatosis to therapy with liposomal doxorubicin. Onkologie. 2004;27:552-6.

22. Mooney EE, Meagher P, Edwards GE, Cahalane SF, Gaffney EF. Fibrosarcoma of the thigh 28 years after excision of fibromatosis. Histopathology 1993;23:498-500.

CHAPTER 45

Devendra K Gupta
M Ragavan

Gastric Teratoma

INTRODUCTION

Teratomas are embryonal neoplasms derived from totipotent germ cells contain tissues from all the three germ layers. These lesions frequently present in infancy and childhood, and may be benign or malignant, and cystic or solid. They can occur anywhere, the common sites being the sacrococcygeal region, the retroperitoneum and the gonads. Gastric teratomas are very rare and account for less than 1 percent of teratomas and 2 percent of abdominal teratoma.

The first gastric teratoma was reported in 1922 by Eusterman and Sentry in a 31-year-old male. It is found exclusively in males, usually in children below 1 year of age. 90 percent of these tumors are seen in neonatal period and infancy.

Gastric teratoma is almost seen only in male infants in contrast to teratoma at other sites where it is more common in girls.[13] Most cases have been reported in infancy.[2,13] Cases of congenital gastric teratomas have been described which were detected prenatally by ultrasound as abdominal calcifications when mothers were investigated for polyhydramnios.[4,8]

The gastric teratoma differs from teratomas arising from other sites. Firstly, overall they are not associated with any congenital anomalies in contrast to 10 to 15 percent incidence at other sites. Secondly, most of the gastric teratomas (> 95%) are seen in males when compared to female preponderance (65-70%) at other sites. Lastly, they are almost always benign in nature as compared to 10 to 39 percent incidence of malignancy at other sites such as the sacrococcygeal region, mediastinum and gonads.[1,5] As a result, they have an excellent prognosis after surgery, compared to teratomas at other sites.

PATHOPHYSIOLOGY

Majority of cases described in infancy and neonatal period, are large enough to cause abdominal distension at the time of detection, and cases detected at birth have almost always been associated with immature elements and or with other congenital anomaly.[4] Therefore, we hypothesize that all gastric teratoma may actually originate in the gestational period. They may be considered to reflect a growth disturbance causing an early arrest in the normal process of differentiation and organogenesis. Such an embryonal tissue when occurring in association with an overgrowth syndrome like Beckwith-Weidmann syndrome may proliferate rather inappropriately leading to very early symptom production and detection.[4] Loss of heterozygosity causing unmasking of recessive mutant alleles may be the basis of formation of embryonal tumor. Alternatively gastric teratomas may arise from incompletely formed monozygotic twin or a fetus in fetu. The tumor can be predominantly exogastric or endogastric. The endogastric type grows into the lumen of the stomach erodes mucosa and vessels and also cause luminal obstruction. The exogastric type grows from the surface of the stomach in the peritoneal cavity or to the lesser sac. This tumor arises most commonly from the posterior wall of the stomach and is exogastric in 58 to 70 percent cases, while it is endogastric in 30 percent cases. Though, gastric teratomas can arise from any part of the stomach, the other common sites where it is encountered are lesser curvature of stomach, antrum and fundus of stomach. Some of these tumors are pedunculated and are attached by a pedicle to the stomach. Large tumor in the lesser curvature can cause obstruction to the common bile duct leading to obstructive jaundice.

CLINICAL FEATURES

The endogastric type is associated with gastric outlet obstruction symptoms, hematemesis and melaena.[5,9] where as the exogastric variant grow from the surface of the stomach most commonly present with abdominal swellings[2,13] with rapid deterioration in general condition. General non-specific symptoms like anemia, malnutrition and fever are also seen as common presentations.[13] Rarely these tumors were the cause of difficulty during childbirth,[9] gastrointestinal bleeding[5,7,15,17] and respiratory distress.[14] Some can present with jaundice due to bile duct compression.

STAGING

In case of malignant teratoma of stomach which is very rare the staging described by children cancer study group and pediatric oncology group for extragonadal teratoma can be used.
Stage I: Complete excision with negative margins, tumor marker positive but fall after to normal and lymph node are negative for tumors.
Stage II: Microscopic residue, lymph nodes are negative, tumor markers negative or positive.
Stage III: Gross residual tumor, nodes positive, and tumor markers positive or negative.
Stage IV: Distant metastasis.

INVESTIGATION

Precise preoperative diagnosis of the origin and nature of the tumor can be very difficult. The calcification can be picked up on plain radiographs in approximately 60 percent of patients with teratomas.[2] The presence of teeth or bone is pathognomic of teratomas but is less frequently seen in teratoma of gastrointestinal region and very rare in gastric teratoma. Plain radiographs show a soft tissue mass with calcification in the upper abdomen. The mass may displace the bowel loops downwards and to the right.

Upper gastrointestinal contrast studies demonstrate gastric deformities or extrinsic pressure on bowel loops. Intraluminal filling defect is said to be characteristic of gastric teratomas. The ultrasonogram of the mass show

cystic mass or heterogeneous mass with solid and cystic areas. The cystic areas are anechoic with or without septation of varying thickness. The solid areas are heterogeneous and may show focal areas of hyperechogenicity with distal shadowing suggestive of calcification. In Computerized tomogram imaging they appear as well encapsulated masses with hypodense solid areas and cystic areas of water attenuation (Fig. 45.1).

The advantages of CT are the demonstration of complete extent of the tumor and its attachments, demonstration of areas of fat, foci of calcification not picked up on X-rays or ultrasound and intraluminal projection of the tumor into the stomach. Involvement of other organs particularly bowel loops is well visualized on CT.[18]

Histopathological examination show several tissues derived from all the three germ layers—skin and its appendages, smooth muscle, fat tissue, cartilage, respiratory epithelium and neural tissue and it is benign most of the time. The neural element can be immature.

DIFFERENTIAL DIAGNOSIS

Large number of tumors thus falls in differential diagnosis of gastric teratomas. These include congenital neuroblastoma, infantile hemangioepithelioma, hepatoblastoma, Wilms' tumor, mesoblastic nephroma, mesenteric lymphangioma and GI duplication cyst, all of which can show calcification and cysts.[12] Because of rarity of tumor and long list of close differential diagnosis, no case reported in literature was diagnosed preoperatively.

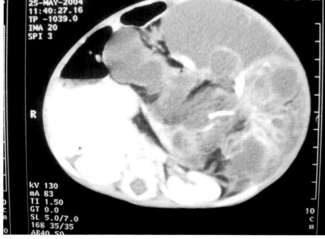

Figure 45.1: CT scan depicting a well encapsulated mass with hypodense solid areas and cystic areas of water attenuation

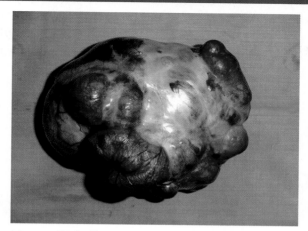

Figure 45.2: Excised specimen of a gastric teratoma

TREATMENT

Operative procedure described includes simple total excision of tumor along with the adherent stomach wall with primary closure of the defect due to essentially benign nature of the tumor. Enucleation of the mass, partial gastrectomy and total gastrectomy has also been described (Fig. 45.2).[13,14]

Most patients recover after surgery. Misdiagnosis due to rarity and complications like hemorrhage had been the usual causes of rare fatal cases. No recurrence has been reported after prolonged follow-up[14] even in immature teratomas.[11] However, occasional case of peritoneal gliomatosis after surgical removal of gastric teratoma has been reported.[3]

Malignancy in gastric teratomas is extremely rare and only two cases have been reported in literature.[1] both were treated by total excision of the tumor occasional cases of immature but benign teratomas treated similarly have also been reported.[4,11] In case of malignant tumors chemotherapy has to be used as for sacrococcygeal teratoma based on the histology.

REFERENCES

1. Balk E, Tuncyurek M, Sayan A, Avanoglu A, Ulman I, Cetinkursun S. Malignant gastric teratoma in an infant. Z Kinderchir 1990;45(6):383-5.
2. Basak D, Das A, Chattered SK, Mukherjee P. Gastric teratoma in children. Ind Pediatr 1992;29:231-4.
3. Couson WF. Peritoneal gliomatosis from a gastric teratoma. Am J Clin Pathol 1990;94(1):87-9.
4. Falik-Borenstein TC, Korenberg JR, Davos I, Platt LD, Gans S, Goodman B, Schreck R, Graham JM Jr. Congenital gastric teratoma in Wiedmann-Beckwith syndrome. Am J Med Genet 1991;3(1):52-7.
5. Gangopadhyay AN, Pandit SK, Gopal CS.Gastric teratoma revealed by gastrointestinal haemorrhage. Ind Pediatr 1992;29:1145-7.
6. Gray SW, Jhonson HC Jr, Skandalakis JE. Gastric teratoma in an adult with review of literature. South Med J 1964;57:1346.
7. Haley T, Dimuler M, Hellier P. Gastric teratoma with gastrointestinal bleeding. J Pediatr Surg 1986;21:949-50.
8. Henderson P, Lake Y. An unusual case of polyhydramnios: Congenital Gastric teratoma. NZ Med J 1994;107:133-4.
9. Matias IC, Huang YC. Gastric teratoma in infancy: Report of a case and review of world literature. Ann Surg 1973;170:631-6.
10. Moriuchi A, Nakayama I, Muta H, Taira Y, Takahara O. Gastric teratoma of children-A case report with review of literature. Acta Pathol Jpn 1977;27(5):749-58.
11. Munoz NA, Takehana H, Komi N, Hizawa K. Immature gastric teratoma in an infant. Acta Pediatr Jpn 1992;34(4):483-8.
12. Niedzwicki G, Wood BP. Radiological case of the month-gastric teratoma. Am J Dis Child 1990;114:1147-8.
13. Purvis JM, Miller RC, Bernard I. Gastric teratoma-First reported case in a female.J.Pediatr Surg 1979;14:86-8.
14. Senokak ME, Kale G, Buyukpakcu N, Hicsonmez A, Ceglar M.Gastric teratoma in children including the third reported female case. J Pediatr Surg 1990;25:681-4.
15. Cairo MS, Grosfeld JL, Wheetman RM. Gastric teratomas: Unusual cause for bleeding of the upper gastrointestinal tract in the newborn. Pediatrics 1981;67:721-4.
16. Mahour GH, Woolley MM, Trivedi SN, Landing BH. Teratomas in infancy and childhood: experience with 81 cases. Surgery 1974;76(2):309-18.
17. Gangopadhyay AN, Pandit SK, Gopal CS. Gastric teratomas revealed by gastrointestinal hemorrhage. Ind. Pediatrics 1992;29:1145-6.
18. Mohan V, Gupta SK, Chooramani S, Arora M. Gastric teratomas in infancy. Ind. Journal of Radiology 1980;36(3):239-41.

CHAPTER 46

Devendra K Gupta
M Ragavan

Mesenchymal Hamartoma of the Liver

INTRODUCTION

Mesenchymal hamartoma of the liver is the second commonest benign hepatic lesion and is seen almost exclusively in children less than 2 years age.[1,2] Benign liver tumors in children can be of epithelial or mesenchymal derivative. Benign mesenchymal tumors are more common and include cavernous hemagioma, hemangioendothelioma and mesenchymal hamartoma. There have been few reports of presentation in older children. It has a predilection for the right lobe but in 5 percent cases may involve both the lobes. Most of the series show a male preponderance. The male female ratio is 1.6:1. However, De Maioribus et al had 18 patients in their series with an equal sex distribution.[1]

ETIOLOGY

The lesion is believed to be the result of aberrant hamatomatous development of primitive mesenchyme in the portal tracts.[3] Biliary ducts and angiomatous tissue constitute the mesenchyme of the portal tracts and Dehner et al have suggested a similar etiopathogenesis for hepatic hemangioendotheliomas.[4] This theory is supported by the predominance of proliferating bile ducts seen on histological examination. The lesion occurs late in embryogenesis as the liver maintains its normal lobular architecture and biliary tree connection. These studies which classified this lesion into a hamartoma are now being questioned by newer studies. Cytogenetic analysis of the mesenchymal hamartoma has revealed a specific translocation involving the long arm of chromosome 19 (19q 13.4).[5,6] Otal et al found a subset of MH patients [2 of 8 patients] with aneuploidy on flow-cytometric analysis.[7] Both these patients were males 2 months of age or younger and one had a highly elevated serum alpha-fetoprotein. There are two confirmed reports of embryonal sarcoma (mesen-chymoma) associated with MH.[8,9] These findings imply that MH may after all be a true neoplasm rather than a developmental anomaly or hamartoma.

PATHOLOGY

Grossly, the lesion is usually well encapsulated and the cut surface shows multiple cysts separated by thin walled septation. Usually no bile staining is seen in the tumor. The cystic cavities contain yellowish or colorless watery or mucoid material.

Microscopically, the lesion shows mesenchymal loose myxoid tissue with branching, proliferating and compressed bile ducts. Islands of hepatocytes can be identified throughout the lesion though normal hepatic architecture is not seen. Vascular spaces including lymphatics are not a prominent feature of the tumor.[1,3,10,11] Dehner et al reported the ultra structural features of the tumor. The loose myxomatous tissue consists of mature collagen fibrils, fibroblast and small vessels. The duct like structures had short non branching microvilli projecting into the lumen and the luminal cells were bound together by juxtaluminal tight junctions. The ductal structures were surrounded by a basal lamina that showed marked reduplication. The hepatocytes in the lesion are arranged in groups and show normal ultrastructural features.[3]

CLINICAL FEATURES

Mesenchymal hamartoma commonly presents with progressive abdominal distension with or without a discrete palpable mass. Stocker and Ishak postulated that the rapid growth of the tumor may be secondary to cystic degeneration of the mesenchyme or destruction and dilatation of lymphatics.[12] The frequent large size of the tumor and the rapid enlargement is responsible for diaphragmatic splinting and respiratory distress. There are two reported cases of prenatally diagnosed MH of the liver.[13] The one reported case of so called MH causing congestive heart failure has different gross and histopathological findings, putting the diagnosis in question.[14]

INVESTIGATION

Ultrasonography is the mainstay in diagnosis. The mass shows cystic spaces with intervening solid septa. The cystic and solid components of the mass may vary and in large predominantly cystic tumors it may be difficult to confirm the hepatic origin of the lesion.[15-17] In such cases a contrast enhanced CT scan is ideal to confirm the diagnosis which show liver lesion (Fig. 46.1). Calcification is rarely present and can be identified on sonography. A sulfur colloid liver scintigraphy reveals a large defect and can be used as an adjunctive modality. Angiographically the mass is hypovascular or vascular though there is no justification in using this investigative modality as the diagnosis of MH can be reliably made by ultrasonography. Serum AFP levels have been measured in 7 of 17 cases reported from Japan. Five cases had high values in the range of 3200 to 6000 ng/ml. Immunohistochemical studies with peroxidase antiperoxidase complex IgG showed that the alpha-fetoprotein was localized in the proliferating liver cells and bile ductal epithelium of this lesion.[18]

DIFFERENTIAL DIAGNOSIS

Liver masses in pediatric age group that can mimic mesenchymal hamartoma are hemagioma, teratomas, simple cysts or the rare cystic hepatoblastoma, mesenchymoma and masses arising in the near by organs. Mesenchymoma is seen in children between 6 and 10 years and hepatoblastoma patients have characteristically high serum alpha-fetoprotein levels. Teratomas and simple cysts usually show calcification on plain X-rays.

TREATMENT

The diagnosis of MH necessitates early surgical excision because the mass has a propensity for rapid growth causing respiratory distress. The four surgical options recommended are:

1. Enucleation—The capsulated MH can be enucleated from normal hepatic tissue minimizing blood loss and parenchymal damage (Figs. 46.2A to C).

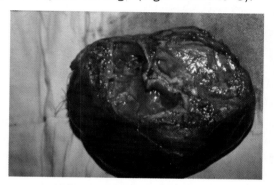

A

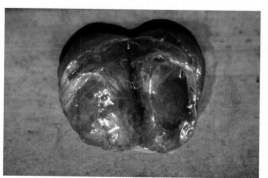

B

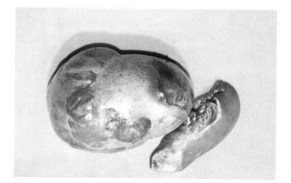

C

Figures 46.2A to C: Excised specimens of mesenchymal hamartomas

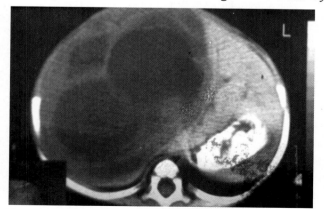

Figure 46.1: CT scan outlining a mesenchymal hamartoma

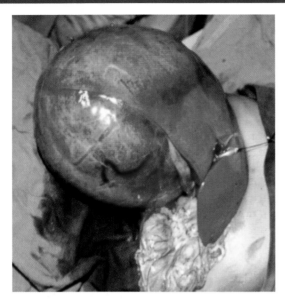

Figure 46.3: Operative photograph of a large mesechymal hamartoma

2. Excision of the hamartoma with a rim of normal tissue is the best alternative keeping in mind the reported association of MH with mesenchymoma.
3. Marsupialization was preferred earlier for large lesions but cannot be recommended as there is a risk of malignant transformation and recurrence.
4. A formal hepatic lobectomy may be needed in cases of large tumors with no well-defined plane between the lesion and normal liver (Fig. 46.3).[1,11,18,19] Rare incidence of malignant angiosarcomatous conversion warrants long-term follow-up.

REFERENCES

1. De Maioribus CA, Lally KP, Simik, et al. Mesenchymal hamartoma of the liver. A 35-year-review. Arch Surg 1990;125;598-600.
2. Balmer B, Le Coultre C, Feldges A. Mesenchymal liver hamartoma in a newborn; Case report. Eur J Pediatr Surg 1996;6:303-5.
3. Dehner LP, Ewing SL, Summer HW. Infantile mesenchymal hamartoma of the liver. Histologic and ultrastructural observations. Arch Pathol 1975;99:379-82.
4. Dehner LP, Ishak KG. Vascular tumors of the liver in infants and children. Arch Pathol 1971;92:101-11.
5. Mascarelio JP, Krous HF. Second reprot of a translocation involving 19q 13.4 in a mesenchymal hamartoma of the liver. Canar Genet Cytogenet 1992;58:141-2.
6. Speleman F, de Telder V, De Potter KR, et al. Cytogenetic analysis of a mesenchymal hamartoma of the liver. Cancer Genet Cytogenet 1989;40:29-32.
7. Otal TM, hendricks JB, Pharis P, et al. Mesenchymal hamartoma of the liver DNA flow cytometric analysis of eight cases cancer 1994;74:1237-42.
8. Corbally MT, Spitz L. Malignant potential of mesenchymal hamartoma: An unrecognized risk. Pediatr Surg Int 1992;7:321-2.
9. De Chadarevian JP, Pawel BR, Falrber EN, et al. Undifferentiated (Ambryjonal) Sarcoma arising in conjunction with mesnechymal hamartoma of the liver. Modern Pathol 1994;7:490-3.
10. Ishida M, Tsuchida Y, Saito S. Mesenchymal hamartoma of the liver: Case report and literature review. Ann Surg 1996;164:175-82.
11. Raffensperger JG, Gazalez - Gussi F, Skeetran T. Mesenchymal hamartoma of the liver. J Pediatr Surg 1983;18:585-7.
12. Stocker JT, Ishak KG. Mesenchymal hamartoma of the liver: Report of 30 cases and a review of the literature. Pediatr Pathol 1983;1:254-67.
13. Rosenbaum DM, Mindell HJ. Ultrasonographic findings in mesenchymal hamartoma of the liver. Radiology 1981;138:425-7.
14. Smith WL, Ballantine TVN, Gonzulez- Crussi F. Hepatic mesenchymal hamartoma causing heart failure in the neonate. J Pediatr Surg 1978;13:183-85.
15. Ros PR, Goodman ZD, Ishak KG, et al. Mesenchymal hamartoma of the liver: Radiologic- pathologic correlation. Radiology 1986;158:619-24.
16. Foucar E, urilliamson RA, Yin-Chin V, et al. Liver identified by fetal sonography. Am J Radiol 140:970-72.
17. Smith WL, Franken EA, Mitros FA. Liver tumors in children. Semin Roentgenol 1983;17:136-48.
18. Ito H, Kishikawa T, Joda T, et al. Hepatic mesenchymal hamartoma of an infant. 1984;19:315-7.
19. Pie rett RV. Mesenchymal hamartoma of the liver in children. Pediatr Surg Int 1995;10:264-6.

CHAPTER 47

Devendra K Gupta
Shilpa Sharma
Gautam Agarwal

Colorectal Carcinoma in Children

Colorectal carcinoma is rare in the pediatric age group with an incidence of 1.3 to 2 cases per million children.[1] The incidence is higher in the US, while it is much lower in india as the incidence of colorectal cancer is also lower in the adults.[1] Most cases have been reported in the second decade of life, though a few have been reported at younger ages. The poor prognosis of pediatric patients is attributed to the advanced stage of the disease at presentation due to a delay in diagnosis and aggressive biological behavior of the disease. The delay in diagnosis is attributable to a lack of awareness.

EPIDEMIOLOGY

Most children develop the carcinoma de novo in a previously normal colon.[2] This is in contrary to adult patients in whom a predisposing history of familial polyposis, ulcerative colitis, or familial colorectal cancer may be positive.[3,4]

Several well-recognized conditions may be associated with the development of colorectal carcinoma in younger patients. Familial polyposis, due to deletion mutation 5P FAP gene is inherited as a dominant trait with 90 percent penetrance. Other syndromes associated with colorectal cancer in young people include Turcot's syndrome (Congenital abnormalities, brain tumors), for which frequent mutation of the adenomatous polyposis coli (APC) gene has been found; Oldfieled's syndrome (Multiple sebaceous cysts, polyposis); and Gardner's syndrome (Multiple sebaceous cysts, exostoses, polyposis). Other predisposing conditions include juvenile polyposis of colon, ulcerative colitis, and family cancer syndrome.[5] Peutz-Jegher syndrome (Muco-cutaneous pigmentation of lips, perioral region, buccal mucosa, polyposis, ovarian granulosa cell tumors) is a hamatomatous polyposis condition with very less risk for malignant conversion.

Colonic cancer is more common in the West due to the relatively long bowel transit time of fecal material with low-fiber diets. Exposure to farm or agricultural chemicals has also been found to be associated in some patients with colorectal carcinomas.[6]

There is no known predisposition of colorectal carcinoma for gender. Most cases that occur in persons younger than 20 years of age occur at the median age of 15 years, though a mucin-secreting adenocarcinoma has been reported in a 9-month-old infant.[7]

PATHOLOGY

In adults, most carcinomas of the colon come from the left-side colon, especially the sigmoid colon and rectum. However in children, there is a regional difference in location of the tumor. While in the west, there appears to be an equal distribution between the right and the left colon, in India, most of the cases have been reported in the left colon.[8-13]

Colorectal carcinoma arises from the mucosal surface of the bowel, generally at the site of an adenomatous overgrowth or polyp. The tumor may extend into the muscularis area, then to the serosa and perforate the serosa into omental fat, lymph nodes, liver, ovaries, and other loops of bowel. Some lesions grow to obstruct the bowel lumen. They may implant along an abdominal scar, at the anastomotic site, or throughout the peritoneum. Early reports of colorectal carcinomas in young patients indicate that obstruction was more frequent at presentation in children than in adults.

Occasionally, more than one cancer is present simultaneously. Two lesions in the large intestine may be seperated by a distance.[2] These lesions may have the same or different histology and be in the same or different stages.

Carcinoma *in situ* may occur in one or more polyps. The principal histologic categories of colorectal cancer are well-differentiated adenocarcinoma, mucinous or colloid adenocarcinoma, signet ring adenocarcinoma, and scirrhous tumors.

Poorly differentiated mucinous adenocarcinoma, which accounts for approximately 5 to 15 percent of adult colorectal carcinomas, is the predominant histologic variety in children and adolescents at the time of diagnosis.[5] Tumors may grow to huge sizes because of the pooling of mucin.

Mucin-producing adenocarcinomas are more aggressive, grow more rapidly and thus have a short clinical course from the onset of the disease to advanced, metastatic disease.[14] Thus, the prognosis with a mucinous carcinoma is very poor. The mucin absorbs water, swells and invades local tissues, thereby promoting spread of malignant cells.[15] It also interferes with the immune recognition of carcinoma cells due to mucopolysaccharide coating.[15] Mucinous carcinoma of rectum are sometimes confused with sarcomas. It is found that tumors expressing hyperdiploid characteristics are more aggressive and should undergo a close watch and regular follow-up for recurrence.[15]

The signet ring cell subtype characterized by diffuse infiltration of the bowel wall by signet-ring-cells has the worst prognosis.

CLINICAL FEATURES

The initial symptoms associated with colorectal carcinoma in the young may be insidious. A change in bowel habits, such as constipation or diarrhea and change in the caliber of the stool may be observed before development of tarry stools or rectal bleeding. With changes in bowel habits, there may be a decrease in appetite followed by loss of body weight.

The child may present with non- specific symptoms like poor appetite, abdominal fullness vague abdominal pain, constipation, vomiting, nausea and occult blood in the stool with chronic anemia rectal bleeding.

The most common symptom of colon cancer in children is chronic persistent abdominal pain. Thus, colon cancer should be included in the differential diagnosis in teenagers with abdominal pain of unknown etiology

Unfortunately, many colon cancers cause periumbilical and epigastric pain that is often indistinguishable from the non-organic recurrent abdominal pain, though some may have right or left lower quadrant pain.

The signs and symptoms of bowel cancer are related to the portion of the large bowel where the primary tumor is located. Tumors of the right colon may cause more subtle symptoms but are often associated with an abdominal mass, weight loss, decreased appetite, and blood in the stools tumors involving the cecum and ascending colon, which may be associated with family colon cancer, may develop into masses of tremendous size before symptoms appear. Tumors of the rectum or sigmoid are generally associated with changes in bowel habits, changes in the caliber of the stool, hematochezia, and dyschezia. Because of the rarity of colorectal carcinoma in patients younger than 20 years, the diagnosis is seldom suspected and often delayed until they present with acute bowel symptoms due to complete intestinal obstruction, at which time bowel perforation may occur with multiple metastatic deposits. Thus most pediatric patients present with advanced metastatic disease, grossly or microscopically. Intestinal obstructions due to tumor occur more frequently in adolescents than in adults.

In advanced cases, an abdominal mass may palpable. Rarely, only tenderness may be elicited on abdominal and rectal palpation without any palpable abdominal mass.[2] Rectal digital examination may also be helpful in evaluation of bleeding or a palpable mass.

INVESTIGATIONS

The hemoglobin level may be low in cases with anemia. The carcinoembryonic antigen (CEA) level may be raised or within normal limits (< 5.0 µg/l).[2] The CEA determination possesses neither sensitivity nor specificity to enable its use as a screening test for suspected colorectal cancer in children.[16,17]

However, increased preoperative CEA levels may be correlated with a higher rate of relapse.[16,17]

Skiagram abomen may be helpful to assess the presence of intestinal obstruction or perforation in cases presenting with acute symptoms.

A noninvasive abdominal ultrasound examination followed by supportive barium enema studies are necessary diagnostic tools in children suffering from persistent abdominal pain with warning signs, like weight loss, anemia, and positive abdominal or rectal tenderness.

Abdominal ultrasound may delineate a "pseudokidney" or target-like lesion on thickened segmental bowel wall with protrusion of the serosa.[2] Ultrasound may also confirm the presence or absence of ascites.

Barium studies may reveal the typical colon lesions. On barium studies, early lesion usually appears as a small polypoid mass, indistinguishable from benign tumors. An upper gastrointestinal barium series with small bowel follow-through study may reveal an advanced lesion as an "apple-core" annular lesion with luminal narrowing where the transition from normal bowel to the tumoral area is usually abrupt.[14] A colonic barium enema study may reveal a stenotic lesion.

Abdominal computed tomography is usual to delineate the thickened wall of the rectum due to carcinoma (Figs 47.1A and B). It may also pick up calcification and edematous swelling of the mesentery. Computed tomography is recommended for preoperative staging and postoperative follow-up.

Colonoscopic examination may help to confirm the diagnosis—an ulcerative tumor or friable polypoid mucosal lesions in the ascending colon may be visualized.

A sigmoidoscopic examination can establish a diagnosis in the left sided lesions.

However, in the west, complete colonoscopic examination is preferred, as half of the colon cancers in children have been seen to arise from the transverse colon and ascending colon in those regions. Colonoscopy has the added advantage of taking a biopsy for pathologic examination from suspicious lesions.

DIFFERENTIAL DIAGNOSIS

Benign colorectal tumors include adenomatous solitary juvenile polyp (commonest), hemangioma, familial adenomatous polyposis coli and hamartomatous polyposis. Solitary adenomatous juvenile polyp is commonly seen in the age group of 3 to 6 years and 90 percent are in the rectosigmoid region. It usually presents with bleeding per rectum, anemia, and prolapsed polyp with pain. Polpectetomy with a snare offers cure. The concern with familial adenomatous polyp is the risk of malignant conversion

Diagnosis of a retrorectal cystic hamartomas may be made when the tumor is large enough to cause pain or intestinal obstruction, or when it becomes infected.[18] Differentiation of benign lesions like colitis cystica profunda from adenocarcinoma by careful histologic evaluation of the epithelium is fundamental in avoiding over treatment.[19]

The presence of multiple clustered polyps in the rectum should alert the radiologist to the possibility of another rare histologic entity, benign lymphoid polyps.[20]

Solitary rectal ulcer and its variants should also be considered in the differential diagnosis.[21] Other rare lesions to be differentiated include congenital fibrolipoma of anal canal and cystic duplication of the rectum.[22,23] A carcinoid in a rectal duplication has also been reported.[24]

An inflammatory pseudotumor involving the ileocecal region in a 16-year-old girl presenting as pyrexia of unknown origin for 4 months followed by

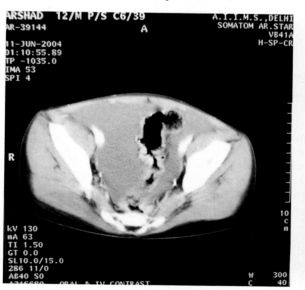 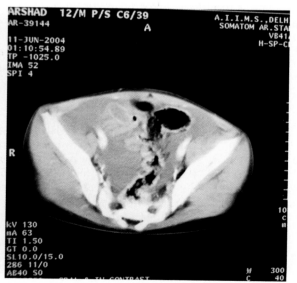

Figures 47.1A and B: CT scan of the pelvis showing the thickened wall of the rectum due to carcinoma

development of a palpable lump in the right iliac fossa has been described. The patient underwent a right hemicolectomy for a presumed ascending colonic neoplasm, and histology revealed that it was an inflammatory pseudotumor.[25]

Malignant lesions that may pose diagnostic difficulties include rare tumors that can involve the large or small bowel, like leiomyosarcoma, malignant fibrous histiocytomas, malignant carcinoid, and metastatic tumor from other sites. All may have similar presentations and metastases and may be identified only by histologic examination of the primary or metastatic sites.

STAGING

In colon cancer, the classical Dukes's classification is still referred to and has prognostic importance.[26] The major contribution of the Astler-Coller system (1954) was stress on the prognostic importance of the level of direct spread in stage C tumors.[27] The Astler-Coller staging system is also popular as an independent factor for prognosis. However, for comparative purposes, the TNM classification of the American Joint Committee on Cancer (1997) is used.[28]

Dukes's Classification

- Dukes's A: invasion of cancer into the bowel wall (no spread beyond muscle layer).
- Dukes's B: invasion through the bowel wall.
- Dukes's C: involvement of local lymph nodes.
- In practice, a modified Dukes's classification is used, which includes Duke's D—that is, presence of distant metastases and is more like the TNM classification.

The Astler-Coller Staging System

This system has five stages, A is limited to the mucosa, B1 involves muscularis propria but does not penetrate it, B2 penetrates the muscularis propria, and C1 and C2 are counterparts of B1 and B2 with nodal metastases.

The TNM Staging System

The TNM system compartmentalizes carcinomas according to the depth of invasion of the primary tumor, the absence or presence of regional lymph node metastases, and the absence or presence of distant metastases (Table 47.1).

MANAGEMENT

Treatment modalities used consists of surgery, chemotherapy and radiotherapy with the aims of cure or palliation depending on the individual case.

Complete removal should be the primary aim but in most instances, this is not possible; removal of large portions of tumor provides little benefit for those with extensive metastatic disease. Most patients with microscopic metastatic disease generally develop gross metastatic disease. Complete resection is the cornerstone of management to improve survival rate. An extended right hemi colectomy is indicated for right-side tumors, and a subtotal colectomy is recommended for left-side tumors. Resection of metastases in the lung or liver, if technically possible, is also advised for advanced diseases. Surgical excision with margin of 2 to 5 centimeter is the treatment of choice.

Palliative ileosigmoidostomy bypass relieves the intestinal obstruction due to diffuse abdominal

Table 47.1: The TNM staging classification for colorectal carcinomas	
TX	Primary tumor cannot be assessed.
T0	No primary tumor identified.
Tis	Carcinoma *in situ* (tumor limited to mucosa).
T1	Involvement of submucosa, but no penetration through muscularis propria.
T2	Invasion into, but not penetration through, muscularis propria.
T3	Penetration through muscularis propria into subserosa (if present), or pericolic fat, but not into peritoneal cavity or other organs.
T4	Invasion of other organs or involvement of free peritoneal cavity.
NX	Nodal metastasis can not be assessed.
N0	No nodal metastasis.
N1	1-3 pericolic/perirectal nodes involved.
N2	4 or more pericolic/perirectal nodes involved.
MX	Distant metastasis cannot be assessed.
M0	No distant metastases.
M1	Distant metastases

carcinomatosis spreading onto the liver surface, diaphragm, and pelvic cavity. Resection even palliative is always preferable to bypass, because it effectively relieves the obstruction and also decreases the tumor load.[15] Surgery should be the first modality of treatment as the disease in children responds poorly to chemotherapy as well to radiotherapy.[15] The role of chemotherapy as a means of palliation has been controversial and responses have been suboptimal.

The outcome of patients correlates with extent of surgery, a lower survival rate in patients in whom only a biopsy/ colostomy/ palliative surgery could be peformed and a better survival with curative resection.[8]

When the primary tumor involves the rectosigmoid area and is considered nonresectable at the time of diagnosis, radiotherapy is often initiated in conjunction with chemotherapy before any surgical procedure. The chemotherapy options are few, including the use of 5-FU with or without leucovorin and one of the nitrosureas (e.g. BCNU, CCNU, or streptozotocin). Some have used a combination of vincristine, methyl-CCNU and 5-fluorouracil.[6] Trials using combination of 5-fluorouracil and methyl-CCNU as adjuvant chemotherapy have shown to double the remission rate in advanced gastrointestinal cancer.[29] Mitomycin C may also produce a favorable response in some of these tumors. Irinotecan, a topoisomerase I inhibitor has also been tried.

Adjuvant use of 5-FU with the immunomodulator levamisole for stage III disease has been found to be useful. Interferon-2α is being used with 5-FU in the treatment of advanced colorectal carcinoma. Interleukin-2 in combination with lymphokine-activated killer cells has been found to be effective in pulmonary and hepatic metastases.

In rectal cancers, preoperative radiotherapy has been utilized extensively to convert unresectable lesions to resectable ones.[8,15] Intraoperative radiation therapy has been advocated for disease known to have metastasized to the mesentery or mesenteric lymph nodes.

Complications

The following complications may be encountered:
1. Gastrointestinal bleeding
2. Tumor recurrence
3. Intractable intestinal obstruction.
4. Acute renal failure may cause mortality
5. Cachexia
6. Sepsis.

PROGNOSIS

The prognosis in adults improves with early diagnosis, surgical resection, and adjuvant therapies. However, in children, the prognosis remains very poor. The 5-year-survival rate was worse in adolescents than in older patients (51 vs. 75%).[4,30]

The factors contributing to this unfavorable prognosis include delay in diagnosis resulting in advanced disease at presentation with up to 60 percent of patients having intestinal obstruction as opposed to 18 percent in adults and majority of the lesions being mucinous adenocarcinomas.[4,31]

A cure is possible only when the cancer is diagnosed and treated at Duke's stage A or B. However, a majority of childhood cases are diagnosed late at Duke's stages C or D, with a poor 5-year-survival of 10 to 20 percent.[4,30]

FOLLOW-UP

Any patient with a solitary adenoma who has multiple polyps, whether adenoma or juvenile polyps, should be observed at appropriate intervals by sigmoidoscopic, roentgenographic and, possibly, colonoscopic examination for development of any suspicious malignant lesion.[32]

Patients with colorectal carcinimas require a close follow up with clinical examinations, appropriate CT scans and serial ESR levels to pick up recurrences. Monitoring of CEA levels is recommended during postoperative follow-up.

CONCLUSION

In conclusion, colorectal carcinoma is relatively rare in children. A high index of suspicion and mandatory diagnostic modalities like abdominal ultrasound, barium studies, and/or colonoscopy can help to identify early lesions for better outcome as the prognosis is poor for advanced disease.

REFERENCES

1. Rao BN, Pratt OB, Fleming ID, Dilawari RA, Green AA, Austin BA. Colon carcinoma in children and adolescents. Cancer 1985;55:1322-6.
2. Shih HH, Lu CC, Tiao M M, Ko SF, Chuang JH. Adenocarcinoma of the Colon in Children Presenting as abdominal Pain: Report of Two Cases. Chang Gung Med J 2002; 25:349-54.
3. Taguchi T, Suita S, Hirata Y. Carcinoma of the colon in children: A case report and review of 41 Japanese Cases. J Pediatr Gastroenterol Nutr 1991;12:394-9.

4. Brown RA, Rode H, Millar AJW. Colorectal carcinoma in children. J Pediatr Surg 1992;27:919-21.

5. Vincente O, Lawrence C, Josefina C, George SL, Pratt CB. The natural history of colorectal carcinoma in adolescents. Cancer 1982;49:1716-20.

6. Pratt CB, Rivera G, Shanks E, Johnson WW, Howarth C, Terrell W, et al. Colorectal carcinoma in adolescents: Implications regarding etiology. Cancer 1977;40:2464-72.

7. Kern WH, White WC. Adenocarcinoma of the colon in a 9-month-old infant: Report of a case. Cancer 1994; 74:1979-89.

8. Bhatia MS, Chandna S, Shah R, Patel DD. Colerectal carcinoma in Indian children. Indian Pediatr 2000; 37:1355-8.

9. Baig SJ, Hui SK, Basu K, Sanyal S, Banerjee S, Chatterjee U. Colorectal carcinoma in children: A report of 2 cases. J Indian Assoc Pediatr Surg 2000;5:26-9.

10. Kumar JK, Rao KVG, Dwarkanath, Kameshwari, Rao KVJ. Colorectal carcinoma in children. J Indian Assoc Pediatr Surg 2000;5:30-2.

11. Agarwal P, Malapure SM, Parelkar SV, Das SA, Mathure AB. Carcinoma rectum in a 9-year-old boy. I Indian Assoc Pediatr Surg 2000;5:33-5.

12. Rao SP, Prabhu VB, Pai GK, Pai PK. Unusual presentation of colonic malignancy in a 10-year-old boy. J Indian Assoc Pediatr Surg 2000;5:36-9.

13. Sarin YK, Jacob S, Prabhakar BR, Shah R. Adenocarcinoma colon. Indian Pediatr 1997;34:345-7.

14. Lamego CMB, Torloni H. Colorectal adenocarcinoma in childhood and adolescent-report of 11 cases and review of the literature. Pediatr Radiol 1989;19:5048.

15. Sarda DK, Kamble AT, Mungate GS, Gosavi A. Mucinous carcinoma of rectum in an 11-year-old child. Indian J Surg 2004;66:236-8.

16. Wanebo HJ, Rao BN, Pinsky CM. Preoperative carcino-embryonic antigen level as a prognostic indicator in colorectal cancer. N Engl J Med 1978;299:448-51.

17. Wolmark N, Fisher B, Wieand S. Prognostic significance of preoperative carcinoembryonic antigen levels in colorectal cancer: Results from the NSABP clinical trials. Ann Surg 1984;199: 375-81.

18. Kovalivker M, Erez I, Lazar L, Motovic A. Retrorectal cystic hamartoma Harefuah 1992;123:394-6, 435.

19. Krummel TM, Bell S, Kodroff MB, Berman WF, Salzberg AM. Colitis cystica profunda: A pediatric case report. J Pediatr Surg 1983;18(3):314-5.

20. Weller MH, Feldman PS.Benign lymphoid polyps of the rectum. Pediatr Radiol 1975;3:209-12.

21. Washington K, Rourk MH Jr, McDonagh D, Oldham KT. Inflammatory cloacogenic polyp in a child: Part of the spectrum of solitary rectal ulcer syndrome. Pediatr Pathol 1993;13: 409-14.

22. Mathur SK, Jindal R, Singh S, Marwah N, Rattan K, Arora B. Congenital fibrolipoma of anal canal. Indian J Pediatr 2003;70:269-70.

23. Kizilcan F, Tanyel FC, Kale G, Hicsonmez A.Duplication of the rectum resembling a juvenile polyp. Turk J Pediatr 1992;34: 193-5.

24. Rubin SZ, Mancer JF, Stephens CA. Carcinoid in a rectal duplication: A unique pediatric surgical problem: Can J Surg 1981;24:351-2.

25. Katara AN, Chandiramani VA, Dastur FD, Deshpande RB. Inflammatory pseudotumor of ascending colon presenting as PUO: A case report. Indian J Surg 2004;66:234-6.

26. Dukes CE. The classification of cancer of the rectum. J Pathol 1932;35:323.

27. Astler VB, Coller FA. The prognostic significance of direct extension of carcinoma of the colon and rectum. Ann Surg 1954;139:846.

28. Colon and rectum. In: American Joint Committee on Cancer: AJCC Cancer Staging Manual (5th ed),. Philadelphia: Lippincott-Raven Publishers, 1997:83.

29. Weber W, Nagel GA. Adjuvant chemotherapy of the colonic and rectal carcinoma: Concepts and upto date results Schweiz Med Wochenschr. 1977;107:840-5.

30. Goldthron JF, Powars D, Hays DM. Adeno carcinoma of the colon and rectum in the adolescent. Surgery 1983;93:409-14.

31. Andersson A, Bergdahl L. Carcinoma of the colon in children: A report of six cases and a review of the literature. J Pediatr Surg 1976;11:967-7.

32. Mazier WP, MacKeigan JM, Billingham RP, Dignan RD.Juvenile polyps of the colon and rectum. Surg Gynecol Obstet 1982;154:829-32.

CHAPTER 48

Devendra K Gupta
M Ragavan

Rare Pediatric Tumors

Apart from the common solid tumors and hematological malignancy it is not uncommon for pediatric surgeon to come across benign and malignant tumors in other location. This chapter describes some of the less frequently encountered neoplastic conditions in pediatric age group. The tumors are discussed in descending anatomic order from head to foot through the trunk and to the skin.

CHEST WALL TUMORS

Benign namely lymphohemangioma, enchondroma, bone cyst, neurofibroma, and lipoma can occur. Malignant tumors namely Ewing's sarcoma, rhabdomyosarcoma, Fibrosarcoma can occur in chest wall (Figs 48.1A to 48.2B).

BREAST TUMORS

Breast enlargement is a common finding in infants, children, and adolescence. In most cases they present either normal variation in endocrine function or benign mass lesion, with malignant lesion rarely being found. The most common cause of breast enlargement in infants and prepubertal female are:
1. Neonatal enlargement due to transplacental hormonal stimulation,
2. Premature thelarche and
3. Precocious puberty: They should be submitted for endocrine and neurological evaluation than biopsy. Those with discrete hard mass should be submitted for biopsy. Gynecomastia in pubertal male child need attention towards body habitus, testicular size and, buccal smear for sex chromatin.

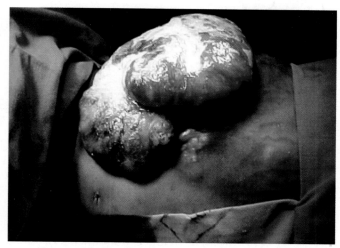

Figure 48.1A: Ewing's sarcoma of the chest wall

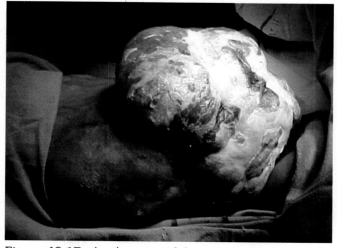

Figure 48.1B: Another view of the same tumor showing the fungating appearance

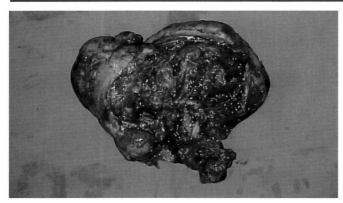

Figure 48.2A: Excised specimen of Ewing's tumor chest wall

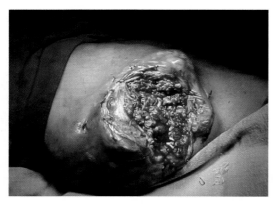

Figure 48.2B: Tumor bed after debulking of the tumor and attaining hemostasis

A wide spectrum of breast disorders occurs in the pediatric and adolescent age groups, but malignant disease is very rare. The relative frequencies of these conditions and their natural history differ substantially from those of adult patients. The gross findings may be very deceptive and mislead the clinician until a histopathological diagnosis is made.[1]

Fibroadenoma is the main cause of unilateral breast mass in teenagers and adolescents. 4 percent of these are a special form described as giant or juvenile fibroadenoma.[2] For primary diagnosis, ultrasound is the method of choice. The MRI allows exact evaluation of size and location. The fibroadenoma must be distinguished from the phylloid tumor, which can be malignant. Although the main reason of an asymmetrical breast enlargement of young girls is a benign mass, an early surgical excision is efficient with regard to the best possible cosmetic outcome.[2]

The common lesions seen in the pediatric age group include:

Benign Tumors

1. *Fibroadenoma:* Most common discrete swelling, in teenagers, slow growing, no malignant potential as such, excision if solitary, careful observation if multiple, recurrent and bilateral.
2. *Fibrocystic disease:* Rarely seen in post-pubertal age due to abnormality in normal development and involution of the breast, present with bilateral lumpiness, cyclical pain and variable finding. Can be managed conservatively.
3. *Cystosarcoma phylloides:* This is a fibro epithelial tumor similar to fibroadenoma but with greater hypertrophy and more cellularity. The terms sarcoma is a misnomer used to refer fleshy appearance of it, cysto for presence of cystic spaces and phylloides for leaf like projection in to the cystic space. It can be benign to malignant. Simple mastectomy and follow-up is needed.
4. *Others:* Include fibroma, lipoma, lymphohemangioma, and intraductal papilloma.

Malignant Tumors

1. *Adenocarcinoma:* Constitute less than 1 percent of pediatric tumors. Histopathology is similar to adult. Axillary node spread and local recurrence are less common on comparison with adult and hence prognosis is good. Breast conservative local excision with radiotherapy offers best outcome. Better to avoid to pregnancy for two years after diagnosis.
2. *Sarcoma:* Even less common than adenocarcinoma. Common types being fibrosarcoma, liposarcoma and metastatic rhabdomyosarcoma. In this case radical breast surgery with chemotherapy for distant lung and liver metastasis is advised.

The most common cause of breast mass seen in the first two decades of life is inflammation.[3] Other causes include asymmetrical gynecomastia, precocious puberty, giant juvenile fibroadenoma, primary rhabdomyosarcoma, lymphoma, and metastatic neuroblastoma.[3]

Though females may develop breast masses early in life, the risk of malignancy is extremely low and the relative composition of the adolescent as compared to the adult breast is different. Thus mammography is not recommended for routine screening or routine imaging of breast masses in adolescents.[4] The prognosis is satisfactory if diagnosed and treated well in time.[5]

BRONCHIAL ADENOMA

Most of the bronchial adenomas are in fact carcinod tumors giving raise to local obstructive symptom and systemic carcinoid syndrome features. Surgical excision is the primary treatment.

BRONCHOGENIC CARCINOMA

Primary pediatric lung cancers are extremely rare; only 100 cases are reported so far. Most of them are adenocarcinoma or undifferentiated type. Common in adolescent age group. Same guidelines that of adults is used for management.

PLEURO PULMONARY BLASTOMA

This tumor is considered to be an embryonal malignancy of mesoblastic tissue with histology showing blastoma and stromal elements. It usually arises in sub pleural location but can be located in intrapulmonary, mediastinal or pleural regions. It is associated with cystic disease of lung. It has ability for local recurrence, sarcomatous differentiation and systemic metastasis. The treatment revolves around surgical excision and chemotherapy.

MESOTHELIOMA

This tumor arises from the mesothelial cells lining the serous cavity namely pleura, pericardium and peritoneal cavity. The etiological factor is exposure to asbestosis. Has ability to spread over the lining surface without invading the underlying tissue but with propensity to have systemic metastasis. Malignant and benign mesothelioma cannot be differentiated on histological backgrounds. Histological staining can demonstrate the typical appearance of the asbestos elements within the tumor. Localized resection is curative, poor prognosis noted in case with diffuse invasion and local recurrence. Chemotherapy with doxorubicin, cisplatinum, 5-FU with leucovorin showed response in advanced cases. Radiotherapy is useful in pain palliation.

THYMIC TUMORS

Primary tumors of thymus include thymoma, lymphoma, germ cell tumor, carcinoid, thymic carcinoma and thymolipoma. All thymic enlargements are not thymoma, which is a primary neoplasm arising from the epithelial elements of the Hassal's corpuscle of the thymus. Less than 20 percent of thymoma occurs in pediatric age group. It is commonly associated with autoimmune disease namely myasthenia gravis, pure red cell aplasia, hypogammaglobulinemia, systemic lupus erythematosis, thyroiditis and Addison's disease. Thymoma is the most frequent tumor of the anterior mediastinum usually slow growing with less potential for distant metastasis to liver, bone and brain. Manifest with cough, dyspnea, chest pain and superior vena cava syndrome. Radiological investigation helps in diagnosis. Surgical excision and radiotherapy is helpful. Doxorubicin and cisplatinum are effective in metastatic disease.

CARDIAC TUMORS

Most of the tumors are metastatic. The common primary tumor is myxoma, other being hemangioma, leiomyoma, rhabdomyoma, teratoma and chondrosarcoma. The metastatic tumors are leukemia, melanoma and rhabdomyosarcoma may involve the pericardium, myocardium and endocardium. The symptoms include arrhythmia, cardiomegaly, pericardial effusion and congestive cardiac failure. The treatment includes pericardiocentesis, irradiation and chemotherapy.

GASTROINTESTINAL TRACT TUMORS

Esophagus

Esophageal tumors are very rare in children. Commonest benign tumor is leiomyoma followed by hemagioma. Most of the malignant tumors are epithelial origin and commonly squamous cell carcinoma. Cases of sarcoma have been reported. The etiologies for cancer esophagus in children are Plummer-Vinson syndrome caustic ingestion, long standing achalasia cardia. Following lye ingestion malignancy occurs after 7-15 years commonly at the level of bronchial division and commonly squamous cell carcinoma. In achalasia cardia commonly seen in middle third followed by lower third.

Esophageal tumors present with dysphagia, weight loss, hematemesis, cough, regurgitation and bone pain. Diagnosis made by endoscopic biopsy. Chemoradiation is main mode of treatment in advanced cases. Early diagnosed lesions have good outcome after surgical excision.

Stomach

Benign tumors of the stomach are hemangioma, leiomyoma, lipoma, teratoma, Peutz-Jeghears polyps and carcinoids. Primary malignant tumors are adenocarcinoma (95%) lymphoma, adenoacanthoma,

and urinary tracts. Inflammatory pseudotumor is an unusual cause of chronic abdominal pain in children. Successful treatment requires careful radiologic and pathologic evaluation to distinguish these from other lesions, along with complete surgical resection. The CT appearance of abdominal inflammatory pseudotumor is variable. The mass may be hypoattenuated or isoattenuated relative to muscle on unenhanced scans, and calcification has been observed within inflammatory pseudotumors of the pancreas, stomach, and liver. Enhancement with contrast material usually occurs but is not pronounced, and a variety of patterns include early peripheral, with delayed central filling heterogeneous; homogeneous; and no enhancement.[24] Larger lesions may have central necrosis. The appearance on MR images is also variable; they are usually hypointense relative to skeletal muscle on T1-weighted images, hyperintense on T2-weighted images, and heterogeneously enhanced after administration of contrast material.[31]

Inflammatory Pseudotumors of the Liver

Inflammatory pseudo-tumor of the liver is a benign encapsulated mass. It is a myofibroblastic proliferation with chronic inflammatory cell infiltration of unknown origin. The majority of hepatic inflammatory pseudotumors occur in children and young adults. They usually arise as solitary solid tumors from the right hepatic lobe though may involve porta hepatis or bile ducts resulting in obstructive jaundice. Other symptoms include abdominal pain and weight loss. Unusual inflammatory or immune responses such as sclerosing cholangitis, phlebitis, and retroperitoneal fibrosis have been found in association with inflammatory pseudotumor.[19,31] Epstein-Barr virus has also been implicated in some of these lesions. Abdominal CT may show slight vascular features and the diagnosis may be made through percutaneous US-guided fine needle biopsy.[32] Spontaneous regression has been reported.[33] The clinical outcome is good.

Inflammatory Pseudotumors of the Spleen

Primary splenic tumors in children are rare and usually benign. Splenic inflammatory pseudotumors, although rare, should be considered in the differential diagnosis of a mass lesion of the spleen in children.[34] Ultrasonographically guided Tru-cut needle biopsy may be done for histopathologic confirmation. Thus, this may avoid even partial splenectomy.[35]

Inflammatory Pseudotumor of the Kidney

Despite its rarity, inflammatory pseudotumor of kidney should be kept in mind in the differential diagnosis of a solitary renal mass.[36] A case of inflammatory pseudotumor of the ureter in a child has been reported.[1]

Gastrointestinal Pseudotumors

Gastrointestinal tract involvement is rare, with ileocecal and gastric tumors in young girls being the most frequently described type. Abdominal pain, a palpable mass, and iron deficiency anemia are the most common presenting symptoms and signs.[37,38] Gastrointestinal inflammatory pseudotumors often have features suggestive of malignancy, including ulceration, infiltration of the wall, and extragastric extension.[38]

An inflammatory pseudotumor involving the ileocaecal region in a 16-year-old girl presenting as pyrexia of unknown origin for 4 months followed by development of a palpable lump in the right iliac fossa has been described. The patient underwent a right hemicolectomy for a presumed ascending colonic neoplasm, and histology revealed that it was an inflammatory pseudotumour.[39]

Gastric Inflammatory Pseudotumor in Children

Gastric inflammatory pseudotumors have radiographic, surgical, and histologic features that simulate malignant tumors. To avoid unnecessary aggressive therapy, it is important to know when to consider this diagnostic possibility preoperatively. The findings may include a gastric mass encompassing an ulcer or a confined gastric perforation.[19] Other unusual inflammatory responses associated with a gastric mass, such as sclerosing cholangitis and retroperitoneal fibrosis may also suggest the diagnosis. The most likely cause of a gastric mass in a child with Castleman syndrome is inflammatory pseudotumor.

A polypoid mass may be seen in the stomach with suspicion of malignancy.[40] The histopathological findings may include fibroblast-like cells with prominent inflammatory reaction inpresence of neutrophils, macrophages, lymphocytes and many plasma cells. Immunohistochemical analysis show positive reactions with smooth muscle actin and vimentin.

Mesenteric Inflammatory Pseudotumor

Recognition of this rare entity is important because the clinical manifestations and radiological features may be indistinguishable from a malignant lymphoproliferative disorder.[41] Apart from presentation as a mass, it may also present with abdominal pain.[42] The histological features may resemble a spindle-cell sarcoma.[41] A rare case of abdominal inflammatory pseudotumor of the sigmoid colon mesentery has been described.[41]

Pseudotumoral Pancreatitis

In the pancreas, a number of non-neoplastic solid masses may mimic cancer. Up to 5 percent of pancreatectomies performed with the preoperative clinical diagnosis of carcinoma turn out to be non-neoplastic by pathologic examination. Chronic inflammatory lesions are the leading cause of pseudotumoral pancreatitis. These include autoimmune and paraduodenal pancreatitis, adenomyomatous hyperplasia of ampulla , accessory spleen, Lipomatous hypertrophy and Hamartomas. Pseudolymphoma forms well-defined nodules composed of hyperplastic lymphoid tissue.[43] Rarely, foreign-body deposits, granulomatous inflammations (such as sarcoidosis or tuberculosis), and congenital lesions may form tumoral lesions. It is vital to recognize the pseudotumors in the pancreas so that they can be distinguished from ductal adenocarcinomas.

PSEUDOTUMORS OF THE BLADDER

Eosinophilic Cystitis

It is an uncommon form of bladder inflammation in children with less than 25 cases described in literature. A case of eosinophilic cystitis mimicking a bladder tumor in a 3 year-old girl with symptoms of urinary frequency has been described.[44] The diagnosis was confirmed histopathology followed by treatment with corti-costeroids.

Schistosomiasis

A tumor-like form of urinary schistosomiasis has been reported.[45] The clinical presentation of hematuria in an endemic area may suggest the diagnosis that may be established by cystoscopy or intraoperatively.

Inflammatory Pseudotumor (IP) of the Bladder

The rare entity of inflammatory pseudotumor (IP) of the bladder may form a huge intravesicular mass and present as acute onset of non-traumatic and painless gross hematuria from exophytic and ulcerated lesions. The gross hematuria may lead to severe anemia and impending hypovolemic shock.[46,47] Other symptoms include frequency of urination and dysuria, and urinary tract obstruction can also occur

Inflammatory pseudotumor should be considered when an enhancing tumor is surrounded by a clot, particularly in young adults though it has been described in a 7-day-old neonate. It is extremely difficult to distinguish from malignant tumors clinically, radiologically, and histologically and may be misdiagnosed as rhabdomyosarcoma . Fine-needle biopsy may fail to yield a sufficient volume of tumor tissue for making a definite diagnosis. Pathological findings may resemble the diagnosis of leiomyoma. The recognition of the benign entity is important to avoid unnecessary radical surgery.[18] Fortunately, spontaneous regression of inflammatory pseudotumor of the bladder has alsobeen described.[48]

REFERENCES

1. Harper L, Michel JL, Riviere JP, Alsawhi A, De Napoli-Cocci S. Inflammatory pseudotumor of the ureter. J Pediatr Surg. 2005;40:597-9.
2. Umiker WO, Iverson LC. Post-inflammatory tumor of the lung: report of four cases simulating xanthoma, fibroma or plasma cell granuloma. J Thorac Surg 1954;28:55-62.
3. Rose AG, McCormick S, Cooper K, Titus JL. Inflammatory pseudotumor (plasma cell granuloma) of the heart. Pathol Lab Med 1996;120:549-54.
4. D'Hermies F, Morel X, Meyer A, Lureau MA, Renard G. Pseudotumor-like superficial conjunctival foreign body J Fr Ophtalmol 1998; 21:78-80.
5. Berard M, Lhuintre Y, Ruchoux M, Dumas-Paoli M, Choux R, Hassoun J. Diagnostic problems posed by inflammatory pseudotumors of the orbit: study of 3 cases J Fr Ophtalmol 1987;10:165-9.
6. Martin CJ. Orbital pseudotumor: case report and overview. J Am Optom Assoc 1997;68:775-81.
7. Zhang H, Song G, He Y. Clinical analysis of 271 cases of orbital inflammatory pseudotumors. Zhonghua Yan Ke Za Zhi. 2002;38:484-7.
8. LD Narla, B Newman, SS Spottswood, S Narla, R Kolli. Inflammatory Pseudotumor Radio Graphics 2003;23:719-29.
9. Mombaerts I, Schlingermann RO, Koorneef L. Are systemic corticosteroids useful in the management of orbital pseudotumors. Ophthalmology 1996;103:521-8.
10. De Vuysere S, Hermans R, Sciot R, Crevits I, Marchal G. Extraorbital inflammatory pseudotumor of the head and neck: CT and MR findings in three patients. AJNR Am J Neuroradiol 1999;20:1133-9.
11. Browne M, Abramson LP, Chou PM, Acton R, Holinger LD, Reynolds M. Inflammatory myofibroblastic tumor (inflammatory pseudotumor) of the neck infiltrating the trachea. J Pediatr Surg 2004;39:e1-4.
12. Ginsty D, Mettoudi JD, Adamsbaum C, Dhellemmes C, Maillet S, Vicens G, Ostermeyer S, Dupuis HJ. Benign tumors and pseudotumor of the maxilla in children Rev Stomatol Chir Maxillofac 1996;97:12-6.
13. Anagnostopoulos D, Miliaras E, Miliaras D, Manios S, Tekneji P. Castleman's pseudotumor in children. Apropos of an unusual case Chir Pediatr 1988;29:269-72.

14. Grossin M, Crickx B, Aitken G, Belaich S, Bocquet L. Subcutaneous localizations of Castleman's pseudo-lymphoma. Review of the literature apropos of a case Ann Dermatol Venereol. 1985;112:497-506.

15. Bark B, Perlick E, Stover B. Thoracic wall crossing (pseudo-?) tumor in a child: abscess-forming thoracic actinomycosis caused by Actinomyces meyeri et israeli Rofo. 2004; 176:125-7.

16. Campanacci M, Gardini GF, Giunti A, Donati U. Pseudo-tumoral ossification of the muscles and/or periosteum. (A study of 57 cases). Ital J Orthop Traumatol. 1980;6:385-93.

17. Bretagne MC, Jolly A, Mouton JN, Metaizeau JP, Beau A, Treheux A. Pseudo-sarcomatous osteomyilitis in the child (author's transl) J Radiol Electrol Med Nucl 1977;58:1-4.

18. Scott L, Blair G, Taylor G, Dimmick J, Fraser G. Inflammatory pseudotumors in children. J Pediatr Surg 1988;23:755-8.

19. Maves CK, Johnson JF, Bove K, Malott RL. Gastric inflammatory pseudotumor in children. Radiology 1989; 173:381-3.

20. Day DL, Sane S, Dehner LP. Inflammatory pseudotumor of the mesentery and small intestine. Pediatr Radiol 1986;16:210-5.

21. Hedlund GL, Navoy JF, Galliani CA, Johnson WH. Aggressive manifestations of inflammatory pulmonary pseudotumor in children. Pediatr Radiol 1999;29:112-6.

22. Hytiroglou P, Brandwein MS, Stauchen JA, Mirante JP, Urken ML, Biller HF. Inflammatory pseudotumor of the parapharyngeal space: case report and review of the literature. Head Neck 1992;14:230-4.

23. Agrons GA, Rosado-de-Christenson ML, Kirejczyk WM, Conran RM, Stocker JT. Pulmonary inflammatory pseudotumor: radiologic features. Radiology 1998; 206:511-8.

24. Rollan Villamarin V, Seguel Ramirez F, Morato Robert P, de Mingo Misena L, Ollero Fresno JC. Pulmonary inflammatory pseudotumor in a child] Cir Pediatr. 2002;15:166-7.

25. Slavotinek JP, Bourne AJ, Sage MR, Freeman JK. Inflammatory pseudotumor of the pancreas in a child. Pediatr Radiol 2000;30:801-3.

26. Hata Y, Sasaki F, Matuoka S, Hamada H, Taguchi K, et al. Inflammatory pseudotumor of the liver in children: report of cases and review of the literature. J Pediatr Surg 1992;27:1549-52.

27. Kim TS, Han J, Kim GY, Lee KS, Kim H, Kim J. Pulmonary inflammatory pseudotumor (inflammatory myofibroblastic tumor): CT features with pathologic correlation. J Comput Assist Tomogr. 2005;29:633-9.

28. Patankar T, Prasad S, Shenoy A, Rathod K. Pulmonary inflammatory pseudotumour in children. Australas Radiol 2000;44:318-20.

29. Soyer T, Ciftci AO, Gucer S, Orhan D, Senocak ME. Calcifying fibrous pseudotumor of lung: a previously unreported entity. J Pediatr Surg. 2004;39:1729-30.

30. Jenkins PC, Dickison AE, Flanagan MF. Cardiac inflammatory pseudotumor: rapid appearance in an infant with congenital heart disease. Pediatr Cardiol 1996;17:399-401.

31. Torzilli G, Inoue K, Midorikawa Y, Hui A, Takayama T, Makuuchi M. Inflammatory pseudotumors of the liver: prevalence and clinical impact in surgical patients. Hepatogastroenterology 2001;48:1118-23.

32. Vanthournout I, Coche G, Sevenet F, Lavenne A, Cordonnier C, Ricard Y, Sevestre H, Pautard B. Inflam-matory pseudotumors of the liver. Apropos of a pediatric case with radiological and ultrasonographic features and anatomopathological correlations J Radiol 1998;79:553-6.

33. Levy S, Sauvanet A, Diebold M, Marcus C, Da Costa N, Thiefin G. Spontaneous regression of an inflammatory pseudotumor of the liver presenting as an obstructing malignant biliary tumor. Gastrointest Endosc 2001;53:371-4.

34. Sarker A, An C, Davis M, Praprotnik D, McCarthy LJ, Orazi A. Inflammatory pseudotumor of the spleen in a 6-year-old child: a clinicopathologic study Arch Pathol Lab Med. 2003;127:e127-30.

35. Yesildag E, Sarimurat N, Ince U, Numan F, Buyukunal C. Nonsurgical diagnosis and management of an inflammatory pseudotumor of the spleen in a child. J Clin Ultrasound. 2003;31:335-8.

36. Tarhan F, Gul AE, Karadayi N, Kuyumcuoglu U. Inflammatory pseudotumor of the kidney: a case report. Int Urol Nephrol 2004;36:137-40.

37. Sanders BM, West KW, Gingalewski C, Engum S, Davis M, Grosfeld JL. Inflammatory pseudotumor of the alimentary tract: clinical and surgical experience. J Pediatr Surg 2001;36:169-73.

38. Estevao-Costa J, Correia-Pinto J, Rodrigues FC, et al. Gastric inflammatory myofibroblastic proliferation in children. Pediatr Surg Int 1998;13:95-99.

39. Katara AN, Chandiramani VA, Dastur FD, Deshpande RB. Inflammatory pseudotumor of ascending colon presenting as PUO: A case report. Indian J Surg 2004;66:234-6.

40. Popova ED, Popov SD.Inflammatory pseudotumor of the stomach in a 12-year old child Arkh Patol. 2005;67:46-7.

41. Uysal S, Tuncbilek I, Unlubay D, Tiras U, Bilaloglu P, Kosar U. Inflammatory pseudotumor of the sigmoid colon mesentery: US and CT findings.(2004:12b). Eur Radiol. 2005;15:633-5.

42. Vaughan KG, Aziz A, Meza MP, Hackam DJ Mesenteric inflammatory pseudotumor as a cause of abdominal pain in a teenager: presentation and literature review. Pediatr Surg Int. 2005; 21:497-9. Epub 2005 Mar 24.

43. Adsay NV, Basturk O, Klimstra DS, Kloppel G. Pancreatic pseudotumors: non-neoplastic solid lesions of the pancreas that clinically mimic pancreas cancer. Semin Diagn Pathol 2004;21:260-7.

44. Guerra LA, Pike J, Filler G, Udjus K, de Nanassy J, Leonard M. Pseudo-tumoral eosinophilic cystitis in a 3 year-old girl. Can J Urol. 2005;12:2846-8.

45. Piarroux R, Garnier JM, Dumon H, Guys JM, Unal D Pseudo-tumoral form of urinary bilharziasis in a child Ann Pediatr (Paris). 1992;39:241-4.

46. Hsieh YJ, Lin KY, Cheng HL, Chen TJ, Chiou YY. Inflammatory pseudotumor of the bladder: a rare cause of hematuria with impending shock in a child. Acta Paediatr Taiwan 2004; 45:350-3.

47. Inoue H, Iwabuchi K, Kuwao S, et al. A case report of inflammatory pseudosarcoma of the urinary bladder. Acta Pathol Jpn 1992;42:760-5.

48. Mochizuki Y, Kanda S, Nomata K, et al. Spontaneous regression of inflammatory pseudotumor of the urinary bladder. Urol Int 1999;63:255-7.

Therapeutic Strategies in Pediatric Surgical Oncology

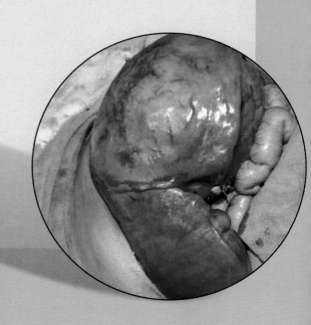

CHAPTER 50

YK Gupta
KH Reeta
S Briyal
V Gupta

Chemotherapy for Pediatric Tumors

INTRODUCTION

Cancers in children are rare, accounting for less than 1 percent of the one million patients diagnosed with cancer.[1] However, cancers in children are important as these are the most common fatal disease in childhood. Nearly every review of the research literature in pediatric oncology describes the significant progress of medical treatment over the past 30 years resulting in the increased survival rate for children and adolescents with cancer. Various factors involving the environment and the genetic makeup of the individual determines the susceptibility of the person for development of cancer. Table 50.1 enumerates the differences between adult and pediatric cancers.

Etiology of cancer

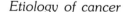

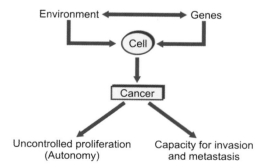

PRINCIPLES OF CHEMOTHERAPY

The objectives of chemotherapy fall into three principle categories: cure, with or without the use of other forms of therapy, palliation and prevention. The prophylactic use of chemotherapeutic agents is still debated because of the concern of efficacy and side effects of the drug. However, prophylactic sunscreens have been shown to prevent skin cancers especially in those patients with xeroderma pigmentosa. Both beta-carotene and 13-cis retinoic acid, a vitamin A analogue have also been shown to produce marked regression of leukoplakia.

All living tissue is composed of cells. Cells grow and reproduce to replace cells lost during injury or normal "wear and tear." The cell cycle is a series of steps that both normal cells and cancer cells go through in order to grow and reproduce to form new cells.[2] There are 5 phases in the cell cycle, designated by letters and numbers:

G_0 = Resting stage
G_1 = RNA and protein synthesis
S = DNA synthesis
G_2 = Construction of mitotic apparatus
M = Mitosis

Each time chemotherapy is given; it involves trying to balance between destroying the cancer cells (in order to cure or control the disease) and sparing the normal cells (to lessen undesirable side effects).

GOALS OF TREATMENT WITH CHEMOTHERAPY

There are 3 possible goals for chemotherapy treatment.[3,4]

• *Cure:* As far as possible, chemotherapy is used to cure the cancer, meaning that the tumor disappears and does not return.

Table 50.1: Differences between pediatric and adult cancer		
	Cancer in children	*Cancer in adults*
Primary sites	Mostly tissue (lymphatic, CNS, hematopoietic, SNS, muscle, bone, etc)	Mostly organs (breast, lung, colon, prostate, uterus, etc)
Histology	Primarily sarcomas (Nonepithelial)	Primarily carcinomas (Epithelial)
Stage at diagnosis	Majority are disseminated	Majority are localized or regional
Early detection	Not routine	Improves with education
Screening test	Not effective or practical, though urinary catecholamines for neuroblastoma are done	Screening can be routinely done, eg mammography, occult blood in stools, pap smear, colonoscopy, self examination, etc
Response to Chemotherapy	Very responsive	Less responsive
Prevention	Unlikely	Many can be prevented, eg discouraging smoking, tobacco chewing, etc.

- *Control:* If cure is not possible, the goal is to control the disease (stop the cancer from growing and spreading) in order to extend life and provide the best quality of life.
- *Palliation:* Sometimes the cancer is at an advanced stage and control is unlikely. At this stage the goal is called palliation, meaning that chemotherapy may be used to relieve symptoms caused by the cancer, thereby improving the quality of life, even though the drugs may not lengthen life.

The response of a patient to any regimen of chemotherapeutic agents depends on a number of factors determined by the host, drug and the tumor (Fig. 50.1).

This chapter will deal with the following medications used to treat pediatric cancers (Table 50.2).

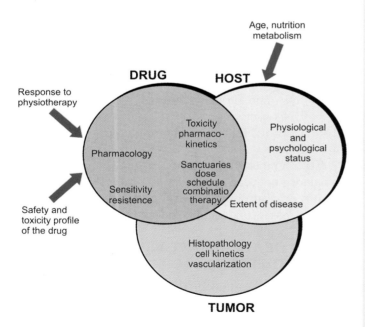

Figure 50.1: Interplay of drug, host and tumor factors in the response to chemotherapeutic agents

Table 50.2: Chemotherapeutic agents used to treat pediatric cancers	
I. Alkylating agents	2. Dactinomycin
1. Cyclophosphamide	3. Doxorubicin
2. Ifosfamide	V. New Intercalating agents
3. Mechlorethamine	1. Bleomycin
4. Chlorambucil	2. Amsacrine
5. Melphalan	VI. Plant Alkaloids
6. Busulfan	1. Vincristine
7. Thiotepa	2. Vinblastine
II. Alkylating-like agents	3. Teniposide, VM-26
1. Cisplatin	4. Etoposide, VP-16
2. Carboplatin	VII. Miscellaneous agents
3. Procarbazine	1. Asparaginase
4. Carmustine	2. Tretinoin
5. Lomustine	3. Mitoxantrone
6. Dacarbazine	4. Irinotecan
III. Antimetabolites	5. Topotecan
1. Methotrexate	VIII. New drugs
2. Mercaptopurine	1. Imatinib
3. Thioguanine	2. Clofarabine
4. Fluorouracil	3. Epothilone
5. Hydroxyurea	4. Nelarabine
6. Cytarabine	5. Betulinic acid
IV. DNA binding agents	6. Liposomal encapsulated drugs
1. Daunorubicin	

ALKYLATING AGENTS

Cyclophosphamide

Mechanism of Action

Cyclophosphamide is a nitrogen mustard type of alkylating agent.[5] An activated form of cyclophosphamide, phosphoramide mustard, alkylates, or binds to DNA. Its cytotoxic effect is mainly due to cross-linking of strands of DNA and RNA, and to inhibition of protein synthesis. Cyclophosphamide does not appear to be cell-cycle specific.

Pharmacokinetics

Interpatient variability in metabolism occurs. The drug is recommended to be taken on an empty stomach, but may be taken with food to decrease GI upset to limited extent. It is metabolised by cytochrome P450 (c-YP) primarily c-YP 2B6 to active metabolites 4-hydroxycyclophosphamide, aldophosphamide, phosphoramide mustard and acrolein.

Indications

The drug can be used in various cancers in different regimens including Ewing's sarcoma, acute myelogenous leukemia, chronic lymphocytic leukemia, chronic myelogenous leukemia, acute lymphocytic leukemia, pediatric acute lymphoblastic leukemia, cutaneous T-cell lymphoma, osteosarcoma, lymphoma, Burkitt's soft tissue sarcoma, Hodgkin's disease; non-Hodgkin's lymphoma, thymoma, lymphoproliferative disease, Waldenstrom's macroglobulinemia, multiple myeloma, Wilm's tumor, mycosis fungoides, neuroblastoma, retinoblastoma, rhabdomyosarcoma.

Dosage in Children

Oral: 50-300 mg/m^2, daily
Intravenous: 250-1800 mg/m^2 for one dose on day 1, day 2, day 3 and day 4 for 3-4 weeks up to 2000-3000 mg/m^2 for one dose on day 1 for 3-4 weeks.

Side Effects

Nausea and vomiting, myelosuppression with platelet sparing, and alopecia occur commonly. Anemia, hemorrhagic myocarditis, pericardial tamponade, dizziness, facial flushing, hyperpigmentation (skin and nails), rash, redness, swelling or pain at injection site, toxic epidermal necrolysis, hyperglycemia, anorexia, diarrhea, hemorrhagic colitis, mucositis, myxedema or sore lips may result from cyclophosphamide treatment. Anaphylactic reaction and nasal congestion can occur when IV doses are administered too rapidly. Cardiotoxicity ranging from minor, transient ECG changes and asymptomatic elevation of cardiac enzymes to fatal myocarditis and myocardial necrosis may occur with high-dose cyclophosphamide. Direct injury to the endothelium by phosphoramide mustard, an active metabolite of cyclophosphamide may be involved in the cyclophosphamide induced cardiac effects. Patients may experience heart failure, arrhythmias, irreversible cardiomyopathy, pericarditis or death as a result of cardiotoxicity. Treatment is supportive. Children on long term or high dose cyclophosphamide therapy may develop hemorrhagic cystitis characterized by nonspecific symptoms such as hematuria, dysuria, urgency and increased frequency of urination and can be confirmed using cystoscopy. Its incidence is reduced by coadministration of mesna. Measures to prevent include encouraging patients to drink plenty of fluids during therapy, to void frequently, and to avoid taking the drug at night. Patients should be well hydrated. As well, cyclophosphamide should be administered as early in the day as possible to decrease the amount of drug remaining in the bladder overnight. Treatment should begin with discontinuation of cyclophosphamide. Fluid intake should be increased and the platelet count should be maintained at >50 000/mm^3 to minimize the extent of bleeding. Hyperuricemia is most likely with highly proliferative tumors of massive burden, such as leukemias, high-grade lymphomas and myeloproliferative diseases. Preexisting renal dysfunction increases the risk. In patients receiving high doses of cyclophosphamide over prolonged periods, interstitial pulmonary fibrosis may occur. Direct injury to the pulmonary epithelium by cyclophosphamide metabolites may be involved. Interstitial pneumonitis has also been reported in patients receiving cyclophosphamide. The drug has to be stopped at the first sign of pulmonary toxicity and all other possible causes of pneumonitis should be ruled out. Nasal stuffiness or facial discomfort has been associated with rapid injection of cyclophosphamide. This may be a mucosal inflammatory response or possibly a cholinergic mechanism may be involved. Slowing down the infusion rate or giving intermittent infusion may help; and analgesics, decongestants, antihistamines, intranasal beclomethasone, or intranasal ipratropium can be used.

Radiation injury to tissues may be enhanced with cyclophosphamide. Though called radiation recall reactions, the timing of the radiation may be before, concurrent with, or after the administration of the cyclophosphamide. SIADH (syndrome of inappropriate secretion of ADH) resulting in hyponatremia, dizziness, confusion or agitation, unusual tiredness or weakness may occur in patients receiving cyclophosphamide. Though this condition is self-limiting, diuretic therapy may be helpful when the patient has stopped urinating. Secondary malignancies including urinary bladder cancer, non-lymphocytic leukemia and non-Hodgkin's lymphoma have been reported in some patients who have had hemorrhagic cystitis. Direct injury to the distal renal tubules and collecting ducts by cyclophosphamide metabolites may be involved.

Ifosfamide

Mechanism of Action

Ifosfamide, a structural analogue of cyclophosphamide has similar mechanism of action as cyclophosphamide.[5-7] Ifosfamide is cell cycle phase-nonspecific.

Indications

Soft tissue sarcoma, cancer of the testis, pediatric brain tumors, Ewing's sarcoma, Hodgkin's disease, leukemias, neuroblastoma, non-Hodgkin's lymphoma, osteogenic sarcoma rhabdomyosarcoma, Wilm's tumor.

Dosage in Children

Intravenous:
- 1.8-2.5 g/m^2/day × 5 consecutive days, three weekly
- 3 g/m^2/day × 2-3 days, 3-4 weekly

Side Effects

Dose-related nausea and vomiting can occur. Urotoxic effects like cystitis can occur. Prophylactic catheter bladder drainage, bladder irrigation, hyperhydration, forced diuresis, morning administration and the administration of mesna have been to reduce this effect. Patients should be observed for the symptoms of dysuria and urinary frequency since this may closely parallel hematuria. Glomerular, proximal or distal tubular impairment may occur. Proximal tubular damage often presents as Fanconi syndrome (hypophosphatemic rickets, growth failure; occasionally renal tubular acidosis or diabetes insipidus). Renal damage does not appear to be reversible. Age less than 5 years (for proximal tubular damage); prior treatment with cisplatin; concurrent use of nephrotoxic drugs, unilateral nephrectomy; and total dose (increased risk with increased cumulative dose) are some of the risk factors for this side effect. Serum phosphate and bicarbonate should be measured during and after ifosfamide therapy and supplements provided as required. Other supplements like calcium, potassium, magnesium and alfacalcidol (1-alpha hydroxyvitamin D) may also be needed. Children appear to be at more risk for nephrotoxicity. Central nervous system toxicity manifesting as mental status changes, cerebellar dysfunction, transient weakness, cranial nerve dysfunction or seizure activity may occur in children. This toxicity appears to be transient and reversible, resolving within 4 days.

Mechlorethamine

Mechanism of Action

Mechlorethamine is an analogue of mustard gas.[4,5] As a polyfunctional alkylating agent, it interferes with DNA replication and RNA transcription through alkylation. Alkylation produces breaks in the DNA molecule as well as cross-linking of its twin strands. Mechlorethamine is cell cycle phase-nonspecific.

Indications

Hodgkin's disease, mycosis fungoides, chronic lymphocytic leukemia, chronic myelogenous leukemia, malignant effusions, medulloblastoma, non-Hodgkin's lymphoma, polycythemia rubra vera.

Dosage in Children

Intravenous: 6 mg/m^2 weekly at 4 weekly interval.

Side Effects

The major acute toxic manifestations include nausea, vomiting, lacrimation and myelosuppression. Leucopenia and thrombocytopenia are dose limiting. Extravasation into subcutaneous tissue causes painful inflammation, and can result in severe, brawny tender induration and sloughing. Mechlorethamine can cause significant sclerosing of the veins through which it is injected, resulting in pain and limitation of movement of the extremities. Application of ice compresses may provide symptomatic relief, and patients should be encouraged to mobilize their arm to avoid limitation of movement. Hyperuricemia developing during treatment can be minimized with allopurinol and hydration. Serious neurotoxicity can occur with high doses. An allergic contact dermatitis to topical mechlorethamine can be seen in some patients. Mechlorethamine should be discontinued if the allergic reaction occurs and depending upon the severity of the allergic reaction, it should be treated with either systemic prednisone or topical glucocorticoids until the reaction has subsided. Mechlorethamine can be restarted at a much more dilute concentration. If no reaction occurs, the dilute solution can be applied daily and the concentration can be gradually increased over the ensuing months back to normal levels as the patient becomes desensitized.

Chlorambucil

Mechanism of Action

Chlorambucil, an aromatic derivative of mechlorethamine, causes alkylation of DNA resulting in breaks in the DNA molecule as well as cross-linking of the twin strands.[5] It thus interferes with DNA replication and transcription of RNA. Chlorambucil is the slowest acting and generally least toxic of the alkylating agents. It is cell cycle phase-nonspecific.

Indications

Chronic lymphocytic leukemia, non-Hodgkin's lymphomas, Hodgkin's disease, multiple myeloma, mycosis fungoides, sezary syndrome, Waldenstrom's macroglobulinemia.

Dosage in Children

Induction: daily: 0.1-0.2 mg/kg or 4.5 mg/m^2 x 3-6 weeks; titrate to response/toxicity
Maintenance: daily: 0.06-0.1 mg/kg

Side Effects

Pancytopenia or bone marrow damage can be seen after prolonged therapy or excessive doses. The disease being treated and the regimen being used determine its effect on the blood count. Hyperuricemia occurring during periods of active cell lysis can be minimized with allopurinol and hydration. Dyspnea, dry cough, fever, rales and tachypnea are usually associated with prolonged therapy and a total dose of >2 g. Within

weeks of discontinuing therapy, partial recovery can be seen. An increased risk of seizures is seen in children with nephrotic syndrome and those receiving high pulse doses.

Melphalan

Mechanism of Action

Melphalan, a phenylalanine derivative of mechlorethamine, causes alkylation of DNA resulting in breaks in the DNA molecules as well as cross-linking of the twin strands. It thus interfering with DNA replication and transcription of RNA.[3,5] Melphalan is cell cycle phase-nonspecific.

Indications

Leukemias, sarcoma, neuroblastoma, rhabdomyosarcoma.

Dosage in Children

Oral: daily: 4-20 mg/m^2 × 1-21 days
Intravenous: 30-45 mg/m^2, 3-4 weekly
Bone marrow transplant: 40-70 mg/m^2/day IV × 3 days or 110-180 mg/m^2 IV × 1 day

Side Effects

Clinical toxicity of melphalan is mostly hematological. Nausea and vomiting are infrequent, but may be more severe with single high oral doses. With high dose therapy gastrointestinal toxicity (mucositis, esophagitis and diarrhea) becomes dose-limiting. Extravasation leading to tissue necrosis may happen days to weeks after the treatment. Patients must be observed for delayed reactions and prior injection sites must be carefully inspected. Bronchopulmonary dysplasia and pulmonary interstitial fibrosis, not related to dose or to duration of therapy, have been reported. Patients either recover with complete resolution of all signs and symptoms of pulmonary toxicity or die from progressive pulmonary disease. Repeated doses of melphalan may cause a cumulative myelosuppression, from which recovery may be prolonged and incomplete.

Busulfan

Mechanism of Action

Busulfan is a bifunctional alkylating agent.[4,5] Following systemic absorption, carbonium ions are rapidly formed, resulting in alkylation of DNA. This causes breaks in the

DNA molecule as well as cross-linking of the twin strands, resulting in interference of DNA replication and transcription of RNA. Busulfan is cell cycle phase-nonspecific.

Indications

Used as a conditioning regimen prior to bone marrow transplant, chronic myelogenous leukemia.

Dosage in Children

Oral: *Initial dose:* 0.06- 0.12 mg/kg or 1.8-4.6 mg/m^2 PO once daily

Maintenance dose: titrate maintenance dose (continuous or intermittent) to maintain WBC from 15-20 × 10^9/L

Bone marrow transplant: 1 mg/kg PO every 6 hours for 4 days for a total of 16 doses

Side Effects

Major toxic effects are related to myelosuppression and prolonged thrombocytopenia may be a hazard. Mucositis/stomatitis, fever, nausea and vomiting, rash, diarrhea and infection occur commonly with BMT doses. Hyperpigmentation involving elbows, knees and skin creases can be seen with busulfan therapy. Symptoms mimic Addison's disease and usually resolve when busulfan is stopped. Hyperuricemia resulting from excessive purine catabolism can be minimized with allopurinol and hydration. Dyspnea, dry cough, fever and rales can occur with busulphan. Thoracic irradiation is a risk factor for busulfan-induced pulmonary toxicity. Most patients progress to pulmonary insufficiency and death. Although no definitive therapy exists, treatment with 50-100 mg of prednisone and discontinuation of busulfan may be of some benefit. Pubertal development and gonadal function in children and adolescents can be adversely affected, sometimes necessitating supplementation with appropriate gonadal hormones. With high doses and concurrent use of multiple alkylating agents, veno-occlusive disease can be seen. Measurement of liver function tests and bilirubin is thus recommended.

Thiotepa

Mechanism of Action

Thiotepa, a polyfunctional alkylating agent chemically related to mechlorethamine, causes alkylation.[5] It thus produces breaks in the DNA molecule as well as cross-linking of its twin strands. Thiotepa is cell cycle phase-nonspecific.

Pharmacokinetics

Oral absorption incomplete. Distribution is rapid and extensive to tissues. It crosses blood brain barrier. It is metabolized in the liver to triethylenephosphoramide (TEPA) and is excreted in the urine (60%) within 72 hours.

Indications

Carcinoma of the urinary bladder, Hodgkin's disease, pediatric brain tumors and relapsed solid tumors.

Dosage in Children

Intravenous: 65 mg/m^2, 3 weekly
Bone marrow transplant: 300-375 mg/m^2 /day IV × 3 days

Side Effects

Include headache, dizziness, nausea and vomiting, stomatitis, diarrhea, type I (anaphylactoid) hypersensitivity, hives, rash, somnolence, seizures, paresthesia, hyperpigmentation, alopecia, myelosuppression, immunosuppression, elevated bilirubin (transient), neoplastic leukemia and hemorrhagic cystitis.

ALKYLATING-LIKE AGENTS

Cisplatin

Mechanism of Action

Cisplatin covalently binds to DNA and disrupts DNA function. After entering the cells, the chloride ligands are replaced by water molecules, resulting in the formation of positively charged platinum complexes that react with the nucleophilic sites on DNA. It prevents DNA, RNA and protein synthesis by forming platinum complexes that covalently bind to DNA bases using intrastrand and interstrand cross-links, thus creating cisplatin-DNA adducts.[5] Cisplatin is cell cycle phase-nonspecific.

Indications

Carcinoma of the bladder, brain cancer, germ cell tumors, head and neck cancer, Hodgkin's lymphoma, non-Hodgkin's lymphoma, mesothelioma, nasopharyngeal cancer, osteosarcoma.

Dosage in Children

Intravenous: 1 week: 30 mg/m^2 IV one dose on day 1

3 weeks: 90 mg/m^2 IV one dose on day 1

3-4 weeks: 60 mg/m^2 IV one dose on day 1 and day 2

Side Effects

Acute nausea and vomiting which may occur within hours after administration of cisplatin can be prevented by pretreatment with a 5-HT$_3$ antagonist (e.g., granisetron, ondansetron) plus a corticosteroid. Delayed nausea and vomiting can occur 24 hours or longer following chemotherapy. Delayed nausea and vomiting is not routinely be treated with 5-HT$_3$ antagonists. Corticosteroids are the cornerstone of the treatment for delayed nausea, although other combinations can also be used. Nephrotoxicity caused by cisplatin may manifest as renal insufficiency, hypokalemia and hypomagnesemia. The risk for these adverse effects is related to the dose and interval of cisplatin and may be minimized by adequate hydration. Anemia observed with cisplatin use may be caused by a decrease in erythropoietin or erythroid stem cells. Serious electrolyte disturbances including hypomagnesemia, hypocalcemia and hypokalemia can occur. These effects are due to renal tubular damage. Cisplatin greatly increases the urinary excretion of magnesium and calcium. Children are at greater risk for developing hypomagnesemia. Sensory peripheral neuropathies (e.g., paresthesias of the upper and lower extremities) can occur. They can also include motor difficulties; reduced or absent deep-tendon reflexes and leg weakness may also occur. Peripheral neuropathy is cumulative and usually reversible, although recovery is often slow. Tinnitus, with or without clinical hearing loss, and occasional deafness have been reported. It results from damage to the inner ear. Ototoxicity may be more severe in children than in adults. Audiograms must be performed prior to initiating therapy and prior to each subsequent dose of drug. Anaphylactoid reactions consisting of facial edema, flushing, wheezing or respiratory difficulties, tachycardia, and hypotension can occur after cisplatin therapy.

Carboplatin

Mechanism of Action

Carboplatin, an analog of cisplatin, contains a platinum atom surrounded in a plane by two ammonia groups and two other ligands in the *cis* position. The other two ligands in carboplatin are present in a ring structure rather than as two chloride atoms in cisplatin, thus making carboplatin more stable with less nephrotoxicity, neurotoxicity, ototoxicity and emetogenesis. By undergoing intracellular activation to form reactive platinum complexes, carboplatin inhibits DNA synthesis by forming interstrand and intrastrand cross-linking of DNA molecules.[5] Carboplatin is a radiation-sensitizing agent. It is cell cycle-phase nonspecific

Indications

Brain tumors, germ cell tumors, head and neck cancer, acute lymphocytic leukemia, Ewing's sarcoma, non-Hodgkin's lymphoma, melanoma, neuroblastoma, osteosarcoma, rhabdomyosarcoma, retinoblastoma, Wilm's tumor.

Dosage in Children

Intravenous: 3-4 weeks: 400 mg/m^2 IV once daily for 2 consecutive days starting on day 1 (total dose per cycle 800 mg/m^2)

4 weeks: 560 mg/m^2 IV for one dose on day 1

4 weeks: 80-216 mg/m^2 IV once daily for 5 consecutive days starting on day 1 (total dose per cycle 400-1080 mg/m^2)

Bone marrow transplant: higher doses are used for tumor ablation prior to bone marrow transplant, e.g.:
100-800 mg/m^2/day IV for 3 days,
250-300 mg/m^2/day IV for 4 days,
250-350 mg/m^2/day IV for 5 days.

Side Effects

Carboplatin is relatively well tolerated. There is less nausea, neurotoxicity, ototoxicity and nephrotoxicity than with cisplatin. Myelosuppression is the dose-limiting toxicity and dose dependent side effect. This usually manifests as thrombocytopenia and less commonly as leucopenia, neutropenia and anemia. Anemia is more common with increased carboplatin exposure and blood transfusions may be needed during prolonged carboplatin therapy. Nausea and vomiting usually begin within hours of administration and may persist up to 24 hours or longer. Acute vomiting can be seen following carboplatin therapy and may be reduced by prophylactic antiemetics. Hypersensitivity including anaphylaxis and anaphylactoid reactions can develop during or several hours to days after carboplatin administration. Management includes prompt treatment of anaphylaxis and oral diphenhydramine for minor delayed reactions. Carboplatin therapy may be continued in some patients with prophylactic corticosteroid and antihistamine and/or desensitization.

Procarbazine

Mechanism of Action

Procarbazine has multiple sites of action. It inhibits incorporation of small DNA precursors, as well as RNA and protein synthesis. Procarbazine can also directly damage DNA through an alkylation reaction. This drug is cell cycle phase-specific (S-phase).

Indications

Hodgkin's disease, brain tumors, non-Hodgkin's lymphoma.

Dosage in Children

- 100 mg/m²/dose po × 7-14 days, 4 weekly
- 75 mg/m²/dose po, 2-4 weekly

Side Effects

Most common toxic effects include leucopenia and thrombocytopenia. Hypersensitivity pneumonitis characterized by nausea, fever, nonproductive cough and dyspnea can occur within hours of ingesting procarbazine. Recover occurs following discontinuation of procarbazine. Procarbazine-induced neurotoxicity may present as altered levels of consciousness, peripheral neuropathy, ataxia or effects of MAO inhibition. The occurrence of frequent nightmares, depression, insomnia, nervousness and hallucinations are distressing to the patient. Paresthesia in hands and feet, decreased deep tendon reflexes and myalgia have also been

reported. Some patients may present with bleeding tendencies (petechiae, nosebleeds, vomiting of blood). The drug can also enhance radiation injury to tissues, weeks to months following radiation.

Carmustine

Mechanism of Action

Carmustine causes alkylation and cross-linking of DNA. It also causes inhibition of DNA repair. It kills cells in all phases of cell cycle. Nitrosoureas generally lack cross-resistance with other alkylating agents.

Indications

Brain tumors, gastrointestinal cancer, Hodgkin's disease, malignant melanoma, multiple myeloma, non-Hodgkin's lymphomas.

Dosage in Children

Initial dose: 60 mg/m² or 2 mg/kg IV
Maintenance: 30-45 mg/m² or 1-1.5 mg/kg IV, 6 weekly
Bone marrow transplant: 300-600 mg/m² IV

Side Effects

This drug causes an unusually delayed myelo-suppression. Effects on bone marrow are dose related and cumulative. Extravasation leading to tissue necrosis may occur weeks to months after the treatment. Patients must be observed for delayed reactions and prior injection sites carefully inspected. Clinical signs associated with carmustine-induced pulmonary toxicity are dyspnea, tachypnea and a dry hacking cough. Nausea and vomiting are variable but may be severe, with an acute onset and lasting several hours. Local burning occurs at the injection site and along the course of the vein. Facial flushing can occur after rapid IV infusion. These effects are probably due to the alcohol diluent. When used in high doses prior to bone marrow transplantation, severe nausea and vomiting, encephalopathy, dose limiting hepatotoxicity and pulmonary toxicity can occur.

Lomustine

Mechanism of Action

Lomustine, a highly lipophilic nitrosourea compound, undergoes hydrolysis to form reactive metabolites which cause alkylation and cross-linking of DNA. Other mechanisms include inhibition of DNA synthesis and some cell cycle phase specificity. It is not cross-resistant with other alkylating agents.

Indications

Brain tumors, Hodgkin's disease, malignant melanoma, multiple myeloma, non-Hodgkin's lymphomas.

Dosage in Children

Dose should be calculated to the nearest 10 mg to accommodate capsule sizes. Oral: 100 mg/m² po, 6 weekly

Side Effects

Nausea and vomiting may be seen after an oral dose and usually abates within 24 hours. Cumulative myelosuppression and pulmonary toxicity has been reported with this drug. Lomustine has a carcinogenic potential and there are reports of acute leukemia and bone marrow dysplasias following its therapy.

Dacarbazine

Mechanism of Action

Dacarbazine functions as a methylating agent after metabolic activation in the liver. However, its primary mode of action appears to be alkylation of nucleic acids. Dacarbazine is cell cycle phase-nonspecific.

Indications

Hodgkin's disease, malignant melanoma, neuroblastoma, soft tissue sarcomas.

Dosage in Children

Intravenous: 375 mg/m², 2 weekly
150-250 mg/m²/day × 5days, 3-4 weekly
750 mg/m², 6-8 weekly

Side Effects

Nausea and vomiting occurs frequently recommending the use of prophylactic and continuing antiemetic medication. Nausea is most severe on the first day of multiple day treatment. Alopecia, diarrhea, anorexia, myelosuppression, facial flushing, photosensitivity, elevated liver function tests, veno-occlusive disease (VOD), allergic vasculitis, type I (anaphylactoid) hypersensitivity, pain on injection, chemical phlebitis, increased BUN and serum creatinine can occur. After large, single doses, a flu-like syndrome consisting of chills, fever, myalgia and malaise may occur.

ANTIMETABOLITES

Methotrexate

Mechanism of Action

Methotrexate, a folate antagonist is converted to tetrahydrofolate by the enzyme dihydrofolate reductase (DHFR). Tetrahydrofolate, the active form of folic acid required for purine and thymidylate synthesis. The cytotoxicity of methotrexate results from inhibition of DHFR, inhibition of thymidylate, and alteration of the transport of reduced folates. Inhibition of DHFR results in a decrease in DNA synthesis, repair and cellular replication.[5] Methotrexate is most active against rapidly multiplying cells because the cytotoxic effects occur primarily during the S phase of the cell cycle.

Pharmacokinetics

Food delays absorption and reduces peak concentration. It is widely distributed with highest concentration in kidneys, gallbladder, spleen, liver, and skin. It does not cross the blood brain barrier. Higher CNS concentrations have been observed in patients with recent cranial irradiation and in patients with primary CNS lymphoma due to disruption of the blood-brain barrier.

Indications

Carcinoma of the bladder, head and neck cancer, leptomeningeal cancer, acute meningeal leukemia; acute lymphoblastic leukemia; acute lymphocytic leukemia; Burkitt's lymphoma, childhood lymphoma, non-Hodgkin's lymphoma, mycosis fungoides; lymphatic sarcoma; osteogenic sarcoma.

Dosage in Children

Oral, Intramuscular, Subcutaneous: 1-2 weeks: 7.5-30 mg/m²
Intravenous: bolus or continuous infusion (6-24 h): 10-33,000 mg/m²
Intrathecal: 6 mg (age <1 yr), 8 mg (age 1 yr), 10 mg (age 2 yr), 12 mg (age > 3 yr)
*Doses above 100 to 300 mg/m², which are usually administered by continuous infusion, must be followed by leucovorin rescue.
*Leucovorin rescue is required in some methotrexate regimens.

Side Effects

The primary toxicities of methotrexate affect the bone marrow and the intestinal epithelium. Anaphylaxis, vasculitis, tinnitus, neutropenia, thrombocytopenia, anemia, hypotension, pericardial effusion, constitutional symptoms, mood alteration; alopecia, dermatitis, erythema multiforme (Stevens-Johnson syndrome), exfoliative dermatitis, toxic epidermis necrolysis, folliculitis, photosensitivity, pigmentary changes, pruritus, rash on extremities, skin necrosis, telangiectasia, urticaria and diabetes can occur. Other effects include abdominal discomfort, anorexia, diarrhea, gingivitis, nausea, dose-related vomiting, petechiae, hematemesis, hematuria, melena, pancreatitis, hyperuricemia, arthralgia/myalgia, hemiparesis, osteoporosis, soft tissue necrosis, mild transient cognitive dysfunction, dizziness, seizure, eye discomfort, severe visual changes, headache, renal dysfunction, secondary malignancy (lymphomas) and acute neurologic syndrome. Life-threatening hepatotoxicity can be seen with both high and low-dose methotrexate. Increased serum aminotransferases and hyperbilirubinemia is seen more often in high-dose methotrexate. The liver enzymes tend to increase with each cycle, and usually return to pretreatment levels once methotrexate has been discontinued for 1 month. Both high and low-dose methotrexate can induce life-threatening pulmonary toxicity. Subacute toxicity, characterized by dyspnea, nonproductive cough, fever, crackles, cyanosis, pulmonary fibrosis, pleural effusions, is the most common. Methotrexate should be discontinued and corticosteroid therapy should be initiated. As methotrexate is mainly eliminated by the kidneys, high-dose methotrexate-induced renal failure is a medical emergency. Renal damage is due to precipitation of methotrexate in the tubules and to tubule injury. Drug precipitation can often be prevented by hydration and alkalization of the urine. Neurotoxicities can be seen with intrathecal injection of methotrexate and with high-dose methotrexate. Aseptic meningitis is the most common toxicity seen after intrathecal (IT) administration, and includes headache, neck rigidity, back pain, nausea, vomiting, fever, and lethargy. The risk of developing this can be decreased by the administration of IT hydrocortisone, or oral corticosteroids. Hyperuricemia may result from cell lysis by cytotoxic chemotherapy and may lead to electrolyte disturbances or acute renal failure. The risk of developing hyperuricemia may be increased in patients with preexisting renal dysfunction, especially ureteral obstruction.

Mercaptopurine

Mechanism of Action

Mercaptopurine, a 6-thiopurine, causes de novo inhibition of purine synthesis and incorporation into DNA. Mercaptopurine is cross-resistant with 6-thioguanine. Cytotoxicity is cell cycle phase-specific (S-phase).

Pharmacokinetics

Oral absorption is incomplete and variable. It is widely distributed to body tissues. CSF concentration is negligible with conventional doses, whereas cytotoxic concentrations are reached with high IV doses. Metabolism is by rapid intracellular activation with the formation of active metabolite(s) (6-thioinosinic acid, 6-thioguanylic acid) and inactive metabolite(s) (6-thiouric acid, 6-methylthiopurine derivatives). At conventional doses clearance is primarily hepatic. Renal clearance may become important at high doses.

Indications

Acute lymphocytic leukemia, acute myelogenous leukemia, chronic myelogenous leukemia, histiocytosis X.

Dosage in Children

Oral: daily: 2.5-5 mg/kg or 70 mg/m^2, preferably at bedtime, decrease dose by 50 percent in children less than 3 months of age
Intravenous: 200 mg/m^2 IV over 20 minutes, then 800 mg/m^2 over 8 hours, 2-5 weekly

Side Effects

The principal toxic effect of mercaptopurine is bone marrow depression leading to thrombocytopenia, granulocytopenia or anemia. Other effects include alopecia, hyperpigmentation, nausea and vomiting, diarrhea, anorexia, stomatitis, pancreatitis, myelosuppression, immunosuppressionskin rash, fever, injection site vein irritation, hematuria and crystalluria. Hyperuricemia can be minimized with allopurinol and hydration. However, with concurrent allopurinol, the dose of mercaptopurine should be reduced to 25 percent of the usual dose. Hepatotoxicity ranging from asymptomatic elevation of liver enzymes with no clinical significance to cholestatic jaundice and liver failure can be seen. Serious toxicity is manifested by rapid onset of cholestatic jaundice, ascites, hepatic encephalopathy and/or elevated liver enzymes, usually associated with hepatic necrosis and severe fibrosis. To prevent hematuria and crystalluria, patients should be hydrated during and after high dose IV mercaptopurine. Mercaptopurine also has the potential to enhance radiation injury to tissues.

Thioguanine

Mechanism of Action

Thioguanine, a 6-thiopurine analogue of the naturally occurring purine bases hypoxanthine and guanine, is incorporated into DNA as a false purine base. It is also incorporated into RNA resulting in an additional cytotoxic effect. Thioguanine is cross-resistant with mercaptopurine. Cytotoxicity is cell cycle phase-specific (S-phase).

Pharmacokinetics

Oral absorption is variable and incomplete. It is metabolized predominantly in liver and other tissues with formation of active metabolite (2-amino-6-methylmercaptopurine) and inactive metabolite(s). Excretion is mainly in urine.

Indications

Acute lymphocytic leukemia, acute myelogenous leukemia, chronic myelogenous leukemia.

Dosage in Children

Doses should be calculated to the nearest 10 mg
Induction: daily: 2-3 mg/kg po until adequate decrease in WBC count

Maintenance:	75-200 mg/m^2/day po × 5-7 days
	2 mg/kg/day po
	300 mg/m^2/day po × 4 days, 8 weekly
Consolidation:	75 mg/m^2/day po × 2-8 weeks

Side Effects

Toxic effects include bone marrow depression and GI effects. Other effects include rash, stomatitis, diarrhea, anorexia, myelosuppression, immunosuppression, elevated liver function tests, veno-occlusive disease, jaundice, loss of vibration sensitivity and unsteady gait. Hyperuricemia can be minimized with allopurinol and hydration. Unlike mercaptopurine, thioguanine's metabolism is not inhibited by the xanthine oxidase inhibitor allopurinol.

Fluorouracil

Mechanism of Action

Fluorouracil, an analog of the pyrimidine uracil acts as a pyrimidine antagonist. The fluorouracil metabolite fluorodeoxyuridine monophosphate (FdUMP) competes with uracil to bind with thymidylate synthetase (TS) and the folate cofactor. This results in decreased thymidine production and therefore decreased DNA synthesis and repair, and ultimately decreased cell proliferation. Additionally, the fluorouracil metabolite fluorodeoxyuridine triphosphate (FdUTP) is incorporated into DNA thus interfering with DNA replication. Finally, the fluorouracil metabolite fluorouridine-5-triphosphate (FUTP) is incorporated into RNA in place of uridine triphosphate (UTP), producing a fraudulent RNA and interfering with RNA processing and protein synthesis. Fluorouracil is cell-cycle specific (S-phase).

Pharmacokinetics

Variations in dihydropyrimidine dehydrogenase (DPD) activity result in differences in toxicity. Oral absorption is erratic; penetrates extracellular fluid and third space fluids (e.g., malignant effusions and ascitic fluid). It crosses the blood brain barrier. 80 percent of the parent drug is degraded in liver by DPD.

Indications

Actinic keratoses (topical fluorouracil), carcinoma of the bladder, esophageal cancer, colorectal cancer, skin cancer, Bowen's disease (topical fluorouracil), head and neck cancer.

Special Precautions

Fluorouracil is contraindicated in patients who have a history of hypersensitivity to fluorouracil or any component of the formulation. It is relatively contra-indicated in patients who have a known hypersensitivity to capecitabine. In patients with dihydropyrimidine dehydrogenase (DPD) deficiency, fluorouracil may result in life-threatening or fatal toxicity.

Dosage in Children

Intravenous: 500 mg/m^2 IV once or daily × 5
800-1200 mg/m^2 IV over 24-120 h
Topical: use and dose as determined by physician

Side Effects

Include febrile neutropenia, myelosuppression, hypotension, somnolence, alopecia, dermatitis, photosensitivity, vein hyperpigmentation proximal to injection sites, anorexia, vomiting, diarrhea, esophagitis, nausea, stomatitis, epithelial ulceration, hepatic toxicity, headache and dyspnea. Patients receiving bolus fluorouracil should undergo 30 minutes of oral cryotherapy to decrease the incidence and severity of fluorouracil-induced stomatitis. The patient is asked to place ice chips into their mouth 5 minutes before injection and swish for 30 minutes. This cooling of the oral cavity leads to vasoconstriction resulting in a lower concentration of fluorouracil reaching the oral mucosa. Acute cerebellar syndrome characterized by an acute onset of ataxia, dysmetria, dysarthria, and nystagmus can occur. These symptoms usually resolve after discontinuation of fluorouracil. Fluorouracil induced cardiotoxicity can present as electrocardiographic changes, angina, myocardial infarction, acute pulmonary edema, arrhythmias, elevated cardiac enzymes, cardiac arrest and pericarditis. Most cases of fluorouracil-induced cardiotoxicities resolve after termination of fluorouracil infusion and/or administration of nitrates or calcium channel blockers. Hand-foot syndrome (palmar-plantar erythrodysesthesia, PPE) may occur in association with the continuous infusion of fluorouracil. PPE may gradually disappear over 5-7 days after discontinuation of fluorouracil therapy. Oral pyridoxine 50–150 mg daily has been tried for treatment of PPE. In patients with dihydropyrimidine dehydrogenase (DPD) deficiency, treatment with fluorouracil can lead to life-threatening complications as fluorouracil clearance is dependent on DPD. Toxicities can include severe diarrhea, stomatitis, and myelosuppression. Nausea, vomiting, rectal bleeding, volume depletion, skin changes, and neurologic abnormalities may also occur. Management includes supportive care with hemodynamic support, parenteral nutrition, antibiotics, and hematopoietic colony stimulating factors. Fluorouracil-induced ocular toxicities include excessive lacrimation, blurred vision, photophobia, and eye irritation. Ice packs can be applied to the eyes before, during, and for 30 minutes after fluorouracil injection may decrease ocular toxicity. Topical application can lead to erythema, vesiculation, erosion, ulceration, necrosis, and epithelization. Pain, pruritus, hyperpigmentation, and burning at the application site are the most frequent local reactions.

Hydroxyurea

Mechanism of Action

Hydroxyurea, an inhibitor of ribonucleotide reductase, leads to depletion of essential DNA precursors. Direct chemical damage to DNA by hydroxyurea or a metabolite may also be involved in its cytotoxicity. It also inhibits repair of DNA damaged by chemotherapy or radiation. Hydroxyurea is cell cycle phase-specific (S-phase).

Indications

Chronic myelogenous leukemia, acute myelogenous leukemia, pediatric brain tumors, head and neck cancer, squamous cell, malignant melanoma, polycythemia rubra vera.

Dosage in Children

CML: daily: 10-20 mg/kg po, adjusted to hematological response
Brain tumors: 1.5-3 g/m^2 po, 2-4 weekly

Side Effects

Hematopoietic depression leading to leucopenia, megaloblastic anemia and thrombocytopenia is the major toxic effect. Recovery occurs on discontinuation of the drug. Interstitial pneumonitis, gastrointestinal disturbances, mild dermatological reactions, stomatitis, alopecia and neurological manifestations can occur. Hyperuricemia can be minimized with allopurinol and hydration. Hydroxyurea also has the potential to enhance radiation injury to tissues.

Cytarabine

Mechanism of Action

Cytarabine after being metabolized intracellularly into its active triphosphate form (cytosine arabinoside triphosphate) damages DNA by multiple mechanisms, including the inhibition of alpha-DNA polymerase, inhibition of DNA repair through an effect on beta-DNA polymerase, and incorporation into DNA. Cytotoxicity is highly specific for the S phase of the cell cycle.

Indications

Acute myelogenous leukemia, meningeal leukemia, acute lymphocytic leukemia, chronic myelogenous leukemia, erythroleukemia, non-Hodgkin's lymphoma.

Dosage in Children

Intravenous: 75-150 mg/m^2/day or 5 mg/kg/day x 5 days, 4 weekly

300 mg/m^2/day, twice weekly x 4 weeks

150 mg/m^2/day x 5 days by continuous IV or SC Infusion, 4 weekly

1-3 g/m^2/dose q12h x 4-12 doses (<3 years: 100 mg/kg/dose) 4 weekly

Intrathecal:

	<1 year	20 mg
	1-2 years	30 mg
	2-3 years	50 mg
	>3 years	70 mg

Bone marrow transplant: 3 g/m^2/dose IV q12h x 12 doses

Side Effects

Myelosuppression leading to severe leucopenia, thrombocytopenia and anemia can occur. High dose regimens can cause hepatotoxicity with significant liver function abnormalities requiring discontinuation of the drug. Pulmonary edema with dyspnea and tachypnea have been reported. It can develop during therapy or within days of discontinuing cytarabine and may be fatal. Cerebellar dysfunction characterized by dysarthria, dysdiadochokinesia, dysmetria and ataxia may follow intrathecal or high dose systemic administration. Cerebral toxicity manifests as somnolence, confusion, cognitive dysfunction, memory loss, psychosis or seizures. A flu-like syndrome characterized by fever, myalgia, bone pain and rash may develop. Symptoms usually disappear when drug is discontinued and may be prevented by pretreatment with corticosteroids. Fever may occur during the administration of cytarabine in the absence of an infection. If fever occurs, the patient should be examined for a potential infectious source. Conjunctivitis occurring with high doses can be minimized by prophylactic use of ophthalmic corticosteroids. Acute arachnoiditis and myelopathic syndromes may occur after intrathecal cytarabine. Adverse effects associated with intrathecal cytarabine include nausea and vomiting, headache and fever.

DNA BINDING AGENTS

Daunorubicin

Mechanism of Action

Daunorubicin, an anthracycline antibiotic, damages DNA by intercalating between base pairs resulting in uncoiling of the helix, ultimately inhibiting DNA synthesis and DNA-dependent RNA synthesis. Daunorubicin may also act by inhibiting polymerase activity, affecting regulation of gene expression and generating free radicals. Cytotoxic activity is cell cycle phase non-specific, although it exerts maximal cytotoxic effects in the S-phase.

Indications

Ewing's sarcoma, acute lymphocytic leukemia, acute myeloid leukemia, chronic myelogenous leukemia, non-Hodgkin's lymphoma, Kaposi's sarcoma, Hodgkin's lymphoma, lymphosacroma, rhabdomyosarcoma, Wilm's tumor.

Dosage in Children

Intravenous: 3-4 weeks: > 2 y old 25-45 mg/m^2 IV, frequency of administration dependent on specific regimen employed < 2 y old or BSA < 0.5 m^2 calculate dose based on BW rather than BSA (mg/kg dose can be approximated by dividing the mg/m^2 dose by 30)

Maximum dose: BW 20 kg: 600 mg/m^2, BW 30 kg: 750 mg/m^2, BW 10 kg: 500 mg/m^2

Side Effects

Include bone marrow depression, stomatitis, alopecia, GI disturbances and dermatological manifestations. Hyperuricemia during periods of active cell lysis can be minimized with allopurinol and hydration. Tissue necrosis may be caused by extravasation of anthracyclines. Flare reaction is a painless local reaction along the vein or near the intact injection of anthracyclines. It is characterized by immediate red blotches, streaks and local wheals, probably due to histamine release. Edema may sometimes occur. Symptoms usually subside with or without treatment 30 minutes after the infusion is stopped. Cardiac toxicity, a peculiar toxicity observed with the anthracycline (doxorubicin, epirubicin, idarubicin, daunorubicin) and anthracenedione (mitoxantrone) classes of drugs, is characterized by tachycardia, arrhythmias, dyspnea, hypotension, pericardial effusion and congestive heart failure. Children with daunorubicin-induced CHF are very sensitive to digitalis.

Dactinomycin

Mechanism of Action

Dactinomycin is a derivative of *Streptomyces*. At low concentrations, it inhibits DNA-primed RNA synthesis by intercalating with guanine residues of DNA. At higher concentrations, it also inhibits DNA synthesis. Dactinomycin causes single strand breaks in DNA, possibly through a free radical or as a result of the action of topoisomerase II. Dactinomycin is cell cycle phase-nonspecific.

Indications

Ewing's sarcoma, rhabdomyosarcoma, Wilm's tumor, germ cell tumors, Kaposi's sarcoma, melanoma, optic nerve glioma, osteogenic sarcoma, testicular cancer.

Dosage in Children

Intravenous: 15 mcg/kg/day x 5 days. Maximum single dose 500 mcg, 5-8 weekly
   45 mcg/kg. Maximum single dose 500 mcg, 3 weekly

Side Effects

Include anorexia, nausea and vomiting usually beginning a few hours after administration. Proctitis, diarrhea, glossitis, cheilitis and ulceration of oral mucosa can also be seen. Extravasation leading to tissue necrosis may happen days to weeks after the treatment. Patients must be observed for delayed reactions and prior injection sites must be carefully inspected. Dactinomycin has the potential to enhance radiation injury to tissues. Hepatotoxicity seen in children may manifest as increased AST (SGOT) and bilirubin levels, ascites and liver enlargement. In some cases, thrombocytopenia may accompany hepatotoxicity.

Doxorubicin

Mechanism of Action

Doxorubicin binds to DNA by intercalating between base pairs on the DNA helix. It also inhibits DNA repair by inhibiting topoisomerase II, resulting in the blockade of DNA and RNA synthesis and fragmentation of DNA. Doxorubicin is also an iron-chelator. The iron-doxorubicin complex can bind DNA and cell membranes producing free radicals that immediately cleave DNA and cell membranes. Although maximally cytotoxic in S phase, doxorubicin is not cell cycle-specific.

Pharmacokinetics

It is not absorbed from GI tract as oral absorption is not stable in gastric acids. It is widely distributed in plasma and in tissues and does not cross blood brain barrier. Children have increased risk for delayed cardiotoxicity.

Indications

Carcinoma of the bladder, multiple myeloma, thymoma, Ewing's sarcoma, head and neck cancer, hepatic carcinoma, Kaposi's sarcoma, acute lymphoblastic leukemia, acute myeloblastic leukemia, Hodgkin's lymphoma, non-Hodgkin's lymphoma, neuroblastomas, osteosarcoma , soft tissue sarcoma, Wilm's tumor.

Dosage in Children

Intravenous: 45-90 mg/m^2 IV continuous infusion (24-96 h)
   30-45 mg/m^2 IV daily x 3 or weekly
1 week: 20-30 mg/m^2 IV for one dose on day 1 (total dose per cycle 20-30 mg/m^2)
3 weeks: 40-75 mg/m^2 IV for one dose on day 1 (total dose per cycle 40-75 mg/m^2)

Side Effects

Myelosuppression presenting as leucopenia, acute arrhythmia, acute transient ECG changes and chronic cardiotoxicity may occur. Anaphylaxis, fever, chills and urticaria and neutropenia have been reported. Complete alopecia, facial flushing, hyperpigmentation of nail beds and dermal creases, soles, palms, photosensitivity, radiation recall reaction, anorexia, diarrhea, stomatitis and esophagitis, nausea and vomiting, ulceration and necrosis of colon, changes in transaminase levels, conjunctivitis and lacrimation, red coloration of urine, secondary acute myelogenous leukemia and acute lymphocytic leukemia may be seen. Pediatric patients are at increased risk for developing later neoplastic disease. Cardiotoxicity thought to be due to free radical damage is cumulative across all anthracyclines and anthracenediones. Treatment includes discontinuation of the drug and standard treatment of CHF. Prevention, monitoring, and early diagnosis are essential. Cardioprotectant therapy with dexrazoxane may be considered for some patients with cumulative doxorubicin dosing. Cardiotoxicity in children increases rapidly at higher cumulative doses. Hyperuricemia risk may be increased in patients with pre-existing renal dysfunction, especially urethral obstruction. Urine should be alkalinized only if the uric acid level is elevated. Extravasation of doxorubicin can occur with or without accompanying stinging or burning sensation and can result in severe ulceration and soft tissue necrosis. Erythematous streaking near the site of infusion (adriamycin flare) is a benign local allergic reaction following therapy with this drug.

NEW INTERCALATING AGENTS

Bleomycin

Mechanism of Action

Bleomycin causes DNA strand scission by interacting with O_2 and Fe^{2+}, resulting in inhibition of DNA synthesis, and to a lesser degree, in inhibition of RNA and protein synthesis. The drug is cell-cycle specific for G_2 phase, M-phase and S phase.

Indications

Cancer of the larynx and paralarynx, Hodgkin's lymphoma, non-Hodgkin's lymphoma, malignant pleural effusion, soft tissue sarcoma, dysplastic oral leukoplakia, head and neck cancer, Kaposi's sarcoma, melanoma, mycosis fungoides, osteosarcoma, skin cancer, craniopharyngioma.

Dosage in Children

10-20 units/m² IV by bolus or infusion, IM, or SC. Intrapleural and intravesicular administration are used.

Side Effects

Cutaneous toxicities are the most frequent adverse effects of bleomycin and include erythema, rash, striae, vesiculation, hyperpigmentation and tenderness of skin. Febrile reactions seen in patients treated with bleomycin can be prevented by hydrocortisone premedication. Hypersensitivity reactions including hypotension, fever, chills, mental confusion, and wheezing can occur immediately or be delayed for several hours. Pulmonary toxicities are the most serious side effects for bleomycin. Nonproductive cough, dyspnea, basal rales, pleuritic chest pain and fever are frequently first signs of toxicity which may progresses to pulmonary fibrosis and death. Pulmonary fibrosis from bleomycin can develop insidiously during treatment. Treatment includes corticosteroids for pneumonitis to prevent pulmonary fibrosis and antibiotics for infectious pneumonitis.

Amsacrine

Mechanism of Action

The mechanism of action of amsacrine, an acridine dye derivative is incompletely defined. Amsacrine can intercalate with DNA, cause double-strand breaks in DNA, and inhibit topoisomerase II. Cytotoxicity is greatest during the S phase of the cell cycle when topoisomerase levels are at a maximum.

Indications

Acute leukemia.

Dosage in Children

150 mg/m²/day IV x 5 days, 2-3 weekly.

Side Effects

Type I hypersensitivity reactions have been reported with rash, pruritus and erythema on the first dose of amsacrine. Extravasation leading to tissue necrosis may occur weeks to months after the treatment. Patients must be observed for delayed reactions and prior injection sites carefully inspected. Hyperuricemia occurring during periods of active cell lysis can be minimized with allopurinol and hydration. Both acute (arrhythmias) and chronic (cardiomyopathies) cardiotoxicities have been documented. The risk of acute congestive heart failure is not conclusively related to increasing cumulative dose. Phlebitis can be reduced by infusing the diluted drug over a period of 60-90 minutes.

PLANT ALKALOIDS

Vincristine

Mechanism of Action

Vincristine, a naturally occurring vinca alkaloid, blocks mitosis by arresting cells in the metaphase. These drugs act by preventing the polymerization of tubulin to form microtubules, as well as inducing depolymerization of formed tubules. Vinca alkaloids are cell cycle phase-specific for M phase and S phase

Indications

Brain tumors, Ewing's sarcoma, Kaposi's sarcoma, acute leukemia, Hodgkin's lymphoma, non-Hodgkin's lymphoma, melanoma, neuroblastoma, osteosarcoma, rhabdomyosarcoma, soft tissue sarcoma, Wilm's tumor, hepatoblastoma, chronic leukemia, multiple myeloma, mycosis fungoides, retinoblastoma, Waldenstrom's macroglobulinemia.

Dosage in Children

Intravenous: 1-3 weeks: 1-2 mg/m^2 for children older than one year
1-3 weeks: 0.03-0.05 mg/kg for children up to one year old
Some regimens limit the total single dose of vincristine to 2 mg, especially on the weekly schedule

Side Effects

Neurotoxicity involving peripheral, autonomic and central neuropathy is the primary and dose-limiting toxicity of vincristine. Most side effects are dose related and reversible, but neurotoxicity can persist for months after discontinuation of therapy in some patients. Infants are at a higher risk for experiencing vincristine-related neurotoxicity. Peripheral neuropathy is the most common type of neuropathy and develops in almost all patients. Loss of deep tendon reflexes, peripheral paresthesias, pain and tingling can occur. With high doses, wrist and foot drop, ataxia, a slapping gait and difficulty in walking can occur. Cranial nerve toxicities may lead to vocal cord paresis or paralysis (hoarseness, weak voice), ocular motor nerve dysfunction (ptosis, strabismus), bilateral facial nerve palsies, or jaw pain. Autonomic neuropathy resulting in constipation, abdominal pain, urinary retention and paralytic ileus can also be seen. Constipation may be associated with impaction of stool in the upper colon. Central neuropathy includes headache, malaise, dizziness, seizures, mental depression, psychosis and SIADH. Hyperuricemia during periods of active cell lysis can be minimized with allopurinol and hydration. Doses of uricosuric drugs, including probenecid and sulfinpyrazone may need to be increased while receiving vincristine therapy.

Vinblastine

Mechanism of Action

Vinblastine binds to the microtubular proteins of the mitotic spindle, leading to crystallization of the microtubule and mitotic arrest or cell death. Vinblastine has some immunosuppressant effect. The vinca alkaloids are considered to be cell cycle phase-specific

Indications

Hodgkin's disease, Kaposi's sarcoma, bladder cancer, germ cell cancer, histiocytosis X, mycosis fungoides, non-Hodgkin's lymphoma.

Dosage in Children

Intravenous: 6.5 mg/m^2, 1 weekly
6 mg/m^2, 2 weekly

Side Effects

Neurotoxicity manifesting as numbness, paresthesia, mental depression, loss of deep tendon reflex, headache, malaise, dizziness, seizures or psychosis can occur. Cranial nerve neuropathy may lead to vocal cord paresis or paralysis, oculomotor nerve dysfunction and bilateral facial nerve palsies. Cranial nerve toxicities tend to be bilateral and reversible when treatment is discontinued. Severe jaw pain can occur within a few hours of the first dose of vinblastine. This can be treated with analgesics. Autonomic neuropathy is manifested as constipation, abdominal pain, urinary retention and paralytic ileus. These gastrointestinal symptoms are seen especially when high doses are used. Hyperuricemia can be minimized with allopurinol and hydration. However, fluid restriction may be required for a patient showing signs of SIADH. Tissue necrosis due to extravasation may happen days to weeks after the treatment. Patients must be observed for delayed reactions and prior injection sites must be carefully inspected.

Teniposide

Mechanism of Action

Teniposide, a semisynthetic podophyllotoxin derived from the root of *Podophyllum*, forms a ternary complex with topoisomerase II and DNA leading to single-strand breaks in DNA. Teniposide also causes DNA damage through activation of oxidation-reduction reactions to produce derivatives that bind directly to DNA. Topoisomerase II carries out breakage and reunion reactions of DNA which are necessary for normal cellular function. Teniposide is cell cycle phase-specific with predominant activity occurring in late S phase and G2.

Indications

Acute lymphocytic leukemia, neuroblastoma, non-Hodgkin's lymphoma, Hodgkin's disease, small cell lung cancer, retinoblastoma.

Dosage in Children

150-165 mg/m^2/dose twice weekly, at 7-10 week interval.

Side Effects

Myelosuppression, nausea and vomiting are its primary toxic effects. There is a significant risk of hypersensitivity reactions in children treated with epipodophyllotoxins. The most common symptoms of hypersensitivity have been flushing and chill. More severe reactions may produce bronchospasm, cyanosis and/or hypotension. Most symptoms can be relieved by discontinuing the teniposide infusion and administering an antihistamine. Rechallenge can be tried after prior treatment with an antihistamine and a corticosteroid. Secondary acute myelogenous leukemia (AML) may follow treatment with teniposide in children.

Etoposide

Mechanism of Action

Etoposide is a semisynthetic derivative of the podophyllotoxins, an epipodophyllotoxin. It inhibits DNA topoisomerase II, thereby inhibiting DNA synthesis. Etoposide is cell cycle dependent and phase specific, affecting mainly the S and G$_2$ phases.

Indications

Acute lymphocytic leukemia, acute nonlymphocytic leukemia, neuroblastoma, sarcomas, testicular tumors, lymphomas, brain tumors.

Dosage in Children

Oral:	4 weeks	50 mg daily for 21 days
Intravenous:	3-6 weeks	60-120 mg/m^2 daily for 3-5 days

Side Effects

The dose limiting toxicity is leucopenia. Thrombocytopenia occurs less frequently. Nausea, vomiting, stomatitis, diarrhea and alopecia can occur. Allergic reactions are rare but can be life threatening. Usually include chest discomfort, dyspnea, bronchospasm, hypotension and/or skin flushing. Treatment is symptomatic and can include pressor agents, corticosteroids, antihistamines, or volume expanders. Higher rates of anaphylactoid reactions are reported in children receiving etoposide infusions at higher than recommended concentrations. Congestive heart failure and myocardial infarction can occur in patients receiving etoposide by continuous IV infusion over 5 days. Hypotension can occur following rapid IV administration. Longer infusion times may be required based on patient tolerance. Hypotension usually responds to stopping the infusion, and administration of IV fluids or other supportive therapy as needed.

MISCELLANEOUS AGENTS

Asparaginase

Mechanism of Action

Asparaginase acts by deaminating extracellular L-asparagine, an amino acid that appears to be essential for protein synthesis by some tumor cells lacking adequate levels of asparagine synthetase. Asparaginase is usually considered to be cell cycle phase-nonspecific, but it may block some cells in G$_1$ or S phase.

Indications

Acute lymphocytic leukemia, acute myeloblastic leukemia, acute myelomonocytic leukemia, chronic lymphocytic leukemia, Hodgkin's disease, melanosarcoma, non-Hodgkin's lymphoma

Dosage in Children

Intramuscular: 6,000 IU/m^2 × 9 doses (some protocols use 200 IU/kg for children <3 years of age) 3 times per week

10,000 IU/m^2/day IV at 7-10 days interval
25,000 IU/m^2/day IM, 1 weekly

Side Effects

Hypersensitivity reactions can occur and can be fatal. Hyperuricemia during periods of active cell lysis can be minimized with allopurinol and hydration. Hepatotoxicity is frequent and can include decreased serum albumin, elevation of transaminase, bilirubin and alkaline phosphatase. Hepatic dysfunction may produce decreased levels of factors II, VII, IX, X and fibrinogen, and thus contribute to coagulation disorders. Liver abnormalities resolve a few days to weeks after therapy. Deficiencies in hemostatic proteins can occur in children receiving asparaginase. Hyperglycemia can occur in leukemic children treated with asparaginase and prednisone. Transient diabetes mellitus may develop. Risk factors in children for the development of hyperglycemia include age >10 years, obesity, family history of diabetes mellitus and Down's syndrome. Symptoms of headache, hemiparesis and seizures may result from intracranial events while extremity thrombi manifest through local pain, swelling and discoloration. Cerebral dysfunction manifested by lethargy, drowsiness, confusion and personality changes can occur. They are seen during the first day of therapy and resolve within a few days to a week after drug discontinuation. A delayed form of organic brain syndrome can occur a week after asparaginase administration and can last several weeks. Pancreatitis can occur during or after therapy, and can be fatal. Serum amylase levels should be obtained prior to each cycle of therapy. Further asparaginase therapy should not be given if pancreatitis is diagnosed.

Tretinoin

Mechanism of Action

Tretinoin is a natural metabolite of retinol and belongs to a class of retinoids, which are structurally related to vitamin.[5] It induces terminal differentiation in several hemopoietic precursor cell lines and in cells from patients with acute promyelocytic leukemia (APL). The exact mechanism of action is not known, but tretinoin induces maturation of leukemic cells and appearance of normal hemopoietic cells.

Indications

Acute promyelocytic leukemia, AIDS-related Kaposi's sarcoma, myelodysplastic syndrome.

Dosage in Children

Oral: 45 mg/m^2/day PO in 2 divided doses
Round dose to the nearest 10 mg. Administer with food.

Side Effects

Tretinoin causes dry skin, cheilitis, reversible hepatic enzyme abnormalities, bone tenderness and hyperlipidemia. Headache occurring several hours after tretinoin ingestion is the most common side effect. It differs from that associated with pseudotumor cerebri in that it is often transient, mild in intensity and well controlled with mild analgesics. Patients usually develop a tolerance with continued tretinoin therapy. Basophilia-associated hyperhistaminemia has been rarely reported. The severity of symptoms depends on the level of plasma histamine. Severe symptoms include tachycardia, shock due to vasodilatation, and gastric and duodenal ulceration. Prophylactic H$_2$- or H$_1$-antagonist has been used to prevent symptoms mediated via H$_2$- and H$_1$-receptors. Pseudotumor cerebri, characterized by signs and symptoms of intracranial hypertension without evidence of infective or space occupying lesions can be seen with tretinoin. Symptoms include severe headache which may be aggravated by analgesic or narcotic overuse, nausea and vomiting, papilledema, retinal hemorrhages, visual changes, ophthalmoplegia. Pseudotumor cerebri is more common in children and may be due to their increased sensitivity to the CNS effects of tretinoin. Narcotic analgesics or temporary discontinuation of tretinoin in non-responding cases may help reduce severe headache, nausea and vomiting. Diuretics or lumbar puncture may reduce CSF pressure. Hyperinflammatory reaction of neutrophil infiltration of the skin and internal organs (Sweet's syndrome) can be seen. Symptoms include fever, painful erythematous cutaneous plaques involving the extremities and the trunk, and prominent musculoskeletal involvement. Retinoic acid syndrome characterized by fever, dyspnea, hypotension, bone pain, respiratory distress, pulmonary infiltrates, hyperleukocytosis, pleural or pericardial effusion, weight gain, lower extremity edema, congestive heart failure, renal failure and multiorgan failure can also occur.

Mitoxantrone

Mechanism of Action

The exact mechanism of action of mitoxantrone, an anthracenedione structurally similar to doxorubicin, is not known but includes intercalation with DNA to cause inter/intrastrand cross-linking. It also causes DNA strand breaks through binding with the phosphate backbone of DNA. Mitoxantrone is cell cycle phase-nonspecific

Indications

Acute myelogenous leukemia, acute nonlymphocytic leukemia, non-Hodgkin's lymphoma, acute lymphocytic leukemia, chronic myelogenous leukemia.

Dosage in Children

Intravenous: 8 mg/m^2/day IV × 5 days, 3-4 weekly

Side Effects

It produces acute myelosuppression, cardiac toxicity and mucositis as its major toxicities. Cardiac monitoring is recommended in patients who have received prior anthracyclines (doxorubicin, epirubicin, daunorubicin, idarubicin) or mediastinal radiotherapy and/or patients with pre-existing cardiac disease as there is a risk of cardiotoxicity. Cardiac monitoring is advisable. Stomatitis is dose-limiting with the 5 day schedule and with the high doses used for bone marrow transplantation. Majority of extravasations of mitoxantrone result in a blue discoloration of the skin which slowly fades.

Irinotecan

Mechanism of Action

Irinotecan is a semisynthetic, water-soluble derivative of camptothecin, which is a cytotoxic alkaloid extracted from plants such as *Camptotheca acuminata*. Irinotecan inhibits the action of topoisomerase I, an enzyme that produces reversible single-strand breaks in DNA during DNA replication. Irinotecan also binds to the topoisomerase I-DNA complex and causes double-strand DNA breakage and cell death. Irinotecan is cell cycle phase-specific (S-phase).

Indications

Currently it is being investigated for use in children. Other indications include glioma, mesothelioma.

Dosage in Children

Irinotecan is currently being studied in children.

Side Effects

The dose limiting toxicity is diarrhea with or without neutropenia. Myelosuppression is the second most common irinotecan associated toxicity. Irinotecan can cause both early and late onset diarrhea. Early onset diarrhea occurs during or within 24 hours of administration of irinotecan. It is usually transient and only infrequently severe. Early onset diarrhea can be treated with atropine as needed. Blood pressure and heart rate should be monitored during atropine therapy. Late onset diarrhea occurs more than 24 hours after administration of irinotecan and can be prolonged, leading to potentially life-threatening dehydration and electrolyte imbalance. Management of diarrhea should include prompt treatment with high dose loperamide. Patients with severe diarrhea should be carefully monitored for dehydration and given fluid and electrolyte replacement as needed. Premedication with loperamide prior to irinotecan treatment is not required. Other side effects include immunosuppression, anemia, leucopenia, thrombocytopenia, arrhythmia, bradycardia, edema, hypotension, chills, fatigue, fever, sweating, constitutional symptoms, weight loss, alopecia, flushing, rash, anorexia, constipation, nausea, vomiting, increased alkaline phosphatase, increased AST, minor infection, insomnia, visual disturbances, abdominal pain or cramping, back pain, headache, cough, dyspnea, rhinitis, secondary malignancy (acute leukemias), dyspnea and reticulonodular pattern on chest X-ray.

Topotecan

Mechanism of Action

Topotecan, a semisynthetic, water-soluble derivative of camptothecin, which is a cytotoxic alkaloid extracted from plants such as *Camptotheca acuminate*, has the same mechanism of action as irinotecan. It inhibits the action of topoisomerase I, an enzyme that produces reversible single-strand breaks in DNA during DNA replication. Topotecan binds to the topoisomerase I-DNA complex and leads to double strand DNA breakage and cell death.[8] Unlike irinotecan, topotecan is found predominantly in the inactive carboxylate form at neutral pH and it is not a prodrug. As a result, topotecan has different antitumor activities and toxicities from irinotecan. Topotecan is a radiation-sensitizing agent. It is cell cycle phase-specific (S-phase).

Indications

Gliomas, acute myelogenous leukemia, multiple myeloma, myelodysplastic syndrome, neuroblastoma, retinoblastoma, rhabdomyosarcoma, Ewing's sarcoma, medulloblastoma.

Dosage in Children

Intravenous: 2 mg/m^2/day (range 1.5-2 mg/m^2/day) IV once daily for 5 consecutive days starting on day 1 (total dose per cycle 10 mg/m^2 [range 7.5-10 mg/m^2]) for 3 weeks.

Side Effects

The dose limiting toxicity with all schedules is neutropenia with or without thrombocytopenia. Other side effects include anemia, leucopenia, fever or infection with severe neutropenia, fatigue, fever, alopecia, rash, anorexia, constipation, diarrhea, nausea, stomatitis, vomiting, elevated bilirubin, elevated hepatic enzymes, headache, sensory neuropathy, abdominal pain, arthralgia, myalgia, body pain, back pain and skeletal pain, cough, dyspnea and acute leukemias.

NEW DRUGS AND APPROACHES

Imatinib

Mechanism of Action

Imatinib interferes with the binding of adenosine triphosphate to *BCR-ABL*, thus blocking the ability of *BCR-ABL* to promote tyrosine kinase phosphorylation. It inhibits the proliferation and induces apoptosis in *BCR-ABL* positive cells including CML.[9,10]

Pharmacokinetics

Imatinib is well absorbed after oral administration with maximum plasma concentrations (Cmax) achieved within 2 to 4 hours and has an absolute bioavailability of 98 percent irrespective of oral dosage form or dosage strength. Food has no relevant impact on the rate or extent of bioavailability. The terminal elimination half-life is approximately 18 hours. Imatinib is approximately 95 percent bound to human plasma proteins, mainly albumin and α 1-acid glycoprotein. The drug is eliminated predominantly via the bile in the form of metabolites, one of which (*CGP 74588*) shows comparable pharmacological activity to the parent drug. The fecal to urinary excretion ratio is approximately 5:1. Imatinib is metabolized mainly by the cytochrome P450 (CYP) 3A4 or CYP3A5 and can competitively inhibit the metabolism of drugs that are CYP3A4 or CYP3A5 substrates.

Indications

Chronic myeloid leukemia, Philadelphia chromosome positive acute lymphoblastic leukemia.

Side Effects

The most frequently reported drug related adverse events are nausea, vomiting, edema, and muscle cramps. Other side effects reported include superficial edema, nausea, muscle cramps, rash and related events, diarrhea, weight gain, vomiting, myalgia, arthralgia, abdominal pain, fatigue, dyspepsia, musculoskeletal pain, headache, pruritus, anemia, thrombocytopenia, leucopenia and neutropenia.

Clofarabine

Mechanism of Action

Clofarabine is a purine nucleoside analog that inhibits DNA synthesis and repair. It acts by inhibiting ribonucleotide reductase and DNA polymerase, depleting dNTPs for DNA replication and premature DNA chain termination. In addition to inhibition of DNA polymerases and DNA synthesis, clofarabine acts as a strong inhibitor of ribonucleotide reductase (RnR), an enzyme involved in regulating intracellular deoxy-nucleotide pools, and has a high affinity to the enzyme deoxycytidine kinase (dCyd), the rate-limiting step in nucleoside phosphorylation. Clofarabine also disrupts the integrity of mitochondrial membranes, resulting in programed cell death.[11,12]

Indications

Approved by the FDA for refractory or relapsed ALL in children.
Combined with cytarabine for initial treatment of older patients with AML.

Side Effects

Include reversible hepatotoxicity and rash, febrile neutropenia, anorexia, hypotension, nausea, hematologic events (including anemia, leukopenia, thrombocytopenia, neutropenia, and febrile neutropenia), gastrointestinal events (including vomiting, nausea, and diarrhea), infections, capillary leak syndrome or systemic inflammatory response syndrome.

Epothilone

Mechanism of Action

Epothilones were first isolated as a fermentation product of the myxobacterium (*Sorangium cellulosum*) and were shown to have taxane-like activity causing microtubule stabilization. Ixabepilone (BMS-247550) is a semisynthetic epothilone B derivative in which the macrolide ring oxygen atom is replaced with a nitrogen atom to give the corresponding macrolactam. Both *in vitro* and *in vivo*, ixabepilone retains cytotoxic activity in tumor cells that are intrinsically insensitive to paclitaxel and in lines selected for acquired resistance to paclitaxel.[13]

Indications

Tried in rhabdomyosarcoma, neuroblastoma, and Wilms' tumor. In addition, it has also been tried in anaplastic astrocytoma and ependymoma xenografts.

Dosage in Children

30 to 40 mg/m^2, 3 weekly

Side Effects

The dose-limiting toxicity was neutropenia. Other side effects include cumulative neuropathy, arthralgia, myalgia, anorexia, nausea, and diarrhea.

Nelarabine (506U78)

It is a pro-drug for ara-G (9-bd arabinoferanosyl-guanine), endogenous toxic compound in T-cells. It is converted to ara-G by adenosine de-aminase. It has completed phase II trials in both children and adults with relapsed or refractory T-ALL. It has FDA approval for refractory T-ALL.[14-16]

Dosage: 900 mg/m^2/day continuous IV infusion × 5 days (children)

Neurotoxicity is the dose-limiting side effect.

Betulinic Acid

Betulinic acid, a natural component isolated from Birch trees, effectively induces apoptosis in neuroectodermal and epithelial tumor cells and exerts little toxicity in animal trials.[17,18] Betulinic acid has been reported to induce apoptosis in human melanoma with in vitro and in vivo model systems. Melanoma, like neuroblastoma, is derived from the neural crest cell. It is proposed that neuroblastoma cells have the machinery for programed cell death and that apoptosis could be induced by betulinic acid. Betulinic acid has been shown to induce apoptosis in neuroblastoma in vitro. It has also been shown that betulinic acid induced marked apoptosis in primary pediatric acute leukemia cells and all leukemia cell lines tested. When compared for in vitro efficiency with conventionally used cytotoxic drugs, betulinic acid was found to be more potent than standard therapeutics and especially efficient in tumor relapse. No cross resistances were found between betulinic acid and any cytotoxic drug. Intracellular apoptosis signaling in leukemia tumor cells paralleled the pathway found in neuroectodermal cells involving caspases, but not death receptors. Betulinic acid potently induced apoptosis in leukemia cells and thus is a candidate for further evaluation as a future drug to treat leukemia.

Liposomal Encapsulated Drugs

Liposomal Vincristine and Daunorubicin, Pegasparaginase or Clofarabine

They offer the ability to infuse higher total doses of the native drug, resulting in greater tumor cell uptake with no increase in neurotoxicity (vincristine) or cardiac toxicity (daunorubicin). They have a prolonged half-life compared with the free drug and preferential uptake into tumor cells. These are in various phases of clinical trials.[19]

Targeting Cyclin D1, A Downstream Effector of INI1/HSNF5

INI1/hSNF5 is a tumor suppressor biallelically inactivated in rhabdoid tumors, one of the aggressive and currently incurable pediatric malignancies. It has been shown that cyclin D1 is a key downstream target of INI1/hSNF5 and genesis and/or survival of rhabdoid tumors in vivo is critically dependent on the presence of cyclin D1. It has been observed in studies that RNA interference of cyclin D1 in rhabdoid cells was sufficient to induce G1 arrest and apoptosis. Furthermore, pharmacological intervention with low micromolar concentrations of N-(4-hydroxyphenyl) retinamide (4-HPR), which downmodulates cyclin D1, induced G1 arrest and apoptosis in rhabdoid cell lines. 4-HPR in combination with 4-hydroxy-tamoxifen (4OH-Tam), synergistically inhibited survival as well as anchorage-dependent and -independent growth of rhabdoid cells and caused synergistic induction of cell cycle arrest and apoptosis. 4-HPR and tamoxifen exhibited synergistic growth inhibition of RTs in xenograft models in vivo. The effects of combination of drugs were correlated to the depletion of cyclin D1 levels both in in vitro and in vivo tumor models.[20] These demonstrate that 4-HPR and tamoxifen are effective chemotherapeutic agents for rhabdoid tumors. Thus cyclin D1 is a potential future target for treatment of certain childhood malignancies.

Other Approaches

Recent approaches that have been the focus of considerable attention in the treatment of adult malignant brain tumors include interstitial administration of chemotherapeutic agents using time-release polymers and convection-enhanced delivery of immunotoxin conjugates targeted to receptors overexpressed in brain tumors relative to normal brain cells. Although it remains to be determined whether these approaches will lead to meaningful improvements in disease control and long-term prognosis in children with brain tumors, the encouraging results from studies in adults support the rationale for further exploring these strategies in the pediatric setting.

The impact of monoclonal antibodies (mAbs) in the treatment of human tumors has greatly increased in recent years. mAb engineering has allowed reducing the immunogenicity of therapeutic antibodies as well as improving their biodistribution. Furthermore, engineered mAbs have been used to vehiculate toxins, drugs and other antineoplastic agents to the tumor site. In the case of neuroblastoma (NB), a pediatric malignancy originating from the neural crest, both murine and chimeric antibodies against the tumor associated antigen GD2 have been tested in clinical trials, either alone or in combination with cytokines. A novel promising approach to mAb engineering is the small immunoprotein (SIP) technique, whereby the variable regions of heavy and light chains of a mAb with a given specificity are connected to the dimerizing CH(3) domain of an immunoglobulin molecule. The SIP technique is being currently studied for neuroblastoma.[21]

Other new biologically based treatment approaches, for example tumor vaccines, differentiating agents, immunotherapy, growth factor inhibitors, gene therapy etc., which promise to provide more rational and selective therapy for childhood cancers are being developed.[22]

The success of chemotherapy in children will ultimately depend on various factors related to the type and stage of tumor, host responses and the drug itself.

REFERENCES

1. Hirschfeld S, Ho PT, Smith M, Pazdur R. Regulatory Approvals of Pediatric Oncology Drugs: Previous Experience and New Initiatives. Journal of Clinical Oncology 2003;21:1066-73.
2. Devita Jr VT, Hellman S, Rosenberg SA. (Eds). Cancer: Principles and Practice of Oncology. 3rd Edition, JB Lippincott Co, Philadelphia, 1989.
3. Haskell CM, (Ed.) Cancer treatment, 3rd ed. Philadelphia: WB Saunders Co, 1990.
4. Pizzo P, Poplack D. (Eds). Principles and Practice of Pediatric Oncology. 4th Edition, Lippincott William and Wilkins, Philadelphia, 2002.
5. Chabner BA, Amrein PC, Druker BJ, Michaelson MD, Mitsiades CS, Goss PE, et al. Antineoplastic agents. In: Brunton LL, (Ed.) Goodman and Gilman's The Pharmacological Basis of Therapeutics. 11th edition. McGraw–Hill, New York 2006:1315-403.
6. Misiura K. Ifosfamide. Metabolic studies, new therapeutic approaches and new analogs. Mini Rev Med Chem 2006;6(4):395-400.
7. Jurgens H, Treuner J, Winkler K, Gobel U. Ifosfamide in pediatric malignancies. Semin Oncol 1989;16(1 Suppl 3):46-50.
8. Bomgaars L, Berg SL, Blaney SM. The development of camptothecin analogs in childhood cancers. Oncologist 2001;6(6):506-16.
9. Durker BJ, Sayers CL, Kantarjian H, et al. Activity of specific inhibitor of the BCR-ABL tyrosine kinase in blast crisis of CML and AML with Philadelphia chromosome. N Engl J Med 2001;344:1038-42.
10. Kantarjian H, Sawyer C, Hochhaus A, et al. Hematological and cytogenetic response to Imatinib mesylate in CML. N Engl J Med 2002;346:645-52.
11. Jeha S, Gaynon PS, Razzouk BI, Franklin J, Kadota R, Shen V, et al. Phase II study of clofarabine in pediatric patients with refractory or relapsed acute lymphoblastic leukemia. J Clin Oncol 2006;24(12):1917-23.
12. Faderl S, Gandhi V, Keating MJ, Jeha S, Plunkett W, Kantarjian HM. The role of clofarabine in hematologic and solid malignancies—development of a next-generation nucleoside analog. Cancer 2005;103(10):1985-95.
13. Peterson JK, Tucker C, Favours E, Cheshire PJ, Creech J, Billups CA. In vivo evaluation of ixabepilone (BMS247550), a novel epothilone B derivative, against pediatric cancer models. Clin Cancer Res 2005;11(19 Pt 1):6950-8.
14. Roecker AM,Allison JC, Kisor DF. Nelarabine: efficacy in the treatment of clinical malignancies. Future Oncol 2006;2(4):441-8.
15. Cohen MH, Johnson JR, Massie T, Sridhara R, McGuinn WD Jr, Abraham S, et al. Approval summary: nelarabine for the treatment of T-cell lymphoblastic leukemia/lymphoma. Clin Cancer Res 2006;12(18):5329-35.
16. Gandhi V, Plunkett W. Clofarabine and nelarabine: two new purine nucleoside analogs. Curr Opin Oncol 2006;18(6):584-90.
17. Ehrhardt H, Fulda S, Fuhrer M, Debatin KM, Jeremias I. Betulinic acid-induced apoptosis in leukemia cells. Leukemia 2004;18(8):1406-12.
18. Schmidt ML, Kuzmanoff KL, Ling-Indeck L, Pezzuto JM. Betulinic acid induces apoptosis in human neuroblastoma cell lines. Eur J Cancer 1997;33(12):2007-10.
19. Pollack IF, Keating R. New delivery approaches for pediatric brain tumors. J Neurooncol 2005;75(3):315-26.
20. Alarcon-Vargas D, Zhang Z, Agarwal B, Challagulla K, Mani S, Kalpana GV. Targeting cyclin D1, a downstream effector of INI1/hSNF5, in rhabdoid tumors. Oncogene 2006;25(5):722-34.
21. Bestagno M, Occhino M, Corrias MV, Burrone O, Pistoia V. Recombinant antibodies in the immunotherapy of neuroblastoma: perspectives of new developments. Cancer Lett 2003;197(1-2):193-8.
22. Balis FM. The challenge of developing new therapies for childhood cancers. Oncologist 1997;2(1):1-11.

CHAPTER 51

GK Rath
Partha Mukhopadhyay
Kalinga K Naik
PK Julka

Radiotherapy in Pediatric Malignancies

BASICS OF RADIATION ONCOLOGY

Radiation oncology is the branch of medicine that is concerned with the treatment of neoplastic diseases and selected benign conditions with ionizing radiation.

The radiation can be divided into:
  i. Electromagnetic radiation and
  ii. Corpuscular radiation

X-rays and gamma rays are forms of electromagnetic radiation, whereas electrons, protons, neutrons, alpha particles, etc are grouped together as corpuscular radiation.

The radiation effect is produced by the energy absorbed on living tissues through the process of ionization and excitation of the atom and molecules that form these tissues. The "radiation dose" is the amount of energy absorbed by the tissues. The radiotherapy can be administered from a distance (i.e. teletherapy) or by placing radiation sources very near or within the tumor (i.e. brachytherapy). This involves expensive and sophisticated machines for planning and execution and both involve certain complexities. However precise is the method of delivery of radiation, it is inevitable that some radiation dose will be delivered to the tissues in the body that are not the intended main targets of treatment. However, the methods of irradiation can be optimized so that the damage to such incidentally irradiated tissues is minimal.

CAUSES OF SUCCESS OR FAILURE OF RADIOTHERAPY

Tumor Factors

  i. *Radiosensitivity* – It is an inherent property of the tumor cells. Tumors vary in radiosensitivity; seminoma and lymphoma are the most radio-sensitive. Gliomas and soft tissue sarcomas are relatively radiononresponsive but radiotherapy is still of value postoperatively for microscopic disease.
  ii. *Tumor volume* – Radiation can eradicate small tumors more easily than large tumors that have more cells, also a higher proportion of hypoxic cells and non-cycling (G0) cells that are less radiosensitive.
  iii. *Tumor site* – The curability of a tumor depends also on the dose permissible to the adjacent normal tissues, since they are inevitably included in the radiation field.

Normal Tissue Factors

An understanding of how radiation can affect normal tissues is crucial to the safe practice of radiotherapy. The most sensitive organs are the bone marrow, gonads, gut mucosa, lymphatic tissue and the lens of the eye. Kidney, liver, lung, skin, breast, gut and marrow tissue are moderately radiosensitive while bone, connective tissue and muscle are relatively insensitive.

TREATMENT PLANNING

Optimization

The practice of radiation oncology has the primary goals of curing disease and sparing normal tissues. However, the therapeutic ratio, i.e. effect on tumor/effect on normal tissue is not large in the treatment of cancer. Thus extreme care must be taken to ensure that the treatment is optimum in order to maintain the gain in therapeutic ratio. Since the dose-response curves for radiation effect are very steep, the first goal is to deliver a homogenous dose into the volume to be treated. If given one small portion of a tumor is significantly underdosed the treatment will fail, on the other hand of a small portion of the treated volume containing a normal tissue is significantly overdosed, a treatment complication may result. Therefore, the challenge is to design radiotherapy treatment, so that the best possibility of tumor cure can be achieved without a significant risk of serious complications. The factors in planning include the volume to be treated and the dose to be given.

Volume

The tolerance to radiation diminishes as the treatment volume increases. The goal is to treat as small a volume as possible, yet adequate enough to treat every tumor cell. Five different types of volumes have been defined.

The gross tumor volume (GTV) denotes the demonstrated tumor. The clinical target volume (CTV) denotes the demonstrated tumor (when present) and also volumes with suspected (subclinical) tumor (e.g. margin around the GTV, and regional lymph nodes, that are considered to need treatment). The planning target volume (PTV) consists of the CTV(s) and a margin to account for variation in size, shape and position relative to the treatment beam(s). It is thus a geometric concept, used to ensure that the CTV receives the prescribed dose. Treated volume (TV) is the volume that receives a dose that is considered significant for local cure or palliation. Irradiated volume (IV) is the volume that receives a dose that is considered significant for normal tissue tolerance.

To limit the dose to normal tissue volumes, the treatment planning must include some method of defining dose volume limitations in the volume outside the target. In practice, the plotting of one or more "limiting isodose" contours can set the limitations of dosage and volume. For the advantage of the radiation oncologist and the physicist, these isodose contours can be defined by values corresponding to the percentage of the maximum dose.

Shrinking Volumes

Knowledge of modern radiobiology allows us to estimate the radiation doses needed to sterilize cells. Since a solid tumor invades and spreads to the adjoining tissues by sending out small number of cancerous cells, we can think of more than one target volume at different dose levels. In the practice of radiation oncology this involves the initial definition of a larger volume that after a certain

dose is given, is reduced to a smaller volume. This concept helps in two ways: it permits a larger than usual treatment volume to be used which enhances the tissue tolerance because of the lower dose to that volume and it permits a higher dose than usual to the second or "cone down": volume which encompasses the more radio-resistant solid central portion of the tumor. This technique often referred to as "field within the field" technique.

Dosage

The term dosage includes all the factors in delivering radiation to a specific point or volume in the patient. These factors include the dose per fraction, the number of fraction, the overall time of treatment and the structure of fractions within the overall time. In the case of brachytherapy, a very important additional factor is dose rate. Dosage schedules are as follows:

- *Normal fractionation* – 5 (range 4-6) fractions per week.
- *Hypofractionation* – less than 4 fractions per week @ one fraction per day.
- *Hyperfractionation* – two or more fraction per day (of reduced size) with overall time similar to normal fractionation.
- *Accelerated hyperfractionation* – two or more fractions per day (of reduced size) with reduced overall time
- *Split course schedule* – generally two abbreviated course of normal fractionation separated by 1 to 2 weeks of rest.

Tumor Lethal Dose

It is a well-known fact that infinitely large tumor dose can cure any cancer, but we are ultimately limited by normal tissue tolerance. Thus, there has developed, by practical experience, a concept of 'tumor dose', which in reality reflects the limit imposed by normal tissue and exposes the best possible dose schedule. From clinical experience and radiobiological assumptions, the dose needed to cure 100% of very small cancers is considerably less where the probability of cure by radical dose of radiation rapidly diminishes when the tumor volumes exceeds 100 cm^3. In addition to numerous other criticisms, the use of empirical equation to calculate tumor dose schedules is seriously limited by this fact. The NSD concept and its corollary TDF system is used to equate different dose schedules (TDF values are valid for overall treatment times between 3 and 6 weeks at the rate of 5 fractions per week). A TDF value between 90 to 100 can cure a majority T1 cancers while for a T3 cancer, a TDF of 110 to 120 may be necessary. Similarly Hodgkin's disease can be cured with a TDF of about 70 and seminomas by a TDF value of 50.

Tolerance Dose

Just as we attempt to estimate the probability of cure with specific doses, it is also important to estimate the probability of complications. An estimate of complication probability should include some geometric value, i.e. volume, area (for the skin) or length (for the spinal cord), as well as dose. In practice, one or more treatment planning contours are taken in the region of interest. The target volume and critical normal organs or tissues (kidney, cord lung for example) are also traced. Thereafter, the clinician traces isodose contours with limiting doses in terms of percentage maximum dose.

Optimization Procedure

The treatment plan should be optimized by giving:
- The highest and most homogenous dose contributions to the target volume.
- The lowest possible dose contributions to the organs at risk outside the target volume.
- The highest possible ratio of integral dose contributions in the target volume to integral dose to tissue outside the volume.

A good plan is usually a simple plan with as few fields as well serve the purpose. The patient treatment position (in which the contours are obtained) should be as comfortable as possible and reproducible. For a given beam, the most efficient path is through the nearest surface, for telecobalt, any path longer than 12 cm is relatively inefficient. Isocentric techniques are easy to set up but an indiscriminate number of beams can be inefficient. Three field techniques may be desirable in many clinician situations but require accurate contour, localization and verification.

Field Arrangements

For single field treatments, an applied dose is used where the radiotherapist wishes to prescribe the dose on the skin surface or a depth dose where the dose must be given a certain depth. With megavoltage beams, the maximum dose is not delivered to the skin but at a level below the skin, which increases with increasing beam energy (Table 51.1).

Table 51.1: Skin depth for delivery of maximum doses for megavoltage beans

Photon beam energy	Depth (cm) for percentages of max dose		
	100%	80%	50%
250 KV	0	3.0	6.8
Co^{60}	0.5	4.7	11.6
4MV	1.0	5.6	13.0
6MV	1.2	6.8	15.6
10MV	2.0	7.8	19.0
25MV	3.0	10.2	21.8

If the radiation oncologist wishes to ensure that part or the entire surface receives the maximum dose, then it is necessary to apply bolus, i.e. tissue equivalent material (wax or wet gauze) of a thickness equivalent to the build up depth for the energy of radiation. This is commonly done where scars needs to be treated or tumor involves skin or is close to the surface. Parallel opposing plain fields are suitable for many clinical situations, e.g. in pelvis, abdomen, head and neck. Where the body contour is not uniform throughout the field, tissue compensation may be necessary. Parallel-unwedged fields are normally used with equal weighting, but the lesions not in the midline (e.g. in brain) 2:1 or 3:1 weighing may be used (from the affected side). Most paired field arrangements, other than parallel fields, will employ the use of wedges, which angles the dose distribution helping to restore the dose homogeneity.

Three-or-four-field plans are commonly used for deep tumors, e.g. esophagus, bladder, prostate, cervix. Higher energy beams have greater skin sparing, better dose at depth, sharper penumbra and greater bone sparing than telecobalt. In parallel opposing fields with separations of 18 cm or more, e.g. in obese patients or in lateral pelvic fields, telecobalt gives too low a dose at the midplane. On the other hand, the higher energy machine is not superior in all clinical situations. For whole brain treatment, with parallel opposing fields, telecobalt gives a superior distribution compared to a higher energy linear accelerator.

The clinical significance of election beams lie in the sharp cut off of dose at a depth. As a rule of thumb, their range in cm is about 50% of their energy in MeV and their 80% isodose curve is about one-third of their energy in MeV.

Shielding blocks are used when a critical organ lies within or close to the treatment volume. They are usually made of lead. Full shields are usually five or six half-value layers while partial transmission shields are one half-value layer.

Thus, essentially we see that the intent of radiation therapy is to treated the tumor along with its microscopic extensions homogeneously to a dose which sterilizes the tumor cells and at the same time does not lead to increased normal tissue complications.

PEDIATRIC RADIATION ONCOLOGY

Cancer by itself accounts for 6.8 cases for 100,000 population below the age of 15 years.[1] The incidence of death due to cancer under 15 years is 1.7 and 0.6% in developed and developing countries.[2] Thus pediatric oncology as a subspecialty is still developing in India and other developing countries. Table 51.2 outlines the relative frequency and survival in childhood malignancy. Table 51.3 gives the adverse effects of radiation treatment of pediatric malignancy.

Table 51.2: Relative frequency and survival in childhood cancer[3]			
Tumor	Incidence/ million year	Total %	5 year survival rate %
Leukemia	30	31	–
ALL	25	NA	70%
AML	05	NA	26%
Brain tumors	20	19	50%
Lymphoma	17	13	–
Hodgkin's	08	NA	88%
NHL	09	NA	70%
Neuroblastoma	08	07	43%
Wilm's tumor	07	06	79%
Soft tissue sarcoma	05	07	61%
Osteosarcoma	03	02	54%
Ewing's sarcoma	02	02	42%
Retinoblastoma	03	03	91%
Germ cell tumors	05	02	84%

Table 51.3: Adverse effects of radiation treatment of pediatric malignancies

1. Stunting
  a. Generalized stunting, e.g. in treatment of gliomas and CNS prophylaxis in ALL due to hypopituitarism.
  b. Localized stunting, e.g. retinoblastoma – RT.
  c. Individual visceral morbidity, e.g. hypodevelopment of breast in mantle field irradiation, kyphoscolios.
2. Intellectual and neuropsychiatric defect.
3. Development of second malignancy.

Pediatric malignancies should be managed in a specialized manner and the successful management of these patients, require a carefully organized centre.[3]

The practice of pediatric oncology requires a team of skillful diagnostic specialists, surgeons, radiation oncologists and pediatric oncologists. As in adult cancers, the main modalities of treatment, i.e. surgery, radiotherapy and chemotherapy remain the same. However their application in children is different. Presently, surgery has a definite role to play on the diagnosis (biopsy) and therapy (organ preserving surgery). The radical and the extraradical surgical techniques are being replaced by conservative surgery in order to minimize the disability and deformity, whereas radiotherapy and chemotherapy have come in a big way in the cancer care of children.

Since the advent of megavoltage teleradiotherapy, the radiation therapy of childhood cancers has become more precise with significant reduction in morbidity.

Radiation is an indispensable part of multidisciplinary cancer management, more so in pediatric oncology. Despite growing concern about long-term effects of irradiation in a child, radiotherapy has not yet been replaced completely. The goal of radiotherapy in pediatric malignancy is to deliver a tumoricidal dose for a particular neoplasm while sparing as much normal tissue as possible. The successfully treated children may be at risk of a variety of organ-related complications. The efforts are on to reduce the radiation dose, alter the fractionation, fraction size and if possible to avoid radiotherapy altogether.

The therapeutic doses of radiation in childhood cancers is 20% less than the adult dose. Weekly tumor dose is reduced to 850-900 cGy per fraction in childhood cancer as compared to conventional 10 Gy in five fractions per week. The reduction in the total dose and fraction size can cement the complication rate.

The vital sensitive structures should be shielded from direct exposure to radiation whenever possible especially the growing epiphyseal ends, gonads, liver, thyroid, spinal cord, pituitary gland, etc. Inclusion of molar teeth area in the radiation field can lead to its maldevelopment. In radiation treatment of head and neck area, especially in maxilla and nasopharynx, the last molar teeth are shielded on the lateral portal. The developmental changes are marked at a dose beyond 45 to 50Gy. The doses of radiation are more fractionated (i.e. the total dose of radiation is given in a more protracted time) to decrease the late morbidity.

Immobilization of the child during radiotherapy is very important for proper and precise delivery of radiation more so in small cranial fields and ophthalmic tumor. The children below the age of 4 are usually apprehensive and phobic and they rarely agree to lie still during radiotherapy on the treatment couch. These children need good anesthetic support during treatment. With the availability of ketamine and propofol anesthesia, repeated anesthetic procedure during radiotherapy is rarely a problem. The immobilization devices used most frequently are head fixation device, immobilization neck rest, arm rest, blocks, mouth bite, etc. Whenever feasible megavoltage beam of 4 to 6MV should be recommended, but telecobalt therapy machines can be used where facilities for linear accelerator are not available. All fields should be treated daily to avoid radiobiological disadvantages. In order to overcome the tissue deficit, appropriate compensators and wedges should be utilized. The gap junctions should be managed with expertise and they should be arranged in such a way that there is no underdosing of tumor and overdosing of critical structures. Use of multiple junctions, double wedge fields and determined gap are a few methods to avoid gap junction problem.

Pediatric Brachytherapy

Many studies have reported improvement of both disease free and actuarial survival rates with the help of brachytherapy. Gerbaulet et al has reported the results of treatment in 45 children with head and neck and pelvic tumors. The patients were treated with iridium-192 interstitial removable implant with or without chemotherapy, partial resection and external radiotherapy. The long-term survival without evidence of disease was 78% and the survival ranged from 2 to 9.5 years.[4]

Most of the complications associated with external beam radiotherapy, i.e. disturbances in growth, development of physiological impairment of the organ function are due to the large treatment volume and high radiation dose. The complication rates are inversely proportional to the age of the child. Brachytherapy has the advantage of very sharp dose fall off thereby having a preferential dose distribution between the tumor and the normal tissue. Thus brachytherapy minimizes radiotherapy related adverse effects both short term and long term. Brachytherapy in conjunction with external radiotherapy and combination chemotherapy can minimize the extent of surgery and late radiation effects. Though brachytherapy has not been used very extensively in pediatric malignancies, the indications include:
1. Tumors of the head and neck.
2. Tumors of female genital organs.

3. Urological malignancies.
4. Locally recurrent pediatric solid tumors.
5. As organ preserving therapy in pediatric sarcomas of head and neck region, trunk or limbs.

The isotopes most commonly used are Iridium-192 and Iodine-125. The optimum dose rates recommended for pediatric tumors are 30 to 60 cGy/hour in temporary (removable) implants and 6 to 8 cGy/hour in permanent implants.

The total dose of an implant depends upon site, size, prior radiation or chemotherapy and the surgical extent. The dose to the normal dose limiting structures, such as skin, spinal cord, rectum, bladder, small bowel, etc are calculated routinely during treatment planning.

RADIOTHERAPY IN LEUKEMIAS

The main role of radiotherapy in the treatment of leukemias lies in the prevention of CNS relapse. At the end of the induction phase the patient are evaluated for remission status both clinically and hematologically. The conventional definition of remission is the achievement of normal blood count (neutrophils >1.0 x 10^9/L, platelets > 100 x 10^9/L), hemoglobin concentration of more than 10 gm/dl, no evidence of extramedullary disease and blast count < 5% in cellular marrow. Now-a-days minimal residual disease can be effectively detected by immunological techniques. As soon as the remission is achieved, CNS prophylaxis is started. The CSF cytology should be negative before CNS prophylaxis is started, but in the current aggressive protocol of ALL management, the remission is not a prerequisite for CNS directed therapy.

It has been postulated that in the absence of CNS directed therapy, leukemia blasts invade the meninges and it has also been suggested that CNS directed radiotherapy early in remission could and eradicate the residual cells and prevent CNS relapse

Without CNS therapy the risk of CNS relapse is between 50 and 75% in both adults and children. The standard treatment practiced worldwide is a combination of whole brain irradiation and intermittent intrathecal methotrexate. The radiotherapy techniques for CNS directed therapy is based on the clinical experience and blood brain barrier making the brain parenchyma a sanctuary site. For the purpose of CNS irradiation a minimum dose of 18 Gy in 10 fractions over 2 weeks is necessary.[5]

Radiotherapy Volume

For preventive CNS therapy, the target volume of cranial irradiation includes the entire intracranial contents and the entire intracranial subarachnoid space.

The cranial margin is at the cranial vault and the caudal margin extends to the bottom of the second cervical vertebra. The anterior margin should include the posterior retina and orbital apex, encompassing the extension of the subarachnoid space along the optic nerves. The posterior margin should cover the entire occipital lobe and the covering meninges. The margins of the base of the skull should cover the cribriform plate and lower limit of the temporal fossa. Proper attention should be given in this margin as it has been shown by CT scan that the position of the cribriform plate relative to the orbital roofs can vary with age and the cribriform plate can be quite low. In order to cover the cribriform plate with a lateral beam it will be necessary, in most children, to encompass part of the superior retina.

When the craniospinal axis irradiation is the aim, the spinal field extends from below 2nd cervical vertebra (C2) upto 2nd sacral vertebra (S2). Currently spinal axis is omitted in the CNS directed therapy and this is substituted by the intrathecal methotrexate. The main purpose of avoiding spinal irradiation below C2 is to prevent late effects on the spinal column (growth retardation and second malignancy).

A parallel-opposed portal encompassing the entire cranium is commonly set up. A telecobalt unit or 4MV X-rays is optimum for treating such fields. At our center, the German helmet technique for irradiation of the whole cranial content upto 2nd cervical vertebra is followed. A posterior tilt of 5° is essential to avoid irradiating the opposite lens. The amount of "flash" beyond the scalp does not appear to be critical for linear accelerator beams.

For Co^{60} teletherapy, "flash" of 1cm or beyond the skull has been recommended. Some clinicians use a "half beam block" technique to avoid the question of divergence of the beams.

Alternatively, a slanting field technique can serve the purpose of taking a field size of 14 x 14 to 16 x 16 cm. The benefit of the German helmet technique is that the meningeal reflections are covered in their entirely. The slanting field does not include the anterior skull base, thus the cribriform plate and the orbital apex does not receive the tumoricidal radiation dose. For appropriate positioning, good head fixation is mandatory or an individualized immobilization cast is mandatory. The head should be kept over a desired headrest for accurate reproducibility of daily treatment set-up. Laser beam alignment is necessary while using isocentric technique. The prescribed dose is calculated at mid-plane.

In CNS preventive treatment, the radiotherapy is supplemented with spinal treatment by intrathecal methotrexate therapy in a dose of 9-12 mg/m^2 biweekly for 6 doses. The radiotherapy is started on the first day of intrathecal methotrexate.

In overt CNS leukemia, the dose of radiation is 24 Gy in 12 fractions.

The complications of CNS prophylaxis are mainly long-term sequelae. The possible consequences of RT to brain are somnolence, microangiopathy, demyelinating leucoencephalopathy and abnormality in the ventricular size. Moreover there is less than 1% chance of second malignancy in patients treated with chemoradiotherapy. Cranial irradiation is one of the most hazardous agent among survivors of leukemia, the other agents being anthracyclines, alkylating agents and epipodophyllotoxins.[5] Cranial irradiation leads to learning deficits, impaired pituitary function and a high risk of brain tumors. An alternative to cranial irradiation are IT MTX regimes, but many trials in this field have been unsatisfactory. Intravenous methotrexate and IT MTX in moderate doses results in higher CNS relapse rates. Cranial irradiation should be avoided under 2 years of age and on these children who are at good risk, only IT MTX alone may be used for CNS prophylaxis.

Testicular Leukemia

Testes are another sanctuary site of ALL where systemic chemotherapy has low penetration. Currently, overt testicular disease is present at diagnosis in approximately 2% of boys with ALL. It appears to respond adequately to systemic chemotherapy, without requiring subsequent testicular irradiation. Fifteen percent of boys with ALL develop testicular relapse. Patients with T-cell ALL and /or high WBC count are more likely to experience testicular relapse. The testicular relapse occuring during the period of therapy has a poorer prognosis as compared to the relapse occuring after the completion of therapy. Bone marrow relapse often follows the testicular relapse within 3 to 6 months. If there is no hematological relapse and the testis is the sole site of relapse than both the testes have to be irradiated.

The tumor volume includes, the entire scrotal region, and epidedymis and the spermatic cord bilaterally upto its entry into the original canal. The site is irradiated as a single enface field.

The dose is calculated at the surface of the testes. A dose of 24 Gy in 12 fractions over 2.5 weeks is usually recommended.[6] A telecobalt and 4MV X-ray or a 12 MeV electron beam can be chosen for this irradiation. Concomitant CNS and marrow relapse has poorer survival when compared to patients having only testicular relapse. Following testicular irradiation, systemic chemotherapy must be employed. For patients developing testicular relapse, it is recommended to switch over to alternative drug regimen.

Radiotherapy in Bone Marrow Transplantation (BMT)

Various preparative regimens are utilized to purge off the whole bone marrow of the cancer cells. Total body irradiation (TBI), usually with high dose cyclophosphamide has been used as a preparation for bone marrow transplantation since the inception of the procedure. With the introduction of fractionated program, TBI has been proven effective and the morbidity of the program has been reduced. There has been, however, considerable impetus to identify alternative, non-radiation programs for BMT preparation particularly in the pediatric population with the hope of reducing late effects of radiation.

International experience has shown that combined treatment strategy of high dose chemotherapy and TBI is probably superior to chemotherapy alone. The TBI fulfills three functions in allogenic bone marrow transplantation.

1. It has a direct, lethal effect on malignant cells.
2. It provides strong immunosuppression and prevents reactivation by donor's hemopoietic stem cells.
3. It creates space in the recipient's bone marrow, enabling the donor bone marrow cells to grow.

There are a large variety of techniques available for the administration of total body irradiation. The techniques include:

a. A lateral approach with patient supine and the collimator of the treatment machine rotated to fit the patient in the beam.
b. A lateral approach with the patient supine and the use of a very extended distance from the treatment machine to the patient so that a rectangular beam may be used.
c. A lateral approach with the patient in a semi-recumbent position and the collimator of the treatment machine rotated to fit the patient in the beam.
d. A specifically prepared TBI suite with one treatment machine mounted the ceiling and one on the floor

– the patient is placed on a treatment couch between the units.
e. A specially prepared TBI suite with two machines mounted at opposite ends of the room – the patient is irradiated in the lateral position while on a treatment couch between the units.
f. A conventional treatment unit is used with the patient on the floor of the treatment room, instead of on the treatment couch, to obtain the necessary extended distance.
g. The patient is seated on a specially designed seat to allow anterior and posterior treatment – some instructions use lung shielding during the proton treatment and then "boost" the ribs with electron beams.

Different method of TBI has been prachced. A single fraction TBI of 10 Gy along with cyclophosphamide has been used. Currently trachomated TBI is being practised to avoid late sequelae. The dose rate in such situation is approximately 5 cSU/min. A total dose of 12 Gy in 6 fraction is delivered by a telecobalt unit. Fractionated TBI requires the patient to be in the same position during radiotherapy to achieve homogenous dose distribution for each fraction.[7]

A randomized study in leukemia patient was conducted to investigate the effects of single dose 10 Gy (dose rate 6 cGy/min) versus fractionaled TBI of 2 Gy x 6, a total dose of 12 Gy at the same dose rate. The study found that during a 10 year observation period, fractionaled TBI could reduce the relapse rate from 22 to 11%.[8] The various complications of TBI are enumerated in Table 51.4.

Table 51.4: Complications of TBI	
Acute	*Late*
Nausea and vomiting	Interstitial pneumonia
Parotitis	Gonadal dysfunction
Mucosctis	Cataract
Diarrhea	Second neoplasm
Veno-occlusive disease	Graft versus
Alopecia	Host reaction

Radiotherapy in Extramedullary Leukemia Deposits

Radiotherapy is also indicated in leukemia patients having extensive malignant cell deposited in the vital structures of the body leading to acute symptoms. For extramedullary leukemia deposit due to ALL, the dose recommended is 6 Gy in 3 fractions or 30 Gy in 10 fractions. In AML deposit, the dose required is higher i.e. in the range of 40 Gy in 15 fractions. The tumor volume encompasses the gross tumor volume (GTV) with 1 to 2 cm margin.

Splenic irradiation

Splenomegaly is a frequent and significant finding in cases of chronic myeloid leukemia (CML). Radiotherapy in very low doses leads to dramatic regression of splenic size and the leucocyte count. Currently, however, the indication of radiotherapy is limited to refractory cases of CML who fail chemotherapy or there is low compliance of the patient to busulfan. Using a megavoltage beam, the spleen is covered partially by a fold size of 15x10 cm by AP-PA port. An incident dose of 25 cGy is prescribed on alternate days till the TLC falls to 10,000/mm^3 and platelets come to 80,000/mm^3. The daily dose may be increased upto 50 to 75 cGy in patients who show slow regression. The leukocyte and platelet count and the splenic size is monitored daily. The total dose required is upto 300 to 400 cGy and very rarely may require a dose upto 800 cGy. The TLC keeps on falling for another 2 weeks after completion of radiotherapy. The main caution for splenic irradiation is disproportionate thrombocytopenia and, hence, a strict vigil is necessary during the treatment.

RADIOTHERAPY IN PEDIATRIC LYMPHOMAS

Hodgkin's Disease

Hodgkin's disease is rare in the pediatric population. The incidence of Hodgkin's disease is patients below the age of 15 years constitutes approximately 10% of the entire population and constitutes 2 to 3% of all cases in children below 5 years of age.[9] It has been observed that HD in children occurs in the higher socioeconomic status group and in more advanced countries. The M:F ratio in children show a higher male preponderance (2.8:1) which decreases to 1.2:1 after adolescence.[10]

Radiotherapeutic Management

The treatment of childhood Hodgkin's disease follows similar guidelines according to stage as practiced in adults.

Success in the radiotherapeutic management of children with HD requires excellent technique. HD is one neoplasm where the outcome is improved due to advancement of the radiotherapy technology. The local control is proportionate to the total dose upto a dose of 3000 cGy and it attains a level of 93% at dose of 3000 cGy. Beyond that dose, there is a plateau in the dose response curve (Kaplan dose response curve). Hence it is unjustified to give a dose beyond 4000 cGy.[11] Therefore in HD, optimum local control can be achieved with a dose range of 3600 to 4000 cGy.

The recommended dose for involved site in 3600 cGy and for uninvolved site 3000 cGy. When radiotherapy is given after chemotherapy, the total dose for involved site in 2500 cGy.

The advent of megavoltage machines, specially the linear accelerator, has dramatically improved the radiation technique and treatment approaches.

The lymphatic involvement in HD is centripetal in distribution and is predictable along the longitudinal extent of the body. A good radiation dose with safe margin leads to improved local control. The radiotherapy can be given as.
1. Extended field radiotherapy, and
2. Involved field radiotherapy.

The extended field radiotherapy involves an extensive area, which includes approximately 50% the total bone marrow. A meticulous monitoring of the blood counts is therefore essential. Such extensive irradiation fields encompass many normal vital structures (lung, larynx, spinal cord, heart, gonads, kidney, etc) and they should be shielded before the threshold dose is reached. The set up reproducibility, choice of right energy and optimization is of great importance in planning RT to these regions.

Extended Field Irradiation

Mantle Field Technique

The mantle field requires meticulous technique because of the distribution of the lymph nodes on close proximity of normal vital structures. This technique involves all nodes from the base of the skull to the nodes at the level of the 10th thoracic vertebral level in a single field. A 4-6 MV linear accelerator or a cobalt unit (80-100 cm SSD) with 35 x 35 cm maximum field size is optimal. In case larger fields are required, the field size can be increased by extended SSD technique.

The mantle field can be simulated with the arms up over the head, or in the akimbo position (i.e. hands on the hips). The former position has the advantage of shifting of the axillary nodes away from the lungs, thus allowing greater and effective lung shielding. However the disadvantage is that the lymph nodes then come in the vicinity of the humeral heads that should be shielded in growing children. The optimum position is chosen after taking into consideration the nodes, the lungs and the humeral heads. The akimbo position has the advantage that the axilla is opened up. Thus exposing the nodes better and without the disadvantage of movement of the nodes nearer to the humeral heads. Equally weighted anterior and posterior fields that are treated daily are used. The dose is calculated at the midplane. When a full mantle is treated, nodes in the neck and axilla receive a higher dose because of the decreased patient thickness compared to the midthorax. Due to this reason, separate axillary, cervical and low mediastinal dosimetry should be performed. Increased source to skin distances decrease dose inhomogeneity in these different areas.

Field Design

Anterior Field

Superior border	: From mid point of chin extends laterally to 2 cm above mastoid tip
Inferior border	: 4 cm above xiphisternum
Lateral border	: Delto-pectoral groove
Inferior axillary border	: 4th costochondral junction
Medial border (upper mediastinum)	: 2-3 cm margin at hilum
Medial border (lower mediastinum)	: Vertebral width with 1.5 cm margin
Upper border of lung block	: 2 cm below clavicle

Posterior Field

Upper border: Thyroid notch
Lower border: Match the anterior field
Lateral border: Match the anterior field

Blocks in Mantle Field Irradiation

From the beginning of treatment	After an elapsed time period
1. Lung shields	1. Cervical spinal cord shield (after 20-30 day)
2. Humeral head	2. Cardiac apical shield
3. Laryngeal shields	
4. Occipital shields	
5. Lip shields	

While applying the shields either at the beginning of treatment or after an elapsed time period the point that must always be kept in mind is that shielding a normal structure should not block a diseased node.

Inverted Technique

For the subdiaphragmatic disease, when the disease is confined to the lower para-aortic and inguinofemoral

nodal areas, the inverted Y irradiation is given alone but it is combined with chemotherapy for unfavorable histological subtype.

Subtotal Nodal Irradiation

The subtotal lymphoid irradiation includes mantle field along with the splenic pedicle and the upper para-aortic nodes upto the lever of L1-L2. Two weeks of rest is advisable between the mantle and sub-diaphragmatic field in STLI.

Total Lymphoid (Nodal) Irradiation

The total lymphoid irradiation involves the fields for STLI + pelvic and inguino-femoral regions. The nodes included are:
  i. Parapharyngeal nodes.
  ii. Jugular nodal chain.
  iii. Axillary nodes.
  iv. Mediastinal nodes.
  v. Posterior intercostal nodes.
  vi. Hilar nodes.
  vii. Juxtavertebral nodes.
  viii. Paraesophageal nodes.
  ix. Diaphragmatic and paracardiac nodes behind xiphisternum.
  x. Splenic nodes, gastrosplenic ligament.
  xi. Hepatic nodes.
  xii. Para-aortic and pelvic nodes.
  xiii. Ilioinguinal and femoral nodes.

While treating the subdiapharagmatic region, the splenic pedicle must be included while minimizing the radiation dose to the kidneys. The upper pole of the left kidney comes into the irradiated volume. At the time of simulation an IVP, a treatment planning CT or a diagnostic CT/MRI are helpful in planing the shields.

While treating the pelvis, the testes and the ovaries should be given adequate attention. The ovaries should be relocated and their new position should be marked by surgical clips thus helping in preparing and placing appropriate shields. The testes receive 5% to 10% of the administered. Pelvic dose which is sufficient to cause transient to permanent azoospermia. The testes can be shielded by external shielding, internal shielding with tungsten, or with the help of multi leaf collimator.

Involved Field Radiotherapy (IFRT)

Involved field radiotherapy (IFRT) is the use of minimal field for the radiotheraputic treatment. The indications of IFRT are for bulky residual disease after completion of effective chemotherapy and for Stage IA disease. (Lymphocyte predominance).

The primary rate with one lymphatic region is incorporated into the target volume. The dose recommended is 3600 cGy in 20 fraction for radiotherapy alone but the dose is reduced to 25 cGy when chemotherapy is followed by radiotherapy.

IFRT is preferable over extended field. RT whenever chemotherapy is used in combination with irradiation.

A linear accelerator with 4-6 MV X-ray energy is preferred for treatment in the region of head and neck and mediastinum, whereas higher energy beams (10-18 MV X-rays) are preferred for para-aortic and pelvic nodal irradiation. Shielding of the sensitive structures (i.e. teeth, epiphyses, uninvolved lung, ear, spinal cord, liver, kidney, gonads, etc) with appropriate shields reduces the chance of late complications.

Consideration of the total dose of radiation is of paramount importance for children suffering from HD. In case of a complete response after 6 cycles of chemotherapy a dose of 15 to 25 Gy is sufficient.[12] Patients who do not show complete response to chemotherapy are more likely to show a persistent disease or local recurrence after radiotherapy. For the children who are treated with radiation alone, the clinically evident disease should receive 30 to 35Gy and the subclinical disease should be treated with a dose of 25 to 30 Gy. This higher dose is also preferred in patient who show residual disease after 6 cycles of chemotherapy. For the majority of patients with pediatric HD, it is now accepted that, 3 to 4 cycles of ABVD chemotherapy followed by 15 to 25 Gy of IFRT is adequate.

Non Hodgkin's Lymphoma

The role of radiotherapy in pediatric NHL is also declining as it is true for all other childhood neoplasms. The indications for radiotherapy in children suffering from NHL are as follows:

1. In localized lesion (I,IE) involving one lymph node regions—curative RT may be recommended.
2. AS IFRT is localized disease (Stage I, II) after chemotherapy.
3. In extramural cord compression—as emergency RT
4. Cranial RT
   - Prophylaxis after induction of remission.
   - Overt CNS leukemia.
   - Carcinomatous meningitis.

- In frank leukemia as a prerequisite for BMT.
- Superior vena caval obstruction.
- Spinal irradiation – in established cases of CNS disease.
- Total Body irradiation – as a prerequisite for BMT.
- Whole abdomen RT – for abdominal lymph nodes.

Currently for localized disease (Stage I-II).

Chemotherapy followed by IFRT is recommended.

Three cycles of chemotherapy followed by IFRT 36 to 40 Gy gives a 10-year survival of approximately 80%.[13]

The cranial irradiation is given by the German Helmet techniques and the recommended dose is 24 Gy in 12 fractions. When intrathecal methotrexate is not used whole cerebrospinal axis need to be irradiated. The incidence of leukoencephalopathy is about 1 to 2% with CSI alone which increases to approximately 15% with the use of both cranial RT and intrathecal MTX.

For abdominal lymphomatous deposit, the whole abdomen is at risk. Hence, the whole abdomen irradiated in a dose of 20 Gy in 20 fraction over 4 weeks. In SVCO, a dose of 7.5 to 15 Gy in 3 fractions is recommended. Bone disease is treated with local radiotherapy to a dose of 30 Gy in 10 fractions. The dose recommended by TBI varies from 8 to 12 Gy with a dose rate of approximately 5 cGy/min. The current protocols of TBI insist on a dose rate of about 2.5 cGy/min from telecobalt unit and 4 cGy/min from linear accelerator. The treatment time varies between 5 to 8 hours. The average total tumor dose at midplane is approximately 9.5 Gy.

WILMS' TUMOR

Children with Wilm's tumor tend to present with more advanced stage disease in less developed nations. The median age at diagnosis is 41.5 months for males with unilateral tumor and 46.9 months for females with unilateral tumors. For bilateral tumors the median age at presentation is 29.5 months for males and 32.6 months for females.

Prognostic Factors

1. Stage of the disease.
2. Favorable or unfavorable histology.
3. Metastases at presentation.
4. Regional lymph node involvement.
5. Hyperdiploidy which correlate well with anaplstic variety.

Management

Treatment Option Overview

Therapy consists of surgery followed by chemotherapy and, in some patients, radiation therapy. Pulmonary nodules not detected on chest radiographs but visible on computed tomography of the chest do not mandate treatment with whole-lung irradiation.

The treatment of WT is multimodal in nature. An optimum balance of surgery, chemotherapy and radiotherapy is of utmost importance and it is essential to offer the correct sequence of therapy. The NWTS, SIOP and the United Kingdom Children's Cancer Study Group (UKCCSG) have gathered a large body of information concerning the clinical management of WT. The most widely and often quoted studies are those of NWTS and SIOP.

The four main aims of NWTS is to:

1. Stratify according to the histologic type.
2. Eliminate radiotherapy as far as possible.
3. Use combination chemotherapy.
4. Identify risk group.

The aim of SIOP is to:

1. Down stage the tumor.
2. Treatment tailored according to the intra-operative findings.

Currently, the recommendation of the NWTS protocols are practiced the world over. Surgery is always the first treatment in operable cases. In case of inoperability due to extensive intra-abdominal disease induction chemotherapy is administered.

The sequencing of treatment is surgery → radiotherapy → chemotherapy in the operable cases or induction chemotherapy → surgery → radiotherapy and chemotherapy in the inoperable cases. The treatment needs to be individualized in case of advanced Stage IV and Stage V disease.

Radiotherapy

Wilm's tumor is highly radiosensitive, and it is possess to achieve a are even without chemotherapy. The radiotherapy dose has varied from 10 Gy to 40 Gy. But over the years, the use of radiation has been reduced. This is due to the awareness and documentation of radiation related late effects (growth disturbances, second cancer) in growing children of WT. The NWTS group has redefined the role of radiotherapy and it has provided specific recommendations so that minimum possible RT dose is administered. The NWTS-3 has documented that there is no survival difference at doses of 10 Gy or 20 Gy in stage III, FH group. The recommended dose per fraction is 1.2 to 1.5 Gy and it should not exceed 1.8 Gy per fraction with concomitant chemotherapy. The current indications of RT are:

1. Stage II,III,IV with unfavorable histology
2. Stage III and IV with favorable histology
3. Metastatic disease
4. CCSK, in all stages

The postoperative radiotherapy is started within 10 days of surgery because delay beyond 10 days leads to tumor cell repopulating and increase in relapse rate. It has been shown that appropriate adjuvant RT reduces the postoperative recurrence to 0-4% in children with favorable histology. The dose of radiotherapy has decreased to approximately 10 Gy from the doses of 25 to 30 Gy that were recommended in the past. In the NWTS-3 patients with group III favorable histology were treated with an external RT dose of 20 Gy or 10 Gy. The control rate and survival were statistically same. Therefore, NWTS-4 has recommended a radiotherapy dose of 1080 cGy is the abdomen for Stage III and IV disease.

NWTS: Volume of radiation fields in Stage III and IV disease

Extent of disease	Volume of radiation field necessary
• Hilar nodes*	Flank RT, crossing midline to
• Gross or microscopic residual disease confined to flank and/or paraaortic nodes	include B/L PA nodes, margins above and below renal poles
• Peritoneal seeding	Whole abdominal RT*
• Gross residual abdominal disease	
• Preoperative/intraoperative rupture	

*Local boost radiotherapy 1080 cGy supplements is be given to volume measuring e" 3 cm in maximum diameter.

TTD	180 cGy/day X 6 days or 150 cGy/day X 7 days 1080 cGy dose coned down boost for residual disease >3 cm.
Gross spillage	1050 cGy, 1500 cGy/ day X 7 days
Pulmonary RT	1200 TTD, 150 cGy/ day X 8 days
Bone metastases	3060 cGy, 180 cGy/ day X 17 fractions

According to the NWT-5 protocol, radiotherapy is advocated for stage II focal and diffuse anaplasia, Stage III, Stage IV, Stage I-IV clear cell sarcoma of kidney and Stage I-IV Rhabdoid tumor of kidney.

Technique of Radiotherapy

The prerequisite for administration of external beam radiotherapy is immobilization and short anesthesia (either Ketamine or Propofol). Cooperative children above approximately 5 years of age can be treated without anesthesia. There after the tumor volume is determined from the CT scan evidence of disease extent, surgical clips, surgico-pathologic findings and clinical examination. The postoperative irradiation portals are either whole abdomen or local blank region.

Field Margins for Local Flank RT

Upper border:	Diaphragm on left side or variable portion of liver on right side
Lower border:	Dictated by preoperative CT scan, 1-2 cm beyond tumor limit
Medial border:	Entire breadth of the vertebral body with adequate C/L extension to include entire paraaortic group of nodes
Lateral border:	1 to 2 cm lateral to the peritoneal reflection

Field Margins for Whole Abdominal RT

Upper border:	Diaphragm
Lower border:	Lower border of obturator foramen
Lateral borders:	1 to 2 cm lateral to the peritoneal reflection

Megavoltage beams (Cobalt-60 or Linear Accelerator 4-6 MV) are preferred. The daily dose as described earlier is limited to 150 to 180 cGy per day. Whenever possible immobilization cast or an alfa-cradle should be used for repositioning. The whole lungs are irradiated in parallel opposed AP-PA portals to a midplane dose of 12 Gy in 8 fractions over 2 weeks. The radiation to the lungs results in 24% cure rate, whereas this increases to 50% with adjuvant chemotherapy.

The indications of radiation therapy in bilateral WT are as follows:

i. When definitive surgery has been accomplished and one or both of the primary tumors are found to be
   a. Stage III favorable histology.
   b. Stages II or III anaplastic tumors.
   c. Stages I to III clear cell sarcoma or rhabdoid tumor.

ii. When preoperative chemotherapy and one or two surgeries have not achieved complete tumor removal then the addition of preoperative low dose irradiation to a tune of 12 to 16 Gy may produce sufficient tumor shrinkage is achieve tumor removal.

According to the NWTS schema of management Stage IV disease with pulmonary metastasis at diagnosis begins with nephrectomy, postoperative chemotherapy, abdominal irradiation if needed and whole lung irradiation. The indication for infra-diaphragmatic irradiation is dictated by the degree of abdominal disease. For patients with pulmonary metastases at diagnosis on chest radiograph, the addition of lung irradiation is a standard approach. Although earlier reports used a dose of 16 to 18 Gy with excellent control, recent reports document impressive results utilizing doses limited to 12 Gy employing 1.5 Gy per fraction. A "boost" to local sites of residual pulmonary nodules is recommended if permitted by the being volumes. Stage IV favorable histology with lung metastases has an 80% 4-year survival rate (NWTS-3) whereas survival for those with Stage IV unfavorable histology is about 55% . On the other hand according to the SIOP protocol, lung irradiation is reserved for those who do not have a complete pulmonary tumor response and are not rendered free of disease by metastatectomy.

One hopes that future studies will help identify those patients with Stage IV disease who on the basis of biologic manners requires whole-lung irradiation and those who may be spared of it. It is also important to take account of prior abdominal irradiation in patients who require thoracic irradiation. One must respect the tolerance of the liver and of the upper pole of the remaining kidney in delineating thoracic irradiation fields in a child with previous abdominal irradiation. Liver metastases may be treated by hepatic irradiation in addition to chemotherapy. Whole liver irradiation is sometimes given for diffuse disease. Whenever possible, however, more limited radiotherapy fields are used if the disease is more localized in the liver.

Late Effects of Treatment

The survival rates of children with Wilm's Tumor has increased dramatically over the last 3 decades and this increase in survival has also made the late effects of treatment more obvious in the survivors. However, the treatment sequelae are becoming less likely with the current multidisciplinary management and this can be attributed to the following:

i. Lower dose of thoracic and abdominal irradiation (in FH)
ii. Less number of patients receiving radiotherapy
iii. Average age of patients receiving radiotherapy is now higher; in fact children below 1 year of age rarely receive RT.

Whole abdominal radiotherapy entails inclusion of almost all intra-abdominal viscera. The liver dose (whole organ) should be limited to 25 Gy. In a review of patients accrued via the German Pediatric Oncology Hematology group to SIOP there were 58 patients who received chemotherapy and abdominal radiation. Eleven of these 58 patients developed signs of hepatotoxicity. There was a predominance of children with right-sided tumors in the group with hepatic injury (9/33 – 27% vs 2/24 - 8%) which was probably due is larger volume of liver irradiated in right-sided tumors.

The kidney dose (whole organ) should be limited to 15 Gy by using beam-modifying devices (shields). After unilateral nephrectomy there is contralateral hypertrophy of the opposite kidney. However, this hypertrophy is not influenced by the adjuvant chemotherapy as evidenced by near normal GFR and effective renal plasma flow of approximately 90% of normal value. On the other hand, the addition of whole abdominal irradiation may cause a late effect of decreased size and impaired creatinine clearance in 19% of patients after a dose of d" 12 Gy and this can progress to chronic renal failure in those who undergo partial nephrectomy. Proteinuria and hypertension may occur even upto 10 to 20 years after nephrectomy with local radiation and chemotherapy for unilateral WT. Another question that frequently arises is the time after diagnosis when renal transplant should be performed for children with renal failure. The consensus is that after a prolonged waiting period of at least 2 years to exclude the relapsed cases, the cases should be selected for transplantation.

In long term survivors of WT, scoliosis and musculoskeletal abnormalities have been found more frequently in irradiated patients than in those patients who did not receive radiotherapy. The most frequent orthopedic abnormalities in patients treated with megavoltage radiation are lower rib hypoplasia and mild scoliosis. On the other hand those treated with orthovoltage radiation the most frequent abnormalities were lower rib hypoplasia (50%), mild scoliosis (40%), severe scoliosis (40%) and limb length inequality (20%). Abdominal radiation can also produce significant reduction in sitting height and a more modest decrease in standing height.

These effects are more pronounced the younger the patient is at the time of radiotherapy. Flank and abdominal radiotherapy doses of 20 to 30 Gy produces a height loss calculated by age at treatment. For child aged 1 year this was 9 cm, age 5 years to 7 cm, age 10 years 5.5 cm.

The second malignant neoplasms (SMNs) can develop in Wilm's Tumor survivors. The NWTS group cohort of patients have shown the associated risk factors for the occurrence of a SMN as radiation therapy, doxorubicin and in a small proportion of patients the causative agents were also AMD and VCR. Most of these tumors are in bone, breast and thyroid. According to a recent report, there is a significant increase in second malignancies as assessed by an observed: expected relative risk ratio (8.4). Patients who received both adriamycin and higher dose irradiation (35 Gy) had the highest relative risk (36.3).

RETINOBLASTOMA

Retinoblastoma is the most common malignant intra-ocular tumor of childhood arising from the nucleated cells of the retina. The retinoblastoma cells are undifferentiated small anaplastic cells that may be round or polygonal. Calcification commonly occurs in the necrotic areas. Histopathologically retinoblastoma is characterized by the presence of Flexner-Wintersteiner rosettes which represent an attempt to differentiate into photoreceptor cells.

Surgery was the earliest form of therapy attempted to provide local control and cure for retinoblastoma. The surgical practice is in the form of enucleation and exenteration.

Enucleation involves removal of the globe after severing the rectus muscles. The optic nerve is then cut near its exit from the socket and keeping a long segment of the nerve is important in the event the tumor is within the nerve.

Exenteration is the removal of the globe, extraocular muscles, lids, nerves and orbital fat. Orbital exenteration is rarely required in the western countries, where as in India majority with advanced tumor need this procedure. The indications are extensive local tumor breaching the globe and recurrence of tumor in the socket after enucleation.

The four local therapies for Retinoblastoma are: (i) Cryotherapy, (ii) Photocoagulation, (iii) Laser hyperthermia, (iv) Radioactive plaque applications.

External Beam Radiotherapy

Orbit is conical in shape and its dimensions in an adult are 3.4 cm (height), 4.1 cm (width), and 5.7 cm (floor length) with a capacity of 30 cc. In children the diameter of the globe ranges from 1.6 to 2.3 cm. The diameter of the lens is 7 mm and thickness is 3 to 4 mm. The distance from the limbus to the anterior surface of the lens is about 2-3 mm and the inter-ora serrata distance is 17 mm. All these measurements both in children and adults are average measurements; the exact measurements in an individual patient can be determined by orbital ultrasound and CT. These dimensions assume importance in RT planning because during external beam radiotherapy if the anterior border of the lateral portal is kept 1.5 mm anterior to the lateral bony canthus then it lies behind the back of the lens.

The indications for curative external beam radiotherapy are as follows:
  i. Multifocal lesions.
  ii. Lesions close to the macula or the optic nerve with the goal of vision preservation.
  iii. Large tumors with vitreous seeding but with an useful vision.

The indications for palliative external beam radiotherapy are as follows:
  i. As a modality for tumor shrinkage in inoperable patients to be followed by assessment for surgery.
  ii. Advanced tumors purely as a palliative modality to prevent the tumor from bursting and hemorrhage.
  iii. For metastatic disease to the bones, brain, spine and lungs.

Principle of EBRT

1. To deliver homogenous tumoricidal dose to the retina and vitreous without compromising normal tissue tolerance.

2. To encompass expansive treatment volume because:
   i. In RB all retinal cells have a genetic neoplastic potential necessitating the treatment of the entire retina.
   ii. In RB vitreous seeding may occur.
   iii. Multiple satellite tumors may arise from a primary RB.
   iv. Tumor may spread via the subretinal space.
   v. Retinal differentiation progresses from posterior to anterior and from superior to inferior, subclinical disease may exist in the immature retina and must be included in the treatment.
3. To deliver the radiation dose after proper immobilization under short general anesthesia (Ketamine or Propofol).
4. To avoid irradiation of the opposite eye as far as possible.

Technique of Irradiation

It was Algernon Reese in the 1930s who first developed technique of irradiation for RB. He used an orthovoltage unit and treatment was delivered through temporal and nasal portals.

In present day practice of radiation oncology there are several methods available to treat patients with RB. However, while treating patients of RB with EBRT two points should be remembered.
   i. Immobilization should be done properly. When a plaster of paris or a thermoplastic head holder is prepared for treatment and the anesthesia gas mask is placed, care must be taken to allow an unobstructed view of the eyes, so that the fields may be correctly set.
   ii. Ketamine anesthesia is known to produce lateral nystagmus. Therefore while using EBRT if a blocking technique is used that relies on the eye being a stable target then ketamine will generally be unacceptable as the anesthetic agent.
   1. *Lateral Beam Megavoltage Technique*: In this technique the anterior border is set at the lateral bony orbit. When the contralateral orbit has been enucleated, a direct lateral field is used but on the contrary if the contralateral globe is in place then the beam is angled about 10 to 15 degree posteriorly so that the contralateral lens does not get the exit dose. It is mostly impractical to treat the entire retina including the edges of the ora serrata and yet spare the lens by this technique resulting in anterior tumor recurrence at or near the ora serrata.

This technique may be useful if there is no gross disease near the ora serrata.

2. *Direct anterior Megavoltage Field*: In this technique the ^{60}Co or the linear accelerator beam treats the entire eye sparing the contralateral eye. The lens cannot be spared leading to inevitable cataract formation, the ipsilateral lacrimal gland is irradiated leading to impaired tear production and there is an exit dose through the brain. However the advantages are that the field is easy to set up and reproducible and homogeneously irradiates the entire vitreous and the retina. The cataract when it forms can be treated surgically.

3. *Half Beam Blocked Lateral Field*: In this technique, the lateral beam is half beam blocked to decrease the penumbra and thus sharpen the field edge. The field edge may be set at the bony orbit or between the bone and the limbus. If the anterior edge is set half way between the limbus and the bony orbit then the ora serrata is covered. In children with unilateral disease, straight lateral fields are replaced with oblique fields. Superior and inferior oblique fields miss the uninvolved eye. In case of an inferior oblique field the exit dose is through the frontal lobe of the brain and in case of a superior oblique field the exit dose is through the maxillary sinus and the mouth. The treatment may be given with a photon beam alone or with a mixed photon/electron straight lateral or lateral oblique fields.

4. *Two field technique with a hanging lens block*: In this technique, a lateral field and an anterior field with a hanging lens block is used with an attempt to achieve a homogeneous retinal dose yet spare the lens. This is by far the commonest technique used. The fields are weighted 75 to 80% from the lateral and 20 to 25% from the anterior. The desired dose distribution can be achieved in the form of two modifications.

i. The lateral field is continued and the anterior photon field is substituted by an anterior electron field with a contact lens mounted lead block for the lens. But small displacements of the contact lens significantly alter the dose from the anterior field.

ii. The second modification uses anterior photons without the hanging eye block that may shield the posterior tumor.

5. *Schipper Technique*: This technique uses a precision lateral technique that calls for a specially devised machine mounted device which, by way of a scale, sets the anterior field edge just behind the lens.

This technique is particularly appropriate for posterior pole lesions. This technique uses a linear accelerator modified with a beam splitting and extended collimation system, to produce a non-divergent and almost penumbra free anterior beam edge. In this technique, the use of an ultrasound is mandatory to measure several intraocular distances, specially the posterior margin of the lens.

6. *McCormick's modification of Schipper technique*: For patients with unilateral tumors, the single oblique field Schipper technique has been modified. This uses a composite arrangement using 3 fields and avoids the uninvolved eye. For the first two-thirds of the treatment, a pair of superior and anterior wedged oblique D shaped fields were used. The superior oblique field is weighted to avoid a significant exit dose to the frontal lobe. For the last one third of the treatment; a d shaped lateral electron beam was used with the anterior border placed 2 to 3 mm behind the limbus.

In general, control of groups I to III with lens sparing external beam irradiation alone is fairly good i.e. 40 to 80%. The addition of salvage therapy in the form of photocoagulation, cryotherapy and plaque therapy results in ultimate eye preservation rate of 67 to 100% for groups I to III. The majority of the failures with lens sparing technique are located anterior in the eye. Due to this reason many radiation oncologists supplement a lateral beam with some dose from an anterior field (80:20, lateral: anterior weighting) to bring up the dose anteriorly. The overall eye preservation rate in patients with anterior failure remains quite good due to the frequent success of focal salvage therapies such as cryotherapy, laser or plaque.

Lateral techniques that utilize a sufficiently anterior placed field border (with or without a lightly weighted anterior beam) or single anterior field are the best techniques to avoid anterior failures. The former technique reduces the risk of anterior structures while the latter one is easy to set up and associated complications are manageable.

Any EBRT technique for treatment of RB should

i. Encompass the entire retinal damage.

ii. Avoid the fellow eye if uninvolved.

iii. Limit the normal tissue dose.

The treatment needs to be individualized that fulfills the aforementioned criteria within the context of the available equipment and expertise.

Dose of Radiotherapy

A large number of dose per fraction schemes have been proposed for EBRT ranging from 2 to 3.8 Gy/fraction to a total dose of 30 to 60 Gy. In our institution the children below the age of 4 years are treated with Ketamine anesthesia or short sedative measures with 3 fractions delivered weekly. A dose of 35 to 45 Gy is delivered over 3 to 5 weeks. For the unilateral group I - III a single lateral field 3 x 3 cm to 4 x 4 cm with a special penumbra trimmer is used.

For patients with obvious anterior extension, an anterior field is added and the lateral field is tilted 5 degrees to 15 degrees to avoid irradiation of the opposite eye. For bilateral disease parallel-opposed temporal portals are used simultaneously within the prescribed isodose level behind the lenses.

For patients with enucleated eye, an anterior portal is added to the lateral portal in order to spare the contalateral eye.

Palliative radiotherapy is planned in case of bulky extraocular involvement or where there is a direct extension into the orbital floor. In case of extension to the maxillary sinus or intracranial extension, anterior and lateral fields are generally planned. The patients with gross intracranial extension and good general condition receive a whole brain dose of 20 to 25 Gy besides the treatment of the primary tumor. The metastatic sites (bones, lungs, and nodes) are treated to a dose of 5 Gy in single fraction or 15 Gy in 5 fractions depending on the merit of each case.

The following conclusions may be drawn:

i. High dose per fraction radiotherapy is associated with an increasing risk of late effects. An increase in the retinopathy has been described at doses greater than and equal to 2.5 Gy per fraction.

ii. With improvement in pediatric anesthesia, the argument that anesthesia is difficult in these cases and, therefore, recommendation of high dose per fraction is not acceptable. RB patients should be treated 5 days per week at less than or equal to 2 Gy per fraction.

iii. The total dose should vary between 40 - 45 Gy @ 1.8 - 2 Gy per fraction, 5 days per week. For large tumor and/or vitreous seeding a higher dose of upto 50 Gy is recommended.

Regression Patterns

Following EBRT, patients should be followed up with ophthalmoscopy and USG at regular intervals. Most of the retinoblastomas have a residual mass after radiotherapy. Five regression patterns are observed ophthalmoscopically.

i. Type 0 Regression: No tumor or tumor less than 5 mm diameter.

ii. Type I Regression: Tumor assumes a cottage cheese appearance (glistening white). They rarely reactivate.

iii. Type II Regression: Fish-flesh appearance (homogeneous gray-translucent) and this is difficult to differentiate from viable tumor.

iv. Type III Regression: This is a combination of Type I and Type II regression. They often reactivate.

v. Type IV Regression: It is usually seen after plaque brachytherapy when there is complete tumor destruction, flattening and scarring.

Complications of Radiotherapy

The aim of radiotherapy is to irradiate the tumor homogeneously with the view of destroying and at the same time to avoid radiation related complications and to preserve vision. The threshold dose of retina is 55 Gy in 25 fractions over a 5-week period.

i. *Radiation Vasculitis*: The retinal vasculature is extremely radiosensitive and, hence radiation vasculitis leads to intra-retinal and pre-retinal fibrosis. The noted incidence of retinal vascular damage and visual loss increases beyond 60 Gy. At times vascular damage leads to vitreous hemorrhage. The macula is highly sensitive and, hence, any complication in this zone leads to total visual loss. Retinal hemorrhage can cause secondary glaucoma. The painful blind eye is an indication for enucleation.

ii. *Cataract*: The lens is highly susceptible to cataract formation even with a dose as low as 4 Gy in a single fraction or 12 Gy in multiple fractions. The direct anterior field without shielding to a dose of more than 25 Gy results in cataract formation within 18 months.

iii. *Keratitis and Keratoconjunctivitis*: They are extremely uncommon when a lateral field is used or when less than 35% of the total dose is delivered by the anterior field. The acute effect of radiation can be minimized by advising the patient to keep the eyes open and look into the beam. In case of anesthetized patients the lid should be kept retracted while treating the anterior field.

iv. *Optic neuritis*: The effect of EBRT on the optic nerve leading to optic atrophy can occur after a dose of more than 68 Gy.

v. *Orbital maldevelopment*: Children treated with enucleation or EBRT for RB are at significant risk for orbital and midfacial growth retardation insofar as their orbital bones are growing during treatment. In long-term survivors of RB, these orbital growth injuries may be apparent. Deformity of the orbit can lead to a 10-30% decrease in orbital volume. Socket contraction is not uncommon in growing child. Enucleation without a properly fitting prosthesis and EBRT can lead to a retardation of bony and soft tissue growth of the midface (orbits, ethmoid bones, nasal bridge), hypotelorism, enophthalmos, depressed temporal bones, atrophy of the temporalis muscle, narrow and deep orbits and a depressed nasion. These effects are accentuated if radiotherapy is used in the very young (<6 months of age) and doses greater than 35 Gy.

vi. *Lacrimal Gland*: Irradiated eyes had a significant lessening of tear production as well as significant reduction in tear protein production when compared with a control group. Although lacrimal gland is shielded whenever possible during EBRT, some long-term survivors of RB will have diminished tear and diminished stability of the tear film making them prone to keratopathies.

vii. *Secondary nonocular tumors*: The relative risk (RR) for death from a second tumor is much higher among patients with bilateral RB (RR=60) than among those with unilateral disease (RR=3.8). The most common secondary malignant neoplasms (SMNs) occurring within the radiation fields in survivors of heritable RB are osteosarcoma, fibrosarcoma, and other spindle cell sarcomas. SMNs developing outside the radiotherapy field also include osteosarcoma, soft tissue sarcomas, malignant melanoma and thyroid carcinoma. In children with hereditary RB treated with EBRT, the incidence of SMNs increases with time. The median latency period is 15 years. At 10 years the incidence is about 10, 20% at 20 years, 25% at 30 years, 51% at 50 years.

Children with heritable RB have a field change rendering them subject to malignant transformation.

Radiotherapy and perhaps chemotherapy adds an additional insult. Radiotherapy shortens the latent period for SMNs, increases the incidence of SMNs and affects the distribution of SMNs.

NEUROBLASTOMA

Neuroblastoma (NB) is an embryonal tumor of the childhood derived from the embryonic neural crest. Neuroblastoma has the broadest spectrum of clinical presentation and paraneoplastic syndromes of any childhood malignancy. It is an enigmatic tumor as there is no clear-cut etiology, disease course, and therapy definitions. Some children may be cured spontaneously or with minimal therapy while others may resist all attempts of disease eradication.

Neuroblastoma constitutes 7 to 10% of all cases of childhood cancer.

Radiation Therapy

Radiotherapy remains one of the main forms of locoregional treatments in the management of neuroblastomas. The use of radiotherapy needs to be optimized stage for stage.

Neuroblastoma cell lines are generally regarded as radiosensitive. Laboratory data suggests that there is a low level of repair capacity of NB cell for the radiation damage as compared to the normal cells. The maximum therapeutic dose for NB is between 15 to 35 Gy, but there is as such no dose response curve and hence the response remains unpredictable. The indications for radiotherapy in the treatment of neuroblastoma are as follows:

- Adjuvant radiation
- Palliative radiation
- Large mediastinal tumor
- Dumb bell-shaped paraspinal tumor.

Acute Infantile Hepatic Enlargement

Adjuvant radiotherapy is beneficial in localized tumor. Thus in Stage I completely excised tumor there is no role of radiotherapy whereas in Stage IIA disease the need for postoperative radiotherapy should be limited to large tumor size with gross surrounding infiltration. The definite indication of postoperative adjuvant radiotherapy is in Stage IIb and III neuroblastoma. In patients with limited spread as in Stage IV S, the healthy child may be considered for induction chemotherapy and radiotherapy followed by surgical extirpation of the localised tumor. Total body irradiation and hemi body irradiation has been tried but with discouraging results. The only role of TBI is in a situation like bone marrow transplantation.

In the case of postoperative radiation, a dose of 15 to 20 Gy in 1.2 to 1.5 Gy per fraction is delivered to an initial volume of tumor bed plus a 2-cm margin. This is followed by a further boost of 5 to 10 Gy in a coned down volume. In infants below the age of 1 year radiotherapy should be avoided as far as possible. In TBI for BMT a dose of 7.5 to 12 Gy is delivered to the whole body in a fractionated manner in a time span of 1 to 5 days. In case of acute distressing hepatomegaly, radiotherapy is indicated. A midplane dose of 6 Gy in 3 fractions by AP-PA portals relieves the distress in majority of the patients. In the case of mediastinal adenopathy and spinal cord compression by a dumb bell-shaped tumor a dose of 15 to 20 Gy in 5 to 10 fractions relieves the symptoms rapidly.

Technique of Radiotherapy

In the case of postoperative radiotherapy being planned to the flank or the hemi-abdomen a 2-cm margin is given around the tumor bed. The field margin should include the vertebral width completely and the opposite kidney and the gonads should be protected. Usually anterior and posterior portals are planned and the dose is calculated at the midplane.

In the case of preoperative radiotherapy being planned for cytoreduction, the radiation fields may be planned by oblique or lateral fields taking into account the kidney. In gross residual tumor or when the patient has extensive intraperitoneal disease, the whole abdomen is treated by anterior and posterior portals. The mediastinal and pelvic sites are also treated by parallel-opposed fields. The spine is treated by direct posterior field or by two oblique fields with wedges. Bone metastases are treated by direct field to the disease site and a dose of 5 Gy in a single fraction or 12 Gy in 4 fractions is recommended.

Targeted radiotherapy or Zetotherapy is a novel method of delivering the therapeutic radiation to the tumor site. The affinity of the tumor towards the agent determines the concentration of the agent at the tumor site. Meta iodo benzyl guanidine (MIBG) is a radioactive iodinated compound strictly metabolized by the neuroblasts. Therapeutic MIBG has got a long biological half-life at the tumor site than the normal cells. Currently MIBG targeted radiotherapy is being advocated on a trial basis in three clinical situations.

1. Treatment of minimal residual disease for cure.
2. Primary inoperable tumors for de bulking.
3. In chemorefractory disease for palliation.

In combination with other chemotherapeutic agents, MIBG shows encouraging results.

RHABDOMYOSARCOMA

Childhood rhabdomyosarcoma, a soft tissue malignant tumor of skeletal muscle origin, accounts for approximately 3.5% of the cases of cancer among children 0 to 14 years and 2% of the cases among adolescents and young adults 15 to 19 years of age.[14] It is a curable disease in the majority of children who receive optimal therapy, with more than 60% surviving 5 years after diagnosis. The most common primary sites for rhabdomyosarcoma are the head and neck (e.g., parameningeal, orbit, pharyngeal, etc.), the genitourinary tract, and the extremities. Other less common primary sites include the trunk, intrathoracic region, the gastrointestinal tract (including liver and biliary tract), and the perineal/anal region.

Management

All children with rhabdomyosarcoma require multimodality therapy. This entails surgical resection, if possible, followed by chemotherapy, followed by second-look surgery for some patients with initially unresected tumors, and, depending on original histologic type, extent of disease and extent of resection, radiation therapy.

Radiation Therapy Management Treatment Options

Standard

Radiation therapy is an effective method for achieving local control of tumor for patients with microscopic or gross residual disease following initial surgical resection or chemotherapy. Patients with completely resected tumors (Clinical Group I) of embryonal histology do well without radiation therapy, but, radiation therapy benefits patients with Clinical Group I tumors with alveolar or undifferentiated histology.[15] As with the surgical management of patients with rhabdomyosarcoma, recommendations for radiation therapy are dependent on the site of primary disease and on the extent of disease following surgical resection.

For optimal care of pediatric patients undergoing radiation treatments, it is imperative to have a radiation oncologist, radiation technicians, and nurses who are experienced in treating children. The facility should be equipped with a linear accelerator as well as capabilities to administer electron beam therapy. Computerized treatment planning, preferably with a 3-dimensional planning system, should be available. Techniques to deliver conformal radiation (e.g., intensity modulated radiation therapy, proton radiation, or interstitial/intracavitary radiation) should be considered.[16]

The radiation therapy dose depends predominantly on the extent of disease following the primary surgical resection. In general, patients with microscopic residual disease (clinical Group II) receive radiation therapy to approximately 4,100 cGy, although doses from 3,000 to 4,000 cGy may be adequate in patients receiving effective multiagent chemotherapy.[15,17] IRS-II patients with gross residual disease (Clinical Group III) who received 4,000 to greater than 5,000 cGy had local/regional relapse rates of over 30%; higher doses of radiation (>6,000 cGy) have been associated with unacceptable long-term toxic effects.[63,64] Patients on the IRS-IV standard treatment arm receive approximately 5,000 cGy.[18]

The treated volume should be determined by the extent of tumor at diagnosis prior to surgical resection and prior to chemotherapy. A margin of 2 cm is generally used, including clinically involved nodes. While the volume irradiated may be modified based on guidelines for normal tissue tolerance, gross residual disease at the time of irradiation should receive full-dose treatment.

The timing of radiation therapy generally allows for chemotherapy to be given for 2 to 3 months prior to the initiation of radiation therapy, with the exception of patients with parameningeal disease and evidence of meningeal extension in whom radiation therapy generally begins at the time of diagnosis.[19] Radiation therapy is usually given for 5 to 6 weeks (e.g., 180 cGy per day for 28 treatment days), during which time chemotherapy is usually modified to avoid the radiosensitizing agent Dactinomycin.

Among the modifications of radiation therapy for specific primary sites recommended for IRS-IV patients are:[18]

1. For patients with orbital tumors, precautions should be taken to shield the lens, cornea, lacrimal gland, and optic chiasm.
2. Patients with bladder/prostate primary tumors that present with a large pelvic mass resulting from a distended bladder from outlet obstruction receive treatment to a volume defined by imaging studies following initial chemotherapy.
3. Patients with parameningeal disease with intracranial extension in contiguity with the primary tumor, and/or cranial base bone erosion, and/or cranial nerve palsy do not require whole-brain irradiation. They should receive irradiation to the site of primary tumor with a 2 cm margin to include the meninges adjacent to the primary tumor 68 and the region of intracranial extension, again with a 2 cm margin, if present. Patients with intracranial extension should begin receiving radiation therapy within 2 weeks after diagnosis.
4. Although a rare occurrence, children who present with tumor cells in the CSF, have other evidence of diffuse meningeal disease, or have multiple intraparenchymal brain metastasis from a distant primary tumor, are treated with whole brain irradiation in addition to the chemotherapy/radiation therapy for the primary tumor. Spinal irradiation may also be given in coordination with other therapies and at the investigator/physician's discretion.

Under Clinical Evaluation

For patients with gross residual tumor following initial surgical excision, the IRS-IV study is comparing conventional radiation therapy with hyperfractionated radiation therapy. Hyperfractionated therapy potentially allows higher total X-ray doses to be given to the tumor without increased normal tissue late toxicity and has been used extensively for patients with central nervous system tumors (especially brain stem gliomas). The hyperfractionated therapy group in IRS-IV received 5,940 cGy (110 cGy fractions given twice daily), and the conventional radiation therapy group received 5,040 cGy (180 cGy fractions daily).

Brachytherapy using either intracavitary or interstitial implants is another method of local control that is under clinical investigation and has been used for children with rhabdomyosarcoma, especially those with primary tumors at vaginal or vulval sites. In a small, single-institution study, this treatment approach was associated with a high survival rate (85%) and with retention of a functional vagina in the majority of patients. Other sites, especially head and neck, pelvis and retroperitoneum have been treated with brachytherapy.

Patients with initial Clinical Group III disease who then have microscopic residual disease after chemotherapy with or without delayed surgery are likely to achieve local control with radiation at doses of 4,000 cGy or more.

Radiotherapy Planning

Preoperative imaging documentation is a must prior to planning of radiotherapy. Surgical clips when added at the time of surgical resection aid in the target volume delineation. The planning needs to be individualised as per the individual site. In the case of orbital RMS antero lateral 60 degree wedged portals usually gives the desired dose distribution when the entire orbital cavity is considered to be the target volume. For parotid tumors a single direct enface electron beam portal (9-12 Mev) is usually sufficient. Parameningeal tumors which usually cross the midline, often require parallel opposed portals; these are rarely resectable and and need higher radiation doses for their control. Pelvic RMS is more ammenable to surgery and radical surgery implies pelvic exenteration along with radiotherapy and/or chemotherapy. Postoperative radiotherapy is delivered by parallel-opposed portals to the whole pelvis. Extensive paratesticular tumors with heavy para-aortic nodal involvement are treated by parallel-opposed portals to the whole abdomen. The total dose in whole abdominal rdaiotherapy should not exceed 30 Gy in a fraction size of 150 to 180 cGy. Vital abdominal organs should be shielded as per their individual tolerances.

EWING'S FAMILY OF TUMORS INCLUDING PRIMITIVE NEUROECTODERMAL TUMOR (PNET)

Ewing's tumors occur most frequently in the second decade of life and account for 4% of childhood and adolescent malignancies. The incidence in boys is slightly higher than in girls (ratio of 1.1:1). Ewing's tumor of Bone is estimated to be 60% of all Ewing's tumors, the sites of origin include extremities, distal (27%) and proximal (25%); pelvis (20%); chest (20%); and spine and skull (9%).[20] For the Extraosseous Ewing's tumors, the most common sites are trunk (32%), extremity (26%), head and neck (18%), retroperitoneum (16%), and all other sites (8%).[21] Common sites for PNET are the chest (44%), abdomen/pelvis (26%), extremities (20%), head and neck (6%), and all other sites (4%).[21] Except for the head and neck, the sites of origin of Extraosseous Ewing's and PNET are similar.

Major prognostic factors include site, tumor volume, and the presence of metastases.

Local control can be achieved by surgery and/or radiation or both. Surgery is generally the preferred approach if the lesion is resectable. If a very young child has an Ewing's tumor of Bone, surgery may be a less

morbid therapy than radiation therapy because of the retardation of bone growth caused by radiation. Another potential benefit for surgical resection of the primary tumor is information concerning the amount of necrosis in the resected tumor. Patients with residual viable tumor in the resected specimen have a worse outcome compared to those with complete necrosis. Radiation therapy should be employed for patients who do not have a surgical option that preserves function and should be used for patients whose tumors have been excised but with inadequate margins.

Radiation therapy should be delivered in a setting in which stringent planning techniques are applied by those experienced in the treatment of Ewing's family of tumors. Such an approach will result in local control of the tumor with acceptable morbidity in a majority of patients. The radiation dose may be adjusted depending upon the extent of residual disease after the surgical procedure. Radiation therapy is usually given in doses of 5600 cGy to the prechemotherapy tumor extent. A randomized study of 40 patients with Ewing's tumor of Bone using 5580 cGy to the prechemotherapy tumor extent with a 2-cm margin compared to the same total tumor dose following 3960 cGy to the entire bone showed no difference in local control or event-free survival. Hyperfractionated radiation therapy was not associated with local control or a decrease in morbidity. Some patients may require surgical resection following radiation therapy.

Radiation Therapy in Ewing's Sarcoma

The sucessful management of a patient with Ewing's sarcoma (ES) requires both local and systemic control. Rdaiation therapy has been used since the 1970s as a component of the multimodality management of ES. Overall tumor control following radiotherapy is 75 to 90% in all the major series. The extremity tumors show a better control with radiotherapy than the pelvic tumors. The factors to be considered in the radiotherapy practice are – treatment technique, dose and the interaction between the radiotherapy and the chemotherapy.

In the earlier days the likelihood of the extension of the ES along the medullary cavity was stressed and the full volume irradiation of tye long and the flat bones was considered mandatory. The full bone was irradiated to a dose of 50 Gy and the local tumor site received a dose of 60 to 65 GY by shrinking field method. This approach resulted in considerable late morbidities in terms of limb length discrepancy, joint deformity, gastrointestinal and bladder toxicities and second malignant lesion notably sarcomas. Thus these older radiotherapy techniques have been questioned in the recent years. Now with the availability of sophisticated imaging modalities like CT scan and MRI provide more accurate tumor definition, permitting more accurate radiation therapy planning resulting in local tumor control with much less morbidities.

Review of literature revealed that there was no great influence of traditional treatment of whole bone radiation versus limited bone irradaition as far as the location of the recurrence was concerned. The distinct advantage of chemotherapy and the knowledge of local failures at the site of primary disease has allowed the radiation oncologist to limit the total dose to 45-50 Gy and to reduce the target volume portal size by sparing the uninvolved distal epiphysis thus lessening the delayed morbidity. The radiotherapy treatment plan should take into account all available radiological tests and include a safe margin of 3-5 cm beyond the tumor extension. The epiphyseal end on the uninvolved side of a long bone and bowel, bladder and other organs in the central axis should be carefully shielded. Although limited volume irradaition has been found effective in localised ES, yet the traditional practice of encompassing the medullary cavity and providing a safe margin should be respected, especially in a bulky tumor with soft tissue extension.

Metastatic Tumors of the Ewing's Family

Prognosis of patients with metastatic disease is poor.

Treatment Options

Standard treatment with alternating vincristine, doxorubicin, cyclophosphamide, and ifosfamide/etoposide combined with radiation therapy to all sites of gross disease and possibly selected surgical excision for patients with metastatic Ewing's tumor of bone/Ewing's tumor of soft tissue often results in complete or partial responses; however the overall cure rate is 20%. For patients with lung/pleural metastases only, cure rates are approximately 30%. Patients who did not receive lung irradiation had a worse outcome than those receiving lung radiation.[22] Patients with only bone/bone marrow metastases have an approximate 20 to 25% cure rate. Patients with combined lung and bone/bone marrow metastases have less than 15% cure rate.

Radiation therapy should be delivered in a setting in which stringent planning techniques are applied by those experienced in the treatment of Ewing's family of tumors.

Such an approach will result in local control of tumor with acceptable morbidity in the majority of patients. Radiation therapy to the primary tumor as well as to the sites of metastatic disease should be considered but may interfere with delivery of chemotherapy if too much bone marrow is included in the field. Metastatic sites of disease in bone and soft tissues should receive radiation therapy of 4500 cGy to 5600 cGy. All patients with pulmonary metastases should undergo whole lung radiation, even if complete resolution of pulmonary metastatic disease has been achieved with chemotherapy.[23] Radiation doses are modulated based on the amount of lung to be irradiated. Doses between 1200 cGy and 1500 cGy are used if whole lungs are treated.

More intensive therapies, many of which incorporate high-dose chemotherapy with or without total-body irradiation in conjunction with stem cell support have not shown improvement in event-free survival rates for patients with bone and/or bone marrow metastases. Secondary leukemias have emerged as a major risk factor in dose-intensive regimens.

Recurrent Tumors of the Ewing's Family

The prognosis for patients with recurrent or progressive Ewing's family of tumors (EFTs) is poor, although the prognosis for patients relapsing off therapy is better than for those patients who relapse while on their initial chemotherapy regimen. The selection of further treatment depends on many factors, including the site of recurrence and prior treatment, as well as individual patient considerations. Ifosfamide and etoposide are active in EFTs and should be considered for patients who have not previously received these agents. Aggressive attempts to control the disease, including myeloablative regimens, may be warranted. Radiation therapy to bone lesions may provide palliation. Residual disease in the lung may be surgically removed.

CHILDHOOD BRAIN TUMORS

Primary brain tumors are a diverse group of diseases that together constitute the most common solid tumor of childhood. Brain tumors are classified according to histology, but tumor location and extent of spread are important factors that affect treatment and prognosis. Immunohistochemical analysis, cytogenetic and molecular genetic findings, and measures of mitotic activity are increasingly used in tumor diagnosis and classification.

Approximately 50% of brain tumors in children are infratentorial, with three fourths of these located in the cerebellum or fourth ventricle. Common infratentorial (posterior fossa) tumors include the following:

1. Cerebellar astrocytoma (usually pilocytic but also fibrillary and high-grade
2. Medulloblastoma (primitive neuroectodermal tumor
3. Ependymoma (low-grade or anaplastic).
4. Brain stem glioma (often diagnosed neuro-radiographically without biopsy; may be high-grade or low-grade).
5. Atypical teratoid.

Supratentorial tumors include those tumors that occur in the sellar or suprasellar region and/or other areas of the cerebrum. Sellar/suprasellar tumors comprise approximately 20% of childhood brain tumors and include the following:

1. Craniopharyngioma.
2. Diencephalic (chiasm, hypothalamic, and/or thalamic) gliomas generally of low-grade.
3. Germ cell tumors (germinoma and non-germinomatous).

Cerebellar Astrocytomas

Untreated Childhood Cerebellar Astrocytoma

Surgical resection is the primary treatment for childhood cerebellar astrocytoma. Complete or near complete removal can be obtained in 90 to 95% of patients with juvenile pilocytic tumors. Diffuse cerebellar astrocytomas may be less amenable to total resection, and this may account for the poorer outcome. The optimal use of radiation therapy is the subject of controversy. Some radiation oncologists advocate the treatment of patients with residual disease, and others withhold treatment until tumor progression has been documented. Chemotherapy may be useful for delaying radiation therapy in the very young child with unresectable, progressive cerebellar astrocytoma.

Recurrent Childhood Cerebellar Astrocytoma

Recurrence may take place in childhood cerebellar gliomas and may develop many years after initial treatment. Disease can be at the primary tumor site or, especially in malignant tumors, at noncontiguous central nervous system sites. Systemic relapse is rare, but may occur.

Patients with cerebellar astrocytoma (pilocytic or diffuse) who relapse after being treated with surgery alone should be considered for another surgical resection. If this is not feasible, local radiation therapy is the usual treatment. If there is recurrence in an unresectable site after irradiation, chemotherapy should be considered.

Medulloblastoma

Two major subclassifications are now being used:
Average risk: Children older than 3 years of age with posterior fossa tumors; tumor is totally or "near-totally" (<1.5 cubic centimeters of residual disease) resected; no dissemination.[24]
Poor risk: Children younger than 3 years of age or those with metastatic disease and/or subtotal resection (>1.5 cubic centimeters of residual disease) and/or non-posterior fossa location.

In the past, treatment has included surgery with radiation therapy. There is evidence to suggest that more extensive surgical resections are related to an improved rate of survival, primarily in children with nondisseminated posterior fossa disease at diagnosis. Chemotherapy has been shown to be active in patients with recurrent medulloblastomas. Adjuvant chemotherapy given during and after radiation therapy may improve overall survival for the subset of children with medulloblastoma who have less favorable prognostic factors, and there has been enthusiasm for exploring the role of chemotherapy in the treatment of childhood brain tumors. Children younger than 3 years of age are particularly susceptible to the adverse effect of radiation on brain development. Debilitating effects on growth and neurologic development have frequently been observed, especially in younger children.[25] For this reason, the role of chemotherapy in allowing a delay in the administration of radiation therapy is under study, and preliminary results suggest that chemotherapy can be used to delay, and sometimes obviate, the need for radiation therapy in children with medulloblastoma.

Untreated Childhood Medulloblastoma

Surgery should be an attempt at maximal tumor reduction; children without disseminated disease at diagnosis have improved progression-free survival if there is minimal residual disease present after surgery. Postoperatively, studies should be conducted to determine if the patient has high risk of relapse. Patients with extensive tumor should be considered at "high risk" for relapse and be treated on protocols specifically designed for them.

Average Risk

The traditional postsurgical treatment for these patients has been radiation therapy consisting of 5,400 to 5,580 cGy to the tumor bed and approximately 3,600 cGy to the entire neuraxis (i.e., the whole brain and spine). The minimal dose of radiation therapy needed for disease control is unknown. Attempts to lower the dose of craniospinal radiation therapy to 2,340 cGy have resulted in an increased incidence of isolated leptomeningeal relapse.[26] Studies are ongoing to determine if a lower dose of radiation therapy, when coupled with chemotherapy, can be used to control disease. Craniospinal irradiation is technically extremely demanding. There is no evidence that adjuvant chemotherapy improves the outcome for patients with average-risk medulloblastoma. However, trials are ongoing to evaluate the possible role of reduced-dose radiation therapy and chemotherapy in these patients.

Poor Risk

In poor-risk patients, the addition of chemotherapy has improved the duration of disease-free survival.[27] Some studies show that approximately 50 to 60% of such patients will experience long-term disease control. These are patients who, at diagnosis, have locally extensive and often unresectable tumor in the posterior fossa, brain stem involvement at diagnosis, and/or noncontiguous metastatic disease within or outside of the central nervous system. Adjuvant chemotherapy has improved progression-free survival for patients with these "poor-risk" parameters at diagnosis.[27] Such patients should be considered for entry into a clinical trial.

Children Younger than 3 Years of Age

Some patients younger than 3 years of age with newly diagnosed medulloblastoma will respond, at least partially, to chemotherapy. Some patients, especially those with minimal residual postoperative disease, may have a long-lasting response. Those children treated with chemotherapy alone may have better neurocognitive outcome than those treated with radiation therapy, with or without chemotherapy. For this reason, strong consideration should be given to entering patients younger than 3 years of age in studies that use chemotherapy to delay, modify, or possibly obviate the need for radiation therapy. High-dose chemotherapy with autologous bone marrow rescue followed by focal radiation therapy has been used with some success in young children with locally recurrent disease for whom primary chemotherapy has failed. Although chemotherapy is being used to prevent neurologic damage caused by radiation therapy in very young patients, neurologic deficits may be present in children prior to the initiation of therapy, and progressive neurologic damage has been noted during therapy.

Recurrent Childhood Medulloblastoma

Recurrence is not uncommon and may develop many years after initial treatment. Disease may recur at the primary tumor site or, especially in malignant tumors, at noncontiguous central nervous system sites. Systemic relapse is rare, but may occur. At time of relapse, a complete evaluation for extent of recurrence is indicated for all malignant tumors and, at times, for more benign lesions. Biopsy or surgical resection may be necessary for confirmation of relapse because other entities such as secondary tumor and treatment-related brain necrosis may be clinically indistinguishable from tumor recurrence. The need for surgical intervention must be individualized on the basis of the initial tumor type, the length of time between initial treatment and the reappearance of the lesion, and the clinical picture. Patients with medulloblastoma that recurs after radiation therapy alone should be considered for treatment with known active agents, which include vincristine, cyclophosphamide, cisplatin, carboplatin, lomustine, and etoposide; although response is seen in more than 50% of patients, long-term disease control is rare. Entry into studies of novel therapeutic approaches including high-dose chemotherapy and autologous stem cell rescue at the time of relapse after radiation therapy alone or radiation therapy and chemotherapy should be considered.

Ependymoma

Ependymomas are divided into the following categories:
- Subependymoma (WHO Grade I)
- Ependymoma (WHO Grade II).
- Variants include cellular, papillary, epithelial, clear cell and mixed.
- Malignant (also known as anaplastic) ependymoma (WHO Grade III).

In the past, treatment has included surgery with radiation therapy. There is evidence to suggest that more extensive surgical resections are related to an improved rate of survival. Chemotherapy has been shown to be active in patients with ependymoma but a small prospective, randomized trial suggests that its activity is limited. Children younger than 3 years of age are particularly susceptible to the adverse effect of radiation on brain development. Debilitating effects on growth and neurologic development have frequently been observed, especially in younger children. For this reason, the role of chemotherapy in allowing a delay in the administration of radiation therapy is under study.[28] Studies are underway evaluating the role of early radiation therapy for local control in infants. Long-term management of these patients is complex and requires a multidisciplinary approach.

Newly Diagnosed Childhood Ependymoma

In the newly diagnosed patient, careful evaluation to fully determine the extent of disease must precede the treatment of ependymoma. Surgery should be performed in an attempt at maximal tumor reduction; children have improved progression-free survival if there is minimal residual disease present after surgery. Postoperatively, studies such as cerebral spinal fluid (CSF) cytological evaluation should be conducted to determine the extent of residual disease and dissemination. Patients with residual tumor or disseminated disease should be considered at high risk for relapse and should be treated on protocols specifically designed for them. Those with no evidence of residual tumor still have an approximately 20 to 40% relapse risk in spite of postoperative radiation therapy.

Post Surgical Treatment Options

Surgery Alone

Limited experience with surgery alone for completely resected supratentorial tumors suggest that, in select cases, this may be an option.

No residual disease, no disseminated disease: The traditional postsurgical treatment for these patients has been radiation therapy consisting of 5,400 to 5,580 cGy to the tumor bed. It is not necessary to treat the entire CNS (whole brain and spine) since these tumors usually recur at the local site. When possible, patients should be treated in a center experienced with this therapy. There is no evidence that adjuvant chemotherapy improves the outcome for patients with ependymoma. Trials are ongoing to evaluate the role of radiation therapy and chemotherapy in these patients.

Residual disease; no disseminated disease: Consideration of re-resection should be made since patients who have

complete resections have better disease control. The traditional postsurgical treatment for these patients has been radiation therapy consisting of 5,400 to 5,580 cGy to the tumor bed. It is not necessary to treat the entire CNS (whole brain and spine) since these tumors usually recur at the local site. When possible, patients should be treated in a center experienced with this therapy. There is no evidence that adjuvant chemotherapy, including high-dose chemotherapy with stem cell rescue, is of any benefit. Trials are ongoing to evaluate the possible role of radiation therapy and chemotherapy in these patients.

Children with CNS disseminated disease: In children with disseminated disease, long-term survivors have been reported and aggressive therapy is warranted. Regardless of degree of surgical resection, these patients require radiation therapy to the entire CNS (whole brain and spine) along with boosts to local disease and bulk areas of disseminated disease. The traditional local postsurgical radiation doses in these patients have been 5,400 to 5,580 cGy. Doses of approximately 3,600 cGy to the entire neuraxis (i.e., the whole brain and spine) should also be administered, but may be modulated depending on the age of the patient. Boosts to bulk areas of spinal disease between 4140 cGy and 5040 cGy should be administered, with doses depending on the age of the patient and the location of the tumor. When possible, patients should be treated in a center experienced with this therapy. Trials are ongoing to evaluate the possible role of radiation therapy and chemotherapy in these patients.

Postsurgical Management of Children Younger than 3 Years of Age

Because of the known effects of radiation on growth and neurocognitive development, its use immediately after surgery in children under 3 years of age is limited. Some patients younger than 3 years of age with newly diagnosed ependymoma will respond, at least partially, to chemotherapy. For this reason, strong consideration should be given to entering patients younger than 3 years of age in studies that use chemotherapy to delay the need for radiation therapy. Although chemotherapy is being used to prevent neurologic damage caused by radiation therapy in very young patients, neurologic deficits may be present in children prior to the initiation of therapy, and progressive neurologic damage has been noted during therapy. The need and timing of radiation therapy for children who have successfully completed chemotherapy and have no residual disease is still to be determined.

Recurrent Childhood Ependymoma

Recurrence is not uncommon in both benign and malignant childhood brain tumors and may develop many years after initial treatment. For ependymoma, delays beyond 10 to 15 years have been reported. Disease generally recurs at the primary tumor site even in children with malignant ependymomas. Systemic relapse is extremely rare. At time of relapse, a complete evaluation for extent of recurrence is indicated for all patients. Patients with recurrent ependymomas who have not previously received radiation therapy and/or chemotherapy, should be considered for treatment with these modalities. Active agents include cyclophosphamide, cisplatin, carboplatin, lomustine, and etoposide.

Brainstem Gliomas

Untreated Childhood Brainstem Glioma

Diffuse intrinsic brainstem gliomas: Conventional treatment for children with diffuse intrinsic brainstem glioma is radiation therapy to involved areas. Such treatment will result in transient benefit for the majority of patients, but over 90% of patients will succumb to the disease within 18 months of diagnosis. The conventional dose of radiation therapy ranges between 5400 cGy and 6000 cGy given locally to the primary tumor site in single daily fractions.

Hyperfractionated (twice daily) radiation therapy techniques have been used to deliver a higher dose, and studies using doses as high as 7800 cGy have been completed. There is no evidence that these increased radiation therapy doses improve the duration or rate of survival for patients with diffuse and/or primary pontine tumors. Studies evaluating the efficacy of various radiosensitizers as a means for enhancing the therapeutic effect of this modality are under study but to date have failed to show significant improvement in outcome.[29]

The role of chemotherapy in the treatment of patients with newly diagnosed brain stem gliomas is limited.

To date neither adjuvant or neoadjuvant chemotherapy nor immunotherapy when added to radiation therapy has been demonstrated to improve survival for children with diffuse intrinsic tumors. Studies using chemotherapy with radiation are ongoing. Children younger than 3 years of age with diffuse intrinsic tumors may benefit from chemotherapy to delay or modify radiation therapy.

Focal or Low-grade Brainstem Gliomas

Selected patients, primarily those with low-grade dorsally exophytic and focal tumors, may be treated surgically. Seven patients with extensive resection may be observed prior to the initiation of further therapy, preferably as part of a prospective clinical study.

Patients with small tectal lesions and hydrocephalus but no other neurological deficits may be treated with cerebrospinal fluid diversion and have follow-up with sequential neuroradiographic studies until there is evidence of progressive disease.

Neurofibromatosis

Children with neurofibromatosis Type I and brain stem gliomas may have a different prognosis than other patients who have intrinsic lesions. Patients with neurofibromatosis may present with a long history of symptoms or be identified on screening tests; a period of observation may be indicated before instituting any treatment. Brainstem gliomas in these children may be indolent and may require no specific treatment for years.

Recurrent Childhood Brainstem Glioma

Recurrence may occur in both benign and malignant childhood brain stem gliomas and may develop many years after initial treatment. Disease may occur at the primary tumor site or, especially in malignant tumors, at noncontiguous central nervous system sites. Biopsy or surgical resection should be considered for confirmation of relapse when other entities such as secondary tumor and treatment-related brain necrosis which may be clinically indistinguishable from tumor recurrence are in the differential. This confirmation is usually not necessary in children with diffuse, intrinsic tumors.

Chemotherapy with agents such as a carboplatin and vincristine may be effective in children with low-grade, recurrent exophytic gliomas. Patients with recurrent diffuse, intrinsic brainstem glioma should be considered for entry into trials of novel therapeutic approaches because there are no "standard" agents that have demonstrated a high degree of activity. Alternatively, palliative care may be indicated for such individuals.

Childhood Cerebral Astrocytoma

According to the most recent classification of the World Health Organization, glial tumors are divided on the basis of histologic criteria into the following subsets: pilocytic astrocytomas, low-grade nonpilocytic astrocytomas, anaplastic gliomas, and glioblastomas multiforme. Various types of nonpilocytic astrocytomas, such as fibrillary protoplasmic and gemistiocytic, have been identified. Both malignant and benign varieties of oligodendrogliomas may occur.

Low-Grade Childhood Cerebral Astrocytoma

The usual treatment for low-grade supratentorial astrocytoma is surgery. There is no evidence that radiation therapy is of benefit for patients with completely resected tumors. For patients with incompletely resected tumor, treatment options include observation, re-resection, radiation, and/or chemotherapy and must be individualized. Radiation therapy is often reserved until progressive disease is documented. Radiation fields encompass the tumor, and doses of 5,400 cGy are common. Evaluation with detailed electro-encephalographic mapping and surgery designed to remove the tumor and adjacent epileptic foci has been recommended for those patients with low-grade tumor and seizures. However, excellent results in tumor and seizure control have been reported with magnetic resonance-based "total" tumor resection. Low-grade tumors may respond to various chemotherapeutic regimens, including carboplatin.[30] Chemotherapy may delay the need for radiation therapy; its role in the treatment of children younger than 5 years of age with newly diagnosed, progressive lesions is under study.[30]

High-Grade Childhood Cerebral Astrocytoma

The therapy for both children and adults with supratentorial high-grade astrocytoma includes surgery, radiation therapy, and chemotherapy. Outcome in high-grade gliomas occurring in childhood may be more favorable than that in adults, but it is not clear if this difference is caused by biologic variations in tumor characteristics, therapies used, tumor resectability, or other factors that are not presently understood. The ability to obtain a complete resection is associated with a better prognosis. Radiation therapy is administered to a field that widely encompasses the entire tumor. Alternatively, it can be administered to the entire brain with a "cone down" to the tumor volume. The radiation therapy dose is usually at least 5,400 cGy. A notable result was seen in children with glioblastoma multiforme who were treated on a prospective, randomized trial with adjuvant lomustine, vincristine, and prednisone. In children with recurrent high-grade gliomas, one study has reported encouraging disease control in those with minimal bulk disease at the time of initiation of chemotherapy. Children younger than 3 years of age may benefit from chemotherapy to delay, modify, or, in selected cases, obviate the need for radiation therapy. Clinical trials that evaluate chemotherapy with or without radiation therapy are ongoing.

Recurrent Low-grade Cerebral Astrocytoma

Systemic relapse is rare, but may occur. At the time of recurrence, a complete evaluation for extent of relapse is indicated for all malignant tumors and, at times, for more benign lesions. Biopsy or surgical resection may be necessary for confirmation of relapse because other entities, such as secondary tumor and treatment-related brain necrosis, may be clinically indistinguishable from tumor recurrence. Patients with recurrent cerebral astrocytoma after maximal surgery and irradiation may benefit from chemotherapy. Drug combinations, such as carboplatin and vincristine, may be useful at the time of recurrence for children with low-grade gliomas.

Recurrent High-grade Cerebral Astrocytoma

Biopsy or surgical resection may be necessary for confirmation of relapse because other entities, such as secondary tumor and treatment-related brain necrosis, may be clinically indistinguishable from tumor recurrence. The need for surgical intervention must be individualized on the basis of the initial tumor type, the length of time between initial treatment and the reappearance of the mass lesion, and the clinical picture.

Patients for whom treatment fails may benefit from additional treatment, including high-dose chemotherapy with bone marrow rescue. They should be considered for entry into trials of novel therapeutic approaches.

REFERENCES

1. Doll R, Muir C, Waterhouse J. Cancer incidence in five continents. Vol.II, New York, Springer-Verlag, 1970.
2. Boffeta P, Parkin DM. Cancer in developing countries CA. Cancer J Clin 1994;44:81-90.
3. Shalet M, Gibson B, Swindell R, Pearson D. Effect of spinal irradium on growth. Arch Dis Child 1987;62:461-4.
4. Gerbault A, Panis X, Flamant F, Chassagne D. Iridium afterloading curietherapy in the treatment of pediatric malignancies. Cancer 1989;56:1274-9.

5. Punkel D. Therapy of acute lymphoid leukemia in children. Leukemia 1992;(Suppl. 2)6:127.

6. Hushe HO, Aur RJA. Extramedullary leukemia. Clin Haematol 1978;7:313-37.

7. Svatin-Tapper G, Nilsson P, Jonsson C, Alvegard T. Calculation and measurements of absorbed dose in total body irradiation. Acta Oncol 1990;29:627-33.

8. Peeg H, Sullivan K, Buckner C et al. Marrow transplantation for acute non-lymphoblastic leukemia in fiest remission: Toxicity and long term follow up of patients conditioned with single dose or fractionated total body irradiation. Bone Marrow Transplant 1986;1:151-7.

9. Mendelhall NP. Hodgkin's disease. In : Cassady RR (ed). Radiation therapy in pediatric oncology. Springer-Verlag Hridelberg 1994;151-74.

10. Parker BR, Casteuino RA, Kaplan HS. Pediatric Hodgkin's disease I. Radiographic evaluation. Cancer 1976;37:2430-35.

11. Kaplan HS. Evidence of tumoricidal dose level in the radiotherapy of Hodgkin's disease. Cancer Res 1966;26:1221-4.

12. Dioner C, Obercin O, Hasrand JL. Initial chemotherapy and low dose radiation in limited fields in childhood Hodgkin's disease. Results of a joint cooperative study by the French society of pediatric oncology (SFOP) and Hospital St. Louis, Paris. Int J Radiat Oncol Biol Phys 1988;15:341-8.

13. Donaldson SS, Whitaker SJ, Plawman PN, Link MP, Malpas JS. Stape I-II pediatric Hodgkin's disease long-term follow up demonstrated equivalent survival rates following different management schemes. J Clin Oncol 1990;8:1128-37.

14. Gurney JG, Severson RK, Davis S, et al. Incidence of cancer in children in the United States: sex-, race-, and 1-year age-specific rates by histologic type. Cancer 1995;75(8):2186-95.

15. Wolden SL, Anderson JR, Crist WM, et al.: Indications for radiotherapy and chemotherapy after complete resection in rhabdomyosarcoma: a report from the Intergroup Rhabdomyosarcoma studies I to III. Journal of Clinical Oncology 1999;17(11):3468-75.

16. Hug EB, Adams J, Fitzek M, et al. Fractionated, three-dimensional, planning-assisted proton-radiation therapy for orbital rhabdomyosarcoma: a novel technique. International Journal of Radiation Oncology, Biology, Physics 2000;47(4):979-84.

17. Mandell L, Ghavimi F, Peretz T, et al. Radiocurability of microscopic disease in childhood rhabdomyosarcoma with radiation doses less than 4,000 cGy. Journal of Clinical Oncology 1990;8(9):1536-42.

18. Maurer HM. Soft Tissue Sarcoma Committee: IRS Study IV: Phase III Comparison of VM (VCR/L-PAM) vs IE (IFF/VP-16) vs ID (IFF/DOX) in Patients with Stage 4 Rhabdomyosarcoma (Summary Last Modified 03/95), IRS-IV-STAGE/GROUP-4, clinical trial, closed, 1995;03:01.

19. Raney RB, Tefft M, Newton WA, et al. Improved prognosis with intensive treatment of children with cranial soft tissue sarcomas arising in nonorbital parameningeal sites: a report from the Intergroup Rhabdomyosarcoma Study. Cancer 1987;59(1):147-55

20. Craft A, Cotterill S, Malcolm A, et al. Ifosfamide-containing chemotherapy in Ewing's sarcoma: The Second United Kingdom Children's Cancer Study Group and the Medical Research Council Ewing's Tumor Study. Journal of Clinical Oncology 1998;16(11):3628-33.

21. Coffin CM, Dehner LP. Neurogenic tumors of soft tissue. In: Coffin CM, Dehner LP, O'Shea PA: Pediatric Soft Tissue Tumors: A Clinical, Pathological, and Therapeutic Approach. Baltimore, Md: Williams and Wilkins, 1997;80-132.

22. Paulussen M, Ahrens S, Craft AW, et al. Ewing's tumors with primary lung metastases: survival analysis of 114 (European Intergroup) Cooperative Ewing's Sarcoma Studies patients. Journal of Clinical Oncology 1998;16(9):3044-52.

23. Madero L, Munoz A, Sanchez de Toledo J, et al. Megatherapy in children with high-risk Ewing's sarcoma in first complete remission. Bone Marrow Transplantation 1998;21(8):795-9.

24. Packer RJ, Siegel KR, Sutton LN, et al. Efficacy of adjuvant chemotherapy for patients with poor-risk medullo-blastoma: a preliminary report. Annals of Neurology 1988;24(4):503-8.

25. Packer RJ, Sutton LN, Atkins TE, et al. A prospective study of cognitive function in children receiving whole-brain radiotherapy and chemotherapy: 2-year results. Journal of Neurosurgery 1989;70(5):707-13.

26. Thomas PR, Deutsch M, Kepner JL, et al. Low-stage medulloblastoma: final analysis of trial comparing standard-dose with reduced-dose neuraxis irradiation. Journal of Clinical Oncology 2000;18(16):3004-11.

27. Johnson DL, McCabe MA, Nicholson HS, et al. Quality of long-term survival in young children with medullo-blastoma. Journal of Neurosurgery 1994;80(6):1004-10.

28. Duffner PK, Horowitz ME, Krischer JP, et al. Postoperative chemotherapy and delayed radiation in children less than three years of age with malignant brain tumors. New England Journal of Medicine 1993;328(24):1725-31.

29. Mandell LR, Kadota R, Freeman C, et al. There is no role for hyperfractionated radiotherapy in the management of children with newly diagnosed diffuse intrinsic brainstem tumors: results of a Pediatric Oncology Group phase III trial comparing conventional vs. hyperfractionated radiotherapy. International Journal of Radiation Oncology, Biology, Physics 1999;43(5):959-64.

30. Packer RJ, Lange B, Ater J, et al. Carboplatin and vincristine for recurrent and newly diagnosed low-grade gliomas of childhood. Journal of Clinical Oncology 1993;11(5): 850-56.

CHAPTER 52

Lalit Kumar
K Ganessan

Bone Marrow Transplantation in Childhood Diseases

INTRODUCTION

High-dose chemotherapy with or without radiotherapy followed by bone marrow or hemopoietic stem cell transplantation (HSCT) is currently an established mode of treatment for a number of malignant and non-malignant diseases (Table 52.1). HSCT refers to intravenous infusion of hemopoietic progenitor cells to re-establish hemopoiesis in a patient with defective or damaged bone marrow (BM).[1-2] For this purpose, hemopoetic progenitor (stem) cells can be obtained either from a genetically identical twin (syngeneic) or from an HLA-identical matched sibling (allogeneic) or patient's own (autologous). For patients who lack an HLA – identical sibling, a number of centers have explored the use of alternative donors, either family members other than HLA–identical siblings or matched voluntary unrelated donors (MUD).[3] Unlike an allogeneic BMT, there is no risk of acute graft versus host disease (GVHD) after autologous transplantation; however, the risk of relapse is increased.

HLA MATCHING

Accurate HLA typing is essential for patients receiving allogeneic transplants. The probability of finding an HLA match in the family is about 25 to 35 percent. Currently, in addition to standard serologic methods using alloantisera for Class 1 (HLA-A,B,C) and Class II (HLA-DR,DQ and DP) antigens, more elaborate techniques – including, one dimensional isoelectric focussing to examine Class I regions, and DNA based techniques such as PCR- with sequence specific oligonucleotide

Table 52.1: Indications of Bone Marrow/Blood Stem cell Transplantation

Condition	Allogeneic	Autologous
Non-malignant		
Severe aplastic anemia	+	–
Fanconi anemia	+	–
Beta thalassemia	+	–
Sickle cell anemia	+	–
Chronic granulomatous diseases	+	–
Immunodeficiency diseases		
SCID	+	–
Wiskott aldrich syndrome	+	–
Chediak–Higashi disease	+	–
Lysosomal storage diseases	+	–
Auto-immune disease	+*	+*
Malignant		
Chronic myeloid leukemia	+	+*
Acute myeloblastic leukemia	+	+
Acute lymphoblastic leukemia	+**	–
Myelodysplastic syndrome	+	+*
Hodgkins disease	–	+
Non-hodgkins lymphoma	–	+
Germ cell tumours of testis	–	+
Neuroblastoma	–	+
Other childhood tumours	–	+*

*Presently experimental, definite evidence of benefit is awaited in randomized trials.

**Not routinely indicated in ALL except in selected cases. SCID-severe combined immunodeficiency disease

probes (PCR-SSOP) for Class II regions are employed. By molecular typing C locus appears to be a significant determinant of graft failure and acute graft versus host disease (GVHD).[4] van Rood has suggested a system for categorizing the degreee of match between the patient and donor.[5] When more than one donor appears suitable for an individual patient, the limiting dilution assay of alloreactive cytotoxic T-lymphocytes precursors in the blood of the prospective donor can aid donor selection.[6] In general, the results of allografting with stem cells from alternative donors are not as good as results of allografting comparable patients with stem cells from HLA-identical siblings.

STEM CELL SOURCE

The stem cells from bone marrow (BM) can renew themselves, proliferate and differentiate into various cell lineages. A transplant of such cells could result in complete reconstitution of hemopoietic and immune systems in the recipient (allogeneic). This reconstitution of hemopoietic system is required especially as support following HD-CT/radiotherapy in autologous setting. As the monocytes produced by the transplanted stem cells can migrate, become macrophages and deliver the deficient enzymes or proteins to the affected tissues, HSCT can be used for the treatment of certain genetic metabolic diseases.[2]

In addition to BM, stem cells can also be obtained from peripheral blood (PB) and umbilical cord (UC). Traditionally, BM has been used as a source of stem cells for allogeneic transplantation. However, recent results from randomized studies in adult patients indicate that peripheral blood stem cells (PBSC) can be used safely in place of BM stem cells without excessive risk of acute GVHD.[7-8] Data from randomized trials in pediatric population is limited. There is some concern that risk of chronic GVHD may be higher with use of PBSC.[8-9] For allogeneic sibling transplantation, if multiple donors are available then donor choice involves donor ABO type, donor age and transfusion history and for female donors, parity.

For use, PBSC have to be mobilized from BM. This is done by giving G-CSF to donor 5-10 mcg/kg/day subcutaneously for 4 to 5 days. On 5th or 6th, PBSC are collected by leukapheresis using cell separator (apharesis) machine. Collections of PBSCs contain substantially more CD-34+ cells and perhaps 10 times more lymphocytes than comparable collections of BM. Recovery of neutrophils and platelet numbers is more rapid in recipients of PB derived allogeneic stem cells than in those receiving marrow derived stem cells. Neither anesthesia nor hospitalization is required for the donor. For autologous transplantation, PB stem cells, rather than BM, are used as a source of stem cells.[10-11]

Umbilical cord (UC) blood is a rich source of most primitive (stem) cells that are able to produce 'in vivo' long term repopulating hemopoietic stem cells compared to adult stem cells. Therefore, these are able to expand rapidly and reconstitute hemopoiesis after myeloablative chemotherapy. Another major advantage of UC blood cells is the relative immaturity of the immune system at birth, resulting in significantly lower risk of acute GVHD compared to adult BM/Blood stem cells. Since, the total yield of stem cells from a single cord blood is limited, presently, UC blood is being used for children weighing up to 25 Kg. Because of ease of procurement, absence of risks to donors, reduced risk of transmitting infection and the prompt availability of cryopreserved samples to transplantation centres, a number of UC blood banks have been set up in North America and Europe. More than 2000 transplants have been performed worldwide, mainly in children using allogeneic HLA matched sibling or matched unrelated UC blood for both non-malignant and malignant conditions.[12-15]

BONE MARROW HARVEST

Marrow is usually harvested under general anaesthesia by repeated aspiration from posterior iliac crest (Fig. 52.1). If there is difficulty in removing adequate number of stem cells from posterior iliac crest, BM can be removed from anterior iliac crest or sternum. The precise number of nucleated marrow cells required is not known. In practice, approximately 3×10^8 nucleated cells/kg of the recipient's body weight (or 5×10^6/kg CD34+ cells are harvested. The harvesting of BM is generally well tolerated. In allogeneic BMT with major ABO incompatibility between donor and recipient, it is necessary to remove mature erythrocytes from graft to avoid a hemolytic transfusion reaction.

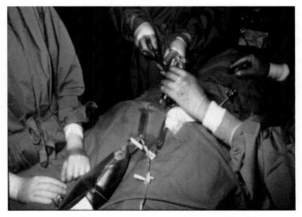

Figure 52.1: Bone marrow harvest iliac crest

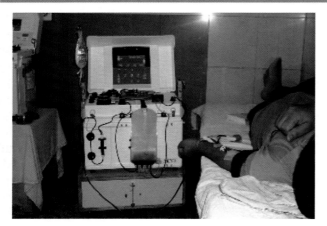

Figure 52.2: Peripheral blood stem cell transplantation

For autologous SCT, PBSCs are harvested with the help of a cell separator either following chemotherapy with growth factors (G-CSF) or G-CSF alone (Fig. 52.2) and Table 52.2. For paediatric population, usually PBSC mobilization is performed with growth factors. A minimum of 5×10^8 per kg mononuclear cells (or 5×10^6/kg CD34 + cells are harvested. These cells are then cryopreserved at –80C using 7.5 percent DMSO or in liquid nitrogen.[16] Following this, patient is administered chemotherapy. Depending upon the halflife of chemotherapy drugs used, PBSC can be re-infused either after 24 hours, e.g. for melphalan or after longer interval (5-7 days). The later requires cryopreservation of stem cells. The primary concern with autologous SCT is relapse due to re-infusion of malignant cells along with progenitor cells (Table 52.2).[17] Various methods including 'in vitro' treatment with chemotherapy drugs, monoclonal antibodies have been developed to remove the contaminating tumour cells (a process called purging). Retrospective analyses have suggested that purging leads to a reduced rate of relapse in patients with AML and non-Hodgkin's lymphoma.[18]

Table 52.2: Allogeneic versus autologous stem cell transplantation

	Allogeneic SCT	Autologous SCT
Regimen related toxicity	+	+
Acute GVHD	++	-
Relapse	+	++
Graft vs leukemia (malignancy) effect	+	-

PREPARATORY REGIMEN

Prior to stem cell transplantation, patients own BM is destroyed by giving HD-CT with or without total body irradiation (TBI). This is done for cytoreduction, to eradicate the malignant cells, and to provide immunosuppression. This prevents rejection and allows normal BM to grow (engraft) in a patient with aplastic anaemia or destroys a dysfunctional BM such as in beta thalassemia and, possibly, creates of space within the BM microenvironment to allow engraftment of the donor stem cells.[1-2]

For autologous transplantation immuno-supression is not required and the preparative regimen is meant to provide maximum dose intensity with a goal of eradicating the malignancy.

For acute and chronic leukemias, most patients have earlier received cyclophosphamide and TBI (Cyclo-TBI) as the preparative regimen. Fractionation of TBI (total dose 1200 to 1500 cGys) is generally used to reduce toxicity to normal tissues. Combination of busulphan (4 mg/kg/day × 4 days = 16 mg/kg) and cyclophosphamide (60 mg/kg/day × 2=120 mg/kg) (Bu-Cy2) is an effective regimen for allogeneic and autologous SCT and has gained popularity in past 2 decades. Two randomized trials evaluating cyclo-TBI vs Bu-Cy as preparative regimen in patients with chronic phase CML revealed equal efficacy.[19-20] Ringden et. al from the Nordic Bone Marrow Transplant Group have reported the results of a randomized trial comparing BuCy2 with Cyclo-TBI as conditioning in 167 allogeneic BMT recipients with leukaemia. The incidence of relapse was not different in two groups. Relapse-free survival was also similar in the two groups on analysis of data from all patients, children, patients with early disease and those with acute myeloblastic leukaemia (AML), acute lymphoblastic leukaemia (ALL) and chronic myelogenous leukaemia (CML). However, in adults (p=0.05) and patients with advanced disease (p<0.005) leukaemia-free survival (LFS) was significantly better in those treated with TBI[21]. Long term follow-up of the French study (median follow up of 10.8 years) has been reported recently; overall survival (59 vs 43%) and event free survival (55 vs 35%, p<.04) was superior for patients receiving Cyclo-TBI compared to Bu-Cy2 prior to allogeneic HLA-identical sibling transplant.[22] One of the recent development has been availability of intravenous busulfan.[23] Oral busulfan has erratic absorption, particularly in children. In general Cyclo-

TBI as preparatory regimen is preferred by many centers for patients with acute leukemia[24] while Bu-Cy is commonly used for CML. The toxicity profile of the two regimens is given in Table 52.3.

Table 52.3: Toxicity profile of conditioning regimens			
	TBI	Chemotherapy alone	Non myeloablative
Mucositis	+	++	+/–
Veno-occlusive disease	+	++	–
Growth retardation	++	+/–	–
Secondary malignancies	++	+/–	?
Cataracts	++	+/–	–
Sterility	++	+	?

For non-malignant conditions like severe aplastic anemia, a combination of cyclophosphamide and anti thymocyte globulin (ATG) or anti-lymphocyte globulin (ALG) is associated with less risk of rejection. Similarly, for beta thalaessemia, combination of Bu-Cy or Bu-Cy plus ATG is used.

Autologous SCT studies have generally used the same regimens developed for allogeneic transplants. For patients with Hodgkin;s disease and non Hodgkins lymphoma, BEAM (BCNU, etoposide, cytosine arabinoside and melphalan) or a combination of BCNU, cyclophosphamide and etoposide has generally been used. Encouraging results have been reported with the use of busulphan and etoposide combination prior to autologous BMT in AML patients.[25] For solid tumours, a combination of carboplatin + VP-16 +/– cyclophosphamide or, ifosphamide, has been used. More recently, monoclonal antibodies like Rituxan or Compath have also been combined with chemotherapy as part of the preparatory regimen for non-Hodgkin's lymphomas.[26]

Non-myeloablative Regimens

In past 5 years, for allogeneic SCT, the focus has shifted from myeloablative (tumoricidal plus immunosuppressive regimen) to simply being immunosuppressive called non-myeloablative or less intensive regimen. Here, 'Graft-versus-Tumor' (GvT) effect plays key role in haematopoietic ablation and subsequent disease elimination. Following infusion of allogeneic stem cells, engraftment results often with state of mixed chimerism. Later, donor lymphocyte infusion is used to augment the GvT effect and to convert the mixed chimeric state into full donor hemopoiesis. Fludarabine, busulfan +/– ATG or a combination of Fludarabine, busulfan + TBI has commonly been used. Initial experience (mainly limited to patients of higher age or those with relapsed / refractory disease or at high risk for GVHD) suggests that this approach is associated with less myelosuppression, allows engraftment to take place and overall is associated with less toxicity. Since there is less organ damage, thus less cytokine release, one would hope that these regimen would be associated with less risk of severe acute GVHD.[27-28] This procedure has been recently performed in children with good results.[29]

COMPLICATIONS

In addition to severe, prolonged mylosuppression, regime related toxicity, graft versus host disease (GVHD), CMV pneumonitis and relapse are main complications seen after SCT (Table 52.4).

Table 52.4: Complications following bone marrow transplantation	
Acute complication	
Infection	
Acute graft versus host disease	
Graft rejection	
Plumonary	Regime related complication
Hemorrhagic cystitis	
Veno-occlusive disease	
Late complications	
Chronic GVHD	
Relapse	
Sterility	
Cataract	
Secondary leukaemia	

Infections

This is one of the most important complications of SCT. The recipients of SCT are at risk of infections at different times of post-transplant period due to immunodeficiency state associated with SCT. Immune system recovery takes place in three phases beginning at day 0, the day of transplant viz- phase I- the pre-engraftment period (<30 days after SCT), phase II- the postengraftment phase (30-100 days after HSCT) and phase III- the late phase (>100 days after HSCT).[30] The immune recovery occurs more quickly and more completely in children than adults.

During the phase I, prolonged neutropenia and breaks in mucocutaneous barrier (secondary to preparative regimens and vascular access) increase the

Cause of infection	Early period (Day 0-30)	Middle period (Day 31-120)	Late period (Day 120[4])
Bacteria	Streptococci Staphylococci Aerobic gram positive rods	Nocardia	Streptococcus pneumoniae Hemophilus influenza
Viruses	Herpes simplex virus	Cytomegalovirus	Varicella-zoster virus
Fungi	Candida aspergillus	Candida Aspergillus	
Parasites		P. carinii T. gondii	P. carinni T. gondii

Table 52.5: Common causes of infections after BMT

risk of infections. The pathogens are usually bacterial — gram-positive and gram-negative and fungal infections (Table 52.5). In this phase the risk of infection is the same for autologous or allogeneic SCT. Additionally, herpes simplex virus reactivation may occur during this period.

The early post-engraftment period is dominated by impaired cell mediated immunity in the recipients. The severity of immune deficiency depends on the presence of GvHD and the use of immunosuppressants among the allogeneic SCT recipients. The predominant infection seen in this period is the cytomegalovirus (CMV). Other infections include *Pneumocystis carinii* and aspergillus species. The risk of *Pnemocystitis carinii* induced interstitial pneumonia may be reduced to <10 percent by chemoprophylaxis with trimethoprim – sulfamethoxazole: one double strength tablet by mouth two or three times per week is given starting after engraftment (when neutrophils are >1000/cmm) and is continued for 6 to 12 months after transplant. In patients allergic to sulfa, pentamidine (300 mg) once a month can be used.

The late post-engraftment period related infections come under late complications of SCT and predominantly seen among allogeneic SCT recipients. The usual infections seen are viral (CMV, HSV, EBV, etc.) and capsulated bacteria due to impaired humoral and cell mediated immunity. The risk increases with the presence of chronic GvHD and the immunosuppressive therapy.

Graft versus Host Disease (GVHD)

GvHD is the principal cause of morbidity and mortality after allogeneic SCT. It is characterized by symptoms and signs associated with skin, gastro-intestinal system and liver. The severity of the condition is graded according to involvement of these organs (Table 52.6). GVHD can be divided into two some what distinct clinical entities : acute GVHD, when it occurs within 100 days after BMT, and chronic GVHD developing after 100 days of BMT.[31,32] The disorder occurs when immunologically competent cells in graft, target antigens on the cells in the recipients. Treatment with cyclosporine – A with or without methotrexate is routinely used for prophylaxis to prevent acute GVHD in the allogeneic BMT recipients. Even with prophylaxis however, most patients develop some degree of acute GVHD after allogeneic BMT. Treatment for established severe acute GVHD include—high doses of corticosteroids, antithymocyte globulin, and monoclonal antibodies.

The clinical features of chronic GVHD are similar to scleroderma.[33] It is most likely to develop in patients with acute GVHD and in older patients. Treatment with prednisolone, cyclosporine A or thalidomide has improved the long term outlook for patient with chronic GVHD.

Higher probability of relapse in chronic phase CML patients allografted with T-cell depleted marrow[34] and in syngeneic transplant recipient compared to recipients of un-manipulated marrow suggest that GVL plays an important role in the cure of leukemia after BMT. It is assumed that this GVL effect is mediated by donor T-lymphocytes that are capable of mediating both GVHD and GVL effect. Whether the same population of T-cells mediates these two diverse effects in not known. The most compelling evidence supporting the powerful and potential curative nature of GVL effect is the observation that complete and durable remissions can be obtained

Table 52.6: Acute graft versus host disease according to organ involvement (From ref. No 31)

Grade	Skin	Liver (serum bilirubin mg/dl)	GIT
1.	Maculopapular rash on <25 percent of body surface	2-3 mg/dl	500-1000 ml liquid stools/day
2.	Maculopapular rash on 25-50 percent of body surface	>3-6 mg/dl	>1000 and <1500 ml liquid stool/day
3.	Generalized erythroderma	>6-15 mg/dl	>1500ml liquid stool/day
4.	Generalized erythrodema with formation of bullous desquamation	>15 mg/dl	severe abdominal pain + ileus

Clinical grade	Skin	Level of injury Liver	GIT
I	1 or 2	0	0
II	1-3	1	1
III	2 or 3	2 or 3	2 or 3
IV	2-4	2-4	2-4

in patients with transfusion of donor lymphocytes without chemotherapy or radiotherapy in patients with CML who have relapsed after allogeneic BMT.[35,36]

Pulmonary Complications

Pulmonary hemorrhage, interstitial pneumonitis, capillary leak syndrome are important respiratory complications seen after BMT. 'Diffuse pulmonary hemorrhage' manifests as fever, hypoxia, and pulmonary infiltrates early after BMT usually during the first 30 days. This syndrome probably related to pulmonary injury from high dose therapy, is most frequently seen in patients who receive autologous BMT and seems to be responsive to corticosteroids.[37]

Interstitial pneumonitis is characterized by high fever, pulmonary infiltrates, hypoxia, and the adult respiratory distress syndrome. This is seen usually during second and third month after allogeneic BMT and is often associated with GVHD. It is most frequently caused by cytomegalovirus (CMV). In CMV seronegative patients use of seronegative blood products has reduced the incidence of CMV pneumonitis. There is evidence that prophylactic acyclovir may reduce CMV infections and pneumonia in seropositive patients. Further, ganciclovir and high-dose immunoglobulin may be beneficial as treatment for early or limited CMV infections. During the third month or later, some patients may develop progressive pulmonary fibrosis. This syndrome can be related to high-dose therapy with carmustine or can be a complication of chronic GVHD. Treatment of this syndrome has generally been disappointing.[38]

A clinical picture like capillary leak syndrome (CLS) may occur frequently following engraftment-during 2nd-3rd week. This is characterised by excessive weight gain, ascites, and edema (a picture similar to non cardiogenic pulmonary oedema) associated with kidney and liver abnormalities suggest a common injury to multiple organs. Cahill et al reviewed clinical courses of 55 allogeneic and autologous marrow transplant recipients with regard to the presentation of a capillary leak syndrome (CLS). Twenty-nine patients (53%) developed non-cardiogenic pulmonary edema with or without concurrent pleural effusions; the incidence was comparable in allogeneic and autologous recipients. Pulmonary features were accompanied by hepatic dysfunction in 28, renal dysfunction in 22, and central nervous system abnormalities in 17. There was a strong correlation between time of engraftment and the first manifestations of CLS, both of which occurred earlier in allogeneic than in autologous transplant recipients. The underlying pathology of this disorder is poorly understood, a pivotal contribution by circulating leukocytes is a possibility.[39]

Graft Rejection

This complication is seen mainly in patients with non malignant conditions, e.g. aplastic anemia, beta thalassemia, Fanconi anemia, lysosomal storage disorders, etc. Predisposing factors include – previous blood transfusions, less intensive preparative regimens, the use of methotrexate rather than cyclosporine to prevent acute GVHD and the removal of

T-cells from graft. Incorporation of anti thymocyte globulin (ATG) into the preparative regimen appears to reduce the incidence of graft rejection for patients with severe aplastic anemia and beta thalassemia.[40]

Hemorrhagic Cystitis

This occurs most often after conditioning regimen containing ifosfamide or cyclophosphamide. A variety of uro-protective measures, e.g. including alkaline diuresis, frequent voiding, urethral catheterization and bladder irrigation and the use of 2-mercaptoethane sulfonate (mesna) (to react with the active urotoxic metabolites of oxazophosphorines) have been utilized to reduce the risk of hemorrhagic cystitis.

Veno-Occlusive Disease (VOD)

VOD of liver, an important regimen related toxicity, is seen in 20-40 percent of patients. VOD is characterized by jaundice (serum bilirubin >2.0 mg %), tender hepatomegaly, ascitis and unexplained weight gain (>2% of base line body weight) within 20 days of BMT.[41-42] Patients with severe VOD may progress to hepatic failure with poor prognosis. Management of established severe VOD is largely unsatisfactory. Recent efforts, therefore, have been directed toward prevention of VOD by using the drugs to interrupt the coagulation cascade or to diminish the influence of factors that favor thrombogenesis. These include – prophylactic use of heparin, prostaglandin EE and recombinant tissue plasminogen factor (ETPA) and oral administration of pentoxyfylline, a tumor necrosis factor alpha (TNF-α)-blocker.

CLINICAL RESULTS

Benign Diseases

Aplastic Anemia

Allogeneic BMT is the treatment of choice for young patients with severe aplastic anemia and it must be done soon after onset before the patients become sensitized by red cell and platelet transfusions.[43] About 80 percent of recipients are long term survivors following transplant. Survival decreases to 10-20 percent when the donor and recipient are mismatched at two or more loci.[44] In the IBMTR study, 3 year probabilities of survival for 1754 HLA-identical sibling transplants performed between 1991 and 1997, were 74 percent +/-3 percent for 978 patients < 20 years of age and 65 +/-3 percent for 776 patients older than 20 years. Results were not so good in unrelated donor transplants; 40 +/– 7 percent in 239 patients < 20 years and 36 percent +/-125 in 71 older patients.[45]

Beta Thalassemia

Allogeneic SCT is the only means of curing thalassemia at present and should be considered if an HLA matched sibling donor is available. The risk is low when transplant is done at an early age. Lucarelli et al. from Pesaro, Italy have recently reported the results on more than 1000 allogeneic BMT recipients for thalassemia. Busulphan and cyclophosphamide were used for preparation. Patients were categorized according to the presence of risk factors (hepatomegaly, portal fibrosis and poor quality of chelation) : Class I-with no risk factor, Class II with one or two and Class III- with all three risk factors. For patients under 16 years of age, for Class I, Class II and III the probabilities of overall survival and of event-free survival were- 95 and 90 percent, 87 and 84 percent, 89 and 64 percent, respectively. For Class III patients they used a more aggressive protocol which had a more favorable outcome.[46] In India, largest experience on thalassemia is from CMC Vellore.[4] The causes of death after SCT for thalassemia are results of iron overload other than the usual events. At present, the major limitation is availability of HLA-matched donors and studies are being conducted with matched unrelated donor transplants and UC blood transplants.

Sickle Cell Anemia

Sickle cell anemia (SCA) is an autosomal recessive disorder characterized by mutation in one of the globulins resulting in red cell sickling in deoxygenated states. At present, allo- SCT offers the only way of cure in these cases. But the selection of cases is still a matter of debate. European centers[48] offer allo-SCT to young patients with symptomatic SCA, before the occurrence of chronic organ damage and before transfusion-related complications. The centers in the US offer for patients fulfilling rigorous selection criteria with severe disorder.[49] Results of allo-SCT are good with overall survival and disease-free survival reaching 90 percent.

Immunodeficiency Diseases

A matched sibling donor transplant is the treatment of choice for patients with severe combined immunodeficiency disease (SCID), Wiscott Aldrich

Syndrome (WAS), or Chediak Higashi syndrome. Fischer et al. for the European Bone Marrow Transplant Group (EBMTG) have reported the results of 183 patients with SCID. Recipients of HLA-identical BMTs (n=70) had a 76 percent probability of survival (median follow up 73 months). HLA-non-identical, T-cell depleted BMT (n=100) gave significantly lower survival 52 percent (median follow up 47 months). Factors associated with poor prognosis were – the presence of lung infection before BMT, the absence of a protected environment, and the use of female donors for male patients. Increased graft failure and Epstein-Barr virus – associated B-cell lympho-profilterative disorders are major problems with T-cell depleted transplants.[50] In a recent EBMTG study, for HLA-identical sibling donor transplant for primary immunodeficiency disease other than SCID, the overall survival was 66 percent.[51]

Fanconi Anemia

Allogeneic transplant can cure some patients with Fanconic anemia. In the IBMTR study, among 215 patients transplanted between 1991 and 1997 from matched siblings, the 3 year survival was 72 percent+/-7 percent.[45] Transplant from other donors have been less successful.[52]

Lysosomal Storage Disorders

Lysosomal storage diseases are heterogenous group of disorders characterized by accumulation of specific substances in the lysosomes of macrophages in the lympho/ hemopoietic systems due to deficiency in lysosomal enzymes. Usually these disorders are progressive and many of them are fatal in childhood or adolescence. Allogeneic SCT is effective by (i) replacing enzymatically deficient cells with normal cells with normal enzyme levels (ii) intercellular transfer of enzymes between normal donor cells and deficient cells (iii) uptake of donor-derived enzymes released into the blood (iv) donor enzymes clear the accumulated substrates.

SCT reduces the storage material in visceral organs in majority of patients, but insufficient to improve the quality of life in patients with severe organ dysfunction. Skeletal deformities are stabilized by SCT. Clear improvement in severe neurological symptoms has not been observed indicating the need for transplants early in the course of the illness.[53-55] Of late, gene therapy has shown lots of promise.

Malignant Diseases

Acute Myeloblastic Leukemia (AML)

The prognosis of children with AML has improved considerably during the last two decades; 80 to 90 percent children achieve remission (CR) and nearly 50 percent are long-term survivors.[56] Cytogenetics is the most important determinant of prognosis in the management of AML. Based on cytogenetics, patients can be subdivided in 3 subgroups.[57] Favourable cytogenetic findings include- t(15;17), t(8;21), and inv 16 or del 16. About 85 percent of adult AML patients with favorable cytogenetics achieve complete remission following standard daunomycin and cytosine arabinoside (3:7) induction chemotherapy. With intensive post remission chemotherapy the overall survival at 5 years exceeds 50 percent. High dose cytosine arabinoside is considered to be critical as part of the post remission therapy.[58] None of the randomized trials[59-62] have demonstrated benefit of allogeneic or autologous BMT in this group of patients.

For patients with intermediate risk cytogenetics (+8, -Y, +6, del (12p, normal karyotype), allogeneic stem cell transplantation may be considered if an HLA identical match is available. The MRC trial reported 3 year survival rate of 65 percent with relapse risk of 18 percent at 3 years.[60] Data regarding autologous transplantation in this subgroup is controversial.

Allogeneic SCT from an HLA – matched sibling must be considered for patients with unfavorable cytogenetics (-5/5q-, t(8;21)with del 9q or complex karyotype, inv(3q), abn 11q23,20q, 21q, del9q,t(6;9),t(9;22), abn 17p, complex karyotypes ($\geq$ 3 abnormalities). In the US Intergroup study, 5 year survival of 44 percent was reported in the transplant group compared to 15 percent in the chemotherapy alone group.[62] Patients in CR2 or those with an untreated relapse are curable with allogeneic SCT with 3 year leukemia-free survival of 22-30 percent. About 10-20 percent of patients with primary chemo-refractory AML can be salvaged with allogeneic transplant.[45]

Allogeneic SCT is not indicated in patients AML with Down's syndrome.[64]

Acute Lymphoblastic Leukemia (ALL)

About 65 percent of children with good risk ALL are cured with standard chemotherapy. Therefore, allogeneic SCT is generally reserved for (i) children below 15 years with cytogenetic abnormalities such as t (4;

malignancies.[82-83] As the number of patients surviving after BMT has increased and the observation period has been extended, new malignancies are indeed recognized in human BMT recipients. The spectrum includes lymphoproliferative disorders, hematopoietic malignancies, and solid tumors.

An increased incidence of MDS has also been reported after autologous transplants for lymphomas[84] and breast cancer. The major factor contributing to the development of MDS or leukemia is the extent of therapy given before BMT. Out of 1,254 patients who had received autologous BMT, generally for Hodgkin's disease or non-Hodgkin's lymphoma, at least 30 had developed MDS. The elapsed time from transplant to the diagnosis of MDS was 2.5 to 8.5 years; the estimated incidences at 3 to 5 years ranged from 4 to 18 percent.[84]

vii. *Nervous System*

Leukoencephalopathy can occur due to damage to the white matter of the brain induced by extensive intrathecal administration of methotrexate alone or combined with cranial irradiation (1800-2400 cGy or even higher doses) and the use of TBI. Other complications like multifocal cerebral demyelination, inflammatory demyelinating polyneuropathy, immune-mediated myelopathy and encephalopathy have also been observed. Patients may also have impaired memory, shortened attention span and defects in verbal fluency. Children, particularly those who also receive cranial irradiation are likely to score lower than controls in visual-motor, processing tasks and various IQ tests.[85-87]

SUMMARY

Marrow and peripheral blood stem cell transplants have developed from a last-ditch effort to a standard and often first-line procedure. The majority of patients who recover from the immediate post-transplant period become healthy long-term survivors and return to a normal life. Some patients, however, develop chronic or delayed problems. Major factors contributing to these problems are pre-transplant therapy, intensive conditioning regimens and chronic GVHD. Thus, managing (and preventing, if possible) post-transplant complications requires careful consideration of transplantation early in treatment planning, development of less toxic conditioning regimens and the prevention of GVHD, particularly in its chronic form.

REFERENCES

1. Armitage JO. Bone Marrow Transplantation. New Eng. J Med 1994;330:827-38.
2. Gross TG, Egeler RM, Smith FO. Pediatric hematopoietic stem cell transplantation. Hemat/Oncol Clin N Am 2001;15:795-808.
3. Kumar I and Goldman JM. Bone Marrow transplantation for patients lacking an HLA-identical sibling donor. Current Opinions in Hematology 1993;234-39.
4. Petersdorf EW, Longton GM, Anasetti C, et al. Association of HLA-C disparity with graft failure after marrow transplantation from unrelated donors. Blood 1997;89:1818-23.
5. Van Rood JJ, Oudshoorn M. An HLA matched donor! What do you mean by an HLA matched donor?. Bone Marrow Transplant 1998; 22(suppl.I) S 83.
6. Spencer A, Brookes PA, Kaminsky E, et al. Cytotoxic T lymphocytes precursor frequency analysis in bone marrow transplantation with volunteer unrelated donors: value in donor selection. Transplantation 1995;59:1302-8.
7. Bensinger WI, Clift R, Martin P et al. Allogeneic peripheral blood stem cell transplantation in patients with advanced hematologic malignancies: A retrospective comparison with bone marrow transplantation. Blood 1996; 88:2796-
8. Korbling M and Anderlini P. Peripheral blood stem cell versus bone marrow allotransplantation: does the source of hemopoietic cells matters?. Review article. Blood 2001;98:2900-8.
9. Levine JE, Wiley J, Kletzel M et al. Cytokine mobilized allogeneic peripheral blood stem cell transplants in children result in rapid engraftment and a high incidence of chronic GvHD. Bone Marrow Transplant 2000;25:13.
10. Kumar L and Gulati SC. Peripheral stem cell transplantation. Lancet 1997;S9:346.
11. Schmitz n, Linch DC, Dreger P et al. Filgastirm mobilized peripheral blood progenitor cell transplantation in comparison with autologous bone marrow transplantation: Results of a randomized phase III trial in lymphoma patients. Lancet 1996;347:353-.
12. Gluckman E, Rocha V, Boyer-Chammard et al. Outcome of cord blood transplantation from related and unrelated donors. N Engl J Med 1997;337:373.
13. Rubinstein P, carrier C, Scaradavou A et al. Outcomes among 562 recipients of placental-blood transplants from unrelated donors. N Engl J Med 1998;339:1565-.
14. Locatelli F, Rocha V, Chastang C et al. factors associated with outcome after cord-blood transplantation in children with acute leukemia. Blood 1999;93:3662-
15. Rocha V, Wagner JE, Sobocinki Ka. Graft-versus-host disease in children who have received a cord-blood or bone marrow transplant from an HLA- identical sibling. N Eng J Med 2000; 342:1846-51.
16. Raju GMK, Kochupillai V, and Kumar L. Storage of haematopoietic stem cells for autologous bone marrow transplantation. Nat Med Jn India. 1995;8:216-21.
17. Brenner MK, Rill DR, Moen RC et al. Gene marking to trace origin of relapse after autologous bone marrow transplantation. Lancet 1993;341:85-6.
18. Gulati SC and Duensing S. Evaluating the benefit of purging in stem cell transplantation Cancer Invest. 1994;12:447-9.
19. Clift RA, Buckner CD, Thomas ED, et al. Marrow transplantation for chronic myeloid leukemia: A randomized study comparing cyclophosphamide and total body irradiation with busulfan and cyclophosphamide. Blood 1994;84:2036-43.
20. Devergie A, Blaise D, Attal M, et al. Allogeneic bone marrow transplantation for chronic myeloid leukemia in first chronic

phase: a randomized trial of busulfan –cytoxan versus cytoxan-total body irradiation as preparative regimen: a report from the French Society of Bone Marrow graft (SFGM). Blood 1995;85:2263-8.

21. Ringden O, Ruutu T, Remberger M et al. A randomized trial comparing busulfan with total body irradiationas conditioning in allogeneic bone marrow transplant recipients with leukemia: a report from the Nordic Bone Marrow Transplantation Group. Blood 1994;83:2723-30.

22. Blaise D, Maraninchi D, Michallet M, et al. Long term follow up of a randomized trial comparing the combination of cyclophosphamide with total body irradiation or busulfan as conditioning regimen for patients receiving HLA-identical marrow grafts for acute myeloblastic leukemia in first complete remission. Blood 2001;97:3669-70.

23. Schuller US, Renner VD, Kroschinsky F, et al. Intravenous busulphan for conditioning before autologous or allogeneic human blood stem cell transplantation. Brit J Haematology 2001; 114:944-50.

24. Davies SM, Ramsay NK, Klein JP, et al. Comparison of preparative regimens in transplants for children with acute lymphoblastic leukemia. J Clin Oncol 2000;18(2):340-7.

25. Linker CA, Ries CA, Damon GD, et al. Autologous bone marrow transplantation for acute myeloid leukemia using busulfan plus etoposide as a preparative regimen. Blood 1993;81:311-8.

26. Vosa MT, Pantel G, Weis M, et al. In vivo depletion of B cells using a combination of high dose cytosine arabinoside/mitoxantrone and rituxan for autografting in patients with non-Hodgkin's lymphoma. Brit J Haematology 2000;110:217-22

27. Barrett AJ, Childs R. Non myeloablative stem cell transplants. Brit J Haematology 2000;111:6-17.

28. Champlin RE, Khouri I, Shimoni A, et al. Harnessing graft versus malignancy: non myeloablative preparative regimens for allogeneic hemopoietic transplantation, an evolving strategy for adoptive immunotherapy. Brit J Haematology 2000;111:18-29.

29. Amrolia P, Gasoar HB, Hassan A et al. Nonmyeloablative stem cell transplantation for congenital immunodeficiencies. Blood 2000;96:1239.

30. Guidelines for prevention of opportunistic infections among Hematopoietic Stem Cell Transplant recipients: Recommendations of Centers for Disease Control, Infectious Disease Society of America and American Society of Blood and Marrow Transplantation. Biol B Marrow Transplant 2001; 6:1-77.

31. Glucksberg H, Storb R, Fefer A, et al. Clinical manifestations of graft versus host disease in human recipients of marrow from HLA matched sibling donors. Transplantation 1974;18:295.

32. Rowlings PA, Przepiorka D, Klein JP et al. IBMTR severity index for grading acute lymphoblastic leukemia graft-versus-host disease: retrospective comparison with Gluksberg grade. Br J Hematol 1997;97:855-64.

33. Atkinson K. Chronic graft versus host disease. Bone Marrow Transplantation 1990;5:69-82.

34. Goldman JM, Gale RP, Horowitz MM et al. Bone marrow transplantation for chronic myelogenous leukemia in chronic phase: Increased risk of relapse associated with T-cell depletion. Ann Int Med 1988;108:806-14.

35. Kumar L. Leukemia Management of relapse after allogeneic bone marrow transplantation. J Clin Oncology 1994;12:1710-17.

36. Peggs KS and Mackinnon S. Cellular therapy: donor lymphocyte infusion. Curr Opin Hematol. 2001;8:349-54.

37. Chao NJ, Duncan SR, Long GD etal. Corticosteroid therapy for diffuse alveolar hemorrhage in autologous bone marrow transplant recipients. Ann Int Med 1991;114:145-6.

38. Crawford SW and Hackman RC. Clinical course of idiopathic pneumonia after bone marrow transplantation. Am Rev Respir Dis 1993;147:1393-1400.

39. Cahill RA, Spitzer TR, Mazumder A. Marrow engraftment and clinical manifestations of capillary leak syndrome. Bone Marrow Transplant 1996;18:177-84.

40. Stucki A, Leisenring W, Sandmaier BM, et al. Decreased rejection and improved survival of first and second marrow transplants for severe aplastic anemia (A 26 year retrospective analysis). Blood 1998;92:2742-9.

41. McDonald GB, Hinds MS, Lloyd RN et al. Veno-occlusive disease of the liver and multiogran failure after bone marrow transplantation: A cohort study of 355 patients. Ann Int Med 1993; 118:255-67.

42. Locasciulli A, Testa M, Valsecchi Mg et al. Morbidity and mortality due to liver disease in children undergoing allogeneic bone marrow transplantation: a 10-year prospective study. Blood 1997; 90:3799-3805.

42. Abkowitz JL. Aplastic anemia: Which treatment ? Ann Int med 2001;135:524-6.

43. Storb R, Leisenring W, Deeg HJ et al. Long term follow up of a randomized trial of graft cyclosporine versus methotrexate alone in patients given marrow grafts for severe aplastic anemia. Blood 1994;83:2749-56.

44. International Bone Marrow Transplant Registry/Autologous Blood and Marrow Transplant Registry (IBMTR/ABMTR) Newsletter. 2000;7(1):3-10.

45. Laucarelll G, Galimberti M, Giardini C, et al. Bone Marrow Transplantation in thalassemia: The experience of Pesaro. Ann NY Acad Sci. 1998;850:270-5.

46. Chandy M, Srivastava A, Dennison D, Mathews V and Geoge B. Allogeneic bone marrow transplantation in the developing world: experience from a center in India. Bone Marrow Transplant 2001;27:785-90.

47. Vermylen C, Cornu G. Bone marrow transplantation in sickle cell anemia. The European experience. Am J Pediatr Hematol Oncol 1994;16:18-21.

48. Walters MC, Patience M, Leisenring et al. Bone marrow transplantation for sickle cell disease. N Engl J Med 1996;335:369-76.

49. Fischer A, Landais B, Freiderich W et al. European experience of Bone Morrow Transplantation for severe combined immunodeficiency. Lancet 1990;336:850-54.

50. Fischer A, Landais P, Friedrich W et al. Bone Marrow Transplantation (BMT) in Europe for primary immunodeficiencies other than severe combined immunodeficiency: A report from the European Group for BMT and the European Group for Immunodeficiency. Blood 1994;83:1149-54.

51. Wagner JE, Davies SM, and Auerbach AD. Haematopoietic stem cell transplantation for Fanconi anemia. In Haematopoietic Cell transplantation ed. SJ Forman, KG Blume and ED Thomas.1997, p1204, Blackwell Science, Malden.

52. Hoogergrugge PM, Valerio D. Lysosomal storage diseases. In the clinical practice of stem-cell transplantation 2001;286-95.

53. Hoogerbrugge PM, Brouwer OF, Bordigoni P, et al for the European Group for Bone Marrow transplantation. Allogeneic bone marrow transplantation for lysosomal storage diseases. Lancet 1995;345:1398-1402.

54. Peters C, Shapiro EG, Anderson J, et al. Hurler syndrome: II. Outcome of HLA-genotypically identical sibling and HLA-haploidentical related donor bone marrow transplantation in fifty-four children. Blood 1998;91:2601-8.

55. Creutzig U. Current controversies: which patients with AML should receive a bone marrow transplantation-a European view. Br J Hematol 2002;118:365-77.

56. Creutz U, Zimmerman M, Ritter J. Definition of standard-risk group in children with AML. Br J Hematol 1999;104:630-39.

57. Stevens RF, Hann IM, Wheatley K, Gray RG. Marked improvement in outcome with chemotherapy alone in pediatric AML: Results of the United Kingdom-MRC 10 AML trial. Br J Hematol 1998; 101:130-40.

58. Harousseau JL, Cahn JY, Pignon B, et al. Comparision of autologous bone marrow transplantation and intensive chemotherapy as post remission therapy in adult acute myeloid leukemia. Blood 1997;90:2978-86.

59. Burnett AK, Goldstone AH, Stevens RMF, et al. Randomized comparision of addition of autologous bone marrow transplantation and intensive chemotherapy as post remission therapy for acute myeloid leukemia in first remission. : Results of MRC AML 10 trial. Lancet 1998; 351:700-708.

60. Cassileth PA, Harrington DP, Appelbaum FR, et al. Chemotherapy compared with autologous or allogeneic bone marrow transplantation in the management of acute myeloid leukemia in first remission. N Eng J Med 1998;339:1649-56.

61. Zittoun RA, Mandelli F, Willemze R et al. Autologous or allogeneic Bone Marrow Transplantation compared with intensive chemotherapy in acute myelogenous leukemia. New Eng J Med 1995; 332:217-23.

62. Slovak ML, Kopecky KJ, Cassileth PA, et al. Karyotypic analysis predicts outcome of preremission and postremission therapy in adult acute myeloid leukemia: A Southwest Oncology Group / Eastern Cooperative Oncology Group study. Blood 2000;96: 4075-83.

63. Ravindranath Y, AbellaE, krischer JP. AML in Down's syndrome is highly responsive to chemotherapy: experience on Pediatric Oncology Group AML study 8498. Blood 1992;40: 2210-14.

64. Arico M, Valsecchi MG, Calmitta B et al. Outcome of treatment in children with Philadelphia Positive Acute lymphoblastic leukemia. N Eng J Med 2000;342:998-1006.

65. Manero GG, Thomas DA. Salvage therapy for refractory or relapsed acute lymphoblastic leukemia. Hematol Oncol Clin North Am 2001;15:163-205.

66. Creutzig U, Ritter J, Zimmerman M et al. Prognosis of children with chronic myeloid leukemia: a retrospective analysis of 75 patients. Klin Padiatr 1996;208:236-41.

67. Hansen JA, Gooley TA, Martin PJ et al. Bone marrow transplants from unrelated donors for Philadelphia positive chronic myeloid leukemia in children. N Eng J Med 1998;338:962-8.

68. Dini G, Rondelli R, Miano M et al. Unrelated-donor bone marrow transplants for Philadelphia positive chronic myeloid leukemia in children: experience of eight European countries. The EBMT Pediatric Diseases working Party. Bone Marrow Transplant 1996;18:80-5.

69. Creutzig U, Bender-Gotze C, Ritter J et al. The role of intensive AML- specific therapy in treatment in children with RAEB and RAEB-t. Leukemia 1998;12:652-9.

70. Ladenstein R, Pearce R, Hartmann O et al. High-dose chemotherapy with autologous bone marrow rescue in children poor risk non Hodgkin's lymphoma: a report from the European Lymphoma Bone marrow Transplant Registry. Blood 1997;90:2921-30.

71. Morrison VA, Peterson BA, High-dose therapy and transplantation in non-Hodgkin's lymphoma. Semin Oncol 1999; 26:84-98.

72. Ladenstein R, Lasset C, hartmann O, et al. Impact of megatherapy on survival after relapse from Stage IV neuroblastoma in patients over 1 year of age at diagnosis: A report from the European Group for Bone Marrow Transplantation. J Clin Oncology 1993;11:2330-41.

73. Matthay KK, Villablanca JG, Seeger RC, et al. Treatment of high-risk neuroblastoma with intensive chemotherapy, radiotherapy, autologous bone marrow transplantation, and 13-cis-retinoic acid. Children's Cancer Group. New Eng J Med 1999;341:1165-73.

74. Ladenstein R, Lasset C, Pinkerton CR et al. Impact of megatherapy in children with high-risk Ewing's tumors in complete remission: A report from the EBMT Solid Tumor Registry. Bone Marrow Transplant 1995;15:697-705.

75. Guruangan S, Dunkel IJ, Goldman S, et al. Myeloablative chemotherapy with autologous bone marrow rescue in young children with recurrent malignant brain tumors. J Clin Oncol 1998; 16:2486-93.

76. Sanders JE. Long-term effects of bone marrow transplantation. Pediatrician 1991;18:76-81.

77. Antin JH. Long term care after hematopoietic cell transplantation in adults. NEJM 2002;347:36-42.

78. Toubert ME, Socié G, Gluckman E, et al. Short- and long-term follow-up of thyroid dysfunction after allogeneic bone marrow transplantation without the use of preparative total body irradiation. Br J Haematol 1997;98:453-7.

79. Brauner R, Adan L, Souberbielle JC, et al. Contribution of growth hormone deficiency to the growth failure that follows bone marrow transplantation. J Pediatr 1997;130:785-92.

80. Thomas BC, Stanhope R, Plowman PN, Leiper AD. Endocrine function following single fraction and fractionated total body irradiation for bone marrow transplantation in childhood. Acta Endocrinologica 1993;128:508-12.

81. Curtis RE, Rowlings PA, Deeg HJ, et al. Solid cancers after bone marrow transplantation. N Engl J Med 1997; 336:897-04.

82. Deeg HJ, Socié G. Malignancies after hematopoietic stem cell transplantation: many questions, some answers. Blood 1998;91:1833-44.

83. Micallef IN, Lillington DM, Apostodilis J, et al. Therapy-related myelodysplasia and secondary acute myelogenous leukemia after high-dose therapy with autologous hematopoietic progenitor cell support for lymphoid malignancies. J Clin Oncol 2000;18:947-55.

84. Molassiotis A, van den Akker OBA, Milligan DW, et al. Quality of life in long-term survivors of marrow transplantation: comparison with a matched group receiving maintenance chemotherapy. Bone Marrow Transplant 1996;17:249-58.

85. Leigh S, Wilson KC, Burns R, Clark RE. Psychosocial morbidity in bone marrow transplant recipients: a prospective study. Bone Marrow Transplant 1995;16:635-40.

86. Duell T, Van Lint MT, Ljungman P, et al. Health and functional status of long-term survivors of bone marrow transplantation. EBMT Working Party on Late Effects and EULEP Study Group on Late Effects. European Group for Blood and Marrow Transplantation. Ann Intern Med 1997;126:184-92.

CHAPTER 53

Mark D Stringer

Liver Transplantation for Liver Tumors

INTRODUCTION

Primary malignant liver tumors make up just over 1 percent of all childhood cancers, with an incidence of approximately 1-1.5 per million children per year in the West.[1] Hepatoblastoma (HB) and hepatocellular carcinoma (HCC) account for the vast majority of such cases, with HB being approximately twice as common as HCC in children in the USA.[2] During the last 30 years, the treatment of children with HB has improved dramatically, largely due to better chemotherapy developed by randomised controlled clinical trials. Advances in surgery have also contributed. In recent years, liver transplantation has played an increasing role in the survival of children with unresectable liver tumors, particularly HB. Table 53.1 lists those pediatric liver tumors where transplantation may be beneficial in selected cases. This chapter reviews the indications for liver transplantation in children with a liver tumor and published outcomes.

INITIAL ASSESSMENT

Most liver tumors present with abdominal distension and/or a mass. Initial investigation using ultrasonography (US) will confirm whether the mass is hepatic, cystic or solid, single or multiple, and provide information about its vascularity. Computerised tomography (CT) of the abdomen and chest and magnetic resonance imaging (MRI) provide additional details about the tumor and any extrahepatic spread. MR angiography is particularly useful when planning surgical resection. Serum alpha-fetoprotein (AFP) is a valuable tumor marker, especially

with HB and HCC. A liver biopsy is recommended in all solid liver tumors in order to characterise the tumor and plan appropriate therapy.[3]

Liver tumors are relatively rare and potentially complex. Diagnostic difficulties are particularly common in young infants.[4] Children with a liver tumor should be managed in a center with appropriate oncological and surgical expertise. Patients with an extensive liver tumor may ultimately require liver transplantation and should be reviewed soon after presentation by a pediatric liver transplant surgeon. In addition to the detailed evaluation of the tumor, the child's nutritional and developmental status and associated conditions/co-morbidity must be taken into account since these can have a significant impact on eventual outcome.

MALIGNANT LIVER TUMORS

Hepatoblastoma

HB is the commonest primary malignant liver tumor in infants and children, with a peak incidence in the first 3 years of life. Most tumors are sporadic but familial cases associated with Beckwith-Wiedemann syndrome or familial adenomatous polyposis are well described. During the past two decades, the incidence of HB in the USA and Japan has increased, particularly among very low-birth-weight babies (< 1500 g).[5]

Hepatoblastoma originates from hepatic progenitor cells. Four histological subtypes are recognized; *fetal* (well-differentiated tumor cells resembling fetal hepatocytes and arranged in cords), *embryonal* (smaller, less well-differentiated cells, loosely arranged and with

Table 53.1: Pediatric liver tumors that may require liver transplantation	
Malignant liver tumors	Hepatoblastoma
	Hepatocellular carcinoma (and fibrolamellar variant)
	Transitional tumors
	Epithelioid hemangioendothelioma
	Undifferentiated embryonal sarcoma
	Other sarcomas, e.g. angiosarcoma
Benign liver tumors	Hemangioendothelioma
	Mesenchymal hamartoma
Other liver tumors	Inflammatory pseudotumor

frequent mitoses), *macrotrabecular* (fetal and/or embryonal cells in cords or plates) and *small cell undifferentiated*. Tumors may have both fetal and embryonal epithelial components and some are mixed with mesenchymal elements. The serum AFP is raised in over 90 percent of cases and is a valuable diagnostic and prognostic marker as well as being helpful in monitoring response to therapy.

Staging

In the USA, the staging of HB and HCC is based on operative findings and histological features, i.e. *postsurgical* (Table 53.2). In Japan, a modified TNM staging system has been used. In Europe, the staging system adopted by the Societe Internationale d'Oncologie Pediatrique (SIOP) is a *pretreatment* grouping (PRETEXT) based on the results of imaging studies.[6] In the latter, the liver is divided into four sections comprising the left lateral section (Couinaud segments II and III), a left medial section (segment IV and left part of I), a right medial section (segments V and VIII and right part of I) and a right posterior section (segments VI and VII). Sectional involvement by the tumor, and the presence of portal vein, vena caval, metastatic, and extrahepatic tumor spread are recorded (Fig. 53.1). The system has been modified in recent SIOPEL studies by the introduction of V1-3 and P1-2 categories to clarify

the extent of hepatic and portal vein involvement, respectively. Imaging studies should include either spiral CT with contrast and/or magnetic resonance imaging.

Treatment

Effective chemotherapy and complete surgical resection of the tumor are the mainstays of therapy.

Chemotherapy

Various chemotherapeutic regimens have been advocated. In the USA, the traditional focus has been on initial laparotomy, surgical resection where possible, and postoperative adjuvant chemotherapy, reserving neoadjuvant chemotherapy for unresectable tumors. The European SIOPEL studies have concentrated on preoperative chemotherapy (Table 53.3):[7,8] all patients except those with small peripheral tumors are treated by preoperative chemotherapy, typically cisplatin and doxorubicin (PLADO). Response to chemotherapy is assessed by radiological imaging and serum AFP levels. Most children are given an initial dose of cisplatin followed by a total of five cycles of PLADO, at 3 weekly intervals, with surgery after the fourth or sixth cycle depending on tumor shrinkage. Preoperative chemotherapy renders most tumors smaller, better demarcated from the surrounding liver, and more likely to be completely resected. HB resectability has

Table 53.2: Intergroup staging system for HB and HCC (Children's Cancer Group/Pediatric Oncology Group)		
Stage	I	Complete resection, negative margins
	II	Resection with microscopic residual disease
		Intrahepatic
		Extrahepatic
	III	Resection with gross residual tumor
		Tumor spill and/or positive lymph nodes
		Incomplete resection of primary tumor
	IV	Distant metastases

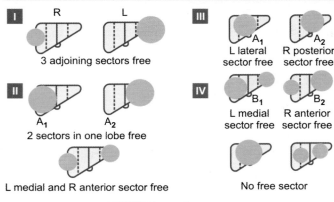

PRETEXT grouping system
In addition, V=Hepatic vein involvement, P=Portal vein involvement, E=Extrahepatic direct spread, M=Metastases

Figure 53.1: SIOPEL pretreatment (PRETEXT) grouping system for malignant liver tumors in children

progressively improved since the introduction of neoadjuvant chemotherapy; between one and two-thirds of patients initially present with unresectable primary tumors or distant metastases and after PLADO therapy 70 to 85 percent of these become operable.

Surgery

The aim of surgery is complete tumor excision. Standard techniques of liver resection are employed. The type of resection is based on the segmental anatomy of the liver (Fig. 53.2).[9] The surgeon should be aware of common variations in vascular and biliary anatomy. Up to 80 percent of the liver can be safely resected in children provided that the remaining parenchyma is healthy and its blood supply and venous drainage are preserved.

Extended right or left hepatectomies (trisectionectomies) can be performed safely in experienced units.[10] Tumor encasement of the retrohepatic vena cava does not preclude radical excision since this portion of the cava can be resected *en bloc* with the tumor and replaced with autologous vein or a prosthetic graft. Occasionally, a central hepatic resection[11] or a non-anatomical resection is indicated. Caudate lobe HBs are typically adherent to the cava and/or porta hepatis and are technically challenging.[12]

In selected cases, intraoperative US imaging is useful to confirm the extent of the tumor and the proximity of major intrahepatic vascular structures. Resection of the HB must be complete but resection margins do not need to be large. In one retrospective study of 23 patients, there was no difference in survival between those with resection margins of 1cm or more compared to those with narrower margins.[13]

Maintenance of a low central venous pressure helps to minimise blood loss during the phase of parenchymal transection. Hilar dissection and hemihepatic vascular occlusion, preferably with extrahepatic control of the relevant hepatic vein, also helps to reduce the need for blood transfusion during standard hemihepatectomies and trisectionectomies. Normothermic total vascular exclusion (TVE) is occasionally valuable for tumors adjacent to the hepatic veins or vena cava; the non-cirrhotic liver will tolerate up to one hour of continuous warm ischemia but severe venous congestion of the gut may be a limiting factor and maintenance of normovolemia is important. TVE requires complete mobilisation of the liver with vascular inflow control (Pringle maneuver), supra and infrahepatic caval

Table 53.3: SIOPEL studies and trials in the treatment of hepatoblastoma[7,8]	
SIOPEL-1 (1990-1994)	Primary chemotherapy Feasibility study - cisplatin + doxorubicin
SIOPEL-2 (1995-1998)	Primary chemotherapy Stratification of HB into 'standard risk' (Cisplatin monotherapy) and 'high risk' (carboplatin + doxorubicin + cisplatin)
SIOPEL-3 (1998-)	Primary chemotherapy 'standard risk'HB: cisplatin + doxorubicin *vs* cisplatin alone 'high risk'HB or HCC: carboplatin + doxorubicin + cisplatin
SIOPEL-4 (2004-)	'high risk' HB: intensified cisplatin + doxorubicin ± carboplatin Liver transplantation for unresectable tumors
Standard risk =	PRETEXT I,II and III with no extrahepatic spread
High risk =	PRETEXT IV and/or evidence of extrahepatic disease Tumor rupture at diagnosis HB with low AFP (<100 ng/ml) at diagnosis

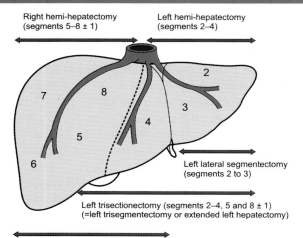

Right hemi-hepatectomy
(segments 5–8 ± 1)

Left hemi-hepatectomy
(segments 2–4)

Left lateral segmentectomy
(segments 2 to 3)

Left trisectionectomy (segments 2–4, 5 and 8 ± 1)
(=left trisegmentectomy or extended left hepatectomy)

Right trisectionectomy (segments 4–8 ± 1)
(=right trisegmentectomy or textended right hepatectomy)

Note: The caudate lobe (segment 1) is not visible

Figure 53.2: Standard liver resections. [Reproduced courtesy of Stringer MD. Hepatobiliary disorders. In *Pediatric Surgery* 2nd edition. Burge DM, Griffiths M, Steinbrecker H, Wheeler R (eds.). Hodder Arnold, London, 2005

clamping and control of the right adrenal vein and any accessory hepatic arteries.

Numerous innovative techniques have been used to treat large central tumors and those involving the hepatic vein confluence or inferior vena cava (Table 53.4).[12,14-19] Hypothermia or cardiopulmonary bypass[20] and *ex-vivo* bench surgery[21] have been advocated in special circumstances but there are only anecdotal reports of these relatively high risk approaches in children and their utility is limited. The techniques listed in Table 53.4 can sometimes be useful when dealing with huge benign tumors or when liver transplantation

is not an option for malignant lesions. However, if liver transplantation is available, heroic attempts to treat a HB of borderline resectability are no longer justified.

Liver Transplantation

HB patients who respond to chemotherapy but have unresectable tumors and no evidence of persistent metastases should be considered for orthotopic liver transplantation (OLT). The following criteria are used by SIOPEL to select potential candidates for OLT:

• Multifocal PRETEXT IV disease, i.e. tumor in all four liver sections (Fig. 53.3)*
• Unifocal PRETEXT IV disease. This is relatively rare but unless pre-operative chemotherapy 'downstages' the tumor to leave a clear margin from the anatomic border of one lateral section (indicating prior compression/displacement rather than tumor invasion), transplantation should be considered.
• PRETEXT III disease where proximity to major vessels makes adequate tumor excision doubtful (Fig. 53.4)**
• Tumor extension into the vena cava and/or all three hepatic veins.
• Invasion of the main and/or both left and right branches of the portal vein.
• Intrahepatic recurrent or residual tumor after previous resection ("rescue" transplant)***

These are useful guidelines but there are areas of uncertainty:

*The current guidelines recommend that all patients with multifocal PRETEXT IV tumors should undergo primary OLT, even if one of the liver sectors is apparently clear after preoperative chemotherapy.[22,23] In support

Table 53.4: Extending the limits of hepatic resection for pediatric liver tumors (excluding total hepatectomy and liver transplantation)[12,14-19]	
Technique	*Comment*
Preoperative portal vein embolization	- Encourages growth of anticipated liver remnant permitting a more extensive hepatic resection to be performed[14]
Caval repair/reconstruction	- Local resection and repair with autologous vein patch/graft- No reconstruction if chronic IVC occlusion[12]
	- Prosthetic replacement
Resection of the hepatic vein confluence	- Extensive resection of segments 2-4 + 7 and 8 possible if there is adequate venous drainage of the remnant liver via retro-hepatic veins[15]
Staged resection	- Allows intervening parenchymal regeneration[16]
	Only applicable to benign liver tumors
Ex-vivo dissection and auto-transplantation	- Total hepatectomy, veno-venous bypass, extracorporeal bench surgery, and autotransplantation[17,18]
Extended hepatic resection with transplant	- Logistics difficult, even with living-related back-up transplantation[19]

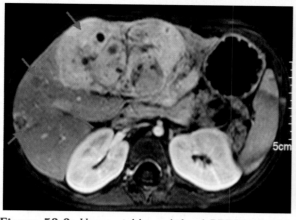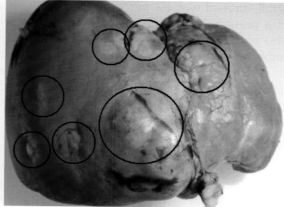

Figure 53.3: Unresectable multifocal PRETEXT IV hepatoblastoma in a 3-year-old child treated by liver transplantation. Magnetic resonance image with gadolinium enhancement and total hepatectomy specimen

of this approach, there are anecdotal reports of the presence of viable tumor foci in sections of total hepatectomy specimens despite the apparent disappearance of tumor nodules from these sites after preoperative chemotherapy.[24] In addition, the results of primary liver transplantation for multifocal PRETEXT IV HB in SIOPEL-1 were excellent: all 6 patients in this category survived.[25] However, some PRETEXT IV multifocal tumors can be successfully downstaged by preoperative chemotherapy allowing long-term survival by partial hepatic resection and chemotherapy.

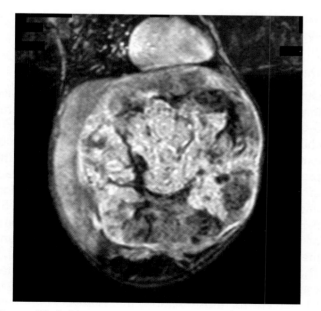

Figure 53.4: Magnetic resonance image of large unresectable PRETEXT III hepatoblastoma in a 7-month-old infant. Only partial response to chemotherapy. Treated by total hepatectomy and liver transplantation

Furthermore, the disappearance of pulmonary metastases with chemotherapy is usually taken to indicate their eradication so why should similar resolution of nodules in the liver not be accepted as successful treatment? The answer to this dilemma lies in the balance of probabilities—the patient with multifocal PRETEXT IV disease is probably more likely to be cured by total hepatectomy and OLT than by partial liver resection.

**The risk of an incomplete resection supports the concept of primary transplantation in these cases. However, the presence of microscopic residual disease at the resection margin does not appear to be a major adverse determinant of survival.[8,26,27] Thus, none of the 11 patients with positive margins in SIOPEL-1 underwent a second resection and all but one was treated by postoperative chemotherapy alone. None developed recurrent tumor and all the survivors were in complete remission after a mean interval of 5 years.[27] Schnater et al (2002) attributed this to the use of the ultrasonic dissector (CUSA) that may ablate a further rim of tissue beyond the actual resection margin of the pathology specimen but they also conceded that any residual tumor may not be viable after preoperative chemotherapy. In SIOPEL-2 microscopic residual disease was noted in 13 children after neoadjuvant chemotherapy and delayed surgery; all survived without recurrent disease.[8] It is likely that the chemosensitivity of the tumor is the key to event-free survival in such cases. Despite these observations, it is inappropriate to embark on a resection where tumor clearance is doubtful and these patients should be treated by primary liver transplantation.

***In their detailed analysis of outcome after transplantation for HB, Otte et al (2004) determined that overall survival was 82 percent in children who received a primary transplant but only 30 percent in those who had undergone a "rescue" transplant after an incomplete resection or intrahepatic recurrence after partial hepatectomy.[25] For some, the concept of rescue transplantation is controversial in the context of a limited supply of donor organs but in the author's opinion it is inappropriate to deny a child this chance of survival.

Absolute contraindications to OLT for unresectable HB include persistent pulmonary metastases and persistent viable extrahepatic tumor not amenable to surgical resection. The tumor should show at least a partial response to chemotherapy (decrease in tumor size and serum AFP); stable or progressive disease is a relative contraindication to OLT.[25,28] Lung secondaries that respond completely to chemotherapy with or without surgical resection do not pose a contraindication to OLT. Similarly, initial involvement of the portal or hepatic veins/vena cava is not a contraindication to OLT—although the outcome is probably worse, long-term survival is still possible in 54 to 77 percent of cases.[25,29]

Potential candidates for OLT not only require careful evaluation of their tumor status but also their overall fitness for transplant. Doxorubicin is cardiotoxic in a cumulative, dose-dependent manner and cisplatin is both nephrotoxic and ototoxic. A detailed echocardiogram and assessment of renal function (including GFR) is essential prior to OLT. The child's pretransplant nutritional status should be optimised, if necessary by supplementary overnight nasogastric feeding. Chemotherapy must be continued up until the time of transplant to maintain control of the tumor. The interval between the last course of chemotherapy and OLT should not be longer than four weeks. If the patient is listed for a deceased donor liver there should be a good chance of obtaining a graft during this period. If it is likely that the waiting period will be significantly longer, a live-related donor liver transplant should be considered.

Otte et al. (2004) recommend that the retrohepatic vena cava should be removed *en bloc* with the liver during the transplant.[25] The cava can be reconstructed using either donor iliac vein (deceased donor OLT) or donor jugular vein (live-related OLT).[30] Other authors maintain that the native retrohepatic vena cava can be retained in selected transplant recipients provided that there is no evidence of tumor involvement.[30]

The potential benefits of OLT must be weighed against the risks of surgical complications and life-long immunosuppression. There is some evidence that less immunosuppression is required after OLT for HB, at least with living-related grafts. Gras et al (2005) compared 12 children who had been transplanted for HB with 12 age-matched children transplanted for benign liver disease.[31] Most patients in both groups had received grafts from a living-related donor. Rejection-free survival was 91 percent in the HB group compared to 58 percent in the controls who had received a similar immunosuppression regimen. Moreover, tacrolimus levels were lower in those transplanted for HB. The authors concluded that less immunosuppression is required after OLT for HB, possibly because of diminished immunity as a result of preoperative chemotherapy. If this is confirmed, giving less immunosuppression could be one way of reducing the combined nephrotoxicity of cisplatin and calcineurin inhibitors in these patients. The situation may be different with deceased donor grafts. Tiao et al (2005) recorded acute cellular rejection in four of eight children transplanted for HB although details of the type of graft and immunosuppression were not given.[32]

The need for post-transplant chemotherapy is at present uncertain. In the world literature review by Otte et al (2004), 65 patients received post-transplant chemotherapy and 82 did not.[25] Their respective survival rates were 77 and 70 percent, not statistically significantly different. The benefits of post-transplant chemotherapy have to be balanced against the additional toxicity risks, although HB chemotherapy is generally well tolerated by the transplanted liver.

Overall survival and prognosis

During the last 30 years, there has been a progressive improvement in the survival of children with HB. Overall 5-year survival in SIOPEL-1, which included 154 children with HB, was 75 percent.[6] In this study, tumor extent at presentation (PRETEXT grouping) and the presence of distant metastases were the most important prognostic variables. Patients with PRETEXT I tumors had a 100 percent 5-year survival compared to 57 percent for those with group IV tumors. The outcome of the 31 patients in SIOPEL-1 presenting with lung metastases was reviewed by Perilongo et al (2000).[33] The presence of metastases at diagnosis was associated with a 57 percent overall 5-year survival compared to 81 percent for those without metastases. Pulmonary metastases can disappear completely with chemotherapy. In those with persistent lesions, an aggressive approach including surgical resection can result in long-term survival.[34,35]

In SIOPEL-2, 77 standard risk HB were compared with 58 high risk HB patients.[8] Tumor resection rates were 97 and 67 percent, respectively and overall 3-year survival was 91 and 53 percent, respectively. A treatment strategy based on cisplatin monotherapy and surgery thus appears effective in standard risk HB but, despite intensified chemotherapy, only half of high-risk HB patients are currently long-term survivors.

Results of Liver Transplantation

The results of liver transplantation in SIOPEL-1 were analyzed by Otte et al (2004).[25] Twelve patients, comprising 8 percent of all HB cases in the study, were transplanted. Of the 7 who received a primary OLT, 6 were long-term survivors; one died from recurrent tumor. However, only 2 of the 5 children who underwent a "rescue" transplant after a previous partial hepatectomy survived; one died from tumor recurrence and two from transplant related complications. The authors went on to review the world experience of transplantation for HB. Of the 147 cases identified, the overall survival rate at 6 years after OLT was 82 percent in the 106 patients who received a primary transplant and 30 percent in the 41 patients who underwent a rescue transplant. Multivariate analysis of the patients undergoing primary OLT showed that only macroscopic venous invasion had a significant adverse impact on overall survival (54% vs 78% survival). Twelve of the transplant patients in this review had pulmonary metastases at presentation and 7 of them survived.[25]

In a recent study from the USA, 30 children treated for HB during a 17-year period were reviewed.[32] Eight were transplanted, 5 as a primary procedure and 3 as a rescue procedure; 7 were alive and well and one died 7 years after transplant from post-transplant lymphoproliferative disease.

Hepatocellular Carcinoma

HCC accounts for about one-third of all primary pediatric malignant liver tumors in Western societies but is much more frequent in Asia, South America and Africa where hepatitis B infection is endemic.[36] HCC typically occurs in older children (10-14 years) and more commonly affects boys. The tumor may arise as a complication of pre-existing liver disease (Table 53.5). In Western children, a smaller proportion of HCCs are associated with cirrhosis but in the Far East, hepatitis B is an important cause of HCC and underlying cirrhosis is very common. In these countries, national hepatitis B

Table 53.5: Examples of hepatic disorders associated with the development of HCC in children
Metabolic
Tyrosinemia
Alpha-1-antitrypsin deficiency
Wilson's disease
Glycogen storage disorders
Galactosaemia
Neonatal iron storage disorders
Infective
Hepatitis B
Hepatitis C
Other
Biliary atresia
Progressive Familial Intrahepatic Cholestasis
Parenteral nutrition associated chronic liver disease
Alagille's syndrome
Androgen therapy
Aflatoxin
Familial adenomatous polyposis

vaccination programs have significantly reduced the incidence of HCC.[37] In tyrosinemia, the incidence of HCC may also have decreased as a result of treatment with NTBC (2-(2-nitro-trifluoromethylbenzoyl)-1,3-cyclohexenedione) but long-term data are needed to determine if treatment actually reduces or just delays the incidence of HCC in these patients.

HCC spreads by lymphatic and vascular invasion. Bilobar, multifocal disease is common and at least half of the affected children have metastases or extrahepatic spread at presentation.[38] Serum AFP is elevated in two-thirds or more of cases but not in the fibrolamellar variant of HCC which typically occurs in adolescents and young adults in the absence of underlying cirrhosis. Fibrolamellar tumors are associated with elevated serum levels of the vitamin B_{12} binding protein, transcobalamin, which can be used to monitor response to treatment.

Treatment

Whilst some HCCs respond to PLADO chemotherapy, the tumor is much more chemoresistant than HB. In the SIOPEL-1 study partial response to PLADO chemotherapy was observed in only half the cases.[39] Complete excision of the tumor offers the only chance of long-term survival but multifocal tumor or distant spread often precludes successful resection. In the SIOPEL-1 study, 51 percent of children with HCC never became operable. Complete tumor resection was achieved in only 36 percent.

Numerous therapies have been used in adults with HCC to achieve palliation and, in some cases, render the tumor resectable. These include ultrasound guided percutaneous intralesional injection of ethanol, radiofrequency thermal ablation and intraoperative cryotherapy; local recurrence is common but survival rates comparable to those of resection have been achieved in the hands of enthusiasts. In children there are a few reports of transarterial chemoembolization[40] and intra-arterial chemotherapy.

Liver Transplantation

The role of liver transplantation in pediatric HCC is controversial. It is not an option for most children with HCC because their disease is too advanced at presentation (Fig. 53.5). However, it should be considered early on in the assessment of patients with unresectable disease with no evidence of extrahepatic spread and macroscopic vascular invasion. Major vascular invasion, as determined by detailed preoperative imaging using spiral CT with dual phase contrast and/or magnetic resonance imaging with gadolinium, is currently a contraindication to transplantation for HCC in children. In the Pittsburgh series, all four children with HCC and major intrahepatic portal venous invasion (without metastases) died from recurrent tumor after transplant.[29] In contrast, three of the four patients with no evidence of major venous invasion or metastases were long-term survivors. All four survivors with T4 tumors in this series had underlying cirrhosis. Lack of response to preoperative chemotherapy is a relative contraindication to OLT since there were no long-term survivors in SIOPEL-1 among those patients who failed to respond to chemotherapy.

In an effort to improve the results of liver transplantation for HCC in adults many units have adopted the Milan criteria. Patients with a low risk of recurrent HCC after liver transplantation are selected on the basis of their preoperative imaging, i.e. the presence of a single tumor 5 cm or less in diameter or no more than three tumor nodules, each measuring 3 cm or less in diameter.[41] Adjuvant treatment is given to limit tumor progression whilst awaiting OLT. However, it should be noted that in the original study reported by Mazzaferro et al (1996), 13 (27%) of the 48 patients who met the Milan criteria on pre-transplant imaging had tumors that exceeded these dimensions on pathological examination of the explanted liver and their recurrence-free 4-year survival was considerably less. Moreover, although 4-year survival rates of 75 percent or more can be achieved in adults transplanted according to the Milan criteria,[42] tumor progression and death on the waiting list result in outcomes that are often inferior to those predicted unless living-related liver transplantation is available. Living donor liver transplantation minimises waiting times and it has been suggested that criteria should be expanded to include larger tumors when this is available. However, the age and size of most patients who require OLT for HCC usually demands the use of a right lobe graft which carries significant risks to the donor and demands a high level of institutional expertise.

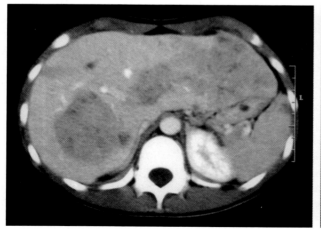 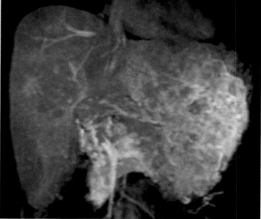

Figure 53.5: Unresectable HCC in a 13-year-old girl with no previous liver disease. PRETEXT IV tumor with extensive vascular invasion

Whether immunosuppression in general, and corticosteroids and calcineurin inhibitors in particular, increase the likelihood of tumor recurrence after OLT for HCC is debatable.[43] This uncertainty has prompted several adult liver transplant centres to use sirolimus with or without calcineurin inhibitors as primary immunosuppression after OLT for HCC. Sirolimus not only functions as an immunosuppressive agent but has been shown to inhibit the growth of a wide variety of cancers.

Overall Survival and Prognosis

Poor prognostic factors for HCC include metastatic spread, large tumor size (PRETEXT grouping), lymph node metastases and macroscopic vascular invasion. In SIOPEL-1, of the 37 children with HCC and adequate follow-up, only 8 (22%) were alive with no evidence of disease at a median of 75 months (Fig. 53.6).[39] None of the 12 patients presenting with lung metasases were long-term survivors. The results of SIOPEL-2 in which chemotherapy was intensified by the addition of carboplatin to PLADO therapy showed no improvement in outcomes compared to SIOPEL-1. In the USA, the Pediatric Oncology Group/Children's Cancer Group reported a similar 19 percent 5-year event-free survival in 46 children and adolescents with HCC; only 8 (17%) underwent primary complete tumor resection and 7 of these survived.[44] A larger study from Taiwan reported only two long-term survivors from a cohort of 55 children with HCC (more than two-thirds of whom were cirrhotic); only 18 percent of tumors were resectable.[38]

The fibrolamellar variant of HCC has traditionally been regarded as having a higher resection rate and a better prognosis compared to typical HCC. These tumors are typically large and solitary and the surrounding liver parenchyma is usually non-cirrhotic. This has encouraged some authors to recommend aggressive surgical treatment, either liver resection or liver transplantation, in patients without evidence of extrahepatic spread or metastases.[45] However, a recent analysis of 10 children with fibrolamellar HCC from the United States showed no difference in outcome compared to typical HCC.[46]

Results of Liver Transplantation

Recent results of liver transplantation for HCC in children are shown in Table 53.6.[29,39,47-52] One of the largest series to date by Reyes et al (2000) was an update of a previous report from Pittsburgh by Tagge et al (1992).[29,53] In this series, 14 of 19 children with HCC had underlying chronic liver disease (e.g. tyrosinemia, progressive familial intrahepatic cholestasis, hepatitis B, etc.). Such children are frequently under regular surveillance allowing detection of their HCC before the onset of symptoms. Children with cirrhosis from biliary atresia, metabolic liver disease and chronic viral hepatitis are also included in many other reports of liver transplantation for HCC in children. However, if the results of OLT for HCC in children are to be properly understood, it is essential that three subgroups of patients are identified and analysed separately: 1) those presenting for the first time with an HCC; 2) those in whom the tumor is detected during surveillance of chronic liver disease; and 3) those in whom an 'incidental' HCC is discovered in the explant when the primary indication for OLT was the liver disease. The latter group of children generally have an excellent prognosis.[54]

If the outcome of children with HCC is to improve, the proportion amenable to resection or transplantation must be increased. This may involve greater use of intra-arterial chemotherapy, chemoembolisation, and/or alternative chemotherapy regimens. The current SIOPEL-5 trial is exploring the utility of the anti-angiogenic agent thalidomide as a supplement to neoadjuvant chemotherapy in children and adolescents with non-cirrhotic HCC.

Other Primary Malignant Liver Tumors

Liver transplantation has occasionally been used in the management of other primary malignant liver tumors in children, all of which are relatively rare. The results have been generally poor.

Undifferentiated (embryonal) sarcoma is a highly malignant mesenchymal tumor that usually affects children aged between 5 and 10 years. Tumors are

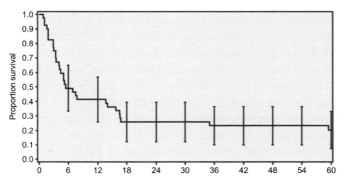

Figure 53.6: Overall survival of children with HCC in the SIOPEL-1 study[39]

Table 53.6: Recent reports of liver transplantation for HCC in children (References 29,39, 47-52)

Author	Year	n	Survival
Yandza et al*	1993	2	Both alive @ 2y
Broughan et al	1994	4	3 (75%) @ mean 63m
Achilleos et al*	1996	2	0 (1 death from recurrence, 1 after OLT)
Otte et al*	1996	5	3 (60%) @ median 49m
Superina and Bilik*	1996	3	3 (100%) @ 1-5y
Reyes et al*	2000	19	79 percent actuarial survival @ 1y, 63 percent @ 5y
Tatekawa et al*	2001	2	Both alive @ 2.8 and 5y, respectively
Czauderna et al*	2002	2	Not stated

*Includes i) patients with HCC discovered incidentally within the explanted liver where the indication for OLT was the underlying liver disease rather than the tumor and/or ii) HCC detected during surveillance of cirrhosis

typically large with areas of necrosis, hemorrhage and cystic change. Until recently the outcome of children with these tumors was poor but long-term survival has now been reported after neoadjuvant multi-agent chemotherapy and partial hepatectomy.[55,56] Otte et al (1996) described two children who underwent OLT for an unresectable sarcoma; both died within 6 months of the transplant, one from tumor relapse and one from viral pneumonia.[50] Dower et al (2000) reported a 6-year-old boy with a non-metastatic undifferentiated sarcoma which was successfully treated by chemotherapy and transplantation.[35] The key factor in this patient appears to have been the chemosensitivity of the tumor.

Hepatic epithelioid hemangioendothelioma (HEHE) is a vascular tumor, distinct from hemangioendothelioma and angiosarcoma. It is most often encountered in young women. It usually behaves as a slow growing malignancy with the potential for distant metastases but it may be a more aggressive tumor in children.[17,57] Most tumors are large and diffuse and unresectable by partial hepatectomy. There is no consistently effective chemotherapy. One child with a slow growing tumor was successfully treated by liver transplantation.[58] However, in a review of 5 children aged between 1 and 12 years of age from 3 European centres both patients who underwent OLT died within a year of transplant, one from viral sepsis and the other from recurrent disease.[17] The role of primary liver transplantation for unresectable HEHE is therefore uncertain.

Angiosarcomas typically present between 3 and 5 years of age. Most are unresectable and lung metastases may be evident from the outset.[59] There are some accounts of probable malignant transformation from a pre-existing hemangioendothelioma[59,60] and there is a

histological overlap with so-called type 2 hemangioendotheliomas. The treatment of this rare high-grade malignant tumor has not been stan-dardised but occasional success after chemotherapy and partial hepatectomy has been reported.[60,61] Two children with unresectable hepatic angiosarcoma and no evidence of extrahepatic spread have been treated by liver transplantation: one died from cytomegalovirus infection 4 months later but had no detectable residual tumor[59] and the other was alive but with pulmonary metastases 14m later[62] Adult experience with liver transplantation for angiosarcoma has also been extremely poor. Penn et al. (1991) reviewed 12 adults from an international registry;[63] there were no long-term survivors and most of the patients died of local recurrence within 2 years of transplant.

There is one report of a 2-year-old boy with an unresectable hepatic yolk sac tumor successfully treated by chemotherapy and liver transplantation.[64]

BENIGN LIVER TUMORS

Mesenchymal hamartoma of the liver (MHL) is the second commonest benign liver tumor in children. Most MHL are large multicystic masses, sometimes reaching 20–30 cm in diameter and weighing up to 3 kg, presenting in the first three years of life. Although classified as a hamartoma, several reports have shown cytogenetic abnormalities in some of these tumors and highlighted an association between MHL and undifferentiated embryonal sarcoma of the liver.[65] MHL are best treated by complete excision.

Very rarely an MHL is unresectable and liver transplantation may have to be considered. Two such children were reported from Pittsburgh.[66] Both had undergone previous partial hepatectomies but had residual pain and progressive liver failure; one died from intraoperative bleeding and the other survived. Bejarano et al. (2003) described an infant who was successfully transplanted for a recurrent MHL after a previous resection.[67] Histology showed a mixed hemangioendothelioma and multicystic MHL.

Hepatic hemangioendotheliomas (HE) are the commonest liver tumors in children. They are typically found in infants, are variable in size and frequently associated with cutaneous hemangiomas.[68] They usually present with asymptomatic hepatomegaly but may be associated with high-output cardiac failure from arteriovenous shunting in the liver or platelet sequestration and consumptive coagulopathy. Two histologic subtypes recognised. Type 1 is the commonest

and consists of irregular vascular channels lined by a single layer of plump endothelial cells separated by fibrous tissue. Type 2 HE are composed of multiple layers of larger more pleomorphic endothelial cells with hypercromatic nuclei forming poorly defined vascular spaces. Type 2 tumors tend to occur in slightly older children than type 1 HE; they can be multicentric and metastasize and generally behave much more aggressively.

Many HE will regress spontaneously. Treatment is indicated if there is cardiac failure, abdominal pain and distension, or other complications such as respiratory compromise. Corticosteroids, alpha-interferon or vincristine may induce or accelerate regression in some but not all cases. Treatment with radiotherapy is controversial. For bilobar disease complicated by cardiac failure, hepatic artery ligation or embolization can be

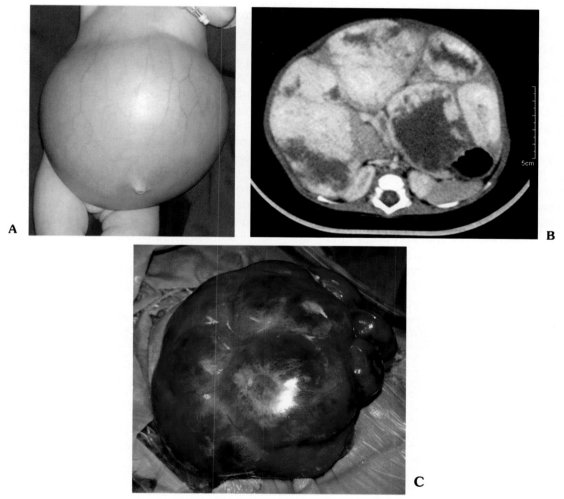

Figure 53.7: Massive hepatic hemangioendothelioma in a 7-month-old infant treated by liver transplantation. (A) Clinical, (B) CT scan, and (C) operative appearances

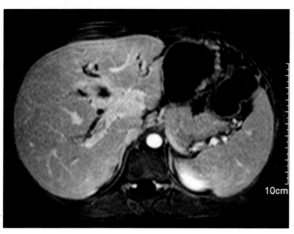 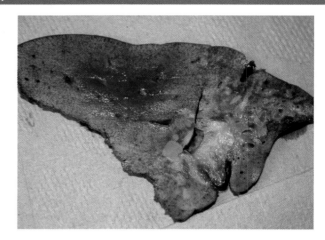

Figure 53.8: (A) Magnetic resonance image of a 7-year-old boy with an aggressive hilar inflammatory myofibroblastic tumor.[73] (B) Gross appearance of resection specimen after hepatectomy and OLT. Note the dense hilar infiltration, left lobe atrophy and satellite nodules

effective. On rare occasions, liver transplantation may be the only therapeutic option when other attempts to control the tumor have failed. There are numerous reports of successful transplantation for massive HE.[69,70-72] The author's unit has experience of a 7 month old infant who failed to respond to medical therapy and underwent OLT (Fig. 53.7); she remains well 21 months later. Not all cases have done well after transplant because of extrahepatic complications (possibly related to an associated vascular malformation in the brain),[66,70] metastases from a type 2 HE,[49] or transplant-related complications.[70]

Inflammatory myofibroblastic tumors, also known as inflammatory pseudotumors are rare proliferative lesions of unknown etiology that can occur at any age and affect almost any organ system, including the liver. Tumors are hard and solid, of a variable size, and are composed of myofibroblasts with an admixture of plasma cells, lymphocytes, and histiocytes in a collagen stroma. Their presentation and imaging characteristics frequently cause confusion with malignancy. Although considered benign, these lesions can have devastating local effects and recurrence after incomplete excision is well described.

Inflammatory myofibroblastic tumors in the liver are solitary and found in the right lobe. Asymptomatic patients can be managed non-operatively and most symptomatic lesions are amenable to resection. However, when these tumors occur at the hilum of the liver, they can cause serious problems including biliary obstruction and occlusive portal phlebitis and present a major therapeutic challenge.[73] Some of these hilar tumors have been successfully resected but others have required management by liver transplantation (Fig. 53.8) (Table 53.7).[66,73-75]

The results of liver transplantation in children have steadily improved during the past 30 years and 5 to 10 year survival in elective cases is now around 90 percent

Table 53.7: Hilar hepatic inflammatory myofibroblastic tumors (IMT) in children treated by liver transplantation (OLT)[66,73-75]			
Heneghan et al. (1984)	8y F, jaundice, lethargy, abdo pain. Portal hypertension	IMT right lobe and hilum	OLT: well 1 yr but later died from post-transplant lymphoproliferative disease
Tepetes et al. (1995)	8y F, recurrent cholangitis and portal hypertension	Unresectable hilar IMT	OLT : died 56m later from fungal sepsis
Kim et al. (1996)	5y F, recurrence of gastric IMT causing jaundice	Recurrence of gastric IMT involving left lobe and hilum	Unsuccessful attempt at ex-vivo left trisectionectomy and reimplantation. Urgent OLT. Well 8m later.
Dasgupta et al. (2004)	7y M, jaundice, diarrhoea, fever, portal phlebitis	Unresectable hilar IMT	Attempted left trisection-ectomy. Urgent OLT. Well 3y later.

in many units. The challenges posed by long-term immunosuppression remain a concern but there is no doubt that liver transplantation is a life-saving procedure for selected children with otherwise unresectable liver tumors.

REFERENCES

1. Mann JR, Kasthuri N, Raafat F, et al. Malignant hepatic tumors in children: Incidence, clinical features and aetiology. Paediatr Perinat Epidemiol 1990;4:276-89.
2. Darbari A, Sabin KM, Shapiro CN, Schwarz KB. Epidemiology of primary hepatic malignancies in U.S. children. Hepatology 2003;38:560-66.
3. Stringer MD. Liver tumors. Sem Pediatr Surg 2000;9:196-208.
4. Von Schweinitz D, Gluer S, Mildenberger H. Liver tumors in neonates and very young infants: diagnostic pitfalls and therapeutic problems. Eur J Pediatr Surg 1995;5:72-6.
5. Reynolds P, Urayama KY, Behren JV, Feusner J. Birth characteristics and hepatoblastoma risk in young children. Cancer 2004;100:1070-76.
6. Brown J, Perilongo G, Shafford E, et al. Pretreatment prognostic factors for children with hepatoblastoma - results from the International Society of Pediatric Oncology (SIOP) study SIOPEL 1. Eur J Cancer 2000;36:1418-25
7. Pritchard J, Brown J, Shafford E, et al. Cisplatin, doxorubicin, and delayed surgery for childhood hepatoblastoma: a successful approach—results of the first prospective study of the International Society of Pediatric Oncology. J Clin Oncol 2000;18:3819-28.
8. Perilongo G, Shafford E, Maibach R, et al. Risk-adapted treatment for childhood hepatoblastoma. final report of the second study of the International Society of Pediatric Oncology-SIOPEL 2. Eur J Cancer 2004;40:411-21
9. Strasberg SM. Terminology of liver anatomy and liver resections: coming to grips with hepatic babel. J Am Coll Surg 1997;184:413-34.
10. Glick RD, Nadler EP, Blumgart LH, LaQuaglia MP. Extended left hepatectomy (left hepatic trisegmentectomy) in childhood. J Pediatr Surg 2000;35:303-8
11. LaQuaglia MP, Shorter NA, Blumgart LH. Central hepatic resection for pediatric tumors. J Pediatr Surg 2002;37:986-9.
12. Takayama T, Makuuchi M, Kosuge T, et al. A hepatoblastoma originating in the caudate lobe radically resected with the inferior vena cava. Surgery 1991; 109:208-213.
13. Dicken BJ, Bigam DL, Lees GM. Association between surgical margins and long-term outcome in advanced hepatoblastoma. J Pediatr Surg 2004;39:721-25.
14. Kaneko K, Ando H, Watanabe Y, et al. Aggressive preoperative management and extended surgery for inflammatory pseudotumor involving the hepatic hilum in a child. Surgery 2001;129:757-60.
15. Superina RA, Bambini D, Filler RM, Almond PS, Geissler G. A new technique for resecting 'unresectable' liver tumors. J Pediatr Surg 2000;35:1294-9.
16. Adam R, Laurent A, Azoulay D, et al. Two-stage hepatectomy: a planned strategy to treat irresectable liver tumors. Ann Surg 2000;232:777-85.
17. Sharif K, English M, Ramani P, et al. Management of hepatic epithelioid hemangio-endothelioma in children: what option? Br J Cancer 2004;90:1498-1501.
18. Fusai G, Steinberg R, Prachalias A et al. Ex-vivo liver surgery for extra-adrenal phaeochromocytoma. Pediatr Surg Int 2006;22:282-5.
19. Millar AJW, Hartley P, Khan D, Spearman W, Andronikou S, Rode H. Extended hepatic resection with transplantation back-up for an "unresectable" tumor. Ped Surg Int 2001;17:378-81.
20. Ein SH, Shandling B, Williams WG, et al. Major hepatic tumor resection using profound hypothermia and circulation arrest. J Pediatr Surg 1981;16:339-42.
21. Pichlmayr R, Grosse H, Hauss J, et al. Technique and preliminary results of extracorporeal liver surgery (bench procedure) and of surgery on the in situ perfused liver. Br J Surg 1990;77:21-6.
22. Czauderna P, Otte JB, Aronson DC, et al. Guidelines for surgical treatment of hepatoblastoma in the modern era – recommendations from the childhood liver tumor strategy group of the International Society of Pediatric Oncology (SIOPEL). Eur J Cancer 2005;41:1031-36.
23. Otte JB, de Ville de Goyet J, Reding R. Liver transplantation for hepatoblastoma: indications and contraindications in the modern era. Pediatric Transplantation 2005;9:557-65.
24. Dall'Igna P, Cecchetto G, Toffolutti T et al. Multifocal hepatoblastoma : is there a place for partial hepatectomy? Med Pediatr Oncol 2003;40:113-7.
25. Otte JB, Pritchard J, Aronson DC, et al. Liver transplantation for hepatoblastoma: results from the International Society of Pediatric Oncology (SIOP) study SIOPEL-1 and review of the world experience. Pediatr Blood Cancer 2004;42:74-83.
26. Stringer MD, Hennayake S, Howard ER, et al. Improved outcome for children with hepatoblastoma. Br J Surg 1995;82:386-91.
27. Schnater JM, Aronson DC, Plaschkes J, et al. Surgical view of the treatment of patients with hepatoblastoma. Results from the first prospective trial of the International Society of Pediatric Oncology Liver Tumor Study Group (SIOPEL-1). Cancer 2002;94:1111-20.
28. Pimpalwar AP, Sharif K, Ramani P, et al. Strategy for hepatoblastoma management: transplant versus nontransplant surgery. J Pediatr Surg 2002;37:240-45.
29. Reyes JD, Carr B, Dvorchik I, et al. Liver transplantation and chemotherapy for hepatoblastoma and hepatocellular cancer in childhood and adolescence. J Pediatr 2000;136:795-804.
30. Chardot C, Martin CS, Gilles A, et al. Living-related liver transplantation and vena cava reconstruction after total hepatectomy including the vena cava for hepatoblastoma. Transplantation 2002;73:90-92.
31. Gras J, Reding R, Brichard B, et al. Optimal therapeutic management of unresectable hepatoblastoma in children: primary liver transplantation with a living related donor graft combined with low immunosuppression. Pediatr Transpl 2005;9 (suppl 6):114.
32. Tiao GM, Bobey N, Allen S et al. The current management of hepatoblastoma: a combination of chemotherapy, conventional resection, and liver transplantation. J Pediatr 2005;146:204-11.
33. Perilongo G, Brown J, Shafford E, et al. Hepatoblastoma presenting with lung metastases: treatment results of the first cooperative, prospective study of the International Society of Pediatric Oncology on childhood liver tumors. Cancer 2000;89:1845-53.
34. Passmore SJ, Noblett HR, Wisehart JD, Mott MG. Prolonged survival following multiple thoracotomies for metastatic hepatoblastoma. Med Pediatr Oncol 1995;24:58-60.

**NB: This chapter is based on a review article by the author due to be published in the Annals of the Royal College of Surgeons of England, 2007.

35. Dower NA, Smith LJ, Lees G, et al. Experience with aggressive therapy in three children with unresectable malignant liver tumors. Med Pediatr Oncol 2000;34:132-5.

36. Moore SW, Hesseling PB, Wessels G, Schneider JW. Hepatocellular carcinoma in children. Pediatr Surg Int 1997;12:266-70.

37. Chang MH. Decreasing incidence of hepatocellular carcinoma among children following universal hepatitis B immunization. Liver Int. 2003;23:309-14.

38. Chen JC, Chen CC, Chen WJ, et al. Hepatocellular carcinoma in children: clinical review and comparison with adult cases. J Pediatr Surg 1998;33:1350-4.

39. Czauderna P, Mackinlay G, Perilongo G, et al. Hepatocellular carcinoma in children: results of the first prospective study of the International Society of Pediatric Oncology Group. J Pediatr Surg 2002;20:2798-2804.

40. Malogolowkin MH, Stanley P, Steele DA et al. Feasibility and toxicity of chemoembolization for children with liver tumors. J Clin Oncol 2000;18:1279-84.

41. Mazzaferro V, Regalia E, Doci R, et al. Liver transplantation for the treatment of small hepatocellular carcinomas in patients with cirrhosis. N Engl J Med 1996;334:693-9.

42. Lo CM, Fan ST. Liver transplantation for hepatocellular carcinoma. Br J Surg 2004;91:131-3.

43. Schwartz M, Konstadoulakis M, Roayaie S. Recurrence of hepatocellular carcinoma after liver transplantation: is immunosuppression a factor? Liver Transplantation 2005;11:494-6.

44. Katzenstein HM, Krailo MD, Malogolowkin MH, et al. Hepatocellular carcinoma in children and adolescents: results from the Pediatric Oncology Group and the Children's Cancer Group Intergroup study. J Clin Oncol 2002;20:2789-97.

45. El-Gazzaz G, Wong W, El-Hadary MK et al. Outcome of liver resection and transplantation for fibrolamellar hepatocellular carcinoma. Transpl Int 2000;13 [Suppl 1]:S406-9.

46. Katzenstein HM, Krailo MD, Malogolowkin MH et al. Fibrolamellar hepatocellular carcinoma in children and adolescents. Cancer 2003;97:2006-12.

47. Yandza T, Alvarez F, Laurent J, Gauthier F, Dubousset AM, Valayer J. Pediatric liver transplantation for primary hepatocellular carcinoma associated with hepatitis virus infection. Transpl Int 1993;6:95-8.

48. Broughan TA, Esquivel CO, Vogt DP, et al. Pretransplant chemotherapy in pediatric hepatocellular carcinoma. J Pediatr Surg 1994;29:1319-22.

49. Achilleos OA, Buist LJ, Kelly DA, et al. Unresectable hepatic tumors in childhood and the role of liver transplantation. J Pediatr Surg 1996;31:1563-7.

50. Otte JB, Aronson D, Vraux H, et al. Preoperative chemotherapy, major liver resection, and transplantation for primary malignancies in children. Transplant Proc 1996;28:2393-4.

51. Superina R, Bilik R. Results of liver transplantation in children with unresectable liver tumors. J Pediatr Surg 1996;31:835-9.

52. Tatekawa Y, Asonuma K, Uemoto S, Inomata Y, Tanaka K. Liver transplantation for biliary atresia associated with malignant hepatic tumors. J Pediatr Surg 2001;36:436-9.

53. Tagge EP, Tagge DU, Reyes J, et al. Resection, including transplantation, for hepatoblastoma and hepatocellular carcinoma: impact on survival. J Pediatr Surg 1992; 27:292-7.

54. Esquivel CO, Gutierrez C, Cox KL, et al. Hepatocellular carcinoma and liver cell dysplasia in children with chronic liver disease. J Pediatr Surg 1994;29:1465-9.

55. Bisogno G, Pilz T, Perilongo G, et al. Undifferentiated sarcoma of the liver in childhood: a curable disease. Cancer 2002;94:252-7.

56. Kim DY, Kim KH, Jung SE, Lee SC, Park KW, Kim WK. Undifferentited (embryonal) sarcoma of the liver: combination treatment by surgery and chemotherapy. J Pediatr Surg 2002;37:1419-23.

57. Makhlouf HR, Ishak KG, Goodman ZD. Epithelioid hemangioendothelioma of the liver: a clinicopathologic study of 137 cases. Cancer 1999;85:562-82.

58. Taege C, Holzhausen H, Gunter G, et al. Malignant epithelioid hemangioendothelioma of the liver - a very rare tumor in children (German). Pathologe 1999;20:345-50.

59. Awan S, Davenport M, Portmann B, Howard ER. Angio-sarcoma of the liver in children. J Pediatr Surg 1996; 31: 1729–32.

60. Kirchner SG, Heller RM, Kasselberg AG, Greene HL. Infantile hepatic hemangioendothelioma with subsequent malignant degeneration. Pediatr Radiol 1981;11:42-5.

61. Gunawardena SW, Trautwein LM, Fineglod MJ, Ogden AK. Hepatic angiosarcoma in a child: successful treatment with surgery and adjuvant chemotherapy. Med Ped Oncol 1997; 28:139–43.

62. Dimashkieh HH, Mo JQ, Wyatt-Ashmead J, Collins MH. Pediatric hepatic angiosarcoma: case report and review of the literature. Pediatr Dev Pathol 2004;7:527-32.

63. Penn I. Hepatic transplantation for primary and metastatic cancers of the liver. Surgery 1991; 110: 726–35.

64. Abramson LP, Pillai S, Acton R, Melin-Aldana H, Superina R. Successful orthotopic liver transplantation for treatment of a hepatic yolk sac tumor. J Pediatr Surg 2005;40: 1185-7.

65. Stringer MD, Alizai NK. Mesenchymal hamartoma of the liver: a systematic review. J Pediatr Surg 2005;40;1681-90.

66. Tepetes K, Selby R, Webb M, Madariaga JR, Iwatsuki S, Starzl TE. Orthotopic liver transplantation for benign hepatic neoplasms. Arch Surg 1995;130:153–6.

67. Bejarano PA, Serrano MF, Casillas J, et al. Concurrent infantile hemangioendothelioma and mesenchymal hamartoma in a developmentally arrested liver of an infant requiring hepatic transplantation. Pediatr Dev Pathol 2003;6:552-7.

68. Davenport M. Hemangiomas and other vascular anomalies. In Howard ER, Stringer MD, Colombani PM (eds.). *Surgery of the Liver, Bile-Ducts and Pancreas in children.* 2nd Edition. Arnold Publishers, London, 2002, pp219-238.

69. Egawa H, Berquist W, Garcia-Kennedy R et al. Respiratory distress from benign liver tumors: a report of two unusual cases treated with hepatic transplantation. J Pediatr Gastroenterol Nutr 1994; 19:114–7.

70. Daller JA, Bueno J, Gutierrez J et al. Hepatic hemangioendothelioma: clinical experience and management strategy. J Pediatr Surg 1999; 34: 98–106.

71. Kasahara M, Kiuchi T, Haga H, et al. Monosegmental living-donor liver transplantation for infantile hepatic hemangioendothelioma. J Pediatr Surg 2003;38:1108-11.

72. Walsh R, Harrington J, Beneck D, Ozkaynak MF. Congenital infantile hepatic hemangioendothelioma type II treated with orthotopic liver transplantation. J Pediatr Hematol Oncol 2004;26:121-3.

73. Dasgupta D, Guthrie A, McClean P, Davison S, Luntley J, Rajwal S, Lodge JPA, Prasad KR, Wyatt JI, Stringer MD. Liver transplantation for a hilar inflammatory myofibroblastic tumor. Pediatr Transpl 2004;8:517-21.

74. Heneghan MA, Kaplan CG, Priebe, Jr CJ, Partin JS. Inflammatory pseudotumor of the liver: a rare cause of obstructive jaundice and portal hypertension in a child. Pediatr Radiol 1984;14:433-5.

75. Kim HB, Maller E, Redd D et al. Orthotopic liver transplantation for inflammatory myofibroblastic tumor of the liver hilum. J Pediatr Surg 1996;31:840-2.

CHAPTER 54

Sandeep Guleria
Arvind Bagga

Pediatric Renal Transplantation

INTRODUCTION AND INCIDENCE OF RENAL FAILURE IN INDIA

Approximately 100,000 patients get renal failure in India every year. Of these 90 percent never see a nephrologist. Of the 10 percent who see a nephrologist renal replacement therapy is offered in 90 percent. 10 percent of these are unable to afford it. Eventually only 17-23 percent of these undergo a renal transplant. (Annually 2,500 to 3,500 transplants every year.)

In children there is even less data available but it is estimated that there are approximately 30,000 children with renal failure and less than 50 transplants are done annually.

ETIOLOGY OF RENAL FAILURE IN INDIA

The cause of renal failure in children has been changing over the years. In 1983 the hemolytic uremic syndrome complicating bacillary dysentery was an important cause. However, currently the major causes are glomerulonephritis and obstructive uropathy (Table 54.1). In a recent study of 2625 children who attended the pediatric nephrology clinic at a tertiary hospital 305 had renal failure. Hemodialysis was undertaken only in 26 percent of patients and transplantation only in 6 percent. CRF in India carries a poor prognosis due to late referral and the limited availability and high cost of renal replacement therapy.

Transplantation is the treatment of choice. It ameliorates uremic symptoms results in improved growth and better psychosocial function. Renal transplantation is thus the goal of children with End Stage Renal Disease. Multidisciplinary inputs from the pediatric nephrologist,

Table 54.I: Causes of renal failure in 305 pediatric patients with renal failure in a tertiary centre

Chronic Glomerulonephritis	27.5%
Obstructive Uropathy	31.8%
Reflex Nephropathy	16.7%
Neurogenic Bladder	4.5%
Renal Dysplasia	4.9%
Hereditary Nephropathy	7.5%
Unknown	5.7%

transplant surgeon, urologist, anesthetist, immunologists, dietician and social worker are imperative in providing optimum care to the transplant patient.

Indications for Transplantation

Children are usually excellent candidates for renal transplantation. Most transplant centers are able to perform the procedure once the child has attained a weight of 10 kg.

Contraindications

There are very few absolute contraindications to renal transplantation
i) Active incurable –HIV nephropathy
ii) Pre-existing metastatic malignancy. Children with a malignancy free period of more than two years can be considered for transplantation
iii) Presence of active vasculitis – anti GBM antibodies
iv) Devastating neurological illness, Gross mental retardation

v) Oxalosis which was once considered as an absolute contraindication due to the risk of recurrence can now be offered a combined liver and kidney transplantation.

RECIPIENT WORK-UP

The recipient needs a good history and physical examination. The family should be counseled about the recurring cost of immunosuppressive drugs post transplantation. A routine blood work up as well as screening for hepatitis and HIV should be done. The neurological status as well as cardiac evaluation should be done.

The lower urinary tract needs special evaluation as this can be a cause for concern in the pediatric population. A complete urological evaluation may include a micturating cystourethrogram, cystoscopy as well a uroflometry.

An ABO blood grouping, HLA tissue typing and screening for cytotoxic antibodies must be done. Before transplantation a final cross match should take place. Active infection like tuberculosis should be excluded and all efforts made to establish the original disease to evaluate the risk of recurrence must be made.

PRE-EMPTIVE TRANSPLANTATION

This may be ideal in children obviating the need for dialysis. There does not appear to be any advantage for children to have dialysis prior to transplantation. Dialysis is accompanied by numerous potential complications not faced by recipients of well functioning grafts. Patient and graft survival rates for transplanted children are similar. The decision to proceed to preemptive transplantation implies that the child has been fully vaccinated and tests for susceptibility to varicella, and other herpes viruses have been carried out.

The bladder, lungs, heart, teeth, sinuses and GIT have been fully evaluated and complete psychological and social evaluation of the child has been completed.

Despite the acceptance of pre-emptive transplantation there will be a segment of children for which this is not indicated. These include children who require native nephrectomies for uncontrolled hypertension, infected urologic systems with hydronephrosis and the presence of the nephritic syndrome due to intractable proteinuria despite a low GFR.

Children in whom compliance will be a problem are particularly not suited for a pre-emptive transplant.

Pre-emptive transplantation is performed worldwide for at least 30 percent of children undergoing a renal transplantation. Graft sand patient survival is as good in this population as in the dialyzed population and this remains an attractive option for children.

DONOR CONSIDERATIONS

In India most of the donors are blood relatives. With the passage of the Human Organ Transplant Bill only the father mother brother sister husband or wife are considered as legal donors. Any other donor will require prior approval from the hospital authorization committee.

In our own series the commonest donor has been the mother and the recipient usually the son. The donor is thoroughly evaluated for any systemic disease including diabetes. Borderline hypertension with no end organ damage is no longer considered a contraindication. The donor's GFR as well as ABO and HLA compatibility are determined and if the cross- match is negative a renal angiogram/spiral CT is done to evaluate the renal anatomy before proceeding for transplantation.

ORGAN PRESERVATION

The essential components of preservation include hypothermia as cooling of the organ markedly reduces the metabolic rate and prolongs the storage time, prevention of cell edema by the use of a hyperosmolar flushing solution, free radical scavengers like gluatathione and allopurinol as well as energy source and lysosomal stabilizers like steroids and magnesium.

In renal transplantation this perfusion solution could be phosphate based sucrose, Hyperosmolar citrate or the University of Wisconsin solution. The mean storage time of kidneys could go upto 72 hours though most centers would transplant a kidney within twenty four hours of harvesting.

OPERATIVE TECHNIQUE

The technique of transplantation in older children and adolescents is similar to that in adults, the only difference being that the vascular anastomosis are more cephalad (Fig. 54.1).

a. *Small children:* In small children the transplantation is done through a midline incision extending from the xiphoid to the pubis. The caecum and the colon are reflected to the left upper quadrant of the abdomen and the anterior wall of the aorta and the vena cava are exposed. The lumbar veins are ligated.

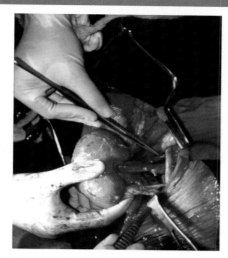

Figure 54.1: The transplant vascular anastomosis

The placement of the anastomosis is usually determined by seeing the lie of the kidney. The venous anastomosis is done by using 6-0 prolene by giving a venotomy that extend from the inferior vena cava to the iliac vein. The arterial anastomosis is usually done to the aorta with one wall continuous and the other interrupted. It is important for the CVP to be more than 12 to 15 cm of water and mannitol as well as a diuretic should be available. Warm saline should be available to warm the patient since an adult kidney uses a significant amount of blood volume aggressive volume replacement is essential at this moment.

The ureteric anastomosis is next done. This is usually done by an onlay extravesical ureteroneocystostomy using 4-0 polydixonane. Reflux has not been a significant problem in our hands provided we have kept the urine sterile. The authors preference it do a suprapubic cystostomy tying the double J stent to the end of the Foleys catheter. The urethral catheter is removed on day one to minimize discomfort to the child. The suprapubic catheter is removed on day five.

b. *Larger Children:* The technique for larger children is similar to that of adults. A modified Gibson incision at the lateral end of the rectus is given. The external iliac vessels are mobilized and the anastomosis can be done either to the common iliac or external iliac artery or vein. The internal iliac artery may be used in larger children if the flow is adequate.

The postoperative care of these patients is critical. Meticulous attention must be paid to fluid and electrolytes. Intravenous fluids are administered to replace urine and to maintain a good CVP. The composition of the fluid given will depend upon the electrolytes that are checked regularly. Replacement therapy is assessed by monitoring pulse rate, blood pressure, peripheral perfusion, arterial blood gases and CVP. No single factor can determine alone the intravascular volume of infants.

Children with adult kidneys that function immediately can require large amount of fluid replacement. Calcium loss is also a frequent problem so calcium levels must be carefully monitored and calcium replaced intravenously as required.

Oliguria must be investigated in an organized fashion. One must check whether the urinary catheter or stent is patent, the volume status must be assessed, an urgent ultrasound must be done to establish that there is no compression of the graft as well as that the flow is normal through the kidney. Close cooperation between a pediatric nephrologist and transplant surgeon is necessary at all times.

Prolonged ileus after an intra-abdominal transplant is common and nasogastric drainage is required.

Volume loading and forced diuresis can often result in hypertension. This may be severe and will require aggressive therapy.

IMMUNOLOGICAL RESPONSE

HLA System

Antigens on the transplant tissues are recognized by the non-identical recipient as foreign. This process of self and non-self recognition initiates rejection. The specificity of the antigens involved in graft rejection is under genetic control. A single chromosomal complex of closely linked genes makes up the code for the major histocompatibility antigens. The major Histocompatibility complex (MHC) in humans is termed the HLA system (Human Leukocyte Antigen), as it was initially detected in leukocytes. This gene is found in the short arm of chromosome 6. It has at least seven loci, A, B, C, D, DR, DQ and DP; each highly polymorphic.

HLA-A, B and C are grouped together as Class I antigens. They are present in virtually all nucleated cells in the body, including Lymphocytes and platelets. They are composed of a heavy (Alfa) chain and light (Beta-2 microglobulin, a non-MHC coded peptide) chain. They act as targets of cytotoxic (CD8) T cells.

Class II antigens include HLA-D (DR, DP and DQ) antigens. They are expressed only on B Lymphocytes, monocytes, activated T lymphocytes and some endothelial cells. They are composed of and alpha and one beta chain. They stimulate the proliferative response of Mixed lymphocyte culture (MLC) and are vital for antigen presentation in vivo. They are preferentially recognized by Helper (CD4) T lymphocytes.

Allograft rejection is a complex event that results from the cytodestructive effects of activated helper T cell, cytotoxic T cells, B-lymphocytes, antibodies and activated macrophages. The initiating event seems to be activation of CD4 cells by class II antigens in the graft. This releases various cytokines, most importantly Interleukin 2 (IL-2). Class I antigens stimulate CD8 T cells to develop IL-2 receptors. In addition, activated macrophages secrete Interleukin 1 (IL-1), which in turn stimulates secretion of IL-2. IL-2 interacts with various IL-2 receptors expressed on T lymphocytes to stimulate their clonal proliferation. In essence, the activation of helper T cells by alloantigens and IL-1 stimulates the release of a variety of lymphokines from CD4 cells and this in turn activates macrophages, CD8 cells and antibody secreting B-lymphocytes. Also, the continued viability of activated T cell clones is IL-2 dependant. Thus, IL-2 is at the centre of all rejection phenomenon and most of the immunosuppressant drugs aim to attack this phenomenon.

Histocompatibility Testing and Cross-match

a. ABO blood group compatibility is considered essential in most of the solid organ transplants, liver being an exception.
b. HLA Histocompatibility testing is done primarily to search for HLA identical siblings. It is not of much value in choosing between parents, offspring, or HLA non-identical siblings as donors. Even in perfect matching of MHC antigens in an HLA identical sibling match, immunosuppression will be required due to incompatibility at minor Histocompatiblity loci. HLA matching is usually not done in cadaver renal transplants. Nevertheless, a six antigen match (at the DR, B and A, in the order of importance, also known as full house match) cadaver kidney donors has a better long-term survival than lesser-matched grades. Currently almost all HLA typing is done by a lymphocyte cytotoxicity procedure. The clinical application of histocompatibility holds great relevance for the transplantation of most solid organs. The presence of HLA antigens on a cell surface can be detected both functionally and serologically. Both tests are frequently performed before transplantation

because the functional method is most specific for class-II antigens while the serologic method detects those in Class I. The serologic method uses antigen-specific antisera that bind to cells expressing that specific antigen. The functional method measures the reactivity of the lymphocytes of a potential recipient to the donor. The responding lymphocytes will proliferate in response to transplantation antigens they recognize as foreign. Only HLA (MHC) antigens can be detected with the functional method. The antigens most effective at generating this response are those of the Class II MHC. However, since Class I antigens also play an important role in transplantation, antisera specific for each of the Class I loci (A, B or C) are also used for serologic typing of a potential donor and recipient.

c. A complement mediated cytotoxic crossmatch with pretransplant recipient sera against non-activated T lymphocytes expressing class I antigens, and not class II, from the potential donor is essential. Presence of IgG antibodies against class I MHC antigens represents a positive test and an absolute contraindication for transplant. This test screens for preformed antibodies in the recipient against donor antigens thus, avoiding Hyperacute reaction.

THE REJECTION PHENOMENON

Rejection is invariable in transplants between non identical twins without immunosuppression. A Perfect HLA match in nonidentical twins is very rare owing to the extreme polymorphism in the HLA system.
The various types of Rejection are:

1. *Hyperacute Rejection (HAR):* It is due to presensitisation of the recipient to an antigen expressed by the donor. The recipient has circulating antibodies prior to transplant owing to prior exposure through pregnancy, previous transplants or blood transfusion to donor alloantigens. A complement-mediated lysis is initiated resulting in immediate graft thrombosis. The graft swells up and becomes blue and hard on the operating table itself. The only measure against it is prevention. The tests used preoperatively are the ABO compatibility and lymphocytotoxicity cross match. They effectively prevent HAR in 99.5 percent of transplants.

2. *Accelerated Rejection (Vascular Rejection):* This is a delayed variant of HAR. The mechanism seems to be presence of alloantibodies at levels undetectable buy the crossmatch assay, in spite of presensitisation.

Sometimes, massive antibody production by T cell dependant B cell activation may cause de novo accelerated rejection. Thus, the graft initially functions well, but deteriorates by day three. Pulse therapy and plasmapheresis may reverse the condition in certain cases.

3. *Acute Rejection (AR):* This is a T cell dependant process and the only variant that can be effectively treated. It commonly occurs within the first six months of transplant. Acute rejection is invariable in transplants between nonidentical twins without immunosuppresion. The incidence of acute rejection declines with decreasing MHC disparity, though even a full house match mandates immunosuppresion. Activation of CD4 T cells leads to IL-2 secretion ultimately resulting in massive infiltration of the graft of mainly CD8 cells and its destruction. A cell-mediated counterpart of HAR is also known; presensitisation at T cell level causing accelerated form of acute rejection mediated by memory T cells. Prompt recognition and treatment leads to graft function retrieval in 90 to 95 percent of patients. Biopsy should be performed in unexplained graft dysfunction. Biopsy would reveal lymphocytic infiltration. In renal transplant, the onset of oliguria, weight gain, hypertension and impaired renal function signals AR. The classic signs of fever, graft enlargement and tenderness are seen infrequently in patients treated with cyclosporine.

The differential diagnoses could be cyclosporine toxicity (Levels are high), Acute tubular necrosis, extrinsic compression on the graft or ureteric obstruction.

Diagnostic modalities include renal diuretic scan with pertechnetate Tc 99, Ultrasound (prominence of renal pyramids and loss of renal sinus fat, hematoma) and MRI (loss of CMD).

4. *Chronic Rejection (Chronic Allograft Nephropathy):* This is a poorly understood process leading to insidious, slow and irreversible graft loss. It usually occurs over a period of months to years. It is not treatable by any method yet. Histologically it is characterized by replacement of graft parenchyma with fibrous tissue with a relatively sparse lymphocyte infiltrate. Non-immunological factors may also play a part. AR may sometimes cause rapid deterioration in a known case of CR and if treated, may lead to partial return of graft function. The only treatment is retransplantation.

IMMUNOSUPPRESSANT DRUGS

Immunosuppresion is a vital part of transplantation. However, it is a double-edged sword, carrying with it the risks of infection and malignancy, apart from the side effects of the drugs itself. The immunosuppression in the initial postoperative period is intense as the chances of rejection are maximum during this period, known as induction immunosuppression. They are also used as Rescue agents, used to reverse an established rejection episode. The dosage of immunosuppressants gradually tapers off, known as maintenance immunosuppression. The various drugs available for immunosuppression are:

1. *Steroids:* The most commonly used steroid is Prednisolone. It alone is ineffective and usually is added to Azathioprine and Cyclosporine in the most commonly used regimen for immunosuppression. The glucocorticoid effect causes a generalized immunosuppression by blunting T-cell proliferation. High dose Methylprednisolone (500-750 mg/day IV bolus X 3-5 days) is used as a rescue agent for reversing acute rejection. Steroids are responsible for cushingoid features like acne, obesity, diabetes and peptic ulceration. They may cause growth retardation in pediatric transplants. The trend now is towards minimal steroid usage and even steroid free immunosuppression.

2. *Azathioprine:* The first immunosuppressive used, it is an antimetabolite. It is a prodrug, which is metabolized to 6-Mercaptopurine and then its derivatives. These then deprive the cell of adenosine, a vital ingredient in DNA synthesis. It is relatively nonspecific acting on all rapidly dividing cells. Its chief use is for maintenance immunosuppression and has no value as induction or rescue agent. The dosage is usually 1-2 mg/kg. The dose limiting side effects are bone marrow depression and hepatotoxicity. Hence, the dose is withheld or reduced if TLC is less than 3000 cells/cc or liver dysfunction is present.

3. *Mycophenolate Mofetil (MMF):* It is also an antimetabolite. It is a reversible inhibitor of IMP dehydrogenase, interfering in Nucleic acid synthesis. It is relatively specific against lymphocytes as they lack the salvage pathway (HGPRT catalyzed GMP production). Both T and B cell proliferation in response to antigen stimulation is blocked. The drug has potential for both induction and maintenance therapy. The side effects, including bone marrow

depression are minimal. It is gradually replacing Azathioprine, especially in patients with high risk of rejection.

4. *Cyclosporine:* Discovered by Borel in 1976, it came into clinical practice in 1983. It is at present the mainstay of maintenance therapy in almost all type of transplants. It is a calcinueurin inhibitor, binding cyclophilin and inhibiting the transcription of IL-2 gene and thus T cell activation. It is remarkably specific against immunocompetent lymphocytes. However, it cannot be used as rescue agent presence of IL-2 in the graft bypasses the drug effect. At present, a microemulsion formulation that has better bioavailability and pharmacodynamics is used. Since most of the metabolism is through the cytochrome P 450 enzyme system, Hepatic dysfunction mandates reduced dosage. The absorbed drug is almost totally metabolized and excreted in bile. Also, drugs influencing the cytochrome enzyme system alter the metabolism of cyclosporine (increased by rifampin, Phenobarbital, Phenytoin, decreased by ketoconazole, erythromycin and calcium channel blockers). The usual dosage is 7.5 to 25 mg/kg. The main toxicity is Nephrotoxicity due to vasoconstrictor effect on proximal renal arterioles. Hyperkalemia, Hemolytic Uremic syndrome, Hypertrichosis, Gingival Hyperplasia, Neurotoxicity are the other side effects seen (Fig 54.2). This mandates strict monitoring of cyclosporine levels to avoid toxicity. Usually the level of cyclosporine 2 hours after intake is measured (C2 levels).

5. *Tacrolimus (FK506):* This is a macrolide calcinuerin inhibitor. It blocks IL-2 translation by binding to FK Binding Protein, the effect and toxicity being additive to cyclosporine. Tacrolimus is 100 times more potent than cyclosporine. However, unlike the latter, it can be used as a rescue agent. The side effect profile is similar to cyclosporine, with more pronounced neurological and diabetogenic effect.

6. *Sirolimus (Rapamycin/Rapamune):* It is the latest immunosuppressant agent for solid organ transplants, prescribed for induction therapy, refractory rejection, steroid withdrawal, and combination therapy. It is an immunophilin binding drug, blocking signal transduction by the IL-2 receptor, hence the response of T-cells to IL-2. It is structurally similar to but antagonizes the action of Tacrolimus and is synergistic with cyclosporine. It is at present in use for renal and heart transplants. The main toxicity of sirolimus is hypertriglyceridemia[1] and pulmonary toxicity.

7. *Monoclonal antibody (muromonab-CD3/OKT3):* They are produced using the Hybridoma technology, developed by Kohler and Milstein in 1970. The immunoglobulin is targeted against the CD3 molecule, part of T Cell Receptor found Thymocytes and mature T cells. It is used for treatment of acute rejection episodes, usually steroid refractory cases. The side effects include a systemic cytokine release syndrome, which can cause hypotension, pulmonary edema, fatal cardiac myodepression and aseptic meningitis. Pretreatment with high dose methylprednisolone, antihistamines and antipyretics reduces the side effects. The usual adult dose is 5 mg/kg/day for 10-14 days. Use of OKT3 is also associated with increased risk of cytomegalovirus, Epstein-Barr and in children, varicella viral infection.

8. *Anti Lymphocyte Globulin/Anti Thymocyte Globulin (ALG/ATG):* This is a polyclonal serum developed by collecting antibodies produced by various animals against human lymphocytes. Most commonly, Horse or rabbit are used. ATGAM is the purified IgG fraction most commonly used. The antibody coats the T cells and promotes its clearance. The drug is most commonly used as part of multidrug induction immunosuppression. Severe thrombocytopenia is occasionally seen. The patient is usually pretreated with antipyretics, antihistamines and antipyretics. Viral infections, both primary and reactivation are seen more frequently in patients treated with this drug.

9. *Anti IL-2 Receptor Antibody (Basiliximab/ Daclizumab):* The chimaeric monoclonal antibody

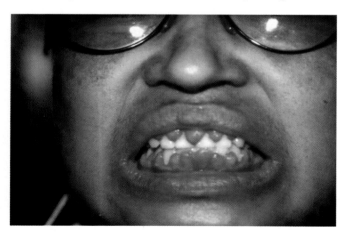

Figure 54.2: Gingival hyperplasia due to cyclosporine

basiliximab specifically binds the alpha subunit of the interleukin-2 (IL-2) receptor on activated T lymphocytes. Renal transplant patients usually receive basiliximab 20 mg 2 hours before and then 4 days after transplantation surgery. These antibodies have been shown to reduce the incidence of acute rejection without increasing the incidence of opportunistic infections or malignancy. Side effects are not very significant. Longer follow up however, is required to fully evaluate the efficacy of these agents.

Newer Agents Recently Approved or in the Pipeline

The transplant community must constantly keep up to date with the fast pace of newer immunosuppressive agents being developed by the pharmaceutical community. Campath-1H® (alemtuzumab; anti-CD52) is a newer anti-T cell agent developed at Cambridge University, which shows prolonged and potent lymphocyte depletion and has promising early results after renal transplantation. FTY720 is a unique agent that traffics lymphocytes to the periphery. Leflunomide is an interesting immunosuppressant that also has anti-viral activity, particularly against BK virus. Myfortic® is a newer enteric coated formulation of mycophenolate mofetil that was intended to have less gastrointestinal side effects but appears to have a similar adverse effect profile while maintaining equivalent efficacy.

Complications of Immunosuppression

Immunosuppression is not obtained without paying a significant price in terms of side effects. Infection and malignancy are the most frequent complications encountered with the use of non-specific immuno-suppressive agent.

a. *Infection:* Transplant recipients who receive immunosuppression encounter a greatly increased incidence of infection, which remains the most common cause of mortality. Most deaths used to be due to invasive infections. These have been controlled by antibiotics. Nowadays most infections are caused by opportunistic pathogens, including fungi, protozoa and viruses, the latter being specially common among kidney transplant patients (Fig. 54.3). Candida albicans and Aspergillus species are the most common fungi

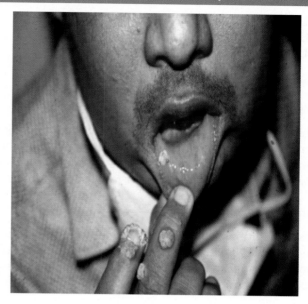

Figure 54.3: Viral warts due to long term immunosuperssion

encountered in transplant patients. The latter produces upper lobe pulmonary cavities. The protozoan *Pneumocystis carinii* is also a frequent cause of pulmonary infection, producing n alveolar infiltrate with severe dyspnea and cyanosis. However, it is seen less often since the use of prophylactic trimethoprim and sulfa-methoxazole in transplant recipients. Among the viruses, cytomegalovirus (CMV) and Epstein-Barr virus (EBV) commonly infect transplant patients. CMV is the most important virus infection seen in immunosuppressed transplant patients. The virus itself produces severe immunosuppression rendering the patient susceptible to bacterial and fungal opportunists.

b. *Malignancy:* Cancer is seen more often in transplant recipients than in the general population. Most cancers that arise in transplanted patients are either epithelia l (carcinomas of the cervix an lip and basal cell carcinomas, constitute about one half of these) or lymphoid (B-cell lymphomas).

Other Complications

These are mostly due to the use of steroids : Cushing's syndrome, cataracts, gastrointestinal bleeding, hypertension, pancreatitis, and avascular necrosis of the femoral heads.

DIAGNOSIS AND TREATMENT OF POSTOPERATIVE ALLOGRAFT DYSFUNCTION

Early Postoperative Period

Pre-Renal

This would include diminished cardiac output or a low central venous pressure, both resulting in diminished renal perfusion. Another important cause is vascular compromise from renal artery or renal vein thrombosis.

Intra-renal Causes

The commonest cause of this would be acute tubular necrosis (ATN) or acute cellular rejection. Causes of ATN include prolonged ischemia time, donor age, drug effects from cyclosporine or reperfusion injury. Both ATN and acute rejection are associated with a poorer long term graft survival.

The treatment of acute rejection should be based on the biopsy findings, as well as on the clinical circumstances. In general mild acute cellular rejection should be treated with high dose steroid boluses given over three consecutive days. In moderate acute interstitial rejection or in the face of vascular rejection OKT3 or a polyclonal antibody is generally used.

The use of OKT3 or ATG is associated with an increased risk of opportunistic infections particularly CMV infections. Most centers would place patients on prophylactic doses of valganciclovir. PCP infection is another common cause of posttransplant infections and patients are routinely placed on *Pneumocystis carnii* prophylaxis.

Postrenal Causes

The most common postrenal cause of allograft dysfunction is obstruction of the ureteric stent or foleys catheter by a blood clot or by kinking. It presents as a sudden drop in urine output despite adequate filling pressure. Checking the foleys catheter for any kinking or gentle flushing with sterile saline will generally alleviate the problem. The catheter may need to be changed in rare cases.

Urinary leak is another important cause of postallograft dysfunction and occurs at the anastomosis between the donor and the recipient. The cause of this is invariably technical and will respond to radiological or surgical interventions.

Late Postoperative Period

Pre-renal Causes

The commonest cause is hypoperfusion due to volume depletion or hypotension. Thus assurance of adequate fluid intake is essential. Renal artery stenosis is another important cause and is usually technical in nature. It can usually be diagnosed by Doppler ultrasound scans where diminished or turbulent flow through the renal artery is seen. Confirmation requires an angiogram and the lesion may be amenable to endovascular repair or in rare cases surgery may be required.

Intrarenal Causes

These are usually related to immunological phenomenon or drug toxicity. Immunological causes would include acute as well as chronic rejection. Other important causes include cyclosporine toxicity or FK 506 toxicity. Thus attention to drug levels is imperative during the long term follow up period.

Infectious Causes of Allograft Dysfunction

Viral infections like CMV or EBV can result in allograft dysfunction. Attention to donor and recipients CMV and EBV titres are important at the time of transplantation.

Urinary tract infection must be considered in the differential diagnosis of allograft dysfunction. This is more crucial in the individual with ESRD with obstructive uropathy or reflux nephropathy.

Recurrence of the Primary Disease

Immunological disease including FSGS and IgA nephropathy as well as MPGN may have high recurrence rates. Treatment of recurrent FSGS has included high dose cyclosporine, pulse steroid therapy or oral cyclophosphamide for twelve weeks as a substitute for azathioprine and plasmaphersis in combination with cyclophosphamide.

Post-Renal Causes of Graft Dysfunction

Stricture of the ureter at the anastomosis as well as stricture of the urethra are important causes. Treatment modalities include dilatation of the stricture through a percutaneous nephrostomy and stenting. If the stricture persists open surgery may be required. Neurogenic bladders are also an important cause and these patients may require self intermittent catheterization.

OUTCOME OF TRANSPLANTATION

With Cyclosporine and Tacrolimus the outcome of transplantation has improved dramatically. The five year graft survival after live related transplantation is around 94 to 97 percent. The Indian literature is scanty and one year grafts survival is around 82 percent. Excellent rehabilitation can be achieved with most children attending school or college normally. Growth is suboptimal but can be improved by the use of recombinant growth hormone.

Pediatric renal transplantation is in its infancy in India as there is lack of awareness and lack of funding from the government. There are inadequate pediatric nephrological facilities in the country and an poorly developed cadaveric transplant program. However, for children with renal failure renal transplantation offers a new lease of life.

THE FUTURE OF SOLID ORGAN TRANSPLANTATION

Newer technologies are likely to change the face of solid organ transplantation in the not too distant future xenotransplantation, i. e. transplantation of tissues from different species other than humans, particularly with tissues derived from swine is also on the horizon. Overcoming the hyperactive rejection due to the alpha-Gal epitope, prevention of human transmission of animal infections and ethical concerns are major obstacles at this time. Tissue engineering strategies to reduce the antigenicity of allografts are also being investigated. Stem cells show great promise in the regeneration of organs, particularly if the issue of teratoma development can be overcome. Therapeutic cloning could become a reality very soon, but ethical concerns are a major issue. It is possible that, in the years to come, transplantation of allogenic human solid organs will cease completely as newer technologies become a reality.

BIBLIOGRAPHY

1. Morris PJ Kidney Transplantation principles and practice, 5th Edition Published by W.B. Saunders company, Philadelphia Pennsylvania.
2. Moudgil A. Renal Transplantation. Indian J Pediatr 2003;70;257-64.
3. Mukta M, Bagga A, Hari P. Renal Replacement therapy, Indian J Pract Pediatr 2002;4:254-62.
4. Phadke K, Ballal S, Venkatesh K, et al. Pediatric renal transplantation- Indian Experience. Indian Pediatrics 1998;35:321-5.
5. Samsonov D, Briscoe DM. Long term care of pediatric renal transplant patients: From bench to bedside. Curr Opin Pediatr 2002;14;205-10.
6. Schurman SJ, Stabien DM, Perlman SA, Warady BA. Center volume effects in pediatric renal transplantation- a report of NAPRTCS. Pediatr. Nephrol 1999;13:730-6.
7. Tejani AH, fine RN Eds in Pediatric Renal transplantation 1994 published by Wiley-LissInc New York.

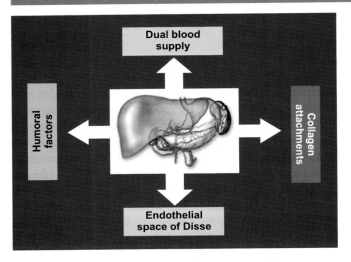

Figure 55.4: Frequent and rare routes of tumor metastases in lung parenchyma

presentation according to the primary tumor. Calcification of nodules is frequently observed in case of osteogenic sarcoma, synovial sarcoma, or chondrosarcoma. Pneumothorax associated with pulmonary metastases usually indicates that an osteosarcoma is the primary site. Hemorrhagic metastases, with a halo of hazy opacity, are most often seen in choriocarcinoma, but also occasionally appear with other vascular tumors such as angiosarcoma or renal cell carcinoma. Solitary pulmonary metastases are uncommon and account for 2-10 percent of all solitary nodules. The primary lesions that are more likely than others to produce solitary metastases include osteosarcoma and carcinoma of the testicle.

The presence of pulmonary metastases is a bad prognostic factor that indicates disseminated disease. The detection and surgical management of pulmonary metastases solely depends on the histologic features of the primary tumor and the response of the primary tumor to combined therapy. Pulmonary metastases should not be approached surgically until the primary tumor is eradicated without evidence of recurrence. Mortality rates depend mainly on the primary tumor. Childhood tumors that are considered for pulmonary metastasectomy are osteogenic sarcoma, soft-tissue sarcoma, and Wilms' tumor.

An important consideration in the surgical management of metastases is the complete resection of all metastases. Wedge resection is generally possible in children with osteogenic sarcoma, however lobectomy

may be more beneficial to totally remove the entire tumor metastases in cases where the primary tumor is unresponsive to chemotherapy or radiation.[1] Advancements in minimal invasive surgical (MIS) allow muscle–sparing techniques for children that require posterolateral thoracotomies.[2] Instrumentation development such as automatic stapler device and the increasing experience of pediatric surgeons in the field of laparoscopy have also shown to be helpful in aiding MIS technique development for this age group.

Osteogenic Sarcoma

Pulmonary metastases should be considered for resection in children with osteogenic sarcoma once the primary lesion has been controlled. The survival rate for children who develop pulmonary metastases is approximately 40 percent. The prognosis for patients with less than four pulmonary nodules is better than those with over four lesions.[3] Although the complete removal of all metastatic pulmonary lesions is of extreme importance to improve the outcome,[4] penetration through the parietal pleura is associated with an adverse prognosis.[5] An aggressive therapy is favored in case of pulmonary metastases regardless of the number of lesions in children with osteogenic sarcoma. Recent data indicate that there is a high rate of contralateral involvement in osteosarcoma patients with unilateral nodules diagnosed by CT scan. Bilateral exploration of unilateral lung metastases is not warranted in all cases. Staged bilateral thoracotomies should be considered in osteosarcoma patients presenting with unilateral pulmonary disease on imaging studies within 2 years of diagnosis.[6] Most patients will have only unilateral disease, and delaying contralateral thoracotomy until disease is detected radiologically does not appear to affect outcome.[7] The thoracoscopic approach to the surgical management of lung nodules in children with osteosarcoma for biopsies as well as the resection of multiple nodules seems to be promising.[8] The data at present indicates an aggressive approach to surgical management of pulmonary metastases in osteogenic sarcoma.

Rhabdomyosarcomas

The time development of pulmonary metastases, number of lesions, and tumor doubling time are important prognostic factors of soft tissue sarcomas. Resection of pulmonary metastases is rarely required in rhabdomyosarcomas,[9] despite an aggressive approach being advocated in the past.[10] Removal of persistant solitary or limited pulmonary metastases after chemotherapy and radiation therapy may result in occasional survival.

Ewing's Sarcoma

In case of Ewing's sarcoma, surgical resection of pulmonary metastases has been advocated only in certain patients, however, without significant improvement in the outcomes.[11] Despite the resection of the pulmonary metastases the survival rate in these patients is remarkably low.[12] Reports have also emerged about patients with lung metastases relapse only without local recurrence of Ewing's sarcoma.[13]

Wilms' Tumor

Resection of pulmonary metastases in children with Wilms' disease is almost not necessary and however, if performed, was found to have no advantage compared with chemotherapy and radiation therapy alone.[14] Recent reports have pointed out that pulmonary metastatectomy may increase survival in carefully selected children, though it is unlikely to cure the patient. Therefore combined therapies such as chemotherapy and/or radiotherapy should be continued in the postoperative period.[15] Since the results of chemotherapy and whole-lung irradiation are excellent for children with Wilms' tumor with pulmonary metastases, pulmonary resection of metastases should be reserved for isolated cases.

LIVER METASTASES

The liver is the second most commonly involved organ by metastatic disease, after the lymph nodes. The dual blood supply and the microvasculature of the liver significantly contribute to the establishment of liver metastases. The liver provides a fertile soil in which metastases can establish, not only because of its rich, dual blood supply but also because of humoral factors that promote cell growth. The fenestrations in the sinusoidal endothelium allow a foothold into the space of Disse for tumor emboli arriving via the blood stream. An intact endothelium prevents the adhesion of tumor emboli, however, stasis-damaged endothelium and normally fenestrated endothelium promote the implantation of tumor emboli. Furthermore, access to underlying collagen in the space of Disse provides

attachment points for cancer emboli arriving at the sinusoid, but not all implanted cancer emboli in the space of Disse progress to develop liver metastases. Many studies have found a great variation in the patterns of liver invasion by different tumor cells, though the initial tumor implantation is similar in all types of tumor cells (Fig. 55.5).

The main factors that determine liver metastases by tumor cells are the following:

(a) The adhesiveness of different types of tumor cells to hepatocytes,
(b) The inability of some tumor cells to remain viable in the bloodstreams for long,
(c) The pressure on the surrounding tissues,
(d) The formation of tumor cell and hepatocyte junction,
(e) Tumor cell kinetic motion, and
(f) Host tissue destruction by enzymes released by tumor cells.

In children, the most common liver metastases are from neuroblastoma, Wilms' tumor or leukemia. Liver involvement at diagnosis indicates a worse prognosis than lung involvement. Wilms' tumor patients with liver metastases should be treated with more intensive regimens than those with lung metastases.[16] Most liver metastases are multiple, involving both lobes and only 10 percent are solitary. Approximately one-half the patients with liver metastases have clinical signs of hepatomegaly or ascites; liver function tests tend to be insensitive and nonspecific.

Six minimally invasive techniques are available for the treatment of primary and metastatic hepatic neoplasms: transcatheter arterial chemoembolization

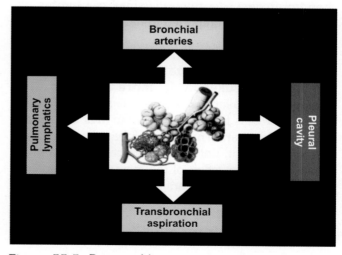

Figure 55.5: Pattern of liver metastases due to supporting factors that encourage hepatic involvement

(TACE); cryoablation; microwave ablation; ethanol ablation, as called percutaneous ethanol injection (PEI); radiofrequency ablation (RFA), and laser ablation.[17,18] Although the indication for surgical resection of the liver metastases must be extremely well calculated depending on the type of primary tumor and the meatstases localization in the liver, open surgical approach in central hepatic resection of malignant tumors or metastases involving segments IV, V, and VIII has been found to be feasible and effective in childhood.[19]

BRAIN METASTASES

In the pediatric age group, metastatic tumors of the brain have been seldom reported. Primary tumors that may metastasize to brain are Wilms' tumor, osteogenic sarcoma, and embryonal rhabdomyosarcoma. Reports of brain metastases in children from hepatoblastoma as well as malignant melanoma have also recently been published.[20,21] Children with metastatic cancer who develop headaches or any other neurologic symptom should be investigated for possible brain metastasis.[22] However, hemorrhage is present in almost up to 15 percent of the cases with generalized focal seizures in almost 20 percent.

OVARIAN METASTASES

Ovarian metastases of tumor is rarely encountered in the pediatric age group. However, neuroblastomas, rhabdomyosarcomas, Ewing's sarcoma, rhabdoid tumor of the kidney, carcinoid tumor of the lung, retinoblastoma, medulloblastoma, osteogenic sarcoma, chondrosarcoma, desmoplastic small cell tumors and leukemia have been reported to have metastases in the ovaries.[23-25]

Ovarian metastasis with leukemia deserves special attention.[26] Ovarian involvement with relapse in lymphocytic leukemia is more common than myelogenous leukemia, because of higher affinity of these tumor cells for the ovaries. Survival in relapsing leukemia with ovarian metastases is based on aggressive chemotherapy and not on the surgical resection of the lesion. Surgical resection of the ovary or other internal genital organs must be carefully evaluated depending on the primary tumor.

TESTICULAR METASTASES

Leukemia and lymphoma have been reported in the literature to be the most common tumors to metastasize

to the testes. However, testicular involvement may be the initial clinical presentation of Burkitt's lymphoma.[27] Testicular metastases in leukemias and lymphomas may be an indication of relapse or persistent disease and has been found in approximately 20 percent of the patients with acute lymphocytic leukemia.[28] However, testicular involvement with acute myeloid leukemias in children has also been reported.[29] It is important to note that the testes offer a sanctuary to tumor cells since the blood-testis barrier prevents chemotherapeutic agents to achieve a direct contact (Fig. 55.6). Therefore, significantly higher false-postive results are obtained in testicular biopsies. As far as the treatment is concerned, chemotherapy combined with radiotherapy has proved promising for the leukemic infiltrates in testicular involvement.[30]

SPLENIC INVOLVEMENT

Splenic involvement is generally seen in the stage III of the Ann Arbor Staging System in Hodgkin's disease. The traditional practice of total splenectomy as part of surgical staging came under scrutiny following reports in the mid 1970s, where noticeable sepsis bouts in children after splenectomy were identified, and the recognition of "Overwhelming Post-splenectomy Infection" was established.[31] Partial splenectomy and the importance of splenic tissue preservation, that is associated with the preservation of humoral immunity towards capsulated microbes, replaced the practise of total splenectomy.[32] Various reports with partial splenectomy subsequently underlined the importance

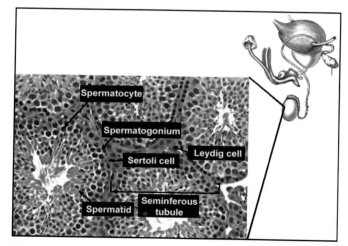

Figure 55.6: The "blood-testis" barrier provides a sanctuary for tumor cells from chemotherapeutic agents

of splenic preservation with reduced morbidity and mortality.[33] However, to date no prospective study has been performed to interpret the use of hemisplenectomy as a staging procedure. Some authors suggest that splenectomy could be avoided if other sites of intra-abdominal involvement are identified during the performance of surgical exploration.[34]

REFERENCES

1. Ballantine TVN, et al. Assessment of pulmonary wedge resection for the treatment of lung metastases. J Pediatr Surg 1975;10:671.
2. Holcomb GW III, et al. Minimally invasive surgery in children with cancer. Cancer 1995;76:121.
3. Roth JA, et al. Differing determinants of prognosis following resection of pulmonary metastases from osteogenic and soft tissue sarcoma patients. Cancer 1985;55:1361.
4. Marina NM, et al. Improved prognosis of children with osteosarcoma metastatic to lung (s) at the time of diagnosis. Cancer 1992;70:27222.
5. Goorin AM, et al. The role of surgical excision in the management of relapsed Wilms' tumor patients with pulmonary metastases: a report from the National Wilms' Tumor Study. J Pediatr Surg 1991;26:728.
6. Su WT, et al. Surgical management and outcome of osteosarcoma patients with unilateral pulmonary metastases. J Pediatr Surg. 39:418,2004
7. Younes RN, et al. Surgical resection of unilateral lung metastases: is bilateral thoracotomy necessary? World J Surg 2002;26:1112.
8. Castagnetti M, et al. Optimizing the surgical management of lung nodules in children with osteosarcoma: Thoracoscopy for biopsies, thoracotomy for resections. Surg Endosc Epub 2004.
9. Hej HA, et al. Prognostic factors in surgery for pulmonary metastases in children. Surgery 1994;115:687.
10. Lembke J, et al. Long-term results following surgical removal of pulmonary metastases in children with malignomas. Thorac Cardiovasc Surg 1986;34:137.
11. Delgado Munoz MD, et al. [Surgery of lung metastasis] Cir Pediatr 2000;13:7.
12. Briccoli A, et al. Surgery for lung metastases in Ewing's sarcoma of bone. Eur J Surg Oncol 2004;30:63.
13. LaQuaglia MP. The surgical management of metastases in pediatric cancer. Semin Pediatric Surg 1993;2:75.
14. Green DM, et al. The role of surgical excision in the management of relapsed Wilms' tumor patients with pulmonary metastases: a report from the national Wilms' tumor study. J Pediatr Surg 1991;26:728.
15. Jimenez RE, et al. Primary Ewing's sarcoma/primitive neuroectodermal tumor of the kidney: a clinicopathologic and immunohistochemical analysis of 11 cases. Am J Surg Pathol 2002;26:320.
16. Varan A. Prognostic significance of metastatic site at diagnosis in Wilms' tumor: results from a single center. J Pediatr Hematol Oncol 2005;27:188.
17. Li XP, et al. Treatment for liver metastases from breast cancer: Results and prognostic factors. World J Gastroenterol. 2005;11(24):3782.
18. Blohm ME, et al. Disseminated choriocarcinoma in infancy is curable by chemotherapy and delayed tumour resection. Eur J Cancer 2001;37(1):72.
19. La Quaglia MP, et al. Central hepatic resection for pediatric tumors. J Pediatr Surg. 2002;37(7):986.
20. Begemann M, et al. Brain metastases in hepatoblastoma. Pediatr Neurol. 2004;30:295.
21. Rodriguez-Galindo C, et al. Brain metastases in children with melanoma. Cancer. 1997;79:2440.
22. Kebudi R, et al. Brain metastasis in pediatric extracranial solid tumors: survey and literature review. J Neurooncol. 2005;71:43.
23. Young RH, et al. Metastatic ovarian tumors in children: a report of 14 cases and review of the literature. Int J Gynecol Pathol 1993;12:8.
24. Young RH, et al. Ovarian involvement by the intra-abdominal desmoplastic small round tumor with divergent differentiation: a report of three cases. Hum Pathol 1992;23:454.
25. Moshfeghi DM, et al. Retinoblastoma metastatic to the ovary in a patient with Waardenburg syndrome. Am J Ophthalmol. 2002;133:716.
26. Pais RC, et al. Ovarian tumors in relapsing acute lymphoblastic leukemia: a review of 23 cases. J Pediatr Surg 1991;26:70.
27. Couper G, et al. Burkitt's tumor of the testicle: an unsual presentation of a lymphamatous process in childhood. Br J Urol 1994;74:124.
28. Bracken RB, et al. Regional lymph nodes in infants with embryonal carcinoma of the testis. Urology 1978;11:376.
29. Dutt N, et al. Secondary neoplasms of the male genital tract with different patterns of involvement in adults and children. Histopathology. 2000;37:323.
30. Askin FB, et al. Occult testicular leukemia: testicular biopsy at three years continuous complete remission of childhood leukemia; a Southwest Oncology Group Study. Cancer 1981;47:470.
31. Chilcote RR, et al. Septicemia and meningitis in children with Hodgkin's disease. N Engl J Med 1976;295:798.
32. Cooney Dr, et al. Relative merits of partial splenectomy, splenic reimplantation, and immunization in preventing post-splenectomy infection. Surgery 1979;86:561.
33. Burrington JD, et al. Surgical repair of a ruptured spleen in children: report of eight cases. Arch Surg 1977;112:417.
34. Hays DM, et al. Postsplenectomy sepsis and other complications following staging laparotomy for Hodgkin's disease in childhood. J Pediatr Surg 1986;21:628.

CHAPTER 56

Amulya K Saxena

Laparoscopy in Pediatric Malignancies

INTRODUCTION

The introduction of minimal access surgery (MAS) as a diagnostic tool in children dates back to the efforts of Gans and Berchi in the 1970s.[1-3] However, it has gained popularity only during the past 10-15 years. This was mainly due to the improvement in video technologies as well as the development of smaller pediatric instruments (Fig. 56.1). The availability of optical devices as small as 2 mm in diameter as well as instruments as delicate as 1.7 to 2.7 mm permits application for neonates (Fig. 56.2). MAS has now been established not only as a method of diagnosis, but also accepted as the preferred method for various surgical pathologies in pediatric age group. Use of these minimally invasive techniques in the pediatric population has lagged behind, especially in pediatric cancer patients. The reasons are diverse and include concerns over loss of tactile ability, familiarity with advanced endoscopic techniques, and lack of equipment appropriate to the pediatric population. Studies suggest that minimal invasive surgery (MIS) results in an overall decrease in pain and need for postoperative narcotics, as well as decreased morbidity with shorter hospital stays and better cosmesis.[4] However, no prospective randomized studies have investigated the utility of MIS in pediatric cancer patients relative to standard open techniques.[5]

Advantages of MAS were realized by the adult surgeons long before it was accepted in the pediatric community. There were many reasons behind this delay in acceptance of MAS in the pediatric age group, the most important being:

a. The widely held belief that children do not experience pain,

b. The cost of laparoscopy was believed to be too high and was not considered feasible for the few patients managed at small MAS centers,

c. Unavailability of equipment for newborns and children,

d. The belief that MAS was too difficult to perform and too difficult to learn,

e. The time to operate the cases was too long during the learning curve,

f. The assumption that MAS was more applicable to the adult population due to frequent application in cases such as cholecystectomy, that is relatively uncommon in children,

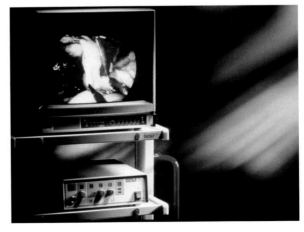

Figure 56.1: Advanced laparoscopy tower with improved video optics and picture quality (*Courtesy:* Richard Wolf GmbH, Germany)

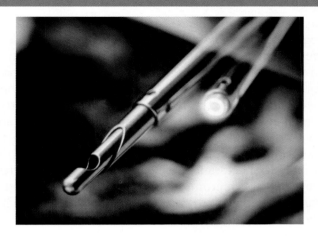

Figure 56.2: Smaller optic without further improved picture quality have reduced the size of the incisions in pediatric laparoscopic surgery (*Courtesy:* Richard Wolf GmbH, Germany)

g. The practice of small incisions already applicable in the pediatric population,
h. Inability to draw comparisons to children from the data acquired from the adults, and
i. Lack of established set of indication to employ MAS in the pediatric population.

PRINCIPLES OF PEDIATRIC MINIMAL ACCESS SURGERY

The principle techniques of pediatric MAS do not differ significantly in the child as compared to the adult. Size and weight are no longer considered contraindications to laparoscopic approach. However, attention must be paid carefully in the pediatric patient with malignancy to the:

a. Pre-existing coagulopathy,
b. Cardiorespiratory condition,
c. Previous extensive abdominal surgery,
d. Anterior abdominal wall infection, and
e. Size of intra-abdominal mass.

All pediatric MAS procedures are performed under general anesthesia. Decompression of the stomach and urinary bladder is generally performed following anesthesia induction. The administration of perioperative antibiotics is not routinely utilized; however, discretion of its administration must be based on the patient's condition and the judicious decision of the surgeon. Although the closed technique using the Veress needle has been employed in the pediatric patient, we strongly discourage it, to eliminate almost completely the risk of intra-abdominal organ injury.[6] The author prefers an open approach with placement of an appropriately sized Hasson trocar under direct visualization. An incision is made in the left or inferior umbilical fold and dissection carried down to the midline fascia. The linea alba and underlying peritoneum are incised longitudinally and a purse-string suture or fascial stay sutures placed to secure the Hasson trocar prior to insufflation.

The initial pressure limits chosen for the abdominal insufflation vary with the size of the child: newborns and small children, 6-8 mm Hg; children, 8-10 mm Hg; adolescents, 12-15 mm Hg. Insertion of work ports is carefully performed under direct visualization depending on the type of procedure. Manual elevation of the abdominal wall during trocar insertion is preferred as it facilitates placement and further minimizes the risk of injury to the intra-abdominal organs.

Removal of specimens in pediatric cases is occasionally complicated by the small size of the ports employed as well as the incisions (Fig. 56.3). However, although a 10-12 mm port can accommodate most specimens; this necessitates use of a smaller laparoscope at a secondary site while the tissue is withdrawn. With larger specimens, a laparoscopic-assisted removal may be employed, enlarging an existing port incision (generally the umbilical fold incision) for withdrawal of the specimen after appropriate positioning. In rare cases, a tissue moreselator may be necessary for piecemeal removal of a specimen.

Following completion of the MAS procedure, the umbilical site fascia and the fascia of all work port sites are closed with absorbable sutures. All incisions are

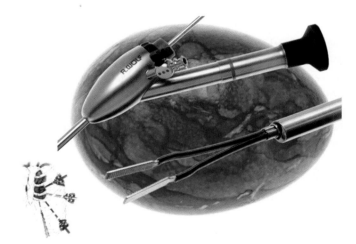

Figure 56.3: Smaller optics have a work channel to further reduce the requirement of accessory work ports. However, to retrieve large specimens the optic work port size may have to be increased during the retrieval phase. (*Courtesy:* Richard Wolf GmbH, Germany)

infiltrated with local anesthetics prior to subcuticular skin closure with absorbable suture. The use of nonabsorbable suture material for skin closure has been discontinued at most of the centers worldwide, and rescues the frightened child from tense moments of suture removal after undergoing MAS.

Postoperative nausea has been controlled with the use of metaclopramide as well as allowing sufficient time for recovery (8-12 hours) before resuming oral intake. A few doses of intravenous narcotic may be needed for postoperative pain management, but oral analgesics are usually adequate when liquids are resumed. Ambulation is encouraged as soon as the child has sufficiently recovered from anesthesia.

MINIMAL ACCESS SURGERY IN MALIGNANCIES

Abdominal tumors that are asymptomatic in the pediatric age group are initially detected by the primary physician. The accurate history and clinical examination along with immediate ultrasound examination gives the primary clues as to the type and localization of the tumor. Advanced and detailed ultrasound examinations, CT and MR provide more details regarding the consistency, vascular manifestation and to some extent initially to the presence of metastasis. Conclusive diagnosis, however, in many cases warrants a biopsy sample for detailed histopathological examination. In some cases, biopsy is performed to reveal clues regarding the prognosis and to determine the course of therapy. Minimal access surgery provides extensive abdominal visualization as well as the possibility to obtain biopsy samples under full vision. Staging can also be performed as part of the MAS while obtaining a biopsy. With increase in the fluency to perform MAS procedures in children, tumor resection, depending on the size and localization, can be performed. However, the trend toward laparoscopic surgery in malignancies has been slower—and more controversial.

MAS FOR TUMOR STAGING

Laparoscopy is an effective tool for the diagnosis and staging of intra-abdominal malignancies; it adds to the information provided by other noninvasive diagnostic modalities and may spare the patient the morbidity of a non-therapeutic laparotomy. The need for laparoscopic tumor staging stems from the fact that radiologic imaging alone is not reliable for the staging of upper abdominal malignancies.[6] Diagnostic laparoscopy provides further more information regarding the spread and resectability of the tumor and can accomplish all components of a staging laparotomy. In the evaluation of neoplasms of the peritoneum and for the evaluation of unclear ascitis, laparoscopy has been found to be even superior to computed tomography.[7] Minimal access staging plays an important role in pediatric patients with Hodgkin's disease to determine the course of therapy. This is helpful in avoiding unnecessary irradiation therapy in children that can result in significant growth deformities in prepubertal children. Radiation therapy furthermore combined with chemotherapy regimes in Hodgkin's disease have been reported to cause a 100 percent sterility in boys and 25 percent in girls.[8] The further advantage in minimal access staging is the avoidance of large-scale postoperative intra-abdominal adhesion that may further render a delayed open surgical resection even more difficult to perform. Unnecessary intra-abdominal related complications such as mechanical ileus due to severe adhesions can be drastically reduced.

Staging laparoscopies of the intestines and the lower pelvis as well as the direct visualization of the upper abdominal organs require no special scopes. However, assessment of difficult to reach places such as the diaphragm or the dome of the liver requires a 30° scope. Alternatively, in case of further access difficulty an additional work port may be placed to permit better visualization. Typically during the staging laparoscopy, fluid is also injected into the abdomen to obtain cytologic wash specimens, a valuable contribution to the staging picture that can help further refine care and identify suitable protocols for individual patients. It is also common during this procedure to place a feeding tube, which provides supportive nutrition to the patient during the course of treatment.

THORACOSCOPY

Primary pulmonary malignancies are rare in children and more often involve metastatic lesions from a distant primary tumor. However, the mediastinum is a common location for primary intrathoracic masses in the pediatric age group of which 40 percent are malignant.[9] Thoracoscopy was introduced in 1910 by Jacobeus with the primary intention of dissecting pleural adhesions in pulmonary tuberculosis,[10] however it was not until 1976 that Rodgers for the first time reported the use of thoracoscopy for diagnosis of thoracic lesions in children.[11] Thorascopy was initially proposed for use in children as a method of obtaining pulmonary biopsy specimens in immunocompromised patients.

In both (a) thoracoscopic evaluation as well as (b) biopsy of mediastinal and pulmonary lesions, preoperative localization and patient positioning are important issues. In cases of mediastinal pathology, imaging studies such as Computerized Tomography (CT) or Magnetic Resonance Imaging (MRI) are important to locate the pathology as well as to establish their relationship to other middle thoracic structures. Gravity should be used to allow the lung and adjacent structures to fall away from the operative site, since a double-lumen endotracheal tube cannot as easily be used in smaller children.[12] Unilateral ventilation, with contralateral mainstream intubation, is helpful for cases requiring extensive mediastinal dissection. Procedures for lung biopsy should be performed in a full lateral decubitus position, whereas anterior mediastinal lesions are best accessed by rolling the patient posteriorly. Children with mediastinal masses should be evaluated with pulmonary function tests and volumetric determination of airway by CT scan prior to performing surgery. The most important factor in estimating whether tracheal compression will occur after induction of anesthesia is the patient's preoperative respiratory status, particularly if he/she can lie flat without symptoms.

Insertion of the thoracoscope is best performed by direct blunt dissection through the chest wall into the thoracic cavity. The initial trocar is placed in the midaxillary line in the fifth or sixth intercostal space. The thoracoscope is passed initially to confirm the correct placement of the trocar. In thoracoscopy it is important to maintain low-pressure insufflation of carbon dioxide of approximately 5 to 8 mm Hg. Despite these lower pressures care should be taken not to create a potentially dangerous controlled tension pneumothorax. Additional work trocars should also be always placed under complete vision. On completion of the procedure, the lung is simply inflated by the anesthetist to evacuate the insufflated carbon dioxide from the thorax; during which the last work trocar should be removed simultaneously without allowing air entry from the outside. Complications after diagnostic thoracoscopy have been quite rare.

Consideration should also be given before biopsy to aspiration of any suspicious lesions to rule out vascular structures. The combination of thoracoscopy and needle localization allows the resection of small nonpalpable pulmonary lesions not visible through the thoracoscope,

thus avoiding the morbidity associated with open thoracotomy.[13] Although lung biopsy specimens may be obtained with the cup biopsy forceps; the use of Endoloop to ligate the lung parenchyma and excise the small lung tissue mass is preferred (Figs 56.4A and B). For the removal of larger specimens, endoscopic GIA stapler is employed through a 12 mm trocar to further facilitates hemostasis and pneumostasis at the biopsy site. Since the stapler requires 5-6 cm of working room in the thorax, it is unsuitable for children under the age of 2 years. The Nd:YAG laser can be used for dissecting or cutting and tends to seal the cut lung tissue by coagulative necrosis.

Mediastinal lesions are approached through the parietal pleura covering the lesion. Generally, lymphatic tumors (Hodgkin's and non-Hodgkin's lymphomas, malignant thymomas or lymphosarcoma) are usually located in the anterior or middle mediastinum, whereas neurogenic tumors (neuroblastoma or ganglioneuroma) arise in the posterior mediastinum. However, germ cell tumors conversely are located in the anterior mediastinum. In case of mediastinal masses, it is important to gain sufficient amount of tissue for histopathological examination. In few cases thoracotomy may be required, when a suspected lesion or lymph node seen on imaging studies is not identified with thoracoscopy. Despite such incidences, minimally invasive surgery is a safe and accurate means of obtaining thoracic tissue in pediatric oncologic patients.[14-16]

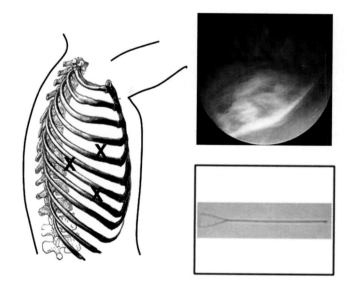

Figures 56.4A and B: Points of trocar insertion (right lateral thorax view). (A) Pulmonary metastases and (B) ENDOLOOP™ (Ethicon Inc.)

LAPAROSCOPY

Splenectomy

There are two main indications for splenectomy in malignancies by children: splenic lymphoma and angiosarcoma. Both of them are primary malignant tumors of the spleen. Lymphomas are the most common malignant tumors involving the spleen.[17] Splenic nodules in cases of Hodgkin's disease are too small to be detected on the present imaging examinations. Non-Hodgkin's lymphoma may be found more commonly as a metastatic disease in children. Angiosarcoma on the other hand are rare, but one-third of the patients present as an emergency case due to spontaneous rupture of the spleen.[18]

Patients are usually placed in a supine position or in a 45° right lateral decubitus position. Typically, 4-5 trocars of varying sizes (5-12 mm) are used. Pneumoperitoneum is created and the intra-abdominal cavity explored. The presence or absence of accessory spleen should be verified. A retractor is inserted to lift the inferior aspect spleen superiorly. It is then important to identify the tail of the pancreas. The spleno-renal and colo-splenic ligaments are divided with sharp dissection (Fig. 56.5A). The dissection is continued superior and lateral to mobilize the entire spleen. It is essential to continue the dissection posterior and inferior to the spleen as far as possible. Its purpose is to sufficiently expose the posterior aspect of the splenic hilum. The short gastric vessels as well as the splenic vessels are then best divided using the ENDOGIA™ Instrument (Fig. 56.5 B). The spleen is placed in the specimen retrieval bag (Figs 56.5C and D). The specimen retrieval bag is closed and brought against the anterior abdominal wall. The spleen is then sectioned in smaller pieces in the specimen retrieval bag and removed with a large clamp. Laparoscopic approach offers a much-improved view without an extensive incision. Most of the dissection has been facilitated by development of better energy modalities and improved stapling devices. The long-term results of pediatric laparoscopic splenectomy have been evaluated and have shown no morbidity in our series.[19]

Liver biopsy

Laparoscopic liver biopsy has many advantages in that through a small incision the color, size, structure and consistency of the entire liver can be evaluated. Optical evaluation further aids in the differentiation of local and diffuse hepatic lesions. In case of focal lesions the biopsy

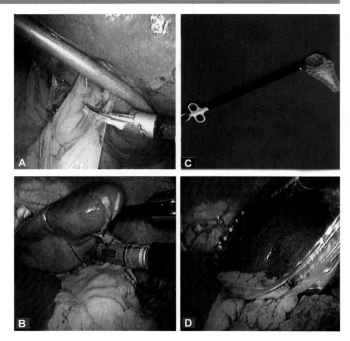

Figures 56.5A to D: Laparoscopic view of the spleen with (A) careful dissection of the attachments using harmonic scalpel, (B) dissection of the splenic vessels using ENDOGIA™, (C) ENDOCATCH BAG™ (Autosuture Inc.), and (D) spleen retrieval using the specimen retrieval bag

can be directed straight to the desired area.[20] Direct visualization prevents injury of blood vessels, neighboring structures as well as the identification of bleeding bile leaks after the biopsy.[21] Liver biopsy is best done through a 3-port technique. After identification of all the structures, biopsy specimens can be taken from the surface lesions using a cup biopsy forceps (Fig. 56.6). After the biopsy is taken, hemostasis is established. Various methods can be employed for hemostasis such electrocautery, laser and even microfibrillar fibrin glue (Fig. 56.7). Wedge resections can also be performed using an endostapler or laparoscopic suturing technique and the wedge specimen can be excised using laser or ultrasonic scalpel.[22,23]

Adnexal Tumors

Determining the frequency of adnexal masses is impossible because most develop and resolve without clinical detection. In girls younger than 9 years, 80 percent of ovarian masses are malignant and generally are germ cell tumors. During adolescence, 50 percent of adnexal neoplasms are adult cystic teratomas. Women with gonads that contain a Y chromosome have a 25

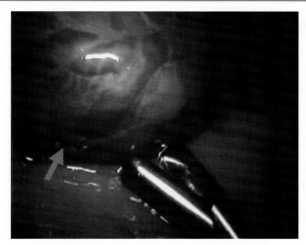

Figure 56.6: Identifications of the vessels (red arrows) allows selection of the biopsy site to reduce injury to the tumor vessels

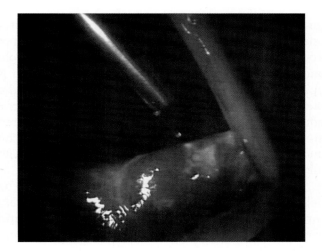

Figure 56.7: Laparoscopic view of application of laser on the hepatic biopsy site for wedge resection

percent chance of developing a malignant neoplasm. Endometriosis is uncommon in adolescent women but may be present in as many as 50 percent of those who present with a painful mass. In sexually active adolescents, one must always consider a tubo-ovarian abscess as the cause of an adnexal mass. Most adnexal masses present as asymptomatic, small, and simple cystic masses, nearly all of which resolve spontaneously. Therefore, care should be taken not to over-react to such a finding because surgeons who rush these women into surgery often create more pathology than they cure. Any surgery performed on adnexal structures can result in impaired fertility. All adnexal masses that are symptomatic or have characteristics of a malignancy must be addressed with surgical removal.[24] Rarely will a functional cyst have either of these features; therefore, few unnecessary surgeries result from this approach. The nature of this approach must be discussed prior to the surgery.

Obvious benign masses can be treated with resection of the mass alone or removal of the adnexal structure. In those cases in which the presence of malignancy is questionable, one should limit the resection to the structures involved unless a preoperative decision has been made that a more aggressive approach should be taken. When an obvious malignancy is encountered, a complete staging protocol must be performed. This generally includes complete exploration of the abdomen and a bilateral salpingo-oophorectomy[25] (Fig. 56.8).

Persistent simple ovarian cysts larger than 5 cm and complex ovarian cysts should be removed surgically. Reserve a laparoscopic approach for patients who have undergone a thorough workup and are thought to not have malignant disease. Such patients include those

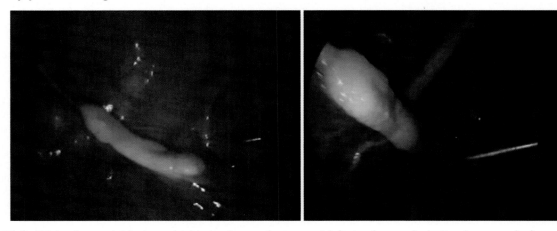

Figure 56.8: Bilateral gonadoblastoma (right streak gonad—top and left streak gonad—bottom) removed after cauterization of the gonadal vessels and using ENDOLOOP™ to perform a bilateral salpingo-oophorectomy

considered to have a dermoid or endometrioma, those with functional or simple cysts that are causing symptoms and have not resolved with conservative management, and those presenting with acute symptoms. In all cases, one should be able to remove the cyst intact. While performing a laparoscopy the goals are as follows:

a. To confirm the diagnosis of an ovarian cyst,
b. To assess whether the cyst appears to be malignant,
c. To obtain fluid from peritoneal washings for cytologic assessment,
d. To remove the entire cyst intact for pathologic analysis, including frozen section, which may mean removing the entire ovary, and
e. To assess the other ovary and other abdominal organs.

Excision of the cyst alone, with conservation of the ovary, may be performed in patients who desire retention of their ovaries for future fertility or other reasons. Included are endometrioma, dermoid, and functional cysts.

Pancreas

Laparoscopic distal pancreatectomy is best suited for endocrine and cystic tumors of the body and tail pancreas. Experience in this procedure has mostly reported in the adult population. However, reports are now emerging on this procedure in the pediatric populations that show successful preservation of the splenic vessels and the spleen in laparoscopic distal pancreatectomy.[26,27]

Laparoscopic central pancreatectomy is a complex operation performed on the pancreas for patients with a pancreatic tumor in the neck of the pancreas. The procedure provides localized removal of the tumor with preservation of the body and tail of the pancreas that would otherwise be removed as part of the distal pancreatectomy that is usually performed for these tumors.[28,29]

Laparoscopic enucleation can be performed for functional pancreatic islet tumors such as insulinoma and gastrinoma. These tumors are often on the surface of the pancreas and have a lining around them that separates them from the pancreas. In this operation the tumor is shelled out from the pancreas without removing any pancreatic tissue.[30]

Miscellaneous tumors

Laparoscopic ligation of the median sacral artery before posterior sagittal resection of type I sacrococcygeal

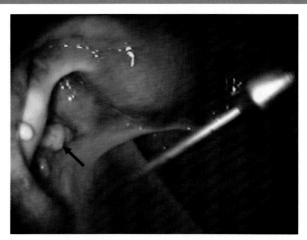

Figure 56.9: Laparoscopic resection of non-Hodgkin's lymphoma manifestation in the lower pelvis, visulalized between the left ovary and uterus

teratoma (SCT) has also been reported.[31] After establishing pneumoperitoneum via an epigastric 5 mm trocar, two additional trocars are inserted in the right and left lower quadrants. The peritoneal reflection is opened to the right of the sigmoid colon, and the presacral space is explored. The large median sacral artery is identified isolated, and divided. The children are placed in a prone position, and the tumors can undergo *en bloc* resection via a Chevron incision with minimal blood loss.

Laparoscopic diagnosis and management can be utilized for the detection of intestinal tumors that are rare in children. However, gastrointestinal and extraparenchymatous manifestations in the abdomen, such as B-non-Hodgkin lymphoma are excellent indications for the laparoscopic approach to obtain biopsies as well as to proceed with resection (Fig. 56.9).[32]

REFERENCES

1. Gans S, et al. Advances in endoscopy of infants and children. J Pediatr Surg 1971;6:199.
2. Gans S, et al. Peritoneoscopy in infants and children. J Pediatr Surg 1973;8:399.
3. Gans S. A new look at pediatric endoscopy. Postgrad Med J 1977;62-91.
4. Chen MK, et al. Complications of minimal-access surgery in children. J Pediatr Surg 1996;31:1161.
5. Ehrlich PF, et al. Lessons learned from a failed multi-institutional randomized controlled study. J Pediatr Surg 2002;37:431.
6. Lavonius MI, et al. Staging of Gastric Cancer: A Study With Spiral Computed Tomography, Ultrasonography, Laparoscopy, and Laparoscopic Ultrasonography. Surgical Laparoscopy, Endoscopy and Percutaneous Techniques 2002;12(2):77.
7. Barth RA, et al. A comparison study of computed tomography and laparoscopy in the staging of abdominal neoplasms. Dig Dis Sci 1981;26:253.

8. Tan HL, et al. Laparoscopic ovariopexy for pediatric pelvic malignancies. Pediatr Surg Int 1993;8:379.

9. Crist WM, et al. Common solid tumors of childhood. N Engl J Med 1991;324:461.

10. Jacobaeus HC. Ueber die moglichkeit die zystoskopie bei untersuchung seroser hohlungnen anzuwenden. Munch Med Wochenschr 1910;40:2090.

11. Rodgers BM, et al. Thoracoscopy for diagnosis of intrathoracic lesions in children. J Pediatr Surg 1976;11:703.

12. Rogers DA, et al. Thoracoscopy in Children: An Initial Experience with an Evolving Technique. J Laparendoscopic Surg 1992;2(1):7-14.

13. Hardaway BW, et al. Needle localization of small pediatric tumors for surgical biopsy. Pediatr Radiol 2000;30:318-22.

14. Waldhausen JHT et al. Minimally invasive surgery and clinical decision-making for pediatric malignancy. Surg Endosc 2000;14(3):250-253.

15. Saenz NC, et al. The Application of Minimal Access Procedures in Infants, Children and Young Infants with Pediatric Malignancies. J Lap and Adv Surg Tech 1997;7(5):289-294.

16. Milanez de Campos JR, et al. Thoracoscopy in Children and Adolescents. Chest 1997;111:494-7.

17. Mauch P, et al. Prognostic factors for positive surgical staging in patients with Hodgkin's disease. J Clin Oncol 1989;8:257.

18. Bakely SS. Disorders of the spleen. In Handin RI, Lux SE, Tossel TP (Eds): Blood: principlea and practice of hematology, Philadelphia, 1995;JB Lippincott.

19. Saxena AK, et al. Long-term evaluation of children after laparoscopic splenectomy. IPEG Annual Meeting. Genoa, Italy. 2002; May 3.

20. Saxena AK, et al. Laparoscopic Pediatric and Neonatal Hepatic Surgery. 3rd International Pediatric Laparoscopic Surgery Workshop, Mumbai: India 2004;November 27-28.

21. Saxena AK, et al. Technical Advances in Pediatric Laparoscopic Hepatic Surgery. Biotechnology Frontiers in Pediatric Surgery Symposium, All India Institute of Medical Sciences, New Delhi: India, 2004;December 13-15.

22. Saxena AK, et al. Mechanism and advantages of fibrin glue spray in laparoscopic hepatic biopsy of oncological patients. 14th Annual Congress for Endosurgery in Children (IPEG); Venice, Italy, 2005; June 1-4.

23. Seki S, et al. Laparoscopic wedge biopsy of the liver with use of an ultrasonically activated scalpel. Digestive Endoscopy 2001;13(1):17-20.

24. van Tuil C, Saxena AK. Laparoscopic management of ovarial cysts: pitfalls teratomas. 14th Annual Congress for Endosurgery in Children (IPEG); Venice, Italy, 2005; June 1-4.

25. van Tuil C, Saxena AK. Laparoscopic resection of bilateral gonadoblastoma in a 6-year old with Frasier syndrome. 13th Annual Congress for Endosurgery in Children (IPEG); Maui, Hawaii, USA, 2004; May 5-8.

26. Sayad P, et al. Laparoscopic distal pancreatectomy for blunt injury to the pancreas. A case report. Surg Endosc 2001; 15(7):759.

27. Carricaburu E, et al. Laparoscopic distal pancreatectomy for Frantz's tumor in a child. Surg Endosc 2003;17(12):2028-31.

28. Warshaw AL, et al. Laparoscopy in the staging and planning of therapy for pancreatic cancer. Am J Surg 1986;151(1):76-80.

29. Ayav A, et al. Laparoscopic approach for solitary insulinoma: a multicentre study. Langenbecks Arch Surg 2005;390(2):134-40.

30. Bax NM, et al. Laparoscopic identification and removal of focal lesions in persistent hyperinsulinemic hypoglycemia of infancy. Surg Endosc 2003;17(5):833.

31. Lukish JR, et al. Laparoscopic ligation of the median sacral artery before resection of a sacrococcygeal teratoma.J Pediatr Surg 2004;39(8):1288-90.

32. Saxena AK, et al. Laparoscopic resection: B-non Hodgkin Lymphoma pelvic infiltrate. 13th Annual Congress for Endosurgery in Children (IPEG); Maui, Hawaii, USA, 2004 May 5-8.

CHAPTER 57

Madhu Bhardwaj
Savita Sapra
Deepika Gupta

Psychosocial Aspects of Pediatric Oncology: An Integrated Approach to Management

Psychology has an important role to play in pediatric cancer. The issue is a sensitive one specially for the parents who have to first cope with the fact that the disease has occurred to their child, come out of their fears and then be strong to face the situation and help their child cope up with the disease and its treatment. Any illness in a child needs special patience and care and especially when it is malignancy, much more attention is required as the parents have to hide their fears of fighting the disease in front of the child. The psychological aspects of pediatric oncology need much more attention than what is currently being given due to the increasing media awareness on the subject and the fact that the parents are aware of the worst outcome possible in the course of the disease and tend to become pessimistic at some stage during the treatment. The whole process from suspicion to diagnosis, treatment and cure is a tragic burden for the hopeful parents who want the best for their child even in the presence of unfavorable circumstances.

The tragic illness occurs during the early stages of the child's growth when at times the child has not even learnt the alphabets. The field has grown rapidly in the past decade of its existence. With the advanced methods of treatment and researches, survival rates have increased in recent times.[1] Emphasis within the field have varied with the times, reflecting advances in medical technology as well as changes in attitudes toward cancer. However, success of treatment is not only measured by how often the disease is eradicated but also by how little it affects the child's opportunity for continued growth and development. Clearly, the work of

psychosocial oncologists has led to important advances in cancer prevention, detection, treatment, and recovery.

Research relating to the effects of cancer and cancer treatment and how they affect the child's ability to carry on a normal life has become increasingly more important. Studies examining child survivors of cancer have described heightened psychological distress.[2-4] More specifically, educational implications of the child's illness have become vital to those who are supporting the children in the transition process from the medical center to the social and family set up and during their growing years.

Children who have to undergo invasive medical or surgical procedures perceive these as a threat or a crisis situation this is further accentuated by the stress of hospital admission and separation from the family. Various studies have been done on different conditions requiring invasive procedures. The diversity of problems exhibited by these children undergoing different procedures requires considerable knowledge of how the child's development can be affected by early childhood experience of various conditions as they not only suffer the pain and trauma of the procedures but also the psychological stress due to various related factors. If such a suspected negative influence can indeed be confirmed, it is necessary to ask whether there is a stable link between the child's disrupted development and his or her expression of psychological adjustment problems later on if not taken preventive measures as later their psychological make up can be affected. Koocher and O'Malley[5] suggested that many survivors of childhood cancer were at increased risk for maladaptive psychosocial sequelae. Other investigations have demonstrated behavioral adjustment problems and preoccupation with somatic concerns,[6,7] lowered self-esteem and, body image,[8,9] and other psychosocial adjustment problems.[10,11]

Children with cancer may experience medical and physical effects, psychological effects, and cognitive and neuropsychological effects, all of which may impact a child's personality and his family. Without intervention, these issues may have negative, long-lasting effects. Investigators have also reported the presence of stress or trauma-related symptoms, such as avoidant behaviors, intrusive thoughts, and heightened arousability in survivors of cancer.[12,13] Estimates from epidemiological studies suggest that on average, approximately 25-33 percent of individuals who are exposed to traumatic events, including cancer, develop PTSD (Stuber M, Nader K, Pynoos R, Cohen S, 1991).[14]

The role of the psychologist is important before, during and as well as after the treatment. The long-term follow up is generally advisable for most of the conditions, as its essential to know the outcome of intervention and more than that if there are any complications or deterioration in the condition after the intervention. In this whole process its not only the child who is being traumatized but parents equally suffer due to various anxieties they have related to the future of the child. It is the lack of knowledge about the condition the child is in, as well as the hows and whys that adds to the parents' misery. It becomes essential to involve psychosocial team in the treatment plan. The approach and content may differ from condition to condition. Thus, it is crucial that comprehensive plans not only focus on child but also involves the family, peers, the teacher, and the other significant people around the child.

Psychosocial aspects of childhood cancer management are important and need to be dealt with by personnel appropriately experienced in psychology, pediatrics, and oncology. Psychosocial support also needs to be accessible to survivors long after the successful completion of their cancer treatment.

Some of the common psychological problems associated with cancer survivor children, which most of the pediatric surgeons would come across in their career are discussed here. This chapter focuses on the common psychological problems associated with cancer survivor children, understanding of symptoms, indications of assessments, and integrated management plan.

INDICATIONS FOR ASSESSMENT

Children affected with malignancy are referred to the psychologist for problems related to adjustment to the diagnosis, side effects of aggressive treatment, their personality development and social difficulties faced by the parents and the family. Psychosocial oncology aims to understand the psychosocial and behavioral factors in cancer etiology, prevention, detection, and treatment, and in long-term physical and emotional recovery from cancer.

Indications of referrals could be:
- Stress in the family upon disclosure of diagnosis
- Behavioral problems in the child due to various reasons
- Progress evaluation of the intervention
- Pain management
- Educational problems
- Personality development
- Mental health issues
- Follow up.

STRESS IN THE FAMILY

Family members of a child with cancer may suffer various forms of distress in regards to the child's illness. The disclosure of diagnosis is devastating for the family and then to watch the side effects of the aggressive treatment on the child. Social stigma becomes the next stress for them. There is significant impact of the disease on the siblings and extended family too. Initial diagnosis is the period of maximum stress. Other problems are:
- Fear of the unknown and uncertainty of the outcome of the illness.
- Frightened by the life threatening prolonged illness.
- Feelings of guilt related to any past errors of omission and commission.
- Lack of information about the condition

Parents may experience wide range of feelings, including anger, sadness, guilt and fear about their child's illness. In the initial stages the most important and useful tool to overcome the anxiety is family counseling. Parents may initially feel reluctant or unwilling to accept the diagnosis. It takes time to adjust to the reality. Overtime, parents come to grips with ways to deal with the situation. Primary goal at this stage is to encourage parents to set realistic expectations from the treatment and their child. Encouraging them to ask questions whenever worries arise can help calm some fears. Parents think that they have major responsibility for protecting their child from danger and harm. Initially, they question what behavior or action of their own may have contributed to their child's life-threatening disease. Sadness and feelings of depression are normal and understandable reactions to a child's cancer diagnosis. Every parent hopes and dreams that life for their child will be healthy, happy and carefree. Cancer and its treatment shatters that dream. Parents must grieve the loss of their hopes. Helping them understand that being overprotective and over sympathetic may create behavioral difficulties.

Parents report feelings of uncertainty, loneliness, low self-esteem, symptoms of PTSD, and distress related to the adjustment of the child's siblings (Kazak et al, 1994; Van Dongen-Melman et al, 1995).[15,16] Child's siblings may experience withdrawal, sleep disturbances, enuresis, excessive crying, etc. due to preferential treatment given to the affected child. At this stage it is important to include them in the discussions and give them correct age appropriate understanding of the disease.

BEHAVIORAL PROBLEMS

The side effects of the treatment are considered at times worse than the disease itself, i.e. growth impairment, neuropsychological squelae. The chronic strains of childhood cancer, such as treatment-related pain; nausea and vomiting; visible side effects such as hair loss, weight gain or loss, and physical disfigurement; and repeated absences from school and peers, interact to negatively impact social and psychological adjustment. The unknown and unfriendly strange hospital environment and fear of pain procedures add to the existing anxiety and other behavioral problems in child. The cancer may also disrupt the normal progression in motor or cognitive areas leading to developmental delay. The young child may treat this experience as a punishment and the fact that parents are witnessing this makes the child confused and frightened. This may further result in developmental regression, which may present in any of the following forms:

- Loss of acquired skills like toilet training, language development, motor growth
- Reappearance of previously discarded habits or development of new ones like thumb sucking, nail biting, eating disorders, clinging behavior, crying spells, etc.
- Later child may have problems in academic achievement, impaired or decreased social relationships, negative self-concept, low self-esteem and chronic pain
- Depression anxiety, post-traumatic symptoms, adjustment disorder, enuresis separation anxiety disorder etc.

EDUCATIONAL PROBLEMS

Factors that may place children and teens at increased risk for difficulties in school
- Diagnosis of cancer at a very young age
- Numerous or prolonged school absences
- Associated learning problems
- Reduced energy levels
- Physical disabilities, e.g. hearing, vision
- Neurological problems.

Common learning problems include:
- Handwriting, Concentration, Attention span, Memory, Spelling, Reading, Vocabulary, Math, Processing, Organization, Problem-solving,

PSYCHOLOGICAL ASSESSMENT

In recent years, there appears to have been a distinction made between testing and assessment, assessment being the broader concept. Psychologists do not just give the test; now they perform assessment. Assessment refers to the procedures and process employed in collecting information about human behavior. In a broader term, it refers to the entire process involved in collecting information through testing, interviewing, observation of behavior in natural or structured settings, and recording of various physiological functions. They are used to make important predictions and inferences. The assessment also provides basis for making decisions concerning the best treatment program, be it hospitalization, the use of medication or psychotherapy, indications for surgery or family counseling. The initial assessment also provides a baseline for comparison, later with other measures obtained following treatment. This is important but forgotten aspect of case management. It makes it possible to check on the effectiveness of an ongoing treatment program, to compare the relative effectiveness of different therapeutic or surgical preventive approaches. This is important not only in treating the individual, but also in conducting the research that can advance our understanding of the disorders themselves, as well as the development of new and more effective assessment and treatment techniques.

This section is focused on evaluation of children. This includes clinical interviews with the parents, the child, and the family; information regarding the child's current school functioning; and a standardized assessment of the child's intellectual level through developmental and mental performance. In some cases neuropsychological assessment are useful. It is mostly advisable to meet with the parents to obtain a full description of current concerns and full description of medical status.

For a complete understanding of children who are just diagnosed with cancer or survivors of cancer, need a thorough and complete assessment. It may also include interviews with teachers, parents, peers and siblings to have a better understanding of the child's behavior and for long term management plan. There are many standardized tests available to assess various areas, however, the scope of present chapter is limited to a brief description of most commonly used tests listed below:

Commonly used tests for children and adolescents are:

DEVELOPMENTAL SCALES AND INTELLIGENCE TESTS

The maturation process in an infant is so rapid that it is not possible to assess child's intellectual potentials in the same way as it is done at late ages. During this early development it is often not easy to differentiate between what is intellectual and what may be neural sensory motor or other aspect of maturing process. For easy comparison of mental growth, developmental schedules are used to assess Motor, Adaptive, Language and Personal-social areas which are considered to be the product of the intellectual potentials of young babies. Some of the development scales and intelligence tests are described below. The score on these developmental scales is not a reliable way to predict a child's future Intelligence Quotient (IQ), however, they are valuable for detecting the delay in development and could be useful as a base line for comparisons in longitudinal studies.

GESELL DEVELOPMENTAL SCHEDULES

These are empirically-derived standardized measures of infant and early childhood development (ages 4 weeks through 6 years) in the areas of motor, adaptive, language, and personal-social functions. The schedules are not really tests, but observations of child's activities, plus information given by the mother or care taker. The child's behavior is compared to established norms. The Gesell[17] scales are most useful as part of an examination for suspected neurological or organic disorders. Murlidharan et al (1971)[18] compared the developmental pattern of Indian children from 30 months to 5 years of age with developmental pattern of the western children using Gesell developmental schedule. Items have been revised and norms have been provided for Indian children for different items.

Bayley Scales of Infant Development—Second Edition (BSID-II)[19]

Ages 1-42 months. The BSID-II can be used to identify children who are developmentally delayed; to chart a child's progress after initiation of an intervention program; as a tool for teaching parents about their infant's development; and as a research tool. It has Mental Scale, the Motor Scale, and the Behavior Rating Scale. Phatak, (1977)[20] revised and standardized this scale for Indian children.

Stanford Binet Test Fourth Edition (SB-IV) 1986

Individual Intelligence test for (2-23 years). In 1916, Lewis Termam, adapted the Binet-Simon scale for American use. This is the Stanford-Binet Intelligence Scale, revised in 1937, in 1960, and again in 1986 (Thorndike et al, 1986b).[21] The Stanford-Binet (4th edition) is appropriate to administer to individuals from age two to adult (32.5 years). Questions on each 15 subtest are divided into age levels, with each age level consisting of two items. Testing begins with the Vocabulary subtest. The new format help educators and psychologists to understand why particular student is having difficulty in school.

Wechsler Intelligence Scales

This is the most widely used test for intelligence. It allows to identify specific areas of deficit and scatter in intellectual abilities as there are multiple breakdowns of the performance and verbal subscales.

Wechsler Preschool and Primary Scale of Intelligence

(WPPSI-R) (3-7 years) (Psychological Corporation, 1989)[22]

Wechsler Intelligence scale for children-revised (WISC-III)

(6-16 years) (Psychological Corporation, 1991)[23]

Peabody Picture Vocabulary (PPVT-R-Dunn & Dunn, 1981)[25] (4 –adult)

Colored Progressive Matrices (1990 Edition),[26] Standard Progressive Matrices (1996 Edition), Advanced Progressive Matrices (1994 Edition): This was originally designed as a test of general intelligence, but is used more as an assessment of perceptual ability and, at the more advanced levels, of spatial logic. It is often included in neuropsychological batteries. The examinee is given a series of designs (matrices) and is asked to indicate from a group of alternatives what the next matrix should be in order to complete the overall set. The RMP is available in three forms, differing in level of difficulty.

Classification of Intelligence by IQ Range

Classification	IQ Range
Profound mental retardation (MR)	Below 29 or 25
Severe MR	20-25 to 35-40
Moderate MR	35-40 to 50-55
Mild MR	50-55 to about 70

According to the fourth edition of Diagnostic and Statistical Manual of Mental Disorders (DSM-IV)[27]

Vineland Adaptive Behavior Scales (Sparrow S, 1984)[28]

This test was developed to assess the developmental level. It can be used for normal or developmentally delayed person from birth to 19 years. The Vineland is available in three versions—two interview versions that entail a semi-structured interview with a parent or caregiver, and a third version, a questionnaire that can be independently completed by the classroom teacher. All three versions measure adaptive behavior in the domain of socialization, communication, daily living skills, and motor skills.

BEHAVIOR CHECKLISTS AND PERSONALITY TESTS

Behavior Assessment System for Children

(BASC-Cecil Reynolds and Randy Kamphaus 1992).[29] This system includes behavior raring scales for parents and teachers and a form for coding and recording direct observations of classroom behavior. It also provides a self-report questionnaire for the children themselves and a structured interview schedule through which parents can provide a developmental history.

Child Behavior Checklist

One of the most commonly used measurements of behavioral problems, can show higher average levels of behavioral and social competence problems in children with cancer and other serious illnesses (Perrin, Stein and Drotar, 1991).[30]

Pediatric Cancer Quality of Life Scale

(Varni, Burwinkle, Katz, Meeske, and Dickinson, 2002).[31]

Pediatric Inventory for Parents

(Tercyak and Kazak, 2001)[32] a measure of stress in parents of children with cancer, and the Psychosocial Assessment Tool (Kazak et al., 2003)[33] a measure to identify psychosocial risk in families of newly diagnosed patients.

Projective Tests

Projective and semi projective tests are commonly used with children to assess the needs, conflicts, and general personality. Commonly used tests are children's apperception test, sentence completion test, etc. The hypothesis is that the child's interpretation of vague and ambiguous stimuli reflects basic characteristics of the child's personality.

Human Figure Drawing (HFD)

(Koppitz E 1968)[34] Can be used as a test of mental maturity and a projective test for children's interpersonal attitudes and concerns.

Machover Draw-A-Person Test (Machover K, 1949)[35]

This test assesses both intelligence and personality characteristics. It is a cathartic type of projective technique that is exploratory as well as therapeutic in nature.

Children Apperception Test (CAT) (Bellak 1993)[36]

Which is an adaptation of the Thematic Apperception Test (TAT). This is designed for children in the age range of 3 to 10 years. There are pictures of animals more like in human situations, e.g. parent-child and sibling issues. The child is asked to describe what is happening and to tell a story about what happens. The Indian version is also available. CAT supplementary cards depict different situations like classroom, interaction in the playground, and reaction to illness.

Sentence Completion Test[37]

Depression scales for children: Anxiety scales for children: Multidimensional Anxiety Scale for Children (MASC).[38]

THERAPEUTIC INTERVENTIONS

Every child is different; therefore they react to their illness in different ways. A nervous child may become more fearful, while a happy child may turn quiet and withdrawn. Some children become aggressive while others cling to their mothers, becoming totally dependent. A child with cancer or any other life threatening prolonged illness should be treated as normally as possible. The child and the family should be reassured and explained through educational and supportive counseling.

The initial focus is usually on assessing the current psychosocial functioning of the family, i.e. family relationship, reaction to the diagnosis and other ongoing stresses. The strategies to cope with the stress have to be planned for each and every family differently according to its needs. In general the support measures for the family may include.

- Educating the child and the family through verbal and printed material to allay the anxiety. The discussion should be frank, open and repetitive. Both the parents should be present along with the child.
- Child and family should be reassured after an interval to evaluate how much knowledge they have gained and understood.
- Parents should be encouraged to communicate the seriousness of the condition to immediate family members, while maintaining the positive attitude about the cure of the disease.
- They should be encouraged to utilize the strength and skill developed and acquired through previous experiences.

The types of interventions used most commonly by health professionals working with cancer patients include education, behavioral training, group interventions, and individual psychotherapy. Approaches that use a combination of cognitive–behavioral approaches are among the most commonly studied (Kazak and Kunin-Batson, 2001)[38] and are regarded as well-established treatments (Powers, 1999).[39]

COUNSELING

Counseling has historically been associated with advice giving. However, its not so, but is actually facilitating the client's efforts to arrive at their own decisions. Counseling in medical set up is more focused on explaining the prevention and management of illness. Coping with the psychological stress and trauma due to the condition. Educating people about the pathology and sources they can get help from. In this situation client is not only the patient but their relatives too.

There are five major goals of counseling:
1. Facilitating behavior change
2. Enhancing coping skills
3. Promoting decision making
4. Improving relationships and
5. Facilitating client potential.

While planning the management of child with malignancy, primary client in counseling is the caretaker, usually parents as they undergo extensive anxiety and are stressed. This in turn reflects on the care of the child. Patient listening to their worries and problems not only create an empathetic relationship with the counselor but also provides them a confidence and an optimistic view for the future of child. It is always advisable to clearly but slowly explain to them about the condition, why it occurs, what are the possible treatment modalities and prognosis. This information should be provided in an understandable and simple language without using medical jargon. Probably keeping their educational background in mind would be useful. The areas to emphasis vary from condition to condition. One of the common goals to be achieved is to convince parents to bring the child for follow up check ups and to explain to them its importance. Individual counseling could be done for the child as he/she grows up. In that case, besides what the child's curiosities are, one may have to assess the areas where child is finding it difficult to cope with, e.g. adjustment inventories could be used to know the areas of maladjustment, i.e. school, home, social, etc.

In counseling cancer patients, multiple modalities of intervention are frequently used to facilitate their adjustment to their illness, and life. An integrated approach using some of the following modalities could be helpful in improving the quality of life of these children.

BEHAVIOR THERAPY

"What is learnt can be unlearnt" is the basis of behavior therapy. The historical roots of behavior therapy are based in the two fundamental learning theories of classical and operant conditioning This therapy has a great success with children. There is a focus on here and now, observable behavior and the avoidance of dynamic formulation. This form of therapy is objective, structured and can be practiced by nurses, parents, spouse, teachers as co-therapists and has been of great success with children.

Steps for Behavioral Training

- ***Behavior analysis:*** It is done to know about the problems and goals of therapy. Information is collected about the child's assets, as well as deficits of adaptive behavior and excess of maladaptive behavior.
- ***Selection of target behavior and reinforcers:*** It is recommended that more than one target behavior (behavior to be modified) be selected so as to allow the parents to be trained in varied techniques and be equipped to deal with a variety of target behaviors. A behavior analysis considers the functional relations between clinical problems and their environmental antecedents (precipitants) and consequences.
- ***Obtaining baseline information:*** Getting the baseline information for the target behavior or training parents to record the information is important for assessing the outcome of the training.

Various treatment methods are used to change the maladaptive behaviors. Some method help to increase the adaptive behavior while others decrease the maladaptive behavior. Commonly used techniques are operant conditioning, social skills training, aversion therapy, desensitization, relaxation training, etc.

COGNITIVE BEHAVIOR THERAPY

It is a short term structured therapy and is a recent development toward the integration of cognitive and behavioral approaches to therapy. It is oriented toward current problems and their resolution. Cognitive-behavioral techniques have proven especially helpful within the crisis-intervention setting. Some of these methods include helping the patient to understand symptoms, teaching effective coping strategies and stress management techniques (such as relaxation training), restructuring cognitions, and providing exposure to opportunities for systematic desensitization of symptoms.

Therapy is usually conducted on an individual basis. It has been mainly applied to depressive disorders. The goal of therapy is to help the patient identify and test negative cognition, to develop alternate schemas and to change the way a person thinks. Methods of assessment used are:
- Behavioral interview
- Self-monitoring
- Self-report
- Information from other family members
- Interviews and monitoring by key people
- Direct observation of behavior in clinical settings
- Physiological measures.

PLAY THERAPY

The essence of this technique is that the child is seen individually for a set period of time, in the same room at the same time each week, from one to five sessions a week, as far as possible the arrangement of furniture in the room is kept the same. The setting offers a reliable framework within which to observe and evaluate the child's actions and responses. Different toys are used depending on the age and problem of the child. The child's play can be observed in detailed sequence for his projected inner feelings. Emotions and conflicts are worked through during the play sessions.

EARLY STIMULATION PROGRAM

Usually children whose minds are slow to develop are slow in learning to use their bodies. They begin later than other children to lift their heads, roll, sit, use their hands, stand, walk, and to do things. The delay could be due to delayed mental development or medical problems. A family member or caretaker when teaching new skills can make a big difference in her whole development. It affects how fast or well child learns the new skill. The goals of early stimulation program are to help the child become as able, self-sufficient, happy, and independent as possible.

STEPS IN DESIGNING A PROGRAM OF EARLY STIMULATION

- Observe the child closely to evaluate what he can and cannot do in each developmental area.
- Notice what things he is just beginning to do or still has difficulty with.
- Decide what new skill to teach or action to encourage that will help the child build on the skills he already has.
- Divide each new skill into small steps; activities the child can learn in a day or two, then go on to next step.

It is important to keep in mind that while teaching the activities one has to be patient and observant. Be orderly and consistent. Respond in the similar way each time to the child's action and needs. Use variety by changing the activities in various ways. You also have to be expressive. Praise and encourage the child often. Be practical and not over enthusiastic.

SUPPORT GROUPS

Support groups also appear to be beneficial for people who experience post-traumatic symptoms. In the group setting, such patients can receive emotional support, encounter others with similar experiences and symptoms thereby validating their own, and learn a variety of coping and management strategies.

Social support can help families cope with the pressures of daily life. There are many ways people can get support. Friends and neighbors can be a great resource. Talking openly with people who are close can bring comfort, relief, and a fresh perspective. Turning to religion or prayer can also provide people with a feeling of hope and a sense that there is some meaning to be gained from difficult experiences. Church offers families a community that is caring and supportive.

MANAGEMENT PLAN

- A follow up psychological assessment after 1, 3, 6 months and every year following intervention. Earlier if need be
- On going parental counseling program before and after therapy
- Play therapy and behavior modification for children with behavior problems
- Rehabilitation program for children
- Individual counseling for children, as they grow older
- Counseling about the physical deformity and delayed development
- Parental training
- Early stimulation training
- Working with common complaints
- Information on signs of identification of any deterioration in condition
- Encouraging care taker to bring child for follow ups
- Referral to rehabilitation services
- Crisis intervention
- Did I cause it? Counseling for parents
- On going counseling for children.

PSYCHOLOGICAL SUPPORT TO THE CHILD

Social and physical stimulation can help the hospitalized child progress through developmental milestones at a normal rate. Older children are usually encouraged to maintain their normal schedule. They should be helped to contact their peers through phone call, letters or visits. Some of the supportive measures like reassuring the child that it is not a punishment, explaining the procedure of therapy. Helping them understand pre and posteffects of the treatment in simple and clear terms. Using rewards and star charts to make child more cooperative. Using distraction techniques, e.g. story telling, video games, during procedures and therapy. If child is concerned, maintaining privacy of child's treatment. Encouraging them to participate in support groups and letting them express their concerns.

Most of the children adjust reasonably well within family and society and adjust to their lifestyle in relation to malignancy when both child and the family get care and proper psychosocial support. Individualized and integrated management plan is the key to psychosocial help for these children.

REFERENCES

1. Bleyer WA. The impact of childhood cancer on the United States and the world. Cancer Journal for Clinicians 1990;40:355-67.
2. Greenberg DB, Goorin A, Gebhardt MC, et al. Quality of life in osteosarcoma survivors. Oncology (Huntington NY) 1994;8(11):19-25.
3. Kornblith AB, Anderson J, Cella DF, et al. Hodgkin disease survivors at increased risk for problems in psychosocial adaptation. Cancer 1992;70(8):2214-24.
4. Koocher G, O'Malley J. The Damocles Syndrome: psychosocial consequences of surviving childhood cancer. New York: McGraw-Hill, 1981.
5. Koocher O'Malley J. The Damocles Syndrome, New York, NY: McGraw Hill; 1981.
6. Mulhern R, Wasserman A, Friedman A, Fairclough D. Social competence and behavioral adjustment of children who are long-term survivors of cancer. Pediatrics1989;83:18-25.
7. Fritz GK, Williams JR. Issues of adolescent development for survivors of childhood cancer. J Am Acad Child Adolesc Psychiatry1988;27:712-15.
8. Neff E, Beardslee CI. Body knowledge and concerns of children with cancer as compared with the knowledge and concerns of other children. J Pediatr Nurs1990;5:179-89.
9. Pendley JS, Dahlquist LM, Dreyer Z. Body image and psychosocial adjustment in adolescent cancer survivors. J Pediatr Psychol1997;22:29-44.
10. Cella DF. Identifying survivors of pediatric Hodgkin's disease who need psychological interventions. J Psychosoc Oncol.1987;5:83-96.
11. Kornblith AB, Herr HW, Ofman US, et al. Quality of life of patients with prostate cancer and their spouses. Cancer 1994;73(11):2791-2802.
12. Ostroff J, Mashberg D, Lesko L. Stress responses among bone marrow transplantation survivors. Psychosomatic Medicine 1989;51:259.
13. Kornblith AB, Anderson J, Cella DF, et al. Hodgkin disease survivors at increased risk for problems in psychosocial adaptation. Cancer 1992;70(8): 2214-24.
14. Stuber M, Nader K, Yasuda P, Pynoos R, Cohen S. Stress responses after pediatric bone marrow transplantation: Preliminary results of a prospective longitudinal study. Journal of the American Academy of Child and Adolescent Psychiatry 1991;30,952-7.

15. Kazak AE. Implications of survival: Pediatric oncology patients and their families. In DJ Bearison, RK Mulhern (Eds): Pediatric psychooncology: Psychological perspectives on children with cancer. 1994;171-93.

16. VanDongen-Melman JE, Pruyn JF, De Groot A, Koot HM, Hahlen K, Verhulst FC. Late psychosocial consequences for parents of children who survived cancer. Journal of Pediatric Psychology 1995;20:567-86.

17. Gesell A, Amatruda CS. Developmental diagnosis (2nd edn). New York: Hoeber-Harper, 1947.

18. Murlidharan R. Motor development of Indian children. Ninth report. National Council of Educational Research and Training, Delhi, 1971.

19. Bayley N. Bayley scales of Infant Development Second Edition: Manual. San Antonio, TX: Psychological Corporation, 1993.

20. Phatak P, Mental and motor growth of Indian babies (1 to 30 months). Final report, Department of Child development, Faculty of Home Sciences, MS University of Baroda, Baroda: India, 1970.

21. Thorndike RL, Hagen EP, Sattler JM. The Stanford-Binet Intelligence Scale: Forth Edition, Technical manual. Chicago: Riverside, 1986b.

22. Wechsler D. WPPSI-R: manual. San Antonio, TX: Psychological Corporation, 1889.

23. Wechsler D. WISC-III. manual. San Antonio, TX: Psychological Corporation, 1991.

24. Wechsler D. WAIS-R: manual: Wechsler Adult Intelligence Scale-Revised. San Antonio, TX: Psychological Corporation, 1981.

25. Dunn L (Loyd) M, Dunn L (Eota) M. Peabody picture vocabulary test-revised: manual for forms L and M. Circle Pines, MN: American Guidance Service, 1981.

26. Raven J, Raven JC, Court JH. Manual for Raven's Progressive Matrices and vocabulary scale- section 1: General Overview (1995 edition). Oxford, England: Oxford Psychologists Press, 1995.

27. American Psychiatric Association: Diagnostic and Statistical Manual of Mental disorders, (4th edn). American Psychiatric Association, Washington, 1994.

28. Sparrow SS, Balla DA, Cicchetti DV. Vineland Adaptive Behavior Scales: Interview edition Survey and Manual. Circle Pines, MN: American Guidance Service, 1984b.

29. Reynolds CR, Kamphaus RW. Behavior Assessment System for children Manual. Circle Pines. MN: American Guidance Service, 1992.

30. Perrin EC, Stein REK, Drotar D. Cautions in using the Child Behavior Checklist: Observations based on research about children with a chronic illness. Journal of Pediatric Psychology 1991;16,411-22.

31. Varni JW, Burwinkle TM, Katz ER, Meeske K, Dickinson P. The PedsQL in pediatric cancer: Reliability and validity of the Pediatric Quality of Life Inventory Generic Core Scales, Multidimensional Fatigue Scale, and Cancer Module. Cancer 2002;94:2090-2106.

32. Derogatis LR, BSI Tercyak, Kazak 2001. Administration, Scoring, and Procedures Manual. Minneapolis, MN: National Computer Systems, Inc.; 1993.

33. Kazak AE, Cant MC, Jensen MM, McSherry M, Rourke MT, Hwang WT, et al. Identifying psychosocial risk indicative of subsequent resource use in families of newly diagnosed pediatric oncology patients. Journal of Clinical Oncology 2003;21,3220-5.

34. Koppitz EM. Psychological evaluation of children's human figure drawings: Boston: Allyn & Bacon, 1968.

35. Machover K. Personality projection in the drawing of the human figure. A method of personality investigation. Springfield, IL: Charles C Thomas, 1949.

36. Bellak AS. The thematic Aapperception test, the children's apperception test, and the senior apperception test in clinical use (5th edn).Boston: Allyn & Bacon, 1993.

37. Rotter JB, Rafferty JE. Manual for the Rotter Incomplete Sentences Blank College Form, New York, Psychological Corporation, 1950.

38. March JS, Parker JDA, Sullivan K, Stallings P, Conners CK. The multidimensional aneexity scale for children (MASC): factor structure, reliability, and validity. Journal of the American Academy of child and Adolscent Psychiatry April 1, 1997;36:554-65.

39. Kazak A, Kunin-Batson A. Psychological and integrative interventions in pediatric procedure pain. In CA Finley, P McGrath (Eds): Acute and procedure pain in infants and children. Seattle, WA: IASP Press, 2001; pp77–100.

40. Powers S. Empirically supported treatments in pediatric psychology: Procedure-related pain. Journal of Pediatric Psychology 1999;24,131-45.

CHAPTER 58

Bharat Agarwal

Role of Biological Therapy for Pediatric Tumors

New tumor-targeted biological approaches to the therapy of childhood solid tumors have the promise to improve the survival of children with advanced or refractory malignancy with less acute and long-term toxicity. The challenge that remains is still similar to that with chemotherapy: identifying metabolic and genetic pathways and targets that are sufficiently different or amplified in the malignant cells to allow interruption without disruption of normal cell processes, and to then synthesize molecules that will inhibit these targets without other non-specific toxicity. Great expectations were raised by the success in two forms of leukemia of agents that target a specific genetic translocation: the older results with induction of remission by all-trans retinoic acid, targeting the retinoic acid receptor, disrupted by the 15;17 translocation in acute promyelocytic leukemia, and the dramatic responses to imatinib, a small molecule targeting the bcr-abl translocation in CML. Thus far, the search for similar "druggable" genetic targets in pediatric cancers has not yet resulted in such dramatic results, though many genetic aberrations that might provide potential targets have been identified, such as the translocation with its cloned EWS-Fli1 protein in Ewing's sarcoma or MYCN gene amplification in neuroblastoma. The far-reaching technologies brought forward by the Human Genome Project of mRNA profiling by micro-arrays now allows description of the gene expression profile of each tumor in great detail, which can then be correlated to biological or clinical characteristics of the tumors to help select new targets.

Biologicals are defined here as agents that are either uniquely or partially tumor-specific, rather than indiscriminately cytotoxic. Such agents may be directed either at the tumor itself, such as a surface receptor, or a unique genetic or metabolic feature within the cell, or at the microenvironment of the tumor. It is now clear that what happens outside the tumor cell boundaries, in the tumor microenvironment, can have a significant impact on tumor progression. A variety of host-derived cells contribute to the tumor microenvironment including endothelial cells, pericytes and smooth muscle cells, fibroblasts and inflammatory cells like neutrophils, tumor associated macrophages, mast cells and T- and B-lymphocytes. Examples of how current pediatric solid tumor studies are exploiting these two approaches are discussed below. Only a few of these studies have yielded results to date, as most of these agents are still in Phase I or early Phase II trials.

EVALUATION BEFORE CLINICAL APPLICATION

The rarity of pediatric cancer as well as ethical considerations necessitate that the agents for testing be carefully and rigorously selected, after both *in vitro* and *in vivo* testing to determine activity as well as the optimal schedule. Current NCI guidelines suggest that a drug that is active against multiple cell lines is likely to be active in xenograft models, and if activity shown *in vivo*, to be clinically active. Agents that fail to demonstrate activity in pre-clinical setting are most likely to fail in the clinical setting. Thus, pre-clinical evaluation enables one to exclude agents and combinations of agents that do not demonstrate effectiveness from entering clinical trials. An analysis of the activity of compounds tested in pre-clinical *in vivo* and *in vitro* assays by the NCIs Developmental Therapeutics Program was reported by Johnson et al.[1] For 39 agents with both xenograft data and Phase II clinical trials results available, *in vivo* activity in a particular histology in a tumor model did not closely correlate with activity in the same human cancer histology, casting doubt on the correspondence of the pre-clinical models to clinical results. However, for compounds with *in vivo* activity in at least one-third of tested xenograft models, there was correlation with ultimate activity in at least some Phase II trials. Thus, an efficient means of predicting activity *in vivo* models remains desirable for compounds with anti-proliferative activity *in vitro*. Using the hollow fiber assay, there was a higher level of predictivity of *in vivo* xenograft activity. Furthermore, potency in a cell line screen had a high correlation with activity in the hollow fiber assay, both for activity and lack of activity.[1] Biologicals present an additional challenge, as they often do not lend themselves to *in vitro* testing, which is more economical, but must be tested directly in animal models.

TARGET: TUMOR

Early approaches to specific targeting of solid tumors utilized monoclonal antibodies. Thus far, in pediatrics, the GD2 disialoganglioside was noted to be a favorable target in neuroblastoma. It is highly expressed and not modulated from the cell surface of virtually all neuroblastoma cells, with only weak expression on a restricted range of normal human tissues (particularly peripheral nerves). This antigen has been exploited for imaging and therapy, both directly and as a vehicle for targeted radiotherapy delivery.[2] As a single agent for patients with relapsed disease, modest response rates of 10–15 percent have been reported.[3-5] More recent attempts to improve these results have included development of a chimeric form of the antibody Ch14.18, and a new humanized form, to reduce the formation of neutralizing antibody (human anti-mouse and human anti-chimeric antibody). Addition of GM-CSF to stimulate ADCC and IL-2 to activate natural killer cells has been tested for feasibility and shown pre-clinical promise.[6,7] Based on promising pre-clinical testing showing ablation of bone marrow and liver metastases in a neuroblastoma model,[8] a Phase I trial of the immunocytokine, Hu14.18-IL2 has recently been completed in the Children's Oncology Group (COG), and a Phase II study is beginning.

Neuroblastoma is a tumor derived from sympathetic nervous system, and therefore expresses high levels of the noradrenalin transporter (NAT), whereby it can internalize and then store catecholamines.[9] Metaiodobenzylguanidine (MIBG) is an analogue of norepinephrine which, when labeled with radioactive iodine, shows high sensitivity and specificity for imaging neuroblastoma, as well as neuroendocrine tumors. ^{131}I-MIBG has shown excellent activity as a targeted radiotherapeutic, with response rates of near 40 percent in relapsed patients[10,11] and promising activity in newly diagnosed patients either alone[12] or given with chemotherapy.[13] Unlike some of the other biologicals, a cytotoxic effect on proliferating hematopoietic precursors often results in significant myelosuppression, due to the non-specific radiation to the red marrow.[14,15]

Tumor differentiation is another approach suggested by the propensity of some tumors to undergo spontaneous differentiation and growth arrest. This characteristic was noted in neuroblastoma, and led to Phase I and II trials,[16] followed by a large randomized study in the Children's Cancer Group testing children in a state of minimal residual disease after induction and consolidation therapy. Treatment with 13-cis-retinoic acid in a more dose intensive schedule developed in pre-clinical testing,[17] resulted in effective plasma concentrations and significantly improved event-free survival in high-risk neuroblastoma.[18] Other retinoids, such as fenretinide, may work via other mechanisms, such as ceramide metabolism,[19] and therefore have a broader application in malignancy.[20] Fenretinide has shown promising activity in pre-clinical studies and is currently being evaluated in Phase I and II trials.[21]

Tyrosine kinase inhibitors are under extensive investigation for treatment of cancer, due to the promising results with imatinib targeting of bcr-abl for CML. Since imatinib also inhibits c-kit and PGDFR, it was postulated that it might have activity in other malignancies than just CML. For that reason, Phase I and II trials in pediatric brain tumors have been undertaken, after a few pre-clinical investigations showed potential activity in Ewing's, medulloblastoma, and neuroblastoma.[22-25] The Trk receptors A, B, and C are highly expressed in neural tumors, and a Phase I study of CEP-701, an oral pan-Trk inhibitor is underway in the New Approaches to Neuroblastoma Consortium (NANT), based on *in vivo* studies showing inhibition of tumor growth in xenograft models.[26] EGFR inhibitors, now approved for treating lung and colon cancer, are also under testing in pediatric cancers. The potential effect of blocking the EGFR pathways is still under pre-clinical investigation in pediatric tumors.[27, 28] A number of these that are currently approved for adult epithelial malignancies, including gefitinib, erlotinib, and cetuximab (a monoclonal antibody against the EGFR), are in Phase I testing in pediatric solid tumors in the COG and the Pediatric Brain Tumor Consortium (PBTC).[29] a novel chimeric protein linking the EGFR binding protein, TGF-α to a pseudomonas exotoxin is also in testing in pediatric brain tumors. Her-2/neu is another tyrosine kinase receptor widely under investigation for therapy of epithelial cancers, which may also have some applicability in pediatric osteosarcoma, where expression has been noted, though the significance remains controversial.[30-34] A phase II window trial in newly diagnosed metastatic osteosarcoma for patients whose tumors express Her-2/neu is currently in progress in the COG.

Manipulation of tumors through alteration of gene expression via farnesyl transferase inhibitors, demethylating agents, histone deacetylase inhibitors (HDACI) or downstream alterations in metabolism is another area of interest. The COG and PBTC has had Phase I and II trials of R115777, the farnesyl transferase inhibitor, for leukemia and CNS tumors. Open trials of HDACI in the COG include valproic acid and depsipeptide, while decitabine combined with chemotherapy is being tested in another Phase I study. Agents which alter glutathione content of tumors may enhance sensitivity to alkylating agents. Pre-clinical and clinical studies of such a compound, buthionine sulfoximine, have shown activity in adult cancers and more recently in neuroblastoma.[35,36] Alterations of ceramide metabolism, as discussed above, may also enhance apoptosis, and new drugs which further synergize with fenretinide in this regard are in pre-clinical development.[37]

TARGET: MICROENVIRONMENT

The microenvironment also provides an interesting biological approach to treating tumors, as angiogenesis, tissue factors involved in invasion and metastasis such as matrix metalloproteinases, integrins and cytokines, and host immunologic response have all been shown to play a role in tumor progression. Anti-angiogenic and anti-metastatic agents have been a major focus in recent trials, since it is widely accepted that tumor growth beyond a few cubic millimeters cannot occur without the induction of a new vascular supply. In theory, inhibiting new blood vessel formation should be relatively selective for tumor cells, since endothelium in normal tissue is usually quiescent. Vascular Endothelial Growth Factor (VEGF) is the best-characterized pro-angiogenic factor. In many pediatric tumors, higher levels have been correlated with more aggressive disease.[38,39] Effective blockade of the VEGF pathway has been demonstrated with multiple agents: neutralizing antibody, receptor tyrosine kinase inhibitors (see above), and ribozyme or anti-sense molecules targeting expression.[40-44] Recent studies of the neutralizing antibody bevacizumab, and small molecule tyrosine kinase inhibitor SU5416, demonstrate that, while unlikely to be effective as monotherapy, incorporation of VEGF blockade into cytotoxic regimens may increase overall response rates. However, incorporation may also produce new toxicities, including thromboembolic complications and bleeding, and there may be other effects in young children on growth and development. Current COG and PBTC trials are testing bevacizumab, lenalidomide (a potent immunomodulatory and anti-angiogenic analog of thalidomide), SU5416, as well as tyrosine kinase inhibitors, and the anti-integrin, cilengitide.

Finally, alteration of the host immune response provides another avenue for overcoming resistance, with monoclonal antibodies (see above), cytokines, and various types of vaccines. Interleukin 2 (IL-2) is the most extensively investigated cytokine in clinical use at present. Interleukin-2 enhances the proliferation, cytokine production and cytolytic activity of T and NK/LAK cell populations, various aspects of monocyte/macrophage function and global measures of immune responsiveness *in vivo*.[45] Although IL-2 has demonstrated pre-clinical anti-tumor activity, it has been disappointing in pediatric clinical trials when used by itself.[46] IL-2 may be more effective in combination with other immunotherapeutic agents, such as the anti-GD2 antibody or other cytokines.[6, 8] Recent preclinical evidence suggests that in combination, IL-12 with IL-2 may possess potent immunomodulatory and anti-tumor activity that exceeds the effect of either agent alone in several murine models.[47, 48] Phase I dose escalation trial of IL-12 combined with IL-2 is now underway in the NANT consortium, based on pre-clinical efficacy against murine neuroblastoma. Pre-clinical and clinical trials are also in progress to try to further enhance the specificity and efficacy of cytokines by using autologous tumor cells transfected with cytokines such as IL-2, IL-12, GM-CSF, interferon gamma, or lymphotactin as vaccines to stimulate the host immune response to solid tumors. Other vaccine approaches include the use of DNA vaccines, or dendritic cell vaccines.

CONCLUSION

Biological therapy of childhood cancer provides a new approach to overcoming resistance by using agents with a different mechanism of action than standard cytotoxic therapy. Better understanding of the genetic pathways and better pre-clinical models to define effective combinations and schedules for the prioritization of clinical testing will increase the likelihood of fulfilling the promise of targeted therapy.

REFERENCES

1. Johnson JI, Decker S, Zaharevitz D, et al. Relationships between drug activity in NCI preclinical *in vitro* and *in vivo* models and early clinical trials. Br J Cancer 2001;84(10):1424-31.
2. Cheung NK, Miraldi FD. Iodine 131 labeled GD2 monoclonal antibody in the diagnosis and therapy of human neuroblastoma. Progress in Clinical and Biological Research 1988;271:595-604.
3. Cheung NK, Kushner BH, Yeh SDJ, et al. 3F8 monoclonal antibody treatment of patients with stage 4 neuroblastoma: a phase II study. Int J Oncol 1998;12(6):1299-306.
4. Handgretinger R, Baader P, Dopfer R, et al. A phase I study of neuroblastoma with the anti-ganglioside GD2 antibody 14.G2a. Cancer Immunol Immunother 1992;35(3):199-204.
5. Yu AL, Uttenreuther-Fischer MM, Huang CS, et al. Phase I trial of a human-mouse chimeric anti-disialoganglioside monoclonal antibody ch14.18 in patients with refractory neuroblastoma and osteosarcoma. J Clin Oncol 1998;16(6):2169-80.
6. Frost JD, Hank JA, Reaman GH, et al. A phase I/IB trial of murine monoclonal anti-GD2 antibody 14.G2a plus interleukin-2 in children with refractory neuroblastoma: a report of the Children's Cancer Group. Cancer 1997;80(2):317-33.
7. Ozkaynak MF, Sondel PM, Krailo MD, et al. Phase I study of chimeric human/murine anti-ganglioside G(D2) monoclonal antibody (ch14.18) with granulocyte-macrophage colony-stimulating factor in children with neuroblastoma immediately after hematopoietic stem-cell transplantation: a Children's Cancer Group Study. J Clin Oncol 2000;18(24):4077-85.
8. Lode HN, Xiang R, Varki NM, et al. Targeted interleukin-2 therapy for spontaneous neuroblastoma metastases to bone marrow. Journal of the National Cancer Institute 1997;89(21):1586-94.
9. Tepmongkol S, Heyman S. 131I MIBG therapy in neuroblastoma: mechanisms, rationale, and current status. Medical and Pediatric Oncology 1999;32(6):427-31;discussion 432.
10. Klingebiel T, Berthold F, Treuner J, et al. Metaiodobenzylguanidine (mIBG) in treatment of 47 patients with neuroblastoma: results of the German Neuroblastoma Trial. Medical and Pediatric Oncology 1991;19(2):84-88.
11. Matthay KK, DeSantes K, Hasegawa B, et al. Phase I dose escalation of 131I-metaiodobenzylguanidine with autologous bone marrow support in refractory neuroblastoma. J Clin Oncol 1998;16:229-36.
12. van Hasselt EJ, Heij HA, de Kraker J, et al. Pretreatment with [131I] metaiodobenzylguanidine and surgical resection of advanced neuroblastoma. Eur J Pediatr Surg 1996;6(3):155-8.
13. Mastrangelo S, Tornesello A, Diociaiuti L, et al. Treatment of advanced neuroblastoma: feasibility and therapeutic potential of a novel approach combining 131-I-MIBG and multiple drug chemotherapy. Br J Cancer 2001;84(4):460-4.
14. Matthay KK, Panina C, Huberty J, et al. Correlation of tumor and whole-body dosimetry with tumor response and toxicity in refractory neuroblastoma treated with (131)I-MIBG. J Nucl Med 2001;42(11):1713-21.
15. Dubois SG, Messina J, Maris JM, et al. Hematologic toxicity of high-dose iodine-131-metaiodobenzylguanidine therapy for advanced neuroblastoma. J Clin Oncol 2004;22(12):2452-60.
16. Villablanca JG, Khan AA, Avramis VI, et al. Phase I trial of 13-cis-retinoic acid in children with neuroblastoma following bone marrow transplantation. J Clin Oncol 1995;13(4):894-901.
17. Reynolds CP, Kane DJ, Einhorn PA, et al. Response of neuroblastoma to retinoic acid *in vitro* and *in vivo*. Progress in Clinical and Biological Research 1991;366:203-11.
18. Matthay KK, Villablanca JG, Seeger RC, et al. Treatment of high-risk neuroblastoma with intensive chemotherapy, radiotherapy, autologous bone marrow transplantation, and 13-cis-retinoic acid. Children's Cancer Group. N Engl J Med 1999;341(16):1165-73.
19. Maurer BJ, Metelitsa LS, Seeger RC, et al. Increase of ceramide and induction of mixed apoptosis/necrosis by N-(4-hydroxyphenyl)-retinamide in neuroblastoma cell lines [see comments]. Journal of the National Cancer Institute 1999;91(13):1138-46.
20. Reynolds CP, Maurer BJ, Kolesnick RN. Ceramide synthesis and metabolism as a target for cancer therapy. Cancer Lett 2004;206(2):169-80.
21. Garaventa A, Luksch R, Piccolo MS, et al. Phase I trial and pharmacokinetics of fenretinide in children with neuroblastoma. Clin Cancer Res 2003;9(6):2032-9.
22. Hotfilder M, Lanvers C, Jurgens H, et al. c-KIT-expressing Ewing tumor cells are insensitive to imatinib mesylate (STI571). Cancer Chemother Pharmacol 2002;50(2):167-9.
23. Chilton-Macneill S, Ho M, Hawkins C, et al. C-kit expression and mutational analysis in medulloblastoma. Pediatr Dev Pathol 2004;7(5):493-8.
24. Ahmed A, Gilbert-Barness E, Lacson A. Expression of c-kit in Ewing family of tumors: a comparison of different immunohistochemical protocols. Pediatr Dev Pathol 2004;7(4):342-7.
25. Beppu K, Jaboine J, Merchant MS, et al. Effect of imatinib mesylate on neuroblastoma tumorigenesis and vascular endothelial growth factor expression. Journal of the National Cancer Institute 2004;96(1):46-55.
26. Evans AE, Kisselbach KD, Yamashiro DJ, et al. Antitumor activity of CEP-751 (KT-6587) on human neuroblastoma and medulloblastoma xenografts. Clin Cancer Res 1999;5(11):3594-3602.
27. Evangelopoulos ME, Weis J, Kruttgen A. Signalling pathways leading to neuroblastoma differentiation after serum withdrawal: HDL blocks neuroblastoma differentiation by inhibition of EGFR. Oncogene 2005;24(20):3309-18.
28. Rickert CH. Prognosis-related molecular markers in pediatric central nervous system tumors. J Neuropathol Exp Neurol 2004;63(12):1211-24.
29. Albanell J, Gascon P. Small molecules with EGFR-TK inhibitor activity. Curr Drug Targets 2005;6(3):259-74.
30. Anninga JK, van de Vijver MJ, Cleton-Jansen AM, et al. Overexpression of the HER-2 oncogene does not play a role in high-grade osteosarcomas. Eur J Cancer 2004;40(7):963-70.

31. Ferrari S, Bertoni F, Zanella L, et al. Evaluation of P-glycoprotein, HER-2/ErbB-2, p53, and Bcl-2 in primary tumor and metachronos lung metastases in patients with high-grade osteosarcoma. Cancer 2004;100(9):1936-42.

32. Gorlick R, Huvos AG, Heller G, et al. Expression of HER2/erbB-2 correlates with survival in osteosarcoma. J Clin Oncol 1999;17(9):2781-8.

33. Thomas DG, Giordano TJ, Sanders D, et al. Absence of HER2/neu gene expression in osteosarcoma and skeletal Ewing's sarcoma. Clin Cancer Res 2002;8(3):788-93.

34. Zhou H, Randall RL, Brothman AR, et al. HER-2/neu expression in osteosarcoma increases risk of lung metastasis and can be associated with gene amplification. J Pediatr Hematol Oncol 2003;25(1):27-32.

35. Anderson CP, Reynolds CP. Synergistic cytotoxicity of buthionine sulfoximine (BSO) and intensive melphalan (L-PAM) for neuroblastoma cell lines established at relapse after myeloablative therapy. Bone Marrow Transplant 2002;30(3):135-40.

36. Anderson CP, Seeger RC, Bailey H, et al. Pilot study of buthionine sulphoximine (BSO) combined with non-myeloablative melphalan (L-PAM) against refractory neuroblastoma (NB). Proc Amer Soc Clin Oncol 2002;21:298a.

37. Maurer BJ, Melton L, Billups C, et al. Synergistic cytotoxicity in solid tumor cell lines between N-(4-hydroxyphenyl) retinamide and modulators of ceramide metabolism. Journal of the National Cancer Institute 2000;92(23):1897-1909.

38. Meitar D, Crawford SE, Rademaker AW, et al. Tumor angiogenesis correlates with metastatic disease, N-myc amplification, and poor outcome in human neuroblastoma. J Clin Oncol 1996;14(2):405-14.

39. Erdreich-Epstein A, Shimada H, Groshen S, et al. Integrins alpha (v) beta 3 and alpha (v) beta 5 are expressed by endothelium of high-risk neuroblastoma and their inhibition is associated with increased endogenous ceramide. Cancer Res 2000;60(3):712-21.

40. Yokoi A, McCrudden KW, Huang J, et al. Blockade of her2/neu decreases VEGF expression but does not alter HIF-1 distribution in experimental Wilms tumor. Oncol Rep 2003;10(5):1271-4.

41. Backman U, Christofferson R. The selective class III/V receptor tyrosine kinase inhibitor SU11657 inhibits tumor growth and angiogenesis in experimental neuroblastomas grown in mice. Pediatr Res 2005;57(5 Pt 1):690-5.

42. Glade-Bender J, Kandel JJ, Yamashiro DJ. VEGF blocking therapy in the treatment of cancer. Expert Opin Biol Ther 2003;3(2):263-76.

43. Kaicker S, McCrudden KW, Beck L, et al. Thalidomide is anti-angiogenic in a xenograft model of neuroblastoma. Int J Oncol 2003;23(6):1651-5.

44. Kieran MW. Anti-angiogenic chemotherapy in central nervous system tumors. Cancer Treat Res 2004;117:337-49.

45. Higashi N, Nishimura Y, Higuchi M, et al. Human monocytes in a long-term culture with interleukin-2 show high tumoricidal activity against various tumor cells. J Immunother 1991; 10(4):247-55.

46. Valteau-Couanet D, Rubie H, Meresse V, et al. Phase I-II study of interleukin-2 after high-dose chemotherapy and autologous bone marrow transplantation in poorly responding neuroblastoma. Bone Marrow Transplant 1995;16(4):515-20.

47. Wigginton JM, Komschlies KL, Back TC, et al. Administration of interleukin 12 with pulse interleukin 2 and the rapid and complete eradication of murine renal carcinoma. Journal of the National Cancer Institute 1996;88(1):38-43.

48. Wigginton JM, Park JW, Gruys ME, et al. Complete regression of established spontaneous mammary carcinoma and the therapeutic prevention of genetically programmed neoplastic transition by IL-12/pulse IL-2: induction of local T-cell infiltration, Fas/Fas ligand gene expression, and mammary epithelial apoptosis. J Immunol 2001;166(2):1156-68.

CHAPTER 59

Chittaranjan Joshi
MK Arora

Relief of Pain in Pediatric Cancer Patients

INTRODUCTION

Cancer is the third leading cause of death in United States in children of 1-4 year old and the second most common cause of death between 5 and 19 year of age. One of the most challenging issues in pediatric pain management is the management of cancer pain, especially in the terminally ill patient. The management of pain in cancer patients requires the understanding of normal childhood development and the natural history and treatment of childhood malignancies. Pain in a cancer patient can result from tumor invasion, procedures, therapy, or other causes unrelated to cancer.

The most common tumors in children are leukemias, lymphomas, brain tumors, neuroblastomas, hepatoblastomas and Ewing's sarcoma. Pain can be visceral, resulting from stretching of abdominal structures by voluminous tumors, it may be present in bones as a consequence of bone marrow expansion, as in leukemia; or pain may be caused by nerve stretching or headache stemming from increased intracranial pressure.

CAUSES AND EFFECTS

Pain management is an important concern for a child with cancer. When a child has cancer one of the child's greatest fears is pain. Every effort should be made to ease the pain during the treatment process. Pain is a sensation of discomfort, distress or agony. Because pain is unique to each individual, a child's pain cannot be evaluated by anyone else. Pain may be acute or chronic. Acute pain is severe and lasts a relatively short time. It is usually a signal that body tissue is being injured in some way, and the pain generally disappears when the injury heals. Chronic pain may range from mild to severe, and is present to some degree for long periods of time. Many people believe that if an individual has been diagnosed with cancer, they must be in pain. This is not necessarily the case, and, when pain is present, it can be reduced or even prevented. Pain management is an important area to discuss with your child's physician as soon as a cancer diagnosis is made or suspected. Pain may occur as a result of the cancer or for other reasons. Children can normally have headaches, general discomfort, pains and muscle strains as part of being a child. Not every pain a child expresses is from the cancer, or is being caused by the cancer. Cancer pain may depend on the type of cancer, the stage (extent) of the disease and your child's pain threshold (or tolerance for pain). Cancer pain that lasts several days or longer may result from:

- Pain from a tumor that is enlarging, or pain from a tumor that is pressing body organs, nerves or bones.
- Poor blood circulation because the cancer has blocked blood vessels.
- Blockage of an organ or tube in the body.
- Metastasis—cancer cells that have spread to other sites in the body.
- Infection or inflammation.
- Side effects from chemotherapy, radiation therapy or surgery.
- Stiffness from inactivity.
- Psychological responses to illness such as tension, depression or anxiety.

ASSESSMENT OF PAIN IN CHILDREN WITH CANCER

According to the consensus report on cancer pain[1], children's pain "should be considered a necessary part of the management of cancer." Pain assessment involves a deliberate and systematic comprehensive approach. Assessment is *deliberate* when an assessment is intentionally focused on the child's pain. Unless pain is unpredictable and/or not well controlled, routine assessments could occur on the vital sign schedule for hospitalized children.

Deliberate and systematic assessments are comprehensive, integrating structured and unstructured information. Structured information results through the use of psychometrically sound tools, whereas unstructured information occurs through more casual and less focused observations. Integration of the structured and unstructured information forms the basis for clinical judgments about pain.

Pain History

Pain assessment begins with a pain history, an approach endorsed by authorities on children's pain.[2] The intent of the pain history is to profile a child's previous pain experiences, identify the child's understanding of pain, and identify preferences for treatment. By using a pain history, the health care professional gets to know the child better, thereby potentially improving the accuracy of assessment. Pain histories proposed by Milch et al[3] and Hester and Barcus[4] are similar, focusing on descriptions of previous pain experiences and how the pain was managed.

The Pain Experience History by Hester and Barcus[4], recommended in the acute pain management clinical practice guidelines, structures this pain history discussion. The Pain Experience History, best used at an initial clinic visit or at admission to the hospital, has two forms, one for the child and the other for the parent. The child form is for verbal children, generally at least 4 years of age. The health care provider asks the child the questions and records the child's responses. The parent form contains parallel questions. The parent can either fill out the form or respond to the questions orally (Table 59.1).

For children with repeated hospitalizations and health care provider visits, previous hospital and clinic records may augment information obtained through the pain history. Too often, however, little information on pain is documented. The chart provides data on the prescription and administration of analgesics and adjuvant drugs.

Self-report

Self-report provides a mechanism to facilitate communication from a verbal child about pain. Since 1974, a myriad of self-report approaches have emerged for use with children. The approaches include interviews,[4,5] diaries,[6] projective tests,[7,8] body maps[9,10] pain words,[10-13] color matching,[12,13] visual analogue scales,[12,13] and graphic rating scales. Graphic rating scales

Table 59.1: Pain experience theory	
Child form	*Parent form*
Tell me what pain is	What word(s) does your child use in regard to pain?
Tell me about the hurt you have had before	Describe the pain experiences your child has had before.
Do you tell others when you hurt? If yes, who?	Does your child tell you or others when he or she is hurting?
What do you do for yourself when you are hurting?	How do you know when your child is in pain?
What do you want others to do for you when you hurt?	How does your child usually react to pain?
What don't you want others to do for you when you hurt?	What do you do for your child when he or she is hurting?
What helps the most to take your hurt away?	What does your child do for him- or herself when he or she is hurting?
Is there anything special that you want me to know about you when you hurt? (If yes, have child describe.)	What works best to decrease or take away your child's pain?
	Is there anything special that you would like me to know about your child and pain? (If yes, describe.)

include numeric rating scales,[14] word-graphic rating scales,[15] pain thermometers[16], and facial scales, including photographic[17,18] and cartoon-face[19,20] scales. Although most self-report approaches were developed for children with pain secondary to diagnostic, monitoring, and surgical procedures, self-report tools with adequate psychometric evidence appear to capture appropriately the pain intensity for children with cancer.

Examples of Self-report Tools

A discussion of selected self-report approaches highlights issues relevant to their use. Included is the measurement of three attributes of pain: intensity, location, and quality. Most tools measure intensity of pain. One of the earliest tools developed, the Poker chip tool[21], measures intensity only. The Poker chip tool consists of four red poker chips that represent *pieces of hurt*. Table 59.2 provides the instructions in both English and Spanish. Children learn to use this tool rapidly. They can either state how many pieces of hurt they have, pick up the chips, or point to the chip in the position representing the number of pieces of hurt.

The Adolescent Pediatric Pain Tool[10,22,23] is similar to the McGill Pain Questionnaire in that it measures intensity, location, and quality. This tool is recommended for children from 8 to 17 years of age.

Behavioral Observation Methods

Behavioral/observation methods are the primary approach to accessing pain information from preverbal and nonverbal children.[24] Unfortunately, development of these methods lags behind self-report approaches.

Physiological Approaches

Physiological approaches generally rely on interpretations of changes in several physiological parameters as indicators of pain. Physiological parameters that have been studied include hormones and metabolites,[25,26] endorphins,[27,28] vital signs (heart/pulse rate, respiration rate, and blood pressure),[29,30] and diaphoresis.[31,32] Substantiation for using these parameters as measures of pain is weak.

SELECTION OF PAIN MEASUREMENT TOOLS

An area of difficulty for many clinicians and researchers is the selection of tools for the measurement of pain. Often researchers and clinicians develop their own tools without attending to what is available. This phenomenon has occurred especially in regard to self-report tools, which have proliferated without attention to their psychometric attributes. Unfortunately, neither of these criteria guarantee that a tool will be appropriate for the intended use. Contended here is that the selection of an approach for measuring pain is a critical decision and that selection should involve the use of guidelines. Thus, guidelines for reviewing and selecting pain measurement approaches are provided in Table 59.3.

TREATMENT

The evaluation of cancer pain requires assessment of the etiology and location of the painful source, qualitative features and intensity of the pain, anticipated course of the painful experience, i.e. the nature of clinical spread of the disease, the nature and efficacy of recent analgesic therapy, the available routes of administration of medication (i.e. central venous access), the psychological state of the child and the family, and an age-appropriate pain evaluation. The World Health Organization has suggested an analgesic stepladder protocol for the management of pain in cancer patients, as shown in Table 59.4.[33]

The analgesic intervention of a child with cancer-associated pain involves a multidisciplinary approach

---

Table 59.2: Poker chip tool instructions

English instructions:

1. Use four red poker chips.
2. Align the chips horizontally in front of the child on the bedside table, a clipboard, or another firm surface.
3. Tell the child, "these are pieces of hurt." Beginning at the chip nearest the child's left side and ending at the one nearest the right side, point to the chips and say, "This [the first chip] is a little bit of hurt and this [the fourth chip] is the most hurt you could ever have." For a young child or for any child who does not comprehend the instructions, clarify by saying, "that means this [the first chip] is just a little hurt; this [the second chip] is a little more hurt; this [the third chip] is more hurt; and this [the fourth chip] is the most hurt you could ever have."
4. Ask the child, "How many pieces of hurt do you have right now?" Children without pain will say they don't have any.
5. Clarify the child's answer by responses such as "Oh, you have a little hurt? Tell me about the hurt." (Use a pain interview.)
6. Record the number of chips selected on the bedside flow sheet.

Table 59.3: Guidelines for critical review of pain measurement tools		
Criteria	*Yes/?/No*	*Comments*
Is pain or a related concept being measured by this tool?		
Is the type of pain (e.g., acute, procedural, chronic malignant) being measured similar to the type of pain I plan to measure?		
Was the tool designed to use with patients like mine?		
Was the tool designed to use in a setting like mine?		
Is the format of the tool appropriate for my patients?		
Is the length of the tool appropriate for my patients?		
Is the readability of the tool appropriate for my patients?		
Is the tool developmentally appropriate for my patients?		
Is the amount of practice time required by the patients appropriate for my patients?		
Would my patients like this tool?		
Is the tool affordable?		
Is the tool readily available?		
Is the tool easily reproducible?		
Is the tool easily transported?		
Is the tool easily disinfected?		
Is the tool easy to score?		
Is the scoring easily interpretable?		
Is the tool appropriate for patients from different cultures?		
Is the estimated reliability adequate?		
Is the estimated validity adequate?		
Are the estimated reliability and validity appropriate for the tool and its intended uses?		
Is the tool sensitive enough to determine differences in pain levels?		
Has additional research been done using this tool?		
Does the additional research support the reliability, validity, and sensitivity of the tool?		
Are other clinical settings using this tool?		
After addressing these criteria, decide whether the tool is adequate for use in your study.		
Adequate: Proceed with clinical application.		
Questionable: Use clinically with caution; pilot-test the tool before adopting it; contact the author and those who have used it clinically or in research to discuss your concerns.		
Inadequate: Do not use		

Table 59.4: World Health Organization cancer pain management
Step 1 Nonopioids and adjuvants
↓   (If pain persists or increases)
Step 2 Weak opioids; Nonopioids and adjuvants
↓   (If pain persists or increases)
Step 3 Potent opioids and adjuvants

(Table 59.5). Multiple methods are available, but they should be chosen on the basis of the treatment modality in managing the pain and the effect it has on the child. Dosing guidelines for analgesics, opioid analgesics and adjuctive drugs are listed in Table 59.6 to 59.8.

Doses are for opioid naïve patient. For infants under 6 months, start at one-fourth to one-third the suggested dose and titrate to effect.

Table 59.5: Analgesic intervention for children with cancer pain

Anticancer therapy:
 Radiotherapy
 Chemotherapy
 Biologic therapy
 Surgery
Analgesic drugs
Non-invasive techniques:
 Transcutaneous electrical nerve stimulation (TENS)
 Physical therapy
 Hypnosis
 Biofeedback
 Relaxation
Neurosurgical interventions
Regional nerve blocks
Supportive counseling

Adapted from WHO. Cancer pain relief and palliative care in children. Geneva: WHO

PRINCIPLES OF OPIOID ADMINISTRATION (WHO)

1. If inadequate pain relief and no toxicity at peak onset of opioid action, increase dose in 50% increments
2. IV and SC are essentially equivalent. Avoid IM administration.
3. Whenever using continuous infusion, hourly prn rescue doses with short-onset opioids should be available. Rescue dose is usually 50-200% of continuous hourly dose. If greater than six rescues is necessary in 24-hours period, increase daily infusion total by the total amount of rescues for previous 24-hours ÷ 24. An alternative is to increase infusion by 50%.

4. To change opioids: Because of incomplete cross-tolerance, if changing between short half-life opioids, start new opioid at 50% of equianalgesic dose. Titrate to effect. If changing from short to long half-life opioid (i.e., morphine to methadone), start at 25% of equianalgesic dose and titrate to effect.
5. To taper opioids: Anyone on opioids over 1 week must be tapered to avoid withdrawal. Taper by 50% for 2 days, then decrease by 25% every 2 days. When dose is equianalgesic to an oral morphine dose of 0.6 mg/kg/day if less than 50 kg or 30 mg per day if greater than 50 kg, it may be stopped.

PAIN TREATMENT DURING TERMINAL ILLNESS

Treatment modalities for cancer and children have improved recently, partly due to a cure-oriented and technology-based health care system. Recently, with the involvement of organizations like hospices, principles of care of terminally ill children have been developed, based on the same philosophy as adults.[34] Pain can be a significant problem in children who require terminal care.

Novel alternative methods for providing analgesia have been used by our pain service for children who do not have intravenous access. Nebulized opioids or the use of transdermal delivery systems have been used in children to offset intractable pain.[35,36] The adverse effects associated with long-term use of opioids include tolerance and withdrawal.[37] Careful rotation of opioids, along with the judicious use of other agents including N-methyl-D-aspartate (NMDA)-receptor antagonists, should be considered in their care.

Several approaches to pain management are taken based on the state of the patient, the involvement of the disease process, and the general state of the

Table 59.6: Non-opioid drugs for relieving cancer pain in children

Drug	Dosage	Comments
Acetaminophen (paracetamol) hematological side effects but	10-15 mg/kg poq 4-6 hours	Lacks gastrointestinal and
Choline magnesium trisalicylate	10-15 mg/kg po, q 8-12 hours	May have minimal antiplatelet effect; lacks gastrointestinal effect
Ibuprofen	10 mg/kg q 6-8 hours	Anti-inflammatory activity but may have gastrointestinal and hematological effect
Naproxen	5 mg/kg q 12 hours	Anti-inflammatory effects but may have gastrointestinal and hematological effect

Adapted from WHO. Cancer pain relief and palliative care in children. Geneva: WHO

Table 59.7: Opioid analgesic dosing							
	Equianalgesic dose	Usual starting dose IV/SC		IV/SC: po	Usual starting dose po		Biological half-life
Drug	Parental	50 Kg	50 Kg	Ratio	50 Kg	50 Kg	Half-life
Short half life Opioids							
Morphine	10 mg	Bolus dose = 0.1mg/kg q2-3 hours, continuous infusion = 0.03-0.05 mg/kg/hour	5-10 mg q2 4 hours	1:3	0.3 mg/Kg q 3-4 hours	30 mg q 3-4 hours	2.5-3 hours
Hydrmorphone	1.5 mg	0.015 mg/kg q 3-4 hours	1-1.5 mg q 3-4 hours	1:5	0.06 mg/Kg 3-4 q hours	4-8 mg q 3-4 hours	2-3 hours
Codeine	130 mg				0.5-1mg/kg q 3-4 hours	60 mg q 3-4 hours	2.5-3 hour
					0.2 mg/kg q 3-4 hours	10 mg q 3-4 hours	1.5 hours
Meperidine	75 mg	0.75 mg/kg q 2-3 hours	75-100 mg q3 hours	1:4	1-1.5 mg/ kg q3-4 hours	50-75 mg q hours	3 hours
Fentanyl	100 μg	0.5-2 μg/kg/ hour as conti- nuous infusion	25-75 μg q1 hour				
Long half-life opioids							
Controlled release morphine					0.6 mg/kg q8 hours or 0.9 mg/kg q 12 hours	30-60 mg q 12 hours	
Methadone	10 mg	0.1 mg/kg q 4-8 hours	5-10 mg q 4-8 hours	1:2	0.2 mg/kg q 4-8 hours	10 mg q 4-8 hours	12-50 hours

caregivers (Table 59.9). Patient-controlled analgesia (PCA) has been used widely in our institution for home-bound patients with terminal cancer.[38,39] Smaller, more user-friendly pumps have been devised for easy programming and they require less frequent changing. In patients who do not have venous access we have recommended the use of subcutaneous PCA. A number of other drugs are very useful in the terminally ill child. NSAIDs and steroids are particularly useful in the management of bone pain from metastasis. Carbamazepine, gabapentin and tricyclic antidepressants (TCAs) are useful for the management of neuropathic pain.[40] Hypnosis, biofeedback and distraction techniques can be used very effectively in children who are not heavily sedated.[41-43]

A child's view of death is very different from that of an adult. There is a consistent progression of the conceptual aspect of death in children as they grow older. The school-age child finally understands the permanence of death. Home care may be very useful for the family to cope with grief and sorrow, and also allows other siblings to spend some time with a loved one. A home

Table 59.8: Adjuvant analgesic drugs		
Drug category	*Drug dosage*	*Indications*
Antidepressants	Amitriptyline, 0.2-0.5 mg/kg. Escalate by 25% every 2-3 days up to 1-2 mg/kg if needed. Alternative: doxepin, imipramine, nortriptyline	Neuropathic pain (vincristine induced)
Anticonvulsants	Carbamazepine, 2 mg/kg p.o.q 12 hours, Phenytoin, 2.5-2 mg/kg p.o.q 12 hours, Clonazepam, 0.01 mg/kg q 12 hours	Neuropathic pain
Neuroleptics	Chlorpromazine, 0.5 mg/kg IV/poq 4-6 hours, promethazine, 0.5-1 mg/kg IV/poq 4-6 hours, Haloperidol, 0.01-0.1 mg/kg IV/po q 8 hours	Nausea, confused child, psychosis, acute agitation
Sedatives, hypnotics, anxiolytics	Diazepam, 0.05-0.1 mg/kg po q 4-6 hours, Lorazepam, 0.02-0.04 mg/kg po/IV q 4-6 hours, Midazolam, 0.05 mg/kg IV q 5 minutes prior to procedure	Acute anxiety, muscle spasm, premedication
Antihistamines	Hydroxyzine, 0.5 mg/kg q 4-6 hours, Diphenhydramine, 0.5-1 mg/kg q 4-6 hours	Opioid induced pruritus, anxiety
Psychostimulant	Dextroamphetamine, methylphenidate, 0.1-0.2 mg/kg twice a day. Escalate to 0.3-0.5 as needed	Opioid induced somnolence
Corticosteroids	Prednisolone, prednisone, dexamethasone dosage depends on clinical situation (i.e., dexamethasone 6-12 mg/m^2/d	Headache from raised ICP, widespread metastases

Adapted from WHO. Cancer pain relief and palliative care in children. Geneva: WHO

Table 59.9: Approaches to pain management in terminally Ill patients

Pharmacological
  — Opioid analgesics
  — Nonsteroidal analgesics
  — Steroids
  — Chemotherapy
Psychological
  — Support
  — Distraction
  — Hypnosis
Anesthetic
  — Regional anesthetics
  — Indwelling epidural and intrathecal catheters
  — Regional blocks
Surgical
  — Neuroablative procedures
  — Tumor debulking to reduce compression
Physical therapy
  — TENS
  — Acupuncture
  — Heat/cooling
  — Exercise

care coordinator should be available for the management of any adverse conditions. Knowing the family helps the coordinator understand their goals. One of the basic tenets of hospice care is to enable the patient to lead a full life, of the best possible quality, for the time remaining. Cooperation between the family and caregiver should allow the child to die with as much dignity as possible. It is the responsibility of the home coordinator to give the caregivers sufficient information on the management of pain. The combination of various techniques for the management of cancer pain should enhance the child's motivation and will to lead as normal a life as the disease state allows.

NERVE BLOCKS FOR CANCER PAIN

Cancer pain can be controlled by opioids in 95% cases; however, circumstances such as intractable neuropathic pain may require specific regional anesthetic technique like continuous brachial plus block.[44] Intraspinal analgesia, which includes either spinal (Subarachnoid) or epidural drug delivery, has been used only sporadically to control pain in terminal pediatric malignancies.[45] Caudal epidural injection is also a useful technique in palliative care, to administer corticosteroid in cases of malignant pain in the pelvis, and local anesthetic for painful procedures.[47]

CONCLUSION

Pediatric pain is mostly a hidden problem. No attempt to meet a need can be begun until the need has been documented. Careful surveys of children in hospitals or in outpatient settings can yield data on prevalence and severity of pain for both professionals and policy makers. A standard of practice in pediatric pain is needed. With the understanding of pain in children and the presence of available professional help, more children can be helped by a chronic pain clinic.

A multidisciplinary approach to pain management helps in determining the course of action and prognosis of the particular patient. When pediatric pain is severe, most management techniques include potent analgesics or the use of narcotics. There is considerable resistance to the use of narcotics in children for fear of addiction or concern about respiratory depression. This may also pose an ethical dilemma to the nursing staff.[48] The use of various methods including physical therapy and the services of the child psychiatry/psychology department can help children cope and overcome persistent pain. Chronic pain can be devastating to a child's morale and should be treated the same way as any other disease symptom is addressed. The key to excellent continuing care for these children is a multidisciplinary approach with a psychologist, physical therapist and a pain management specialist.

REFERENCES

1. McGrath PJ, Beyer J, Cleeland C, Eland J, McGrath PA, Portenoy R. Report of the subcommittee on assessment and methodologic issues in the management of pain in childhood cancer. *Pediatrics* 1990;86:814-7.
2. Acute Pain Management Guideline Panel. Acute pain management in infants, children, and adolescents: operative and medical procedures. Quick reference guide for clinicians, AHCPR publ. no. 92-0020. Rockville, MD: Agency for Health Care Policy and Research, Public Health Service, U.S. Department of Health and Human Services, 1992.
3. Milch RA, Freeman A, Clark E. Palliative pain and symptom management for children and adolescents. Division of Maternal and Child Health, US Department of Health and Human Services, 1982.
4. Hester NO, Barcus CS. Assessment and management of pain in children. *Pediatr Nurs Update* 1986;1:1-8.
5. McGrath PA. Pain in children: nature, assessment, and treatment. New York: Guilford Press, 1990.
6. McGrath PJ, Unruh AM. Pain in children and adolescents. Amsterdam: Elsevier, 1987.
7. Eland JM, Anderson JE. The experience of pain in children. In: Jacox AK, ed. Pain: a sourcebook for nurses and other health professionals. Boston: Little, Brown, 1977:453-73.
8. Hester NKO. The preoperational child's reaction to immunization. Nurs Res 1979; 28:250-54.
9. Eland JM. The effectiveness of transcutaneous electrical nerve stimulation (TENS) with children experiencing cancer pain. In: Funk SG, Tornquist EM, Champagne MT, Copp LA, Wiese RA, eds. Key aspects of comfort: management of pain, fatigue, and nausea. New York: Springer, 1989:87-100.
10. Savedra MC, Tesler MD, Holzemer WL, Ward JA. Adolescent pediatric pain tool (APPT): preliminary user's manual. San Francisco: University of California, 1989.
11. Abu-Saad HH. Toward the development of an instrument to assess pain in children: Dutch study. In: Tyler DC, Krane EJ, eds. Advances in pain research and therapy, volume 15: pediatric pain. New York: Raven Press, 1990:101-6.
12. Varni JW, Walco GA, Katz ER. Assessment and management of chronic and recurrent pain in children with chronic diseases. Pediatrician 1989;16:56-63.
13. Villarruel AM, Denyes MJ. Pain assessment in children: theoretical and empirical validity. Adv Nurs Sci 1991; 14:32-41.
14. McGrath PJ, Unruh AM. Pain in children and adolescents. Amsterdam: Elsevier, 1987.
15. Tesler MD, Savedra MC, Holzemer WL, Wilkie DJ, Ward JA, Paul SM. The word-graphic rating scale as a measure of children's and adolescents' pain intensity. Res Nurs Health 1991;14:361-71.
16. Katz ER, Kellerman J, Siegel SE. Behavioral distress in children with cancer undergoing medical procedures: developmental considerations. J Consult Clin Psychol 1980;48:356-65.
17. Beyer JE. The oucher: a user's manual and technical report. Denver, CO: University of Colorado Health Sciences Center; 1989.
18. Weekes DP, Savedra MC. Adolescent cancer: coping with treatment-related pain. J Pediatr Nurs 1988;3:318-28.
19. Jay SM, Elliott C. Behavioral observation scales for measuring children's distress: the effects of increased methodological rigor. J Consult Clin Psychol 1984; 52:1106-7.
20. Kuttner L, Bowman M, Teasdale M. Psychological treatment of distress, pain, and anxiety for young children with cancer. Dev Behav Pediatr 1988;9:374-81.
21. Hester NKO. The preoperational child's reaction to immunization. Nurs Res 1979;28:250-54.
22. Savedra MC, Tesler MD, Holzemer WL, Wilkie DJ, Ward JA. Pain location: validity and reliability of body outline markings by hospitalized children and adolescents. Res Nurs Health 1989; 12:307-14.
23. Savedra MC, Tesler MD, Holzemer WL, Wilkie DJ, Ward JA. Testing a tool to assess postoperative pediatric and adolescent pain. In: Tyler DC, Krane EJ, eds. Advances in pain research and therapy, volume 15: pediatric pain. New York: Raven Press, 1990:85-94.
24. Johnston CC. Pain assessment and management in infants. Pediatrician 1989;16:16-23.
25. Anand KJS, Brown MJ, Causon RC, Christofides ND, Bloom SR, Aynsley-Green A. Can the human neonate mount an endocrine and metabolic response to surgery? J Pediatr Surg 1985;20:41-8.
26. Anand KJS, Phil D, Hickey PR. Pain and its effects in the human neonate and fetus. N Engl J Med 1987;317:1321-48.
27. Katz ER, Sharp B, Kellerman J, Marston AR, Hershman JM, Siegel SE. B-Endorphin immunoreactivity and acute behavioral distress in children leukemia. J Nerv Ment Dis 1982;170:72-7.
28. Olness K, Wain HJ, Ng L. A pilot study of blood endorphin levels in children using self-hypnosis to control pain. Dev Behav Pediatr 1980;1:187-8.
29. Abu-Saad H. Assessing children's response to pain. Pain 1984;19:163-71.
30. Abu-Saad H, Holzemer WL. Measuring children's self-assessment of pain. Issues Comprehensive Pediatr Nurs 1981;5:337-49.
31. Harpin VA, Rutter N. Development of emotional sweating in the newborn infant. Arch Dis Child 1982;57:691-5.

32. Melamed BG, Siegel LJ. Reduction of anxiety in children facing hospitalization and surgery by use of filmed modeling. J Consult Clin Psychol 1975;43:511-21.

33. Fiselier T, Monnens L, Moerman E, et al. Influence of the stress of venipuncture on basal levels of plasma renin activity in infants and children. Int J Pediatr Nephrol 1983;4:181-185.30a Foster RL. Coping strategies of the child with leukemia: the stress of invasive procedures. Master's Thesis, University of Colorado, Denver, 1981.

34. Fowler-Kerry S. Adolescent oncology survivors' recollection of pain. In: Tyler DC, Krane EJ, eds. Advances in pain research and therapy, volume 15: pediatric pain. New York: Raven Press, 1990:365-72.

35. Gauvain-Piquard A, Rodary C, Rezvani A, Lemerle J. Pain in children aged 2-6 years: a new observational rating scale elaborated in a pediatric oncology unit=mpreliminary report. Pain 1987;31:177-88.

36. Gordin PC. Assessing and managing agitation in a critically ill infant. Maternal Child Nurs J 1990;15:26-32.

37. Grunau RVE, Craig KD. Pain expression in neonates: facial action and cry. Pain 1987;28:395-410.

38. Grunau RVE, Johnston CC, Craig KD. Neonatal facial and cry responses to invasive and non-invasive procedures. Pain 1990;42:295-305.

39. Gunnar MR, Fisch RO, Korsvik S, Donhowe JM. The effects of circumcision on serum cortisol and behavior. Psychoneuroendocrinology 1981;6:269-75.

40. Hester NKO. The preoperational child's reaction to immunization. Nurs Res 1979;28:250-54.

41. Hester NO. Comforting the child in pain. In: Funk SG, Tornquist EM, Champagne MT, Copp LA, Weise RA, Eds. Key aspects of comfort: management of pain, fatigue, and nausea. New York: Springer, 1989:290-98.

42. Hester NO, Barcus CS. Assessment and management of pain in children. Pediatr Nurs Update 1986;1:1-8.

43. Hester NO, Barcus CS. The human experience of pain for hospitalized children. Research study funded by Intramural Research Award, School of Nursing, University of Colorado Health Sciences Center, 1984-7.

44. Cooper MG, Keneally JP, Kinchington D. Cotinuous brachial plexus neural blockade in a child with cancer pain.[Review]. J Pain Symptom Manage 1994;9(40):277-81.

45. JM Saroyan, WS Schechter, ME Tresgallo, L. Granowetter. Journal of Clinical Oncology 2005, 23(6):1318-21.

46. Wood PE, Rushby CL, Ahmedzai S. Epidural steroid injections for malignant pain. J Cancer Care 1992;1:139-44.

47. Hester NO, Davis RC, Hanson SH, Hassanein RS. The hospitalized child's subjective rating of painful experiences. Kansas City, KS: University of Kansas, 1978.

CHAPTER 60

Bharat Agarwal

Use of Biological Agents in Supportive Care

Dose and schedule are important factors in the therapy of cancer. Animal model and clinical data show that there is a significant correlation between dose-intensity nd survival; moreover, the shortening of interval between chemotherapy cycles prevents from tumor regrowth and maximize the effect of chemotherapy on cancer cells.[1] Most of anti-cancer drugs are non-selective and act indiscriminately on dividing cells. Hematological toxicity is one of the most important limiting factor for the protocols that are based on the dose-escalation or the dose-density of chemotherapy. This result in peripheral blood cytopenia (neutropenia, anemia and thrombocytopenia), higher transfusion requirement, severe infectious complications, prolonged hospitalization and higher health care expenses. The use of hematopoietic growth factors such as the granulocyte colony-stimulating factors (G-CSF) filgrastim or lenograstim and erythropoietin represented a step forward to reduce the hematological toxity of high-dose chemotherapy and to manage the frequent infectious complications.

CHEMOTHERAPY INDUCED NEUTROPENIA: USE OF G-CSF

G-CSF is a natural cytokine that acts on committed myeloid progenitor cells. Its secretion is stimulated by infections or by the reduction of mature myeloid cells, as a result of bacterial lipolysaccharides and chemotherapy, respectively;[2] so the serum G-CSF concentration increase from approximately 25 pg/ml of healthy people to 1,000 pg/ml of patients with severe infections or after stem-cell transplantation.[3]

Several studies showed a clear benefit of the use of G-CSF in terms of reduction of length of severe neutropenia, incidence of infections, use of intravenous antibiotic and duration of hospitalizations. Overall, G-CSF facilitates the delivery on time of chemotherapy planned dose but the high costs of acquisition raised the issue of its appropriate use. The guidelines of The American Society of Clinical Oncology (ASCO), updated in 2000, indicated the settings where the use G-CSF is recommended as primary prophylaxis of febrile neutropenia in patients with an expected incidence of chemotherapy-induced neutropenia greater than or equal to 40%; in the treatment febrile neutropenia in patients at high risk of severe infections (sepsis, pneumonia, fungal infections); after high-dose chemotherapy with autologous progenitor stem-cell rescue; in the mobilization of peripheral blood progenitor cells (PBPCs); in patients with acute myeloid leukemia to reduce the neutropenia of the post-induction chemotherapy; and in patients with acute lymphoblastic leukemia to reduce the neutropenia that follows the induction chemotherapy. The adult indications of the use of G-CSF are generally extended to pediatric patients, though less data are available.[4]

Recently, new interest in G-CSF therapy has been obtained with the introduction of pegfilgrastim, the pegylated form of filgrastim.[5] Filgrastim, the recombinant human G-CSF, is a relatively small protein that is rapidly eliminated from the body via the kidneys. The short half-life, about 3.5 hours, requires its daily administration by intravenous or subcutaneous injection until the recovery to normal values of the absolute neutrophil count. Pegfilgrastim consists of a 20-kDa polyehylene glycol molecule covalently bound to the N-terminal amino group of filgrastim molecule. Polyethylene glycol molecule are pH-neutral, non-toxic, water soluble polymers that confers to pegfilgrastim a larger volume and a slower renal clearance; as a result the half-life of pegfilgrastim is 35 hours. The most important route of elimination of pegfilgrastim is the so-called neuthrophil-mediated clearance: after binding with the G-CSF receptor on surface of neutrophils, the molecule is removed from circulation and the resulting molecule-receptor complex is internalized and metabolized. The neutrophil-mediated clearance is a process slower than renal clearance and in healthy volunteers this molecule produced a sustained neutrophil count for 9-10 days.[6] The study performed on neutropenic cancer patients showed that pegfilgrastim reached a peak approximately 24 hours after injection, remained high for all the neutropenic period without daily fluctuation and declined as the patient recovered the baseline count of neutrophils. This favorable kinetic provides a patient's tailored protection from severe neutropenia and a smooth recovery of neutrophil levels.

Several phase II-III studies with pegfilgrastim has been performed in lung cancer, breast cancer, and lymphoma[5, 8-10] and the results are summarized as follows: a) the fixed dose of 6 mg (or 100 μg/kg) of pegfilgrastim, administered once per chemotherapy cycle, is equivalent to the 5 μg/kg-daily-dose of filgrastim, administered for 10-11 days, with respect to the incidence and duration of severe neutropenia, and the median time to absolute neutrophil count recovery; b) no dose-limiting toxicities were observed with pegfilgrastim, and the safety profile or the incidence of adverse events was similar to that of filgrastim, including bone pain; c) no effect of body weight was found on duration of severe neutropenia; d) a lower risk of febrile neutropenia was observed in patients who received pegfilgrastim than those given daily filgrastim: 11 vs 19% (relative risk 0.56, CI 0.35-0.89, p<0.005); f) a trend towards a lower risk of hospitalization and use intravenous antibiotics was observed in patients treated with pegfilgrastim. A recent randomized study in breast cancer patients who underwent moderately myelosuppressive chemotherapy regimen showed that the use of pegfilgrastim compared to placebo was associated to a lower incidence of febrile neutropenia (1% vs 17%), febrile-neutropenia-related hospitalization (1% vs 14%) and intravenous antibiotic use (2% vs 10%). These findings demonstrated that the use of

pegfilgrastim reduced significantly the incidence of infectious complications also in the patients with a moderate risk of febrile neutropenia (10-20%) and raised the issue of its use as primary prophylaxis out of the current guidelines of ASCO.[11] Phase II studies recently reported that pegfilgrastim ws effective both in mobilizing a sufficient number of CD34+peripheral stem cell in patients with myeloma and lymphoma[12,13] and in decreasing the duration severe neutropenia and febrile neutropenia after autologous peripheral blood stem cell transplantation.[14] These data deserve a further validation by prospective randomized study. In conclusion, pegfilgrastim offers a simplified dosing regimen that is more convenient for nurse and patients but its potentiality warrants further investigation especially in setting where no data are still not available or conclusive (children, stem cell mobilization, autologous stem cell transplantation).

ANEMIA: USE OF ERYTHROPOIETIN (EPO)

Anemia is a common complication in patients treated with chemotherapy for cancer. Its occurrence may delay the chemotherapy schedule, affect negatively the quality of life (QoL) and compromise the anti-tumor activity of radiotherapy and chemotherapy.[15-16] Prior to 1980s, the treatment od cancer-related anemia was based only on red blood cell (RBC) transfusion when the hemoglobin levels fell below 8-9 g/dl. The introduction of recombinant human erythropoietin in the '80s gave the opportunity to reduce the need for RBC transfusions and to improve overall QoL and possibly prognosis of patients. EPO is a protein synthesised in the kidney and, to a lesser extent, in the liver that binds erythopoietin receptors on surface of bone marrow red cell precursors (BFU-e, CFU-e, erythroblsts) and promotes erythropoiesis. This glycoprotein hormone has a molecular weight of 34 kDa and consists of 165 amino acids carbohydrates represent around the 40% of the molecule. Three recombinant human EPO has been approved for anemia in cancer: epoetin alfa, epoetin beta and darbepoetin alfa.[17] Evidence-based guidelines have been published by ASCO and EORTC about the use of the recombinant human erythropoietin in patients with cancer. The major goals of the erythropoietin therapy is the correction of chemotherapy-related anemia (defined as Hb level < 9-11 g/dl), prevent transfusions and possibly improve the QoL. The recommended dose of epoetin alfa and beta is 150 IU/ kg three times a week for a minimum of 4 weeks that can escalated to 300 IU/kg three times a week for other 4-8 weeks in those patients who do not respond to the initial regimen. An alternative schedule is the administration of 30-40,000 IU once a week in order to improve patient compliance.[18,19] Darbepoetin alfa is a biochemically distinct erythropoietin characterized by an increased carbohydrate content, a major number of sialic acid molecules and a higher molecular weight; these properties determine a longer hal-life (about 49 hours) and an increased biological activity compared to epoetin alfa or beta. The recommended dose of darbepoetin is 2.25 μg/kg per week but a dose finding study in patients with solid tumors showed that the most effective weekly dose is 4.5 μg/kg.[20] In the same study, the administration of 9 ug/kg every 2 weeks had a comparable efficacy to the weekly dose of 4.5 ug/kg. Other authors found that the doses of 12 ug/kg and 15 ug/kg of darbepoetin alfa allow to maintain the efficacy of darbepoetin despite a longer interval of administration, 3 and 4 weeks, respectively.[21,22] A recent meta-analyses including 27 prospective randomized trials published between 1985 and 2002 demonstrated that the use of recombinant human erythropoietin reduced significantly the risk of RBC transfusion, mainly in patients with solid tumors and gives some evidence for improving QoL and survival.[23] Despite these favorable data, recombinant human erythropoietin is not routinely used in cancer patients for several reasons: limited data (children), best dosing schedule not defined yet, slow onset of response, costs, no clear impact on survival and risk of thrombovascular events when used to correct Hb levels beyond anemia.

In conclusion, the development of long-acting darbepoetin gives the opportunity to simplify the management of chemotherapy-related anemia but more data are needed to assess the real cost/benefit ratio and impact on outcome.

REFERENCES

1. Gregory SA, Trumper L. Chemotherapy dose intensity in non-Hodgkin's lymphoma: is dose intensity an emerging paradigm for better outcomes? Ann Oncol 2005; 2 (epub ahead).
2. Lieschke GJ, Burgess AW. Granulocyte colony-stimulating factor and granulocyte-macrophage colony-stimulating factor. N Engl J Med 1992;327:99-106.
3. Kawakami M, Tsutsumi H, Kumakawa T, et al. Levels of serum granulocyte colony-stimulating factor in patients with infections. Blood 1990;76:1962-4.
4. Ozer H, Armitage JO, Bennett CL, et al. 2000 update of recommendations for the use of hematopoietic colony-stimulating factors: evidence-based, clinical practice guidelines. J Clin Oncol 2000;18:3558-85.
5. Waladkhani AW. Pegfilgrastim: a recent advance in the prophylaxis of chemotherapy-induced neutropenia. Eur J Cancer care 2004;13:371-9.
6. Molineux G, Kinsler O, Briddel B, et al. A new form of filgrastim with sustained duration of and enhanced ability to mobilize PBPC in both mice and humans. Experimental hematology 1999;27:1724-34.
7. Biganzoli L, Untch M, Skacel T, Pico JL. Neulast (pegfilgrastim): a once-percycle option for the management of chemotherapy-induced neutropenia. Sem Oncol 2004;31(S8):27-34.
8. Holmes FA, O'Shaughnessy J, Vukelja S, et al. Blinded, randomized, multicenter study to evaluate single administration of peg-filgrastim once per cycle versus daily filgrastim as an adjunct to chemotherapy in patients with high-risk stage II or stage III/IV breast cancer. J Clin Oncol 20:727-31.
9. Green MD, Koebl H, Baselga J, et al. A randomized, double-blind, multicenter, phase 3 study of fixed-dose, single administration pegfilgrastin vs daily filgrastim in patients receiving myelosuppressive chemotherapy. Ann Oncol 2003;14:29-35.
10. Siena S, Piccart MJ, Holmes FA, et al. A combined analysis of two pivotal randomized trials of a single dose of pegfilgrastim per chemotherapy cycle and daily filgrastim in patients with stage II-IV breast cancer. Oncology Reports 2003;10:715-24.
11. Vogel CL, Wojtukiewicz MZ, Carroll RR, et al. First and subsequent cycle use of pegfilgrastim prevents febrile neutropenia in patients with breast cancer: a multicenter, double-blind, placebo-controlled phase III study. J Clin Oncol 2005;23:1178-84.
12. Isidori A, Tani M, Bonifazi F, et al. Phase II study of a single pegfilgrastim injection as an adjunct to chemotherapy to mobilize stem cells into the peripheral blood of pretreated lymphoma patients. Haematologica 2005;90:225-31.
13. Steidl U, Fenk R, Bruns I, et al. Successful transplantation of peripheral blood stem cells mobilized by chemotherapy and a single dose of pegylated G-CSF in patients with multiple myeloma. Bone Marrow Transplant 2005;35:33-6.
14. Staber PB, Holub R, Linkesch W, et al. Fixed-dose single administration of pegfilgrastim vs daily filgrastim in patients with haematological malignancies undergoing autologous peripheral blood stem cell transplantation. Bone Marrow Transplant 2004;35:889-93.
15. Ludwig H, Fritz E. Anemia in cancer patients. Semin Oncol 1998;25:2-6.
16. Crawford J, Cella D, Cleeland CS, et al. Relationship between changes in hemoglobin level and quality of life during chemotherapy in anemic cancer patients receiving epoetin therapy. Cancer 2002;95:888-95.
17. Egert A. Recombinant human erythropoietin in oncology: current status and further developments. Ann Oncol 2005; June 15 (epub ahead).
18. Rizzo JD, Lichtin AE, Woolf SH, et al. Use of epoetin in patients with cancer:evidence-based clinical practice guidelines of the American Society of Clinical Oncology and the American Society of Hematology. J Clin Oncol 2002;19:4083-107.
19. Bokemeyer C, Apro MS, Courdi A, et al. EORTC guidelines for the use of erythropoietic proteins in anaemic patients with cancer. Eur J Cancer 2004;40:2201-16.
20. Glaspy JA, Jadeja JS, Justice G. Darbepoetin alfa given every 1 or 2 weeks alleviates anemia associated with cancer chemotherapy. Br J Cancer 2002;87:268-76.
21. Kotasek D, Albertsson M, John Mackey J, et al. Randomized, double-blind, placebo-controlled, dose-finding study of darbepoetin alfa administered every 3 (Q3W) or 4 (Q4W) weeks in patients with solid tumours. Proc Am Soc Clin Oncol 2002; (abstr 1421).
22. Glaspy JA, Jadeja JS, Justice G, et al. A randomized, active control, pilot trial of front-loaded dosing regimens of darbepoetin-alfa for the treatment of patients with anemia during chemotherapy for malignant disease. Cancer 2003;97:1317-20.
23. Bohlius J, Langensiepen S, Schwarzer G, et al. Recombinant human erythropoietin and overall survival in cancer patients: results of a comprehensive mata-analysis. J Natl Cancer Inst 2005;97:489-98.

Shilpa Sharma
Devendra K Gupta

CHAPTER 61

Acute Crisis Management in Pediatric Oncology

Children with malignancy fall prey to critical conditions at sometime in their life that need to be recognized in time for favourable outcome. These children are at increased risk for acute life-threatening situations as a direct result of the underlying disease or as a result of the treatment. Early diagnosis and needful management are important to avoid crisis that may prove fatal.

The primary etiologies that underlie most emergencies that occur in the field of pediatric oncology have been shown in Table 61.1.

ACUTE INFECTION

Immunosuppression is the primary predisposing factor for development of infection in children suffering from malignancy. The source may originate from bacteria, parasites, mycoplasma, viruses, and fungi. Patients are variably subjected to decreases in T-cell function, granulocyte function (neutropenia), B-cell function (hypogammaglobulinemia), splenic function, and immunologic and integument barriers. Alteration of the typical flora can lead to overgrowth of pathogenic organisms. Immunocompromised children are susceptible to systemic dissemination of endogenous bacteria and fungi colonizing skin and gastrointestinal tract, reactivation of endogenous viruses (e.g. herpes), or reactivation of latent cysts (e.g. *Pneumocystis carinii*).[1] They are also at increased risk of systemic infection from aerosolized viruses, *Legionella* species, and fungal spores. Formation of evidence-based practice guidelines commissioned to provide assistance to clinicians when making decisions on treating specific conditions by panel members representing experts in infectious diseases and oncology may help in prevention and treatment of many infectious complications.[2]

Table 61.1: Causes of acute crisis in pediatric oncology	
Acute infection and inflammation	Bacterial
	Fungal
Hematologic	Bone marrow depression
	Anemia
	Febrile neutropenia
	Thrombocytopenia
	Hypogammaglobulinemia
	Severe external tumor bleeding
Severe pain	
Respiratory	Airway obstruction
	Pneumonitis
	Transfusion-related acute lung injury (TRALI)
	Pneumothorax
	Pleural Effusion
Cardiothoracic	SVC/ Superior mediastinal syndrome
	Cardiac temponade
	Pericardial effusion
	Pneumomediastinum
Abdominal	GI bleeding
	GI obstruction
	Gastroenteritis
	Enterocolitis
	Internal tumor bleeding
	Severe hepatomegaly (Neuroblastoma IV S)
	Ascitis
	Pancreatitis
Genitourinary	Oliguria
	Hypertension
	Hemorrhagic cystitis
Neurologic emergencies	Spinal cord compression
	Cerebral herniation
Metabolic emergencies	Hyponatremia
	Hypoglycemia
	Adrenal failure
	Lactic acidosis
Side effects of chemotherapy	Extravasation
	Hypersensitivity

HEMATOLOGIC ABNORMALITIES

Hematological conditions requiring emergent treatment result from hematopoiesis or coagulopathy. Abnormal hematopoiesis may result from underproduction or overproduction, underproduction being more common. Underproduction may be a result of malignant bone marrow infiltration, bone marrow failure, or treatment-related myelotoxicity causing anemia, thrombocytopenia, neutropenia, or a combination of the three. Overproduction of hematopoietic tissue primarily is observed in the form of leukocytosis associated with acute leukemia. Coagulopathy manifests as hemorrhage, thrombosis, or both. Coagulopathy may result from primary consequence of disease, treatment toxicity or secondary to other known complications.

Bone Marrow Depression

Bone marrow depression results in anemia, thrombocytopenia, and neutropenia. These are best treated with supportive care. Transfusion of individual blood components like red cells, platelets, and granulocytes can be done. Judicious use of blood products decreases infectious risks. These products can be irradiated to prevent the lethal complication of graft versus host disease.

Severe Anemia

A drastic fall in the hemoglobin levels may result from tumor hemorrhage or as a side effect of chemotherapy or radiotherapy (Fig. 61.1). Severe anemia in a girl with wilm's Tumur presenting with hematuria. Reduced erythropoietin may also add to anemia in renal tumors. Very severe anemia may present with shock, myocardial insufficiency, or altered sensorium.

Usually, anemia in pediatric patients who are not critically ill is well tolerated and does not require transfusion unless the hematocrit level is less than 20 to 25 percent. Transfusion of packed red blood cells may also be necessary to maintain optimal intravascular volume. The use of recombinant erythropoietin is limited by weeks of therapy necessary to increase hemoglobin (Hb) levels significantly. Once developed, severe anemia usually requires transfusion.

Early identification of the source of bleeding and slow transfusion of packed cells is life saving. Packed RBCs are the blood product of choice for treatment of patients with anemia. Generally, 10-15 ml of Packed RBCs per kilogram can be transfused safely over 2-4

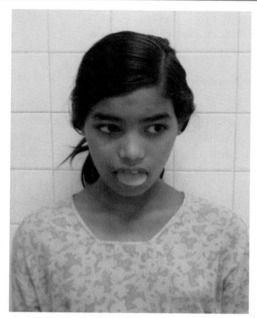

Figure 61.1: Severe anemia in a girl with Wilms' Tumor presenting with haematuria

hours. Rate of transfusion should be decreased by at least 50 percent in patients with heart failure or severe chronic anemia in whom the Hb level is less than or equal to 5 g/dl.

Neutropenia

Neutropenia commonly is defined as an ANC less than 500/mm.[3] It is the primary risk factor for bacterial infections. Neutropenia is the most common toxic result of myelosuppressive chemotherapy but may result from failure or suppression of the bone marrow.

Neutropenia extending beyond two weeks is associated with increased risk of systemic fungal infection. Prolonged neutropenia resulting from myelotoxic chemotherapy is treated primarily with myeloid growth factors, granulocyte colony-stimulating factor (GCSF) and granulocyte-macrophage colony-stimulating factor (GMCSF). Neutropenia associated with bone marrow failure syndromes may respond to immunosuppressive therapy alone or in combination with androgens and growth factors. Although granulocyte transfusion is a viable therapeutic modality, no reliable criteria exist that predict which patients are likely to benefit from this moderately toxic and expensive therapy. Pediatric patients with cancer, fever, and treatment-induced neutropenia who present with high fever or prolonged CFT are at increased risk of developing life-threatening illnesses requiring administration of critical care therapies, independent of hematologic factors, type of cancer, or other physiologic signs of sepsis.[3]

Febrile Neutropenia

The incidence of bacterial infections increases as the absolute neutrophil count (ANC) decreases from 1000/mm[3] to 100/mm[3]. The most common etiologic agents are bacteria that colonize the skin and gastrointestinal tract of the host. Fever is the most common presenting symptom

For febrile neutropenia, fever is defined as a temperature greater than 38.0°C twice within 24 hours or a temperature greater than 38.3 to 38.5°C once. Such patients require complete evaluation. Inspection of central venous catheter sites, skin, oropharynx, and perirectal areas is necessary. Cultures of the blood, skin lesions, and diarrheal stool, chest radiographs, complete blood counts, blood urea nitrogen, creatinine, transaminase, and serum electrolyte levels are recommended. Pediatric patients with higher fever or prolonged CFT are at increased risk of developing life-threatening illnesses requiring administration of critical care therapies, independent of hematologic factors, type of cancer, or other signs of sepsis.[1]

Institution of empiric antibiotic therapy for febrile neutropenia has decreased infection-related mortality rates, particularly due to gram-negative organisms.

An extensive diagnostic evaluation identifies an established or occult infection in fewer than 48-60 percent of patients. Bacteremia is present in 10 to 20 percent of patients with neutropenia who are febrile. Gram-positive organisms account for approximately 60 to 70 percent of microbiologically identified organisms, and antibiotic resistance has been increasing among isolated organisms. The most common gram-positive organisms are *Staphylococcus aureus, Staphylococcus epidermidis, S. pneumoniae, Streptococcus pyogenes and Enterococcus faecalis.* Gram-negative isolates of *E. coli, P. aeruginosa,* and *Klebsiella* species are more common. Anaerobic cocci and bacilli are other common bacteriologic isolates.

Initial antibiotic therapy for febrile neutropenia should consist of broad-spectrum monotherapy using cefepime, ceftazidime, or imipenem. Dual therapy consisting of an aminoglycoside in combination with an anti-pseudomonal beta-lactam is an equivalent alternative and should be considered, particularly when the patient's presentation suggests gram-negative bacteremia or

sepsis.[2] Initial empiric use of vancomycin in combination with single or dual therapy is appropriate in the setting of severe mucositis, quinolone prophylaxis, known colonization with resistant strains of *S aureus* or *S pneumoniae,* catheter-related infections, and hypotension/sepsis syndrome. Vancomycin should be discontinued after 48 to 72 hours if warranted by clinical course or culture results. A confirmed infectious focus may also require antibiotics beyond empiric coverage. Typhlitis or perirectal abscess requires coverage for anaerobic organisms. *C. difficile* enterocolitis requires either metronidazole or oral vancomycin. Additional coverage should be guided by culture results.

Empiric antibiotics typically are discontinued when the patient is afebrile and has an ANC greater than 500/mm[3] if both occur within the first seven days of therapy. Continuation of antibiotics usually is recommended regardless of fever when neutropenia is profound, which is indicated by an ANC less than 100/mm[3].

Antibiotic chemoprophylaxis for patients with profound neutropenia to selectively decontaminate the gut with orally administered absorbable antibiotics, such as trimethoprim-sulfamethoxazole and quinolones, are preferable to nonabsorbable polymyxin, aminoglycosides, or vancomycin secondary to the increasing incidence of resistant bacteria to the latter two drugs. Antibiotic prophylaxis during neutropenia results in fewer bacterial infections. However, increased bacterial resistance and lack of reduction in mortality rates argues against antibiotic prophylaxis as a routine practice.[4]

Blood cultures should be obtained from all catheter lumens in a febrile patient with cancer without neutropenia. In the absence of an obviously infectious site, a broad-spectrum third-generation cephalosporin may be commenced for 24 to 72 hours and patients with positive culture results may be treated with a full course of appropriate antibiotics.

In a patient with neutropenia, persistent or recurrent fever after defervescence despite broad-spectrum antibiotic therapy, invasive fungal disease should be suspected. Fungal infections may present as focal or disseminated disease. *Candida* and *Aspergillus* species are the most common cause of fungal infections in immunocompromised hosts. Corticosteroid therapy, antibiotics and neutropenia predispose to fungal infections.

Empiric antifungal therapy is recommended after 4-7 days of persistent unexplained fever, despite broad-spectrum antibiotic therapy, or new fever after defervescence to antibiotics. Amphotericin B is the drug of choice for established fungal infections though its use is limited by substantial nephrotoxicity and infusion-associated toxicity. A dose of 0.5-0.7 mg/kg/d is appropriate when targeting *Candida* species, but 1 mg/kg/d is appropriate to target *Aspergillus* species and other molds. Amphotericin B also has been used intranasally to decrease the rate of fatal infections by *Aspergillus* species in patients undergoing bone marrow transplant, but the use is not widespread. Fluconazole may be considered if there is a suspicion for susceptible *Candida* species, as expected after only 7-10 days of neutropenia, colonization with *C albican without* prior fluconazole prophylaxis.

Thrombocytopenia

Thrombocytopenia may result from underproduction or excessive consumption of platelets. Platelet transfusions remain the primary treatment to treat bleeding and also as prophylaxis. However, it should be avoided in the absence of bleeding if thrombocytopenia is secondary to platelet consumption. Surgical microvascular bleeding usually requires platelet transfusion with a platelet count less than 50,000/mm^3. An incremental increase of 40,000-45,000/mm^3 is sufficient to attain hemostasis in patients with active bleeding from thrombocytopenia.

A rise of less than 5000 to 6500/mm^3 for each transfused unit/m^2 on 2 consecutive transfusions suggests active destruction resulting from alloimmunization, which can be confirmed by a low posttransfusion platelet count obtained 15 to 20 minutes after platelet transfusion and by presence of antiplatelet antibodies that precipitate platelet destruction more rapidly than other forms of consumption. Alloimmunization requires either cross-matching or HLA typing of platelets prior to transfusion.

Hyperleukocytosis

It is defined as a peripheral leukocyte count greater than 100,000/mm^3. Hyperleukocytosis is seen most children in chronic phase of CML and few cases of ALL and ANLL. Clinical manifestations result from anaerobic metabolism and proliferation of blast cells within the microvasculature. Physical findings result from increased viscosity associated with blast cell aggregates and thrombi along with damage to vessels and secondary hemorrhage. Resultant clinical findings include respiratory and neurologic signs like dyspnea, hypoxia, focal deficit, ataxia, agitation, confusion, delirium, and stupor. Other signs include plethora, cyanosis, papilledema, and

distension of retinal artery or vein. Mortality may be caused by CNS hemorrhage or thrombosis, pulmonary leukostasis and metabolic derangements accompanying tumor lysis. Treatment is directed toward decreasing the peripheral leukocyte count and specific therapeutic stategies to control metabolic, hemorrhagic, and thrombotic risks. Packed RBC transfusions increase blood viscosity and should be avoided. The haemoglobin level should not be raised above 10gm/dl, most children are asymptomatic with haemoglobin level of 7gm/dl. Platelet transfusions do not significantly change the viscosity and may be transfused safely if indicated. Specific antileukemic therapy is the treatment of choice for decreasing the peripheral leukocyte count. In absence of definitive therapy, leukophoresis or exchange transfusion may be considered[5].

Coagulopathy

Pediatric malignancy patients may have significant abnormalities in procoagulation, inhibitors of coagulation, and fibrinolysis that result in hypocoagulable and hypercoagulable conditions leading to hemorrhage or thrombosis. Hemorrhage predominates in hyperleukocytosis secondary to relative excess of fibrinolytic proteases, compared to prothrombotic thromboplastic materials, released from blast cells, consumption of coagulation factors or from underproduction of necessary coagulation factors.

Disseminated Intravascular Coagulation

Disseminated intravascular coagulation (DIC) is characterized by excessive activation of blood coagulation with consumption of clotting factors. DIC causes hemorrhage, microangiopathic hemolytic anemia, and thrombosis. It is commonly seen with ANLL induction chemotherapy in which thromboplastic materials are released from leukemic blast cells, in presence of sepsis or rarely in widely disseminated solid tumors.

Diagnosis is made by elevated PT, elevated aPTT, decreased platelet counts and decreased fibrinogen levels with concomitant elevation of fibrin monomers or fibrin degradation products. Primary therapy is directed towards supportive care. Low-dose heparin therapy may be beneficial. Thrombocytopenia is treated with platelet transfusion. Fibrinogen is replaced using cryoprecipitate, 1 unit (bag)/10 kg. Hyperfibrinolysis, as evidenced by low antiplasmin levels, is treated with aminocaproic acid in absense of hematuria.

Thrombosis

Thrombosis is commonly seen in presence of hyper-leukocytosis and ALL treated with L-asparaginase in which *severe cerebral venous sinus thromboembolism* is reported. L-asparaginase therapy is associated with decreased plasminogen, antithrombin III, protein C and protein S levels. Symptomatic thrombosis may be associated with central venous catheters.

Clinical presentation of sagittal sinus thrombosis varies from asymptomatic to life threatening situations. Most patients present with seizure, focal motor deficits or cognitive deficits including aphasia. Treatment is supportive with good long-term recovery.

Severe Tumor Bleeding

Tumors on the surface like sacrococcygeal teratoma may undergo superficial ulceration with impending rupture of the tumor (Fig. 61.2). Such cases need to operated upon on emergency basis with arrangement of adequate blood for transfusion as a life saving measure. Some tumors like wilms' Tumor may bleed massively internally and present with hematuria, sock and severe anemia. After initial stablization, investigations like ultra-sonography and CT scan may be helpful for the diagnosis (Fig 61.3 A-C). In certain situations if the bleeding does not stop, emergency nephroureterectomy is mandatory as a life saving procedure (Fig. 61.4 and

61.5). If it is not possible to remove the tumor completely, debulking may be done followed by appropriate chemotherapy.

SEVERE PAIN

Large tumors may cause pain due to due abdominal distension, stretching of the capsule, clot colic and setting in of infection due to tumor necrosis. Metastasis to the bone are a common cause of pain in lukemia and neuroblastoma (Fig. 61.6). Intraspinal extension in cases of neuroblastoma is very painful. Cachexic patients may require dose adjustment for pain management due to their moribound condition. This has been dealt in detail on the chapter on pain management.

RESPIRATORY EMERGENCIES

Airway Obstruction

Obstruction to the airway is the primary respiratory emergency in pediatric oncology patients and can occur at the level of larynx, trachea, or bronchi. Airway obstruction is the most common complication in pediatric patients presenting with a mediastinal mass and has been reported in 60 percent patients.[6] Leukemia, lymphoma, Hodgkin disease, rhabdomyosarcoma, and neuro-blastoma are the most common causes (Fig. 61.7 and 61.8). Laryngeal obstruction though uncommon in pediatric patients may occur due to vocal cord paralysis. Airway compromise has been reported in hemangioma, lymphangioma, teratoma (cervical and mediastinal), respiratory papillomatosis, thymoma, and other head and neck tumors.

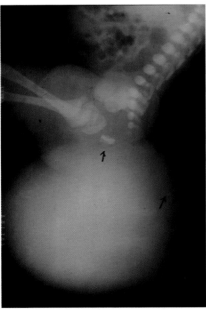

Figure 61.2: Sacrococcygeal tumor in a newborn that presented with superficial ulceration

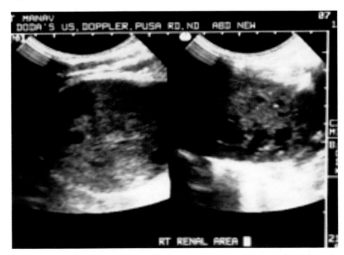

Figure 61.3A: Ultrasonography image in a 11 month old male child with right Wilms' Tumor showing internal hemorrhage

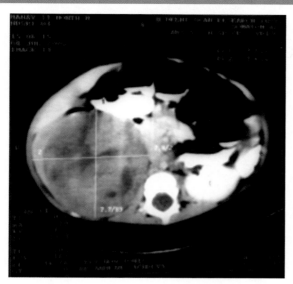

Figure 61.3B: CT scan image of the same child showing the tumor

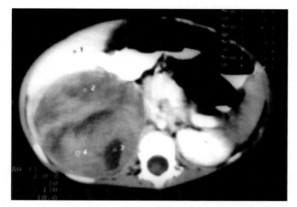

Figure 61.3C: CT scan showing the internal hemorrhage within the tumor mass

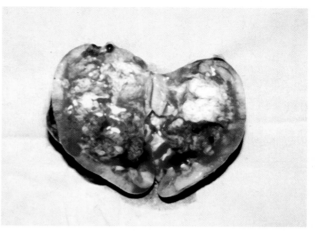

Figure 61.5: Resected specimen of Wilms' tumor operated in emergency due to tumor bleed

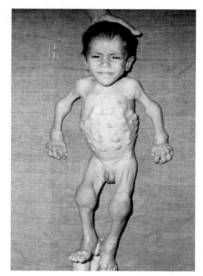

Figure 61.6: A case of neuroblastoma stage IV-S with subcutaneous nodules and bony pains due to metastasis

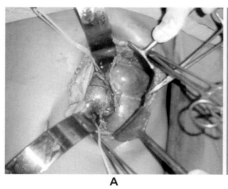

A

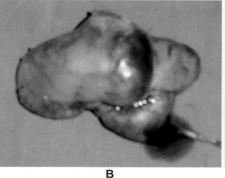

B

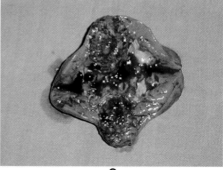

C

Figure 61.4A: Operative photograph in a case of Wilms' tumor with internal hemorrhage showing the pelvis full of blood

Figure 61.4B: Resected specimen of nephrouretenectomy showing the pelvis full of blood

Figure 61.4C: Cut section of the tumor with blood clots in the pelvicalxceal system

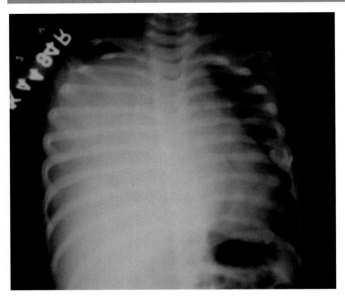

Figure 61.7: Skiagram chest in a case of massive thoracic neuroblastoma causing respiratory compromise

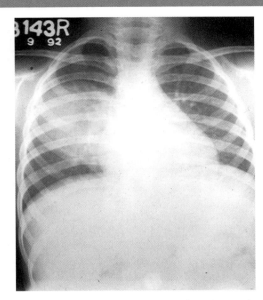

Figure 61.8: Skiagram chest in a case of mediastinal teratoma presenting with respiratory distress

Clinical symptoms depend on the level of obstruction. Stridor is associated with extrathoracic obstruction, and a hoarse voice suggests unilateral vocal cord paralysis. Increased obstruction of the trachea or mainstem bronchi may manifest as wheezing, dyspnea, orthopnea, or increased effort of breathing. Rapid CT scan is the preferred imaging study for children. More than 30 percent of symptomatic patients with a mediastinal mass have a 35-90 percent decrease in tracheal cross-sectional area as measured using CT scans. The diagnosis may be established by node or needle biopsy under local anesthesia, and general anesthesia is preferably deferred until the compromised airway is alleviated by radiation and chemotherapy.[6]

Occassionally, symptomatic airway obstruction may occur as a complication of refractory disease. Prompt diagnosis and institution of appropriate antitumor therapy is the optimal treatment strategy. Local radiotherapy may be used but can induce inflammation that worsens symptoms transiently. Symptomatic relief is the primary objective for patients with airway obstruction as a terminal medical complication and may require a multimodality approach with radiotherapy, surgery, and chemotherapy.

Pneumonitis

Noninfectious pneumonitis is a complication of radiation therapy, chemotherapy, stem cell transplantation, and transfusion.[7] The spectrum of clinical presentation varies and ranges from asymptomatic to respiratory failure. Chest radiographs may demonstrate interstitial infiltrates. Bronchoalveolar lavage is performed to exclude infectious etiologies and typically reveals a lymphocytic infiltrate. Pulmonary function tests demonstrate decreased compliance and decreased diffusion capacity. Corticosteroid therapy is the primary treatment.

Whole-lung or high-dose partial-lung irradiation directly damages alveolar type II cells and capillary endothelial cells; weeks later, the damage results in alveolar hyalinization and reactive pulmonary infiltrates. Decreased pulmonary function and pulmonary fibrosis are consequent to these early effects and often are demonstrated within 12 months of radiation.. Subacute pneumonitis or late fibrosis occurs in 5-10 percent of patients receiving whole-lung irradiation of 18 to 20 Gy. Specific chemotherapeutic agents are associated with acute lung injury. Bleomycin is most commonly associated with pneumonitis and fibrosis. Other drugs frequently reported to cause pulmonary injury are carmustine, mitomycin and methotrexate[8].

Acute respiratory distress syndrome is a rare complication following intrathecal injection of methotrexate in acute lymphoblastic leukemia patients.[8] Histopathologic study of the lungs has revealed a pattern of diffuse alveolar damage with interstitial cellular infiltration. The pulmonary infiltrates have been found to resolve gradually following treatment with corticosteroids.[8]

The use of all-trans retinoic acid (ATRA) to induce hematologic remission in patients with acute promyelocytic leukemia is associated with a pneumonitis syndrome that consists of fever and respiratory distress, which may include hypoxia and pulmonary infiltrates.[9] ATRA syndrome responds well to dexamethasone therapy. Pneumonitis and pulmonary fibrosis are complications of hematopoietic stem cell transplantation and may occur in several settings. Acute noninfectious pneumonitis is associated with high-dose chemotherapy regimens.

Transfusion-related Acute Lung Injury (TRALI)

Transfusion-related acute lung injury (TRALI) is a hazardous but little-known complication of blood transfusion, characterized by non-cardiogenic lung oedema after blood transfusion.[10] It is characterized by noncardiogenic pulmonary edema variably associated with respiratory distress and hypoxia following transfusion of a blood product. TRALI results from granulocyte-agglutinating anti-HLA antibody-induced pulmonary leukoagglutination.[10] Leucoagglutinating antibodies in the donor plasma are considered to play a central role in the pathogenesis of TRALI but no recommended procedure currently exists for their detection, and most of them have not yet been well characterized. TRALI is associated not only with donor- but also with recipient-related leucocyte antibodies.[10] In addition to leucoagglutinating antibodies, non-agglutinating granulocyte-specific antibodies can be also involved. For immunodiagnosis, sera from both must be investigated by a combination of granulocyte and lymphocyte (HLA) antibody screening tests and leucocyte incompatibility verified by crossmatching.[10] TRALI typically occurs within 6 hours of transfusion and is a potentially life-threatening condition. Mechanical ventilation may be necessary for respiratory support.

Pneumothorax

A case has been reported of recurrent Wilms' tumour presenting with bilateral pneumothorax, 10 years following initial treatment.[11]

Hemothorax

Haemothovax may develop in uses of melignancies like leukemia (Fig. 61.9 A-C). Tube Thoracostomy with adequate blood replacement is required.

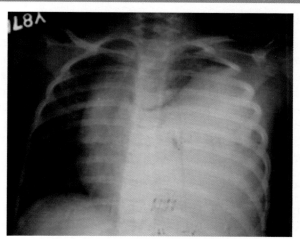

Figure 61.9A: Skiagram chest showing pacity in the left hemithorax due to haemothorax in a case of acute lymphocytic leukemia

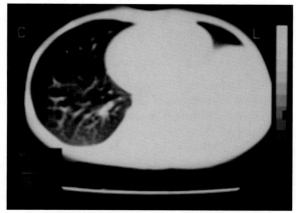

Figure 61.9B: CT scan image of the same child showing opacity in the left hemithorax

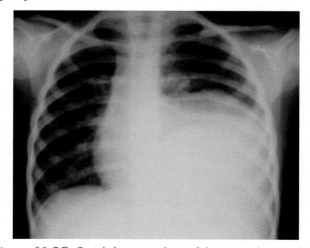

Figure 61.9C: Serial skiagram chest of the same showing little improvement in the amount of haemothorax

Hemoptysis

The most common etiology for hemoptysis in children is aspiration of blood from epistaxis, the most common cause being invasive pulmonary aspergillosis. Treatment includes localization of the site of bleeding and prevention of asphyxiation. If the site of bleeding is localized, postural drainage by lying on the side of haemorrhage is recommended to prevent collection of blood into the normal lung.

CARDIOVASCULAR EMERGENCIES

Cardiovascular emergencies are not so common in pediatric patients. They may result from compromise in cardiac function or vascular flow. Anthracycline chemotherapy may depress myocardial contractility and result in long-term medical complications. Rarely, vessel compression from a tumor mass may precipitate a medical emergency. Cardiac tamponade may result from malignant or reactive pericardial effusion.

Superior Vena Cava Syndrome

Obstruction of the superior vena cava (SVC) may result from external compression or internal thrombosis. The term superior mediastinal syndrome is used when there is associated tracheal compression. SVC syndrome is found in about 10 percent of pediatric patients with a large anterior mediastinal mass. Thrombosis of the SVC in pediatric patients is unusual and most likely is a result of extension from an indwelling central venous catheter.[11] Obstruction of the superior vena cava is rare in childhood and adolescence and its etiology is now mainly iatrogenic.[12] The most common mediastinal tumors presenting with the SVCS are the lymph node tumors and especially the lymphosarcomas.[12]

Symptoms include dyspnea, cough, hoarse voice, chest pain, dysphagia, and orthopnea and progress to headache, confusion, altered vision, and syncope. Symptoms are aggravated in the supine position or on performing the Valsalva maneuver. Signs of SVC syndrome are swelling and plethora of the head, neck, and upper extremities. Blood flow within the SVC and presence of a thrombus are best assessed using ultrasound. Removal of the indwelling catheter and short-term anticoagulation therapy usually is sufficient to treat a thrombus. Rapid CT is recommended for evaluation of a mediastinal mass and assess the extent of tracheal compression. The mass in children with SVC syndrome is usually in the anterosuperior mediastinum.

Pleural or pericardial effusions are more common in NHL.[12] A skiagram chest may show tracheal deviation. Patients with tumors larger than 45 percent of the transthoracic diameter are more likely to be symptomatic than those with ratios of less than 30 percent.[12,13] An echocardiogram should be obtained in cases of pericardial effusion.

In emergency situations, establishing a tissue diagnosis may be impossible and empiric therapy may be medically necessary to cause a rapid shrinking of the tumor.[12] Treatment should consist of a combination of radiation therapy, chemotherapy, and steroids.[12] Surgery should be limited to obtaining tissue for diagnosis, except when the tumor is localized to the mediastinum and is completely resectable.[12] Improvement has been reported after emergent radiotherapy within 12 hours in cases of radiosensitive tumors like NHL.[14] However, prebiopsy irradiation may render the specimen uninterpretable.[15] Also, tracheal swelling after irradiation may cause respiratory deterioration. Thus, emergent local radiotherapy usually can be avoided for a short time in pediatric patients in favor of supportive medical treatment. However, in cases of renal failure, irradiation may be given in preference to chemotherapy in SVC syndrome to avoid tumor lysis syndrome.

Diagnosis using tissue samples and initiation of definitive anticancer therapy are the objectives if SVC syndrome results from external compression from a tumor mass. Chemotherapy is indicated in ALL accompanied by a high leucocyte count and a mediastinal mass causing SCV syndrome.

Cardiac Tamponade

Cardiac tamponade is the inability of the ventricle to maintain normal cardiac output due to extrinsic pressure or intrinsic mass. Cardiac temponade is a rare complication of pediatric malignancy and may develop following compression by leukemic infilteration, inflammation, or infection of the pericardium, constrictive fibrosis from previous irradiation or occlusion from tumors of the cardiac muscle or endocardium.[16] Infectious pericarditis or myocarditis is the most common cause of temponade in immunocompromised children. Pericardial effusion and tamponade has been reported in pediatric age group in AML, ALL, Hodgkin disease, B-cell lymphoma, medulloblastoma, desmoplastic small round cell tumor and rhabdomyosarcoma.[16,17] Effusion volume ranged from 82 to 500 ml. The quantity of fluid required to induce tamponade depends on the rate of accumulation. A Wilms' tumor thrombus can extend from the renal vein through the tricuspid valve to fill the right cardiac chambers.

Clinical findings of impending tamponade mimic heart failure and include chest pain, cough, dyspnea, hiccups, nonspecific abdominal pain, and a pulsus paradoxus greater than 10 mm Hg. Chest radiographs may reveal cardiomegaly. ECG may demonstrate low-voltage QRS complexes and flattened or inverted T waves. Echocardiography is the best single study used, and it demonstrates pericardial effusion and atrial or ventricular collapse with hemodynamic compromise. Percutaneous catheter drainage is the treatment of choice for pediatric oncology patients and may be performed under echocardiographic or fluoroscopic guidance.[18] Pericardial fluid may contain malignant cells and should be evaluated accordingly. Resolution of the effusion is expected with treatment of the underlying malignancy. In cases of Wilms' tumor with intracardiac thrombus, if the mass does not occlude the chambers, chemotherapy has been reported to reduce the thrombus size in one week.

Hypertensive Crisis

Tumors like adrenal carcinoma may present with hypertensive crises (Fig. 61.10, 61.11). This requires stabilization with medical treatment before operative inervention.

SEVERE ABDOMINAL DISTENSION

Large tumors may cause severe abdominal distension that may require debulking in emergency due to respiratory compromise (Fig. 61.12). A Benign intrahepatic cyst may also present with gross abdominal distension necessitating an urgent removal (Fig. 61.13). Large tumors may occupy the whole of the abdomen and displace the intestine to one side (Fig. 61.14 A,B)

GASTROINTESTINAL TRACT OBSTRUCTION

Gastrointestinal tract obstruction in children though not so common may occur secondary to intussusception in which a neoplasm within the bowel wall creates a lead point to initiate the process. Intussusception has been reported in patients with Burkitt lymphoma in the terminal ileum, adenomyoma of the Meckel diverticulum, hamartoma of the ileum, acute lymphoblastic leukemia, leiomyosarcoma, and following resection of

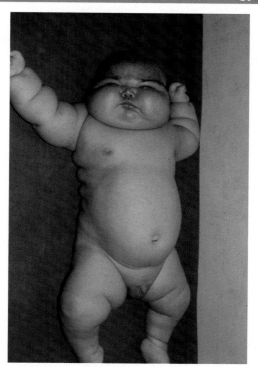

Figure 61.10: Photograph of a child with inoperable adrenal carcinoma presenting with respiratory distress and hypertensive crisis

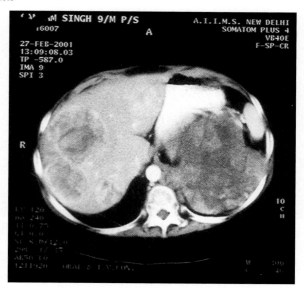

Figure 61.11: CT scan image of a child with left adrenal carcinoma and secondaries liver who also had hypertensive crisis

a Wilm's tumor.[18-21] Gastrointestinal tract obstruction also has been reported following a volvulus resulting from a mesenteric lymphangioma. Obstruction of the large colon primarily occurs in large pelvic tumors and

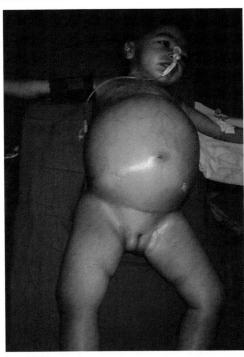

Figure 61.12: Photograph of a girl with a huge neuroblastoma causing abdominal distension that required debulking of the tumor

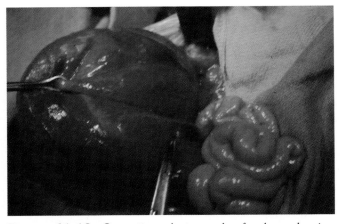

Figure 61.13: Operative photograph of a huge benign intrahepatic cyst

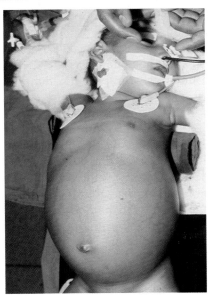

Figure 61.14A: Photograph of a child with large mesenchymal hamartoma causing massive abdominal distension

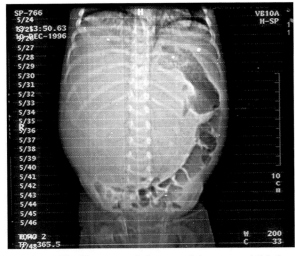

Figure 61.14B: Skiagram abdomen of the same child showing the displaced bowel loops

as a complication of constipation/obstipation induced by chemotherapy (e.g. vincristine), narcotic analgesia, or both. A temporary ileus also may be precipitated by typhlitis, sepsis, or other severe illness.

The complete clinical intussusception triad of cramping abdominal pain, palpable abdominal mass, and currant jelly stool may not be present in pediatric patients with malignancy; symptoms may be atypical and limited to abdominal pain and emesis. Nonreducible intussusception and intussusception outside the expected pediatric age range are also suggestive of a pathologic lead point.

Abdominal ultrasound or fluoroscopy with air-soluble or water-soluble contrast is the recommended diagnostic procedure. Fluoroscopic procedures also may be therapeutic. Surgery may be necessary for reduction, tissue diagnosis, or both. Reduction of the intussusception and treatment of the primary pathology are the principal approaches. In general, large tumor masses that cause gastrointestinal tract obstruction via external compression are best treated with chemotherapy, surgery, radiation, or a combination of the three. Treatment-related complications respond to gastrointestinal decompression and supportive medical treatment.

PANCREATITIS

Pancreatitis may occur following immunosuppressive therapy particularly with L-asparaginase chemotherapy and systemic steroids. The primary symptom is severe abdominal pain that may or may not be associated with vomiting. Serum amylase levels may not be raised. Reported mortality rate is 5 to 15 percent.

Physical examination of patients with pancreatitis requires close attention to respiratory and cardiovascular status and abdominal examination. Severity of illness as measured by either Ranson's criteria or the revised Acute Physiology and Chronic Health Evaluation (APACHE II) correlates with outcome. Laboratory evaluation of patients should include complete blood counts and amylase, lipase, blood urea nitrogen, serum electrolyte, creatinine, glucose, lactate dehydrogenase, transaminase, and calcium levels. Abdominal ultrasound is the initial radiographic evaluation and should be obtained within 24-48 hours of hospitalization. Abdominal computed tomography (CT) scan is recommended for patients with severe pancreatitis. In the absence of renal insufficiency, IV contrast is recommended.

Treatment primarily is supportive with an emphasis on bowel rest, fluid resuscitation, and close electrolyte monitoring, particularly for hypocalcemia. Principal complications of pancreatitis include pseudocyst formation in approximately 17 percent of patients without trauma and bacterial infection in 20 to 30 percent of patients. Alterations in diet, total parenteral nutrition, proton pump inhibitors, H2-blocking agents and octreotide have been used in the medical treatment of these patients.

NEUROLOGIC EMERGENCIES

The main neurologic mechanical emergencies requiring acute medical treatment manifest as spinal cord compression, increased intracranial pressure (ICP) in association with cerebral herniation, and status epilepticus.

Spinal Cord Compression

Impingement of the spinal cord may occur due to an intramedullary primary CNS tumor or a tumor in the epidural space by direct extension of metastases in the vertebral bone or from tumor growth through intervertebral foramina.

Pain is the first symptom of spinal cord compression and may occur hours or months prior to neurologic dysfunction. Pain associated with epidural spinal cord compression is exacerbated in recumbent position and improves in upright position. Radicular pain is less common but important localizing symptom. Weakness usually occurs after the onset of pain followed by sensory complaints.

Magnetic resonance imaging (MRI) is the best diagnostic test to localize the disease and distinguish between tumor, abscess, hematoma, and disc herniation.

Spinal cord compression requires rapid intervention to minimize irreversible dysfunction. Acute treatment requires a combination of corticosteroids, radiation, surgery and chemotherapy.

Apart from appropriate analgesia, corticosteroid therapy is the usual initial treatment, particularly in presence of paresis. Use of systemic steroids is however contraindicated in favor of local radiation if symptoms are suspected to arise from an undiagnosed lymphoproliferative disease. Otherwise, high-dose or moderate-dose dexamethasone is the preferred treatment. Dexamethasone may be used in combination with radiotherapy and surgery as appropriate.

Local radiotherapy alone may be used for patients who are ambulatory and is determined by quantity of prior local radiation, tumor type, and the tissue field requiring radiation. Systemic chemotherapy is appropriate for responsive tumors.

Surgical intervention as a primary treatment for cord compression is restricted to an unstable spine, bony compression of the spinal cord, previously irradiated areas and no prior history of cancer.

Cerebral Herniation

Cerebral herniation may result from a tumor mass, hemorrhage, thrombosis, abscess, or infarction leading to expansion within the cranial vault or obstruction of cerebrospinal fluid circulation. Impending herniation may lead to impaired consciousness, abnormal extraocular movements, pupil size abnormality, nausea, emesis, and stiff neck. Papilledema is a more common finding if the presentation is subacute. Cushing reflex of hypertension and bradycardia are late signs of increased ICP.

If evidence exists of impending cerebral herniation, immediate treatment and diagnostic efforts are

A compensatory down-regulation of serum calcium often is present in patients with hyperphosphatemia. Administration of exogenous calcium should be avoided unless the ionized calcium is reduced significantly, since a product of greater than 50 to 60 when the serum calcium level is multiplied by the serum phosphate level may lead to precipitation, particularly in renal tubules. The potential for precipitation is increased due to the elevated urine pH level that is necessary to minimize uric acid precipitation. Treatment is critically dependent on adequate renal function. Acute renal failure and active TLS require early initiation of renal dialysis and appropriate modification of chemotherapeutic agents.

Hyperkalemia

It is severe if more than >6 mEq/L and rapid rate of rise or ECG changes and mild to moderate if more than >5.5 mEq/L or there is a rapid rate of rise. Potassium is removed from all IV fluids and ECG and cardiac monitoring is essential. Calcium gluconate may be given. Sodium bicarbonate is given in a dose of 1 to 2 mEq/kg IV over 5 to 10 min. seperately. If hyperkalemia persists, Insulin and glucose (0.1 U/kg regular insulin IV with 2 ml/kg 25 percent glucose q30-60 min) may be given with monitoring. Other options include Furosemide and sodium polystyrene resin in the dose of 1-2 g/kg with 3 ml sorbitol per gram resin PO q6h after sensitivity testing. Potassium binding resins may also be given in the form of rectal enemas.

Hyperphosphatemia

It can be treated with aluminum hydroxide (50-150 mg/kg/d divided q4-6h) or Isotonic sodium chloride solution bolus and IV mannitol 0.25 to 1.0 g/kg IV push. Dialysis may be required if >10 mg/dl or there is poor renal function. Compensatory hypocalcemia may coexist

Elevated Uric Acid

Hyperhydration along with Allopurinol is given in a dose of 300 mg/m^2/d PO/IV. Alkalinization of urine with sodium bicarbonate is done. Dialysis may be required if >10 mg/dl or there is renal failure. Best treatment is prophylaxis

METABOLIC EMERGENCIES

Hypercalcemia

Hypercalcemia refers to a serum calcium level greater than 10.5 mg/dl and usually results from increased bone resorption. It may be seen acute lymphoblastic leukemia,

non-Hodgkin lymphoma, pediatric renal tumors, astrocytoma, desmoplastic round cell tumor, solid tumors with significant bone metastasis and as a dose-limiting toxicity in 13-*cis*-retinoic acid treatment of patients with neuroblastoma.

In the absence of elevated serum protein levels, disturbances to other organ systems are observed at levels greater than 12.0-13.0 mg/dl; levels greater than 20 mg/dl may be fatal.

Clinical manifestations include neuropsychological, neuromuscular, gastrointestinal, cardiac, and renal symptoms like confusion, psychosis, seizure, obtundation, stupor, coma, fatigue, muscle weakness, hypotonia, hyporeflexia, nausea, vomiting, constipation, obstipation, ileus, bradycardia, atrial or ventricular arrhythmia and polyuria. ECG may show prolonged PR interval, shortened QT interval, and wide T wave

Pediatric patients with hypercalcemia may also present with bone pain. Bone pain may result from significant bone marrow infiltration by disease, pathologic fracture of severely demineralized bone, or direct osteolysis of bone caused by metastatic disease.

The pathophysiology underlying malignant hypercalcemia is excessive osteoclast-mediated bone resorption resulting from direct dysregulation of normal calcium homeostasis. Normal bone resorption is stimulated by parathyroid hormone (PTH), prostaglandin E_2, osteoclast-activating factor, other polypeptide growth factors, and osteoclasts derived from mononuclear phagocytes.

Blast cells from patients with ALL and AML have been shown to produce PTH in vitro. Hypercalcemia also has also been reported in presence of elevated prostaglandin E_2 levels in infants with mesoblastic nephroma or malignant rhabdoid tumor of the kidney. Elevated prostaglandin E_2 production also was suggested in a patient with primary disseminated Ewing sarcoma with hypercalcemia that improved following indomethacin treatment.

Transforming growth factor alpha is released as a result of osteoclast activity and increases PTHrP production by tumor cells. Tumor necrosis factor and interleukin 6 (IL-6) levels that are often increased in malignancy tend to increase osteoclast production and differentiation.

Treatment includes forced diuresis, calcitonin, corticosteroids, and mithramycin use. Recently, bisphosphonates which are potent inhibitors of osteoclast-mediated bone resorption have been found useful. They are safe, effective and appear to be useful for pain and osteoporosis as well. Treatment with bisphosphonates should be considered with a corrected serum calcium level greater than or equal to 12 mg/dl (3.0 mmol). Pamidronate which is 1000 times more potent than etidronate is used in a pediatric dose of 1 to 2 mg/kg/dose IV over 3 to 24 hr in malignancy-induced hypercalcemia, malignancy-induced bone pain, Paget disease and osteoporosis.

Hyponatremia

Severe hyponatremia (Serum Na < 125 mEq/L) can result from systemic illness, syndrome of inappropriate secretion of antidiuretic hormone (SIADH), or iatrogenically. Early mild hyponatremia may be asymptomatic. Symptoms of hyponatremia include anorexia, nausea, malaise that progress to headache, confusion, lethargy, seizure, coma, and death. Care should be taken that rapid changes of 1-2 mEq/L/h lead to cerebral edema and neurologic dysfunction. Severe life-threatening symptoms are seen at a serum sodium concentration of less than 105 mEq/L, or even if the level falls to 120 mEq/L within 24 hours.

Hyponatremia most often results from water retention combined with administration of normal or excessive amounts of fluid. Water retention is a consequence of antidiuretic hormone (ADH) release induced by decreased effective circulating intravascular volume.

Hyponatremia associated with edematous states is more common in patients with cancer and may result from liver disease, veno-occlusive disease, infection, drug toxicity, or multiple other etiologies. Hyponatremia associated with true volume depletion is less common and a consequent to identifiable fluid losses. Thus, hyponatremia results from disproportionate accumulation of water from administered hypotonic fluids.

Patients usually are oliguric with urine sodium levels less than 15 mEq/L. Excessive renal salt wasting also may cause hyponatremia and can result from drug-induced nephropathy, adrenal insufficiency, or use of thiazide diuretics. Patients with renal-induced hyponatremia usually are nonoliguric and have inappropriately high urine sodium levels.

Abnormal release of ADH also may result in hyponatremia, as in SIADH. Hyponatremia is secondary both to dilution of sodium from retention of free water and to progressive increase in urinary loss of sodium. SIADH is defined by an inappropriately elevated urine

osmolality in the context of decreased serum osmolality, and it frequently is associated with a urine sodium concentration greater than 20 mEq/L. The rate of development of hyponatremia depends on the rate and volume of fluid administration.

Cyclophosphamide is most commonly associated with impaired renal excretion of water. To a lesser extent, vincristine, vinblastine, melphalan, and thiotepa have had similar effects. SIADH associated with vincristine therapy may be coincident with severe vincristine neurotoxicity. Chemotherapy-induced nausea and emesis also produce a significant increase in plasma ADH levels independent of changes in serum osmolality or blood pressure. Therefore, highly emetogenic chemotherapy regimens, particularly when administered with hypotonic fluid hyperhydration, may lead to significant hyponatremia. SIADH has been reported to follow both major and minor surgical procedures, and 18 to 27 percent of patients may be affected following surgery of the head and neck. CNS tumors in the pediatric population are most commonly associated with SIADH. Failure to administer stress-dose levels of glucocorticoids to patients who are adrenally suppressed also results in hyponatremia.

Treatment is symptomatic and depends on underlying pathophysiology. In an asymptomatic patient, serum sodium concentrations should be corrected at a rate of less than or equal to 0.5 mEq/L/h during the first 24 hours of intervention or 12 mEq/L total. A more rapid correction of 1-2 mEq/L/h in the serum sodium concentration is indicated only if a patient is symptomatic. In symptomatic patients, rapid correction is indicated only for the first 1 to 3 hours of therapy, with a goal to improve the serum sodium concentration 12 to 15 mEq/L in the first 24 hours.

Management of fluid volume depends on underlying pathophysiology. In the setting of true extracellular hypovolemic hyponatremia, saline administration corrects hyponatremia and suppresses ADH secretion, thereby improving free water excretion. In patients with evidence of fluid retention, such as edema or ascites, treatment consists of salt and water restriction, improvement of effective intravascular volume, and direct treatment of any underlying disorder. Primary therapy for asymptomatic patients with SIADH is water restriction; however, administration of hypertonic 3 percent saline 2-4 mL/kg/dose with or without furosemide 1 mg/kg should be considered if CNS symptoms are present. Chronic SIADH may be managed using furosemide with or without salt tablets. Demeclocycline induces nephrogenic diabetes insipidus and can be used if control of SIADH is still inadequate.

Hypoglycemia

Hypoglycemia is defined as a serum glucose level of less than 40 mg/dl. Initial symptoms may occur at higher levels if the blood glucose level is decreased rapidly. Symptoms are worse in the early morning and may include weakness, dizziness, diaphoresis, and nausea. They may progress to diffuse neurologic deficits, seizure, coma, and death.

Hypoglycemia most commonly results from insulin-producing islet cell tumors that occur alone or as part of multiple endocrine neoplasia syndrome. Symptomatic hypoglycemia also may result from tumor production of compounds with low molecular weight with nonsuppressible insulinlike activity. These include insulinlike growth factor-1, insulinlike growth factor-2 (IGF-2), somatomedin A, and somatomedin C. Production of these substances extends beyond islet cell tumors as evidenced by the report of IGF-2–induced hypoglycemia by a pediatric renal tumor. Although excessive glucose use by large tumors is a possible cause of hypoglycemia, few data support this as an etiology in pediatric patients with malignancies.

Mild hypoglycemia may be managed best by increased frequency of feedings. More severe or symptomatic hypoglycemia may require corticosteroid and glucagon administration. Diazoxide is useful therapy for known hyperinsulinemia. Regardless of the type of treatment used, IV infusion of dextrose-containing solutions provides temporary support, and specific treatment of the underlying tumor provides definitive therapy.

Adrenal Insufficiency

Adrenal insufficiency though rare in pediatric oncology is secondary to adrenal suppression resulting from extended use of glucocorticoids at supraphysiologic doses combined with abrupt termination of therapy. Symptoms of adrenal insufficiency are exaggerated in the setting of physiologic stress and can manifest as mild acidosis, hyponatremia, and hypokalemia. Severe circulatory collapse and shock are uncommon.

Lactic Acidosis

Lactic acidosis is rare in pediatric patients and most frequently is associated with hypoperfusion and tissue hypoxia, as seen in patients with sepsis, low cardiac output, or extreme anemia. Treatment is directed at the underlying etiology. Serum lactate level greater than 4 mEq/L is associated with a poor prognosis.

EXTRAVASATION

Extravasation of chemotherapy products is reported to occur in 0.1-6.5 percent of chemotherapy infusions and may cause severe, irreversible, local injury. Chemotherapeutic agents may be classified as irritant, vesicant, or nonvesicant based on the local toxicity to subcutaneous tissues. Irritant drugs cause pain at the injection site and may be associated with local inflammation. Vesicant drugs cause local tissue necrosis or induce blister formation. Nonvesicant drugs produce acute reactions only occasionally.

Tissue damage from extravasation occurs via several mechanisms. Anthracycline drugs are absorbed by local cells, induce cell death through DNA damage, then are released to similarly affect other cells. Significant anthracycline levels are locally present for weeks to months following extravasation. Local tissue damage from vinca alkaloids and epipodophyllotoxins results from the lipophilic solvents used in the drug preparations and is treated more easily. Ulcers have been reported following extravasation of vinblastine and dacarbazine [Adamai].

In general, residual drugs should be aspirated from the infiltrated area, and antidotes, if available, should be administered soon after extravasation. Table 61.2 gives an outline for the management for some agents. Direct pressure should be avoided on the local site to minimize risk of spread to a broader area. Heat or cold may be applied appropriately. Ice packs may be applied for Mitomycin C extravasation.[22] Warm packs should be applied locally for extravasation of Vinca alkaloids and concentrated epipodophyllotoxins.[22] Hyaluronidase may be used for vinca alkaloids, epipodophyllotoxins, and paclitaxel.[22] Daily evaluation of the effected area is recommended. Prevention is the best cure for extravasation and for this utmost nursing care is required.[23]

HYPERSENSITIVITY REACTIONS

Hypersensitivity reactions may occur following administration of some chemotherapy agents like taxanes and L-asparaginase, and their administration requires the use of premedication to prevent these reactions.[22] Once a reaction has occurred, therapy may

Table 61.2: Guidelines for extravasation of some chemotherapeutic agents

Agent	Antidote

Anthracyclines
  • Doxorubicin
  • Daunorubicin
	Dimethyl sulfoxide topically 6 hourly for 2-4 days

Plant alkaloids
  • Vinca alkaloids
    (Vincristine, Vinblastine)
  • Epipodophyllotoxins
    (Etoposide)
	Hyaluronidase 150-900 U SC/IDin isotonic saline injected intolocal site

Other
  • Mechlorethamine
  • Cisplatin
	Sodium thiosulfate (10%) 4 ml with 5 ml sterile water injected into local site

be continued by using an analog drug or by the administration of premedication as prophylaxis if the reaction was minor.

TOXICITIES DUE TO BIOLOGICAL AGENTS

It is pertinent to be acquainted with the emergencies induced by biological agents, taking into consideration their increasing usages. These include interferons, interleukin-2 (IL-2), cytokine-toxin fusion proteins (DAB3891L-2) and monoclonal antibodies

REFERENCES

1. West, Daniel C, Marcin, James P, et al. Children With Cancer, Fever, and Treatment-Induced Neutropenia: Risk Factors Associated With Illness Requiring the Administration of Critical Care Therapies. Pediatric Emergency Care 2004;20:79-84.
2. Hughes WT, Armstrong D, Bodey GP, et al. 1997 guidelines for the use of antimicrobial agents in neutropenic patients with unexplained fever. Infectious Diseases Society of America. Clin Infect Dis 1997;25:551-73.
3. Quadri TL, Brown AE. Infectious complications in the critically ill patient with cancer. SeminOncol 2000;27:335-46.
4. Klaassen R J, Allen U, Doyle J. Randomized Placebo-Controlled Trial of Oral Antibiotics in Pediatric Oncology Patients at Low-Risk With Fever and Neutropenia. Journal of Pediatric Hematology/Oncology 2000;22:405-11.
5. Bunin NJ, Pui CH. Differing complications of hyperleukocytosis in children with acute lymphoblastic or acute nonlymphoblastic leukemia. J Clin Oncol 1985;3:1590-5.
6. Azizkhan RG, Dudgeon DL, Buck JR, et al. Life-threatening airway obstruction as a complication to the management of mediastinal masses in children. J Pediatr Surg 1985;20:816-22.
7. Cohen IJ, Loven D, Schoenfeld T, et al. Dactinomycin potentiation of radiation pneumonitis: a forgotten interaction. Pediatr Hematol Oncol 1991;8:187-92.
8. Dai MS, Ho CL, Chen YC, et al. Acute respiratory distress syndrome following intrathecal methotrexate administration: a case report and review of literature. Ann Hematol 2000;79:696-9.
9. Frankel SR, Eardley A, Lauwers G, et al. The "retinoic acid syndrome" in acute promyelocytic leukemia. Ann Intern Med 1992;117:292-6.
10. Bux J, Becker F, Seeger W, et al. Transfusion-related acute lung injury due to HLA-A2-specific antibodies in recipient and NB1-specific antibodies in donor blood. Br J Haematol 1996;93: 707-13.
11. Gordon J, Akhtar S, Thorpe A. Recurrent Wilms tumour presenting as bilateral pneumothoraces. Eur J Cardiothorac Surg. 2003;23:645-6.
12. Janin Y, Becker J, Wise L, et al. Superior vena cava syndrome in childhood and adolescence: a review of the literature and report of three cases. J Pediatr Surg 1982;17:290-5.
13. King DR, Patrick LE, Ginn- Pease ME, et al. Pulmonary function is compromised in children with mediastinal lymphoma. J Pediatr Surg 1997;32:294.
14. Maity A, Goldwein JW, Lange BJ, et al. Mediastinal masses in children with Hodgkin's disease. Cancer 1992;69:2755.
15. Bertsch H, Rudoler S, Needle MN, et al. Emergent/ urgent therapeutic irradiation in pediatric oncology: patterns of presentation, treatment and outcome. Med Pediatr Oncol 1998; 30:101.
16. Loeffler JS, Leopold KA, Recht A, et al. Emergency prebiopsy radiation for mediastinal masses. Impact on subsequent pathologic diagnosis and outcome. J Clin Oncol 1986;4:716.
17. da Costa CM, de Camargo B, Gutierrez y Lamelas R, et al. Cardiac tamponade complicating hyperleukocytosis in a child with leukemia. Med Pediatr Oncol 1999;33:120-3; discussion 124.
18. Medary I, Steinherz LJ, Aronson DC, La Quaglia MP. Cardiac tamponade in the pediatric oncology population: treatment by percutaneous catheter drainage. J Pediatr Surg 1996;31:197-9; discussion 199-200.
19. Yao JL, Zhou H, Roche K, et al. Adenomyoma arising in a meckel diverticulum: case report and review of the literature. Pediatr Dev Pathol 2000;3:497-500.
20. Furuta GT, Bross DA, Doody D, Kleinman RE. Intussusception and leiomyosarcoma of the gastrointestinal tract in a pediatric patient. Case report and review of the literature. Dig Dis Sci 1993;38:1933-7.
21. Hulbert WC Jr, Valvo JR, Caldamone AA, et al. Intussusception following resection of Wilms tumor. Urology 1983;21:578-80.
22. Albanell J, Baselga J. Systemic therapy emergencies. Semin Oncol 2000;27:347-61.
23. Adami N P, Rivero M G, Montosa S, Magalhães E P. Risk management of extravasation of cytostatic drugs at the Adult Chemotherapy Outpatient Clinic of a university hospital. Journal of Clinical Nursing 2005;14:876.

Long-term Results in Pediatric Surgical Oncology

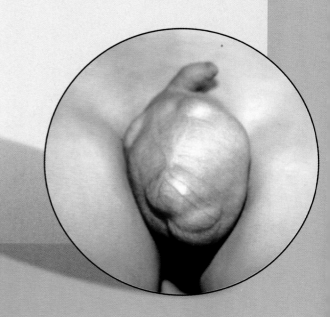

CHAPTER 62

Scong Min Kim
Seung Hoon Choi

Long-term Follow-up of Wilms' Tumor

Wilms' tumor is a primary renal tumor of embryonic origin and usually presents in childhood. It makes up about 5-6 percent of all pediatric malignant neoplasms. Wilms' tumor is the fifth most common pediatric tumor, after CNS tumors, lymphoma, neuroblastoma, and soft tissue sarcomas. Unlike other malignant neoplasms, Wilms' tumors usually have a potential for cure. During the past twenty years, the treatment outcomes have improved, mostly due to the refinement of surgical technique and multimodal treatment regimen, including perioperative adjuvant chemotherapy and radiotherapy. We retrospectively studied pathologically confirmed Wilms' tumor patients at Yonsei University Medical Center Severance Hospital who underwent a nephrectomy during a 20-year period, from March 1986 to March 2005. Specific operations performed included ipsilateral nephrectomy and lymph node sampling for unilateral Wilms' tumor, and ipsilateral nephrectomy and contralateral partial nephrectomy or biopsy. We followed the NWTS (National Wilms' Tumor Study Group) protocol recommendation regarding chemotherapy, using EE-4A (pulse-intensive vincristine + actinomycin D for 18 weeks). If the tumor showed unfavorable histology, doxorubicin was added to the regimen (DD-4A, including doxorubicin for 24 weeks). If the tumor recurred after the initial course of chemotherapy, we adopted the ICE regimen (ifosfamide + carboplatin +VP-16). Postoperative radiation therapy was performed if the tumor was incompletely resected, or in the case of distant metastasis, tumor cell anaplasia, postoperative local relapse, the bilateral Wilms' tumor, or gross tumor cell emboli. We retrospectively analyzed

the patients (based on admission records) in terms of their gender, age at operation, clinical signs and symptoms, associated anomalies, pathologic findings, clinical stage, postoperative morbidity and mortality, overall five-year survival rate, and disease-free survival rate. In addition, we also analyzed risk factors affecting tumor recurrence and patient survival. During the twenty-year period, 68 patients were pathologically diagnosed with Wilms' tumor after receiving a nephrectomy for a primary renal tumor. Those patients with clear cell sarcomas or rhabdoid tumors were excluded from this study. Mean age at diagnosis was 25 months (range: 2-130 months). Forty patients (58.8%) were male, and 28 (41.2%) were female. Male-to-female ratio was 1.4:1. Primary signs and symptoms included a palpable abdominal mass in 62 patients (91.2%), gross hematuria in 14 (20.6%), severe low abdominal pain in eight (11.8%), fever in six (8.8%), and one case of nausea and vomiting (1.5%). None of the patients diagnosed with Wilms' tumor in this study were asymptomatic, and none were diagnosed as the result of an incidental finding. In terms of associated anomalies, two patients demonstrated cryptorchidism (3.0%). Five other patients were found to have anomalies including ureteral duplication, congenital blindness, horseshoe kidney, hypospadias, and nephroblastomatosis. Primary tumors were discovered in the right kidney of 25 patients (36.8%), in the left kidney of 39 (57.4%), and bilaterally in four (5.9%). In terms of histologic findings, 53 demonstrated the favorable type (77.9%), while 15 demonstrated the unfavorable type (22.1%). At the time of diagnosis, 60 patients presented did not present with distant metastasis (88.2%). Five patients presented with lung metastasis (7.4%), and three presented with liver metastasis (4.4%). Clinically, 19 patients were classified as stage I (27.9%), 25 as stage II (36.8%), 12 as stage III (17.6%), eight as stage IV (11.8%), and four as stage V (5.9%) (Table 62.1).

Twenty-seven patients received preoperative neoadjuvant chemotherapy (39.7%), whereas 41 patients received a primary nephrectomy without chemotherapy (60.3%). Twenty-seven patients (39.7%) received radiation therapy. The median follow-up period after operation was eight years and two months (range: 24 days – 18 years and 6 months). The overall five-year survival and five-year disease-free survival rate was 87.0 percent and 76.9 percent, respectively (Fig. 62.1). During the follow-up period, 12 patients (17.6%) died: disease-specific in nine, disease-unrelated in three (Table 62.2). Univariate survival analysis showed that significant prognostic factors affected survival, including the age of the patient (two years of age, $p=0.0287$), tumor rupture during operation ($p=0.0134$), tumor cell anaplasia ($p=0.0414$), and the pathologic stage of the tumors ($p=0.0132$) (Fig. 62.2). Multivariate survival analysis showed that tumor rupture during operation was the most important prognostic factor affecting patient survival (Exp(^{2} P;â–) = 4.455) (Table 62.3). The overall five-year survival of the 33 patients who received an operation for Wilms' P;â– tumor between 1986 and 1995 was 78.1 percent, while the overall five-year survival of the 35 patients who received an operation for Wilms P;â– tumor between 1996 and 2005 was 96.0 percent. The difference in survival rate based on treatment period proved to be statistically significant (Fig. 62.3) ($p=0.0232$).

The treatment of Wilms' tumor is divided into two protocols: one is that of the International Society of Pediatric Oncology (SIOP), and the other is that of the National Wilms' Tumor Study (NWTS) Group. The protocol of the SIOP is composed of initial clinical staging by physical examination, radiologic evaluation, and neoadjuvant chemotherapy. The tumor burden is reduced after preoperative chemotherapy, facilitating resection of the tumor and reducing the total amount of postoperative chemotherapy and radiotherapy. In addition, if complete remission of a metastatic lesion does occur after neoadjuvant chemotherapy, SIOP protocol can downstage the tumor, which may already present distant metastasis at initial diagnosis. Nevertheless, peritumoral adhesion secondary to

necroinflammatory changes after neoadjuvant chemotherapy makes precise dissection between tumor and normal tissue more difficult. However, it is that adhesion that also minimizes the likelihood of tumor rupture during operation and subsequent peritoneal tumor seeding and local recurrence. The SIOP protocol has a few pitfalls: neoadjuvant chemotherapy is performed without histopathologic confirmation, so there is a possibility that a patient with a benign or borderline tumor may receive chemotherapy. Likewise, patients with a more serious tumor (or tumors with highly malignant potential) may be undertreated, instead receiving a reduced dosage of chemotherapy. In the results of SIOP-9, 2 percent of the patients who received neoadjuvant chemotherapy without tumor biopsy did indeed have a benign tumor, and 3 percent were found to have a malignant renal tumor other than a Wilms' tumor. Therefore, transcutaneous tumor biopsy is highly, recommended in cases where preoperative neoadjuvant chemotherapy will be used as a treatment modality. The protocol for NWTS is composed of an initial nephrectomy and lymph node sampling, histological confirmation of the tumor, and pathologic staging followed by postoperative adjuvant chemotherapy. NWTS protocol has the advantage of proper chemotherapy relevant to stage of the tumor. However, if the tumor size is very large, or if the tumor has formed an adhesion to adjacent great vessels or other organs, resection is often impossible, and the chance of postoperative complications (such as intraoperative tumor rupture) increases. In this study, we did not solely follow either the SIOP or NWTS protocol. Our treatments were divided into either initial nephrectomy or initial neoadjuvant chemotherapy. The latter therapy was adopted for stage IV patients who presented with either a distant metastatic lesion at the time of diagnosis, encasement of great vessels by the tumor, tight adhesion of the tumor to adjacent organs, or a large tumor not amenable to resection. For these tumors, we were able to perform a safer nephrectomy after initial neoadjuvant chemotherapy. One of the problems of the SIOP protocol is overstaging. First, lymph node enlargement in radiologic study is often discovered intraoperatively to be secondary to nonspecific lymphadenopathy rather than metastasis of the tumor. Second, even if the tumor seems to be tightly adhered to an adjacent organ and determined unresectable upon radiologic evaluation, the tumor may in fact be easily separated from the adjacent organ, mainly because often the adhesion is actually a result of

Table 62.1: Patient (n=68) demographics and clinical parameters	
Demographics, clinical parameters	*Number (%)*
Gender	
Male 40 (58.8%)	
Female	28 (41.2%)
Age at diagnosis (years)	
< 2 33 (48.5%)	
2–4	19 (27.9%)
> 4 16 (23.5%)	
Initial clinical presentation	
Palpable abdominal mass	62 (91.2%)
Gross hematuria	14 (20.6%)
Abdominal pain	8 (11.8%)
Fever 6 (8.8%)	
Nausea/vomiting	1 (1.5%)
Asymptomatic	0 (0.0%)
Associated anomaly	
Cryptorchidism	2 (3.0%)
Ureter duplication	1 (1.5%)
Congenital blindness	1 (1.5%)
Horseshoe Kidney	1 (1.5%)
Hypospadia	1 (1.5%)
Nephroblastomatosis	1 (1.5%)
Tumor characteristics	
Laterality	
Right	25 (36.8%)
Left	39 (57.4%)
Bilateral	4 (5.9%)
Histology	
Favorable	53 (77.9%)
Unfavorable	15 (22.1%)
Initial metastasis	
No	60 (88.2%)
Lung 5 (7.4%)	
Liver 3 (4.4%)	
Clinical stage	
I	19 (27.9%)
II	25 (36.8%)
III	12 (17.6%)
IV	8 (11.8%)
V	4 (5.9%)

Table 62.2: Mortality cases after surgery (n=12)

Sex	Age (months)	Histology	Initial meta.	Pathologic staging	Late meta.	Neoadj. CTx	LR	Cause of death	Duration (months)
Disease specific death (n=9)									
F	60	Anaplasia	No	II (sp.)	No	No	Yes	LR	22
F	120	FH	No	III (sp.)	Liver	No	Yes	LR, liver	18
F	30	FH	No	II	Liver	Yes	Yes	LR, liver	15
M	99	Anaplasia	No	III (sp.)	Brain, lung	No	Yes	Brain, lung	32
M	50	Anaplasia	Liver	IV	Liver, testis	No	No	Liver	28
M	102	FH	No	II (sp.)	Lung	Yes	No	Lung	63
M	7	UH	No	III	Lung	No	No	Lung	11
M	2	FH	No	III (sp.)	No	No	Yes	LR	54
M	78	FH	Liver	IV	Lung	No	No	Lung	10
Disease unrelated death (n=3)									
M	49	UH	Lung	IV	No	Yes	No	D-CMP	28
M	31	FH	No	I	No	No	No	ALL (L-2)	162
M	5	FH	No	V	No	No	No	ARF	0.8

Abbreviations: Meta., Metastasis; Neoadj. CTx, Neoadjuvant chemotherapy; LR, Locoregional recurrence; Sp., Tumor spillage or rupture during surgery; FH/UH, Favorable histology/unfavorable histology;

D-CMP, Dilated cardiomyopathy; ALL, Acute lymphocytic leukemia; ARF, Acute renal failure

Table 62.3: Multivariate analysis of prognostic factors affecting overall survival of Wilms' tumor patients (Cox regression analysis)

	B	df	Sig.	Exp (B)	95% CI for Lower	Exp (B) Upper
Age (>2yr or <2yr)	1.25	1	0.273	3.494	0.373	32.752
Tumor spillage	1.494	1	0.031	4.455	1.145	17.341
Tumor anaplasia	1.412	1	0.070	4.104	0.891	18.905
Pathologic stage	0.630	1	0.091	1.877	0.905	3.892

Abbreviations: df., Degree of freedom; Sig., Significance; CI, Confidence interval;

[†]Tumor spillage was also the most important factor in recurrence-free survival

inflammation rather than tumor advancement. In this study, tumors were larger than those reported in other studies for a relative number of patients in clinical stages I and II. The median age at the time of operation was 25 months. These are due to earlier diagnosis of Wilms' tumor than in other studies. Thirty-three patients (48.5%) demonstrated a discrepancy between clinical stage and pathologic stage. These were divided into two groups: 18 patients had downstaging of tumor pathologic stage and 15 had upstaging of tumor pathologic stage (Table 62.4). The former condition was due to downstaging of the tumor after successful neoadjuvant chemotherapy or after a radiologically overstaged tumor was proven to be less advanced. The latter condition was due to overstaging of the tumor in the case of intraoperative tumor dissemination, or if the tumor cell showed unfavorable histology. In these circumstances, postoperative adjuvant therapy should be adopted as protocol dictates. In this study surgical rupture of the tumor was the most important prognostic factor affecting survival and recurrence (Relative risk = 4.5).

Surgical rupture is defined as intraoperative tumor transection and/or peritoneal dissemination of tumor

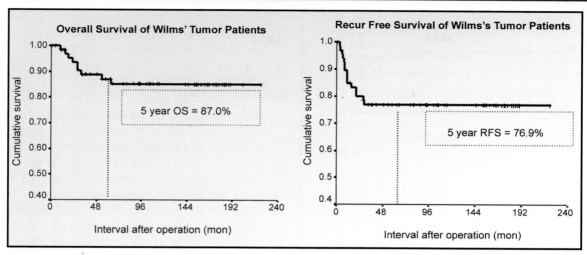

Figure 62.1: Overall survival (OS) and recurrence-free survival (RFS) of 68 Wilms' tumor patients (Overall five-year survival = 87.0 percent, five-year recurrence-free survival = 76.9 percent)

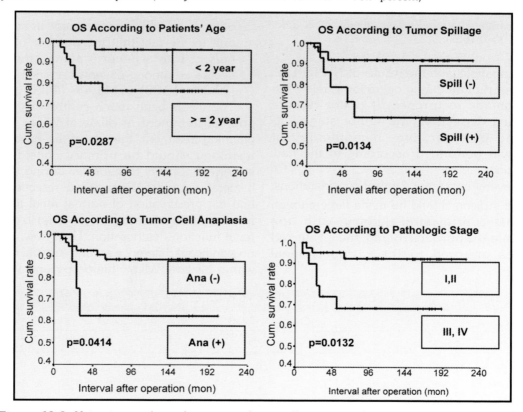

Figure 62.2: Univariate analysis of prognostic factors affecting overall survival (OS) of Wilms' tumor patients (using Log rank test) according to patients' age, tumor spillage, tumor cell anaplasia, and pathologic stage

cells during operation. However, it does not imply tumor dissemination after preoperative tumor biopsy or minimal tumor spillage. In general, tumor rupture seems to be highly related to local recurrence. In our multivariate survival analysis, tumor rupture was also the most important independent prognostic factor affecting local recurrence and survival of the patients. Considering tumor histology and pathologic stage,

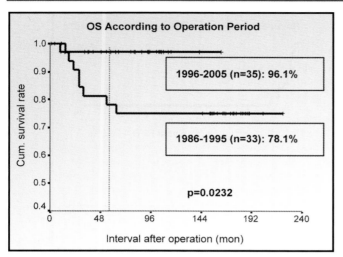

Figure 62.3: Five-year overall survival (OS) of the Wilms' tumor patients according to the operation period (using Log rank test *p*=0.0232). Five-year recurrence-free survival (not shown) also demonstrated a trend toward improvement (from 69.6% to 84.5%, *p*=0.1667).

which were compatible with the results of NWTS-1, 2, 3 in which tumor rupture during operation is related to infra-diaphragmatic recurrence. If tumor rupture occurred during dissection, the tumor stage was upgraded, and postoperative chemotherapy or radiotherapy was performed according to the new pathologic staging.

There are several important surgical considerations:

1. A transverse incision should be made large enough to see the contralateral kidney with the transperitoneal approach being the preferred method (as opposed to the retroperitoneal approach).

2. Initial ligation of the proximal portion of renal vessels decreases blood loss during operation and minimizes the chance of hematolymphangitic metastasis.

3. Capsular tearing causes tumor cells to disseminate into the peritoneal cavity; and

4. Formal lymph node dissection of the perirenal, periaortic area is unnecessary and even harmful (e.g. causing formation of chylous ascites), though it helps to select proper chemotherapeutic agents. In this study, the overall five-year survival was increased from 76 percent (between 1986 and 1995, n=33, early period) to 96 percent (between 1996 and 2005, n=35, later period). The pathologic stage and frequency of neoadjuvant chemotherapy were not statistically different in each period. This improved survival may introduce study bias, as the patients in the later period had a shorter follow-up period as compared with patients in the earlier period. On the other hand, this improvement in survival may be due to the fact that the number of patients who present with a tumor rupture during surgery has decreased among patients classified in a later stage (30.3% (10/33) vs. 11.4% (4/35), *p*=0.054).

There has been much controversy regarding the optimal treatment of bilateral Wilms' tumor. When planning treatment, the age of the patients and tumor histology should be primary considerations. Two important aspects to consider during surgery for the bilateral tumor are the complete resection of the tumor and the preservation of normal renal tissue and renal function during dissection (if possible) in order to prevent renal function deterioration. Until now, there has been no significant difference among survival rates of patients with a bilateral Wilms' tumor, patients who underwent

		Pathologic stage					
		I	*II*	*III*	*IV*	*V*	*Total*
	I	13	6	0	0	0	19(27.9%)
Clinical	II	9	7	9	0	0	25(36.8%)
stage	III	1	7	4	0	0	12(17.6%)
	IV	0	1	0	7	0	8(11.8%)
	V	0	0	0	0	4	4(5.9%)
Total		23(33.8%)	21(30.9%)	13(19.1%)	7(10.3%)	4(5.9%)	68

Table 62.4: Clinical stage and pathologic stage of the 68 patients

Clinical stage is based on preoperative ultrasonography (US), computerized tomography (CT), and physical examination. Pathologic stage is based on tumor histopathology after operation

		Pre-op				Post-op		Post-op				RFS	
Sex	Age (months)	bx.	Neo	RK	LK	Histology CTx				Recur (months)	Survival	(months)	Remark
F	38	+	+	Tot	Par	FH	+	+	LK, Lung	142	28		
F	40	+	+	Par	Tot	FH	+	+	-	95	95	Horseshoe kidney
M	5	-	-	Par	Tot	FH	-	-	-	-	-	Death from ARF
F	10	+	+	Par†	Par	FH	+	+	-	5	5	

Table 62.5: Bilateral Wilms' tumor patients (n=4)

Abbreviations: Pre-op bx., Preoperative biopsy; Neo, Neoadjuvant chemotherapy; RK, Right kidney; LK, Left kidney; Post-op CTx, Postoperative chemotherapy; Post-op. RTx, Postoperative radiotherapy; RFS, Recurrence-free survival; Tot, Total nephrectomy; Par, Partial Nephrectomy; †Resection margin positive

an initial tumor biopsy and received neoadjuvant chemotherapy and surgery, and the patients who received an initial nephrectomy followed by postoperative adjuvant chemotherapy. We recommend an initial tumor biopsy with neoadjuvant chemotherapy, followed by surgery. After neoadjuvant chemotherapy, the tumor should be reevaluated for any changes in tumor diameter or changes in tumor advancement. If the size of the tumor remains unchanged, then surgery should be performed, i.e., a partial nephrectomy, including tumor or wedge resection.

Postoperative radiation therapy for the patients with a bilateral Wilms' tumor is selectively performed according to the effectiveness of previous therapy. In our study, four patients who were diagnosed with a bilateral Wilms' tumor (Table 62.5) were treated with an initial unilateral nephrectomy and contralateral partial nephrectomy or wedge biopsy, followed by postoperative adjuvant chemotherapy. Partial nephrectomies should be performed only if postoperative deterioration of renal function is unlikely. If postoperative renal failure dose occur, peritoneal dialysis and renal transplantation should be considered.

Recently, organ preservation surgery has been favored over aggressive surgery, even in the treatment of selective malignant neoplasms. The use of a partial nephrectomy in the treatment of Wilms' tumor has been a matter of debate. NWTS-5 does not recommend a partial nephrectomy, but patients with a unilateral, small-sized tumor diagnosed early may benefit from a partial

nephrectomy, which is comparable to a conventional en-bloc resection of the tumor.

Benefits and toxicities of perioperative chemotherapeutic agents have long been debated, especially in cases involving young infants diagnosed before 12 months of age. The dosage should be reduced to half of the proper dosage. Dose reduction of chemotherapeutic agents in young infants not only reduced toxicity, but also maintained a treatment outcome comparable to conventional dosage. Regular liver function tests should be performed after chemotherapy treatment because veno-occlusive disease may occur following chemotherapy. Most of the patients with intestinal obstruction secondary to adhesion improve by non-operative management. One patient in our study received an operation for intestinal obstruction. This case comprises 1.5 percent of the total patients, and comprises 3.7 percent of patients who received adjuvant chemotherapy. This still represents a lower incidence rate than evident in other reports. Three patients in our study died after multimodal treatment secondary to causes other than cancer: one patient as a result of a dilated cardiomyopathy, one due to acute renal failure, and one due to acute lymphoblastic leukemia. Cardiomyopathy is related radiation therapy and/or doxorubicin toxicity. Acute renal failure is related to the abrupt reduction and deterioration of renal function after surgery. The incidence of a secondary malignancy increases during or after treatment, and is usually associated with the intensity of radiation therapy, doxorubicin use, and/or genetic predisposition.

CHAPTER 63

PA Kurkure
B Arora

Late Effects in Childhood Cancer Survivors: Current Scenario and Future Challenges

INTRODUCTION

Not long ago, it could be said that 'If some one lived long enough to develop long-term complications after childhood cancer, we would jump for joy and treat the complication.' Much has changed since then. Survival after the diagnosis of cancer in children has become a rule rather than an exception. Currently, more than 70 percent of children with cancer in developed countries survive at least 5 years and most survivors are cured.[1] For most childhood cancers, survival without relapse for 5 years after diagnosis means cure. More than 90 percent patients, who are relapse-free at 5 years after diagnosis survive after 15 years of follow-up and are cured.[2] Consequent to this success arise challenges inherent in coordinating life long health care for a high risk group of patients predisposed to a variety of cancer related complications. Cancer-related sequelae that persist or develop 5 years after the cancer diagnosis are termed late effects. As there is a burgeoning population of vulnerable aging adult survivors, there is a pressing need to study the late effects of childhood cancer and adverse health outcomes in the context of organ senescence.

An awareness of the potential long-term complications is important not only for optimizing health care of the current survivors but also for modifying future treatment protocols to avoid therapies that are associated with unacceptable morbidity and mortality. In this article we attempt to summate the current evidence relating to late consequences of cure, burden of problem in our country, future challenges and possible strategies for long-term follow-up of this growing population with unique health care needs.

MAGNITUDE OF BURDEN

It has been estimated that in USA, the prevalence of childhood cancer survivors is expected to increase from 1 in 900 among young adults to 1 in 250 persons by 2010.[3] It is estimated that approximately 30 to 40,000 new cases of childhood cancer occur in India annually. Even with conservative estimates of 10-20 percent long-term cure, approximately 3.5 to 7,000 survive.[4] This is 8 to 10 times the annual number of survivors in UK.[5]

Two-third of survivors are known to have at least one late effect of their cancer therapy and of these, one third have serious or life threatening complications.[6] More than 50 percent of survivors have at least one major adverse outcome of their health status due to cancer therapy, which compromises their quality of life. The incidence of most late effects increases with age, often becoming clinically apparent decades after therapy.[7]

This high-risk highly heterogeneous population is catered by a wide array of health care professionals apart from oncologists including physicians, pediatricians, psychiatrists and surgeons, many of whom may not be adequately sensitized to the unique health care needs of this group. Since many of the potential late effects can be ameliorated by prevention or early diagnosis with therapeutic intervention, a specialized and structured plan for life-long surveillance and prevention based on risks inherent to primary cancer and cancer therapy is required for each survivor.

DETERMINANTS OF LATE EFFECTS

Management of a child with cancer is always a balancing act, weighing the need for cure against the risk of late effects. Accordingly, the cure and late effects share a common foundation i.e. treatment intensity. The degree of late effects is essentially a function of 3 types of factors (Fig. 63.1) which include (a) Tumor related factors such as histology, site and biology (b) Treatment related factors such as type of radiation therapy(dose/ fraction size/volume/machine energy), chemotherapy (type/ dose/ schedule), and surgery (site / technique) and (c) Host related factors such as developmental status, genetic predisposition, organ function, premorbid state, inherent tissue sensitivity and capacity of normal tissue repair. Organ senescence in aging survivors may accelerate the presentation of health conditions in survivors with subclinical organ dysfunction resulting form cancer treatment. Health behaviors such as dietary intake, physical activity, tobacco and alcohol use, sun exposure may also impact upon the adverse health outcomes of cancer treatment. Lastly, sociodemographic factors such as income, educational attainment and socioeconomic status may influence access to health care services.

Consequences of Cure: In the following section, the more common or serious problems experienced by the survivors with a focus on each therapeutic modality and its attendant complications are discussed:

Radiation Therapy (RT): Apart from attacking the malignant tissues, ionizing radiation may destroy the normal surrounding tissue also. It is particularly toxic to the rapidly growing organs of children and young adults. The degree and spectrum of RT-related late effects depends upon many factors including; site of RT, type of radiation used, age of the patient, total dose and fraction size, tissue volume, machine energy and delivery techniques. The prime determinant of type of RT-related toxicity is the site of radiation therapy and the effects are described below in major RT sites.

Head and Neck Radiation therapy: The common solid tumors in this region requiring RT are brain tumors, soft tissue sarcomas, retinoblastoma and nasopharyngeal carcinomas. Dose and volume of RT varies for different tumor types and location.

Major side effects include:

Neurocognitive Sequelae

Many studies evaluating brain tumours survivors have found cognitive deficits in a variety of areas including general intelligence, academic achievement, visual as well as perceptual motor skills, non-verbal or verbal memory, language and attention span.[8,9] Younger age at the time of treatment, high dose of cranial RT, tumor site in cerebral hemisphere, and presence of hydrocephalus with a shunt have been found to be adverse risk factors for cognitive deficits.[10] A correlation has been demonstrated between volume of white matter loss and intelligence quotient (IQ).[11] After 36 Gy cranial RT, approximately 75 percent survivors may have sub-optimal IQ (< 80).[12] A childhood cancer survivors study (CCSS) found that brain tumor survivors are less likely to complete school and college and more likely to require special educational services than siblings.[13]

Neuroendocrine Problems

Approximately 60 to 80 percent of pediatric brain tumor patients receiving cranial RT >30 Gy develop growth hormone deficiency within 5 years of treatment (Figs 63.2A and B).[14] Additionally, there is higher incidence of gonadotropin deficiency, precocious puberty, obesity and short stature in young girls with brain tumors.[15,16] Central hypothyroidism may occur in 65 percent of patients with brain tumour or nasopharyngeal carcinoma after radiation therapy.[17] Radiation to thyroid may also cause primary hypothyroidism and incidence may be 50 percent in those receiving more than 45 Gy RT to thyroid.[18] Figure 63.3 shows a patient who developed hyperthyroidism after neck P-T.

Psychosocial and Other Effects

Approximately 25 to 93 percent of survivors in different studies have been found to have psychological

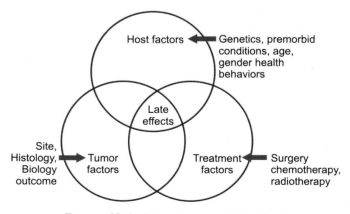

Figure 63.1: Determinants of late effects

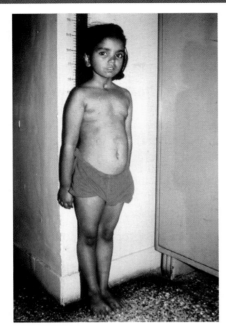

Figure 63.2A: Hypopituitarism in a survivor of childhood nasopharyngeal carcinoma after radiation therapy

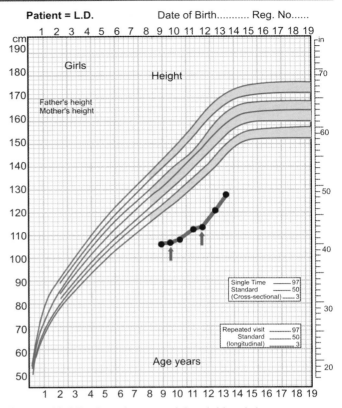

Figure 63.2B: Growth curve of the child with hypopituitarism showing response to hormonal therapy

maladjustment.[19] There is also high incidence of post-traumatic stress disorder in survivors and their parents.[20] Furthermore, cranial RT may also increase the risk of second malignant neoplasms (meningiomas and gliomas),[21] cataract,[22] dental problems[23] and hearing problems.[24] Doses exceeding 20 Gy to developing teeth may cause root shortening, abnormal curvature, dwarfism and hypocalcification.[23] More than 85 percent patients with head and neck sarcomas have dental problems including mandibular or maxillary hypoplasia, increased caries, hypodontia, root stunting and xerostomia.[25] Salivary gland irradiation may cause significant xerostomia as well as dental caries.[26]

Chest Radiation Therapy

RT to chest is used in cases of sarcomas overlying chest and in metastases of Wilms' tumor or sarcomas to lungs. RT to chest can increase the risk of breast cancer, cardiac disease and pulmonary disease. Incidence of breast cancer after exposure to RT is high if patient is treated before 21 years of age and continues to increase with age. Early diagnosis with screening mammography is likely to improve the outcome of breast cancer in this group.[27] RT damages the vasculature of heart and can cause coronary artery disease (CAD), pericarditis, pancarditis with endocardial fibroelastosis, myopathy,

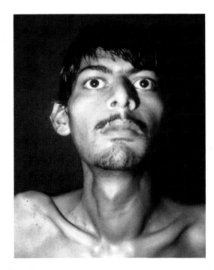

Figure 63.3: Hyperthyroidism in a survivor after Neck RT

valvular injury and conduction defects.[28] It has been suggested that cardiac radiation of < 25 Gy may be safe for the heart.[29] In addition, other risk factors for CAD such as obesity, hypertension, smoking, diabetes and hypercholestremia are likely to impact upon the frequency of cardiac morbidity in these patients.[30] RT exacerbates the anthracycline-induced cardiac toxicity in children.

RT-induced pulmonary toxicity may present as acute pneumonitis after doses exceeding 40 Gy when given alone or at lower doses, if given along with dactinomycin or anthracyclines. Furthermore, chronic lung dysfunction in the form of abnormal diffusion capacity, decreased vital capacity and obstructive or restrictive flow pattern has been seen in wilms' tumor survivors given RT of 12-14 Gy.[31] In CCSS study, survivors had increased risk of long fibrosis, recurrent pneumonia, chronic cough, pleurisy, use of supplemental oxygen, bronchitis and exercise-induced shortness of breath compared to their siblings with relative risk ranging from 1.2 to 13.[32] Lung cancer is infrequent after chest RT in non-smoking patients.[33]

Abdomino-pelvic Radiation Therapy

Major organs affected by abdomino-pelvic RT include liver, spleen, gastrointestinal tract (GIT), genitourinary tract and gonads.

Hepatic Toxicity

Cumulative dose, volume of liver irradiated and concomitant use of chemotherapy are important risk factors for RT induced hepatopathy. Radiation hepatopathy can occur with doses of 30 to 40 Gy to entire liver but focal RT is generally safe.[34] In a study of children with Wilms' tumor, neuroblastoma and hepatoma treated with RT and chemotherapy, fractionated doses of 12 to 25 Gy caused abnormalities in liver function or radionuclide scans in 50 percent patients, 25 to 35 Gy caused abnormalities in 63 percent cases and more than 35 Gy was toxic in nearly 80 percent patients.[35] In national Wilm's tumor study (NWTS), 5.3 percent patients receiving abdominal RT had liver toxicity with right flank or whole abdominal RT found to be associated with highest risk of hepatopathy.[36]

GIT Toxicity: RT induced vascular injury can cause digestive tract toxicity which may manifest as necrosis, ulceration, stenosis or perforation and is characterized by pain, diarrhea(enteritis), malabsorbtion, bowel obstruction and infection.[37] Generally, doses less than 30 Gy are safe while doses more than 40 Gy can cause bowel obstruction and chronic enterocolitis. The incidence of small bowel fibrosis is 5 percent after 40-50 Gy and may be up to 40 percent when RT doses are more than 60 Gy.[38] In a study of Wilms' tumor survivors, bowel obstruction was seen in 9.5, 13 and 17 percent patients respectively at a follow up of 5, 10 and 15 years respectively.[39] RT may be involved in increased risk of GI cancers in survivors. These cancers develop at relatively younger age in this population.[21,40] RT doses of more than 30 Gy to spleen may cause functional asplenia requiring lifelong special care of these patients.[41]

Genitourinary Tract Damage

Radiation nephropathy is dose related. Doses of 12-14 Gy may cause some renal injury in children while doses more than 25 Gy to both kidneys can cause renal failure within 6 months of therapy.[42,43] Concomitant treatment with radiomimetic drugs like doxorubicin and dactinomycin or other nephrotoxic agents may exacerbate the damage to kidney.[44] In studies of Wilms' tumor survivors, incidence of renal failure ranged from 0.6-1 percent for unilateral disease and 5.5 -13 percent for bilateral disease.[42,45]

Pelvic RT of more than 45 Gy may affect bladder capacity and function by inducing fibrosis and cystitis. Incidence of cystitis is limited to 5 percent at doses less than 45 Gy. Also, concomitant RT along with cyclophosphamide or ifosfamide for pelvic tumors may cause secondary bladder malignancies.[46,47]

Gonadal Dysfunction and Infertility: Treatment with RT may have adverse effects on germ cell survival, fertility and health of offspring. The effect of RT on ovarian function is related to dose, schedule and age. Younger girls are more resistant to RT than adolescents. Radiation doses > 8 Gy might be associated with ovarian ablation. Abdominal RT > 20 Gy may lead to ovarian failure in > 70 percent of women.[48,49] Additionally, this can also lead to reduced uterine volume and elasticity which may cause increased risk of spontaneous miscarriage, IUGR and prematurity.[50] Radiation doses of > 4 Gy lead to permanent azoospermia. Doses more than 20 Gy can cause Leydig cell failure in most prepubescent boys and doses exceeding 30 Gy lead to leydig cell failure at all ages.[48] Abdominal radiation can also cause germ cell dysfunction in many patients due to scatter effect.

The fertility of survivors compared to their siblings is impaired. In a landmark study of approximately 2,200 patients, survivors who received abdominal irradiation were 25 percent less fertile than their siblings. Male survivors receiving alkylating agents were 60 percent less fertile than siblings. Females, who received only alkylating agents experienced no appreciable affect on fertility.[51] Studies have shown a 7 to 15 percent fertility loss and 42 percent incidence of premature menopause in female survivors treated with alkylating agents with abdominal RT.[52] Fertility may also be impaired by abnormalities in uterine size or vascular abnormalities in females receiving abdominal RT. Currently, semen cryopreservation should be offered to all young men at significant risk of infertility. In females, all potential methods of preservation are experimental. In CCSS study of >4,000 pregnancies, female survivors were less likely to have live births, and more likely to have medical abortions or low birth weight babies.[53] Similarly, male survivors were also found to have less likelihood of live births.[54] There is no increase noticed in frequency of congenital anomalies or risk of cancer and genetic diseases in offspring of survivors in most of the studies.[55,56]

Musculoskeletal Side Effects

Radiation therapy can affect skin, muscles and bones. Factors affecting the severity of musculoskeletal toxicity include total dose of RT, dose per fraction, dosimetry (asymmetry and inhomogenity), age and inclusion of epiphyses in the RT field. RT doses of > 20 Gy to young children can cause muscular hypoplasia, which in addition to muscle loss during surgery may produce asymmetry in muscle mass, decreased range of motion, stiffness and pain in affected areas.[57] RT doses of > 20 Gy to hemiabdomen or spine may cause spinal abnormalities (kyphosis, scoliosis, lordosis and decreased sitting height) leading to back pain, hip pain, rib hump, uneven shoulder and gait abnormalities. Similar doses to growing epiphyses may lead to limb length discrepancy leading to lower back or hip pain and limp, which may warrant contralateral epiphysiodesis in severe cases (Figs 63.4A and B). RT doses more than 40 Gy to long bones can cause pathological fracture. Bone mineral density has been found to be reduced in survivors of childhood ALL, Wilms' tumor, CNS tumors and osteogenic sarcoma. This is more likely to be seen in female gender, increased age, corticosteroid use, cranial RT and growth hormone deficiency. Additionally, avascular necrosis may develop after long term use of steroids mainly in adolescent children.[58,59]

CHEMOTHERAPY

Present multimodal approach and risk adapted treatment strategies in pediatric cancers provide optimal balance of cure with toxicity. Increasing appreciation of unique toxicity of each chemotherapy agent has been pivotal in modification of contemporary chemotherapy regimens. Salient toxic profile of each group of chemotherapeutic agents is detailed below:

Alkylating Agents

These agents form part of majority of pediatric protocols. These are highly mutagenic and carcinogenic agents. These include cyclophosphamide, ifosfamide, melphelan, nitrosureas, and busulphan.

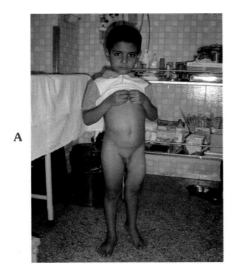

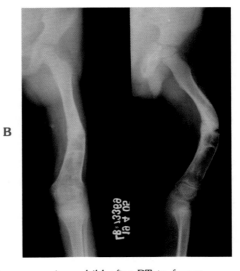

Figures 63.4A and B: Limb deformity and length discrepancy in a child after RT to femur

Common late toxicities include secondary cancers, gonadal toxicity, pulmonary and genitourinary toxicity.

Available data suggests that males who receive < 4 gm/m^2 of cyclophosphamide without other agents or RT are likely to retain their fertility. Conversely, doses > 9 gm/m^2 generally lead to sterility. The data related to long-term gonadal toxicity of ifosfamide is limited. Ifosfamide doses of 42 to 60 g/m^2 are associated with high risk of azoospermia in osteosarcoma survivors.[60-61] Pelvic radiation may enhance the alkylator-related germ cell damage. Chemotherapy with alkylating agents in girls can lead to amenorrhea and ovarian failure. However, prepubescent females may tolerate cumulative doses as high as 25 gm/m^2. Recovery of ovarian function is unlikely if menstrual periods do not return with in 3 months of treatment.[62]

Alkylator therapy can lead to myelodysplastic syndrome (MDS), acute myeloid leukemia (AML) as well as solid tumors in survivors. Alkylator-related secondary AML is associated with antecedent MDS, chromosomal 5 and 7 abnormalities and has a latent period of 5 to 7 years. Most potent leukemogenic agent is nitrogen mustard (NM) with a 15-year incidence rate of 4.8 percent for secondary AML compared to 1 percent after cyclophosphamide therapy.[63] Alkylator-related pulmonary fibrosis is commonly seen with nitrogen mustard (NM) or busulphan and rarely with high dose cyclophosphamide and ifosfamide used in pediatric solid tumors.[64]

Alkylator-associated hemorrhagic cystitis is seen in 5 to 10 percent patients after high dose cyclophosphamide and 20 to 40 percent patients after high dose ifosfamide.[47,65] Alkylator nephropathy is seen with high doses of ifosfamide. It is more common at doses exceeding 60 gm/m^2 and in preschool age group.[65,66] It may manifest as proximal tubular dysfunction (Fanconi-like syndrome), reduced glomerular function and proteinurea. Acute reversible nephropathy occurs in majority of children. However, chronic nephrotoxicity is seen in 1.4 to 30 percent of childhood cancer survivors treated with ifosfamide.[67]

Anthracyclines

Most worrisome late effect of anthracyclines is cardiac toxicity. Anthracyclines directly cause free-radical damage to cardiac myocytes. Increased risk of anthracycline-related cardiomyopathy is associated with female sex, cumulative dose exceeding 300 mg/m^2, younger age at the time of exposure and previous chest RT.[66,69] The impact of infusion time on cardiotoxicity is unclear at the moment.[70] Studies evaluating cardiac function by exercise stress tests in survivors have found abnormalities in exercise tolerance, cardiac output, aerobic capacity and ectopic rhythms;[71,72] however, the clinical impact of these findings is still not clear. A systematic review of cardiotoxicity in survivors found that 15.5 to 27.8 percent patients receiving anthracycline doses of more than 300 mg/m^2 and 0-15 percent patients receiving doses less than 300 mg/m^2 develop sub-clinical left ventricular (LV) dysfunction.[73] A study of Wilms' tumor survivors revealed a cumulative risk of congestive heart failure (CHF) of 4.4 percent at 20 years after treatment in anthracycline-naïve patients and 17.4 percent in anthracycline pretreated patients. This study reported that relative risk (RR) of CHF is 3.3 for every 100 mg/m^2 of anthracycline use.[74] It has been observed that LV function deteriorates for first 2 years followed by partial recovery over next 3 to 4 years and then progressive deterioration after 7 years of completion of treatment.[75] Dexrazoxane, a chelating agent may help to prevent anthracycline-related cardiotoxicity;[76] however ACE inhibitors have not succeeded in retarding the progression of LV dysfunction in these patients.[77]

PLATINUMS

Cisplatin and carboplatin are alkylating agents. They can cause nephrotoxicity, ototoxicity and neurotoxicity in long-term survivors. Nephrotoxicity is the most important toxicity which is dose-dependent. This is manifested by tubular dysfunction in the form of electrolyte wasting and azotemia. Some cases may manifest as hypomagnesemia, hypocalciurea, and hypokalemic metabolic alkalosis.[78,79] Renal dysfunction is generally acute and irreversible. It is enhanced by concomitant use of ifosfomide and amino-glycosides.[67,78,79] Cisplatin related ototoxicity manifests as high frequency hearing loss and is generally seen at doses exceeding 400 $mg/m.^2$ It is largely irreversible with increased risk seen in younger age, brain tumor patients, and with concomitant use of ifosfamide or cranial RT.[79,80] Neurotoxicity presents as sensory neuropathy commonly after cumulative doses of cisplatin exceed more than 300 $mg/m.^2$ More than 30 percent of patient may develop permanent neuropathic changes.[79,81] Carboplatin may cause similar spectrum of side effects but they tend to be infrequent and milder than cisplatin.[82]

Topoisomerase Inhibitors

Teniposide and etoposide are two most commonly used topoisomerase-II inhibitors. Both can cause secondary AML (M_4 or M_5-) in a non-dose dependent fashion. This secondary AML has a lag period of 2 to 3 years is associated with 11q23 (MLL gene) mutations and has no antecedent MDS phase. Although risk is not clearly dose-dependent but doses less than 5 gm/m^2 are relatively safer. Intermittent weekly or biweekly schedules increase the risk of secondary AML.[83]

Corticosteroids

Corticosteroids used in histiocytic disorders and brain tumour patients can cause cushingoid habitus with centripetal obesity, proximal myopathy, osteopenia, hypertension, psychiatric disturbances, immuno-suppression and avascular necrosis. Prolonged use may cause suppression of hypothalamic-pituitary-adrenal axis for many months after usage and requires reinstitution of rescue steroids in times of stress.[84]

SURGICAL MORBIDITY

In past, aggressive surgical treatment of childhood solid tumors led to significant long-term morbidities. However, the development of effective systemic therapy, better diagnostic imaging, advanced radiation therapy techniques and multimodal approach in treatment are slowly replacing aggressive surgeries with organ and limb conservation techniques. This is clearly exemplified in increasing usage of limb-sparing surgeries in extremity sarcomas, organ conservation in bladder, prostate, vaginal and uterine sarcomas, replacement of staging laparotomy with imaging-based staging, nephron-sparing surgery in bilateral Wilms' tumor, globe and vision preservation in retinoblastoma and fertility preserving surgeries in pediatric germ cell tumors.

Splenectomy in children may increase the risk of overwhelming sepsis with life time risk of 2.4 percent. These survivors need penicillin prophylaxis and vaccination against encapsulated organisms such as pneumococci, hemophilus influenzae and meningococci. Any febrile episode should be managed as medical emergency in these children.[85,86] Nephrectomy may lead to increased risk of hypertension, hyperfilteration injury of other kidney and renal failure in 1 percent cases of unilateral Wilms' tumor and 5.5 to 13 percent cases of bilateral tumors.[42,45,87] Bladder surgeries, e.g. total cystectomy with urinary diversion may increase the risk

of urinary tract infections and hydronephrosis. Partial cystectomy may increase the risk of functional bladder problems such as contracture or incontinence.[88] Retroperitoneal lymph node dissection may cause neural damage and lead to retrograde ejaculation in male survivors.[89] Amputation may be associated with stump pain, bony overgrowth and phantom pain in long-term survivors. Survivors undergoing limb-conserving surgeries may have endoprosthetic fracture, aseptic loosening, limb-length discrepancy, non-union and poor joint movement leading to compromised quality of life.[90] Increasing appreciation of long-term morbidity and mortality due to surgery in long-term survivors demands that treatment team of pediatric oncologist, surgeon and radiation oncologist make therapy recommendations after consideration of acute and long-term health risks.

STRATEGIES FOR DELIVERY OF LONG-TERM CARE FOR SURVIVORS

Many of the late effects can be lessened by prevention or early diagnosis with therapeutic intervention. Hence, there is a increasingly felt need for optimal delivery of health care to this growing, vulnerable population. The common approach is to adopt an individualized life long health care plan for each survivor encompassing screening, surveillance and prevention that incorporates risks based on previous cancer, cancer therapy, genetic predisposition, life style and comobidities. This model targets the health care of whole person and his family; provides longitudinal life long care by a single health care provider leading a multidisciplinary term and believes in comprehensive anticipatory care using preventive strategies. This modal is remarkable in its ability to provide optimal delivery of care, to facilitate transition of survivors care from pediatric treatment centre to community physicians and to simultaneously support investigations of late cancer related mortality and morbidity.[91,92]

On the pattern of care established at St. Jude Children Research Hospital, USA, a similar follow-up clinic for long-term survivors of childhood cancer was initiated at Tata Memorial Hospital in February 1991. This clinic was appropriately named after Completion of Therapy (ACT) clinic to emphasize that ACTs are needed beyond therapy to achieve ²CURE² in its full dimensions. The aims of the clinic are to monitor growth, development, and sexual maturation as well as the somatic late effects of therapy and to apply corrective measures whenever feasible. Other objectives are to rehabilitate survivors for productive adulthood and collect data for future protocol modification so as to minimize late effects. A wealth of information already exists in literature regarding expected consequences of multimodality treatment in pediatrics cancers. However, this is a service-oriented clinic rather than a mere fact-finding unit. Our ACT model has 3 basic facets; providing longitudinal care at a tertiary are centre by a single physician coordinator integrates patient care, education and research; second, ongoing communication with primary care provider ensures continuity of follow-up and finally education and empowerment of survivors sensitizes them towards the potential of late effects, need for continued surveillance and a healthy life style.[93,94]

Lessons learned through years of collaboration in pediatric oncology have generated a substantial body of evidence regarding damage to innocent bystander organs by non-selective cytotoxic hits. However, it must be realized that most late-effect studies are retrospective studies and are a reflection of past treatments, many of which have been replaced by safer, more efficacious therapies at present. Hence, provision of optimal treatment with minimal late effects is a constantly moving target. There are still many unanswered questions and unmet needs relating to the effects of childhood cancer and its treatment in India. Creation of nation wide ACT clinics with tight linkage to primary care providers would be the right beginning. Furthermore, there is a urgent need for national and international prospective multicenter studies, national population cohort studies,

and randomized clinical trials designed to evaluate not only the survival and long term toxicities but more importantly, interventions to prevent, treat or modify late effects in our young survivors. It is time, all health care workers involved in the care of pediatric oncology patients realize that 'biological cure is not enough.' One should strive towards 'Meaningful cure i.e., complete restoration of physical, mental and social wellbeing and not merely absence of disease' (Fig. 63.5).

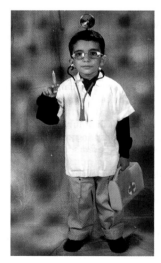

Figure 63.5: Today's survivors shall shape the destiny of the nation

REFERENCES

1. Gatta G, Capocaccia R, Coleman MP, Ries LA, Berrino F. Childhood cancer survival in Europe and the United States. Cancer 2002;15;95:1767-72.
2. Meadows AT, Hobbie WL. The medical consequences of cure. Cancer 1986;15;58:524-8.
3. Li FP, Myers MH, Heise HW, Jaffe N. The course of five-year survivors of cancer in childhood. J Pediatr 1978;93:185-7.
4. Indian Council of Medical Research. (2004). National Cancer Registry Programme. Consolidated Report of the Population Based Cancer Registries 1997-1998: Incidence and distribution of cancer. Indian Council of Medical Research, New Delhi.
5. Wallace WH, Blacklay A, Eiser C, Davies H, Hawkins M, Levitt GA, Jenney ME; Late Effects Committee of the United Kingdom Children's Cancer Study Group (UKCCSG). Developing strategies for long-term follow-up of survivors of childhood cancer. BMJ 2001;323:271-4.
6. Oeffinger KC, Hudson MM. Long-term complications following childhood and adolescent cancer: Foundations for providing risk-based health care for survivors. CA Cancer J Clin 2004;54:208-36.
7. Hudson MM, Mertens AC, Yasui Y, et al. Health status of adult long-term survivors of childhood cancer: a report from the Childhood Cancer Survivor Study. JAMA 2003;290:1583-92.
8. Duffner PK, Cohen ME: The long-term effects of central nervous system therapy on children with brain tumors. Neurol Clin 1991;9:479-95.
9. Packer RJ, Meadows AT, Rorke LB, et al. Long-term sequelae of cancer treatment on the central nervous system in childhood. Med Pediatr Oncol 1987;15:241-53.
10. Reimers TS, Ehrenfels S, Mortensen EL, et al. Cognitive deficits in long-term survivors of childhood brain tumors: Identification of predictive factors. Med Pediatr Oncol 2003;40:26-34.
11. Reddick WE, White HA, Glass JO, et al. Developmental model relating white matter volume to neurocognitive deficits in pediatric brain tumor survivors. Cancer 2003;97:2512-9.
12. Hoppe-Hirsch E, Renier D, Lellouch-Tubiana A, et al. Medulloblastoma in childhood: progressive intellectual deterioration. Childs Nerv Syst 1990;6:60-65.
13. Mitby PA, Robison LL, Whitton JA, et al. Utilization of special education services and educational attainment among long-term survivors of childhood cancer: A report from the Child-hood Cancer Survivor Study. Cancer 2003;97:1115–26.
14. Merchant TE, Goloubeva O, Pritchard DL, et al. Radiation dose-volume effects on growth hormone secretion. Int J Radiat Oncol Biol Phys 2002;52:1264-70.
15. Shalet SM, Brennan BM. Puberty in children with cancer. Horm Res 2002;57:39-42.
16. Lustig RH, Post SR, Srivannaboon K, et al. Risk factors for the development of obesity in children surviving brain tumors. J Clin Endocrinol Metab 2003;88:611-6.

LATE EFFECTS OF SURGERY

The late effects of surgery are mutilation with loss of function and/or poor cosmesis; growth disturbances; intra-abdominal adhesions with the risk of intestinal obstruction (15%, Paulino, 2000).[17]

Central venous access systems deserve special attention. External catheters or subcutaneous (internal) Port-a-Cath reservoirs for administration of cytotoxics, parenteral nutrition and withdrawal of blood, have facilitated the treatment of children with cancer but carry complications like infection, thrombosis and unsightly scars. Children with malignancies are more prone to venous thrombosis (Bazjar, 2006).[18] The most reliable method to diagnose venous thrombosis is by venography. At present, there are few prospective studies using venography as golden standard to detect the incidence of thrombosis (Barnes, 2002).[19] The PARKAA study found that 36.7 percent of the children with ALL and a central venous line, had thrombotic events (Mitchell, 2003, Male 2003).[20,21] Mortality directly attributable to thromboembolic disease in the Canadian Childhood Thrombophilia Registry was 2.2 percent, all of whom had central venous line-associated thrombosis. Morbidity was substantial, with 8.1 percent recurrent thrombosis and 12.4 percent postphlebitic syndrome (Monagle, 2000).[22] This latter cohort comprises also patients with CVL for other indications than malignancies.

The long-term consequences of thrombosis of central veins in children are only partially known. Initially, symptoms may be mild but complications may become manifest later in life (Goldenberg, 2005).[23]

Subclavian vein stenosis after catheterisation for hemodialysis has been reported in up to 40 percent of cases (Toepfer, 2000).[24] The risk of thrombosis after insertion of central venous catheters into the femoral vein was found to be 21.5 percent versus 1.9 in the subclavian. Jugular vein catheters are associated with a four times greater risk than subclavian vein catheters (McGee, 2003).[25]

In many of these studies, all patients undergoing long-term central venous access, irrespective of age or underlying disease, are grouped together and not easy to separate. The message is, that central venous access carries considerable risk, both short term and long term, and should not be undertaken lightly.

LATE EFFECTS OF CHEMOTHERAPY

Many adverse side-effects have been reported (Bhatia; Bath; etc).[26,27] Some examples are listed in Table 64.2.

Most of these effects are dose-related, e.g. the cardiotoxic effect of anthracyclines and careful monitoring of total doses is required. Other side effects, like vincristin-induced neuropathy, was found not to be dose-related (Hartman, 2006).[28] Adequate supportive treatment may reduce the risk of veno-occlusive disease of the liver due to actinomycin-D, which can be induced by dehydration. Protective measures, like hyperhydration, cardioxane (in treatment with anthracyclines), MESNA (in treatment with cyclophosphamide) are strongly recommended.

LATE EFFECTS OF RADIOTHERAPY

Profound long-term effects on many organs have been reported, some of which are presented in Table 64.3. It is occasionally possible to prevent these harmful effects by surgical measures, like transposition of the ovaries outside the radiation field.

LATE EFFECTS OF TREATMENT ACCORDING TO SPECIFIC TYPES OF PRIMARY CHILDHOOD CANCER

Wilms' Tumor

As radical excision of the tumor is the mainstay of surgical treatment, nephrectomy is performed in more than 90 percent of the patients with unilateral Wilms' tumor. The main point of concern is the function of the remaining kidney.

Compensatory hypertrophy occurs in the majority of patients, and is responsible for an ultimate kidney function that equals 75 percent of the normal function (Provoost, 1990).[29] Baudouin followed 111 patients for up to 50 years after nephrectomy (14 had Wilms' tumor) and showed that renal function after more than 25 years has a tendency to deteriorate, with an increase of proteinuria and decrease of GFR; however, only three patients had a GFR <60 ml/min/1.73 m2 (Baudouin, 1993).[30] These patients did not undergo radiotherapy, but it is known that irradiation of the kidney may hamper compensatory hypertrophy, particularly if dosages of more than 1200 cGy have been delivered.

Wilms' tumor patients in general have a low (0.6%) risk of end-stage renal failure but this risk is significantly increased in patients with syndromes, like WAGR (36%), Denys Drash (75%) or urogenital malformations (6.7%) in the NWTS (Breslow, 2005).[31]

Although renal function may initially be sufficient in the small child, this may deteriorate during growth and the child may outgrow its kidney function. Careful and long-term follow-up of these patients is therefore

Table 64.2: Late effects of chemotherapy agents on organs

Organ	Cytotoxic drugs	Potential Effects
Central nervous system	Intrathecal chemotherapy	Cognitive dysfunction
	High dose methotrexate	Leukencephalotpathy
Ears	platinums	Hearing loss
Heart	Anthracyclines	Cardiomyopathy
		arrhythmias
Lung	Bleomycin	Restrictive lung diases
		nitrosureas
Liver	Methotrexate	Liver dysfunction
	Thioguanine	Veno-occlusive disease
	Dactinomycin	
	Mercaptopurin	
Kidney	platinums	Renal failure
	High dose methotrexate	
	Ifosfamide	Electrolyte wasting
Bladder	Cyclophosphamide	Hemorrhagic cystitis
	Ifosfamide	Second bladder cancer
Gonads	Alkylating agents	Ovarian failure
	Nitrosureas	Testicular failure, Leydig
		cell dysfunction
SMN	Etoposide	
	Anthracyclines	
	Alkylating agents	Leukaemia
	Topoisomerase inhibitors	
	platinums	
	Cyclophosphamide	Transitional bladder carcinoma

Table 64.3: Late effects of radiotherapy on organ systems

Organ system	Potential effects
Central nervous system	Precocious puberty, Growth hormone deficiency and other pituitary dysfunction stroke, blindness, cognitive dysfunction, leukoencephalopathy
Eye	Cataract, optic neuropathy
Heart	Cardiomyopathy reinforced by cytotoxics like doxorubicin; coronary artery disease Valvular disease, pericarditis
Lung	Lung fibrosis after more than 30Gy
Thyroid	hypothyroidism, nodules, cancer
Musculo-skeletal system	muscular hypoplasia, impaired growth leading to leg length discrepancy, kyphosis, iliac wing hypoplasia and scoliosis (Paulino)
Endocrine system	
Hypophysis	Hypopituitarism with growth hormone deficiency (Bos 2004) and subsequent increased risk of cardiovascular disease (Heikens, 2000),
Thyroid	Hypothyroidism,
Gonads	ovarian failure oligo-/azoospermia Leydig cell dysfunctiom
Liver	Fibrosis, after more than 12 Gy
Kidneys	Nephritis, after more than 20 Gy.
SMN	any organ in the radiation is at risk for SMN Sarcomas, CNS tumors, breast and thyroid cancer

mandatory. In 28 out of 81 survivors of irradiated bilateral Wilms' tumor, between 3 and 100 months after treatment, elevated BUN and/or creatinine levels were found, 18 had moderate and 10 marked renal failure due to the combined effects of radiation and surgery (Smith, 1998).[32]

Late effects in children with Wilms' tumor treated with radiation therapy were reported by Paulino et al (2000).[17] Forty-two survivors were examined, 13 of them (31%) had no late effects. Scoliosis occurred in 18 (43%), but only one needed orthopedic intervention Bowel obstruction was seen in 17 percent after 15 years of follow-up. Three second malignancies developed, one leukaemia and two solid tumors in the radiation field. (For SMN in WT survivors: see also Breslow 1995, Carli, 1997; Friedman, 2002; Nelson, 2005).[33-36]

Rhabdomyosarcoma

Over 600 survivors in the Childhood Cancer Survivor Study completed questionnaires and were compared with 3701 siblings. They had various localisations of the tumor and different stages; most side effects occurred within 5 years, but after 5 years there was an increased rate of visual impairment, endocrine disturbances (growth hormone, thyroid hormone), delayed puberty, cardiopulmonary, and neurological problems (Punyko, 2005).[37]

Sklar and LaQuaglia (1998) found on examination that bilateral retroperitoneal lymphnode dissection leads to retrograde ejaculation, but after unilateral or limited dissection this occurred only in one our of 32.[38] Similar problems can be expected after cystoprotatectomy.

A comparable 'conservative' management protocol of bladder-prostate RMS resulted in normal bladder function in three out of eight, four had minor problems and one patient needed deviation because of disabling dysuria (Soler, 2005).[39] Nonaggressive management is not always feasible. Others have reported a higher rate of radical operations with permanent urinary diversion as long term solution. Bladder augmentation was also necessary because of bladder contraction after chemotherapy and radiation. These procedures have several late sequellae, like infections, stone formation and perforations (Filipas, 2004).[40]

Neuroblastoma

A retrospective study of 63 survivors of high-risk neuroblastoma (stage 3 and 4) at a median follow-up of 7 years after surgery and chemotherapy (100%), radiotherapy (89%) and autologous stem cell transplant (56%) showed late complications in 95 percent, but the majority were mild and only 4 percent life-threatening (Laverdiere, 2005).[41]

Kiely (1997) reported on the late effects of neuroblastoma operations. After excision of thoracic tumors: Horner syndrome can be expected; neurological deficits can occur after removal of tumor invading the spinal canal.[42]

Radical excision of abdominal tumors may involve bilateral adrenalectomy, but this is rarely necessary; similarly, unilateral nephrectomy is unusual but postoperative loss of renal function may occur because of vascular impairment after extensive dissection of the renal vessels. Retroperitoneal dissection may cause a sympathectomy effect with vasodilatation of the lower half of the body; there are no reports that this may also lead to ejaculatory problems in the patients.

Extensive dissection causes denervation of GI-tract, which leads to chronic diarrhea in 30 percent of cases; it is uncertain whether there may be an increased risk of gallstones.

Liver Tumors

After major resection, the liver regenerates within 4 to 6 weeks. There is no evidence that cytotoxic treatment impairs regeneration (Tagge, 1998).[43]

Liver transplantation has been applied for irresectable for hepatoblastoma, and has long term implication beyond the scope of this chapter (Otte, 2004).[44]

Sacrococcygeal Teratoma

Neonatal SCT is usually mature, therefore benign, if removed early in life, as is the case in Altman type I or II. Because of uncertain reasons, neurogenic bladder develops in about 25 percent of the patients.

Ozkan (2006) analyzed 14 patients with neurogenic bladder that were referred to a tertiary center, and found both upper and lower motor neuron dysfunction.[45] This may be caused by the tumor or by the treatment, Therefore, they stress the importance of pre- and postoperative urodynamic assessment in these patients.

Secondary Malignant Neoplasms (SMN's)

Special Attention has to be Given to Second Malignant Neoplasms (SMN's)

Research in this field is hampered by selection and publication biases. Analysis of the real incidence depends on the completeness of long-term follow-up. Furthermore, the risk of SMN increases annually, to a cumulative incidence of 3.2 percent after 20 years, and it is uncertain if and when a plateau will be reached (Neglia, 2001).[46]

It has to borne in mind that pediatric cancer can be due to several underlying factors and that these factors may also increase the risk of a second tumor.

Genetic and environmental factors have been implicated. Retinoblastoma is a good example: About 7 percent of survivors of RB and 0.5 percent of survivors of other childhood cancers are affected by bone cancer within 20 years of diagnosis of the original cancer. Both constitutional mutations in the RB gene and exposure of bone to radiotherapy and alkylating agents are held responsible (Wallace, 2001).[10]

Certain genetic syndromes, like Li-Fraumeni, Beckwith-Wiedeman and MEN, are associated with an increased risk of tumors of kidneys, liver and endocrine organs.

Radiation is also known as a causative factor. Chernobyl survivors have an increased risk of leukaemia and thyroid cancer. Even diagnostic radiology has been implicated in increased cancer risks later in life. Abdominal CT-scan in the first year of life leads to a cancer risk late in life of 1 in 500. The increased risk of hepatoblastoma in very low birth weight infants is attributed to the high number of X-rays that are made of these babies (Don, 2004).[47] Children represent a special case in radiation induced cancer. First , they are more sensitive to radiation than adults by a factor 10. Second, radiation scattered is more important in a small body. Third, there is the question of genetic susceptibility to irradiation (Hall, 2006).[48]

There is conflicting evidence about the role of toxic substances. Daughters born of mothers who were treated with DES have an increased risk of vaginal carcinoma. On the other hand, a study into the risk of cancer in children born of mothers who received cytotoxic drugs during pregnancy, reported no increased risk of malignancy nor of congenital malformations.[49] However, children born after treatment of infertility, with high doses of hormones, may have an increased risk of certain tumors, like retinoblastoma.[50]

The combined effects of chemotherapy and irradiation lead to an increased risk of leukaemia, lymphoma and cancer of the breast. Although chemotherapy alone may not increase the risk of SMN, it may potentiate the effects of radiotherapy.[51] The risk of all types of SMN in a childhood cancer survivor is 4

to 8 percent, resulting in six times the expected number of cancers.[10] After a median follow-up of 14.1 yrs after treatment for Hodgkin's lymphoma, the overall RR to develop a SMN was 7.0. The risk to develop leukaemia, and non-Hodgkin lymphoma was resp 37.5 and 21.5 (Aleman, 2000, van Leeuwen, 2000).[52,53] The time interval between treatment and development of SMN varies for different types of SMN. The risk to develop breast cancer starts to increase only after 15 years. This study confirms the findings of others that the curves have not reached a plateau and that the risk continues to increase with mre extended follow-up (Breslow, 1995; Bhatia, 2003).[4,33]

Young age at first treatment for Hodgkin's disease increased the relative risk of gastro-intestinal, lung, breast and bone and soft tissue cancer more than in patients treated at older ages, although the absolute excess risks were greater in older patients. The mixed-modality treatment was considered responsible for gastro-intestinal and lung cancers, whereas radiotherapy was related to increased breast cancer risks.[46,54]

Certain types of treatment are associated with SMN's more than others. A recent CCSS report found that the risk of thyroid cancer increased with radiation doses up to 20 – 29 cGy (O.R. 9.8), but fell at greater irradiation doses. There was no association with chemotherapy for the first cancer. The O.R. was even higher in patients receiving treatment before the age of 10 years. They also found that this increased risk continues for 30 years, and emphasize the need for long-term follow-up.[55] The benefit of follow-up for thyroid cancer, which carries a favorable prognosis, even when detected late, remains open for debate.

The Standardised Incidence Ratio (SIR). in Wilms' tumor patients treated according to the NWTS protocols is 8.4, more or less similar to the risk in the early SIOP studies when 80 percent of the patients underwent radiotherapy: SIR 7.32. In the SIOP VI protocol, with only 40 percent receiving radiotherapy, the SIR decreased to 2,56.[33,34] Doxorubicin is known to reinforce the irradiation effect, leading to a SIR. of 36 in Wilms' tumor patients (Breslow, 1995).[33]

Survivors of neuroblastoma have a SIR of 24 of a carcinoma, and the risk of developing renal cell carcinoma is 329 fold increased.[56]

Radiotherapy on the chest increases the risk of breast cancer. A twenty-fold increase in the incidence of breast cancer compared to age- and race-matched controls has been reported. After Hodgkin lymphoma the risk has been found 75 times higher.[53,57] The CCSS reported a

SIR of 24.7 in women with various primary malignancies receiving chest radiotherapy.[58] Radiotherapy at any age below 20 years leads to increased risk of breast cancer (Ronckers, 2005).[59]

Women treated for cancer during childhood have a increased risk to develop breast cancer, that is related to the radiation dosage: each Gray unit received by any breast increased the excess relative risk by 0.13. After treatment for Hodgkin's disease the relative risk is 7.0 which is considered to be due not only to higher radiation dose to the breasts, but also to a specific susceptibility (Guibout, 2005).[60]

Recommendations for screening for breast cancer have been proposed by the CCSS and include, apart from regular self-examination, also mammography (Tables 64.4A and B).

Long-term follow-up will also have to be directed at early detection of these malignancies.

FERTILITY

The combined effects of chemotherapy and irradiation have a negative impact on fertility, depending on gender and age at which the noxe was administered.

In girls, the prepubertal ovaries are relatively radioresistent compared to the postpubertal situation. Irradiation doses between 12 and 50Gy on the prepubertal ovaries will result in amenorrhea and delayed onset of puberty in 68 percent. Alkylating cytotoxics are particularly harmfull to the gonads. In girls, the loss of endocrine function occurs concomitant with germ cell failure. As a consequence, prepubertal cancer treatment may result in high FSH and LH levels, with low oestradiol and delayed onset of puberty. Postpubertal treatment in girls will lead to a- or oligomenorrhea and/or early menopause (Byrne, 2004).[61]

The prepubertal testes are more radio-sensitive than postpubertal: 20Gy or more to the prepubertal testes will lead to gonadal failure in the majority, but after puberty more than 30Gy will lead to failure in 'only' 50 percent. Sertoli cells are more sensitive than Leydig cells. As a result, prepubertal treatment can cause high FSH and LH, low testosteron levels and delayed onset of puberty, whereas postpubertal treatment may be associated with high FSH and LH levels but without clinical symptoms.[2,62]

Sperm banking has to be considered but requires careful psychological preparation in young boys to reduce anxiety and reinforce motivation.[63]

Table 64.4A: Suggested screening of females who are long-term survivors of childhood cancer	
Age	*Action*
Initial diagnosis of childhood cancer <10 years following initial diagnosis or puberty, whichever comes first	Education of second malignancy risks breast self examination
10 years after initial diagnosis	Baseline digital mammography and clinical examination
>10 years after initial diagnosis to age 30	Yearly clinical examination, digital mammogram every 3 years
>30 years of age	Clinical examination every 6 months, yearly digital mammogram
Ref. Powers (MPO, 2000)[57]	

Table 64.4B: Summary of ukccsg guidelines for breast cancer screening	
Age	*Action*
<25 years	No imaging
25 – 29 years	Annual MRI or Ultrasound if MRI contraindicated
30 – 50 years	Annual 2 view mammography, + MRI/US if dense breast tissue
>50 years	3 yearly 2 view mammography
(Ref. www.ukccsg.org.uk)	

One study has demonstrated no deleterious effects on spermatozoal DNA, which means that ICSI may be a good option in men with reduced fertility.[64]

The outcome of pregnancy in women who have been treated for cancer depends on the nature of the tumor and the treatment given. In general, the outlook is less favourable than in the normal population. The chance of a live born child is reduced to between 0.55 and 0.87, there is an increased risk of preterm develivery (RR 2.0). Radiotherapy of spinal column or pelvis increases the risk of abortion to 1.6 and 3.6 respectively. In a cohort of Wilms' tumor survivors, Paulino et al reported 3 pregnancies in 25 irradiated survivors, 2 of which were at term and one six weeks premature; 15 women had regular menstrual cycles (Paulino, 2000).[17]

Even in spouses of men who have been treated for cancer, there is a reduced chance of a live-born child (RR 0,79). (Nagarajan, 2005, Kalapurakal, 2004).[65-66]

QUALITY OF LIFE

Although the research into Quality of Life is hampered by many biases (Parsons),[67] some results deserve to be mentioned here.

Both the physical effects of cancer treatment, the psychological consequences of a life-threatening illness and the sense of vulnerability are reasons to expect an impaired quality of life (Langeveld).[68]

Research by means of questionnaires has not produced significant differences between childhood cancer survivors and their peers with regards to overall quality of life, self-esteem and worries. In some areas, cancer survivors were even less worried about health than controls. Specific concerns were more often present about fertility, getting a job and obtaining insurance (Langeveld, 2004a).[69]

Although the proportion of cancer survivors reporting post-traumatic stress disorder (PTSD) is not different from the proportion found in the general population, certain risk factors for PTSD were identified: being female, unemployed, having lower education, and having severe late effects and/or health problems. Early identification and treatment of PTSD symptoms can enhance quality of life for survivors of childhood cancer (Langeveld, 2004b).[70]

Although enlistment in military service is reduced, those who participate, do not perform worse than their peers (Latheenmaki, 1999).[71]

ORGANIZATION OF CHILDHOOD CANCER SURVIVORSHIP CARE

Several barriers exist to delivering health care to survivors. One of the survivor-related barriers is the lack of knowledge among survivors about their tumor, the treatemt and the subsequent risks. Physician-related barriers are the lack of capacity among health care providers (Oeffinger 2006; Ginsberg, 2006).[11,72]

Long-term effects have to be recorded by all pediatric and 'adult' specialists taking care of childhood cancer survivors. Until now, this is not done in a systematic way in many countries (Taylor, 2004).[73] Systems have been developed for this follow-up and require wide-spread application. Specialists for adults play a vital role in this respect (Jaspers, 2000, Bos, 2004).[74,75] They have to give feed-back to the paediatricians, radiotherapists and paediatric surgeons about late effects of their treatments.

Improvements in the outcome of cancer in adolescents and young adults is lagging behind the progress made in young children. As mentioned above, a number of SMN's after childhood cancer treatment develops in adolescents and young adults. The need for adolescent oncology has been recognized, as adult oncologists are untutored in arranging ancillary medical, psychological and educational supports, whereas pediatric oncologists have little or no experience in epithelial tumors (Bleyer, 2002).[76]

A multidisciplinary tumor board for adolescent and young adults with cancer has been started in Amsterdam several years ago.

ETHICAL ISSUES

The above mentioned data raise the issue of moral justification of submitting a, sometimes very young, child to the various forms of cancer treatment. Many children will be too young when cancer is diagnosed, to be able to express their own will. But a reasonable proportion will be at an age when they can participate in decision-making. They and their parents need an expert advice on which to base their decisions.

No general answer can be given to the question whether total effort is warranted under all circumstances or to be reserved in applying treatment modalities that may result in physical mutilation, failure of one or several organ systems and psychosocial dysfunctioning.

Factors that are determining are: the type and stage of tumor and the prognosis, including the side effects that can reasonably be expected to occur. But also the previous history and psychosocial situation taken into account. Decisions will have to be made by the doctors in close rapport with the patient and the parents. When obtaining informed consent is absolutely vital that the information is given by the treating physician, rather than collected haphazardly from the internet.

FUTURE DIRECTIONS

According to Osler, 'Medicine is a science of uncertainty and an art of probability.' Much of the information presented here is the result of retrospective studies that are inherently biased by selection of data and publications, incomplete follow-up and relatively small numbers. Also, we have to realize that we are seeing now the late effects of treatments given 15 or 20 years ago. Conditions may have improved in the meantime, and the outcomes therefore changed.

Systematic follow-up of all childhood cancer survivors is hampered by: patient uncertainty about the need for follow-up, patient unwillingness and difficulties in locating adult survivors or medical records. Minority participation continues to challenge investigators. Several projects are running. The National Wilms Tumor Study has a late effects study; the US Childhood Cancer Survivor Study follows a retrospective cohort of five-year survivors of childhood cancer in 25 institutions in North America. The British Childhood Cancer Survivors Study has a similar aim.

The Children's Oncology Group has developed long-term follow-up guidelines for survivors of childhood , adolescent and young adult cancers. The risk-based guidelines are intended to promote earlier detection of and intervention for complications that may arise (Landier, 2003). They can be downloaded from <www.survivorshipguidelines,org>

Prospective registrations like the above mentioned will have to provide the evidence for long-term follow up policies. Cost-benefit analyses will have to made to support the prevailing wisdom among many paediatric oncologists and haematologists that all survivors of childhood cancer should be follow up for life. There is a group of survivors for whom the benefit of clinical follow-up is not established and for whom postal or telephone follow up may be all that is needed (Wallace 2001).[10] Questionnaires into self-reported disease-specific and generic measures of health and quality of life have been found to correlate well with physician's reports (Friedman, 2002).[35]

Risk stratification, has been proposed by Skinner (2006).[77] For example level 1 patients with Wilms' tumor

stage I or II, who were operated and received low risk chemotherapy, can be followed every 1 or 2 years by post or telephone. Level 2 patients, who received chemotherapy and low-dose cranial radiotherapy (e.g. ALL), can be seen by a nurse or primary care physician at two-yearly intervals. Only level 3 patients, with intensive treatment schedules, e.g. brain tumors, bone-marrow transplants or metastatised disease, require annual follow-up in a physician-led clinic.

Genetics may help to identify those at risk of side effects (Mertens, 2004).[78] A recent conference, at Niagara on the Lake (9-10 June 2006), chaired by Daniel Green, was dedicated to this subject. A few publications have appeared and more will be forthcoming. The risk of intellectual impairment after treatment of ALL with chemotherapy and cranial radiotherapy, was found to be related to polymorphisms of genes controlling homocystein levels (Krajinovic, 2005).[79]

Also, the timing of ALL relapse may be genetically determined. Matched-pair analysis revealed significant differences in expression of genes involved in cell-cycle regulation, DNA-repair and apoptosis of patients with early relapse of ALL compared to late relapses (Bhojwani, 2006).[80]

REFERENCES

1. Steliarova-Foucher E, Stiller C, Kaatsch P, Berrino F, Coebergh J-W, Lacour B, Parkin M. Geographical patterns and time trends of cancer incidence and survival among children and adolescents in Europe since the 1970s (the ACCIS project): An epidemiological study. The Lancet 2004;364:2097- 2105.
2. Bhatia S, Landier W. Evaluating survivors of pediatric cancer. Cancer J 2005;11:340-54.
3. Landier W, Bhatia S, Eshelman DA, Forte KJ, Sweeney T, Hester AL, Darling J, et al. Development of risk-based guidelines for pediatric cancer survivors: the Children's Oncology Group long-term follow-up guidelines from the Children's Oncology Group Late Effects Committee and Nursing Discipline. J Clin Oncol 2004;22:4979-90.
4. Bhatia S, Yasui Y, Robison LL, et al. High risk of subsequent neoplasms continues with extended follow-up of childhood Hodgkin's disease: report from the Late Effects Study Group. J Clin Oncol 2003;21:4386-94.
5. Lackner H, Benesch M, Schagerl S, Kerbl R, Schwinger W, Urban C. Prospective evaluation of late effects after childhood cancer therapy with a follow-up over 9 years. Eur J Pediatr 2000;159:750-8.
6. Aziz NM, Rowland JH. Trends and advances in cancer survivorship research: Challenge and opportunity. Seminars Radiation Oncol 2003;13:248-66.
7. Curry HL, Parkes SE, Powell JE, Mann JR. Caring for survivors of childood cancers: The size of the problem. Eur J Cancer 2006;42:501-8.
8. Mertens AC, Yasui Y, Neglia JP, Potter JD, Nesbit ME, Ruccione K, Smithson WA, Robison LL. Late mortality experience in five-year survivors of childhood and adolescent cancer: The Childhood Cancer Survivor Study. J Clin Oncol 2001;19:3163-72.

9. Cardous-Ubbink MC, Heinen RC, Langeveld NE, et al. Long-term cause specific mortality among five-year survivors of childhood cancer. Pediatr Blood Cancer 2004;42:563-73.

10. Wallace WHB, Blacklay A, Eiser C, Davies H, Hawkins M, Levitt GA, Jenney MEM. Developing strategies for long term follow up of survivors of childhood cancer. BMJ 2001;323:271-4.

11. Oeffinger KC, Wallace HB. Barriers to follow-up care of survivors in the United States and the United Kingdom. Pediatr Blood Cancer 2006;46:135-42.

12. Randolph J. Warfare against Wilms' tumor: reconnaissance, individual heroes, a unified army and victory. In: Brooks BF: Malignant Tumors of Childhood, pp 5-16, University of Texas Press, Austin, 1986 ISBN 0-292-75082-X.

13. Shamberger RC, Guthrie KA, Ritchey ML, Haase GM, Takashima J, Beckwith JB, D'Angio GJ, Green DM, Breslow NE. Surgery – related factors and local recurrence of Wilms' tumor in National Wilms Tumor Study 4. Ann Surg 1999;229:292-7.

14. Lemerle J, Voute PA, Tournade MF, Delemarre JF, Jereb B, Ahstrom L, Flamant H, Gerard-Marchant R. Preoperative versus postoperative radiotherapy, single versus multiple courses of actinomycin D in the treatment of Wilms' tumor. Preliminary results of a controlled clinical trial conducted by the International Society of Pediatric Oncology (SIOP). Cancer 1976;38:647-54.

15. Tournade MF, Com-Nougue C, de Kraker J , Ludwig R, Rey A, Burgers JMB, Sandstedt B, Godzinski J, Carli M, Potter R, Zucker JM. Optimal duration of preoperative chemotherapy in unilateral and nonmetastatic Wilms' tumour in children older than 6 months: Results of the ninth SIOP Wilms' Tumour trial and study. J Clin Oncol 2001;19:488-500.

16. de Kraker J de, Graf N, van Tinteren H, for the International Society of Pediatric Oncology Nephroblastoma Trial Committee. Reduction of postoperative chemotherapy in children with stage I intermediate-risk and anaplastic Wilms' tumor (SIOP 93-01 trial): a randomised controlled trial. Lancet 2004;364:1229-35.

17. Paulino AC, Wen BC, Brown CK, Tannous R, Mayr NA, Zhen WK, Weidner GJ, Hussey DH. Late effects in children treated with radiation therapy for Wilms' tumor. Int J Radiation Oncology Biol Phys 2000;46:1239-46.

18. Bajzar L, Chan AK, Massicotte MP, Mitchell G. Thrombosis in children with malignancy. Curr Opin Pediatr 2006;18: 1-9.

19. Barnes C, Newall F, Monagle P. Thromboembolic complications related to indwelling central venous catheters in children with oncological/haematological diseases: a retrospective study of 362 catheters. Support Care Cancer 2002;10:256-7.

20. Mitchell LG . A prospective cohort study determining the prevalence of thrombotic events in children with acute lymphoblastic leukaemia and a central venous line who are treated with L-asparaginase. Cancer 2003;97:508-16.

21. Male C, Chait P, Andrew M, Hanna K, Julian J, Mitschell L. Central venousd line-related thrombosis in children: association with centra; venous line location and insertion technique. Blood 2003;101:4273-8.

22. Monagle P, Adams M, Mahoney M, Kaiser A, Barnard D, Bernstein M, Brisson L et al. Outcoem of pediatric thromboembolic disease: a report from the Canadian Childhood Thrombophilia Registry. Pediatr Res 2000;47:763-6.

23. Goldenberg NA. Long-term outcomes of venous thrombosis in children. Curr Opin Hematol 2005;12:370-6.

24. Toepfer JG, Wills EM, Lamarche MB. Subclavian vein stenosis revisited. Nephrol Nursing J 2000;27:69-71.

25. McGee DC, Gould MK. Preenting complications of central venous catheterization. N Engl J Med 2003;348:1123-33.

26. Bhatia S, Meadows AT. Long-term follwo-up of childhood cancer survivors: future directions for clinical care and research. Pediatr Blood Cancer 2006;46:143-8.

27. Bath L, Pritchard J, Wallace H. Treatment of cancer with chemotherapy and radiotherapy. In: Stringer MD, Oldham KT, Mouriquand PDE, Howard ER. Pediatric surgery and urology: long term outcomes. Pp 645-659. WB Saunders Copany Ltd, London 1998 ISBN 0-7020-2190-3.

28. Hartman A, van den Bos C, Stijnen T, Pieters R. Decrease in motor performance in children with cancer is independent of the cumulative dose of vincristine. Cancer 2006; 106:1395-1401.

29. Provoost, Baudouin P, Keijzer MH de, et al. The role of nephron loss in the prognosis of renal failure: experimental evidence. Am J Kidney Dis 1991;17:27-32.

30. Baudouin P, Provoost AP, Molenaar JC. Renal function up to 50 years after unilateral nephrectomy in children. Am J Kidney Dis 1993;21:603-11.

31. Breslow NE, Collins AJ, Ritchey ML, Grigoriev YA, Peterson SM, Green DM. End stage renal disease in patients with Wilms' tumor: results from the NWTS group and the United States renal data system. J Urol 2005;174:1972-5.

32. Smith GR, Thomas PRM, Ritchey M, Norkool P. Long-term renal function in patients with irradiated bilateral Wilms' tumor. Am J Clin Oncol 1998;21:58-83.

33. Breslow NE, Takashima JR, Whitton JA, Moksness J, D'Angio GJ, Green DM. Second malignant neoplasms following treatment for Wilms' tumor: A report from the NWTS Group. J Clin Oncol 1995;13:1851-59.

34. Carli M, Frascella E, Tournade MF, de Kraker J, Rey A, Guzzinati S, Burgers JMV, Delemarre JFM, Masiero L, Simonato L. Second malignant neoplasms in patients treated in SIOP Wilms Tumour Studies and trials 1,2,5 and 6. Med Pediatr Oncol 1997;29: 239-44.

35. Friedman DL, Meadows AT. Late effects of childhood cancer therapy. Pediatr clin N Am 2002;49:1083-1106.

36. Nelson MB, Meeske K. Recognizing health risks in childhood cancer survivors. J Am Acad Nurse Practitioners. 2005;17:96-103.

37. Punyko JA, Mertens AC, Gurney JG, Yasui Y, Donaldson SS, Rodeberg DA, Raney RB, Stovall M, Sklar C, Robison LL, Baker KS. Long-term medical effects of childhood and adolescen rhabdomyosarcoma: A report form the childhood cancer survivor study. Pediatr Blood Cancer 2005;44:643-53.

38. Sklar C, LaQuaglia MP. Rhabdomyosarcoma. In: Stringer MD, Oldham KT, Mouriquand PDE, Howard ER. Pediatric surgery and urology: Long term outcomes. Pp 688-701. WB Saunders Copany Ltd, London 1998 ISBN 0-7020-2190-3.

39. Soler R, Macedo A, Bruschini H, Puty F, Caran E, Petrilli A, Garrone G, Srougi M, Ortiz V. Does the less aggressive multimodal approach of treating bladder-prostate rhabdomyosarcoma preserve bladdrr function? J Urol 2005;174:2343-6.

40. Filipas D, Fisch M, Stein R, Gutjahr P, Hohenfellner R, Thuroff JW. Rhabdomyosarcoma of the bladder, prostate or vagina: The role of surgery. BJU International 2004;93:125-9.

41. Laverdiere C, Cheung NKV, Kushner BH, Kramer K, Modak S, LaQuaglia MP, Wolden S, Ness KK, Gurney JG, Sklar CA. Lomg-term complications in survivors of advanced stage neuroblastoma. Pediatr Blood Cancer 2005;45:324-32.

42. Kiely E. Neuroblastoma. In: Stringer MD, Oldham KT, Mouriquand PDE, Howard ER. Pediatric surgery and urology: long term outcomes. Pp 660-664. WB Saunders Copany Ltd, London 1998 ISBN 0-7020-2190-3.

43. Tagge EP. Liver tumors and resections. In: Stringer MD, Oldham KT, Mouriquand PDE, Howard ER. Pediatric surgery and urology: Long term outcomes. Pp 702-712. WB Saunders Copany Ltd, London 1998 ISBN 0-7020-2190-3.

44. Otte JB, Pritchard J, Aronson DC, Brown J, Czauderna P, Maibach R, Perilongo G, Shafford E, Plaschkes J. Liver transplantation for hepatoblastoma: results from the SIOP study SIOPEL-1 and review of the world experience. Pediatr Blood Cancer 2004;42:74-83.

45. Ozkan KU, Bauer SB, Khoshbin S, Borer JG. Neurogenic bladder dysfunction after sacrococcygeal teratoma resection. J Urol 2006;175:292-6.

46. Neglia JP, Friedman DL, Yasui Y et al. Second malignant neoplasms in five-year survivors of childhood cancer: Childhood Cancer Survivor study. J Natl Cancer Instit 2001;93:618-29.

47. Don S. Radiosensitivity of children: potential for overexposure in CR and DR and magnitude of doses in ordinary radiographic examinations. Pediatr Radiol 2004;34 (Suppl 3) S167-72.

48. Hall EJ. The inaugura Frank Ellis Lecture – Iatrogenic cancer: the impact of intensity-modulated radiotherapy. Clin Oncol 2006 (The Royal Coll Radiologists) epub/ in press.

49. Gwyn K. Children exposed to chemotherapy in utero. J Natl Cancer Instit Mongraphs 2005;34:69-71.

50. Ayhan A, Salman MC, Celik H, Dursun P, Ozyuncu O, Gultekin M. Association between fertility drugs and gynaecologic cancers, breast cancer, and childhood cancers. Acta Obstet Gynecol Scand 2004;83:1104-11.

51. Garwicz S, Anderson H, Olsen JH, et al. second malignant neoplasms after cancer in childhood and adolescence: a population-based case-control study in the five Nordic countries. Int J Cancer 2000;88:672-8.

52. Aleman BMP, Klokman WJ, van Leeuwen FE. Tweede primaire tumoren bij mensen die op jonge leeftijd zijn behandeld voor de ziekte van Hodgkin; conseuqnties voor de follow-up. Ned Tijdschr Geneeskd 2000;144:1517-20.

53. Van Leeuwen FE, Klokman WJ, Veer MB van 't, Hagenbeek A, Krol ADG, Vetter UAO, Schaapveld M, Heerde P van, Burgers JMV, Somers R. Long-term risk of second malignancies in survivors of Hodgkin's disease treated during adolescence or young adulthood. J Clin Oncol 2000;18:487-97.

54. Swerdlow AJ, Barber JA, Vaughan Hudson G et al. Risk of second malignancy after Hodgkin's disease in a collaborative British cohort: the relation to age at treatment. J Clin Oncol 2000;13:498-509.

55. Sigurdson AJ, Ronckers CM, Mertens AC, Stovall M, Smith SA, Liu Y, Berkow RL, Hammond S, Neglia JP, Meadows AT, Sklar CA, Robison LL, Inskip PD. Primary thyroid cancer after a first tumour in childhood (the Childhood Cancer Survivor Study): A nested case-control study. The Lancet 2005;2014-23.

56. Bassal M, Mertens AC, Taylor L, Neglia JP, Greffe BS, Hammond S, et al. Risk of selected subsequent carcinomas in survivors of childhood cancer: a report from the Childhood Cancer Survivor Study. J Clin Oncol 2006;24:476-83.

57. Powers A, Cox C, Reintgen DS. Breast cancer screening in childhood cancer survivors. Med Pediatr Oncol 2000; 34:210-12.

58. Kenney LB, Yasui Y, Inskip PD, Hammond S, Neglia JP, Mertens AC, Meadows AT, Friedman D, Robison LL, Diller L. Breast cancer after childhood cancer: A report from the childhood Cancer Survivor Study. Ann Intern Med 2004;141:590-7.

59. Ronckers CM, Land CE, Neglia JP, Meadows AT. Breast Cancer. The Lancet 2005;366:1605-6.

60. Guibout C, Adjadj E, Rubino C, Shamsaldin A, Grimaud E, Hawkins M, Mathieu MC et al. Malignant breast tumors after radiotherapy for a first cancer during childhood. J Clin Oncol 2005;23:197-204.

61. Byrne J, Fears TR, Mills JL, Zeltzer LK, Sklar C, Nicholson HS, Haupt R, Reaman GH, Meadows AT, Robison LL. Fertility in women treated with cranial radiotherapy for childhood acute lymphoblastic leukaemia. Pediatr Blood Cancer 2004;42:589-97.

62. Hobbie WL, Ginsberg JP, Ogle SK, Carlson CA, Meadows AT. Fertility in males treated for Hodgkins disease with COPP/ABV hybrid. Pediatr blood Cancer 2005;44:193-6.

63. Edge B, Holmes D, Makin G. Sperm banking in adolescent cancer patients. Arch Dis Child 2006;91:149-52.

64. Thomson AB, Campbell AJ, Irvine DS, Anderson RA, Kelnar CJH, Wallace WHB. Semen quality and spermatozoal DNA integrity in survivors of childhood cancer: A case-control study. The Lancet 2002;360:361-7.

65. Nagarajan R, Robison LL. Pregnancy outcomes in survivors of childhood cancer. J Natl Cancer Instit Monographs 2005;34:72-6.

66. Kalapurakal JA, Peterson S, Peabody EM, Thomas PRM, Green DM, D'Angio GJ, Breslow NE. Prenancy outcomes after abdominal irradiation that included or excluded the pelvis in childhood Wilms tumor survivors: a report from the NWTS, Int J Radiat Oncol Biol Phys 2004;58:1364-8.

67. Parsons SK, Brown AP. Evaluation of quality of life of childhood cancer survivors: a methodological conundrum. Med Pediatr Oncol 1998; suppl 1: 46-53.

68. Langeveld NE, Stam H, Grootenhuis MA, Last BF. Quality of life in young adults survivors of childhood cancer: a literature review. Supportive Care in Cancer 2002;10:579-600.

69. Langeveld NE, Grootenhuis MA, Voute PA, de Haan RJ, van den Bos C. Quality of life, self esteem and worries in young adult survivors of childhood cancer. Psycho-oncology 2004;13:867-81.

70. Langeveld NE, Grootenhuis MA, Voite PA, de Haan RJ. Posttraumatic stress symptoms in adult survivors of childhood cancer. Pediatr Blood Cancer 2004;42:604-10.

71. Lahteenmaki PM, Salmi HA, Salmi TT, Helenius H, Makipernaa A, Lanning M, Perkkio M, Siimes M. Military service of male survivors of childhood malignancies. Cancer 1999;85:732-40.

72. Ginsberg JP, Hobbie WL, Carlosn CA, Meadows AT. Delivering long-term follow-up care to pediatric cancer survivors: Transitional care issues. Pediatr Blood Cancer 2006;46:169-73.

73. Taylor A, Hawkins M, Griffiths A, Davies H, Douglas C, Jenney M, Wallace WHB, Levitt G. Long-term follow-up of survivors of childhood cancer in the UK. Pediatr Blood Cancer 2004;42: 161-8.

74. Jaspers MW, Caron H, Behrendt H, van den Bos C, Bakker P, van Leeuwen F. The development of a new information model for a pediatric cancer registry on late treatment sequelae in The Netherlands. Stud Health Technol Inform 2000;77:895-9.

75. Bos C van den, Heinen RC, Sukel M, Pal HJH van der, Geenen MM. Screening for late effects in survivors of childhood cancer: Growth hormone deficiency from a pediatric oncologist's point of view. Growth Hormone and IGF Research 2004;14: S125-8.

76. Bleyer A. Older adolescents with cancer in NorthAmerica. Deficits in outcome and research. Pediatr Clin N Am. 2002;49:1027-42.

77. Skinner R, Wallace WHB, Levitt GA, on behalf of the UK Children's Cancer Study Group (UKCCSG) late effects group (LEG). Long-term follow-up of people who have survived cancer during childhood. Lancet Oncol 2006; 7:489-98.

78. Mertens AC, Mitby PA, Radioff G, Jones IM, Perentesis J, Kiffmeyer WR, Neglia JP, et al. XRCC1 and glutathione-s-transferase gene polymorphisms and susceptibility to radiotherapy-related malignancies in survivors of Hodgkin disease. Cancer 2004;101:1463-72.

79. Krajnovic M, Robaey P, Chiasson S, et al. Polymorphisms of genes controlling homocysteine levels and IQ score following the treatment for childhood ALL. Pharmacogenomics 2005;6:293-302.

80. Bhojwani D, Kang H, Moskowitz NP et al. Biologic pathways associated with relapse in childhood acute lymphoblastic leukaemia: a Children's Oncology Group study. Blood 2006;108:711-7.

Appendices

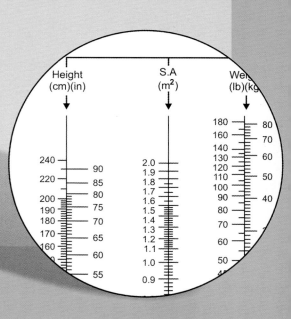

APPENDIX I–CHEMOTHERAPY PROTOCOLS

The chemotherapy protocols described here are those in use at the Department of Pediatric Surgery, All India Institute of Medical Sciences, New Delhi.

Chemotherapy regimens for the following tumors are detailed here:

Neuroblastoma
      Stage I, IIA
      Stage IIB, III, IV
      Stage IV-S
Wilms' tumor
      Stage I, II FH and I anaplasia (focal/diffuse)
      Stage III, IV FH, and II, III, IV focal anaplasia
      Stage II-IV diffuse anaplasia
Clear cell sarcoma of the kidney
Rhabdoid tumor of the kidney
Hepatoblastoma
Malignant germ cell tumor
Rhabdomyosarcoma
      Stage I, II
      Stage III, IV
Ewing's sarcoma family of tumors
Salvage regime for solid tumors

CHEMOTHERAPY REGIME FOR NEUROBLASTOMA

Chemotherapy Regime for Neuroblastoma Stage I, IIA

Drug Doses and Administration

Cyclophosphamide (CTX): 150 mg/m^2/day × 7 days IV in the first cycle and orally thereafter. Prehydrate for 2 hours with 200 ml/m^2/hr of N/3 saline +1 ml/100 ml KCl. Daily dose to be dissolved in 200 ml/m^2 of 5 percent dextrose and given over 60 minutes. Continue hydration with 125 ml/m^2/hr of N/2 saline + 1 ml/100 ml KCl for 6 hours.

Doxorubicin (DOX): 35 mg/m^2/dose IV bolus over 10 to 15 min. Total dose not to exceed 175 mg/m^2.

Antiemetic: Ondansetron or metoclopramide

Antibiotics: All patients to receive BACTRIM PO BD as trimethoprim 5 mg/kg/dose for the duration of chemotherapy administration. If fever/ neutropenia then add gentamycin 5 mg/kg/day in three divided doses.

Road map

Week	0	1	3	4	6	7	9	10	12	13
CTX	■		■		■		■		■	
DOX		■		■		■		■		■

Chemotherapy regime for Neuroblastoma Stage IIB, III, IV

Drug Doses and Administration

Cyclophosphamide (CTX): 150 mg/m^2/day × 7 days IV in the first cycle and orally thereafter. Prehydrate for 2 hours with 200 ml/m^2/hr of N/3 saline +1 ml/100 ml KCl. Daily dose to be dissolved in 200 ml/m^2 of 5 percent dextrose and given over 60 minutes. Continue hydration with 125 ml/m^2/hr of N/2 saline + 1 ml/100 ml KCl for 6 hours.

Cisplatinum (CDDP): (Total dose not to exceed 540 mg/m^2). Pre-hydrate for 2 hours with 250 ml/m^2/hr of N/3 saline +1 ml/100 ml KCL + 8 mEq/L(1 gm/L) of magnesium sulfate. Via the second IV line give Mannitol 10 gm/m^2 (total). Inj. Cisplatinum 90 mg/m^2/day to be dissolved in a total fluid of 1000 ml/m^2 of N/3 saline + 0.5 ml/100 ml KCl and this to be given over 6 hours. Via the second IV line continue infusing mannitol 10 gm/m^2 (total) over these 6 hours. After completing Cisplatinum continue hydration @ 125 ml/m^2/hr of N/2 saline + 1 ml/100 ml KCl for 18 hours and then 65 ml/m^2/hr. Maintain urine output >150 ml/m^2. If less than give mannitol 200 mg/kg in 25 ml of normal saline over 15 min. If still urine output is less then give inj. Lasix 0.5 mg/kg IV bolus.

Doxorubicin (DOX): 35 mg/m^2/dose IV bolus over 10 to 15 min. Total dose not to exceed 175 mg/m^2.

Etoposide (VP-16): 100 mg/m^2/day × 2 days. Dissolve to make a concentration of 0.4 mg/ml of N/2 saline in 5% dextrose + 1 ml/100 ml KCl and give this over 1 hour.

Antiemetic: Ondansetron or metoclopramide

Antibiotics: All patients to receive BACTRIM PO BD as trimethoprim 5 mg/kg/dose for the duration of the chemotherapy administration. If fever/neutropenia then add gentamicin 5 mg/kg/day in three divided doses.

Magnesium gluconate: 3 gm/m^2/day (6 tabs/m^2) in 2 to 3 divided doses orally.

2. All patients to undergo tumor bed irradiation irrespective of stage. All metastatic sites to be irradiated also.

3. Tumor bed irradiation is to start as soon as possible postoperative (once the patient is stable and there is no ileus). Administration of VCR should continue during the RT.

Road map

Week	0	1	2	3	4	5	6	7	8	9	10	12	13	15	18	21	24
VCR		■	■		■	■	■	■	■		■	■*	■*		■*		■*
CTX				■*			■			■*		■		■*	■	■*	■
DOX	■						■					■			■		■
VP-16				■					■					■		■	

CHEMOTHERAPY REGIME FOR RHABDOID TUMOR OF THE KIDNEY—RTK REGIME

Drug Doses and Administration

Carboplatin (CBDCA): 16.7 mg/kg/day × 2 days IV bolus (the dose is 500 mg/m²/day × 2 days for those more than 30 kg).

Etoposide (VP-16): 3.3 mg/kg/day × 3 days in 200 ml/m² of N/2 saline as IV infusion over 1 hour daily. The dose is 100 mg/m²/day × 3 days for those more than 30 kg.

Cyclophosphamide (CTX): Prehydration with 200 ml/m²/hr of N/2 saline for two hours followed by 14.7 mg/kg/day × 3 days in 200 ml/m² of N/2 saline as IV infusion over 1 hr daily. Continue hydration with 125 ml/m²/hr of N/2 saline for 6 hrs. The dose is 440 mg/m²/day × 3 days for patients who weigh more than 30 kg.

Mesna: 3 mg/kg/dose × 4 doses (at 0,3,6,9 hrs after cyclophosphamide) in 10 ml over 15 minutes. The dose should be 90 mg/m²/dose for those more than 30 kg.

G-CSF: 5 micrograms/kg/day subcutaneously starting 24 hours after the last dose of cyclophosphamide and given until ANC > 10,000.

Antiemetic: Ondansetron or metoclopramide

Antibiotics: All patients to receive BACTRIM PO BD as trimethoprim 5 mg/kg/dose for the duration of the chemotherapy administration. If fever/ neutropenia then add gentamycin 5 mg/kg/day in three divided doses.

RT: To be given at week 6.

Guidelines:

1. Babies < 12 months should receive ONE-HALF of the recommended dose of all chemotherapeutic agents. Full dose should be given when the child is > 12 months of age.

2. All patients to undergo tumor bed irradiation irrespective of stage. All metastatic sites to be irradiated also.

3. Tumor bed irradiation is to start as soon as possible postoperative (once the patient is stable and there is no ileus). Administration of VCR should continue during the RT.

Road map

Week	0	3	6	9	12	15	18	21	24
CBDCA	■	■		■	■		■	■	
VP-16	■	■		■	■		■	■	
CTX			■			■			■

CHEMOTHERAPY REGIME FOR HEPATOBLASTOMA—PLADO REGIME

Drug Doses and Administration

Cisplatinum (CDDP): 25 mg/ m²/day × 3 days as IV infusion. Prehydration with 200 ml/m²/hr of N/3 saline + 1 ml/100 ml of KCl for two hours. Then cisplatin dose dissolved in 200 ml/m² of N/3 saline to be given over 60 minutes. After this hydration to be continued with 125 ml/ m² of N/3 saline + KCl for at least 6 hours.

Doxorubicin (Dox): 20 mg/m²/day × 3 days as IV infusion in 200 ml/m²/hr of N/3 saline over one hour.

Oral Magnesium gluconate: 3 gm/m²/day in 2 divided doses.

Antiemetic: Ondansetron or metoclopramide

Antibiotics: All patients to receive BACTRIM PO BD as trimethoprim 5 mg/kg/dose for the duration of the chemotherapy administration. If fever/neutropenia then add gentamycin 5 mg/kg/day in three divided doses.

Guidelines:

1. Dosages to be reduced ONE-HALF in children less than 12 months of age and made full once they are >12 months old.

2. Reduce dosage to 50 percent in TLC 2500 to 4000 and withhold chemotherapy if TLC <2500.

3. MUGA scan to be performed before starting of therapy and after 6th and 15th week doses.

Road map

Week	0	3	6	9	12	15
CDDP	■	■	■	■	■	■
Dox	■	■	■	■	■	■

CHEMOTHERAPY REGIME FOR MALIGNANT GERM CELL TUMORS—PEB REGIME

Drug Doses and Administration

Cisplatinum (CDDP): 35mg/ m^2/day × 3 days as IV infusion. Prehydration with 200 ml/m^2/hr of N/3 saline+ 1 ml/100 ml of KCl for two hours. Then cisplatin dose dissolved in 200 ml/m^2 of N/3 saline to be given over 60 minutes. After this hydration to be continued with 125 ml/ m^2 of N/3 saline+ KCl for at least 6 hours.

Etoposide(VP-16): 120 mg/m^2/day × 3 days in 200 ml/m^2 of N/2 saline as IV infusion over 1 hour daily.

Bleomycin (Bleo): 15 mg/m^2 day 2 (IV infusion over 1 hr).

Antiemetic: Ondansetron or metoclopramide

Antibiotics: All patients to receive BACTRIM PO BD as trimethoprim 5 mg/kg/dose for the duration of the chemotherapy administration. If fever/neutropenia then add gentamycin 5 mg/kg/day in three divided doses.

Road map

Week	0	3	6	9
CDDP	■	■	■	■
VP-16	■	■	■	■
Bleo	■	■	■	■

CHEMOTHERAPY REGIME FOR RHABDOMYOSARCOMA

RMS Stage I, II—VA Regime

Drug Doses and Administration

Vincristine (VCR): 0.05 mg/kg IV push (maximum dose – 2.0 mg) starting day 21 (week 3). The dose of VCR is 1.5 mg/m^2 IV push for all patients who weigh more than 30 kilograms, but no single dose to exceed 2.0 mg.

Dactinomycin (ACD): 45 µg/kg/dose IV push (maximum dose—2.3 mg), beginning week 1. The dose will be 1350 µg/m^2 IV push for all patients who weigh more than 30 kilograms, but no single dose to exceed 2300 µg.

Guidelines:
1. Day of excision is day 0, week 0.
2. Dosages to be reduced ONE-HALF in children less than 12 months of age and made full once they are >12 months old.
3. If postoperative radiation is to be given, it should begin concomitantly with the first course of chemotherapy.

Road map

Week	1	2	3	4	5	6	7	8	9	10	11	12	13	14	15	16	17	18	19	20	21
VCR			■	■	■	■	■	■	■	■	■	■	■	■	■	■	■	■	■	■	■
ACD	■									■						■					

Road map continued

Week	22	23	24	25	26	27	28	29	30	31	32	33	34	35	36	37	38
VCR	■	■	■	■	■	■	■	■	■	■	■	■	■	■	■	■	■
ACD	■					■						■					

Road map continued

Week	39	40	41	42	43	44	45	46	47	48	49	50	51	52	53	54	55
VCR	■	■	■	■	■	■	■	■	■	■	■	■	■	■	■	■	■
ACD	■					■						■					

RMS Stage III, IV—VAC Regime

Drug Doses and Administration

Vincristine (VCR): 0.05 mg/kg IV push (maximum dose — 2.0 mg). The dose of VCR is 1.5 mg/m^2 IV push for all patients who weigh more than 30 kilograms, but no single dose to exceed 2.0 mg.

Dactinomycin (ACD): 45 µg/kg/dose IV push (maximum dose — 2.3 mg), beginning within 5 postoperative days (week 0). The dose will be 1350 µg/m^2 IV push for all patients who weigh more than 30 kilograms, but no single dose to exceed 2300 µg.

Cyclophosphamide (CTX): Prehydration with 200 ml/m^2/hr of N/2 saline for two hours followed by cyclophosphamide 2.2 gm/m^2 in 200 ml/m^2 of N/2 saline as IV infusion over 1 hr. Continue hydration with 125 ml/m^2/hr of N/2 saline +1 ml/100 ml of KCl for 6 hrs.

Mesna: 500 mg/m^2/dose × 3 doses at 0,3,6, hrs after cyclophosphamide, in 125 ml/m^2/hr of N/2 saline +1 ml/100 ml of KCl given over 1 hour.

G-CSF: 5 micrograms/kg/day subcutaneously starting 24 hours after dose of cyclophosphamide and given until ANC > 10,000.

Antiemetic: Ondansetron or metoclopramide

Antibiotics: All patients to receive BACTRIM PO BD as trimethoprim 5 mg/kg/dose for the duration of the chemotherapy administration. If fever/neutropenia then add gentamycin 5 mg/kg/day in three divided doses.

Radiotherapy: RT is given to the tumor bed as well as the metastatic sites starting week 9.

Guidelines:

1. Dosages to be reduced ONE-HALF in children less than 12 months of age and made full once they are >12 months old.

2. Cyclophosphamide should be omitted on days 42 and 63 in children who have urinary bladder included in the radiation portal, or who will have large volumes of bone marrow irradiated, such as irradiation to the whole abdomen, including the pelvis.

Road map

Week	0	1	2	3	4	5	6	7	8	9	10	11	12	16	20	21	22
VCR	■	■	■	■	■	■	■	■	■	■	■	■	■	■	■	■	■
ACD	■			■			■			■					■		
CTX	■			■			■			■			■	■	■		

Road map continued

Week	23	24	25	29	30	31	32	33	34	38	39	40	41	42	43
VCR	■	■	■	■	■	■	■	■	■	■	■	■	■	■	■
ACD	■			■			■			■			■		
CTX	■			■			■			■			■		

CHEMOTHERAPY REGIME FOR EWING'S SARCOMA FAMILY OF TUMORS (EWING'S AND PNET)—VDC-IE REGIME

Drug Doses and Administration

Vincristine (VCR): 0.05 mg/kg IV push for children < 3 years old or older but with surface area < 0.6 m^2 (maximum dose – 2.0 mg). The dose of VCR is 1.5 mg/m^2 IV push for all other patients, but no single dose to exceed 2.0 mg.

Doxorubicin (Dox): 2.5 mg/kg for children < 3 years old or older but with surface area < 0.6 m^2. The dose is 75 mg/m^2 for all other children. Total dose is dissolved in IV in 200 ml/m^2/hr of N/2 saline over 48 hours. Maximum dose not to exceed 300 mg/m^2.

Cyclophosphamide (CTX): Prehydration with 200 ml/m^2/hr of N/2 saline for two hours followed by cyclophosphamide dissolved in 200 ml/m^2 of N/2 saline as IV infusion over 1 hr. Continue hydration with 125 ml/m^2/hr of N/2 saline +1 ml/100 ml of KCl for 6 hrs. Dose of cyclophosphamide is 40 mg/kg for children < 3 years old or older but with surface area < 0.6 m^2. The dose is 1.2 gm/m^2 for all other children.

Mesna: 360 mg/m^2/dose × 3 doses at 0, 3, 6, 9 hours after cyclophosphamide, in 125 ml/m^2/hr of N/2 saline +1 ml/100 ml of KCl given over 1 hour.

Etoposide (VP-16): 3.3 mg/kg/day × 5 days for children < 3 years old or older but with surface area < 0.6 m^2, dissolved in 200 ml/m^2 of N/2 saline as IV infusion over 1 hour daily. The dose is 100 mg/m^2/day × 5 days for all other children.

Ifosphamide (IFOS): Prehydrate patient with 200 ml/ m^2/hr of N/2 saline +1 ml/100 ml of KCl for 2 hours. Ifosphamide should be dissolved in 200 ml/m^2 of N/2 in 5 percent dextrose and given over 1 hour. Posthydration to be given with 125 ml/m^2/hour of N/2 saline in 5 percent dextrose +1 ml/100 ml of KCl for the remaining of 24 hours. Dose is 60 mg/kg/day × 5 days for children < 3 years old or older but with surface area < 0.6 m^2. For all others the dose is 1.8 gm/m^2/day IV × 5 days.

G-CSF: 5 micrograms/kg/day subcutaneously starting 24 hours after dose of cyclophosphamide or ifosphamide and given until ANC > 10,000.

Antiemetic: Ondansetron or metoclopramide

Antibiotics: All patients to receive BACTRIM PO BD as trimethoprim 5 mg/kg/dose for the duration of the chemotherapy administration. If fever/ neutropenia then add gentamycin 5 mg/kg/day in three divided doses.

Radiotherapy: RT is given to the tumor bed as well as the metastatic sites starting week 12.

Guidelines:
1. Dosages to be reduced ONE-HALF in children less than 12 months of age and made full once they are >12 months old.
2. If cardiac irradiation has occurred then omit doxorubicin at weeks 21 and 27.
3. Surgical resection should be considered around week 30 or 33 after proper re-evaluation.

Road map

Week	0	3	6	9	12	15	18	21	24	27	30	33	36	39	42	45	48
VCR	■		■		■			■		■		■		■		■	■
DOX	■		■		■			■		■							
CTX	■		■		■			■		■		■		■		■	■
IFOS		■		■		■	■		■		■		■		■		
VP16		■		■		■	■		■		■		■		■		

SALVAGE REGIME RECURRENT OR NON-RESPONSIVE SOLID TUMORS—ICE REGIME

Drug Doses and Administration

Ifosphamide (IFOS): 1.5 gm/m^2/day IV × 3 days (day 1-3). Prehydrate patient with 200 ml/ m^2/hr of N/2 saline +1 ml/100 ml of KCl for 2 hours. Ifosphamide to be dissolved in 200 ml/m^2 of N/2 in 5% dextrose and given over 1 hour. Posthydration to be given with 125 ml/m^2/ hour of N/2 saline in 5% dextrose +1 ml/100 ml of KCl for the remaining of 24 hours.

Mesna: 500 mg/m^2/dose at 0,3,6 hours after ifosphamide infusions. Each dose to be given over 1 hour dissolved in 125 ml/m^2/hour of N/2 saline in 5% dextrose.

Carboplatin (CBDCA): 635 mg/m^2 IV on day 3. Carboplatin to be dissolved in 200 ml/m^2 of N/2 saline and infused over 1 hour.

Etoposide (VP-16): 100 mg/m^2/day IV × 3 days. Etoposide to be dissolved in 200 ml/m^2 of N/2 in 5 percent dextrose and given over 1 hour.

GCSF: 5 microgram/kg/day subcutaneously starting 24 hours after dose of ifosphamide and given until ANC > 10,000.

Antiemetic: Ondansetron or metoclopramide

Antibiotics: All patients to receive BACTRIM PO BD as trimethoprim 5 mg/kg/dose for the duration of the chemotherapy administration. If fever/ neutropenia then add gentamycin 5 mg/kg/day in three divided doses.

Guidelines:
1. Dosages to be reduced ONE-HALF in children less than 12 months of age and made full once they are >12 months old.
2. Reduce dosage to 50 percent in TLC 2500 to 4000 and withhold chemotherapy if TLC < 2500.

Road map

Week	0	3	6	9	12	15
IFOS	■	■	■	■	■	■
CBDCA	■	■	■	■	■	■
VP-16	■	■	■	■	■	■

APPENDIX II—NORMOGRAMS

CHART FOR CALCULATION OF BODY SURFACE AREA (BSA)

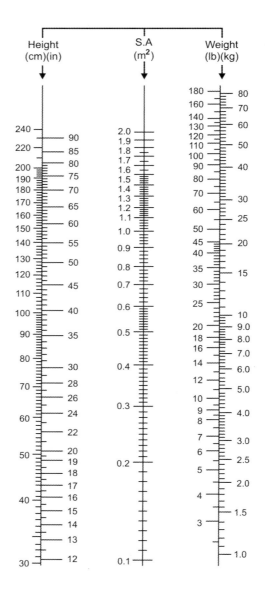

NORMAL VALUES OF TUMOR MARKERS

	Term	
Alpha fetoprotein	Term	*10,000 – 120,000 ng/ml* *(Usually < 70,000)* *(Increased in prematures)*
	2 months	30 - 400 ng/ml
	2-11 months	15 - 30 ng/ml
	12 months	3 - 15 ng/ml
	> 1 year	≤ 10ng/ml
Beta-hCG		< 5 miu/ml
Alkaline phosphatase	Adult	20-125 U/L (72.5)
	Children	40-400 U/L (220)
Lactic acid dehydrogenase	Adult	0-250 U/L (125)
Placental alkaline phosphatase (PLAP)		0.1-0.4 U/L
Neuron specific enolase (NSE)		0-12.5 ng/ml
Chromogranin (Cg A)		0-5 nmol/ml
	Men	< 76 ng/ml
	Women	< 51 ng/ml
Neuropeptide (NpY)		0-8 pmol/ml
VMA		0-35 mmols/L/24 hr
HVA		0-40 mmols/L/24 hr
Thyroglobulin		< 10 ng/ml
Beta 2 microglobulin		< 2.5 microgm/ml
Calcitonin	Children	3-26 pg/ml
5-hydroxyindoleacetic acid (5-HIAA)		(< 10 mg)
Carcinoembryonic antigen (CEA)		< 5 ng/ml
Prolactin		0-14 ng/ml
CA 19-9		< 40 U/ml
CA-125		< 35 U/ml
CA 15-3		5- 15 units/ml
Prostate-specific antigen (PSA)		0-4 ng/ml
Renin		160- 220 microunits/ml
Prorenin		70- 120 microunits/ml

EDIBLE THAT HELP TO COMBAT CANCER

Fruits: apricots, blueberries, cherries, grapefruit, grapes, mangoes, oranges, peaches, strawberries.

Vegetables: beans, beets, broccoli, cabbage, carrots, cauliflower, chilli peppers, figs, garlic, lemons, mushrooms, onions, sweet potatoes, tomatoes.

Cereals: rice, oats, wheat germ, wheat bran.

Nuts: peanuts, chestnuts, walnuts.

Others: fish, green tea, olive oil, water.

APPENDIX III—SUPPORT GROUPS FOR CHILDREN WITH CANCER

Support Groups for Children with Cancer

Children with cancer have support groups where kids can talk about things that are specific to their age group. Adolescents may particularly benefit from groups since they are mature enough to share verbally their concerns. Being independent, planning for the future, and dealing with friends and family are some of the topics that young people discuss. If children are younger, groups engage in art and play activities that relate to their illness, rather than sitting around talking about it. Some are offered in hospitals and clinics, and others through local and national organizations.

Childhood Cancer

- *Group Loop* - Provides an online support for teens with cancer and their parents.
- *The Never-Ending Squirrel Tale* - Offers practical support and encouragement to the parents of kids with cancer.
- *Orphans of the Cancer Storm* - Provides support and information for families and individuals dealing with either retinoblastoma or optic glioma, two rare tumors of childhood.
- *Outlook Portal* - Addresses the needs of survivors of childhood cancer and their families. Includes history, insurance and financial issues, health, education, and job concerns.
- *Ped-Hospice@Listserv* - For parents whose child with cancer is currently in hospice care or seeking care. Group provides support, comfort, ideas and information. Archives included.
- *Ped-Onc@Listserv* - Information on how to join The Pediatric Cancers Online Support Group. Includes archives.
- *Ped-Onc-Survivors@Listserv* - Discussion group for parents and family members of childhood/adolescent cancer survivors to share ideas, information and support.
- *Super Sibs* - Supports and recognizes brothers and sisters of children with cancer.
- *Teens Living with Cancer* - Offers information and resources about cancer, treatments, and support network presented by teens for teens.

- CALM (Children's Cancer and Leukaemia Movement) - *www.calmcharity.org*. Cares for the needs of families of children with cancer or leukaemia within the Swindon Health District, Wiltshire.
- CanTeen Ireland - *www.canteen.ie*. CanTeen Ireland is a nationwide support group for young people who have or have had cancer.
- CCLASP (Children with Cancer and Leukaemia Advice and Support for Parents) - *www.cclasp.co.uk*. Based in Edinburgh, the charity supports families affected by cancer and leukaemia in Scotland.
- CHICS - *www.chics.org.uk* provides support and information for parents of children with cancer in Merseyside the Wirral and North Wales.
- CLIC Sargent *www.clicsargent.org.uk*. Charity providing information and support for all family members affected by childhood cancer.
- *www.click4tic.org.uk*. Up to date information for teenagers with cancer and their families.
- Help Adolescents with Cancer (HAWC) *www.hawc-co-uk.com*. National support group for adolescents with cancer.
- gaps:line - *www.gapsline.org.uk*. Support line for parents and carers of children with cancer and leukemia.
- National Alliance of Childhood Cancer Parent Organisations (NACCPO) - *www.naccpo.org.uk*. Formed by UK parent organisations NACCPO has shared aims of working with families and professionals to support children with cancer.
- Neuroblastoma Society - *www.nsoc.co.uk*. Funds research into causes of neuroblastoma and provides support to affected families.
- OSCAR (Offering Support to Children and Relatives) for children with brain or spinal tumors *www.support-oscar.org*. Support group at the Radcliffe Infirmary, Oxford for families affected by brain and spinal tumors.
- PASIC (Parents Association for Seriously Ill Children) - *www.pasic.org.uk*.
- Parent support group for families of children with cancer and leukemia across the East Midlands.

- Siblinks - *www.siblinks.org.* Support network for young people aged 13 to 25 who are siblings or sons and daughters of people affected by cancer.
- SuperSibs - *www.supersibs.org.* American organizaiton devoted to providing services specifically to support the needs of siblings of children with cancer.
- Tak Tent Cancer Support Scotland - *www.taktent.org.uk.* Youth project provides support/ recreational activities to young people affected by cancer.
- Tayside Children with Cancer and Leukaemia - *www.tccl.org.uk.* Supports families in Tayside and North Fife with a child under 21 affected by cancer or leukemia.
- Teenage Cancer Trust - *www.teencancer.org.* Designs and builds dedicated adolescent cancer units in hospitals and funds and organizes support and information services for patients, their families, schools and health professionals.
- The Cancer Counselling Trust - *www.cctrust.org.uk.* Counseling service for individuals, families and friends affected by cancer.
- Wilms at Home *www.wilmsineurope.net.* Website by families for families affected by Wilms' tumor living in Europe.
- Courage India cancer Foundation *www.courageindia.org/* Works for the poor cancer patients and gives them direct financial aid, and psychological support.

- CPAA *www.cpaaindia.org/aboutus/ourbranches.htm.* India based NGOs dedicated to Cancer Awareness, Cancer Care and Cancer
- National Cancer Institute (NCI) *www.cancer.gov/nci.*

Bone Marrow Transplant

- *Andrews Helpful Hands Foundation Inc* - A Massachusetts based organization that helps families with children who are going through the bone marrow transplant process.
- *BMT Support Online* - An online support organization for people facing or recovering from Bone Marrow Transplantation, their family members, caregivers and friends.
- *Bone Marrow Transplant Support Group* - Information and links to resources for BMT, Leukemia, Lymphoma, fatigue, and stem cell. Patient stories, message board, and a glossary of terms available.
- *The Bruce Denniston Bone Marrow Society* - A registered charity raising money to help match donors to patients needing bone marrow transplants. It also assists patients with transplant-related expenses. Information on the society, its history and activities

Websites with Useful Information for Childhood Cancer Survivors and Caretakers

- www. sign.ac.uk
- www.nice.org.uk
- www.ukccsg.org.uk
- www.childrensoncologygroup.com
- www.survivorship-guidelines.org

Index